THE WASHINGTON MANUAL® OF MEDICAL THERAPEUTICS

Second South Asian edition

THE WASHINGTON MANUAL® OF MEDICAL THERAPEUTICS

Second South Asian edition

Editors

Zachary Crees, MD

Cassandra Fritz, MD

Alonso Heudebert, MD

Jonas Noé, MD

Arvind Rengarajan, MD

Xiaowen Wang, MD

SAE Editor

Archith Boloor, MD (Internal Medicine)
Additional Professor, Department of Medicine
Kasturba Medical College, Mangalore
Manipal Academy of Higher Education,
Karnataka

This work is an adaptation of the *The Washington Manual® of Medical Therapeutics, 1st SAE and 37th International Edition.* Authorized for sale only in South Asia.

Wolters Kluwer

Publishing Manager: Ruchi Chawla
Development Editor: Megha Saini
Production Editor: Pooja Chauhan
Asstt. Manager Manufacturing: Sumit Johry

3rd Floor, Tower B, Building No. 10, Phase II, DLF Cyber City,
Gurugram, Haryana - 122002

First South Asian Edition, 2022
Second South Asian Edition, 2024

Print ISBN: 978-81-97137-70-9
E-ISBN: 978-81-97137-71-6

Authorised for sale only in South Asia

Published by Wolters Kluwer (India) Pvt. Ltd., New Delhi
Compositor: B2K - Bytes 2 Knowledge
Printed and bound at Sterling Graphics Pvt. Ltd.

To download our latest price list or contact us, please visit https://www.wolterskluwer.com/en-in/solutions/lwwindia. For any other queries, email us at ggm-india.support@wolterskluwer.com.

Dedicated to those
who tirelessly seek healing,
to the minds that push the boundaries
of medical knowledge and to the
hearts that care for the well-being of
others.

Preface

When the previous edition of this book was being written, we were in the midst of a raging pandemic. The trials that the medical fraternity endured during the COVID-19 crisis may have traumatized an entire generation of upcoming doctors, but it is safe to say that we did an exceptional job. Doctors from around the world mobilized themselves—in mind, spirit and hope—to stave off an unprecedented healthcare disaster that quite possibly may be the greatest medical event in history since the Great Plague. Five years later, we have comfortably returned to our normal lives; less masks, more tasks. At this point it is perhaps prudent to ask: what have we, the global community of healthcare personnel, learnt from our experience?

It is, of course, hard to pin-point one specific lesson that anyone learnt during the pandemic. But I do know one thing: we were not able to learn fast enough. At the turn of every week, there was a new variant. The new variant had to be combatted by a new vaccine. The drugs that were part of our daily protocols during the first wave became either obsolete ornaments or last resort lifesavers during the last wave. Journals were churning out research, and it still wasn't fast enough for us to keep up with the disease. The demand for up-to-date information at the fingertips of doctors became rather apparent. However, it also became even more apparent that no matter how much we knew, nature was always one move ahead of us. Like I have said before, the purity of medicine lies in the way it treats those who yearn to study it. Doctors around the world remain united through their pursuit of knowledge—the knowledge to fend off a disease that was alive and evolving.

With the idea of perpetual evolution in mind, I have compiled the second edition of the South Asian edition of the Washington Manual of Medical Therapeutics. Written as an everyday handbook for residents and junior faculty, *The Washington Manual® of Medical Therapeutics* has occupied a place of pride in most personal libraries of internists across the globe. We have worked to retain all the positive feedback that was received in the first edition. The heart of the manual continues to remain the same; it has simply evolved to meet the needs of the modern-day physician.

Some much-needed updates were covered, especially in the Primary Care Medicine section on medical emergencies. The entire chapter on COVID-19 from the previous book has now been merged into the infectious diseases section—a win for science as well as for us physicians. Sections on tropical diseases, maternal medicine, geriatrics, palliative and end-of-life care have been updated, along with the latest reviews of disease pathophysiology and evidence-based explanations of current therapeutic protocols in a no-nonsense format—a quality that has defined the essence of this book for years.

The demand to be precise has always been the bane of a doctor's existence. However, looking back, I realize how far we have come. All the knowledge in the world is now available at our fingertips. But for us doctors, both information and misinformation find their way into our lives rather easily. That is probably why, even through a pandemic, we relied on the integrity of books.

Learning is a continuum—a process that never stops, involving many parts. The second edition of this book is yet another cogwheel in the grand system that aims to help the current generation of physicians with their day-to-day practice and educate the next in their quest for knowledge.

Archith Boloor, MD

Preface to the First South Asian Edition

When I embarked on my rather long and arduous journey to become a doctor, I had a rose-tinted view of what my everyday would be like—the glorious life of a physician with a snazzy white coat, a stethoscope adorning my neck, perhaps a pager, and a notepad. I am not going to say it is not any of that, but I definitely did not see myself (or any other doctor) spending as much time with books as we do. Even during this raging pandemic, when our healthcare system was undergoing its harshest trial yet, the one thing that kept the doctors united were the books—information that is hand-picked, jotted down, or spoken out in the hope that it may someday help someone. Even the tiniest of information is important—a small hand-written mnemonic passed down through generations of students, a little black and white illustration that quickly adds sense to the ocean of text next to it, and the infinite books you can lay your hands on. The purity of medicine has always been in the way it has treated those who yearn to study it.

To follow in the footsteps of stalwarts who have walked before you is a daunting task. Written as an everyday handbook for residents and junior faculty, *The Washington Manual®* *of Medical Therapeutics* has occupied a pride of place in most personal libraries of internists across the globe. With the release of South Asian edition of this much-loved book, I hope to retain the succinctness and quick referencing style that has been the hallmark of this book while adding relevant text.

Sections on tropical diseases, maternal medicine, geriatrics, and palliative care have been added along with concise reviews of disease pathophysiology, evidence-based explanations of current therapeutic protocols in a no-nonsense format—a quality that has for years defined the essence of this book.

As I write this, struggle with the pandemic continues. Modern medicine has never been under the microscope as much as it is today. All it took was a virus to upend the system that took centuries to learn and build. Every day has been as uncertain as the day before, and yet, we have remained united–united in our efforts to understand the disease, united in our quest to prevent it from consuming us whole, and united in our attempts to minimize our losses. When the pandemic struck, our need for knowledge transcended geographical boundaries, went beyond hierarchy, and involved the combined efforts of many disciplines of health. Learning is a continuum—a process that never stops, involving many gears and wheels, and parts. Even in our current predicament, we continue to learn something that helps us in our everyday life as a doctor despite being overworked, understaffed, tested, and sidelined.

The medical fraternity has been many things: overworked, understaffed, pressurized, politicized, tested, sidelined—but it has also always been united. This book is just that: a rose-tinted symbol of our unity.

As we look forward to better and brighter days, this edition will remain a testimony to the team efforts of an amazing group of physicians, the likes of whom can fend off a pandemic.

Archith Boloor, MD

Acknowledgments

The Washington Manual® of Medical Therapeutics was the preferred handbook that I used to carry every day to my residency, streaming through the pages to refer in times of crisis and even otherwise. Little did I know then that in a decade I would be editing its South Asian edition for the second consecutive edition. It came as a real surprise, when I received a call offering me the privilege to edit this book. It was an uphill task but with the pitching in of my colleagues all across India, the process got smoother than I imagined.

Firstly, I would like to thank my family, my mom, and my sisters—the unwavering pillars of my strength through all the challenges. My friends, colleagues, and well-wishers who have always supported my work were not an exception this time too. I also want to thank all my students, each and every one, because without their unrelenting urge to learn, I would not have the drive to teach.

The modifications that this book had to undergo to become a cohesive second edition undoubtedly needed lots of research and data. I am thankful to all my friends whose contribution and knowledge flowed seamlessly at a very short notice. I thank Dr. Nikhil Kenny Thomas, Dr. Mohamed Faizan Thouseef, Dr. Mohammed Shaheen, Dr. Madhav H Hande, Dr. Vivek K Koushik, Dr. Anudeep Padakanti, Dr. Mahesha Padyana, Dr. Sunil Karanth, Dr. Jalli Sai Nithin Reddy, Dr. Isha Tiwari, Dr. Jeco Jacob Kuttykandathil, Dr. Gauri Malavalli Girish, Dr. Shishir M Upadya, Dr. Sohan M, Dr. Anudeep Gaddam, Dr. Suraj Utmani, Dr. Mounika R N, Dr. Aashna Pankaj Gandhi, Dr. Navyashree H C, Dr. Hasmukh Jain, Dr. Ashwini M V, Dr. Athulya G Asokan, Dr. Harsha Sagar, Dr. G G Akshay Prabhu, Dr. Sheetal Raj M, Dr. Murali Mohan Rama Krishna Reddy, Dr. Vidarshan Mathavan, Dr. Kunal Seth, Dr. Vivek S Dandin, Dr. Anjali Sahni, Dr. Pranavjith A, Dr. Rajaram Prasad A, and Dr. Abu Thajudeen, for their contribution.

I am grateful to my department, my college Kasturba Medical College, Mangalore and my university, the Manipal Academy of Higher Education (MAHE), Manipal for supporting my endeavors. I was made here and every achievement of mine is made here as well.

A very special gratitude goes out to all my teachers, who are solely responsible for what I am today and for having ignited the passion of teaching and writing in me.

I would like to thank my publisher, Wolters Kluwer India, in particular, Ms. Megha Saini (Content Management Analyst-Health), Ms. Ruchi Chawla (Content and Publishing Consultant), Ravi Vishwakarma (Senior Content and Publishing Analyst-Health), and Sheenam Aggarwal (Associate Director, Content Mgt & Publishing) for their unwavering support during the process of developing this project.

Lastly, I thank my guiding force, Mother Goddess for what was, what is, and what will be.

May this book serve as a beacon of insight and guidance on the journey towards better health for all.

From all of me, to all of you

Archith Boloor, MD

Contributors to the South Asian Edition

Nikhil Kenny Thomas, MD, DM
Consultant, Department of Medical Gastroenterology and Hepatology
St. Luke Hospital, Pathanamthitta
Dr. K M Cherian Institute of Medical Sciences, Chenganur
Futureace Hospital, Kochi, Kerala

Madhav H Hande, MD, DrNB
Associate Consultant
Department of Nephrology
Manipal Hospital, Whitefield
Bangalore, Karnataka

Vivek K Koushik, MD, DrNB
Consultant Nephrologist
Prashanth Hospitals, Kolathur
Chennai, Tamil Nadu

Mohammed Shaheen
Resident,
Department of Emergency Medicine
Hamad Medical Corporation
Doha, Qatar

Anudeep Padakanti, MD
Senior Resident
Department of Medical Oncology
MNJ Institute of Oncology and Regional Cancer Centre
Hyderabad, Telangana

Mahesha Padyana, MD, FNB
Consultant Critical Care Medicine
Manipal Hospitals
Bengaluru, Karnataka

Sunil Karanth, MD, FNB. FCICM
Chairman of Critical Care Services
Manipal Health Enterprises Pvt Ltd
Bengaluru, Karnataka

Athulya G Asokan, MD
Assistant Professor
Department of Internal Medicine
Government Medical College
Kottayam, Kerala

Anudeep Gaddam, MD, DM
Associate Professor
Department of Endocrinology
Kasturba Medical College, Manipal
Manipal Academy of Higher Education, Karnataka

Mohamed Faizan Thouseef, MD
Senior Resident
Department of Internal Medicine
Kasturba Medical College, Mangalore
Manipal Academy of Higher Education, Karnataka

Navyashree H C, MD
Consultant, Internal Medicine
Manipal Hospitals, HAL road
Bengaluru, Karnataka

Suraj Utmani, MD
Assistant Professor
Department of Internal Medicine
Kasturba Medical College, Mangalore
Manipal Academy of Higher Education, Karnataka

Jalli Sai Nithin Reddy, MD
Senior Resident
Department of Internal Medicine
Kasturba Medical College, Mangalore
Manipal Academy of Higher Education, Karnataka

Isha Tiwari, MD
Senior Resident
Department of Medical Oncology
MS Ramaiah Medical College
Bangalore, Karnataka

Jeco Jacob Kuttykandathil, MD
Senior Resident
Department of Internal Medicine
Kasturba Medical College, Mangalore
Manipal Academy of Higher Education, Karnataka

Gauri Malavalli Girish, MD
Senior Resident
Department of Internal Medicine
Kasturba Medical College, Mangalore
Manipal Academy of Higher Education, Karnataka

Shishir M Upadya, MD
Senior Resident
Department of Internal Medicine
Kasturba Medical College, Mangalore
Manipal Academy of Higher Education, Karnataka

Sohan M, MD
Senior Resident
Department of Internal Medicine
Kasturba Medical College, Mangalore
Manipal Academy of Higher Education, Karnataka

Mounika R N, MD
Senior Resident
Department of Pathology
Kasturba Medical College, Mangalore
Manipal Academy of Higher Education, Karnataka

Aashna Pankaj Gandhi, MD
Consultant, Infectious Diseases
Amar Nursing Home – Medical
Kandivali West
Mumbai, Maharashtra

Vidarshan Mathavan
Resident
Department of Internal Medicine
Kasturba Medical College, Mangalore
Manipal Academy of Higher Education, Karnataka

Kunal Seth
Resident
Department of Internal Medicine
Kasturba Medical College, Mangalore
Manipal Academy of Higher Education, Karnataka

Vivek S Dandin
Resident
Department of Internal Medicine
Kasturba Medical College, Mangalore
Manipal Academy of Higher Education, Karnataka

Anjali Sahni
Resident
Department of Internal Medicine
Kasturba Medical College, Mangalore
Manipal Academy of Higher Education, Karnataka

Murali Mohan Rama Krishna Reddy
Resident
Department of Internal Medicine
Kasturba Medical College, Mangalore
Manipal Academy of Higher Education, Karnataka

Sheetal Raj M, MD
Associate Professor
Department of Internal Medicine and Program Director—Geriatric Medicine Fellowship
Kasturba Medical College, Mangalore
Manipal Academy of Higher Education, Karnataka

Hasmukh Jain, MD, DM
Professor
Department of Medical Oncology
Tata Memorial Centre, Homi Bhabha National University
Mumbai, Maharashtra

Pranavjith A
Resident
Department of Internal Medicine
Kasturba Medical College, Mangalore
Manipal Academy of Higher Education, Karnataka

M Harsha Sagar, MD, DM
Consultant Cardiologist
Varam Hospital
Hosur, Tamil Nadu

Ashwini M V, MD
Senior Resident
Department of Cardiology
Kasturba Medical College, Manipal
Manipal Academy of Higher Education, Karnataka

G G Akshay Prabhu, MD
Senior Resident
Department of Cardiology
Sri Jayadeva Institute of Cardiovascular Sciences and Research
Bangalore, Karnataka

Abu Thajudeen, MD
Department of Neurology
Father Muller Medical College Mangalore, Karnataka

Rajaram Prasad A, MD, DM, FSCAI
Consultant Interventional Cardiologist
Aasai Specialty Clinic
Salem, Tamil Nadu

Contents

1 Inpatient Care in Internal Medicine

Mark Thoelke, Eric Johnson, Crystal Atwood, Jalli Sai Nithin Reddy, and Madhav H. Hande

General Care of the Hospitalized Patient

GENERAL PRINCIPLES

- Although a general approach to common problems can be outlined, **therapy must be individualized.** All diagnostic and therapeutic procedures should be explained carefully to the patient, including the potential risks, benefits, and alternatives.
- The period of hospitalization represents a complex interplay of multiple caregivers that subjects the patient to potential harm by **medical errors and iatrogenic complications.** Every effort must be made to minimize these risks. Basic measures include the following:
  - Use of standardized abbreviations and dose designations
  - Excellent communication between physicians and other caregivers
  - Institution of appropriate prophylactic precautions
  - Prevention of nosocomial infections, including attention to hygiene and discontinuation of unnecessary catheters
  - Medicine reconciliation at all transfers of care
- **Hospital orders**
  - Computer order entry offers admission order sets that should be entered promptly after evaluation of a patient. A contact number should be made available.
  - Daily rounds should include assessment for ongoing need of IV fluids, telemetry, catheters, and supplemental oxygen, all of which can limit mobility.
  - Routine daily labs, such as complete blood count (CBC) and basic metabolic panel (BMP), should be discouraged because significant iatrogenic anemia may develop.
- **Discharge**
  - **Discharge planning** begins at the time of admission. Assessment of the patient's social situation and potential discharge needs should be made at this time.
  - **Early coordination** with nursing, social work, and case coordinators/managers facilitates efficient discharge and a complete post discharge plan.
  - **Patient education** should occur regarding changes in medications and other new therapies. Compliance with treatment is influenced by the patient's understanding of that treatment.
  - **Prescriptions** should be written for all new medication, and the patient should be provided with a complete medication list including instructions and indications.
  - **Communication** with physicians who will be resuming care of the patient is important for optimal follow-up care and should be a component of the discharge process.

PROPHYLACTIC MEASURES

Venous Thromboembolism Prophylaxis

GENERAL PRINCIPLES

Epidemiology

Venous thromboembolism (VTE) is a preventable cause of death in hospitalized patients. In the largest observational study to date attempting to risk-stratify medical patients,

1.2% of medical patients developed VTE within 90 days of admission. A total of 10%–31% of patients were deemed to be at high risk for VTE, defined as having **two or more points** by weighted risk factors below.[1]

- Three points: previous VTE, thrombophilia
- One point: cancer, age >60
- The addition of D-Dimer (≥ 2 × the upper limit of normal) improved VTE risk discrimination and reclassification. The modified IMPROVE VTE score with an elevated D-dimer identified a nearly threefold higher VTE risk.[2]

Prevention

- **Ambulation** several times a day should be encouraged.
- **Pharmacologic prophylaxis** results in a 50% decrease in VTE risk, although this includes many asymptomatic calf vein thromboses that do not progress. No overall mortality benefit from prophylaxis has been demonstrated.
- Acutely ill patients at high risk of VTE, without bleeding or high risk of bleeding, should be treated with low-dose unfractionated heparin (UFH), 5000 units SC q12h or q8, or low-molecular-weight heparin (LMWH); enoxaparin, 40 mg SC daily, or dalteparin, 5000 units SC daily; or fondaparinux, 2.5 mg SC daily.
- Rivaroxaban is a direct oral anticoagulant (DOAC) approved for use in hospitalized acutely ill medical patients who are not at high risk of bleeding. The recommended dosage is 10 mg daily for a total of 31–39 days, provided the patient's CrCl is >30 mL/min/1.73 m^2. Extended-duration rivaroxaban reduced the risk of venous thromboembolism.[3]
- Aspirin alone is not sufficient for prophylaxis in hospitalized patients.[4]
- At-risk patients with contraindications to anticoagulation prophylaxis may receive mechanical prophylaxis with intermittent pneumatic compression or graded compression stockings, although evidence of benefit is lacking.[5] Intermitted pneumatic compression is an effective method and was found to reduce the risk of DVT in stroke patients.[6]

Decubitus Ulcers

GENERAL PRINCIPLES

Epidemiology

Decubitus ulcers typically occur within the first 2 weeks of hospitalization and can develop within 2–6 hours. Once they develop, decubitus ulcers are difficult to heal and have been associated with increased mortality.[7] More than 100 risk factors for the development of decubitus ulcers have been identified; the most important include immobility, malnutrition, reduced skin perfusion, and sensory loss.[8]

Prevention

Prevention is the key to management of decubitus ulcers. It is recognized that not all decubitus ulcers are avoidable.[9] Preventative measures include the following:

- **Risk prediction** using the Norton or Braden scales scores immobility, activity levels, incontinence, impaired nutritional status, impaired circulation, and altered level of consciousness to identify patients at risk for pressure injury.
- **Advanced static mattresses or** overlays should be used in at-risk patients.[10]
- **Skin care**, including daily inspection with particular attention to bony prominences including heels, minimizing exposure to moisture, and applying moisturizers to dry sacral skin.
- **Nutritional supplements** may be provided to patients at risk.
- **Frequent repositioning** (minimum of every 2 h, or every 1 h for wheelchair-bound patients) is suggested.
- **Multilayer foam dressings** have been shown to reduce the rates of pressure injuries.[11]

DIAGNOSIS

National Pressure Ulcer Advisory Panel Staging:

- **Suspected deep tissue injury:** Purple or maroon localized area of discolored intact skin or blood-filled blister because of damage of underlying soft tissue from pressure and/or shear. The area may be preceded by tissue that is painful, firm, mushy, boggy, warmer, or cooler as compared with adjacent tissue.
- **Stage I:** Intact skin with nonblanchable redness of a localized area usually over a bony prominence. Darkly pigmented skin may obscure findings.
- **Stage II:** Partial thickness loss of dermis presenting as a shallow open ulcer with a red pink wound bed without slough. May also present as a blister.
- **Stage III:** Full thickness tissue loss. Subcutaneous fat may be visible, but the bone, tendon, or muscle is not exposed. Slough may be present but does not obscure the depth of tissue loss. May include undermining and tunneling.
- **Stage IV:** Full thickness tissue loss with exposed bone, tendon, or muscle. Slough or eschar may be present on some parts of the wound bed. Often includes undermining and tunneling.
- **Unstageable:** Full thickness tissue loss in which the base of the ulcer is covered by slough (yellow, tan, gray, green, or brown) and/or eschar (tan, brown, or black) in the wound bed.

TREATMENT

Optimal treatment of pressure ulcers remains poorly defined. There is evidence to support the following[12]:

- **Hydrocolloid or foam** dressings may reduce wound size.
- **Protein or amino acid supplementation** is recommended, although there are insufficient data to recommend a specific supplement regimen.[13]
- **Electrical stimulation** may accelerate healing.
- **Other adjunctive therapies** with less supporting evidence include radiant heat, negative pressure, and platelet-derived growth factor. Topical agents (silver sulfadiazine) may optimizing healing or lead to minor slough debridement (Santyl, Xenaderm).
- There is no role for antibiotics to aid healing of a noninfected ulcer.
- **Adequate pain relief:** Oral nonopioid pain medications are recommended for mild pain, while opioid analgesics are reserved for moderate-to-severe pain. Topical analgesics has shown minimal benefit.[14]
- **Redistribution of pressure and proper positioning:** Utilize powered mattresses to aid in healing, though studies showing certain benefits are lacking.[15]

OTHER PRECAUTIONS

- **Fall precautions** should be written for patients who have a history of falls or are at high risk of a fall (e.g., dementia, weakness, orthostasis). Falls are the most common accident in hospitalized patients, frequently leading to injury. **Fall risk should not be equated with bed rest**, which may lead to debilitation and higher risk of future falls.
- **Seizure precautions**, which include padded bed rails and an oral airway at the bedside, should be considered for patients with a history of seizures or those at risk of seizing.
- **Restraint orders** are written for patients who are at risk of injuring themselves or interfering with their treatment because of disruptive or dangerous behaviors. Physical restraints may exacerbate agitation. Bed alarms, sitters, and sedatives are alternatives in appropriate settings.

ACUTE INPATIENT CARE

An approach to selected common complaints is presented in this section. An evaluation should generally include a directed history and physical examination, review of the medical problem list (including chronic conditions), review of medications with attention to recent medication changes, and consideration of recent procedures.

Chest Pain

GENERAL PRINCIPLES

Common causes of chest pain range from life-threatening causes such as myocardial infarction (MI) and pulmonary embolism to other causes including esophageal reflux, peptic ulcer disease, pneumonia, costochondritis, shingles, trauma, and anxiety.

DIAGNOSIS

History and Physical Examination

- History should include previous cardiac or vascular disease history, operative or procedural history, cardiac risk factors, and factors that would predispose the patient to a pulmonary embolus.
- Pain characteristics and associated symptoms help point toward etiology.
- Physical examination is ideally conducted during an episode of pain and includes vital signs (bilateral blood pressure [BP] measurements if considering aortic dissection), cardiopulmonary and abdominal examination, and inspection and palpation of the chest.

Diagnostic Testing

Assessment of oxygenation status, chest radiography, and ECG is appropriate in most patients. Serial cardiac biomarkers should be obtained if there is suspicion of ischemia. Spiral CT and ventilation/perfusion scans are employed to diagnose pulmonary embolus.

TREATMENT

- If cardiac ischemia is a concern, see Chapter 4, Ischemic Heart Disease, for details.
- Control of blood pressure in aortic dissection with beta-blockers (esmolol or labetalol) and vasodilators (nitroprusside) while awaiting endovascular or surgical interventions.
- If a gastrointestinal (GI) source is suspected, Maalox, viscous lidocaine, and hyoscyamine (1:1:1 mix) can be administered.
- Musculoskeletal pain typically responds to acetaminophen or NSAID therapy.
- Prompt empiric anticoagulation if there is high suspicion for MI or pulmonary embolism.

Dyspnea

GENERAL PRINCIPLES

Dyspnea is most commonly caused by a cardiopulmonary abnormality, such as congestive heart failure (CHF), cardiac ischemia, bronchospasm, pulmonary embolus, infection, mucus plugging, and aspiration. Dyspnea must be promptly and carefully evaluated.

DIAGNOSIS

History and Physical Examination

- Initial evaluation should include a review of the medical history for underlying pulmonary or cardiovascular disease and a directed history.
- A detailed cardiopulmonary examination should take place, including vital signs.

Diagnostic Testing

- Oxygen assessment by pulse oximetry or arterial blood gas and chest radiography are useful in most patients.
- Other diagnostic measures should be directed by the findings in the initial evaluation.

TREATMENT

Oxygen should be administered promptly if needed. Other therapeutic measures should be directed by the findings in the initial evaluation.

Acute Hypertensive Episodes

GENERAL PRINCIPLES

- Acute hypertensive episodes in the hospital are most often caused by inadequately treated essential hypertension. If there is evidence of end-organ damage, IV medications are indicated. Oral agents are more appropriate for hypertensive urgency without end-organ damage.
- Hypertension associated with withdrawal syndromes (e.g., alcohol, cocaine) and rebound hypertension associated with sudden withdrawal of antihypertensive medications (i.e., clonidine, α-adrenergic antagonists) should be considered. These entities should be treated as discussed in Chapter 3, Preventive Cardiology.
- Volume overload and pain may exacerbate hypertension and should be recognized appropriately and treated.

Fever

GENERAL PRINCIPLES

Fever accompanies many illnesses and is a valuable marker of disease activity. Infection is a primary concern. Drug reaction, malignancy, VTE, vasculitis, central fever, and tissue infarction are other possibilities but are diagnoses of exclusion.

DIAGNOSIS

History and Physical Examination

- History should include chronology of the fever and associated symptoms, medications, potential exposures, past medical history, and a complete social and travel history.
- Physical examination should include oral or rectal temperature. In the hospitalized patient, special attention should be paid to any IV lines, asymmetric edema, a thorough skin exam, and indwelling devices such as urinary catheters.
- For management of neutropenic fever see Chapter 22, Cancer.

Diagnostic Testing

- Testing includes blood and urine cultures, CBC with differential, serum chemistries with liver function tests, urinalysis, and stool cultures if appropriate.
- Diagnostic evaluation generally includes chest radiography.
- Cultures of abnormal fluid collections, sputum, cerebrospinal fluid, and stool should be sent if clinically indicated. Cultures are ideally obtained prior to initiation of antibiotics; however, antibiotics should not be delayed if serious infection is suspected.
- Testing should also cover the local endemic diseases such as tuberculosis, malaria, dengue, and leptospirosis in South Asian countries as per the disease profile and climate.
- During epidemics, the disease of concern should be tested.

TREATMENT

- Antipyretic drugs may be given to decrease associated discomfort. Aspirin, 325 mg, and acetaminophen, 325–650 mg PO or PR q4h, are the drugs of choice.
- Empiric antibiotics should be considered in hemodynamically unstable patients in whom infection is a primary concern, as well as in neutropenic and asplenic patients.
- Heat stroke and malignant hyperthermia are medical emergencies that require prompt recognition and treatment (see Chapter 26, Medical Emergencies).

Pain

GENERAL PRINCIPLES

Pain is subjective, and therapy must be individualized. Chronic pain may not be associated with any objective physical findings. Pain scales can be employed for quantitation. Quick assessment may be done by the OPQRST checklist.

TREATMENT

- Treatment should be individualized toward the type and intensity of pain.
- Acute pain usually requires short-term therapy. Multimodal analgesia postoperatively improves pain management and reduces opioid requirements.
- **Chronic pain requires multimodality management to keep opioid use to a minimum to prevent risk of dependence and subsequent escalation of opioid doses.** Higher doses of opioids have been shown to increase the risk of overdose without providing increased pain relief.[16]
- If pain is refractory to medical therapy, then nonpharmacologic modalities, such as nerve blocks, sympathectomy, and cognitive behavioral therapy, may be appropriate.

Nonopioid Analgesics

- Acetaminophen
  - Effects: Antipyretic and analgesic actions; no anti-inflammatory or antiplatelet properties.
  - Dosage: 325–1000 mg q4–6h (maximum dose, 4 g/d), available in oral, IV, and rectal suppository. Dosage in patients with liver disease and older adults should not exceed 2 g/d.
  - Adverse effects: The *principal* advantage of acetaminophen is its lack of gastric toxicity. Hepatic toxicity may be serious, and acute overdose with 10–15 g can cause fatal hepatic necrosis (see Chapter 19, Liver Diseases, and Chapter 26, Medical Emergencies).
- Aspirin
  - Effects: Aspirin has analgesic, antipyretic, anti-inflammatory, and antiplatelet effects. Aspirin should be used with caution in patients with hepatic or renal disease or bleeding disorders, those who are pregnant, and those who are receiving anticoagulation therapy. Antiplatelet effects may last for up to 1 week after a single dose.
  - Dosage: 325–650 mg q4h PRN (maximum dose, 4 g/d), available in oral and rectal suppository. Enteric coated formulation may minimize GI side effects.
  - Adverse effects: Dose-related side effects include tinnitus, dizziness, and hearing loss. Dyspepsia and GI bleeding can develop and may be severe. Hypersensitivity reactions, including bronchospasm, laryngeal edema, and urticaria, are uncommon, but patients with asthma and nasal polyps are more susceptible. Chronic use can result in interstitial nephritis and papillary necrosis.
- NSAIDs
  - Effects: NSAIDs have analgesic, antipyretic, and anti-inflammatory properties mediated by inhibition of cyclooxygenase. All NSAIDs have similar efficacy and toxicities,

with a side effect profile similar to that of aspirin. Patients with allergic or bronchospastic reactions to aspirin should not be given NSAIDs. See Chapter 25, Arthritis and Rheumatologic Diseases, for further information on NSAIDs.

- Anticonvulsants (e.g., gabapentin, pregabalin, carbamazepine, oxcarbazepine), tricyclic antidepressants (e.g., amitriptyline), and serotonin-norepinephrine reuptake inhibitors (duloxetine, milnacipran, and venlafaxine) are PO agents that can be used to treat neuropathic pain.
- Topical anesthetics (e.g., lidocaine, capsaicin patch) may provide analgesia to a localized region (e.g., postherpetic neuralgia).
- Benzodiazepines and muscle relaxants should not be used for pain control.

Opioid Analgesics

Effects: Opioid analgesics are pharmacologically similar to opium or morphine and are indicated for moderate to severe pain, particularly when there is a contraindication to NSAIDS.

- Dosage: Table 1-1 lists equianalgesic dosages.
- For acute pain management, the **lowest effective dose of immediate-release opioids** should be given. Use of nonopioid pain medications and nonpharmacological pain management strategies to minimize opioid needs is encouraged.
- When changing to a new narcotic because of poor response or patient intolerance, the new medication should be started at 50% the equianalgesic dose to account for incomplete cross-tolerance.
- Parenteral and transdermal administration are useful in the setting of dysphagia, emesis, or decreased GI absorption.
- Agents with short half-lives, such as morphine, should be used. Narcotic-naïve patients should be started on the lowest possible doses, whereas patients with demonstrated tolerance will require higher doses.
- Patient-controlled analgesia often is used to control pain in a postoperative or terminally ill patient. Opioid-naïve patients should not have basal rates prescribed because of risk of overdose.
- If a patient requires continuous (basal) analgesia, supplementary PRN doses for breakthrough pain at doses of roughly 5%–15% of the daily basal dose can be provided. If frequent PRN doses are required, the maintenance dose should be increased, or the dosing interval should be decreased.

TABLE 1-1 Equipotent Doses of Opioid Analgesics

Drug	Onset (min)	Duration (h)	IM/IV/SC (mg)	PO (mg)
Fentanyl	7–8	1–2	0.1	NA
Levorphanol	30–90	4–6	2	4
Hydromorphone	15–30	2–4	1.5–2.0	7.5
Methadone	30–60	4–12	10	20
Morphine	15–30	2–4	10	30[a]
Oxycodone	15–30	3–4	NA	20
Codeine	15–30	4–6	120	200
Tramadol	30–60	4–6	100	300

[a]An IM:PO ratio of 1:2 to 1:3 used for repetitive dosing.
Note: Equivalences are based on single-dose studies.
NA, not applicable.

- Severe pain uncontrolled with large doses of opiates, particularly while using patient-controlled analgesia with basal rates, may warrant consultation with a pain specialist.
- Selected opiates
  - **Tramadol** is an opioid agonist and a centrally acting nonopioid analgesic that acts on pain processing pathways.
    - Dosage: 50–100 mg PO q4–6h can be used for acute pain. For elderly patients and those with renal or liver dysfunction, dosage reduction is recommended.
    - Adverse effects: Concomitant use of alcohol, sedatives, or narcotics should be avoided. Nausea, dizziness, constipation, and headache may also occur. Respiratory depression has not been described at prescribed dosages but may occur with overdose. Tramadol should not be used in patients who are taking a monoamine oxidase inhibitor, as it can contribute to serotonin syndrome.
  - **Tapentadol** is a mixed-mechanism opioid with a higher affinity for the mu opioid receptor than tramadol (though weaker than pure mu agonists), along with noradrenergic reuptake inhibition. It is the only opioid with a specific US-FDA indication for neuropathic pain, particularly in its ER form for painful diabetic neuropathy.
    - Dosage: For acute pain, administer 50–100 mg PO q4-6h. For neuropathic pain, prescribe 50 mg PO q12h with ER tablets. Dosage reduction is recommended for elderly patients and those with renal or liver dysfunction.
  - Codeine is usually given in combination with aspirin or acetaminophen.
  - Oxycodone and hydrocodone are both available orally in combination with acetaminophen; oxycodone is available without acetaminophen in immediate-release and sustained-release formulations. Care should be taken to avoid acetaminophen overdose with these formulations.
  - Morphine sulfate preparations include both immediate release and sustained release. The liquid form can be useful in patients who have difficulty in swallowing pills. Morphine should be used with caution in renal insufficiency.
  - Methadone is very effective when administered orally and suppresses the symptoms of withdrawal from other opioids because of its extended half-life. Despite its long elimination half-life, its analgesic duration of action is much shorter.
  - Hydromorphone is a potent morphine derivative, five to seven times the strength of morphine, and caution should be used when ordering this medication.
  - Fentanyl is available in a transdermal patch with sustained release over 72 hours. Initial onset of action is delayed. Respiratory depression may occur more frequently with fentanyl.
- Precautions
  - Opioids are relatively contraindicated in acute disease states in which the pattern and degree of pain are important diagnostic signs (e.g., head injuries). They also may increase intracranial pressure.
  - Opioids should be used with caution in patients with hypothyroidism, Addison disease, hypopituitarism, anemia, respiratory disease (e.g., chronic obstructive pulmonary disease [COPD], asthma, kyphoscoliosis, severe obesity), severe malnutrition, debilitation, or chronic cor pulmonale.
  - Opioid dosage should be adjusted for patients with impaired hepatic or renal function.
  - Drugs that potentiate the adverse effects of opioids include phenothiazines, antidepressants, benzodiazepines, and alcohol.
  - Tolerance develops with chronic use and coincides with the development of physical dependence, which is characterized by a withdrawal syndrome (anxiety, irritability, diaphoresis, tachycardia, GI distress, and temperature instability) when the drug is stopped abruptly. It may occur after only 2 weeks of therapy.
  - Administration of an opioid antagonist may precipitate withdrawal after only 3 days of therapy. Tapering the medication slowly over several days can minimize withdrawal.

- The quantity of opioid tablets prescribed at discharge should not exceed the expected duration of pain. A quantity to cover 3 days or less should be sufficient. **Prescribing a quantity at discharge to cover more than 7 days duration of pain should not be necessary and is discouraged.**[16]

- Adverse and toxic effects
  - Central nervous system (CNS) effects include sedation, euphoria, and pupillary constriction.
  - **Respiratory depression** is dose related and pronounced after IV administration.
  - Cardiovascular effects include **peripheral vasodilation** and hypotension.
  - GI effects include **constipation, nausea,** and **vomiting.** Stool softeners and laxatives should be prescribed to prevent constipation. Opioids may precipitate toxic megacolon in patients with inflammatory bowel disease.
  - Genitourinary effects include **urinary retention.**
  - **Pruritus** occurs most commonly with spinal administration.
  - **Opioid overdose**
    - Naloxone, an opioid antagonist, should be readily available for administration in the case of accidental or intentional overdose. For details of administration, see Chapter 26, Medical Emergencies.
    - Naloxone home rescue kits have been shown to reduce opioid overdose mortality.[17] **Patients being discharged home on more than 50 morphine milligram equivalents per day have a higher risk of overdose** and may benefit from a prescription for intranasal naloxone at discharge.

Altered Mental Status

GENERAL PRINCIPLES

Mental status changes have a broad differential diagnosis that includes neurologic (e.g., stroke, seizure, delirium), metabolic (e.g., hypoxemia, hypoglycemia), toxic (e.g., drug effects, alcohol withdrawal), and other etiologies. Infection (e.g., urinary tract infections, pneumonia) is a common cause of mental status changes in the elderly and in patients with underlying neurologic disease. Sundown syndrome refers to the appearance of worsening confusion in the evening and is associated with dementia, delirium, and unfamiliar environments.

DIAGNOSIS

History and Physical Examination

- Focus particularly on medications, underlying dementia, cognitive impairment, neurologic or psychiatric disorders, as well as any history of alcohol and/or drug use. Additionally, conduct a review of their current medications.
- Family and nursing personnel may be able to provide additional details.
- Physical examination generally includes vital signs, a search for sites of infection, a complete cardiopulmonary examination, and a detailed neurologic examination including mental status evaluation.

Diagnostic Testing

- Testing includes blood glucose, serum electrolytes, creatinine, CBC, urinalysis, and oxygen assessment.
- Other evaluation, including lumbar puncture, toxicology screen, cultures, thyroid function tests, noncontrast head CT, electroencephalogram, chest radiograph, or ECG should be directed by initial findings.

TREATMENT

- Withdrawal of the offending medication contributing to altered mental status.
- First-line management would be the use of supportive and nonpharmacological therapies to reorient the patient before considering pharmacological interventions.

Medications

Agitation and psychosis may be features of a change in mental status. The antipsychotic haloperidol and the benzodiazepine lorazepam are commonly used in the acute management of these symptoms. Second-generation antipsychotics (risperidone, olanzapine, quetiapine, clozapine, ziprasidone, aripiprazole, paliperidone) are alternative agents that may lead to decreased incidence of extrapyramidal symptoms. All of these agents pose risks to elderly patients and those with dementia if given long term.

- Haloperidol is the initial drug of choice for acute management of agitation and psychosis. The initial dose of 0.5–5 mg (0.25 mg in elderly patients) PO and 2–10 mg IM/IV can be repeated every 30–60 minutes. Haloperidol has fewer active metabolites and fewer anticholinergic, sedative, and hypotensive effects than other antipsychotics but may have more extrapyramidal side effects. In low dosages, haloperidol rarely causes hypotension, cardiovascular compromise, or excessive sedation.
- Prolongation of the QT interval. Use should be discontinued with prolongation of QTc >450 ms or 25% above baseline.
- Postural hypotension may occasionally be acute and severe after administration. IV fluids should be given initially for treatment. If vasopressors are required, dopamine should be avoided because it may exacerbate the psychotic state.
- Neuroleptic malignant syndrome (see Chapter 27, Neurologic Disorders).
- Lorazepam is a benzodiazepine that is useful for agitation and psychosis in the setting of hepatic dysfunction and sedative or alcohol withdrawal. The initial dose is 0.5–1 mg IV. Lorazepam has a short duration of action and few active metabolites. Excessive sedation and respiratory depression can occur.

Nonpharmacologic Therapies

Patients with delirium of any etiology often respond to frequent reorientation, observance of the day–night light cycle, maintain hydration, avoid restraints, manage pain, mobilization, bedside sitters, and maintenance of a familiar environment.

Insomnia and Anxiety

GENERAL PRINCIPLES

- Insomnia and anxiety may be attributed to a variety of underlying medical or psychiatric disorders, and symptoms may be exacerbated by hospitalization.
- Causes of insomnia include environmental disruptions, mood and anxiety disorders, substance abuse disorders, common medications (i.e., β-blockers, steroids, bronchodilators), sleep apnea, hyperthyroidism, and nocturnal myoclonus.
- Anxiety may be seen in anxiety disorder, depression, substance abuse disorders, hyperthyroidism, and complex partial seizures.

DIAGNOSIS

The diagnosis of insomnia and anxiety is a clinical one. No laboratory or imaging tests help in establishing the diagnosis; however, they can help to rule out other etiologies.

TREATMENT

Provide education on sleep hygiene and keeping the sleep environment quiet and dark.

Benzodiazepines

Benzodiazepines are frequently used in management of anxiety and insomnia. Table 1-2 provides a list of selected benzodiazepines and their common uses and dosages.

TABLE 1-2 Characteristics of Selected Benzodiazepines

Drug	Route	Common Uses	Usual Dosage	Half-Life (h)[a]
Alprazolam	PO	Anxiety disorders	0.75–4.0 mg/24 h (in three doses)	12–15
Chlordiazepoxide	PO	Anxiety disorders, alcohol withdrawal	15–100 mg/24 h (in divided doses)	5–30
Clonazepam	PO	Anxiety disorders, seizure disorders	0.5–4.0 mg/24 h (in two doses)	18–28
Diazepam	PO	Anxiety disorders, seizure disorders, preanesthesia	6–40 mg/24 h (in one to four doses)	20–50
	IV		2.5–20.0 mg (slow IV push)	20–50
Estazolam	PO	Insomnia	1–2 mg	10–24
Flurazepam	PO	Insomnia	15–30 mg at bedtime	50–100
Lorazepam[b]	PO	Anxiety disorders	1–10 mg/24 h (in two to three doses)	10–20
	IV or IM	Preanesthetic medication	0.05 mg/kg (4 mg max)	10–20
Midazolam	IV	Preanesthetic and intraoperative medication	0.01–0.05 mg/kg	1–12
	IM		0.08 mg/kg	1–12
Oxazepam[b]	PO	Anxiety disorders	10–30 mg/24 h (in three to four doses)	5–10
Temazepam[b]	PO	Insomnia	15–30 mg at bedtime	8–12
Triazolam	PO	Insomnia	0.125–0.250 mg at bedtime	2–5
Quazepam	PO	Insomnia	7.5–15 mg at bedtime	39
Etizolam	PO	Anxiety, Insomnia	1–3 (in single or divided doses)	4–8

[a]Half-life of active metabolites may differ.
[b]Metabolites are inactive.

- Pharmacology: Most benzodiazepines undergo oxidation to active metabolites in the liver. Lorazepam, oxazepam, and temazepam undergo glucuronidation to inactive metabolites; therefore, these agents may be particularly useful in the elderly and in those with liver disease. Benzodiazepines with long half-lives may accumulate substantially in the elderly, in whom the half-life may be increased manyfold.
- Dosages: Relief of anxiety and insomnia is achieved at the doses outlined in Table 1-2. Therapy should be started at the lowest recommended dosage with intermittent dosing schedules.
- Side effects include drowsiness, dizziness, fatigue, psychomotor impairment, and anterograde amnesia. Benzodiazepine toxicity is heightened by malnutrition, advanced age, hepatic disease and concomitant use of alcohol, other CNS depressants, and CYP3A4 inhibitors. The elderly may experience falls, paradoxical agitation, and delirium.
  - IV administration of diazepam and midazolam can be associated with hypotension, bradycardia, and respiratory or cardiac arrest.
  - Respiratory depression can occur even with oral administration in patients with respiratory compromise.
  - Tolerance to benzodiazepines can develop and dependence may develop after only 2–4 weeks of therapy.
  - Seizures and delirium may also occur with sudden discontinuation of benzodiazepines. A *withdrawal syndrome* consisting of agitation, irritability, insomnia, tremor, palpitations, headache, GI distress, and perceptual disturbance begins 1–10 days after a rapid decrease in dosage or abrupt cessation of therapy. Short-acting and intermediate-acting drugs should be decreased by 10%–20% every 5 days, with a slower taper in the final few weeks. Long-acting preparations can be tapered more quickly.
- Overdose: **Flumazenil**, a benzodiazepine antagonist, should be readily available in case of accidental or intentional overdose. For details of administration, see Chapter 26, Medical Emergencies.

Trazodone

- Trazodone is a serotonin receptor antagonist antidepressant that may be useful for the treatment of severe anxiety or insomnia. Common dosing is 50–100 mg at bedtime.
- It is highly sedating and can cause postural hypotension. It is rarely associated with priapism.
- Levels may be substantially increased when used with CYP3A4 inhibitors.

Doxepin

- Low-dose doxepin, at 3–6 mg, is approved for the treatment of sleep maintenance insomnia.
- Doxepin is a tricyclic antidepressant with antihistaminic activity that enhances sleep maintenance. It exhibits high selectivity for postsynaptic histamine H_1 receptors.
- At low doses, its activity at other receptors is limited, resulting in fewer associated side effects.
- Common side effects include sedation, nausea, and upper respiratory tract infection. It should be avoided in cases of angle-closure glaucoma, urinary retention, and when used concomitantly with MAO-I drugs.

Nonbenzodiazepine Hypnotics

These agents appear to act on the benzodiazepine receptor and have been shown to be safe and effective for initiating sleep. All should be used with caution in patients with impaired respiratory function.

- Zolpidem is an imidazopyridine hypnotic agent that is useful for the treatment of insomnia. It has no withdrawal syndrome, rebound insomnia, or tolerance. Side effects include headache, daytime somnolence, and GI upset. The starting dose is 5 mg PO every night at bedtime.

- Zaleplon has a half-life of approximately 1 hour and no active metabolites. Side effects include dizziness and impaired coordination. The starting dose is 10 mg PO at bedtime (5 mg for the elderly or patients with hepatic dysfunction).
- Eszopiclone offers a longer half-life compared to the previous agents. Side effects include headache and dizziness. Starting dose is 1 mg PO at bedtime.
- Ramelteon is a melatonin analog. The usual dose is 8 mg PO at bedtime.

Dual Orexin Receptor Antagonists

- These agents target the orexin receptors (OX1R and OX2R), facilitating sleep by reducing wake drive. They are indicated for insomnia characterized by difficultly with sleep onset and/or sleep maintenance. The drugs should be given at least 7 hours before the planned time of awakening.
- These drugs have significant drug-drug interactions with CYP3A4 inhibitors and inducers, requiring dose modification or avoidance.
- Lemborexant is administered at a dose of 5–10 mg before bedtime. When used in combination with mild inhibitors of CYP3A4, the recommended dose is 5 mg. Avoid use with moderate and strong inhibitors and inducers of CYP3A4.
- Suvorexant is started at a dose of 10–20 mg within 30 minutes of bedtime. If used in combination with moderate inhibitors of CYP3A, the recommended dose is 5 mg; it may increase to 10 mg. Strong inhibitors or inducers of CYP3A should be avoided.
- Daridorexant is administered at 25–50 mg within 30 minutes of bedtime. When used in combination with moderate inhibitors of CYP3A, the recommended dose is 25 mg. Strong inhibitors or moderate/strong inducers of CYP3A should be avoided.
- Common side effects are somnolence and dose-dependent driving impairment in the morning. They do not cause respiratory depression.

Antihistamines

Over-the-counter antihistamines can be used for insomnia and anxiety, particularly in patients with a history of drug dependence. Anticholinergic side effects limit the utility, especially in the elderly.

Constipation

- Constipation is frequently encountered in hospital settings and can have potentially serious consequences but is often unrecognized and undertreated. The prevalence among inpatients over 65 years is estimated at 50%.[18] Opioid-induced constipation is a common cause of constipation in hospitalized patients.
- Constipation assessment should be routinely done.
- The treatment of constipation is further discussed in Chapter 18, Gastrointestinal Diseases.

PERIOPERATIVE MEDICINE

The role of the medical consultant is to estimate the level of risk associated with a given procedure, determine the need for further evaluation based on this risk estimate, and prescribe interventions to mitigate risk. Although preoperative consultations often focus on cardiac risk, it is essential to remember that poor outcomes can result from significant disease in other organ systems. Evaluation of the entire patient is necessary to provide optimal perioperative care.

Preoperative Cardiac Evaluation

GENERAL PRINCIPLES

Perioperative cardiac complications are generally defined as cardiac death, MIs (both ST and non-ST elevation), CHF, and clinically significant rhythm disturbances.

Myocardial injury after noncardiac surgery (MINS)—defined as the peak elevation of the fourth-generation troponin T assay >0.03 ng/mL—is the most common major vascular complication following surgery and is associated with a marked increase in 30-day mortality. According to Vascular Events in Noncardiac Surgery Patients Cohort Evaluation (VISION) study, the prevalence of MINS is 8%.

Epidemiology

- Overall, an estimated 50,000 perioperative infarctions and one million other cardiovascular complications occur annually.[19] Of those who have a perioperative MI, the risk of in-hospital mortality is estimated at 10%–15%.[20]
- Perioperative MI (PMI) is believed to occur via two distinct mechanisms. Type I PMI results from erosion or rupture of unstable atherosclerotic plaque, leading to coronary thrombosis and subsequent myocardial injury. Type II PMI occurs when myocardial oxygen demand exceeds supply in the absence of overt thrombosis.
- Although angiographic data suggest that existing stenoses may underpin some perioperative events, a significant number of PMIs are "stress" related (Type II) and not because of plaque rupture.[21,22]
- Autopsy data indicate that fatal PMIs occur predominantly in patients with multivessel and especially left main coronary artery disease, via the same mechanism as non-PMIs.[23]

DIAGNOSIS

Clinical Presentation

History

The aim is to identify patient factors and comorbid conditions that will affect perioperative risk. Current guidelines focus on identification of active cardiac disease and known risk factors for perioperative events, which include:

- Unstable coronary syndromes including severe angina
- Recent MI (defined as >7 but <30 days)
- Decompensated CHF (New York Heart Association class IV, worsening or new-onset heart failure [HF])
- Significant arrhythmia including nonsinus rhythm (rate controlled and stable)
- Severe valvular disease
- Clinical risk factors for coronary artery disease (CAD)
- Preexisting, stable CAD
- Compensated or prior CHF
- Diabetes mellitus
- Prior cerebrovascular accident (CVA) or transient ischemic attack (TIA)
- Chronic kidney disease
- Poorly controlled hypertension
- Abnormal ECG (e.g., left ventricular hypertrophy, left bundle branch block, ST-T wave abnormalities)
- Age >70 years identified in several studies as a significant risk factor but not uniformly accepted as independent.[24,25]

Physical Examination

Specific attention should be paid to the following:

- Vital signs, with particular evidence of hypertension. Systolic blood pressure (SBP) <180 and diastolic blood pressure (DBP) <110 are generally considered acceptable. The management of stage III hypertension (SBP >180 or DBP >110) is controversial. However, postponing elective surgery to allow adequate BP control in this setting seems reasonable; how long to wait after treatment is implemented remains unclear.
- Evidence of **decompensated CHF** (elevated jugular venous pressure, rales, S3, edema).
- **Murmurs suggestive of significant valvular lesions**. According to the 2014 American Heart Association (AHA)/American College of Cardiology (ACC) Guideline for the Management of Patients with Valvular Heart Disease, the risk of noncardiac surgery is increased in all patients with significant valvular heart disease, although symptomatic aortic stenosis (AS) is thought to carry the greatest risk. The estimated rate of cardiac complications in patients with undiagnosed severe AS undergoing noncardiac surgery is 10%–30%. However, aortic valve replacement is also associated with considerable risk. Risk–benefit analysis appears to favor proceeding to intermediate-risk elective noncardiac surgery (see below) with appropriate intra- and postoperative hemodynamic monitoring (including intraoperative right heart catheter or transesophageal echocardiogram) as opposed to prophylactic aortic valve replacement in the context of asymptomatic severe disease. The same recommendations (albeit with less supporting evidence) apply to asymptomatic severe mitral regurgitation, asymptomatic severe AR with normal ejection fraction, and asymptomatic severe mitral stenosis (assuming valve morphology is not amenable to percutaneous balloon mitral commissurotomy, which should otherwise be considered to optimize cardiac status prior to proceeding to surgery). Symptomatic severe valvular disease of any type should prompt preoperative cardiology consultation. See the section on Valvular Heart Disease in Chapter 6, Pericardial and Valvular Heart Disease.
- In patients with moderate-to-severe rheumatic MS and symptoms or SPAP >50 mm Hg, valve intervention (PMC or surgery) is recommended before elective intermediate or high-risk surgery (Class I).

Diagnostic Criteria

The 2014 ACC/AHA Guideline on Perioperative Cardiovascular Evaluation and Management of Patients Undergoing Noncardiac Surgery offers a stepwise approach to preoperative evaluation and risk stratification (Figure 1-1).

- Step 1: Establish the urgency of surgery. Many surgeries are unlikely to allow for a time-consuming evaluation.
- Step 2: Assess for active cardiac conditions (see History, above).
- Step 3: Determine the surgery-specific risk as follows:
  - Low-risk surgeries (<1% expected risk of adverse cardiac events) include superficial procedures, cataract/breast surgery, endoscopic procedures, and most procedures that can be performed in an ambulatory setting.
  - Intermediate-risk surgeries (1%–5% risk of adverse cardiac events) include carotid endarterectomy, intraperitoneal/intrathoracic surgery, orthopedic surgery, head and neck surgery, and prostate surgery.
  - Vascular surgery involving extremity revascularization or aortic repair generally carries the highest risk (>5% risk of adverse cardiac events).
- Step 4: Assess the patient's functional capacity.

Poor functional capacity (<4 metabolic equivalents [METs]) is associated with an increased risk of perioperative cardiac events.[26,27] Although exercise testing is the gold standard, functional capacity can be reliably estimated by patient self-report.[28] Examples of activities that suggest at least moderate functional capacity (>4 METs) include climbing

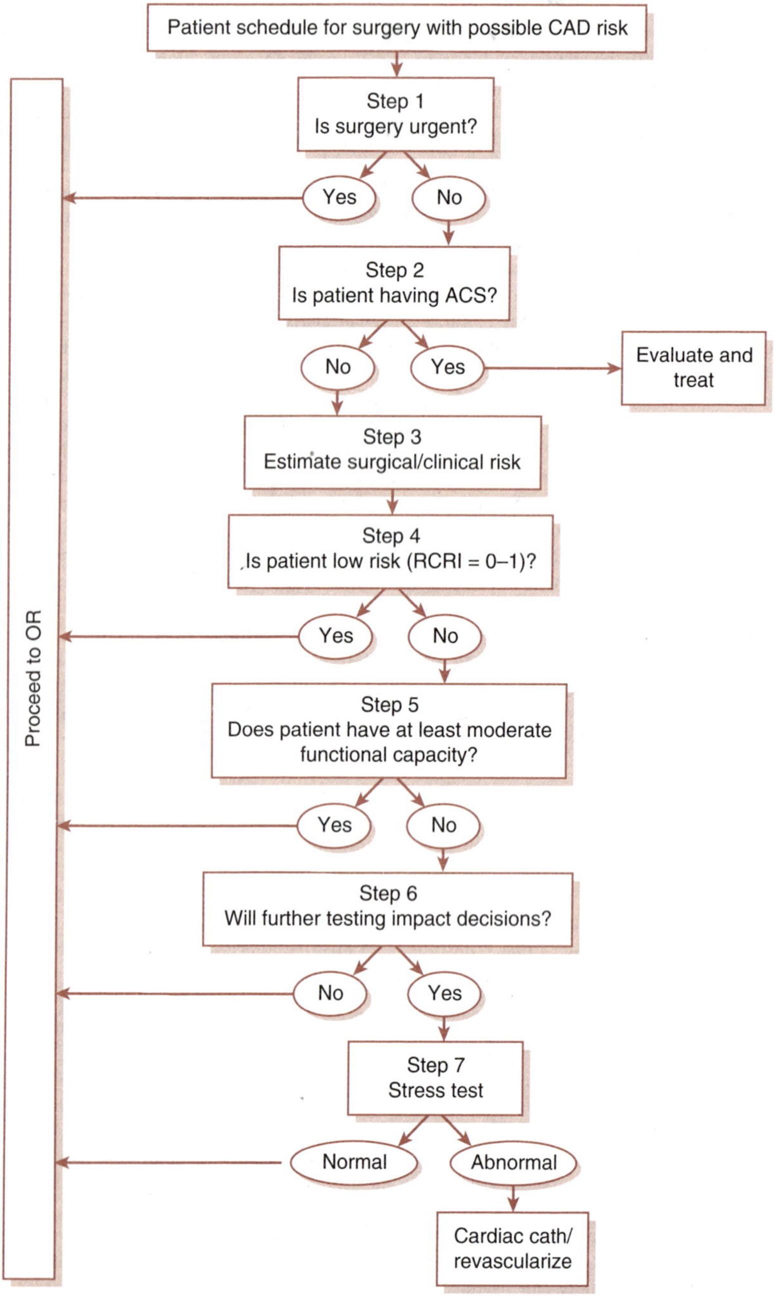

Figure 1-1 Cardiac evaluation algorithm for noncardiac surgery. (Modified from *Circulation*. 2014;130:e278–e333.)

one to two flights of stairs or walking a block at a brisk pace. Patients with a functional capacity of >4 METs without symptoms can proceed to surgery with relatively low risk.

- Step 5: Assess the patient's clinical risk factors.
  - The number of risk factors combined with the surgery-specific risk (intermediate vs. vascular) determines further management. The following risk factors are adapted from the Revised Cardiac Risk Index (RCRI)[29]
    - Ischemic heart disease
    - History of TIA or CVA
    - History of CHF
    - Preoperative serum creatinine ≥2 mg/dL
    - Diabetes mellitus requiring insulin
- Patients with no clinical risk factors are at inherently low risk (<1% risk of cardiac events) and may proceed to surgery without further testing. Patients with one or two clinical risk factors are generally at intermediate risk and may proceed to surgery, although stress testing might help refine risk assessment in selected cases. Patients with three or more clinical risk factors are at high risk of adverse cardiac events, particularly when undergoing vascular surgery. In this population especially, stress testing may provide a better estimate of cardiovascular risk and may be considered if knowledge of this increased risk would change management.[30] A positive stress test in a high-risk patient portends a substantially increased risk of a perioperative cardiac event, whereas a negative study suggests a lower risk than that predicted by clinical factors alone.[24]

2017 CCS STEPWISE APPROACH TO RISK STRATIFICATION

The 2017 Canadian Cardiovascular Society Guidelines on perioperative cardiac risk assessment and management for patients who undergo noncardiac surgery offer a stepwise approach to preoperative evaluation and risk stratification:

- **Step 1**. Assess for risk factors.
- **Step 2**. Establish the urgency of surgery. Urgent or emergency surgery, usually performed for organ- or life-threatening conditions, should not be delayed as benefits outweigh preoperative cardiac risk stratification concerns. Preoperative cardiac risk assessment should, however, be performed in patients undergoing urgent or semiurgent surgery whose history or physical examination indicates elevated risk of cardiovascular disease, such as severe obstructive intracardiac abnormality, severe pulmonary hypertension, or other cardiovascular condition.
- **Step 3**. Estimate surgical risk with RCRI.
  - **RCRI** contains six variables, each worth one point (i.e., history of ischemic heart disease, cerebrovascular disease, congestive heart failure, preoperative insulin usage, preoperative creatinine 177 mmol/L, and high-risk surgery), is easy to use, and discriminates moderately well between high-risk and low-risk patients undergoing mixed noncardiac surgery.
- **Step 4**. Measurement of N-terminal pro–B-type natriuretic peptide (NT-proBNP) or BNP should be performed in patients 65 years of age or older, 45–64 years of age with significant cardiovascular disease, or RCRI score ≥1, whenever available. The threshold values of ≥300 ng/L for NT-proBNP and ≥92 mg/L for BNP were found to be strongly associated with major cardiac events and death in patients undergoing in-hospital noncardiac surgery.

Diagnostic Testing

- **12-Lead ECG**. The value of a routine ECG is controversial. As per the ACC/AHA guidelines (level of evidence: B):

- ECG is "reasonable" in patients with known CAD, significant arrhythmia, peripheral arterial disease, cerebrovascular disease, or other significant structural heart disease prior to intermediate-risk surgery and above (Class IIa);
- "May be considered" for asymptomatic patients without known coronary heart disease prior to intermediate- and high-risk surgery (Class IIb);
- Is "not useful" for asymptomatic patients undergoing low-risk surgical procedures (Class III).

- **12-lead ECG:** As per the ESC 2022 guidelines, in patients who have known CVD or CV risk factors (including age >65 years) or symptoms or signs suggestive of CVD, 12-lead ECG and measurement of hs-cTnT or hs-cTnI is recommended before intermediate and high-risk surgery (Class I).[31]
- **Resting echocardiogram.** In general, the indications for preoperative echocardiographic evaluation are no different from those in the nonoperative setting. Murmurs found on physical exam suggestive of significant underlying valvular disease (see above) should be evaluated by echocardiogram. Assessment of left ventricular function should be considered when there is clinical concern for underlying undiagnosed CHF or if there is concern for deterioration since the last exam.
- **Noninvasive stress testing.** The decision to pursue a stress evaluation should be guided by an assessment of preoperative risk as detailed above. For further details on stress testing see Chapter 4, Ischemic Heart Disease.

Special Considerations

- Patients with drug-eluting coronary stents: see Perioperative Anticoagulation and Antithrombotic Management.
- Multiple studies have reported a correlation between delayed repair of hip fracture and increased morbidity and mortality.[32,33] For urgent surgical procedures (i.e., those that should be done within 48 hours of diagnosis), the value of additional testing is typically outweighed by the risk of worsened short- and long-term outcomes incurred with surgical delay. Unnecessary preoperative cardiac testing may be an independent risk factor for postoperative complications in hip fracture patients.[34] In such cases, it is advisable to optimize the patient's medical status and modifiable risk factors and then proceed to the operating room.
- For patients with an acute coronary syndrome (ACS), elective noncardiac surgery is typically postponed to manage the ACS effectively and minimize the risk of perioperative myocardial infarction (MI) and mortality. As per the 2022 European Society of Cardiology guidelines (ESC), for patients who underwent stenting, nonemergency, noncardiac surgery, it is deferred for at least 6 and 12 months after an ACS. For patients in whom delaying the surgery outweighs the benefits, surgery should be deferred by at least 1–3 months.
- Patients with newly diagnosed HFrEF surgery should be postponed by at least 3 months to allow medical stability.
- For patients with decompensated HFrEF or new or decompensated HF with preserved ejection fraction, delay elective surgery for at least 1 month to allow adequate optimization of therapy and stabilization of clinical status.
- In patients with atrial fibrillation with acute or worsening hemodynamic instability, emergency electrical cardioversion is recommended. Patients with symptomatic, monomorphic, sustained VT associated with myocardial scar, recurring despite optimal medical therapy, ablation of arrhythmia is recommended (Class I).

TREATMENT

- **General risk reduction strategies:** According to the ESC 2022 guidelines, smoking cessation >4 weeks before noncardiac surgery (Class I recommendation).

- Control of cardiovascular risk factors, including blood pressure, dyslipidemia, and diabetes (Class I recommendation).

Medications

- **β-Blockers**
  - Multiple studies have provided support for perioperative β-blockade in patients with or at risk for CAD undergoing noncardiac surgeries. The most pronounced benefit has been observed in high-risk patients undergoing vascular surgery where β-blocker dose was titrated to heart rate control.[30,35] However, a subsequent analysis has called into question the role of dose titration.[36] Although reduction in perioperative cardiac events has been observed consistently, it warrants mentioning that few data support the effectiveness of perioperative β-blockade in reducing mortality.
  - According to the 2014 ACC/AHA guidelines:
    - In patients with three or more RCRI risk factors (see above) or evidence of myocardial ischemia on preoperative stress testing, starting preoperative β-blockade is reasonable (level of evidence: B).
    - β-blockade should not be started on the day of surgery, as it is at minimum ineffective and may actually be harmful (level of evidence: B).
    - Patients already taking β-blockers should be continued on their medication (level of evidence: B).
- **Statins**
  - Statins are believed to improve cardiovascular outcomes by enhancing endothelial function, reducing vascular inflammation, and stabilizing atherosclerotic plaque in addition to their lipid-lowering effects. Multiple trials have shown a decrease in perioperative cardiac events and/or mortality with statin use in patients undergoing vascular surgery. Moreover, a recent cohort study of statin therapy in patients undergoing intermediate-risk noncardiac, nonvascular surgery revealed a fivefold reduced risk of 30-day all-cause mortality along with a statistically significant reduction in the composite end point of 30-day all-cause mortality, atrial fibrillation (AF), and nonfatal MI.[37]
  - Per the ACC/AHA guidelines:
    - Patients currently taking statins should be maintained on therapy (level of evidence: B).
    - Patients undergoing vascular surgery, and those with risk factors undergoing intermediate-risk surgery, may benefit from initiation of statin therapy perioperatively (level of evidence: B and C, respectively). Optimal dose, duration of therapy, and target low-density lipoprotein (LDL) levels for perioperative risk reduction are unclear.
    - Non-statin lipid lowering agents, such as niacin and fibric acid derivatives may cause rhabdomyolysis. Hence, they should be stopped one day before surgery and resumed after surgery.
- **Aspirin**
  For discussion, see Perioperative Anticoagulation and Antithrombotic Management.
- **Angiotensin-converting enzyme inhibitors (ACE-I)/angiotensin receptor blockers (ARB)**
  - ACE-I/ARB should be withheld 24 hours preceding noncardiac surgery and restarted 48 hours following surgery if the patient is hemodynamically stable.
  - **Diuretics:** Transient discontinuation on the day of surgery (Class IIa), unless prescribed for heart failure. Continuation can lead to hypotension and hypovolemia.
  - **SGLT2 inhibitors:** For patients on SGLT2 inhibitors, the drug should be stopped at least 3 days before intermediate or high-risk noncardiac surgery (Class IIa).

Revascularization

- The best available data on preoperative revascularization come from the Coronary Artery Revascularization Prophylaxis (CARP) trial, a prospective study of patients scheduled to undergo vascular surgery.[38] Patients with angiographically proven significant CAD were randomized to revascularization versus no revascularization. There was no difference between the groups in the occurrence of MI or death at 30 days or in mortality with long-term follow-up. Patients with three or more clinical risk factors and extensive ischemia on stress testing were evaluated in a separate small study.[39] High event rates were seen in both study arms, and no benefit was seen with revascularization. Taken together, these studies suggest that the risk of adverse cardiac events is not altered by attempts at preoperative revascularization, even in high-risk populations. A notable possible exception are patients with left main disease, who appeared to have benefited from preoperative revascularization in a subset analysis of the CARP trial data.[40]

- Based on these cumulative results, a strategy of routinely pursuing coronary revascularization as a method of decreasing perioperative cardiac risk cannot be recommended. However, careful screening of patients is still essential to identify those high-risk subsets who may obtain a survival benefit from revascularization independent of their need for noncardiac surgery.

MONITORING/FOLLOW-UP

Postoperative Infarction and Surveillance

- Myocardial injury after noncardiac surgery (MINS): The diagnosis of myocardial injury after noncardiac surgery requires that two criteria are met:
    - The presence of noncardiac surgery in the last 30 days with an elevated troponin level indicative of acute injury (e.g., fall, rise).
    - Nonischemic causes (e.g., sepsis, pulmonary embolism, cardioversion) of troponin elevation are reasonably excluded.
- Most events will occur within 48–72 hours of surgery, with the majority in the first 24 hours.[41]
- Most are not heralded by chest pain and may be **clinically asymptomatic.**[42] Although overall 30-day mortality has been linked to postoperative troponin elevation, the cause of death is not predictable, and no specific course of therapy may be offered.[43]
- The American Heart Association scientific statement on the diagnosis and management of patients with MINS recommends that high-risk individuals undergoing noncardiac surgery should have serial cardiac troponin measurements during the first 48–72 hours postoperatively while hospitalized.[44]
- The European Society of Cardiology guidelines recommend measurement of high-sensitivity troponin before intermediate- and high-risk noncardiac surgery and at 24–48 hours after surgery in patients who have cardiovascular risk factors (including age ≥65 years).[45]
- Patients with postoperative STEMI, NSTE-ACS, acute HF, and arrythmias should be treated in accordance with standard therapy (see Chapter 4, Ischemic Heart Disease), after considering bleeding risks with anticoagulants.
- As per 2017 CCS guidelines, postoperative ECG is recommended in patients with elevated NT-proBNP/BNP before surgery, those in whom NT-proBNP/BNP is not assessed prior to surgery, those with RCRI ≥1, those who are 45–64 years of age with significant cardiovascular disease, or patients 65 years of age or older.

Perioperative Anticoagulation and Antithrombotic Management

GENERAL PRINCIPLES

- Patients on chronic anticoagulation for AF, VTE, or mechanical heart valves often need to undergo procedures that pose risk of bleeding.

- The indication for anticoagulation and risk of interruption must be weighed against the risk of bleeding of the procedure (including possible neuraxial anesthesia).
- Until better research is available, decisions regarding perioperative anticoagulation will have to be made with the help of guidelines with relatively weak strength of evidence.[46]

TREATMENT

- Recommended management varies according to the indication for anticoagulation, medication used, and surgical bleeding risk.
- For patients being treated with oral anticoagulants/vitamin K antagonists (VKA):
    - **Low bleeding risk** procedures permit continuation of **oral anticoagulation** through the perioperative period (e.g., minor dental and dermatologic procedures, cataract extraction, endoscopy without biopsy, arthrocentesis). Pacemaker and implantable cardioverter defibrillator (ICD) placement lead to less hematoma if anticoagulation is not interrupted.[47]
    - **Significant bleeding risk procedures** require the anticoagulation to be discontinued.
        - Although the international normalized ratio (INR) at which surgery can be safely performed is subjective, an INR of <1.5 is typically a reasonable goal.
        - The VKA (e.g., warfarin) will typically need to be stopped 5 days preoperatively.
        - The INR should be checked the day before surgery. If a level <1.5 is not obtained, 1–2.5 mg oral vitamin K effectively achieves an INR <1.5 on the day of surgery.
        - The VKA can generally be resumed 12–24 hours postoperatively if postoperative bleeding has been controlled.[46]
    - **High bleeding risk procedures** (e.g., intracranial or spinal) with potential catastrophic outcomes because of bleeding will preclude any anticoagulation in the perioperative period. Other procedures with high bleeding risk (e.g., sessile polypectomy; bowel resection; kidney, liver, or spleen biopsy; extensive orthopedic or plastic surgery) should lead to a delay of at least 48 hours prior to resumption of anticoagulation.
- **Bridging therapy** refers to the administration of an alternative anticoagulation during the time the INR is anticipated to be below the therapeutic range. The potential decrease in thrombosis must be weighed against the increased risk of bleeding.[48]
- **High thrombotic risk patients** below should typically be treated with bridging therapy. Bridge with LMWH at therapeutic dose 3 days before surgery, with last preoperative dose 24 hours before surgery.
    - Mechanical mitral valve
    - Older-generation mechanical valve (e.g., Starr-Edwards ball-in-cage valve)
    - Any mechanical valve with a history of cardioembolism within the preceding 6 months
    - Nonvalvular AF with either a history of embolism in the last 3 months or $CHADS_2$ score ≥5 (see Chapter 7, Cardiac Arrhythmias)
    - Valvular AF
    - Recent VTE (<3 months)
    - Known thrombophilic state (e.g., protein C deficiency)
- For **moderate thrombotic risk patients** as below, bridging may be considered in patients with low bleeding risk. Deep venous thrombosis (DVT) prophylaxis dosing is acceptable.
    - Mechanical aortic valve (bileaflet) with one or more associated risk factors: AF, CHF, hypertension, age ≥75, DM, and prior CVA or TIA
    - History of VTE within preceding 3–12 months
    - Non–high-risk thrombophilia (e.g., heterozygous factor V Leiden mutation)
    - History of recurrent VTE
    - Active malignancy
- **Low thrombotic risk** patients are **not** believed to require bridging therapy. Treatment with DVT prophylaxis doses of LMWH or UFH is an alternative. This group includes patients with:

- Mechanical aortic valve (bileaflet) without associated risk factors, as above
- AF with a $CHADS_2$ score < 4, or history of prior embolism[49]
- Prior VTE >12 months prior (without history of recurrent VTE or known hypercoagulable state)

Decision regarding anticoagulation is discussed in Table 1-3.

TABLE 1-3 Anticoagulation Based on Risk of Thromboembolism and Bleeding Risk

	Minimal Bleeding Risk	Low Bleeding Risk	High Bleeding Risk
Low risk for thromboembolism	Do not interrupt oral anticoagulation May consider interrupting DOAC therapy on the day of the procedure	DOAC users: Interrupt DOAC therapy 1 day before the procedure Warfarin users: Warfarin should be interrupted ~5 days before the procedure and reinitiated within 24 hours after the procedure, provided that adequate hemostasis is present	DOAC users: Interrupt DOAC therapy 2 days before procedure and restart 24 hours after procedure Warfarin users: Warfarin should be interrupted ~5 days before the procedure and reinitiated within 24 hours after the procedure, provided that adequate hemostasis is present
Moderate risk for thromboembolism	Do not interrupt oral anticoagulation May consider interrupting DOAC therapy on the day of the procedure	DOAC users: Interrupt DOAC therapy Warfarin users: Warfarin should be interrupted ~5 days before the procedure and reinitiated within 24 hours after the procedure, provided that adequate hemostasis is present	DOAC users: Interrupt DOAC therapy Warfarin users: Warfarin should be interrupted ~5 days before the procedure and reinitiated within 24 hours after the procedure, provided that adequate hemostasis is present May administer prophylactic-dose LMWH for VTE prevention
High risk for thromboembolism	Do not interrupt oral anticoagulation May consider interrupting DOAC therapy on the day of the procedure	DOAC users: Interrupt DOAC therapy Therapeutic-dose heparin bridging should be administered	DOAC users: Interrupt DOAC therapy Therapeutic-dose heparin bridging therapy may be administered

DOAC, direct oral anticoagulant; LMWH, low-molecular-weight heparin; VTE, venous thromboembolism.

- **Choices for bridging therapy** are generally the LMWHs and UFH, including patients with mechanical heart valves.[46] ESC 2022 guidelines suggest LMWH for bridging in patients with mechanical heart valves and high surgical risk (Class I recommendation). There is less experience in this setting with other agents (e.g., fondaparinux), and their use cannot be considered routine.
  - **LMWHs** have the advantages of relatively predictable pharmacokinetics and ability to be administered SC. Monitoring of anticoagulant effect is typically not required. Renal dosing is available for patients not on dialysis. Subcutaneous administration allows for outpatient therapy in appropriate patients. This decreases the length and cost of hospitalization. The last dose should be given 24 hours prior to surgery.
  - **UFH** is the agent of choice for patients with end-stage renal disease (ESRD). It is typically administered IV and requires frequent monitoring of the activated partial thromboplastin time. UFH should be stopped at least 4 hours prior to the planned surgical procedure to allow the anticoagulant effect to wane. Fixed-dose subcutaneous UFH has been proven efficacious for treatment of VTE and may be considered as an option.[50]
  - **Novel oral anticoagulants** have relatively short half-lives (dabigatran = 14 h, rivaroxaban = 9 h, apixaban = 12 h), obviating the need for bridging anticoagulation. Agents should be held for two or three half-lives for low bleed risk procedures and three or four half-lives for high bleed risk procedures, keeping in mind the effects of renal function on clearance.
  - **Reversal agents** may be used if urgent surgery is required before this washout period.
  - **Idarucizumab** reverses dabigatran, **Andexanet alfa** reverses all Xa inhibitors.

  Summary of novel oral anticoagulant usage perioperatively is summarized in Table 1-4.
- **Patients being treated with antiplatelet agents**
  - Continuing antiplatelet agents perioperatively carries a risk of bleeding, whereas discontinuation may increase cardiovascular events. Irreversible agents must be withheld for 5–7 days before effects fully abate. Clinicians are again left with little evidence and sometimes conflicting guidelines.
- **Aspirin**
  - Perioperative ischemic evaluation-2 (POISE-2) trial found that perioperative aspirin increased bleeding risk but did not improve cardiovasculaı or mortality outcomes.
  - **Low bleeding risk procedures** (e.g., minor dermatologic or dental procedures) allow continuation of aspirin (acetylsalicylic acid [ASA]) being given for secondary prevention of cardiovascular disease.
  - For patients undergoing high bleeding risk surgery (e.g., intracranial, spinal or vitreoretinal eye surgery), it is recommended to stop aspirin for atleast 7 days preoperatively.
  - **Noncardiac surgery patients** should generally have clopidogrel (or other thienopyridines) held 5 days preoperatively. Prompt reinitiation with a loading dose of 300 mg should take place postoperatively. Further stratification drives decisions regarding ASA:
    - **Moderate to high cardiac risk**, in which case ASA should be continued perioperatively
    - **Low cardiac risk**, in which case ASA should be held 7 days preoperatively
- **Coronary artery bypass graft** candidates should generally continue ASA perioperatively and have clopidogrel held 5 days preoperatively.
- **Coronary stents** pose a particular risk of in-stent thrombosis and infarction if dual antiplatelet therapy is prematurely withheld. Whenever possible, surgery should be deferred until the minimum period of dual antiplatelet therapy is completed (balloon angioplasty without stent, 14 days; drug-eluting stents, 6 months; bare metal stents, 30 days).
- **Urgent surgeries** within the previous time frames should proceed with continued dual antiplatelet treatment, if possible. If the bleeding risk is felt to be high, ASA alone should be continued. Heparin bridging has not been shown to be of benefit. Bridging with IV glycoprotein IIb/IIIa antagonists or reversible oral agents (e.g., ticagrelor) is not routinely recommended.[51]

TABLE 1-4 Perioperative Usage of Novel Anticoagulant Agent

Anticoagulant	Renal Function CrCl (mL/min)	Withholding: Last Dose		Restarting		Reversal Antidotes for Major Bleeding
		Low Bleeding Risk Surgery	High Bleeding Risk Surgery	Minimal Low Bleeding Risk Surgery	High Bleeding Risk Surgery	
Dabigatran	>50	2 days before surgery	3 days before surgery	Resume ~24 hours after procedure	Resume 48–72 hours postprocedure	Idarucizumab alternative: Four-factor PCC tranexamic acid hemodialysis
	30–50	3 days before surgery	4–5 days before surgery			
Apixaban	>50	2 days before surgery	3 days before surgery	Resume ~24 hours after procedure	Resume 48–72 hours postprocedure	Andexanet alfa alternative: PCC factor VIIa tranexamic acid
	30–50	2 days before surgery	3 days before surgery			
	15–29.9	Individualized on the basis of patient and procedural factors for bleeding and thrombosis	Individualized on the basis of patient and procedural factors for bleeding and thrombosis			
Rivaroxaban	>50	2 days before surgery	3 days before surgery	Resume ~24 hours after procedure	Resume 48–72 hours postprocedure	Andexanet alfa alternative: Four-factor PCC factor VIIa tranexamic acid
	30–50	2 days before surgery	3 days before surgery			
	15–29.9	Individualized on the basis of patient and procedural factors for bleeding and thrombosis	Individualized on the basis of patient and procedural factors for bleeding and thrombosis			
Edoxaban	>50	2 days before surgery	3 days before surgery	Resume ~24 hours after procedure	Resume 48–72 hours postprocedure	PCC factor VIIa tranexamic acid

CrCl, creatinine clearance; PCC, prothrombin complex concentrate.

TABLE 1-5 Perioperative Usage of Other Antiplatelet Agents

Antiplatelet Agent	When to Cease Antiplatelet Therapy (If Required)	
	Elective Surgeries	Semiurgent CABG
Clopidogrel	7 days	48–72 hours
Prasugrel	7 days	5 days
Ticagrelor	5 days	48–72 hours
Ticlopidine	10–14 days	-

CABG, coronary artery bypass grafting.

Recommended time interval between discontinuation of antiplatelet agents prior to procedure is discussed in Table 1-5.

PERIOPERATIVE MANAGEMENT OF SPECIFIC CONDITIONS

Hypertension

GENERAL PRINCIPLES

- **Severe hypertension** (BP >180/110) preoperatively often results in wider fluctuations in intraoperative BP and has been associated with an increased rate of perioperative cardiac events (see the previous section, Preoperative Cardiac Evaluation).
- Antihypertensive agents that the patient has taken prior to admission for surgery may have an impact on the perioperative period.
  - When the patient is receiving β-blockers or clonidine chronically, withdrawal of these medications may result in tachycardia and rebound hypertension, respectively.
  - Evidence suggests that holding ACE-I and angiotensin II receptor blockers on the day of surgery may reduce perioperative hypotension. These agents should not be held if given for CHF.

DIAGNOSIS

BP monitoring should be done as part of a patient's routine vital signs. A portable or wall blood pressure cuff should be used. In the setting of severe hypertension, BP should be checked in both arms and with suitably sized BP cuffs to ensure accuracy.

TREATMENT

- Hypertension in the postoperative period is a common problem with multiple possible causes.
  - All **remediable causes of hypertension**, such as pain, agitation, hypercarbia, hypoxia, hypervolemia, and bladder distention, should be excluded or treated.
  - Poor control of essential hypertension secondary to discontinuation of medications the patient was previously taking in the immediate postoperative period is not uncommon; thus, reviewing the patient's home medication list is recommended.
  - A rare cause of perioperative hypertension is **pheochromocytoma**, particularly if its presence was unrecognized. Patients can develop an acute hypertensive crisis perioperatively

which should be treated, with **phentolamine** or **nitroprusside** recommended in this situation. When the diagnosis of pheochromocytoma is suspected, preoperative treatment to minimize risk is recommended and can be classically accomplished by titration of **phenoxybenzamine** preoperatively.

- Many parenteral antihypertensive medications are available for patients who are unable to take medications orally. Transdermal clonidine also is an option, but the onset of action is delayed.

Pacemakers and ICDs

GENERAL PRINCIPLES

- The use of electrocautery intraoperatively can have adverse effects on the function of implanted cardiac devices.
- A variety of errors can occur, from resetting the device to inadvertent discharge of an ICD.
- Complications are rare but are more likely with abdominal and thoracic surgeries.
- The type of device (i.e., pacemaker or ICD) and manufacturer should be determined.
- The initial indication for placement and the patient's underlying rhythm should be determined. Ideally, this can be determined from the history and an ECG.
- The device should be interrogated within 3–6 months of a significant surgical procedure.

TREATMENT

- **If the patient is pacemaker dependent, the device should be reprogrammed to an asynchronous mode (e.g., VOO, DOO) for the surgery.**
- The application of a magnet will cause most pacemakers to revert to an asynchronous pacing mode; however, if this is the planned management, it should be tested preoperatively, especially in the pacemaker-dependent patient.
- It should be noted that the effect of a magnet on ICDs is typically different from the effect on pacemakers in that it affects the antitachycardia function but does not alter the pacing function of most models. If the pacing function of an ICD needs to be altered perioperatively, the device will need to be reprogrammed.
- The antitachycardia function of an ICD will typically need to be programmed off for surgical procedures in which electrocautery may cause interference with device function, leading to the potential for unintentional discharge. The effect of a magnet on this function is variable, so programming is the preferred management. Continuous monitoring for arrhythmia is essential during the period when this function is suspended.
- Continuous ECG and pulse monitoring is recommended during surgery. Pulse monitoring should not be affected by electrocautery interference.
- Postoperative interrogation may be necessary, particularly if the device settings were changed perioperatively or if the patient is pacemaker dependent.
- **Consultation with an electrophysiologist** is strongly recommended if there is any uncertainty regarding the perioperative management of a device.

Pulmonary Disease and Preoperative Pulmonary Evaluation

GENERAL PRINCIPLES

Postoperative pulmonary complications are the second most common postoperative complication; their incidence ranges from 2% to 5.6% in the general surgical population.[52] Postoperative pulmonary abnormality that produces identifiable disease or dysfunction that is clinically significant and adversely affects the clinical course. Clinically significant pulmonary complications include atelectasis, pneumonia, bronchospasm, exacerbation of preexisting chronic lung disease, and respiratory failure.[53] Postoperative respiratory failure, defined as ventilator dependency for more than 48 hours or unplanned reintubation, carries a 30-day mortality rate as high as 26.5%.[54]

Risk Factors

Both patient-dependent and surgery-specific risk factors determine overall risk.[55]

- **Surgical site** is generally considered the greatest determinant of risk of pulmonary complications, with proximity to the diaphragm correlating with increasing risk.[56] Neurosurgery and surgeries involving the mouth and palate also impart increased risk.[54,57]
- **Duration of surgery** also correlates strongly with risk.[58–60]
- Regional anesthesia may reduce risk of pneumonia and respiratory failure as compared with **general anesthesia**, though it is difficult to draw firm conclusions.[61–64] Prolonged **neuromuscular blockade** is also strongly associated with postoperative pulmonary complications.[65]
- **COPD** is a well-known risk factor, with disease severity associated with risk of serious complications.[66] They have higher risk of postoperative pneumonia, prolonged ventilation, and reintubation. Patients with severe COPD (forced expiratory volume in 1 second [FEV1] <40% predicted) are 6 times more likely to have a major postoperative complication. Similarly, an FEV1 <60% predicted was found to be an independent predictor of increased mortality in patients undergoing coronary artery bypass graft (CABG) procedures. However, even patients with advanced lung disease can safely undergo surgery if deemed medically necessary; in contradistinction to hepatic disease (see "Liver Disease"), there is no identified threshold that precludes surgery.[67,68]
- **Interstitial lung disease** places patients at elevated risk for surgical lung biopsy and resection of malignancy but is not as well studied in patients undergoing general surgery.[69–71]
- **Pulmonary hypertension** is associated with significant morbidity in patients undergoing surgery.[72,73]
- Conversely, treated asthma and restrictive physiology associated with obesity do not appear to be significant risk factors.[55,74]
- **Congestive heart failure** may increase the risk of pulmonary complications to an even greater degree than that seen with COPD.[75]
- Multiple indices of general health status including **degree of functional dependence** and **American Society of Anesthesiologists class** have been linked to poor pulmonary outcomes.[75,76] ASA class >2 confers a 4.87-fold increase in risk.[77] Odds ratios for postoperative respiratory failure of 2.53 and 2.29 were observed for **hypoalbuminemia** (<3 g/dL) and **azotemia** (BUN > 30 mg/dL), respectively, in a large cohort.[57]
- **Age > 50 years** has been identified as an independent predictor of postoperative pulmonary complications. Risk increases linearly with age, in contrast to postsurgical cardiac risk (see "Preoperative Cardiac Evaluation"). Large observational studies informing currently used risk prediction models (see "Risk Stratification" below) have further validated these observations.
- **Smoking** is a well-established risk factor for both postoperative pulmonary and nonpulmonary complications.[78] As with malignancy, risk appears to be dose-dependent and associated with active use.[60,79]
- **Obstructive sleep apnea** (OSA) is increasingly being recognized as a risk factor for both cardiac and pulmonary complications.[80,81] OSA increases the odds of postoperative complications two- to fourfold.[82] Unrecognized OSA may pose an even greater risk; it is estimated that over 50% of patients with OSA presenting for surgery are undiagnosed.[83–85] The need for postoperative opioids is an important risk factor for oxygen desaturation and apnea in patients with OSA.
- Compared with patients solely diagnosed with OSA, patients with obesity hypoventilation syndrome (characterized by persistent daytime hypercapnia with $PaCO_2$ >45 mm Hg)

and those with overlap syndrome (chronic obstructive pulmonary disease [COPD] plus OSA) have an additional increased risk of pulmonary and cardiac complications, intensive care transfer, and length of stay.
- Neurologic impairment: Patients with impaired sensorium or residual deficits from a previous stroke have an increased risk of postoperative pneumonia and respiratory failure.[86]
- Immunosuppression: Chronic steroid use is associated with an increased risk of postoperative pneumonia. Daily use of alcohol within 2 weeks of surgery is associated with an increased risk of postoperative pneumonia and respiratory failure. Insulin-treated diabetes is associated with an increased risk of postoperative respiratory failure.
- Obesity and asthma have not been found to increase postoperative complications.

DIAGNOSIS

Clinical Presentation

History

Preoperative pulmonary evaluation should focus on the above-mentioned patient-dependent risk factors.
- Is there a history of lung disease? If so, what is the patient's baseline (e.g., level of exertional tolerance, degree of hypoxemia)? Is there evidence of recent deterioration (e.g., increased cough, sputum production)? Though not an absolute contraindication to surgery, it may be prudent to postpone an elective procedure until an exacerbation is treated or a superimposed upper respiratory tract infection has resolved.
- A full smoking history should be obtained.
- Screening for OSA should be undertaken. The STOP-Bang questionnaire (see "Obstructive Sleep Apnea–Hypopnea Syndrome", Chapter 10) can be implemented to determine risk of OSA.
- As nonpulmonary comorbidities impact the likelihood of pulmonary complications, (as delineated above), review of other organ systems is mandatory.

Physical Examination

- Vital signs can be helpful in determining pulmonary risk. Both **body mass index (BMI)** and **blood pressure** are components of the STOP-Bang questionnaire. Though hypoxemia itself does not appear to be a significant independent predictor of risk **oxygen saturation by pulse oximetry** may assist in risk stratification.[52,87]
- High **Mallampati class** (see "Obstructive Sleep Apnea–Hypopnea Syndrome", Chapter 10) may corroborate clinical suspicion for OSA. A study of 137 adults being evaluated for OSA found that every 1-point increase in Mallampati class increased the odds of OSA by 2.5.[88]
- **Stigmata of chronic lung disease** (e.g., increased anteroposterior dimension of the thorax, digital clubbing, adventitious lung sounds) should be actively sought along with **signs of decompensated heart failure** (jugular venous distention, rales, pretibial edema).

Risk Stratification

- Several validated risk indices have been developed for quantitating risk of postoperative pulmonary complications. Of these, the Arozullah respiratory failure index offers both practicality (in terms of a clearly defined outcome) and ease of use. It consists of six factors for which point scores are assigned based on multivariate analysis to stratify patients into five classes of postoperative respiratory failure risk (ranging from 0.5% to 26.6%).[57,87,89–90]
- Other risk assessment tools include the ARISCAT Risk Index, which predicts the overall incidence of postoperative pulmonary complications, by assigning a point score to seven independent risk factors.

- Gupta calculator for postoperative respiratory failure and pneumonia predicts the risk of failure to wean from mechanical ventilation within 48 hours of surgery or unplanned intubation/reintubation postoperatively.

Diagnostic Testing

- Routine laboratory testing
  - As mentioned earlier, underlying chronic kidney disease and hypoalbuminemia portend increased risk of postoperative pulmonary complications. The addition of **serum bicarbonate 28 mmol/L or above** to a STOP-Bang score of three or above increases the specificity for detecting moderate to severe OSA from 30% to 82%, though sensitivity is accordingly reduced.[91]
- Chest radiography (CXR)
  - As many findings deemed abnormal on routine CXR are chronic and do not alter management, imaging is recommended only if signs or symptoms (e.g., unexplained dyspnea) warrant.[92,93]
- Arterial blood gas (ABG) analysis
  - No data exist that suggest that ABG results contribute to risk estimation beyond the variables delineated earlier. Nevertheless, ABG may be helpful in certain circumstances (e.g., to determine whether a patient's known chronic lung disease is compensated). See "Respiratory Failure", Chapter 8.
- Pulmonary function testing (PFTs)
  - The value of preoperative PFTs is at best debatable outside of lung resection surgery, where its role is relatively well defined (see Chapters 9, "Chronic Obstructive Pulmonary Disease", and 22, "Lung Cancer"). However, they may be considered in further evaluation of selected patients with unexplained dyspnea or exertional impairment or for those with known lung disease with unclear baseline.
  - Exercise testing: Cardiopulmonary exercise testing (CPET) is used to assess patients with abnormal PFTs to determine the safety of planned lung resection surgery. Alternatively, the six-minute walk test can be performed.

TREATMENT

- Preoperative treatment should focus on those risk factors which are modifiable.
- The effect of preoperative smoking cessation on pulmonary complications has been largely described in cardiothoracic surgeries, where a **benefit to quitting smoking at least 2 months prior to surgery** has been shown.[94] Though the effect on a general surgical population is less clear, pooled data show a significant reduction in pulmonary complications.[95] Maximizing the preoperative smoking cessation period appears to minimize complications. Though it is unknown whether smoking cessation is beneficial within 2 weeks of surgery, previous concerns about a paradoxical increase in complications appear unfounded.[96,97]
- COPD and asthma therapy should be optimized (see Chapter 9, Obstructive Lung Disease), and respiratory tract infections should be treated. Indeed, risk of postoperative pulmonary complications is increased in the month following a respiratory tract infection.[98] Nonemergency surgery may need postponement to allow recovery of pulmonary function to baseline.
- OSA should be treated prior to elective high-risk surgery when feasible. Though evidence from randomized controlled trials remains limited, a recent cohort study revealed a significant reduction in cardiovascular complications (primarily cardiac arrest and shock) between undiagnosed and diagnosed OSA after prescription of CPAP.[99] A subsequent meta-analysis of 904 patients failed to show a significant difference in postoperative adverse events despite statistically significant reduction in apnea-hypopnea index with

postoperative use of CPAP, a finding attributed to overall poor compliance.[100] Patients with known OSA should be continued on CPAP perioperatively.[101]

- Educating patients on inspiratory muscle training and pulmonary rehabilitation has shown to decrease complications and length of stay in patients undergoing AAA repair, CABG, and lung resection.[102–104]
- Alternative procedures with reduced pulmonary risk should be considered for high-risk patients. Laparoscopic procedures may yield fewer pulmonary complications; regional nerve block appears to be associated with decreased risk as well.[105,106] If general anesthesia (particularly with neuromuscular blockade) is absolutely necessary, duration should be minimized to the degree possible.

Anemia and Transfusion Issues in Surgery

GENERAL PRINCIPLES

Preoperative anemia is present in 5%–35% of patients depending on the definition of anemia and type of surgery studied. Both anemia and its treatment by allogeneic red cell transfusion have been associated with increased mortality and morbidity. There is no standardized preoperative evaluation for anemia.

- For low-risk procedures, there is no evidence that routine testing of asymptomatic individuals before low-risk procedures increases safety.[107]
- For higher risk procedures, particularly those with higher bleeding risk, a baseline CBC and coagulation profile are typically obtained. Further testing should be performed as indicated.

DIAGNOSIS

- A history of anemia, hematologic disease, or bleeding diathesis should be noted on history or review of medical records.

  Any clinical signs of anemia (e.g., pallor) or coagulopathy (e.g., petechiae) should prompt further evaluation. Strategies to reduce perioperative transfusions in noncardiac surgery are discussed in Table 1-6.

TABLE 1-6 Interventions to Reduce Perioperative Transfusions

Evaluations	Interventions for Individuals with Relevant Findings
Preoperative	
Screen for anemia (to be done 4 weeks before planned surgery)	• Address treatable causes of anemia, such as iron deficiency or vitamin B_{12} deficiency • Determine need for erythropoietin • Delay elective high blood loss surgery (anticipated >500 mL) until cause of anemia can be addressed and appropriate therapy instituted
For patients receiving anticoagulants, determine thrombotic and bleeding risks	• Follow current recommendations for anticoagulant discontinuation and reinitiation

(Continued)

TABLE 1-6 Interventions to Reduce Perioperative Transfusions (Continued)

Evaluations	Interventions for Individuals with Relevant Findings
Determine expected blood loss	• Prepare to use intraoperative blood salvage for those with expected blood loss >1000 mL
Intraoperative	
All patients	• Maintain euvolemia (large volumes of crystalloid solution are typically avoided) • Avoid hypothermia • Use meticulous hemostatic technique • Topical hemostatic agents when appropriate
Expected large surgical blood loss >1000 mL	• Use intraoperative blood salvage if appropriate • Administer an antifibrinolytic agent if appropriate
Postoperative	
All patients	• Minimize blood sampling
Excessive bleeding	• Early surgical re-exploration for those with localized internal bleeding • Cell salvage in selected cases with large external blood loss • Laboratory testing and hematology input for those with diffuse bleeding

Modified from Graetz ATJ, Nuttall G, Shander A. Perioperative blood management: Strategies to minimize transfusions. 2020;1–28. https://www.uptodate.com/contents/perioperative-blood-management-strategies-to-minimize-transfusions

TREATMENT

- Patients undergoing emergency procedures should proceed with surgery with the option of blood transfusions as necessary.
- Elective surgeries may be delayed until the cause of anemia is determined, and appropriate treatment is provided.
- Volume resuscitation and control of active bleeding are the initial therapy of anemia, particularly in the perioperative period when acute blood loss is a common occurrence.
  - A restrictive RBC transfusion threshold of 7 g/dL and a target of 7–9 g/dL are recommended for patients undergoing orthopedic surgery, those undergoing cardiac surgery, and those with preexisting cardiovascular disease.[108]

SPECIAL CONSIDERATIONS

Patients with sickle cell anemia should generally be transfused to a hemoglobin of 10 g/dL preoperatively to decrease the incidence of complications.[109]

Platelet transfusions may be required for invasive procedures if the thrombocytopenia is severe, if there is insufficient time to use other therapies to raise the platelet count and if the risks of bleeding are high. Platelet transfusion is considered based on the type of surgery when it's below the threshold.

- Neurosurgery or ocular surgery: <100,000/μL
- Endoscopic procedures: <50,000/μL for therapeutic procedures; 20,000/μL for low-risk diagnostic procedures
- Bronchoscopy with bronchoalveolar lavage (BAL): <20,000–30,000/μL
- Central line placement: <20,000/μL
- Lumbar puncture: <10,000–20,000/μL in patients with hematologic malignancies and <40,000–50,000 μL in patients without hematologic malignancies; lower thresholds may be used in patients with ITP.
- Neuraxial analgesia/anesthesia: <80,000/μL
- Bone marrow aspiration/biopsy: <20,000/μL

Liver Disease

GENERAL PRINCIPLES

Patients with liver disease face increased operative morbidity and mortality in comparison to those with normal hepatic function. Not only does the stress of surgery place them at risk for acute hepatic decompensation, the myriad systemic effects of liver disease result in an increased frequency of complications to multiple other organs as well. Emergency surgery confers four to five times higher mortality, and certain surgeries, such as cardiac surgeries with cardiopulmonary bypass, are to be avoided even in patients with Child–Turcotte–Pugh (CTP) class B. Emergency surgeries should be deferred if possible, and, with meticulous optimization of medical management, the semielective surgery should be arranged. The preoperative consultant's role is to minimize these risks.

Classification

- Both the older CTP and more recent Model for End-stage Liver Disease (MELD) classification schemes (see Chapter 19, "Liver Diseases") are well-validated statistical models for predicting surgical risk in patients with cirrhosis.
  - Two different studies separated by 13 years revealed strikingly similar results: a mortality rate of 10% for patients with CTP class A, 30% for class B, and 76%–82% for class C cirrhosis.[110,111] Accordingly, it has been suggested that patients with CTP class A cirrhosis can safely undergo elective surgery in general, and those with class C cirrhosis should not under any circumstances.[112] However, the distinction is less clear for class B cirrhosis, and the inherent subjectivity of the CTP system limits its discriminatory ability.[113]
  - MELD offers several advantages for calculation of 30-day mortality:
    - Variables are both objective and weighted.
    - It includes serum creatinine, which has been shown to correlate with postoperative mortality.[114]
    - Predictive performance is equal to if not better than that of CTP.[115-117]
    - Patients with a MELD (or MELD-Na) score less than 10 can undergo elective surgery, those with a MELD score of 10–15 may undergo elective surgery with caution, and those with a MELD score >15 should not undergo elective surgery.
  - Because CTP includes ascites, which is also correlated with poor prognosis in general surgical patients, the two scoring systems could be considered complementary rather than mutually exclusive.[118,119]
- American Society of Anesthesiologists (ASA) class appears to be the strongest predictor of 7-day mortality in cirrhotic patients undergoing surgery.[120] All 10 patients with ASA class V disease died, indicating that ASA class V should be a contraindication to surgery other than liver transplantation.[121]
- Patients with cirrhosis have increased morbidity and mortality associated with abdominal (especially cholecystectomy, gastric resection, or colectomy), cardiac, hepatic resection, bariatric, and emergency surgeries.

- Surgery is contraindicated in settings with an unacceptable risk of surgical mortality such as acute alcoholic hepatitis, acute liver failure, acute viral hepatitis, severe chronic hepatitis, severe coagulopathy (platelet <50,000 or PT >3 seconds despite vitamin K administration), and severe extrahepatic complications.

DIAGNOSIS

Clinical Presentation

Significant hepatic disease that greatly impacts surgical risk (e.g., acute liver failure, advanced cirrhosis) is usually clinically obvious (scleral icterus, abdominal distention from ascites, florid encephalopathy). For milder disease, however, more subtle findings such as spider nevi, palmar erythema, and testicular atrophy may be the only clues. Historical details such as family history of hepatic disease, current or prior alcohol and/or intravenous drug abuse, and transfusion history may increase clinical suspicion. See Chapter 19, "Liver Diseases" for further details.

Diagnostic Testing

- Because of the exceedingly low yield of laboratory testing (0.14% in one prospective study enrolling 7620 patients), routine preoperative assessment of hepatic function is not recommended unless clinical findings dictate.[112,122]
- Those with suspected or known hepatic disease should undergo thorough laboratory evaluation including hepatic enzyme levels, albumin and bilirubin measurement, and coagulation studies along with renal function and electrolytes. If significant laboratory abnormalities (e.g., unexplained transaminase elevation greater than 3 times upper limit of normal) are found in patients without known liver disease, surgical intervention may need to postponement to allow further workup, as the incidence of undiagnosed cirrhosis in this population may be 6% or even higher.[112,123]

TREATMENT

- Historically, patients with acute viral or alcoholic hepatitis have been observed to tolerate surgery poorly and delaying surgery until clinical and biochemical recovery is recommended.[112,124,125]
- Patients with mild chronic hepatitis without associated cirrhosis generally tolerate surgery well.[126]
- For patients with cirrhosis, several steps should be taken to optimize preoperative status:
  - Coagulopathy should be treated to minimize risk of hemorrhage. Vitamin K supplementation may be helpful if the INR is elevated. However, in the context of marked hepatic synthetic dysfunction, administration of fresh frozen plasma and/or cryoprecipitate may be necessary. Marked thrombocytopenia should be corrected via transfusion. (See section on Liver Disease in Chapter 20, Disorders of Hemostasis and Thrombosis.)
  - As cirrhosis is associated with renal dysfunction, intravascular hypovolemia, and extravascular fluid retention, careful attention to volume status is crucial. Nephrotoxic agents should be used with extreme caution if at all, and free water restriction may be required in patients with serum sodium below 130. However, judicious use of diuretics and/or timely paracentesis may be required to control ascites, particularly if abdominal surgery is being considered.[127] Administration of large amounts of crystalloid should be avoided. Despite theoretical benefits, strong evidence for preoperative TIPS to reduce portal hypertension prior to major abdominal surgery remains lacking but may be considered in select circumstances.[119]
  - Close attention to nutritional status is warranted in light of the very high incidence of malnutrition in this population.[128] In particular, deficiencies of fat-soluble vitamins,

thiamine, magnesium, and phosphorus are common. See Chapter 2, Nutrition Support.

- Patients with known esophageal varices should receive appropriate prophylactic treatment.
- Transjugular intrahepatic portosystemic shunt can be considered to reduce portal hypertension prior to the nonhepatic abdominal surgery. Laparoscopic surgery should be performed whenever possible, as it is associated with less tissue trauma, traction of the abdominal viscera, and risk of bleeding and infection.
- Nutrition. Patients with cirrhosis are often malnourished and may have sarcopenia (loss of muscle mass). Perioperative nutritional support can reduce the frequency of postoperative complications and short-term mortality; its benefit on long-term survival is uncertain.[129]
- Finally, encephalopathy (see Chapter 19, "Hepatic Encephalopathy") frequently complicates surgical intervention.[130] Lactulose should be titrated to three to four bowel movements per day, and concurrent rifaximin therapy should be strongly considered.[131] Opioid use should be minimized because of its propensity to engender constipation and ileus, and dose reduction considered in light of expected reduced hepatic clearance.
- Following surgery, patients with liver disease should be observed closely for hepatic decompensation, which often presents with worsening jaundice, encephalopathy, and ascites. The best biochemical measures of liver function are probably the PT/INR and serum bilirubin concentration.

Diabetes Mellitus

GENERAL PRINCIPLES

- Medical and surgical patients with hyperglycemia are at increased risk for poor outcomes.[132]
- The fact that hyperglycemia is a marker for poor outcomes appears to be relatively clear. However, whether aggressive management truly improves outcomes is uncertain. Trial results have been mixed.

TREATMENT

- The goals of perioperative diabetic management include avoidance of hypoglycemia, prevention of ketoacidosis, maintenance of fluid and electrolyte balance, and avoidance of marked hyperglycemia.
- Elective surgery in patients with uncontrolled diabetes mellitus should preferably be scheduled after acceptable glycemic control has been achieved.
- The American Diabetes Association (ADA) suggests a target glucose range between 80 and 180 mg/dL perioperatively.
- If possible, the operation should be scheduled for early morning to minimize prolonged fasting.
- Frequent monitoring of blood glucose levels is required in all situations.
- Type 1 diabetes
    - Some form of basal insulin is required at all times.
    - On the evening prior to surgery, the regularly scheduled basal insulin should be continued. If taken in the morning, it is still recommended to give the regularly scheduled basal insulin without dose adjustment.[133] However, patients who are very tightly controlled may be at increased risk for hypoglycemia and will need to be monitored closely. A decrease in the last preoperative basal insulin dose may be considered in this circumstance.
    - Glucose infusions (e.g., D5-containing fluids) can be administered to avoid hypoglycemia while the patient is NPO and until tolerance of oral intake postoperatively is established.

    - For complex procedures and procedures requiring a prolonged NPO status, a continuous insulin infusion will likely be necessary.
    - **Caution should be exercised with the use of subcutaneous insulin** in the intraoperative and critical care settings, as alterations in tissue perfusion may result in variable absorption.
- **Type 2 diabetes**
    - Treatment of type 2 diabetics varies according to their preoperative requirements and the complexity of the planned procedure.[134]
    - **Diet-controlled type 2 diabetes** can generally be managed without insulin therapy. Glucose values should be checked regularly and elevated levels (>180 mg/dL) can be treated with intermittent doses of short-acting insulin.
    - **Type 2 diabetes managed with oral therapy**
        - **Short-acting sulfonylureas and other oral agents** (e.g., DPP-4 inhibitors) should be withheld on the operative day.
        - **Metformin and long-acting sulfonylureas** (e.g., chlorpropamide) should be withheld 1 day before planned surgical procedures. Metformin is generally held for 48 hours postoperatively provided there is no acute renal injury. Other oral agents can be resumed when patients are tolerating their preprocedure diet.
    - SGLT2 inhibitors should be withheld 3–4 days before surgery due to increased risk of UTI and hypovolemia. Also increased association of postoperative euglycemic ketoacidosis has been described.
    - Daily GLP-1 receptor agonists (e.g., liraglutide) should be withheld on the morning of surgery. Weekly once GLP-1 based therapies should be withheld one week prior to surgery.
        - Glucose values should be checked regularly and elevated levels (>180 mg/dL) can be treated with intermittent doses of short-acting insulin.
    - **Type 2 diabetes managed with insulin**
        - Long-acting insulin (e.g., glargine insulin) if normally given in morning, it can be given at 50% of the usual dose the day of surgery. If it is administered in the evening, then reduce the dose of basal insulin by 10–25% on the evening prior to surgery.
        - If patients are on basal-bolus regimen, then the prandial insulin should be omitted once the fasting for surgery begins. Basal insulin should be continued as mentioned earlier in the chapter.
        - Intermediate-acting insulin (e.g., NPH), can be given at one-half to two-thirds of the usual morning dose.
        - Dextrose-containing IV fluids may be required to avoid hypoglycemia.
        - The usual insulin treatment can be reintroduced once oral intake is established postoperatively.
- **Target glucose levels**
    - There are no generally agreed-upon target glucose levels applicable to the entire postsurgical population.
    - Pending further research, a goal of maintaining glucose levels <180 mg/dL in the postoperative setting seems reasonable. It should be noted that this may still require intensive treatments such as insulin infusion.
    - In patients treated with sliding scale insulin, it is essential to monitor the response to therapy. Patients who are hyperglycemic consistently are unlikely to have adequate glucose control with intermittent treatment alone, and a basal/bolus regimen should be introduced if hyperglycemia is persistent.[135]
- Patient requiring emergency surgery with high glucose levels (>250) should be started on IV insulin infusion. If the patient was on basal insulin or short-acting insulin, it should be continued along with the insulin infusion.

Thyroid Disease

GENERAL PRINCIPLES

The prevalence of patients with abnormal thyroid function is considerable. It is higher in women and it increases with age. Thus, a substantial number of patients undergoing surgery may have concomitant thyroid disease. Preoperative thyroid function testing is not routinely recommended. It is reasonable, however, if the history and physical examination are suggestive of thyroid disease, as it may have an effect on perioperative care.

Acutely/severely ill hospitalized patients may suffer from nonthyroidal illness which may be differentiated from central hypothyroidism. In such patients nonurgent surgeries should ideally be postponed and thyroid functions should be monitored every 4–6 weeks.

If the surgery is urgent, treat it with thyroid hormone replacement in the pre- and perioperative periods if there is clinical evidence to suggest a diagnosis of moderate-to-severe hypothyroidism (e.g., bradycardia and hypothermia along with slow mentation, puffy face, a possible personal or strong family history of thyroid disease, or personal history of hypothalamic or pituitary disease or cranial irradiation).

HYPOTHYROIDISM (TABLE 1-7)

TABLE 1-7 Perioperative Recommendations for Hypothyroidism

	Surgical Outcomes	Management
Subclinical/mild hypothyroidism • Normal serum free T4 with elevated serum TSH	No significant differences in major adverse cardiovascular events or other outcomes	Surgery need not be postponed
Overt hypothyroidism • Elevated TSH • Low free T4 • Without features of severe hypothyroidism	Higher frequency of perioperative and postoperative ileus, hypotension, hyponatremia, impaired wound healing, prolonged mechanical ventilation or reintubation, prolonged inotropic support, and central nervous system dysfunction	Elective surgery should be postponed till euthyroid state is achieved. However, urgent surgery may be done and minor perioperative complications should be anticipated and managed, if they occur Oral thyroxine 1.6 micro gram/kg to be initiated
Severe hypothyroidism • Patients with myxedema syndrome may experience altered sensorium, pericardial effusion, or heart failure	Intraoperative hypotension; cardiovascular collapse; extreme sensitivity to opioids, sedatives, and anesthesia; and higher mortality rate	Elective surgery should be delayed until hypothyroidism has been treated If emergency surgery must be performed in a patient with severe hypothyroidism, the patient should be treated as soon as the diagnosis is made

(Continued)

TABLE 1-7 Perioperative Recommendations for Hypothyroidism (Continued)

	Surgical Outcomes	Management
• Very low total T4 (<1 μg/dL) or free T4 (<0.5 ng/dL)		Loading dose of levothyroxine (200–300 μg) is given intravenously followed by 50 μg daily. *Or* loading dose of T3 (5–20 μg intravenously) is given simultaneously, followed by 2.5–10 μg every 8 hours depending on the patient's age and coexistent cardiac risk factors Hydrocortisone, 50 mg IV q8h, is recommended to prevent adrenal crisis. Postoperatively, fluid and electrolyte status should be closely monitored

HYPERTHYROIDISM (TABLE 1-8)

TABLE 1-8 Perioperative Recommendations for Hyperthyroidism

	Features	Management
Subclinical hyperthyroidism	Clinical: Asymptomatic Laboratory: Low TSH with normal free T4 and T3	Surgery need not be postponed Unless contraindicated, administer beta-blocker preoperatively to older patients (>50 years) or younger patients with cardiovascular disease and taper after recovery
Overt hyperthyroidism	Clinical: May be symptomatic Laboratory: Elevated free T4 and/or T3, suppressed TSH	Elective surgery should be postponed till euthyroid state is achieved (3–8 weeks). However, urgent surgery may be done Preoperative treatment of hyperthyroidism should be initiated as soon as possible. Patient should be evaluated for cardiopulmonary disease, and monitored for the development of arrhythmias, cardiac ischemia, and congestive heart failure Preoperative preparation is as described for thyroid surgeries and includes a combination of β-blockers, antithyroid agents, and iodine to control the resting heart rate to less than 90 bpm, as well as prophylactic corticosteroid supplementation to prevent thyroid storm

Modified from Palace MR. Perioperative management of thyroid dysfunction. *Health Serv Insights*. 2017;10:117863291668967.

Adrenal Insufficiency and Corticosteroid Management

GENERAL PRINCIPLES

- Surgery is a potent activator of the hypothalamic–pituitary axis, and patients with adrenal insufficiency may lack the ability to respond appropriately to surgical stress.
- Patients receiving corticosteroids as anti-inflammatory therapy may rarely develop postoperative adrenal insufficiency. Case reports of presumed adrenal insufficiency from the 1950s led to the widespread use of perioperative "stress-dose" steroids in this population.[136,137]
- The dose and duration of exogenous corticosteroids required to produce clinically significant tertiary adrenal insufficiency is highly variable, but general principles can be outlined.[134]
  - Daily therapy with 5 mg or less of prednisone (or its equivalent), alternate-day corticosteroid therapy, and any dose given for <3 weeks should not result in clinically significant adrenal suppression.
  - Patients receiving >20 mg/d prednisone (or equivalent) for >3 weeks and patients who are clinically "cushingoid" in appearance can be expected to have significant suppression of adrenal responsiveness.
  - The function of the hypothalamic–pituitary axis cannot be readily predicted in patients receiving doses of prednisone 5–20 mg for >3 weeks.

DIAGNOSIS

Cosyntropin stimulation test may also be performed to determine adrenal responsiveness, measuring a single cortisol level at 60 minutes after 250 μg of cosyntropin. This can be done any time of day and there is no need for baseline cortisol. Levels >18 μg/dL at 30 minutes generally suggest an intact hypothalamic–pituitary axis.

TREATMENT

- If there is concern for secondary adrenal insufficiency, it is reasonable **to simply continue to provide baseline steroid supplementation** perioperatively.[138] It may be prudent to switch to an IV formulation to ensure it is not withheld while the patient is NPO.
- For patients with primary adrenal insufficiency, a stress stratification scheme has been developed, based on expert opinion. Please refer to Chapter 24, Endocrine Diseases, for details of treatment.

Chronic Renal Insufficiency and ESRD

GENERAL PRINCIPLES

- **Chronic renal insufficiency** (CRI) is an independent risk factor for **perioperative cardiac complications**, so all patients with renal disease need appropriate cardiac risk stratification.[24]
- **Patients with ESRD** have a substantial mortality risk when undergoing surgery.[139]
- Most general anesthetic agents have no appreciable nephrotoxicity or effect on renal function other than that mediated through hemodynamic changes.[140]
- Avoid nephrotoxic agents by substituting or dosage adjustments, these include NSAIDs, muscle relaxants, sedatives, antibiotics, and radiocontrast material.

TREATMENT

- **Correction of Volume status**
  - Every effort should be made to **achieve euvolemia** preoperatively to reduce the incidence of volume-related complications intraoperatively and postoperatively.[141]
  - Although this typically entails removing volume, some patients may be hypovolemic and require hydration.
  - Ringer lactate should be avoided as it can cause hyperkalemia.
  - Patients with CRI not receiving hemodialysis may require treatment with loop diuretics.
  - Patients being treated with **hemodialysis** should undergo dialysis preoperatively, which is commonly performed on the day prior to surgery. Hemodialysis can be performed on the day of surgery as well, but the possibility should be considered that transient electrolyte abnormalities and hemodynamic changes post dialysis can occur.
- Patients with peritoneal dialysis who are undergoing abdominal surgery should be switched to hemodialysis until wound healing is complete. Peritoneal dialysis should be continued for those undergoing nonabdominal surgery.
- **Electrolyte abnormalities**
  - **Hyperkalemia** in the preoperative setting should be treated, particularly because tissue breakdown associated with surgery may elevate the potassium level further postoperatively.
    - For patients on dialysis, preoperative dialysis should be utilized.
    - For patients with CRI not undergoing dialysis, alternative methods of potassium excretion will be necessary.
      - **Loop diuretics** can be utilized, particularly if the patient is also hypervolemic.
      - **Sodium polystyrene sulfonate (SPS) resins** can also be utilized. The possibility that **intestinal necrosis** with SPS resins occurs more frequently in the perioperative setting has been suggested.[142]
  - Although chronic **metabolic acidosis** has not been associated with elevated perioperative risk, some local anesthetics have reduced efficacy in acidotic patients. Preoperative metabolic acidosis should be corrected with sodium bicarbonate infusions or dialysis.

Blood Pressure

- Ensure adequate blood pressure control. Ideal BP <140/90 mm Hg. Antihypertensives should be continued up to the morning of surgery. Elective surgery can proceed if BP is <180/110 mm Hg, unless end-organ damage is present.

Anemia

- Correct anemia with the use of recombinant erythropoietin and iron transfusion such that an ideal hemoglobin of 10–11.5 g/dL is achieved.
- **Bleeding diathesis**
  - **Platelet dysfunction** has long been associated with uremia.
    - The value of a preoperative bleeding time in predicting postoperative bleeding has been questioned.[143] A preoperative bleeding time is, therefore, not recommended.
    - Patients with evidence of perioperative bleeding should, however, be treated.
      - **Dialysis** for patients with ESRD will improve platelet function.
      - **Desmopressin** (0.3 μg/kg IV or intranasally) can be utilized.
      - **Cryoprecipitate,** 10 units over 30 minutes IV, is an additional option.
      - In patients with coexisting anemia, **red blood cell transfusions** can improve uremic bleeding.
      - For patients **with a history of prior uremic bleeding,** preoperative desmopressin or **conjugated estrogens** (0.5 mg/kg per day IV for 5 days) should be considered.
  - **Heparin** given with dialysis can increase bleeding risk. Heparin-free dialysis should be discussed with the patient's nephrologist when surgery is planned.
- Check INR (warfarin), thrombin time (dabigatran), or anti-Xa levels (Xa inhibitors) if high risk.

- The effectiveness of acetylcysteine and sodium bicarbonate use prophylactically for the prevention of kidney injury in patients receiving contrast is still controversial, as no rigorous clinical trials are available. But these are still in use in clinical practice.

Acute Renal Failure

GENERAL PRINCIPLES

Surgery has been associated with an increased risk of **acute renal failure** (ARF).[141]

- Patients with **CRI** are at increased risk of ARF.
- ARF among patients with normal preoperative renal function is a relatively rare event but is associated with increased mortality when it occurs.[144]
- AKI was reported in 6.8% of patients in a study leading to a 13.3% hospital mortality rate.[145]

DIAGNOSIS

- The approach to ARF in the perioperative setting is not substantially different from that in the nonoperative setting (see Chapter 13, Renal Diseases). However, in the setting of surgery, creatinine levels may not begin to rise until GFR has decreased by half, and urine output is usually decreased for various reasons.
- However, certain additional factors have to be considered when evaluating the cause in the perioperative setting:
    - **Intraoperative hemodynamic changes**, particularly hypotension, should be considered.
        - Intraoperative factors associated with ARF postoperatively include vasopressor use and diuretic use.[144]
        - A careful review of the operative record is advised.
    - Certain procedures can have an adverse effect on the renal function (e.g., aortic clamping procedures). Therefore, careful attention to the details of the procedure is necessary.
    - The possibility that bleeding is responsible for a prerenal state deserves special attention.
    - The identification of AKI is now possible using several novel biomarkers. They are surrogates of early stress on the renal tubules. They are mobilized secondary to cardiopulmonary bypass and surgical stimulation and reflect underlying mechanisms of renal injury since different biomarkers are released in response to specific insults.
    - Tissue-inhibitor of metalloproteinase-2 (TIMP-2) and insulin-like growth factor-binding protein-7 (IGFBP-7) biomarkers are predictive of major adverse kidney events, including death, persistent renal dysfunction, and need for dialysis.[146]
    - NGAL prevents bacteria from absorbing iron, which inhibits their growth and multiplication. In AKI, NGAL levels are elevated in both plasma and urine up to 24 hours before elevated plasma creatinine levels.[147]
    - Cystatin C is a tiny, charged molecule entirely filtered at the glomerulus, where it is catabolized in proximal tubule cells. Consequently, cystatin C is virtually absent in the urine of healthy individuals.

However, further research and studies are required before these biomarkers can be used in clinical practice.

TREATMENT

For a detailed discussion regarding the management of ARF, please refer to Chapter 13, Renal Diseases.

TABLE 1-9 Recommendations for Other Common Medications

Medication Class	Recommendation
Oral contraceptives, hormone replacement, and SERMs	These drugs are associated with increased risk of venous thromboembolism. May discontinue 4 weeks before surgery only in patients at high risk for perioperative venous thromboembolism; otherwise continue Hormone replacement stopped 2 weeks prior to surgery in patients with high risk of VTE and resume once risk is reduced; otherwise continue Raloxifene stopped 3 days before surgery Tamoxifen taken for breast cancer prevention should be discontinued 2 weeks prior; if taken for cancer, treatment should be continued.
Psychotropic agents	Continue SSRIs Continue tricyclic antidepressants, benzodiazepines, lithium, and antipsychotics Usually discontinue MAOIs 10–14 days before surgery
Chronic opioids	Continue; substitute equianalgesic or higher doses for surgical pain
Rheumatologic agents	Continue methotrexate Discontinue other DMARDs and anticytokines about 2 weeks before surgery Continue hypouricemic agents
Neurologic agents	Continue antiseizure medications Continue antiparkinsonian agents Continue agents for myasthenia gravis

DMARDs, disease-modifying antirheumatic drugs; MAOIs, monoamine oxidase inhibitors; SERMs, selective estrogen receptor modulators; SSRIs, selective serotonin reuptake inhibitors.

MISCELLANEOUS

Patients are commonly on multiple medications. The recommendations, perioperatively for continuation of commonly prescribed drugs, are summarized in Table 1-9.

Postoperative Issues in the Elderly

- Confirm and document patient goals and treatment preferences, including advance directives (living will, durable power of attorney, do not resuscitate, and do not intubate).
- Confirm and document the patient's healthcare proxy or surrogate decision maker.
- In patients with existing advance directives, discuss new risks associated with the surgical procedure and an approach for potentially life-threatening problems consistent with the patient's values and preferences ("required reconsideration"). The preventive strategies are summarized in Table 1-10.

TABLE 1-10 Postoperative Concerns in Elderly

Daily Evaluation	Prevention/Management Strategies
Delirium/cognitive impairment	Provide adequate analgesia Optimize physical environment (e.g., sleep hygiene, sleep protocol, encourage family at bedside) Vision and hearing aids accessible Remove catheters Monitor for substance withdrawal syndromes Minimize sedatives and other psychoactive medications Avoid potentially inappropriate medications (e.g., Beers' criteria medications)
Perioperative acute pain	Directed pain history Multimodal, individualized pain control Vigilant dose titration
Pulmonary complications	Chest physiotherapy and incentive spirometry Early mobilization/ambulation. Aspiration precautions
Fall risk	Universal fall precautions Vision and hearing aids accessible. Scheduled toileting Appropriate treatment of delirium. Early mobilization/ambulation Early physical/occupational therapy if indicated Assistive walking devices
Ability to maintain adequate nutrition	Resume diet as early as feasible. Dentures made available. Supplementation if indicated Avoid dehydration
Urinary tract infection prevention	Daily documentation of Foley catheter indication Catheter care bundles, hand hygiene, barrier precautions
Functional decline	Early mobilization and/or physical therapy/occupational therapy. Family participation Nutritional support
Pressure ulcers	Reduce/minimize pressure, friction, humidity, and shear force Maintain adequate nutrition Wound care

Summary

- In-patient care in medicine demands a customized approach that takes into account the patient's underlying condition and needs. Besides treating the disease, it's crucial to take measures that prevent any additional problems such as venous thromboembolism, decubitus ulcers, falls, and constipation.
- Common problems encountered in the wards include dyspnea, fever, pain, and altered mental status. A comprehensive history and physical examination are imperative to identify the underlying problem and devise specific actions to address it.
- Preoperative medicine necessitates a thorough assessment of the patient's risk factors and the surgical risks to create a management plan that reduces postoperative mortality, morbidity, and the length of hospital stay.

- This involves adequately controlling conditions such as hypertension, diabetes, hypo/hyperthyroidism, and kidney disease before surgery, as well as correcting anemia and thrombocytopenia.
- Cardiac and pulmonary evaluation should be carried out based on the patient's risk factors and comorbidities, and a 12-lead ECG is strongly recommended for patients undergoing intermediate and high-risk procedures. Preoperative pulmonary rehabilitation can significantly reduce postoperative morbidity.
- A meticulous review of the patient's medications is also necessary, and any medications that increase the risk of bleeding, cause dehydration, or can cause electrolyte abnormalities should be withheld before surgery.

Scan the QR code to access chapter references.

2 Nutrition Support

Dominic Reeds and Mohamed Faizan Thouseef

NUTRIENT REQUIREMENTS

General Principles

ENERGY

- **Total daily energy expenditure** (TEE) is composed of resting energy expenditure (normally ~70% of TEE), the thermic effect of food (normally ~10% of TEE), and energy expenditure of physical activity (normally ~20% of TEE).
- It is impossible to determine **daily energy requirements** precisely with predictive equations because of the complexity of factors that affect the metabolic rate. Judicious use of predictive equations can provide a reasonable estimate that should be modified as needed based on the patient's clinical course.
- **Malnutrition and hypocaloric feeding** may decrease resting energy expenditure to values 15%–20% below those expected for actual body size, whereas metabolic stressors, such as inflammatory diseases or trauma, often increase energy requirements (usually by ~30%–50% of preillness values).
- The **Harris–Benedict equation** provides a reasonable estimate of resting energy expenditure (in kilocalories [kcal] per day) in healthy adults. The equation takes into account the effect of body size and lean tissue mass (which is influenced by gender and age) on energy requirements and can be used to estimate total daily energy needs in hospitalized patients (where W is the weight in kilograms, H is the height in centimeters, and A is the age in years).[1]
  - Men = $66 + (13.7 \times W) + (5 \times H) - (6.8 \times A)$
  - Women = $665 + (9.6 \times W) + (1.8 \times H) - (4.7 \times A)$
  - **Revised Harris–Benedict equation** to calculate basal metabolic rate (BMR) is given as follows:
    - Men BMR = (10 × weight [kg]) + (6.25 × height [cm]) − (5 × age [years]) + 5.
    - Women BMR = (10 × weight [kg]) + (6.25 × height [cm]) − (5 × age [years]) − 161.
  - To calculate total energy expenditure (TEE):
    - The BMR may be multiplied by a factor that approximates an individual's physical activity level (PAL) to estimate his/her TEE. The PAL for sedentary/light activity, moderate activity, and vigorous activity is 1.53, 1.76, and 2.25, respectively.
- Energy requirements per kilogram of body weight are inversely related to body mass index (BMI) (Table 2-1). The lower range within each category should be considered in insulin-resistant, critically ill patients unless they are depleted in body fat.
- **Ideal body weight** can be estimated based on height, and calculated as follows:
  - Males: IBW (kg) = 50 kg + 2.3 kg for each inch over 5 ft.
  - Females: IBW (kg) = 45.5 kg + 2.3 kg for each inch over 5 ft.
  - Calculating IBW is the first step in determining an "adjusted body weight (ABW)" used for dosing of some medications in patients who are obese.
  - ABW, also known as "adjusted dosing weight," is calculated using the formula: ABW = IBW + (0.4 × [actual weight − IBW]).

TABLE 2-1 Estimated Energy Requirements for Hospitalized Patients Based on Body Mass Index

Body Mass Index (kg/m²)	Energy Requirements (kcal/kg/d)
15	35–40
15–19	30–35
20–24	20–25
25–29	15–20
≥30	<15

Note: A safe starting point for most critically ill patients is approximately 8–10 kcal/kg/day. Attempting to achieve a goal of 25–30 kcal/kg of dosing weight per day after 1 week is reasonable for most stable patients.

A goal of 35 kcal/kg/day is an acceptable goal if weight gain is desired in a relatively stable patient; weight gain should not be attempted until the patient is stable and in a lower inflammatory state. We keep the caloric goal at 25 kcal/kg/day or less if extubation is imminent.

PROTEIN

- Protein intake of 0.8 g/kg/d meets the requirements of 97% of the adult population.
- Protein requirements are affected by several factors, including the amount of nonprotein calories provided, overall energy requirements, protein quality, baseline nutritional status, and the presence of inflammation and metabolic stressors (Table 2-2).
- Inadequate amounts of any of the essential amino acids result in inefficient utilization.
- Illness increases the efflux of amino acids from skeletal muscle; however, increasing protein intake to >1.2 g/kg/d of prehospitalization body weight in critically ill patients may not reduce the loss of lean body mass.[2]

ESSENTIAL FATTY ACIDS

- The liver can synthesize most fatty acids, but humans lack the desaturase enzyme needed to produce the ω-3 and ω-6 fatty acids. Therefore, linoleic acid should constitute at least 2% and linolenic acid at least 0.5% of the daily caloric intake to prevent deficiency.
- The plasma pattern of increased triene-to-tetraene ratio (>0.4) can be used to detect essential fatty acid deficiency.

TABLE 2-2 Recommended Daily Protein Intake

Clinical Condition	Protein Requirements (g/kg IBW/d)[a]
Normal	0.8
Metabolic stress (illness/injury)	1.0–1.5
Acute renal failure (undialyzed)	0.8–1.0
Hemodialysis	1.2–1.4
Peritoneal dialysis	1.3–1.5

[a]Additional protein intake may be needed to compensate for excess protein loss in specific patient populations such as those with burn injury, open wounds, and protein-losing enteropathy or nephropathy. Lower protein intake may be necessary in patients with chronic renal insufficiency who are not treated by dialysis and certain patients with hepatic encephalopathy.

IBW, ideal body weight.

CARBOHYDRATE

Certain tissues, such as bone marrow, erythrocytes, leukocytes, renal medulla, eye tissues, and peripheral nerves, cannot metabolize fatty acids and require glucose (~40 g/d) as a fuel. Endogenous protein and glycerol from lipid stores can undergo gluconeogenesis to supply glucose-requiring organs. Carbohydrates should make up 45%–65% of the total caloric intake.

MAJOR MINERALS

Major minerals such as sodium, potassium, and chloride are important for ionic equilibrium, water balance, and normal cell function.

MICRONUTRIENTS (TRACE ELEMENTS AND VITAMINS)

Trace elements and vitamins are essential constituents of enzyme complexes. Trace elements are naturally occurring, homogeneous, and inorganic substances required in humans in amounts less than 100 mg/day.

The recommended dietary intake for trace elements, fat-soluble vitamins, and water-soluble vitamins is set at 2 standard deviations above the estimated mean as to meet the needs of 97% of the healthy population. See Table 2-3 for specifics regarding the assessment of micronutrient nutritional states as well as signs and symptoms of micronutrient deficiency and toxicity.

SPECIAL CONSIDERATIONS

- Both the amount and location of prior gut resection influence nutrient needs. Patients with a reduced length of functional small bowel may require additional vitamins and minerals if they are not receiving parenteral nutrition. Table 2-4 provides guidelines for supplementation in these patients.
- Ileal inflammation, resection, inflammatory bowel disease (IBD), and bypass (ileojejunal bypass) can cause B_{12} deficiency and bile salt loss. Diarrhea in this setting may be improved with oral cholestyramine.
- Proximal gut resection (stomach or duodenum) via partial gastrectomy, Billroth I and II, duodenal switch/biliopancreatic diversion, Roux-en-Y gastric bypass, pancreaticoduodenectomy (Whipple), and sleeve gastrectomy may impair absorption of divalent cations such as iron, calcium, and copper. Copper deficiency is extremely common in post–gastric bypass patients who do not receive routine supplementation.[30]
- Patients with excessive gastrointestinal (GI) tract losses require additional fluids and electrolytes. An assessment of fluid losses due to diarrhea, ostomy output, and fistula volume should be made to help determine fluid requirements. Intestinal mineral losses may be calculated by multiplying the volume of fluid loss by the fluid electrolyte concentration (Table 2-5).

ASSESSMENT OF NUTRITIONAL STATUS

General Principles

- Patients should be assessed for protein–energy malnutrition as well as specific nutrient deficiencies.
- A thorough history and physical examination combined with appropriate laboratory studies is the best approach to evaluate nutritional status.

Diagnosis

HISTORY

- Assess for changes in diet pattern (size, number, and content of meals). If present, the reason(s) for altered food intake should be investigated.
- **Unintentional weight loss** of >10% body weight in the last 6 months is associated with a poor clinical outcome but may not be due directly to malnutrition but rather to the underlying illness.[31]
- Look for evidence of **malabsorption** (diarrhea, weight loss).
- For symptoms of specific **nutrient deficiencies**, see Table 2-3.
- Consider factors that may increase metabolic stress (e.g., infection, inflammatory disease, malignancy).
- Assess the patient's functional status (e.g., bedridden, suboptimally active).

PHYSICAL EXAMINATION

- According to the criteria by the World Health Organization (WHO) (Table 2-6), patients can be classified by BMI as underweight (<18.5 kg/m^2), normal weight (18.5–24.9 kg/m^2), overweight (25.0–29.9 kg/m^2), class I obesity (30.0–34.9 kg/m^2), class II obesity (35.0–39.9 kg/m^2), or class III obesity (≥40.0 kg/m^2).[32] These cutoffs underestimate the risk in the Asian and South Asian population; the WHO and the NIH guidelines for Asians define overweight as a BMI between 23 and 24.9 kg/m^2 and obesity as a BMI >25 kg/m^2. Some investigators employ four classes of obesity such that class 3 is defined as BMI 40–49.9 kg/m^2 and super obesity is defined as BMI ≥50 kg/m^2.
- Patients who are **extremely underweight** (BMI <15 kg/m^2) or those **with rapid, severe weight loss** (even with supra-normal BMI) have a high risk of death and should be considered for admission to the hospital for nutritional support.
- Diagnostic criteria for **malnutrition**.
  - According to the Global Leadership Initiative on Malnutrition (GLIM), 2018, the diagnosis requires the combination of at least one phenotype and one etiologic criterion, such as the following:
    - Phenotype criteria: Nonvolitional weight loss, low BMI, or reduced muscle mass.
    - Etiologic criteria: Reduced food intake or absorption, or underlying inflammation due to acute disease/injury or chronic disease.
- Look for **tissue depletion** (loss of body fat and skeletal muscle wasting in major muscle groups).
- Assess **muscle function** (strength testing of individual muscle groups).
- **Fluid status:** Evaluate patients for dehydration (e.g., hypotension, tachycardia, mucosal xerosis) or excess body fluid (edema or ascites).
- Evaluate patients for sources of protein or nutrient losses: large wounds, burns, nephrotic syndrome, surgical drains, etc. Quantify the volume of drainage and the concentration of fat and protein content in the fluid losses.
- Evidence that a patient has malnutrition includes poor nutritional intake accompanied by unintentional weight loss or low body weight.
  - Criteria include a BMI less than 18.5 kg/m^2, the unintentional loss of more than 2.3 kg or 5% of the body weight over 1 month, or the unintentional loss of more than 4.5 kg or 10% of the body weight over 6 months.

TABLE 2-3 Trace Minerals, Fat-Soluble Vitamins, and Water-Soluble Vitamins: Recommended Daily Intake, Deficiency, at-Risk Populations, Toxicity, and Status Evaluation

Nutrient	Recommended Daily Enteral Intake[3]/ *Parenteral Intake*[4]	Signs and Symptoms of Deficiency[5]	Populations at Risk for Deficiency[3,5]	Signs and Symptoms of Toxicity[5]	Status Evaluation[5–16]
Chromium (Cr^{3+})	30–35 µg/ ***10–15 µg***	Glucose intolerance, peripheral neuropathy[a]	None[a,5]	PO: gastritis IV: skin irritation Cr^{6+}: (steel, welding) lung carcinogen if inhaled	Chromium[s]
Copper (Cu^{2+})	900 µg/ ***300–500 µg***	Hypochromic normocytic or macrocytic anemia (rarely microcytic), neutropenia, thrombocytopenia, diarrhea, osteoporosis/pathologic fractures Intrinsic: Menkes disease[17]	Chronic diarrhea, high-zinc/low-protein diets[18,19]	PO: gastritis, nausea, vomiting, coma, movement/neurologic abnormalities, hepatic necrosis Intrinsic: Wilson disease	Copper[s,u] Ceruloplasmin[p]
Iodine (I_)	150 µg/***70–140 µg (not routinely added)***	Thyroid hyperplasia (goiter) + functional hypothyroidism Intrinsic in utero: cretinism, poor CNS development, hypothyroidism	Those without access to fortified salt, grain, milk, or cooking oil[20]	Deficiency: causes hypothyroidism Excess: acutely causes hypothyroidism; chronic excess: hyperthyroidism	TSH_s, $iodine_u$ (24-h intake and iodine: Cr ratio are more representative than a single sample) $Thyroglobulin_s$[12]

(Continued)

TABLE 2-3 Trace Minerals, Fat-Soluble Vitamins, and Water-Soluble Vitamins: Recommended Daily Intake, Deficiency, at-Risk Populations, Toxicity, and Status Evaluation (Continued)

Iron ($Fe^{2+,3+}$)	8 mg/***1.0–1.5 µg (not routinely added)***	Fatigue, hypochromic microcytic anemia, glossitis, koilonychia	Reproductive-age females, pregnant females, chronic females, chronic anemias, hemoglobinopathies, post–gastric bypass/duodenectomy, alcoholics	PO or IV: hemosiderosis, followed by deposition in liver, pancreas, heart, and glands Intrinsic: Hereditary hemochromatosis	$Ferritin_s$, $TIBC_s$, % transferrin saturation[c], $iron_s$
Manganese (Mn^{2+})	2.3 mg/***60–100 µg***	Hypercholesterolemia, dermatitis, dementia, weight loss[b]	Chronic liver disease, iron-deficient populations	PO: None[b] Inhalation: hallucination, Parkinsonian-type symptoms[21]	No reliable markers $Manganese_s$ does not reflect bodily stores, especially in the CNS
Selenium (SeO_4^{2-})	55 µg/***20–60 µg***	Myalgias, cardiomyopathy[a] Intrinsic: Keshan disease (Chinese children), Kashin–Beck disease, myxedematous endemic cretinism	Endemic areas of low soil content include certain parts of China and New Zealand[22]	PO: Nausea, diarrhea, AMS, irritability, fatigue, peripheral neuropathy, hair loss, white splotchy nails, halitosis (garlic-like odor)	Selenium[s], glutathione peroxidase $activity_b$

(Continued)

TABLE 2-3 Trace Minerals, Fat-Soluble Vitamins, and Water-Soluble Vitamins: Recommended Daily Intake, Deficiency, at-Risk Populations, Toxicity, and Status Evaluation (Continued)

Nutrient	Recommended Daily Enteral Intake[3]/ *Parenteral Intake*[4]	Signs and Symptoms of Deficiency[5]	Populations at Risk for Deficiency[3,5]	Signs and Symptoms of Toxicity[5]	Status Evaluation[5–16]
Zinc (Zn^{2+})	11 mg/***2.5–5.0 mg***	Poor wound healing, diarrhea (high fistula risk), dysgeusia, teratogenicity, hypogonadism, infertility, acro-orificial skin lesions (glossitis, alopecia), behavioral changes Intrinsic: Acrodermatitis enteropathica	Chronic diarrhea, cereal-based diets, alcoholics, chronic liver disease, sickle cell, HIV, pancreatic insufficiency/any intestinal malabsorptive states, fistulas/ostomies, nephrotic syndrome, diabetes, post–gastric bypass/duodenectomy, anorexia, pregnancy[23] Intrinsic: Acrodermatitis enteropathica	PO: Nausea, vomiting, gastritis, diarrhea, low HDL, gastric erosions Competition with GI absorption can precipitate Cu^{2+} *deficiency* Inhaled: Hyperpnea, weakness, diaphoresis	$Zinc_{s,p}$, alkaline phosphatase[s] (good for those on TPN, but in general $Zincs_{s,p}$ hair, RBC, WBC levels can be misleading) Zinc radioisotope studies (most accurate tests at present; limited by cost and availability)[11]

(Continued)

TABLE 2-3 Trace Minerals, Fat-Soluble Vitamins, and Water-Soluble Vitamins: Recommended Daily Intake, Deficiency, at-Risk Populations, Toxicity, and Status Evaluation (Continued)

Molybdenum	45 μg/***45 μg***	CNS toxicity, hyperoxypurinemia, hypouricemia, low urinary sulfate excretion[a],[24] (also reported with parenteral sulfite infusion) Intrinsic: Molybdenum cofactor deficiency, isolated sulfite oxidase deficiency	None[a]	PO or any exposure: Hyperuricemia + gout Inhaled: Pneumoconiosis (industrial exposure)	$Molybdenum_b$
Vitamin A *Retinol*	900 μg/***3300 IU***	Conjunctival xerosis, keratomalacia, follicular hyperkeratosis, night blindness, *Bitot's spots*, corneal + retinal dysfunction	Any malabsorptive state involving proximal small bowel, vegetarians, chronic liver disease	Acute: Teratogenic, skin exfoliation, intracranial hypertension, hepatocellular necrosis Chronic: Alopecia, ataxia, cheilitis, dermatitis, conjunctivitis, pseudotumor cerebri, hyperlipidemia, hyperostosis	$Retinol_s$, retinol $esters_p$, electroretinogram, liver biopsy (diagnostic for toxicity), retinol binding protein (useful in ESRD; accurately assesses blood levels)[25]

(Continued)

TABLE 2-3 Trace Minerals, Fat-Soluble Vitamins, and Water-Soluble Vitamins: Recommended Daily Intake, Deficiency, at-Risk Populations, Toxicity, and Status Evaluation (Continued)

Nutrient	Recommended Daily Enteral Intake[3]/ *Parenteral Intake*[4]	Signs and Symptoms of Deficiency[5]	Populations at Risk for Deficiency[3,5]	Signs and Symptoms of Toxicity[5]	Status Evaluation[5–16]
Vitamin D *Ergocalciferol*	5–15 μg/***200 IU***	Rickets/osteomalacia	Any malabsorptive state involving proximal small bowel, chronic liver disease Of note: Those with higher skin melanin content (i.e., darker skin) have low baseline 25-OH vitamin D levels; it is unclear whether this merits their inclusion as an "at-risk" population[26]	Hypercalcemia, hyperphosphatemia, which can lead to $CaPO_4$ precipitation, systemic calcification +/– AMS +/– AKI	25-OH vitamin D_s Of note: lively debate between IOM and Endocrine Society regarding definitions of deficiency, goal serum 25-OH levels, and at-risk populations[26,27]

(Continued)

TABLE 2-3 Trace Minerals, Fat-Soluble Vitamins, and Water-Soluble Vitamins: Recommended Daily Intake, Deficiency, at-Risk Populations, Toxicity, and Status Evaluation (Continued)

Vitamin E (α,γ)-*Tocopherol*	15 mg/***10 IU***	Hemolytic anemia, posterior column degeneration, ophthalmoplegia, peripheral neuropathy Seen in severe malabsorption, abetalipoproteinemia	Any malabsorptive state involving proximal small bowel, chronic liver disease	Possible increased risk in hemorrhagic CVA, functional inhibition of vitamin K–mediated procoagulants	Tocopherol Must account for cholesterol/triglyceride ratio: otherwise, higher cholesterol/triglyceride ratio overestimates vitamin E, lower cholesterol/triglyceride ratio underestimates vitamin E[2,c]
Vitamin K *Phylloquinone*	120 μg/***150 IU***	Hemorrhagic disease of newborn, coagulopathy	Any malabsorptive state involving proximal small bowel, chronic liver disease	In utero: Hemolytic anemia, hyperbilirubinemia, kernicterus IV: flushing, dyspnea, hypotension (possibly related to dispersal agent)	Prothrombin time[p]
Vitamin B_1 *Thiamine*	1.2 mg/***6 mg***	Irritability, fatigue, headache *Wernicke encephalopathy, Korsakoff psychosis, "wet" beriberi, "dry" beriberi*	Alcoholics, severely malnourished	IV: Lethargy and ataxia	RBC transketolase activity$_b$, thiamine$_{b\&u}$

(Continued)

TABLE 2-3 Trace Minerals, Fat-Soluble Vitamins, and Water-Soluble Vitamins: Recommended Daily Intake, Deficiency, at-Risk Populations, Toxicity, and Status Evaluation (Continued)

Nutrient	Recommended Daily Enteral Intake[3]/ *Parenteral Intake*[4]	Signs and Symptoms of Deficiency[5]	Populations at Risk for Deficiency[3,5]	Signs and Symptoms of Toxicity[5]	Status Evaluation[5–16]
Vitamin B_2 *Riboflavin*	1.3 mg/***3.6 mg***	Cheilosis, angular stomatitis, glossitis, seborrheic dermatitis, normocytic normochromic anemia	Alcoholics, severely malnourished	None[b]	RBC glutathione reductase activity$_p$
Vitamin B_3 *Niacin*	16 mg/***40 mg***	*Pellagra* dysesthesias, glossitis, stomatitis, vaginitis, vertigo Intrinsic: Hartnup disease	Alcoholics, malignant carcinoid syndrome, severely malnourished	Flushing, hyperglycemia, hyperuricemia, hepatocellular injury[b]	N-methyl-nicotinamide
Vitamin B_5: *Pantothenic acid*	5 mg/***15 mg***	Fatigue, abdominal pain, vomiting, insomnia, paresthesias[b]	Alcoholics[5]	PO: Diarrhea	Pantothenic acid$_u$
Vitamin B_6 *Pyridoxine*	1.3–1.7 mg/***6 mg***	Cheilosis, stomatitis, glossitis, irritability, depression, confusion, normochromic normocytic anemia	Alcoholics, diabetics, celiac sprue, chronic isoniazid or penicillamine use[5]	Peripheral neuropathy, photosensitivity	Pyridoxal phosphate$_p$
Vitamin B_7 *Biotin*	30 µg/***60 µg***	Mental status changes, myalgias, hyperesthesias, anorexia[c,28] (excessive egg white consumption results in avidin-mediated biotin inactivation)	Alcoholics[29]	None[b,16]	Biotin$_p$, methyl-citrate$_u$, 3-methyl-crotonyglycine$_u$, 3-hydroxyisovalerate$_u$

(Continued)

TABLE 2-3 Trace Minerals, Fat-Soluble Vitamins, and Water-Soluble Vitamins: Recommended Daily Intake, Deficiency, at-Risk Populations, Toxicity, and Status Evaluation (Continued)

Vitamin B_9 *Folic acid*	400 μg/***600 μg***	Bone marrow suppression, macrocytic megaloblastic anemia, glossitis, diarrhea Can be precipitated by sulfasalazine + phenytoin	Alcoholics, celiac or tropical sprue, chronic sulfasalazine use[5]	PO: May lower seizure threshold in those taking anticonvulsants	Folic $acid_s$, RBC folic $acid_p$
Vitamin B_{12} *Cobalamin*	2.4 μg/***5 μg***	Bone marrow suppression, macrocytic megaloblastic anemia, glossitis, diarrhea, posterolateral column demyelination, AMS, depression, psychosis	Vegetarians, atrophic gastritis, pernicious anemia, celiac sprue, Crohn disease, patients postgastrectomy or ileal resection	None[b]	Cobalamin $(B_{12})_s$, methylmalonic $acid_{s\&p}$
Vitamin C *Ascorbic acid*	90 mg/***200 mg***	*Scurvy*, ossification abnormalities Tobacco lowers plasma and WBC vitamin C[2] Sudden cessation of high-dose vitamin C can precipitate scurvy	Fruit-deficient diet, smokers,[3] ESRD[28]	Nausea, diarrhea, increased oxalate synthesis (theoretical nephrolithiasis risk)	Ascorbic $acid_p$, leukocyte ascorbic acid

[a]Only reported in patients on long-term TPN.
[b]Never demonstrated in humans.
[c]Only able to induce under experimental conditions and/or only been able to induce in animals.
AKI, acute kidney injury; AMS, altered mental status; CNS, central nervous system; CVA, cerebrovascular accident; ESRD, end-stage renal disease; IOM, Institute of Medicine; GI, gastrointestinal; HDL, high-density lipoprotein (cholesterol); RBC, red blood cell; TIBC, total iron bonding capacity; TPN, total parenteral nutrition; TSH, thyroid-stimulating hormone; WBC, white blood cell.
Subscript: b, blood; c, calculated; p, plasma; s, serum; u, urine.

TABLE 2-4 Guidelines for Vitamin and Mineral Supplementation in Patients With Severe Malabsorption

Supplement	Dose	Route
Prenatal multivitamin with minerals[a]	1 tablet daily	PO
Vitamin D[a]	50,000 units 2–3 times per week	PO
Calcium[a]	500 mg elemental calcium tid–qid	PO
Vitamin B_{12}[b]	1 mg daily	PO
	100–500 μg q1–2 mo	SC
Vitamin A[b]	10,000–50,000 units daily	PO
Vitamin K[b]	5 mg/d	PO
	5–10 mg/wk	SC
Vitamin E[b]	30 units/d	PO
Magnesium gluconate[b]	108–169 mg elemental magnesium qid	PO
Magnesium sulfate[b]	290 mg elemental magnesium 1–3 times per week	IM/IV
Zinc gluconate or zinc sulfate[b]	25 mg elemental zinc daily plus 100 mg elemental zinc per liter intestinal output	PO
Ferrous sulfate[b]	60 mg elemental iron tid	PO
Iron dextran[b]	Daily dose based on formula or table	IV

[a]Recommended routinely for all patients.
[b]Recommended for patients with documented nutrient deficiency or malabsorption.

TABLE 2-5 Electrolyte Concentrations in Gastrointestinal Fluids

Location	Na (mEq/L)	K (mEq/L)	Cl (mEq/L)	HCO_3 (mEq/L)
Stomach	65	10	100	–
Bile	150	4	100	35
Pancreas	150	7	80	75
Duodenum	90	15	90	15
Mid–small bowel	140	6	100	20
Terminal ileum	140	8	60	70
Rectum	40	90	15	30

TABLE 2-6 Body Mass Index (BMI) in kg/m² Categories

Classification	WHO General Population	Asian
Underweight	<18.5	<18.5
Normal	18.5–24.9	18.5–22.9
Overweight	25–29.9	23–24.9
Obese Class 1	30–34.9	25–29.9
Obese Class 2	35–39.9	>30
Obese Class 3	≥40	

DIAGNOSTIC TESTING

- Perform laboratory studies to determine specific nutrient deficiencies only when clinically indicated because the plasma concentration of many nutrients may not accurately reflect body stores (Table 2-3).
- Plasma albumin and prealbumin concentrations should **not** be used to assess patients for protein–calorie malnutrition or to monitor the adequacy of nutrition support. Although levels of these plasma proteins correlate with clinical outcome, inflammation and injury can alter their synthesis and degradation, limiting their usefulness for nutritional assessment.[33,34]
- Most hospitalized patients are vitamin D deficient, and caregivers should have a low threshold for checking plasma 25-OH vitamin D levels.[35]

ENTERAL NUTRITION

General Principles

Indications for nutritional support are as follows:

- Severely malnourished patients on admission to hospital.
- Moderately malnourished patients who are not expected to eat for more than 3–5 days (because of their physical illness).
- Normally nourished patients not expected to eat for more than 5 days or to eat less than half their intake for more than 8–10 days.

Prerequisite: Patients must have a functioning GI tract. Patients who are not able to swallow may need artificial nutritional support (e.g., after acute stroke or throat surgery, or long-term neurological disorders such as motor neuron disease and multiple sclerosis).

Whenever possible, the enteral route is preferred to parenteral feeding because of the following:

- Intake easily/accurately monitored.
- Provides nutrition when oral intake is not possible or adequate.
- Less cost than parenteral nutrition.
- Readily available.
- Reduces risks associated with disease state.
- Preserves gut integrity and immunologic function.
- Decreases likelihood of bacterial translocation.
- Increased compliance with intake.
- Decreases the risk of multiorgan failure in intensive care patients.

TYPES OF FEEDINGS

Hospital diets include a regular diet and those modified in either nutrient content (amount of fiber, fat, protein, or sodium) or consistency (liquid, puréed, soft). There are ways that food intake can often be increased:

- Provide assistance at mealtime.
- Allow some food to be supplied by relatives and friends.
- Limit missed meals for medical tests and procedures.
- Avoid unpalatable diets. Milk-based formulas (e.g., Carnation Instant Breakfast™) contain milk as a source of protein and fat and are more palatable than many other formula diets.
- Use of calorically dense supplements (e.g., Ensure™, Boost™).

Defined Liquid Formulas (Table 2-7)

- **Polymeric formulas** (e.g., Osmolite™, Jevity™) are appropriate for most patients. They contain nitrogen in the form of whole proteins and include blenderized food, milk-based, and lactose-free formulas. Other formulas are available with modified content including high-nitrogen, high-calorie, fiber-enriched, and low-potassium/phosphorus/magnesium.
- **Semielemental *oligomeric* formulas** (e.g., Peptamen™) contain hydrolyzed protein in the form of small peptides and free amino acids. Although these formulas may have benefit in those with exocrine pancreatic insufficiency or short gut, pancreatic enzyme replacement is a less expensive and an equally effective intervention in most patients.
- **Elemental monomeric formulas** (e.g., Vivonex™, Glutasorb™) contain nitrogen in the form of free amino acids and small amounts of fat (<5% of total calories) and are hyperosmolar (550–650 mOsm/kg). These formulas are not palatable and therefore require either tube feeding or mixing with other foods or flavorings for oral ingestion. Furthermore, these formulas have not been shown to be clinically superior to oligomeric

TABLE 2-7 Enteral Feeding Formulas: Comparing Composition

Formula	kcal/mL	% Protein	% Lipid	% Carbohydrate	K^+ (mEq/L)	PO_4^{3-} (mg/L)	Purpose/Niche
Osmolite	1.0	16.7	29	54.3	40.2	760	Standard polymeric
Jevity	1.5	17	29	53.6	40.2	1200	Standard polymeric
TwoCal HN	2	16.7	40.1	43.2	62.6	1050	Volume restricted
Nepro with Carb Steady	1.8	18	48	34	27.2	700	ESRD
Glucerna	1.2	20	45	35	51.8	800	Glucose intolerance/diabetes
Promote	1.0	25	23	52	50.8	1200	High protein
Peptamen AF	1.2	25	39	36	41	800	Short gut, exocrine pancreatic insufficiency
Vivonex RTF	1.0	20	10	70	31	670	Fat malabsorption
Oxepa	1.5	16.7	55.2	28.1	50.1	1060	SIRS, ARDS, sepsis

Table adapted from Barnes-Jewish Hospital Enteral Nutrition Formulary (8/2009).
ARDS, acute respiratory distress syndrome; ESRD, end-stage renal disease; SIRS, systemic inflammatory response syndrome.

or polymeric formulas in patients with adequate pancreatic digestive function and are much more expensive than polymeric formulas.
- **Oral rehydration solutions** stimulate sodium and water absorption by taking advantage of the sodium–glucose cotransporter present in the brush border of intestinal epithelium. Oral rehydration therapy (using 90–120 mEq/L solutions to avoid intestinal sodium secretion and negative sodium and water balance) can be especially useful in patients with short bowel syndrome.[36] The characteristics of several oral rehydration solutions are listed in Table 2-7.

Tube Feeding

- Tube feeding is useful in patients who have a **functional GI tract** but who cannot or will not ingest adequate nutrients.
- The type of tube feeding approach selected (nasogastric, nasoduodenal, nasojejunal, gastrostomy, jejunostomy, pharyngostomy, and esophagostomy tubes) depends on physician experience, clinical prognosis, gut patency and motility, risk of aspirating gastric contents, patient preference, and anticipated duration of feeding.
- Short-term (<6 weeks) tube feeding can be achieved by placement of a soft, small-bore nasogastric or nasoenteric feeding tube. Although, nasogastric feeding is usually the most appropriate route, orogastric feeding may be needed in those who are intubated or those with nasal injury or deformity. **Nasoduodenal and nasojejunal feeding tubes** can be placed at the bedside with a success rate approaching 90% when inserted by experienced personnel.
- Long-term (>6 weeks) tube feeding usually requires a **gastrostomy or jejunostomy** tube that can be placed percutaneously by endoscopic or radiographic assistance. Alternatively, they can be placed surgically, depending on the clinical situation and local expertise.

Feeding Schedules

Patients who have feeding tubes in the stomach can often tolerate intermittent bolus or gravity feedings, in which the total amount of daily formula is divided into four to six equal portions. It is determined by the medical status, feeding route, and volume and nutritional goals.
- **Bolus feedings** are given by syringe as rapidly as tolerated. Total 300–400 mL rapid delivery is done via syringe several times daily.
- **Gravity feedings** are infused over 30–60 minutes.
- The patient's upper body should be elevated by 30–45 degrees during feeding and for at least 2 hours afterward. Tubes should be flushed with water after each feeding. Intermittent feedings are useful for patients who cannot be positioned with continuous head-of-the-bed elevation or who require greater freedom from feeding. Patients who experience nausea and early satiety with bolus gravity feedings may require continuous infusion at a slower rate.
- **Continuous feeding** can often be started at 20–30 mL/h and advanced by 10 mL/h every 6 hours until the feeding goal is reached. Patients who have gastroparesis often tolerate gastric tube feedings when they are started at a slow rate (e.g., 10 mL/h) and advanced by small increments (e.g., 10 mL/h every 8–12 hours). Patients with severe gastroparesis may require passage of the feeding tube tip past the ligament of Treitz. Continuous feeding should always be used when feeding directly into the duodenum or jejunum to avoid distention, abdominal pain, and dumping syndrome.
- Jejunal feeding may be possible in closely monitored patients with mild to moderate acute pancreatitis.[37]

CONTRAINDICATIONS TO ENTERAL FEEDING

The intestinal tract cannot be used effectively in some patients because of the following:
- Persistent nausea or vomiting
- Postprandial abdominal pain or diarrhea

- Mechanical obstruction or severe hypomotility
- Malabsorption
- Absent gag reflex/dysphagia
- Presence of high-output fistula

COMPLICATIONS

- Mechanical complications
  - Nasogastric feeding tube misplacement occurs more commonly in unconscious patients. Complications include intubation of the tracheobronchial tree and intracranial placement can occur in patients with skull fractures.
  - Erosive tissue damage can lead to nasopharyngeal erosions, pharyngitis, sinusitis, otitis media, pneumothorax, and GI tract perforation.
  - Tube occlusion is often caused by inspissated feedings or pulverized medications given through small-diameter (<#10 French) tubes. Frequent flushing of the tube with 30–60 mL of water and avoiding administration of pill fragments or "thick" medications help to prevent occlusion. The techniques used to unclog tubes include the use of a small-volume syringe (10 mL) to flush warm water or pancreatic enzymes (Viokase™ dissolved in water) through the tube.
- Hyperglycemia
  - The precise level at which glucose should be maintained in hospitalized patients remains controversial.
  - Subcutaneously administered insulin can usually maintain good glycemic control. IV insulin drip protocols should be used to control blood glucose in critically ill patients with anasarca or hemodynamic instability to ensure adequate insulin absorption.
  - Short-acting (e.g., lispro™) or, in stable patients, intermediate-duration insulin (e.g., NPH) can be used once tube feedings reach 1000 kcal/d. Long-duration insulin (e.g., detemir, glargine) should be used with caution on patients because changes in clinical status may affect pharmacokinetics and increase the risk of sustained hypoglycemia.
  - Patients who are receiving bolus feeds should receive short-acting insulin at the time of the feed.
  - Patients who are being given continuous (24 hours per day) feeding should receive intermediate-duration insulin every 8 hours when clinically stable. If tube feeds are interrupted and insulin has been given, an infusion of dextrose-containing fluid should be given at a rate to match the infusion rate of the scheduled tube feeds until the insulin has worn off.
- Pulmonary complications
  - The etiology of **pulmonary aspiration** can be difficult to determine in tube-fed patients because aspiration can occur from refluxed tube feedings or oropharyngeal secretions that are unrelated to feedings. Recent evidence suggests that oral secretions play a far greater role in the development of ventilator-associated pneumonia than aspiration of tube feedings.[38]
  - The addition of food coloring to tube feeds **should not be used** for the diagnosis of aspiration. This method is insensitive for diagnosis, and several case reports suggest that food coloring can be absorbed by the GI tract in critically ill patients and can lead to serious complications and death.[39]
  - Gastric residuals are poorly predictive of aspiration risk.
  - Prevention of reflux: Decrease gastric acid secretion with pharmacologic therapy (H2 blocker, proton pump inhibitor), elevate head of bed during feeds, and avoid gastric feeding in high-risk patients (e.g., those with gastroparesis, frequent vomiting, gastric outlet obstruction).
- GI complications
  - Nausea, vomiting, and abdominal pain are common.

  - Diarrhea is often associated with antibiotic therapy and the use of liquid medications that contain nonabsorbable carbohydrates, such as sorbitol. If diarrhea from tube feeding persists after proper evaluation of possible causes, a trial of antidiarrheal agents or fiber is justified. Diarrhea is common in patients who receive tube feeding and occurs in up to 50% of critically ill patients.
  - Diarrhea in patients with short gut, who do not have other causes such as *Clostridium difficile* infection, may be minimized by the use of small, frequent meals that do not contain concentrated sweets (e.g., soda). Intestinal transit time should be maximized to optimize nutrient absorption using a tincture of opium, loperamide, or diphenoxylate. Low-dose clonidine (0.025–0.05 mg orally bid) may be used to reduce diarrhea in hemodynamically stable patients with short bowel syndrome.[40] Intestinal ischemia/necrosis has been reported in patients receiving tube feeding. These cases have occurred predominantly in critically ill patients receiving vasopressors for blood pressure support in conjunction with enteral feeding. There are no reliable clinical signs for diagnosis, and the mortality rate is high. **Caution should be used when enterally feeding critically ill patients requiring vasopressors.**

PARENTERAL NUTRITION

General Principles

Parenteral nutrition should be considered if energy intake cannot, or it is anticipated that it cannot, be met by enteral nutrition (<50% of daily requirements) for more than 7–10 days. This guideline originates from two intensive care unit (ICU)-focused meta-analyses citing increased complications[41] and increased overall mortality[42] in ICU patients receiving early parenteral nutrition (i.e., within 7 days of admission), compared with those receiving no nutrition support. Recent studies have found that critically ill patients who are unable to meet caloric goals by enteral nutrition alone for the first 8 days of hospitalization have longer durations of stay and greater mortality rates than those in whom total parenteral nutrition (TPN) is withheld for the first 8 days after admission.[43]

- Indications for total parenteral nutrition are as follows:
  - GI nonfunctioning
  - Nil per oral >5 days
  - GI fistula
  - Acute pancreatitis
  - Short bowel syndrome
  - Malnutrition with >10%–15% weight loss
  - Nutritional needs not met

CENTRAL PARENTERAL NUTRITION (CPN)

- The infusion of hyperosmolar (usually >1500 mOsm/L) nutrient solutions requires a large-bore, high-flow vessel to minimize vessel irritation and damage.
- Percutaneous subclavian vein catheterization and peripherally inserted central venous catheterization (PICC) are the most commonly used techniques for CPN access. The internal jugular, saphenous, and femoral veins are also used, although they are less desirable because of decreased patient comfort and difficulty in maintaining sterility. Tunneled catheters are preferred in patients who are likely to receive >8 weeks of TPN to reduce the risk of mechanical failure.

- PICCs (which reduce the risk of pneumothorax) are increasingly used to provide CPN in patients with adequate antecubital vein access. These catheters are not suitable for patients in whom CPN is anticipated to be necessary for an extended duration (>6 months).

CPN MACRONUTRIENT SOLUTIONS

- Crystalline **amino acid solutions** containing 40%–50% essential and 50%–60% nonessential amino acids (usually with little or no glutamine, glutamate, aspartate, asparagine, tyrosine, and cysteine) are used to provide protein needs (Table 2-2). Infused amino acids are oxidized and should be included in the estimate of energy provided as part of the parenteral formulation.
- Some amino acid solutions have been modified for specific disease states such as those enriched in branched-chain amino acids for use in patients who have hepatic encephalopathy and those that contain mostly essential amino acids for use in patients with renal insufficiency.
- **Glucose** (dextrose) in IV solutions is hydrated; each gram of dextrose monohydrate provides 3.4 kcal. Although there is no absolute requirement for glucose in most patients, providing >150 g of glucose per day maximizes protein balance.
- **Lipid emulsions** are available as a 10% (1.1 kcal/mL) or 20% (2.0 kcal/mL) solution and provide energy as well as serve as a source of essential fatty acids. Emulsion particles are similar in size and structure to chylomicrons and are metabolized like nascent chylomicrons after acquiring apoproteins from contact with circulating endogenous high-density lipoprotein cholesterol particles. Lipid emulsions are as effective as glucose in conserving body nitrogen economy once absolute tissue requirements for glucose are met. The optimal percentage of calories that should be infused as fat is not known, but 20%–30% of total calories are reasonable for most patients. The rate of infusion should not exceed 1.0 kcal/kg/h (0.11 g/kg/h) because most complications associated with lipid infusions have been reported when providing more than this amount.[44] A rate of 0.03–0.05 g/kg/h is adequate for most patients who are receiving continuous CPN. Lipid emulsions should not be given to patients who have triglyceride concentrations of >400 mg/dL. Moreover, patients at risk for hypertriglyceridemia should have serum triglyceride concentrations checked at least once during lipid emulsion infusion to ensure adequate clearance. Underfeeding obese patients by the amount of lipid calories that would normally be given (e.g., 20%–30% of calories) facilitates mobilization of endogenous fat stores for fuel and may improve insulin sensitivity. IV lipids should still be administered twice per week to these patients to provide essential fatty acids.

PERIPHERAL PARENTERAL NUTRITION

- Peripheral parenteral nutrition is often considered to have limited usefulness because of the high risk of thrombophlebitis.
- Appropriate adjustments in the management of peripheral parenteral nutrition can increase the life of a single infusion site to >10 days. The following guidelines are recommended:
  - Provide at least 50% of total energy as a lipid emulsion piggybacked with the dextrose–amino acid solution.
  - Add 500–1000 units of heparin and 5 mg of hydrocortisone per liter (to decrease phlebitis).
  - Place a fine-bore 22- or 23-gauge polyvinylpyrrolidone-coated polyurethane catheter in as large a vein as possible in the proximal forearm using sterile technique.

- ◦ Place a 5-mg glycerol trinitrate ointment patch (or 0.25 in of 2% nitroglycerin ointment) over the infusion site.
- ◦ Infuse the solution with a volumetric pump.
- ◦ Keep the total infused volume <3500 mL/d.
- ◦ Filter the solution with an inline 1.2-m filter.

LONG-TERM HOME PARENTERAL NUTRITION

- Long-term home parenteral nutrition is usually given through a tunneled catheter or an implantable subcutaneous port inserted in the subclavian vein.
- Nutrient formulations can be infused overnight to permit daytime activities in patients who are able to tolerate the fluid load. IV lipids may not be necessary in patients who are able to ingest and absorb adequate amounts of fat.
- Patient selection for appropriate patients for home TPN is crucial due to the high rates of complications (~50% at 6 months). The risk factors for complications include the use of a nontunneled or multilumen catheter, blood being drawn from the catheter, infusion of nonparenteral medications, use of lipid infusions, anticoagulation, older age, and open wounds.[45]

COMPLICATIONS

Common complications encountered with parenteral nutrition are listed in Table 2-8.

Mechanical Complications

- Complications at time of line placement include pneumothorax, air embolism, arterial puncture, hemothorax, and brachial plexus injury.
- Thrombosis and pulmonary embolus: Radiologically evident subclavian vein thrombosis occurs commonly; however, clinical manifestations (upper extremity edema, superior vena cava syndrome) are rare. Fatal microvascular pulmonary emboli can be caused by nonvisible precipitate in parenteral nutrition solutions. Inline filters should be used with all solutions to minimize the risk of these emboli.

TABLE 2-8 Complications of Parenteral Nutrition

	Mechanical	Metabolic/GI	Infectious
First 48 hours	Malposition, hemothorax, pneumothorax, air embolism, blood loss, puncture of subclavian/carotid artery	Fluid overload, hypoglycemia, hypophosphatemia, hypokalemia, hypomagnesemia, refeeding syndrome	—
First 2 weeks	Catheter displacement, thrombosis, occlusion, air embolism	Hypoglycemic coma, acid–base and electrolyte imbalance	Catheter-induced sepsis, exit-site infection
3 months onwards	Tear of catheter, catheter thrombosis, air embolism, blood loss	Essential FA deficiency, vitamins or trace element deficiency, metabolic bone disease, liver disease	Tunnel infection, catheter-induced sepsis, exit-site infection

Metabolic Complications

- Fluid overload
- Hypertriglyceridemia
- Hypercalcemia
- Specific nutrient deficiencies. Consider providing supplemental **thiamine** (100 mg for 3–5 days) during initiation of CPN in patients at risk for thiamine deficiency (e.g., alcoholism).
- Hypoglycemia
- Hyperglycemia. In most patients, attempts should be made to maintain a blood glucose concentration of 140–180 mg/dL during TPN infusion. Management of patients with hyperglycemia or type 2 diabetes can be performed in several ways:
  - If blood glucose is >200 mg/dL, consider obtaining better control of blood glucose before starting CPN.
  - If CPN is started, (1) limit dextrose to <200 g/d, (2) add 0.1 unit of regular insulin for each gram of dextrose in CPN solution (e.g., 15 units for 150 g), (3) discontinue other sources of IV dextrose, and (4) order routine, regular insulin with blood glucose monitoring by finger stick every 4–6 hours or IV regular insulin infusion with blood glucose monitoring by finger stick every 1–2 hours.
  - In outpatients who use insulin, an estimate of the reduction in blood sugar that will be caused by the administration of 1 unit of insulin may be calculated by dividing 1500 by the total daily insulin dose (e.g., for a patient receiving 50 units of insulin as an outpatient, 1 unit of insulin may be predicted to reduce plasma glucose concentration by 1500/50 = 30 mg/dL).
  - If blood glucose remains >200 mg/dL and the patient has been requiring SC insulin, add 50% of the supplemental short-acting insulin given in the last 24 hours to the next day's CPN solution and double the amount of SC insulin sliding-scale dose for blood glucose values >200 mg/dL.
  - The insulin-to-dextrose ratio in the CPN formulation should be maintained while the CPN dextrose content is changed.

Infectious Complications

- Catheter-related sepsis is the most common life-threatening complication in patients who receive CPN and is most commonly caused by skin flora: *Staphylococcus epidermidis* and *Staphylococcus aureus.*
- In **immunocompromised patients** and those with long-term (>2 weeks) CPN, *Enterococcus*, *Candida* species, *Escherichia coli*, *Pseudomonas*, *Klebsiella*, *Enterobacter*, *Acinetobacter*, *Proteus*, and *Xanthomonas* should be considered.
- The principles of **evaluation and management** of suspected catheter-related infection are outlined in Chapter 14, Treatment of Infectious Diseases.
- Use of sterile technique during connection of TPN, avoiding accessing the TPN lumen of the central catheter for other uses, and ensuring that TPN is never disconnected and then restarted can reduce the risk of infection.

HEPATOBILIARY COMPLICATIONS

Although these abnormalities are usually benign and transient, more serious and progressive disease may develop in a small subset of patients, usually after 16 weeks of CPN therapy or in those with a short bowel syndrome.

- Biochemical: Elevated aminotransferases and alkaline phosphatase are commonly seen.
- Histologic alterations: Steatosis, steatohepatitis, lipidosis, phospholipidosis, cholestasis, fibrosis, and cirrhosis have all been seen.

- Biliary complications as listed below usually occur in patients who receive CPN for >3 weeks:
  - Acalculous cholecystitis
  - Gallbladder sludge
  - Cholelithiasis
- Routine efforts to prevent hepatobiliary complications in all patients receiving long-term CPN include providing a portion (20%–40%) of calories as fat, cycling CPN so that the glucose infusion is stopped for at least 8–10 hours per day, encouraging enteral intake to stimulate gallbladder contraction and maintain mucosal integrity, avoiding excessive calories, and preventing hyperglycemia.
- If abnormal liver biochemistries or other evidence of liver damage occurs, evaluation for other possible causes of liver disease should be performed.
- If mild hepatobiliary complications are noted, parenteral nutrition need not be discontinued, but the same principles used in preventing hepatic complications can be applied therapeutically.
- When cholestasis is present, copper and manganese should be deleted from the CPN formula to prevent accumulation in the liver and basal ganglia. A 4-week trial of metronidazole or ursodeoxycholic acid has been reported to be helpful in some patients.

METABOLIC BONE DISEASE

- Metabolic bone disease has been observed in patients receiving long-term (>3 months) CPN.
- Patients may be asymptomatic. Clinical manifestations include bone fractures and pain. Demineralization may be seen in radiologic studies. Osteopenia, osteomalacia, or both may be present.
- The precise causes of metabolic bone disease are not known, but several mechanisms have been proposed, including aluminum toxicity, vitamin D toxicity, and negative calcium balance.
- Several therapeutic options should be considered in patients who have evidence of bone abnormalities.
- Remove vitamin D from the CPN formulation if the parathyroid hormone and 1,25-hydroxy vitamin D levels are low.
- Reduce protein to <1.5 g/kg/d because amino acids cause hypercalciuria.
- Maintain normal magnesium status because magnesium is necessary for normal parathormone action and renal conservation of calcium.
- Provide oral calcium supplements of 1–2 g/d.
- Consider bisphosphonate therapy to decrease bone resorption.

Contraindications to Nutrition Support in Critically Ill Patients

Enteral Nutrition

- Hemodynamic instability/shock: Patients may be predisposed to bowel ischemia
- Bowel obstruction
- Severe and protracted ileus
- Major upper gastrointestinal bleeding
- Intractable vomiting
- Gastrointestinal ischemia
- High-output gastrointestinal fistula
- Abdominal compartment syndrome

Parenteral Nutrition

- Severe hyperglycemia
- Severe electrolyte abnormalities

- Volume overload
- Inadequate intravenous access
- Inadequate attempts to feed enterally

SPECIAL CONSIDERATIONS

- Monitoring nutrition support
  - Adjustment of the nutrient formulation is often needed as medical therapy or clinical status changes.
  - When nutrition support is initiated, other sources of **glucose** (e.g., peripheral IV dextrose infusions) should be stopped and the volume of other IV fluids adjusted to account for CPN.
  - Vital signs should be checked every 8 hours.
  - In certain patients, body weight, fluid intake, and fluid output should be followed daily.
  - Serum electrolytes (including phosphorus) should be measured every 1–2 days after CPN is started until the values are stable and then rechecked weekly.
  - Serum glucose should be checked up to every 4–6 hours by finger stick until blood glucose concentrations are stable and then rechecked weekly.
  - If lipid emulsions are being given, **serum triglycerides** should be measured during lipid infusion in patients at risk for hypertriglyceridemia to demonstrate adequate clearance (triglyceride concentrations should be <400 mg/dL).
- Careful attention to the catheter and catheter site can help to prevent **catheter-related infections.**
  - Gauze dressings should be changed every 48–72 hours or when contaminated or wet, but transparent dressings can be changed weekly.
  - Tubing that connects the parenteral solutions with the catheter should be changed every 24 hours.
  - A 0.22-μm filter should be inserted between the IV tubing and the catheter when **lipid-free CPN** is infused and should be changed with the tubing.
  - A 1.2-μm filter should be used when a total nutrient admixture containing a **lipid emulsion** is infused.
  - When a **single-lumen** catheter is used to deliver CPN, the catheter should not be used to infuse other solutions or medications (with the exception of compatible antibiotics) and should not be used to monitor central venous pressure.
  - When a **triple-lumen** catheter is used, the distal port should be reserved solely for the administration of CPN.

REFEEDING THE SEVERELY MALNOURISHED PATIENT

Refeeding syndrome may occur after initiating nutritional therapy in patients who are severely malnourished and have had minimal nutrient intake. It is a syndrome consisting of metabolic disturbances that occur as a result of reinstitution of nutrition to patients who are starved or severely malnourished. It usually occurs within 4 days of restarting the nutritional support.

Initial features may be nonspecific. Later, the refeeding syndrome can lead to rhabdomyolysis, leukocyte dysfunction, hypotension, arrhythmias, seizures, respiratory and cardiac failure, coma, and sudden death.

- **Hypophosphatemia, hypokalemia, and hypomagnesemia:** Rapid and marked decreases in these electrolytes occur during initial refeeding because of insulin-stimulated increases in cellular mineral uptake from extracellular fluid. For example, plasma phosphorus concentration can fall below 1 mg/dL and cause death within hours of initiating nutritional therapy if adequate phosphate is not given. Suggested replacement guidelines are reviewed in several sources.[46]

- **Fluid overload and congestive heart failure** are associated with decreased cardiac function and insulin-induced increased sodium and water reabsorption in conjunction with nutritional therapy containing water, glucose, and sodium. Renal mass may be reduced, limiting the ability to excrete salt or water loads.
- **Cardiac arrhythmias:** Patients who are severely malnourished often have bradycardia. Sudden death from ventricular tachyarrhythmias can occur during the first week of refeeding in severely malnourished patients and may be associated with a prolonged QT interval and electrolyte abnormalities. Patients with ECG changes should be monitored on telemetry, possibly in an ICU.
- **Glucose intolerance:** Starvation causes insulin resistance such that refeeding with high-carbohydrate meals or large amounts of parenteral glucose can cause marked elevations in blood glucose concentration, glycosuria, dehydration, and hyperosmolar coma. In addition, carbohydrate refeeding in patients who are depleted in thiamine can precipitate Wernicke encephalopathy.

MANAGEMENT OF SEVERE MALNUTRITION

- Careful **evaluation** of cardiovascular function and plasma electrolytes (history, physical examination, ECG, and blood tests) and correction of abnormal plasma electrolytes are **important before initiation of feeding.**
- Refeeding by the oral or enteral route involves the frequent or continuous administration of small amounts of food or an isotonic liquid formula.
- Parenteral supplementation or complete parenteral nutrition may be necessary if the intestine cannot tolerate feeding.
- During initial refeeding, fluid intake should be limited to approximately 800 mL/d plus insensible losses. Adjustments in fluid and sodium intake are needed in patients who have evidence of fluid overload or dehydration.
- Changes in body weight provide a useful guide for evaluating the efficacy of fluid administration. Weight gain >0.25 kg/d or 1.5 kg/wk probably represents fluid accumulation in excess of tissue repletion. Initially, approximately 15 kcal/kg, containing approximately 100 g carbohydrate and 1.5 g protein per kilogram of actual body weight, should be given daily.
- The rate at which the caloric intake can be increased depends on the severity of the malnutrition and the tolerance to feeding. In general, increases of 2–4 kcal/kg every 24–48 hours are appropriate.
- Sodium should be restricted to approximately 50 mEq/m^2 body surface area/day, but liberal amounts of phosphorus, potassium, and magnesium should be given to patients who have normal renal function.
- All other nutrients should be given in amounts needed to meet the recommended dietary intake (Table 2-9).
- Body weight, fluid intake, urine output, plasma glucose, and electrolyte values should be **monitored daily** during early refeeding (first 3–7 days) so that nutritional therapy can be appropriately modified when necessary.

Protein–Energy Malnutrition

Protein–energy malnutrition or protein–calorie malnutrition includes marasmus, kwashiorkor, and intermediate states of marasmus–kwashiorkor (Table 2-10).

TABLE 2-9 Major Mineral Daily Requirements, Deficiency, Toxicity, and Diagnostic Evaluation

Mineral	Recommended Daily Enteral[3] Intake/Parenteral[4] Intake	Signs and Symptoms of Deficiency	Signs and Symptoms of Toxicity	Diagnostic Evaluation
Sodium	1.2–1.5 g[47,a]/**1–2 mEq/kg**	Encephalopathy, seizure, weakness, dehydration, cerebral edema	Encephalopathy, seizure	$Sodium_p$ (correct for hyperglycemia) $Sodium_u$ (will often only provide a rough estimate [i.e., too low, too high])
Potassium	4700 mg[48,a]/**1–2 mEq/kg**	Abdominal cramping, diarrhea, paresthesias, QT prolongation, weakness	QRS widening, QT shortening (sine wave morphology in extreme cases), peaked T waves	$Potassium_{w,b}$
Calcium	1000–1200 mg/**10–15 mEq**	QRS widening, paresthesias (Trousseau sign), tetany (Chvostek sign), osteomalacia	Encephalopathy, headache, abdominal pain, nephrolithiasis, metastatic calcification	$Calcium_{w,b}$, 24-h $calcium_u$ (correct for $albumin_s$)
Magnesium	420 mg/**8–20 mEq**	Tachyarrhythmia, weakness, muscle cramping, peripheral and central nervous system overstimulation (seizure, tetany)	Hyporeflexia, nausea, vomiting, weakness, encephalopathy, decreased respiratory drive, hypocalcemia, hyperkalemia, heart block	$Magnesium_s$, $magnesium_u$
Phosphorus	700 mg/**20–40 mmol**	Weakness, fatigue, increased cell membrane fragility (hemolytic anemias, leukocyte + platelet dysfunction), encephalopathy	Metastatic calcification, theoretic higher risk of nephrolithiasis, secondary hyperparathyroidism	$Phosphorus_p$

[a]*Note*: Adequate daily intake.
Subscript: b, blood; p, plasma; s, serum; u, urine; w, whole blood.

TABLE 2-10 Distinguishing Features of Marasmus vs Kwashiorkor

Features	Marasmus	Kwashiorkor
Height and weight	• Wasting • Stunting, if chronically malnourished	• Weight for age is abnormal. • Low height for age (stunting) if also chronically malnourished.
Head	Appears large relative to body, with staring eyes	Moon face with or without facial edema. May appear plump.
Extremities	Emaciated arms, thighs, and buttocks, with loose folds due to loss of subcutaneous fat.	Edema
Behavior	Typically irritable, fretful	Typically apathetic, listless; may be irritable when handled.
Abdomen		Distended, dilated intestinal loops; hepatomegaly.
Skin	Thin, dry skin.	Thin, dry and peeling skin, with areas of hyperkeratosis and hyperpigmentation (flaky paint dermatosis).
Hair	Thin, sparse hair that is easily plucked.	Dry, dull, and hypopigmented hair that falls out or is easily plucked. Hypopigmentation may occur in stripes if malnutrition has been intermittent ("flag sign").

- **Marasmus** develops due to inadequate intake of protein and calories. It is characterized by emaciation with apparent muscle wasting and loss of body fat. There is no edema. The hair is thin and dry. Diarrhea is frequent and there may be signs of infection.
- **Kwashiorkor** develops due to an inadequate protein intake with reasonable caloric (energy) intake. In kwashiorkor, marked protein deprivation causes hypoalbuminemia leading to generalized or dependent edema. Kwashiorkor has characteristic skin lesions. This consists of alternating zones of hyperpigmentation and hypopigmentation, producing "flaky paint" appearance. The hair is dry and sparse. There may be loss of color or alternating bands of pale and darker hair (flag sign).

Treatment of protein–energy malnutrition includes provision of protein and energy supplements and control of infection.

OBESITY

General Principles

Obesity is defined as the accumulation of excess body fat, that is, adipose tissue that is of sufficient magnitude to impair health.

TYPES OF OBESITY

- Central obesity: Fat accumulation in the trunk/abdominal cavity (in the mesentery, around viscera) associated with increased waist: hip ratio. Central obesity is defined according to the WHO criteria: Waist circumference (WC) ≥90 cm for men and ≥80 cm

for women or waist-to-hip ratio (WHR) ≥0.90 in men and ≥0.85 in women and a waist-to-height ratio (WHTR) of >0.50.
- Generalized obesity: Excess fat accumulation occurs diffusely in subcutaneous tissue.

Etiology

- Genetics: Hereditary—usually a polygenic disorder. Rarely monogenic—usually a cause of childhood obesity. Includes mutations in leptin gene, leptin receptor gene, proopiomelanocortin (POMC), and melanocortin-4 receptor (Mc4R). Few genetic conditions such as Prader–Willi syndrome and Laurence–Moon–Biedl syndrome are associated with obesity.
- Environmental factors: These include increased consumption of food and decreased physical activity.

Reversible causes of obesity are as follows:
- Endocrine factors: Hypothyroidism, Cushing syndrome, insulinoma, Stein–Leventhal syndrome, hypothalamic damage (trauma/tumor), etc.
- Drug-induced: Psychiatric/neurologic medications—atypical antipsychotics (olanzapine), pizotifen, sodium valproate, and flunarizine. Steroid hormones—progesterone, corticosteroids, and OC pills. Antidiabetic medications—insulin, sulfonylureas, and thiazolidinediones. Antihypertensive medications—α-adrenergic blockers and β-adrenergic blockers.

ETIOLOGIC CLASSIFICATION OF OBESITY

Iatrogenic

- Drugs that cause weight gain (Table 2-11)
- Hypothalamic surgery

Dietary Obesity

- Infant feeding practices
- Progressive hyperplastic obesity
- Frequency of eating
- High-fat diets
- Overeating

Neuroendocrine Obesities

- Hypothalamic obesity
- Hypothyroidism
- Seasonal affective disorder
- Cushing syndrome
- Polycystic ovary syndrome
- Hypogonadism
- Growth hormone deficiency
- Pseudohypoparathyroidism

Social and Behavioral Factors

- Socioeconomic status
- Ethnicity

Psychological Factors

- Restrained eaters
- Night eating syndrome
- Binge eating
- Sedentary lifestyle

TABLE 2-11 Drugs Causing Weight Gain and Alternatives That Can Be Used

Drug Class	Weight Gain	Alternatives
Antipsychotic	Clozapine, risperidone, olanzapine, quetiapine, haloperidol, perphenazine	Ziprasidone, aripiprazole
Antidepressants/mood stabilizers: Tricyclic antidepressants	Amitriptyline, doxepin, imipramine, nortriptyline, trimipramine, mirtazapine	Bupropion, nefazodone, fluoxetine (short term), sertraline (<1 year)
Antidepressants/mood stabilizers: SSRIs	Paroxetine, fluvoxamine	
Antidepressants/mood stabilizers: MAOIs	Phenelzine, tranylcypromine	
Antiseizure medications	Carbamazepine, gabapentin, valproate	Topiramate, zonisamide
Diabetes drugs	Insulin (weight gain differs with type and regimen used), sulfonylureas, thiazolidinediones, metiglinide	Metformin, acarbose, miglitol, pramlintide, edenatide, liraglutide
OCPs	Progestational steroids, hormonal contraceptives containing progestational steroids	Barrier methods, IUDs
Steroid hormones	Corticosteroids, progestational steroids	NSAIDs

IUD, intrauterine device; MAOI, monoamine oxidase inhibitor; NSAIDs, nonsteroidal anti-inflammatory drugs; OCP, oral contraceptive pills; SSRI, selective serotonin reuptake inhibitor.

- Enforced inactivity (postoperative)
- Aging

Genetic (Dysmorphic) Obesities

- Autosomal recessive traits
- Autosomal dominant traits
- X-linked traits
- Chromosomal abnormalities

Other

- Low birth weight

Complications of Obesity

All the systems are affected by the effects of obesity. Table 2-12 lists the systemwise effects and complications of obesity.

MANAGEMENT OF OBESITY

Goals are as follows:

- To reduce weight by about 10% from baseline.
- Reduce weight of about 0.5–1 kg/week for 6 months.

TABLE 2-12 Complications of Obesity

Risk Factors/System Involved	Outcomes
Metabolic syndrome	
• Type 2 diabetes	Coronary heart disease, ischemic heart disease
• Hypertension	Stroke
• Hyperlipidemia	Diabetes complications
Cardiovascular	Heart failure, arrhythmias
Gastrointestinal	Gastroesophageal reflux disease Hiatus hernia
Hepatobiliary	Nonalcoholic steatohepatitis, NAFLD
	Cirrhosis
	Gallstones
Pulmonary disease Restricted ventilation	Exertional dyspnea, breathlessness
	Obstructive sleep apnea
	Obesity hypoventilation syndrome (Pickwickian syndrome)
Mechanical effects of weight	Urinary incontinence
	Osteoarthritis of knees and hips
	Varicose veins
Endocrine manifestations (increased peripheral steroid interconversion in adipose tissue)	Menstrual abnormalities Hormone-dependent cancers (breast, uterus) Polycystic ovarian syndrome (infertility, hirsutism)
Neurological	Stroke Depression Entrapment neuropathies Sleep disturbances
Others	Accident proneness Psychological morbidity (low self-esteem, depression) Socioeconomic disadvantage Postoperative problems Increased cancer risk—colorectal, prostate, ovary, esophagus, gallbladder cancer Skin infections (groin and submammary candidiasis, hidradenitis), acanthosis, striae

NAFLD, nonalcoholic fatty liver disease.

Identify Candidates

- Low risk: Individuals with a BMI between 25 and 29.9 kg/m^2, who do not have risk factors for CVD or other weight-related comorbidities, may be described as having low risk, particularly if they are older. They should receive counseling on prevention of weight gain, including advice on dietary habits and physical activity.
- Moderate risk: Individuals with a BMI between 25 and 29.9 kg/m^2 and with one or more risk factors for CVD (diabetes, hypertension, dyslipidemia), or with a BMI of 30–34.9 kg/m^2, are at moderate risk. Such patients should be offered or referred to

intensive, multicomponent behavioral intervention. This includes tools and strategies to make dietary changes, increase physical activity, and support and maintain weight loss. Pharmacologic therapy should also be considered.
- High risk: Individuals with a BMI of 35-40 kg/m^2 are at high risk, especially those ages 20–39, as well as those with a BMI above 40 kg/m^2. Individuals in the highest-risk categories should receive the most aggressive treatment (intensive, multicomponent behavioral intervention, pharmacologic therapy, and bariatric surgery).

Lifestyle Modifications

- Diet : A low-calorie diet low in saturated fats and dense foods, with normal protein intake and increased fiber, can be effective. A 1000 kcal deficit can lead to a 1 kg weight loss per week. However, total fasting is not recommended as it can cause diuresis, natriuresis, and nutritional deficiencies. It also poses the risk of refeeding syndrome, which is a severe and potentially fatal electrolyte, fluid, and metabolic imbalance.
- There are several options for diets, including balanced low-calorie, low-fat/low-calorie, moderate-fat/low-calorie, or low-carbohydrate diets, as well as the Mediterranean diet. These diets can be consumed conventionally or on a time-restricted basis, such as intermittent fasting.
- Metabolic studies using state-of-the-art techniques have shown that most adults will lose weight when fed fewer than 1000 kcal/day.
- Physical activity: Regular physical activity is recommended and it should be supervised. Moderate physical exercise should be done for 30 minutes or more for 5–7 days/week.
- Behavior modification: Behavior modification, also known as behavior therapy, is one cornerstone in the treatment for obesity. The primary objective of behavioral therapy is to assist patients in making long-term changes in their eating habits. This involves the adjustment and monitoring of food intake, modification of physical activity, and management of environmental cues and stimuli that trigger eating behaviors.

Pharmacotherapy

- Recommended if BMI ≥27 with weight-related comorbidities or BMI ≥30.

Centrally and peripherally acting drugs available for treatment are listed in Table 2-13.

TABLE 2-13	Drugs Available for Treatment of Obesity
Sibutramine	Centrally acting monoamine reuptake inhibitor (mainly serotonin and norepinephrine)—causing sympathetic stimulation and increase in BMR, causing decrease in appetite 10–15 mg once daily
Rimonabant	Endocannabinoid (CB1) receptor blocker—it has both central and peripheral receptor actions, and reduces weight and weight-related metabolic factors Not FDA approved (depression, anxiety, and suicidal tendencies)
Orlistat	Nonsystemic reversible inhibitor of gastric and pancreatic lipases by forming a covalent bond with serine residue. It acts on stomach and intestine 120 mg BD/TID with meals
Olestra	Synthesized using a sucrose molecule, can support six to eight fatty acid chains arranged radially like an octopus. This molecule is too large to move through the intestinal wall and be absorbed

(Continued)

TABLE 2-13	Drugs Available for Treatment of Obesity (Continued)
Phentermine	Amphetamine-like drug Acts centrally to reduce appetite Low addictive potential, modest efficacy, and modest CVS side effects
Metformin	Decreases appetite Good choice for T2DM as most patients are obese
Tesofensine	Norepinephrine, dopamine, and serotonin reuptake inhibitor Appetite suppressant
Betahistine	Stimulates histamine-1 receptor and reduces craving for food (especially fatty food) Not FDA approved
Amylin (pramlintide)	Part of endocrine pancreas Contributes to glycemic control Functions as synergistic partner to insulin
Liraglutide	GLP-1 agonist 1.8–3 mg daily
Lorcaserin	Serotonin agonist

Devices

- Devices may be considered for use in patients for whom medications prove ineffective or are not tolerated. Additionally, they may be suitable for individuals who are unable or unwilling to undergo bariatric surgery, or as a bridging therapy prior to bariatric surgery.
- Intragastric balloon systems: With these techniques, saline-filled balloons are placed in the stomach to take up space and produce a sensation of satiety. These systems are recommended for weight reduction in conjunction with diet and exercise for adult patients with a BMI of 30–40 kg/m^2 and one or more obesity-related comorbid conditions. They are also suitable for adult patients with obesity who have not achieved weight reduction through diet and exercise alone.
- Gastric emptying (aspiration) systems: Using a surgically placed gastrostomy tube, these systems drain a portion of the stomach contents after every meal, reducing the absorption of calories. These are intended to assist in weight loss in patients aged 22 and older with a BMI of 35–55 kg/m^2, and who have not succeeded in achieving and maintaining weight loss through nonsurgical weight-loss therapy. These devices are contraindicated in patients with eating disorders.
- Hydrogels: Recognizing as medical devices, hydrogels are orally administered products taken twice daily before meals. They expand in the stomach and intestines, generating a feeling of satiety. They are not systemically absorbed and are eliminated through the feces. Hydrogels are recommended as weight management aids for adults with a BMI of 25–40 kg/m^2, intended to be used alongside diet and exercise.
- Bariatric endoscopy: Bariatric endoscopy includes the placement of gastric balloons as well as endoscopic sleeve gastroplasty (a procedure which uses a suturing device which creates a tubular shape similar to the sleeve gastrectomy).

Surgery

Indications

- BMI >35 with type 2 diabetes mellitus or a BMI >40.
- Repeated failures of other therapeutic approaches.
- Capability of tolerating surgery.

Types of surgeries:

- **Restrictive surgeries** limit the amount of food the stomach can hold and slow the rate of gastric emptying.
- **Malabsorptive surgeries** to reduce the amount of absorption
  - Laparoscopic gastric band (LAGB).
  - The Roux-en-Y gastric bypass.
  - Biliopancreatic diversion with duodenal switch.
  - Biliopancreatic diversion with vertical-banded gastroplasty.
  - Biliopancreatic diversion.
- **Combined**—both restrictive and malabsorptive surgeries.

Summary

- Nutritional assessment allows us to systematically assess the overall nutritional status of patients, diagnose malnutrition, identify underlying pathologies that lead to malnutrition, and plan necessary interventions.
- Malnutrition risk screening should be performed on all patients needing healthcare services, whether in a hospital, community, long-term care, or home setting.
- Obesity has become the world's most extensive pandemic, and its prevalence, distribution, and costs continue to rise.
- Malnutrition is a significant contributor to ICU morbidity and mortality, manifesting in terms of increased susceptibility to ICU-acquired weakness, pressure areas, poor wound healing, poor immune function, and many other problems.
- Latest guidelines recommend supplemental parenteral nutrition after 7–10 days, "if unable to meet 60% of energy and protein requirements by the enteral route alone."
- Unlike energy-protein undernourishment, the health impacts of micronutrient deficiency are not always acutely visible. Micronutrient deficiency is therefore sometimes termed "hidden hunger."

Scan the QR code to access chapter references.

3 Preventive Cardiology

Angela L. Brown, Dominique S. Williams, Johnathan Seth Parham, Anne C. Goldberg, Rajaram Prasad A., and Vidarshan Mathavan

Hypertension

GENERAL PRINCIPLES

Hypertension is defined as the presence of a blood pressure (BP) elevation to a level that places patients at increased risk for target organ damage in several vascular beds including the retina, brain, heart, kidneys, and large conduit arteries (Table 3-1).

Classification

- **Normal BP** is defined as systolic blood pressure (SBP) <120 mm Hg and diastolic blood pressure (DBP) <80 mm Hg; pharmacologic intervention is not indicated.
- Classification and stages of hypertension are as defined in the recent American College of Cardiology (ACC) guidelines.
- **Elevated blood pressure** is defined as SBP of 120–129 mm Hg and DBP of <80 mm Hg. These patients should engage in comprehensive lifestyle modifications to delay progression or prevent the development of hypertension.
- **In stage 1 hypertension** (SBP 130–139 mm Hg or DBP 80–89 mm Hg), pharmacologic therapy should be initiated in addition to lifestyle modification in patients with diabetes mellitus (DM), chronic kidney disease (CKD), clinical cardiovascular disease (CVD),

TABLE 3-1 Manifestations of Target Organ Disease

Organ System	Manifestation
Large vessel	Aneurysmal dilation Accelerated atherosclerosis Aortic dissection
Cardiac	*Acute:* Pulmonary edema, myocardial infarction *Chronic:* Clinical or ECG evidence of CAD; LVH by ECG or echocardiogram Heart failure, both reduced ejection fraction (systolic) and preserved ejection fraction (diastolic) Atrial fibrillation
Cerebrovascular	*Acute:* Intracerebral bleeding, coma, seizures, mental status changes, TIA, stroke, hypertensive encephalopathy *Chronic:* TIA, stroke
Renal	*Acute:* Hematuria, azotemia *Chronic:* Serum creatinine >1.5 mg/dL, proteinuria >1+ on dipstick
Retinopathy	*Acute:* Papilledema, hemorrhages *Chronic:* Hemorrhages, exudates, arterial nicking

CAD, coronary artery disease; LVH, left ventricular hypertrophy; TIA, transient ischemic attack.

or age ≥65 years to lower BP <130/80 mm Hg. In patients age ≥65, treatment to a BP goal of <130/80 mm Hg is recommended if therapy is tolerated without adverse side effects. In patients ≤65 years of age without DM, CKD, or clinical CVD, pharmacologic therapy should be initiated in addition to lifestyle modifications for primary prevention of CVD if the 10-year atherosclerotic cardiovascular disease (ASCVD) risk is ≥10%.[1]

- **In stage 2 hypertension** (SBP ≥140 mm Hg or DBP ≥90 mm Hg), pharmacologic therapy should be initiated in addition to lifestyle modification to lower BP to <130/80 mm Hg. Patients with BP levels >20/10 mm Hg above their treatment target will often require more than one medication to achieve adequate control, and a two-drug regimen may be initiated as initial therapy. Patients with an average BP of 180/120 mm Hg or greater require immediate therapy and, if symptomatic end-organ damage is present, hospitalization.[1,2]
- The recent **ESC/ESH guidelines came out in 2023** and defined hypertension as follows:
  - Optimal: SBP less than 120 mm Hg and DBP less than 80 mm Hg.
  - Normal: SBP 120–129 mm Hg and/or DBP 80–84 mm Hg.
  - High normal: SBP 130–139 mm Hg and/or DBP 85–89 mm Hg.
  - Grade 1 hypertension: SBP 140–59 mm Hg and/or DBP 90–99 mm Hg.
  - Grade 2 hypertension: SBP 160–179 mm Hg and/or DBP 100–109 mm Hg.
  - Grade 3 hypertension: SBP greater than or equal to 180 mm Hg and/or DBP greater than or equal to 110 mm Hg.

Comparison of various guidelines on normal BP and definition of hypertension is described in Table 3-2.

- **Hypertensive crisis** includes hypertensive emergencies and urgencies. It usually develops in patients with a previous history of elevated BP but may arise in those who were previously normotensive. The severity of a hypertensive crisis correlates not only with the absolute level of BP elevation but also with the rapidity of development because autoregulatory mechanisms have not had sufficient time to adapt.
  - **Hypertensive urgencies** are defined as a substantial increase in BP, usually with a DBP >120 mm Hg, and occur in approximately 1% of hypertensive patients. Hypertensive urgencies (i.e., upper levels of stage 2 hypertension, hypertension with optic disk edema, progressive end-organ complications rather than damage, and severe perioperative hypertension) warrant BP reduction within several hours to 48 hours and close follow-up over several days.[3,4]
  - **Hypertensive emergencies** include **accelerated hypertension**, typically defined as an SBP >180 mm Hg and DBP >120 mm Hg presenting with headaches, blurred vision, or focal neurologic symptoms and **malignant hypertension** (which requires the presence of papilledema). Hypertensive emergencies with acute emergency like aortic dissection require the blood pressure to be lowered to below 140 mm Hg in the first hour require immediate BP reduction by 20%–25% over the first hour to prevent or minimize end-organ damage (i.e., hypertensive encephalopathy, intracranial hemorrhage, unstable angina [UA] pectoris, acute myocardial infarction [MI], acute left ventricular failure with pulmonary edema, dissecting aortic aneurysm, progressive renal failure, or eclampsia) and then to 160/100 over the next 2–6 hours, and then gradually to normal over 2 days.[5]
  - **Isolated systolic hypertension,** defined as an SBP ≥130 mm Hg and DBP <90, occurs frequently in the elderly (beginning after the fifth decade and increasing with age). It can also be seen in young and very young individuals (ISHY), more commonly in male individuals. Nonpharmacologic therapy should be initiated with medications added as needed to lower SBP to the appropriate level based on age and comorbidities.
- ESC/ESH recommendations also shed light on **home (HBPM) and ambulatory BP measurements (ABPM)** and the following cutoffs were given:
  - Daytime (or awake) SBP greater than or equal to 135 mm Hg and/or DBP greater than or equal to 85 mm Hg.

TABLE 3-2 Comparison of New Definition of Hypertension

Current classifications of high blood pressure

SBP [mm Hg]		DBP [mm Hg]	ESH/ESC 2023	AHA/ACC 2019	Position of the DHL, 2017	NICE 2023
<120	and	<80	Optimal	Normal	Optimal	Normal
120–129	and	<80	Normal	Elevated	Normal	Normal
130–139	or	80–89	Upper range of normal	Grade I hypertension	Upper range of normal	Upper range of normal
140–159	or	90–99	Grade I hypertension	Grade II hypertension	Grade I hypertension	Grade I hypertension (≥135/85 mm Hg)*
160–179	or	100–109	Grade II hypertension	Grade II hypertension	Grade II hypertension	Grade II hypertension (≥150/95 mm Hg)*
≥180	or	≥110	Grade III hypertension	Grade II hypertension	Grade III hypertension	Severe hypertension

A comparison of the new definitions of normal blood pressure and the different grades of high blood pressure by the American Heart Association (AHA) and American College of Cardiology (ACC) with the definitions by the European Society of Cardiology (ESC) and European Society of Hypertension (ESH), as well as the most recent position of the German Hypertension League (*Deutsche Hochdruckliga*, DHL) and the National Institute for Health and Care Excellence (NICE) of the United Kingdom.
The lowering of cutoff values led to an increase in the prevalence of hypertension in the USA from 32% to 46%.
*The values refers to further measurements in the outpatient setting or at home.
DBP, diastolic blood pressure: SPB, systolic blood pressure

  - Night-time (or asleep) SBP greater than or equal to 120 mm Hg and/or DBP greater than or equal to 70 mm Hg.
  - Twenty-four hours mean SBP greater than or equal to 130 mm Hg and/or DBP greater than or equal to 80 mm Hg.
  - Home SBP greater than or equal to 135 mm Hg and/or DBP greater than or equal to 85 mm Hg.
- **Resistant hypertension** is defined as an office BP ≥140/90 in hypertensive patients on ≥3 antihypertensive agents, one of which is a diuretic at maximally recommended/tolerated doses or controlled BP on ≥4 antihypertensive agents. Causes of resistant hypertension include inaccurate BP measurement, inadequate regimen, nonadherence, ingestion of exogenous substances (e.g., decongestants, oral contraceptives, appetite suppressants, sympathomimetics, venlafaxine, tricyclic antidepressants, monoamine oxidase inhibitors [MAOIs], chlorpromazine, some herbal supplements [ma huang], steroids, NSAIDs, cyclosporine, caffeine, thyroid hormones, cocaine, alcohol use, erythropoietin) and secondary causes of hypertension.[1]

- **White coat hypertension** is an office BP 130/80 mm Hg or more but less than 160/100 mm Hg which comes down to 130/80 mm Hg or less after at least 3 months of antihypertensive therapy. ABPM or HBPM is usually necessary for this diagnosis.
- **Masked hypertension** is an elevated office systolic BP 120–129 mm Hg and diastolic BP less than 80 mm Hg but raised BP on ambulatory or home measurements (130/80 mm Hg or more).

Epidemiology

- The **public health burden** of hypertension is enormous. In 2019, the worldwide prevalence of hypertension was 32% in women and 34% in men.[4] For nonhypertensive individuals aged 55–65 years, the lifetime risk of developing hypertension is 90%.[6] The prevalence of prehypertension and hypertension among South Asian adults (18–49 years) is 43.2% and 14.9% in India, 35.1% and 19.8% in Bangladesh, and 25.2% and 13.8% in Nepal, respectively.[7] Hypertension was found to be higher in the studies conducted in urban areas than in rural areas.
- Data derived from the Framingham Study have shown that hypertensive patients have a *fourfold* increase in cerebrovascular accidents and a *sixfold* increase in congestive heart failure (CHF) when compared with normotensive control subjects.
- Disease-associated morbidity and mortality, including ASCVD, stroke, heart failure (HF), and renal insufficiency, increase with higher levels of SBP and DBP.
- Over the last three decades, aggressive treatment of hypertension has resulted in a substantial decrease in death rates from stroke and coronary heart disease (CHD). Although the incidence of end-stage renal disease (ESRD) has stabilized and hospitalizations for CHF have overall decreased,[8] BP control rates remain poor, with 53% of treated hypertensive patients with BP above target goal.[9]

Etiology

- BP rises with age. Other contributing factors include overweight/obesity, increased dietary sodium intake, decreased physical activity, increased alcohol consumption, and lower dietary intake of fruits, vegetables, and potassium.
- Of all hypertensive patients, more than 90% have primary or essential hypertension. The remainder have secondary hypertension. Causes of secondary hypertension are described in Table 3-3.

DIAGNOSIS

Clinical Presentation

- BP elevation is usually discovered in asymptomatic individuals during routine health visits.
- Optimal detection and evaluation of hypertension require accurate noninvasive BP measurement, which should be obtained in a seated patient with the arm resting level with the heart. A calibrated, appropriately fitting BP cuff (inflatable bladder encircling at least 80% of the arm) should be used because falsely high readings can be obtained if the cuff is too small.
- Two readings should be taken, separated by 2 minutes on 2 separate occasions. SBP should be noted with the appearance of Korotkoff sounds (phase I) and DBP with the disappearance of sounds (phase V).
- In certain patients, the Korotkoff sounds do not disappear but are present at 0 mm Hg. In this case, the initial muffling of Korotkoff sounds (phase IV) should be taken as the DBP. One should be careful to avoid reporting spuriously low BP readings because of an auscultatory gap, which is caused by the disappearance and reappearance of Korotkoff

TABLE 3-3 Causes of Secondary Hypertension

Renal • Parenchymal (2%–3%): CKD, polycystic kidney disease, chronic glomerulonephritis, and obstructive uropathy • Renovascular (1%–2%): Atherosclerosis (older individuals), fibromuscular dysplasia (women) Takayasu arteritis, scleroderma, vasculitis (PAN)
Endocrine • Adults ◦ Cushing syndrome, primary aldosteronism, pheochromocytoma, hyperthyroidism, hypothyroidism, hyperparathyroidism, and acromegaly • Children ◦ CAH—11-beta-hydroxylase deficiency, 17-alpha-hydroxylase deficiency, Liddle syndrome
Medications (contraceptive drugs, NSAIDs, erythropoietin, nasal decongestants with adrenergic effects, MAOIs, steroids, methamphetamine, and cocaine)
Obstructive sleep apnea
Coarctation of aorta
Pre-eclampsia, eclampsia
Neurological—dysautonomia, raised intracranial tension, lead poisoning, GB syndrome, and porphyria

CAH, congenital adrenal hyperplasia; PAN, polyarteritis nodosa.

sounds in hypertensive patients and may account for up to a 25-mm Hg gap between true and measured SBP.

- Hypertension should be confirmed in both arms, and the higher reading should be used.

History

- History should seek to discover secondary causes of hypertension and note the presence of medications and supplements that can affect BP (e.g., decongestants, oral contraceptives, appetite suppressants, sympathomimetics, venlafaxine, tricyclic antidepressants, MAOIs, chlorpromazine, some herbal supplements [ma huang], steroids, NSAIDs, cyclosporine, caffeine, thyroid hormones, cocaine, alcohol use, erythropoietin).
- A diagnosis of **secondary hypertension** should be considered in the following situations:
  - Age at onset younger than 30 years.
  - Onset of diastolic hypertension in persons older than 55 years.
  - Hypertension that is difficult to control after therapy has been initiated.
  - Stable hypertension that becomes difficult to control.
  - Resistant hypertension.
  - Clinical occurrence of a hypertensive crisis.
  - The presence of signs or symptoms of a secondary cause such as hypokalemia or metabolic alkalosis that is not explained by diuretic therapy.
  - Significant elevation of plasma creatinine with the use of ACE inhibitors.
- In patients who present with significant hypertension at a young age, a careful family history may give clues to forms of hypertension that follow simple Mendelian inheritance.

Physical Examination

Physical examination should include investigation for target organ damage or a secondary cause of hypertension by noting the presence of carotid bruits, an S_3 or S_4, cardiac murmurs, neurologic deficits, elevated jugular venous pressure, rales, retinopathy, unequal pulses, enlarged or small kidneys, cushingoid features, and abdominal bruits.

Differential Diagnosis

- Hypertension may be partly due to withdrawal from drugs, including alcohol, cocaine, and opioid analgesics. Rebound increases in BP may be seen in patients who abruptly discontinue antihypertensive therapy, particularly β-adrenergic antagonists and central α_2-agonists (see Complications).
- Cocaine and other sympathomimetic drugs (e.g., amphetamines, phencyclidine hydrochloride) can produce hypertension in the setting of acute intoxication and when the agents are discontinued abruptly after chronic use. Hypertension is often complicated by other end-organ insults, such as ischemic heart disease, stroke, and seizures. Phentolamine is effective in acute management, and sodium nitroprusside or nitroglycerin can be used as an alternative. β-Adrenergic antagonists should be avoided because of the risk of unopposed α-adrenergic activity, which can exacerbate hypertension.

Diagnostic Testing

- Tests are needed to help identify patients with possible target organ damage, to assess cardiovascular risk, and to provide a baseline for monitoring the adverse effects of therapy.
- Basic laboratory data should include urinalysis, hematocrit, plasma glucose, serum potassium, serum creatinine, calcium, uric acid, and fasting lipid levels.
- Other testing includes ECG and chest radiography. Echocardiography may be of value for certain patients to assess cardiac function or detection of left ventricular hypertrophy (LVH).
- Clinical clues and diagnostic testing in suspected cases of secondary hypertension are discussed in Table 3-4.

TREATMENT

- The goal of treatment is to prevent long-term sequelae (i.e., target organ damage) while controlling other modifiable cardiovascular risk factors. BP should be reduced to a goal of <130/80 mm Hg. Discretion is warranted in prescribing medication to lower BP that may affect cardiovascular risk adversely in other ways (e.g., glucose control, lipid metabolism, uric acid levels).
- In the absence of hypertensive crisis, BP should be reduced gradually to avoid end-organ (e.g., cerebral) ischemia.
- Lifestyle modifications should be encouraged in all hypertensive patients regardless of whether they require medication (Table 3-5). These changes may have beneficial effects on other cardiovascular risk factors.
- Barring an overt need for immediate pharmacologic therapy, most patients should be given the opportunity to achieve a reduction in BP over an interval of 3–6 months by applying nonpharmacologic modifications and pharmacologic therapies.

MONITORING/FOLLOW-UP

- BP measurements should be performed on multiple occasions under nonstressful circumstances (e.g., rest, sitting, empty bladder, comfortable temperature) to obtain an accurate assessment of BP in a given patient.
- Hypertension should not be diagnosed based on one measurement alone, unless it is >180/120 mm Hg or accompanied by target organ damage (i.e., hypertension urgency

TABLE 3-4 Guide to Evaluation of Secondary Hypertension

Diagnosis	Clinical Clues	Specific Investigation
Renal parenchymal hypertension	Estimated GFR <60 mL/min/1.73 m^2 Urine albumin-to-creatinine ratio ≥30 mg/g	Renal ultrasonography Azotemia
Renovascular disease	New elevation in serum creatinine, marked elevation in serum creatinine with initiation of ACEI or ARB, refractory hypertension, flash pulmonary edema, abdominal bruit	Magnetic resonance or CT angiography, invasive angiography
Coarctation of the aorta	Arm pulses > leg pulses, arm BP > leg BP, chest bruits, rib notching on chest radiography	Magnetic resonance imaging, aortography
Primary aldosteronism	Hypokalemia and refractory hypertension	Plasma renin and aldosterone, 24-hour urine potassium, adrenal CT, adrenal vein sampling
Cushing syndrome	Truncal obesity, wide and blanching purple striae, and muscle weakness	Plasma cortisol, urine cortisol after dexamethasone, and adrenal CT
Pheochromocytoma	Headaches, paroxysmal hypertension, palpitations, perspiration, pallor, and diabetes	Plasma metanephrine and normetanephrine, 24-hour urine catecholamines, adrenal CT
Obstructive sleep apnea	Loud snoring, daytime somnolence, obesity, and large neck	Sleep study/Polysomnography
Hypothyroidism Hyperthyroidism	Thyromegaly, weight loss/gain Tachycardia/bradycardia, eye signs	Thyroid-stimulating hormone (TSH), free thyroxine (FT4) and free triiodothyronine (FT3) RAIU (radioiodine uptake) scan

TABLE 3-5 Lifestyle Modifications and Effects

Modification	Approximate SBP Reduction (mm Hg)
Weight reduction (for every 10-kg weight loss)	5–20
Adoption of DASH eating plan	8–14
Dietary sodium reduction (intake <2 g/d)	2–8
Physical activity (150 min/wk)	4–9
Moderation of alcohol consumption (intake <2 drinks/d)	2–4

DASH, dietary approaches to stop hypertension; SBP, systolic blood pressure.

or emergency). Two or more abnormal readings should be obtained, preferably over a period of several weeks, before therapy is considered.

- Care should also be used to exclude pseudohypertension, which usually occurs in elderly individuals with stiff, noncompressible vessels. A palpable artery that persists after cuff inflation (**Osler sign**) should alert the physician to this possibility.
- Home and ambulatory BP monitoring can be used to assess a patient's true average BP, which correlates better with target organ damage.[10-12] Circumstances in which ambulatory BP monitoring might be of value include the following:
  - Suspected "white coat hypertension" (increases in BP associated with the stress of physician office visits), which should be evaluated carefully.
  - Evaluation of possible drug resistance, where suspected.

Medications

- Initial drug therapy
  Drug interactions, cost, and coexistent factors such as age, race, angina, HF, renal insufficiency, LVH, obesity, hyperlipidemia, gout, and bronchospasm should be considered in initial drug choice. The BP response is usually consistent within a given class of agents; therefore, if a drug fails to control BP, another agent from the same class is unlikely to be effective. At times, however, a change within drug class may be useful in reducing adverse effects. The lowest possible effective dosage should be used to control BP, adjusted every 1–2 months as needed (Table 3-6).
- In most patients, treatment should be initiated with a single pill combination (SPC) of two drugs to improve the speed, efficiency, and predictability of BP control.
- Although several two-drug combinations can be used, the preferred two-drug combinations should be a RAS blocker with a CCB or a thiazide/thiazide-like diuretic.
- A BB can be used at any step of combination with any drug from the other major drug classes as GDMT or in several other conditions.
- Initial monotherapy is recommended for very-high-risk patients with a high-normal BP as well as (for cautionary reasons) for very old and frail patients. It may also be considered in low-risk patients with stage 1 hypertension whose SBP is more modestly elevated (<150 mm Hg).
- An SPC comprising of RAS blocker with CCB and thiazide/thiazide-like diuretic, should be used if two-drug combinations do not achieve BP control (at the maximum tolerated doses) and a BB is not indicated.
- Regardless the initial treatment choice, ultimately most patients should be on combination treatment, using SPC whenever possible
- In the general black population, including those with diabetes, a diuretic or CCB can be considered for first-line therapy. Data from the ALLHAT trial have shown decreased cardiovascular and cerebrovascular morbidity and mortality with the use of thiazide diuretics or CCB over an ACE inhibitor.[13]
- In patients with chronic kidney disease stage 3 or higher, or CKD with albuminuria (>300 mg/d), initial or combination therapy with an ACE inhibitor or ARB is recommended.[1]
- **Additional therapy:** When a second drug is needed, it should generally be chosen from among the other first-line agents.
- **Adjustments of a therapeutic regimen:** Before considering a modification of therapy because of inadequate response to the current regimen, other possible contributing factors should be investigated. Poor patient compliance, use of antagonistic drugs (i.e., sympathomimetics, venlafaxine, tricyclic antidepressants, MAOIs, chlorpromazine, some herbal supplements [ma huang], steroids, NSAIDs, cyclosporine, caffeine, thyroid hormones, cocaine, erythropoietin), inappropriately high sodium intake, or increased alcohol consumption may be the cause of inadequate BP response. Secondary causes of hypertension

TABLE 3-6 Commonly Used Antihypertensive Agents by Functional Class

Drugs by Class	Properties	Initial Dose	Dosage Range (mg)
β-Adrenergic Antagonists			
Atenolol[a]	Selective	50 mg PO daily	25–100
Betaxolol[a]	Selective	10 mg PO daily	5–40
Bisoprolol[a]	Selective	5 mg PO daily	2.5–20
Metoprolol	Selective	50 mg PO bid	50–450
Metoprolol XL	Selective	50–100 mg PO daily	50–400
Nebivolol[a,b]	Selective with vasodilatory properties	5 mg PO daily	5–40
Nadolol[a]	Nonselective	40 mg PO daily	20–240
Propranolol	Nonselective	40 mg PO bid	40–240
Propranolol LA	Nonselective	80 mg PO daily	60–240
Timolol	Nonselective	10 mg PO bid	20–40
Pindolol	ISA	5 mg PO daily	10–60
Labetalol	α- and β-antagonist properties	100 mg PO bid	200–1200
Carvedilol	α- and β-antagonist properties	6.25 mg PO bid	12.5–50
Carvedilol CR[b]	α- and β-antagonist properties	10 mg PO daily	10–80
Acebutolol[a]	ISA, selective	200 mg PO bid, 400 mg PO daily	200–1200
Calcium Channel Antagonists			
Amlodipine	DHP	5 mg PO daily	2.5–10
Diltiazem		30 mg PO qid	90–360
Diltiazem LA		180 mg PO daily	120–540
Diltiazem CD		180 mg PO daily	120–480
Diltiazem XR		180 mg PO daily	120–540
Diltiazem XT		180 mg PO daily	120–480
Isradipine	DHP	2.5 mg PO bid	2.5–10
Nicardipine[b]	DHP	20 mg PO tid	60–120
Nifedipine	DHP	10 mg PO tid	30–120
Nifedipine XL (or CC)	DHP	30 mg PO daily	30–90
Nisoldipine	DHP	20 mg PO daily	20–40
Verapamil		80 mg PO tid	80–480
Verapamil SR		120 mg PO daily	120–480
Angiotensin-Converting Enzyme Inhibitors[c]			
Benazepril		10 mg PO bid	10–40
Captopril		25 mg PO bid–tid	50–450
Enalapril		5 mg PO daily	2.5–40

(Continued)

TABLE 3-6 Commonly Used Antihypertensive Agents by Functional Class (Continued)

Drugs by Class	Properties	Initial Dose	Dosage Range (mg)
Fosinopril		10 mg PO daily	10–40
Lisinopril		10 mg PO daily	5–40
Moexipril		7.5 mg PO daily	7.5–30
Quinapril		10 mg PO daily	5–80
Ramipril		2.5 mg PO daily	1.25–20
Trandolapril		1–2 mg PO daily	1–4
Perindopril		4 mg PO daily	2–16
Angiotensin II Receptor Blockers[c]			
Azilsartan[b]		40 mg PO daily	40–80
Candesartan		8 mg PO daily	8–32
Eprosartan		600 mg PO daily	600–800
Irbesartan		150 mg PO daily	150–300
Olmesartan[b]		20 mg PO daily	20–40
Losartan		50 mg PO daily	25–100
Telmisartan		40 mg PO daily	20–80
Valsartan		80 mg PO daily	80–320
Direct Renin Inhibitor[c]			
Aliskiren[b]		150 mg PO daily	150–300
Diuretics[c]			
Chlorthalidone	Thiazide diuretic	25 mg PO daily	12.5–50
Hydrochlorothiazide	Thiazide diuretic	12.5 mg PO daily	12.5–50
Hydroflumethiazide[b]	Thiazide diuretic	50 mg PO daily	50–100
Indapamide	Thiazide diuretic	1.25 mg PO daily	2.5–5
Methyclothiazide	Thiazide diuretic	2.5 mg PO daily	2.5–5
Metolazone	Thiazide diuretic	2.5 mg PO daily	1.25–5
Bumetanide	Loop diuretic	0.5 mg PO daily (or IV)	0.5–5
Ethacrynic acid[b]	Loop diuretic	50 mg PO daily (or IV)	25–100
Furosemide	Loop diuretic	20 mg PO daily (or IV)	20–320
Torsemide	Loop diuretic	5 mg PO daily (or IV)	5–10
Amiloride	Potassium-sparing diuretic	5 mg PO daily	5–10
Triamterene[b]	Potassium-sparing diuretic	50 mg PO bid	50–200
Eplerenone	Aldosterone antagonist	25 mg PO daily	25–100
Spironolactone	Aldosterone antagonist	25 mg PO daily	25–100

(Continued)

TABLE 3-6 Commonly Used Antihypertensive Agents by Functional Class (Continued)

Drugs by Class	Properties	Initial Dose	Dosage Range (mg)
α-Adrenergic Antagonists			
Doxazosin		1 mg PO daily	1–16
Prazosin		1 mg PO bid–tid	1–20
Terazosin		1 mg PO at bedtime	1–20
Centrally Acting Adrenergic Agents			
Clonidine		0.1 mg PO bid	0.1–1.2
Clonidine patch		TTS 1/wk (equivalent to 0.1 mg/d release)	0.1–0.3
Guanfacine		1 mg PO daily	1–3
Guanabenz		4 mg PO bid	4–64
Methyldopa[a]		250 mg PO bid–tid	250–2000
Direct-Acting Vasodilators			
Hydralazine[a]		10 mg PO qid	50–300
Minoxidil		5 mg PO daily	2.5–100
Miscellaneous			
Reserpine		0.5 mg PO daily	0.01–0.25

[a]Adjusted in renal failure.
[b]Available only in brand name. Assume all drugs are available in generic form unless otherwise denoted by superscript "*b*."
[c]Renal function should be considered for all angiotensin-converting enzyme inhibitors before initiation.
DHP, dihydropyridine; ISA, intrinsic sympathomimetic activity; TTS, transdermal therapeutic system.

should be considered when a previously effective regimen becomes inadequate and other confounding factors are absent.

- **Diuretics** (see Table 3-6) are effective agents in the therapy of hypertension and have been shown to reduce the incidence of stroke and cardiovascular events. Several classes of diuretics are available, generally categorized by their site of action in the kidney.
- **Thiazide** and thiazide-like diuretics (e.g., hydrochlorothiazide, chlorthalidone) block sodium reabsorption predominantly in the distal convoluted tubule by inhibition of the thiazide-sensitive Na/Cl cotransporter. Thiazide diuretics can produce weakness, muscle cramps, and impotence. Metabolic side effects include hypokalemia, hypomagnesemia, hyperlipidemia (with increases in low-density lipoproteins [LDLs] and triglyceride levels), hypercalcemia, hyperglycemia, hyperuricemia, hyponatremia, and rarely azotemia. Thiazide-induced pancreatitis has also been reported. Metabolic side effects may be limited when thiazides are used in low doses (e.g., hydrochlorothiazide, 12.5–25.0 mg/d).
- **Loop diuretics** (e.g., furosemide, bumetanide, ethacrynic acid, torsemide) block sodium reabsorption in the thick ascending loop of Henle through inhibition of the Na/K/2Cl cotransporter and are the most effective agents in patients with renal insufficiency

(estimated glomerular filtration rate [GFR] <30 mL/min/1.73 m^2). Loop diuretics can cause electrolyte abnormalities such as hypomagnesemia, hypocalcemia, and hypokalemia and can also produce irreversible ototoxicity (usually dose related and more common with parenteral therapy).

- **Spironolactone and eplerenone, potassium-sparing agents,** act by competitively inhibiting the actions of aldosterone on the kidney. Triamterene and amiloride are potassium-sparing drugs that inhibit the epithelial Na^+ channel in the distal nephron to inhibit reabsorption of Na^+ and secretion of potassium ions. Potassium-sparing diuretics are weak agents when used alone; thus, they are often combined with a thiazide for added potency. Aldosterone antagonists reduce morbidity and mortality in heart failure with reduced ejection fraction and may have an additional benefit in improving myocardial function; this effect may be independent of its effect on renal transport mechanisms. Spironolactone and eplerenone can produce hyperkalemia. The gynecomastia that may occur in men and breast tenderness in women are not seen with eplerenone. Triamterene (usually in combination with hydrochlorothiazide) can cause renal tubular damage and renal calculi. Unlike thiazides, potassium-sparing and loop diuretics do not cause adverse lipid effects.
- **Calcium channel antagonists** (see Table 3-6) generally have no significant central nervous system (CNS) side effects and can be used to treat diseases, such as angina pectoris, which can coexist with hypertension. **Because of the concern that the use of short-acting dihydropyridine calcium channel antagonists may increase the number of ischemic cardiac events, they are not indicated for hypertension management**[14]; long-acting agents are considered safe in the management of hypertension.[15,16]
    - **Classes of calcium channel antagonists** include diphenylalkylamines (e.g., verapamil), benzothiazepines (e.g., diltiazem), and dihydropyridines (e.g., nifedipine). The dihydropyridines include many newer second-generation drugs (e.g., amlodipine, felodipine, isradipine, and nicardipine), which are more vasoselective and have longer plasma half-lives than nifedipine. Verapamil and diltiazem have negative cardiac inotropic and chronotropic effects. Nifedipine also has a negative inotropic effect, but in clinical use, this effect is much less pronounced than that of verapamil or diltiazem because of peripheral vasodilation and reflex tachycardia. Less negative inotropic effects have been observed with the second-generation dihydropyridines. All calcium channel antagonists are metabolized in the liver; thus, in patients with cirrhosis, the dosing interval should be adjusted accordingly. Some of these drugs also inhibit the metabolism of other hepatically cleared medications (e.g., cyclosporine). Verapamil and diltiazem should be used with caution in patients with cardiac conduction abnormalities, and they can worsen HF in patients with decreased left ventricular function.
    - **Side effects** of verapamil include constipation, nausea, headache, and orthostatic hypotension. Diltiazem can cause nausea, headache, and rash. Dihydropyridines can cause lower extremity edema, flushing, headache, and rash. Calcium channel antagonists can also cause gingival hyperplasia. They have no significant effects on glucose tolerance, electrolytes, or lipid profiles.
- **Inhibitors of the renin–angiotensin system** (see Table 3-6) include ACE inhibitors, ARBs, and a direct renin inhibitor.
    - **ACE inhibitors** may have beneficial effects in patients with concomitant HF or kidney disease. One study has also suggested that ACE inhibitors (ramipril) may significantly reduce the rate of death, MI, and stroke in patients without HF or low ejection fraction.[17] Additionally, they can reduce hypokalemia, hypercholesterolemia, hyperglycemia, and hyperuricemia caused by diuretic therapy and are particularly effective in states of hypertension associated with a high renin state (e.g., scleroderma renal crisis). **Side effects** associated with the use of ACE inhibitors are infrequent. They can cause a dry cough (up to 20% of patients), angioneurotic edema, and hypotension, but they do not cause levels of lipids, glucose, or uric acid to increase. ACE inhibitors that contain

a sulfhydryl group (e.g., captopril) may cause taste disturbance, leukopenia, and a glomerulopathy with proteinuria. Because ACE inhibitors cause preferential vasodilation of the efferent arteriole in the kidney, worsening of renal function may occur in patients who have decreased renal perfusion or who have preexisting severe renal insufficiency. ACE inhibitors can cause hyperkalemia and should be used with caution in patients with a decreased GFR who are taking potassium supplements or who are receiving potassium-sparing diuretics.

  ◦ **ARBs** are a class of antihypertensive drugs that are effective in diverse patient populations.[18] ARBs are useful alternatives in patients with HF who are unable to tolerate ACE inhibitors.[19] **Side effects** of ARBs occur rarely but include angioedema, allergic reaction, and rash.
  ◦ The **direct renin inhibitor** class consists of one agent, aliskiren, which is indicated solely for the treatment of hypertension (see Table 3-6). It may be used in combination with other antihypertensive agents; however, combined use with ACE inhibitors or ARBs is contraindicated in patients with diabetes and increases the risk of hyperkalemia[18,19] (Food and Drug Administration [FDA] Drug Safety Communication, April 2012).

- **β-Adrenergic antagonists** (see Table 3-6) are part of medical regimens that have been proven to decrease the incidence of stroke, MI, and HF. β-Adrenergic antagonists work via competitive inhibition of the effects of catecholamines at β-adrenergic receptors, which decreases heart rate and cardiac output. These agents also decrease plasma renin and cause a resetting of baroreceptors to accept a lower level of BP. β-Adrenergic antagonists cause release of vasodilatory prostaglandins, decrease plasma volume, and may also have a CNS-mediated antihypertensive effect.
  ◦ **Classes of β-adrenergic antagonists** can be subdivided into those that are cardioselective, with primarily β_1-blocking effects, and those that are nonselective, with β_1- and β_2-blocking effects. At low doses, the cardioselective agents can be given with caution to patients with mild chronic obstructive pulmonary disease, DM, or peripheral vascular disease. At higher doses, these agents lose their β_1 selectivity and may cause unwanted effects in these patients. β-Adrenergic antagonists can also be categorized according to the presence or absence of partial agonist or intrinsic sympathomimetic activity (ISA). β-Adrenergic antagonists with ISA cause less bradycardia than do those without it. In addition, there are agents with mixed properties having both α- and β-adrenergic antagonist actions (labetalol and carvedilol). Nebivolol is a highly selective β-adrenergic antagonist that is vasodilatory through an unclear mechanism.
  ◦ **Side effects** include high-degree atrioventricular block, HF, Raynaud phenomenon, and impotence. Lipophilic β-adrenergic antagonists, such as propranolol, have a higher incidence of CNS side effects including insomnia and depression. Propranolol can also cause nasal congestion. β-Adrenergic antagonists can cause adverse effects on the lipid profile; increased triglyceride and decreased high-density lipoprotein (HDL) levels occur mainly with nonselective β-adrenergic antagonists but generally do not occur when β-adrenergic antagonists with ISA are used. Pindolol, a selective β-adrenergic antagonist with ISA, may increase HDL and nominally increase triglycerides. Side effects of labetalol include hepatocellular damage, postural hypotension, a positive antinuclear antibody (ANA) test, a lupus-like syndrome, tremors, and potential hypotension in the setting of halothane anesthesia. Carvedilol appears to have a similar side effect profile to other β-adrenergic antagonists. Both labetalol and carvedilol have negligible effects on lipids. Rarely, reflex tachycardia may occur because of the initial vasodilatory effect of labetalol and carvedilol. Because β-receptor density is increased with chronic antagonism, abrupt withdrawal of these agents can precipitate angina pectoris, increases in BP, and other effects attributable to an increase in adrenergic tone.
- **Selective α-adrenergic antagonists** such as prazosin, terazosin, and doxazosin have replaced nonselective α-adrenergic antagonists such as phenoxybenzamine (see Table 3-6)

in the treatment of essential hypertension. Based on the ALLHAT trial, these drugs appear to be less efficacious than diuretics, CCBs, and ACE inhibitors in reducing primary end points of CVD when used as monotherapy.[13]

- **Side effects** of these agents include a "first-dose effect," which results from a greater decrease in BP with the first dose than with subsequent doses. Selective α_1-adrenergic antagonists can cause syncope, orthostatic hypotension, dizziness, headache, and drowsiness. In most cases, side effects are self-limited and do not recur with continued therapy. Selective α_1-adrenergic antagonists may improve lipid profiles by decreasing total cholesterol and triglyceride levels and increasing HDL levels. Additionally, these agents can improve the negative effects on lipids induced by thiazide diuretics and β-adrenergic antagonists. Doxazosin specifically may be less effective at lowering SBP than thiazide diuretics and may be associated with a higher risk of HF and stroke in patients with hypertension and at least one additional risk factor for coronary artery disease (CAD).[13]

- **Centrally acting adrenergic agents** (see Table 3-6) are potent antihypertensive agents. In addition to its oral dosage forms, clonidine is available as a transdermal patch that is applied weekly.
  - **Side effects** may include bradycardia, drowsiness, dry mouth, orthostatic hypotension, galactorrhea, and sexual dysfunction. Transdermal clonidine causes a rash in up to 20% of patients. These agents can precipitate HF in patients with decreased left ventricular function, and abrupt cessation can precipitate an acute withdrawal syndrome (AWS) of elevated BP, tachycardia, and diaphoresis. Methyldopa produces a positive direct antibody (Coombs) test in up to 25% of patients, but significant hemolytic anemia is much less common. If hemolytic anemia develop's secondary to methyldopa, the drug should be withdrawn. Severe cases of hemolytic anemia may require treatment with glucocorticoids. Methyldopa also causes positive ANA test results in approximately 10% of patients and can cause an inflammatory reaction in the liver that is indistinguishable from viral hepatitis; fatal hepatitis has been reported. Guanabenz and guanfacine decrease total cholesterol levels, and guanfacine can also decrease serum triglyceride levels.
- **Direct-acting vasodilators** are potent antihypertensive agents (see Table 3-6) now reserved for refractory hypertension or specific circumstances such as the use of hydralazine in pregnancy.
  - Hydralazine in combination with nitrates is useful in treating patients with hypertension and HF with reduced ejection fraction (see Chapter 5, Heart Failure and Cardiomyopathy). **Side effects** of hydralazine therapy may include headache, nausea, emesis, tachycardia, and postural hypotension. Asymptomatic patients may have a positive ANA test result, and a hydralazine-induced systemic lupus-like syndrome may develop in approximately 10% of patients. Patients at greater risk for the latter complication include those treated with excessive doses (e.g., >400 mg/d), those with impaired renal or cardiac function, and those with the slow acetylation phenotype. Hydralazine should be discontinued if clinical evidence of a lupus-like syndrome develops and a positive ANA test result is present. The syndrome usually resolves with discontinuation of the drug, leaving no adverse long-term effects.
  - **Side effects** of minoxidil include weight gain, hypertrichosis, hirsutism, ECG abnormalities, and pericardial effusions.
- **Reserpine, guanethidine, and guanadrel** (see Table 3-6) were among the first effective antihypertensive agents available. Currently, these drugs are not regarded as first- or second-line therapy because of their significant side effects.
  - **Side effects** of reserpine include severe depression in approximately 2% of patients. Sedation and nasal stuffiness also are potential side effects. Guanethidine can cause severe postural hypotension through a decrease in cardiac output, a decrease in peripheral resistance, and venous pooling in the extremities. Patients who are receiving

guanethidine with orthostatic hypotension should be cautioned to arise slowly and to wear support hose. Guanethidine can also cause ejaculatory failure and diarrhea.

- **Parenteral antihypertensive agents** are indicated for the immediate reduction of BP in patients with hypertensive emergencies. Judicious administration of these agents (Table 3-7) may also be appropriate in patients with hypertension complicated by HF or MI. These drugs are also indicated for individuals who have perioperative hypertensive urgency or are in need of emergency surgery. If possible, an accurate baseline BP should be determined before the initiation of therapy. In the setting of hypertensive emergency, the patient should be admitted to an intensive care unit for close monitoring, and an intraarterial monitor should be used when available. Although parenteral agents are indicated as a first-line treatment in hypertensive emergencies, oral agents may also be effective in this group; the choice of drug and route of administration must be individualized. If parenteral agents are used initially, oral medications should be administered shortly thereafter to facilitate rapid weaning from parenteral therapy.
  - **Sodium nitroprusside,** a direct-acting arterial and venous vasodilator, is the drug of choice for most hypertensive emergencies (see Table 3-7). It reduces BP rapidly and is easily titratable, and its action is short lived when discontinued. Patients should be monitored very closely to avoid an exaggerated hypotensive response. Therapy for more than 48–72 hours with a high cumulative dose or renal insufficiency may cause accumulation of thiocyanate, a toxic metabolite. Thiocyanate toxicity may cause paresthesias, tinnitus, blurred vision, delirium, or seizures. Serum thiocyanate levels should be kept at <10 mg/dL. Patients on high doses (>2–3 mg/kg/min) or those with renal dysfunction should have serum levels of thiocyanate drawn after 48–72 hours of therapy. In patients with normal renal function or those receiving lower doses, levels can be drawn after 5–7 days. Hepatic dysfunction may result in accumulation of cyanide, which can cause lactic acidosis, dyspnea, vomiting, dizziness, ataxia, and syncope. Hemodialysis should be considered for thiocyanate poisoning. Nitrites and thiosulfate can be administered intravenously for cyanide poisoning.
  - **Nitroglycerin** given as a continuous IV infusion (see Table 3-7) may be appropriate in situations in which sodium nitroprusside is relatively contraindicated, such as in patients with severe coronary insufficiency or advanced renal or hepatic disease. It is the preferred agent for patients with moderate hypertension in the setting of acute coronary ischemia or after coronary artery bypass surgery because of its more favorable effects on pulmonary gas exchange and collateral coronary blood flow. In patients with severely elevated BP, sodium nitroprusside remains the agent of choice. Nitroglycerin reduces preload more than afterload and should be used with caution or avoided in patients who have inferior MI with right ventricular infarction and are dependent on preload to maintain cardiac output.
  - **Labetalol** can be administered parenterally (see Table 3-7) in hypertensive crisis, even in patients in the early phase of an acute MI, and is the drug of choice in hypertensive emergencies that occur during pregnancy. When given intravenously, the β-adrenergic antagonist effect is greater than the α-adrenergic antagonist effect. Nevertheless, symptomatic postural hypotension may occur with IV use; thus, patients should be treated in a supine position. Labetalol may be particularly beneficial during adrenergic excess (e.g., clonidine withdrawal, pheochromocytoma, postcoronary bypass grafting). Because the half-life of labetalol is 5–8 hours, intermittent IV bolus dosing may be preferable to IV infusion. IV infusion can be discontinued before oral labetalol is begun. When the supine DBP begins to rise, oral dosing can be initiated at 200 mg PO, followed in 6–12 hours by 200–400 mg PO, depending on the BP response.
  - **Esmolol** is a parenteral, short-acting, cardioselective β-adrenergic antagonist (see Table 3-7) that can be used in the treatment of hypertensive emergencies in patients in whom β-blocker intolerance is a concern. Esmolol is also useful for the treatment of

TABLE 3-7 Commonly Used Antihypertensive Agents by Functional Class

Drug	Administration	Onset	Duration of Action	Dosage	Adverse Effects and Comments
Fenoldopam	IV infusion	<5 min	30 min	0.1–0.3 μg/kg/min	Tachycardia, nausea, vomiting
Sodium nitroprusside	IV infusion	Immediate	2–3 min	0.5–10 μg/kg/min (initial dose, 0.25 μg/kg/min for eclampsia and renal insufficiency)	Hypotension, nausea, vomiting, apprehension; risk of thiocyanate and cyanide toxicity is increased in renal and hepatic insufficiency, respectively; levels should be monitored; must shield from light
Diazoxide	IV bolus	15 min	6–12 h	50–100 mg q5–10 min, up to 600 mg	Hypotension, tachycardia, nausea, vomiting, fluid retention, hyperglycemia; may exacerbate myocardial ischemia, heart failure, or aortic dissection
Labetalol	IV bolus	5–10 min	3–6 h	20–80 mg q5–10 min, up to 300 mg	Hypotension, heart block, heart failure, bronchospasm, nausea, vomiting, scalp tingling, paradoxical pressor response; may not be effective in patients receiving α- or β-antagonists
	IV infusion			0.5–2 mg/min	
Nitroglycerin	IV infusion	1–2 min	3–5 min	5–250 μg/min	Headache, nausea, vomiting. Tolerance may develop with prolonged use
Esmolol	IV bolus	1–5 min	10 min	500 μg/kg/min for first 1 min	Hypotension, heart block, heart failure, bronchospasm
	IV infusion			50–300 μg/kg/min	
Phentolamine	IV bolus	1–2 min	3–10 min	5–10 mg q5–15 min	Hypotension, tachycardia, headache, angina, paradoxical pressor response

(Continued)

TABLE 3-7 Parenteral Antihypertensive Drug Preparations (Continued)

Drug	Administration	Onset	Duration of Action	Dosage	Adverse Effects and Comments
Hydralazine (for treatment of eclampsia)	IV bolus	10–20 min	3–6 h	10–20 mg q20 min (if no effect after 20 mg, try another agent)	Hypotension, fetal distress, tachycardia, headache, nausea, vomiting, local thrombophlebitis. Infusion site should be changed after 12 h
Methyldopate (for treatment of eclampsia)	IV bolus	30–60 min	10–16 h	250–500 mg	Hypotension
Nicardipine	IV infusion	1–5 min	3–6 h	5 mg/h, increased by 1.0–2.5 mg/h q15 min, up to 15 mg/h	Hypotension, headache, tachycardia, nausea, vomiting
Clevidipine	IV infusion	2–4 min	5–15 min	1–2 mg/h, double dose every 90 seconds up to 16 mg/h	Hypotension, reflex tachycardia
Enalaprilat	IV bolus	5–15 min	1–6 h	0.6255 mg q6h	Hypotension

aortic dissection. β-Adrenergic antagonists may be ineffective when used as monotherapy in the treatment of severe hypertension and are frequently combined with other agents (e.g., with sodium nitroprusside in the treatment of aortic dissection).
  - **Nicardipine** is an effective IV calcium channel antagonist preparation (see Table 3-7). Side effects include headache, flushing, reflex tachycardia, and venous irritation. Nicardipine should be administered via a central venous line. If it is given peripherally, the IV site should be changed q12h. Fifty percent of the peak effect is seen within the first 30 minutes, but the full peak effect is not achieved until after 48 hours of administration. **Clevidipine**, an IV calcium channel antagonist, has a quicker onset of action and shorter half-life than nicardipine.
  - **Enalaprilat** is the active de-esterified form of enalapril (see Table 3-7) that results from hepatic conversion after an oral dose. Enalaprilat (as well as other ACE inhibitors) has been used effectively in cases of severe and malignant hypertension. However, variable and unpredictable results have also been reported. ACE inhibition can cause rapid BP reduction in hypertensive patients with high renin states such as renovascular hypertension, concomitant use of vasodilators, and scleroderma renal crisis; thus, enalaprilat should be used cautiously to avoid precipitating hypotension. Therapy can be changed to an oral preparation when IV therapy is no longer necessary.
  - **Diazoxide and hydralazine** are only rarely used in hypertensive crises and offer little or no advantage to the agents discussed previously. It should be noted, however, that hydralazine is a useful agent in pregnancy-related hypertensive emergencies because of its established safety profile.
  - **Fenoldopam** is a selective agonist to peripheral dopamine-1 receptors, and it produces vasodilation, increases renal perfusion, and enhances natriuresis. Fenoldopam has a short duration of action; the elimination half-life is <10 minutes. The drug has important application as parenteral therapy for high-risk hypertensive surgical patients and the perioperative management of patients undergoing organ transplantation.
- **Oral loading of antihypertensive agents (captopril, clonidine, hydralazine, nifedipine)** has been used successfully in patients with hypertensive crisis when urgent but not immediate reduction of BP is indicated.

  Oral clonidine loading is achieved by using an initial dose of 0.2 mg PO followed by 0.1 mg PO q1h to a total dose of 0.7 mg or a reduction in diastolic pressure of 20 mm Hg or more. BP should be checked at 15-minute intervals over the first hour, 30-minute intervals over the second hour, and then hourly. After 6 hours, a diuretic can be added, and an 8-hour clonidine dosing interval can begin. Sedative side effects are significant. Sublingual nifedipine has an onset of action within 30 minutes but can produce wide fluctuations and excessive reductions in BP. Because of the potential for adverse cardiovascular events (stroke/MI), sublingual nifedipine should be avoided in the acute management of elevated BP. Side effects include facial flushing and postural hypotension.

SPECIAL CONSIDERATIONS

- **Hypertensive crisis:** In hypertensive emergency, control of acute or ongoing end-organ damage is more important than the absolute level of BP. BP control with a rapidly acting parenteral agent should be accomplished as soon as possible (within 1 hour) to reduce the chance of permanent organ dysfunction and death. A reasonable goal is a 20%–25% reduction of mean arterial pressure over a period of minutes to hours and then a reduction to normal BP over 24–48 hours. A precipitous fall in BP may occur in patients who are elderly, volume depleted, or receiving other antihypertensive agents. BP control in hypertensive urgencies can be accomplished more slowly and with use of oral antihypertensives. Excessive or rapid decreases in BP should be avoided to minimize the risk of cerebral hypoperfusion or coronary insufficiency. Normal BP can be attained gradually over several days as tolerated by the individual patient.

- **Aortic dissection**
  - All patients with aortic dissection, including those treated surgically, require acute and chronic antihypertensive therapy to provide initial stabilization and to prevent complications (e.g., aortic rupture, continued dissection). Medical therapy of chronic stable aortic dissection should seek to maintain SBP ≤120 mm Hg and heart rate <60 bpm if tolerated.[22] Antihypertensive agents with negative inotropic properties, including calcium channel antagonists, β-adrenergic antagonists, methyldopa, clonidine, and reserpine, are preferred for management in the postacute phase.
  - **β-Blockers** are considered the initial drug of choice and should precede vasodilator therapy. β-Blockers are effective in lowering the heart rate and counteracting the reflex tachycardia and increased inotropy seen with vasodilator therapy. **IV labetalol** has been used successfully as a single agent in the treatment of acute aortic dissection. Labetalol produces a dose-related decrease in BP and lowers contractility. It has the advantage of allowing for oral administration after the acute stage of dissection has been managed successfully. **Esmolol**, a cardioselective class intravenous β-adrenergic antagonist with a very short duration of action, may be preferable, especially in patients with relative contraindications to β-antagonists. If esmolol is tolerated, a longer-acting β-adrenergic antagonist should be used. In patients intolerant of β-blockade, CCBs diltiazem and verapamil may be used.
  - **Vasodilator therapy** in combination with β-blockade allows for more effective and rapid reduction in BP. **Sodium nitroprusside** is considered the initial vasodilator drug of choice because of the predictability of response and absence of tachyphylaxis. Nitroprusside alone causes an increase in left ventricular contractility and subsequent arterial shearing forces, which contribute to ongoing intimal dissection. Thus, when using sodium nitroprusside, adequate simultaneous **β-adrenergic antagonist therapy** is essential. Nicardipine, clevidipine, nitroglycerin, enalaprilat, and fenoldopam may also be used.
- **The elderly hypertensive patient** (age >65 years) is generally characterized by increased vascular resistance, decreased plasma renin activity, and greater LVH than in younger patients. Often, elderly hypertensive patients have coexisting medical problems that must be considered when initiating antihypertensive therapy. SBP <140 mm Hg has been associated with decreased major adverse cardiovascular events.[23,24]

  Drug doses should be increased slowly to avoid adverse effects and hypotension. Diuretics as initial therapy have been shown to decrease the incidence of stroke, fatal MI, and overall mortality in this age group.[25] Calcium channel antagonists decrease vascular resistance, have no adverse effects on lipid levels, and are also good choices for elderly patients. ACE inhibitors and ARBs may be effective agents in this population.
- **African American hypertensive patients** generally have a lower plasma renin level, higher plasma volume, and higher vascular resistance than do Caucasian patients. Thus, African American patients respond well to diuretics, alone or in combination with calcium channel antagonists. ACE inhibitors, ARBs, and β-adrenergic antagonists are also effective agents in this population, particularly when combined with a diuretic.
- **The obese hypertensive patient** is characterized by more modest elevations in vascular resistance, higher cardiac output, expanded intravascular volume, and lower plasma renin activity at any given level of arterial pressure. Weight reduction is the primary goal of therapy and is effective in reducing BP and causing regression of LVH.
- **The diabetic patient** with nephropathy may have significant proteinuria and renal insufficiency, which can complicate management (see Chapter 13, Renal Diseases). Control of BP is the most important intervention shown to slow down loss of renal function. In the setting of proteinuria, ACE inhibitors should be used as first-line therapy because they have been shown to decrease proteinuria and to slow down progressive loss of renal function independent of their antihypertensive effects. ACE inhibitors may also be beneficial in reducing the rates of death, MI, and stroke in diabetics who have cardiovascular

risk factors but lack left ventricular dysfunction. Hyperkalemia is a common side effect in diabetic patients treated with ACE inhibitors, especially in those with moderate to severe impairment of their GFR. ARBs are also effective antihypertensive agents and have been shown to slow down the rate of progression to ESRD, thus supporting a renal protective effect.[26]

- **The patient with chronic renal insufficiency** has hypertension that usually is partially volume dependent. Retention of sodium and water exacerbates the existing hypertensive state, and diuretics are important in the management of this problem. When estimated GFR is <30–35 mL/min/1.73 m^2, loop diuretics are the most effective class. In the presence of proteinuria, ACE inhibitors/ARBs should be considered because higher urinary excretion of protein is associated with a more rapid decline in GFR, regardless of the cause of renal insufficiency.
- **The hypertensive patient with LVH** is at increased risk for sudden death, MI, and all-cause mortality. Although there is no direct evidence, regression of LVH could be expected to reduce the risk for subsequent complications. Aggressive BP control and renin–angiotensin system blockade with ACE inhibitors/ARBs appear to have the greatest effect on regression.[27-29]
- **The hypertensive patient with CAD** is at increased risk for UA and MI. β-Adrenergic antagonists can be used as first-line agents in these patients because they can decrease cardiac mortality and subsequent reinfarction in the setting of acute MI and can decrease progression to MI in those who present with UA. β-Adrenergic antagonists also have a role in secondary prevention of cardiac events and in increasing long-term survival after MI. Care should be exercised in those with cardiac conduction system disease. ACE inhibitors are beneficial in patients with CAD and decrease mortality in individuals who present with acute MI, especially those with left ventricular dysfunction.[30-33]
- **The hypertensive patient with heart failure with reduced ejection fraction** (HFrEF) is at risk for progressive left ventricular dilatation and sudden death. Patients should be prescribed guideline-directed medical therapy to attain a BP <130/80 mm Hg. In this population, ACE inhibitors decrease mortality,[31] and in the setting of acute MI, they decrease the risk of recurrent MI, hospitalization for HF, and mortality.[34] ARBs have similar beneficial effects, and they appear to be an effective alternative in patients who are unable to tolerate an ACE inhibitor.[19] β-Adrenergic antagonist therapy has been shown to decrease morbidity and mortality. Agents shown to have proven benefit include metoprolol succinate, carvedilol, and bisoprolol.[15,35,36] Nitrates and hydralazine also decrease mortality in patients with HF irrespective of hypertension, but hydralazine can cause reflex tachycardia and worsening ischemia in patients with unstable coronary syndromes and should be used with caution. Mineralocorticoid receptor antagonists have been shown to decrease mortality in patients with HFrEF. Nondihydropyridine calcium channel antagonists should generally be avoided.
- **The hypertensive patient with heart failure with preserved ejection fraction** (HFpEF) may present with signs of volume overload and thus diuretics may be used as initial therapy. The optimal treatment regimen for hypertension in patients with HFpEF is unclear. ACE inhibitors/ARBs have the greatest effect on regression of LVH and thus may improve diastolic function.[37]
- **In the pregnant patient with hypertension**, there is concern for potential maternal and fetal morbidity and mortality associated with elevated BP and the clinical syndromes of preeclampsia and eclampsia. The possibility of teratogenic or other adverse effects of antihypertensive medications on fetal development also should be considered.
  - **Classification of hypertension** during pregnancy has been proposed by the American College of Obstetrics and Gynecology.[38]
    - **Preeclampsia–eclampsia:** Diagnosis is established if there is *new-onset* hypertension after 20 weeks of gestation and the presence of proteinuria. Elevated SBP ≥140 mm Hg

or DBP ≥90 mm Hg on two occasions at least 4 hours apart or a one-time measurement of SBP ≥160 mm Hg or DBP ≥110 mm Hg qualifies as hypertension. If no proteinuria is present, then hypertension along with one of the following qualifies: platelets <100,000/μL, creatinine >1.1 mg/dL (or doubling from baseline), liver transaminases greater than twice the normal, pulmonary edema, or cerebral/visual symptoms. Eclampsia encompasses these parameters in addition to generalized seizures.

    - **Chronic (preexisting) hypertension:** This disorder is defined by a BP ≥140/90 mm Hg before the 20th week of pregnancy.
    - **Chronic hypertension with superimposed preeclampsia:** This classification is used when a woman with chronic hypertension develops worsening hypertension and new proteinuria and/or other features of preeclampsia as outlined previously.
    - **Gestational hypertension:** This disorder is defined by a BP ≥140/90 mm Hg after the 20th week of pregnancy without proteinuria or other features of preeclampsia.
  - **Therapy:** Treatment of hypertension in pregnancy should begin if SBP is ≥160 mm Hg or DBP is ≥100 mm Hg.
    - Nonpharmacologic therapy, such as weight reduction and vigorous exercise, is not recommended during pregnancy.
    - Alcohol and tobacco use should be strongly discouraged.
    - Pharmacologic intervention with labetalol, nifedipine, or methyldopa is recommended as first-line therapy because of its proven safety. Other antihypertensives have theoretical disadvantages, but none except the ACE inhibitors have been proven to increase fetal morbidity or mortality.
    - If a patient is suspected of having preeclampsia or eclampsia, urgent referral to an obstetrician who specializes in high-risk pregnancy is recommended.
- **MAOIs:** MAOIs used in association with certain drugs or foods can produce a catecholamine excess state and accelerated hypertension. Interactions are common with tricyclic antidepressants, meperidine, methyldopa, levodopa, sympathomimetic agents, and antihistamines. Tyramine-containing foods that can lead to this syndrome include certain cheeses, red wine, beer, chocolate, chicken liver, processed meat, herring, broad beans, canned figs, and yeast. Nitroprusside, labetalol, and phentolamine have been used effectively in the treatment of accelerated hypertension associated with MAOI use (see Table 3-7).

Selection of Antihypertensive Agent

An initial 3-drug regimen is recommended that consists of maximally tolerated doses of ACE-I or ARB, calcium channel blocker and diuretic. If target blood pressure goals are not met, sequential drug addition can be considered as outlined below.

- Substitution of the diuretic:
  - Previously used diuretic may be substituted with a thiazide - like diuretic (such as indapamide or chlorthalidone) if eGFR ≥30 mL/min/1.73 m^2, or with a loop diuretic if eGFR <30 mL/min/1.73 m^2.
  - Addition of mineralocorticoid receptor antagonist (spironolactone/eplerenone) if eGFR ≥30 mL/min/1.73 m^2 and absence of hyperkalemia
- Addition of a beta blocker (such as metoprolol succinate or bisoprolol), combined alpha-/beta blocker (such as carvedilol or labetalol), an alpha blocker (such as doxazosin), or central alpha agonist (such as clonidine).
- Addition of hydralazine; requires concomitant use of beta blocker and diuretic
- Substitution of minoxidil for hydralazine; requires concomitant use of beta blocker and diuretic

However, therapy should be individualized, as discussed in Table 3-8.

TABLE 3-8 Individualizing Antihypertensive Therapy

Compelling indications (major improvement in outcome independent of blood pressure)	
Diabetes mellitus	ACE inhibitor or ARB
Heart failure with reduced ejection fraction	ACE inhibitor or ARB, β-blocker, diuretic, aldosterone antagonist
Postmyocardial infarction	ACE inhibitor or ARB, β-blocker, aldosterone antagonist
Proteinuric chronic kidney disease (nondiabetic)	ACE inhibitor or ARB
Angina pectoris	β-Blocker, calcium channel blocker
Atrial fibrillation/flutter rate control	β-Blocker, nondihydropyridine calcium channel blocker
Previous CVA/TIA	ACE inhibitor ± diuretic
Antihypertensive agents with a favorable effect on symptoms in comorbid conditions	
Benign prostatic hyperplasia	α-Blocker
Essential tremor	β-Blocker (noncardioselective)
Hyperthyroidism	β-Blocker
Migraine	β-Blocker, calcium channel blocker
Osteoporosis	Thiazide diuretic
Raynaud phenomenon	Dihydropyridine calcium channel blocker
Contraindications	
Angioedema	Avoid ACE inhibitor
Peripheral vascular disease	Avoid β-blocker
Bronchospasm	Avoid nonselective β-blocker
Liver disease	Avoid methyldopa
Pregnancy	Avoid ACE inhibitor, ARB, or renin inhibitor
Second- or third-degree heart block	Avoid β-blocker, nondihydropyridine calcium channel blocker unless a functioning ventricular pacemaker
Bilateral renal artery stenosis	Avoid ACE inhibitors/ARB/renin inhibitor
Drug classes that may have adverse effects on comorbid conditions	
Depression	Avoid β-blocker, central alpha-2 agonist
Gout	Avoid loop or thiazide diuretic
Hyperkalemia	Avoid aldosterone antagonist, ACE inhibitor, ARB, renin inhibitor
Hyponatremia	Avoid thiazide diuretic
Renovascular disease	Avoid ACE inhibitor, ARB, or renin inhibitor

ACE, angiotensin-converting enzyme; ARB, angiotensin receptor blocker; CVA, cerebrovascular accident; TIA, transient ischemic attack.

Withdrawal syndrome associated with discontinuation of antihypertensive therapy: In substituting therapy in patients with moderate-to-severe hypertension, it is reasonable to increase doses of the new medication in small increments while tapering the previous medication to avoid excessive BP fluctuations. On occasion, an antihypertensive withdrawal syndrome (AWS) develops, usually within the first 24–72 hours. Occasionally, BP rises to levels that are much higher than those of baseline values. The most severe complications of AWS include encephalopathy, stroke, MI, and sudden death. AWS is associated most commonly with centrally acting adrenergic agents (particularly clonidine) and β-adrenergic antagonists but has been reported with other agents as well, including diuretics. Discontinuation of antihypertensive medications should be done with caution in patients with preexisting cerebrovascular or cardiac disease. Management of AWS by reinstitution of the previously administered drug is generally effective.

Dyslipidemia

GENERAL PRINCIPLES

- Lipids are sparingly soluble macromolecules that include cholesterol, fatty acids, and their derivatives.
- Plasma lipids are transported by lipoprotein particles composed of **apolipoproteins**, **phospholipids**, **free cholesterol**, **cholesterol esters**, and **triglycerides**.
- Human plasma lipoproteins are separated into **five major classes** based on density:
  - Chylomicrons (least dense)
  - Very-low-density lipoproteins (VLDLs)
  - Intermediate-density lipoproteins
  - LDLs
  - HDLs
- A sixth class, lipoprotein(a) [Lp(a)], resembles LDL in lipid composition and has a density that overlaps LDL and HDL.
- Physical properties of plasma lipoproteins are summarized in Table 3-9.

TABLE 3-9 Physical Properties of Plasma Lipoproteins[a]

Lipoprotein	Lipid Composition	Origin	Apolipoproteins
Chylomicrons	TG, 85%; chol, 3%	Intestine	A-I, A-IV; B-48; C-I, C-II, C-III; E
VLDL	TG, 55%; chol, 20%	Liver	B-100; C-I, C-II, C-III; E
IDL	TG, 25%; chol, 35%	Metabolic product of VLDL	B-100; C-I, C-II, C-III; E
LDL	TG, 5%; chol, 60%	Metabolic product of IDL	B-100
HDL	TG, 5%; chol, 20%	Liver, intestine	A-I, A-II; C-I, C-II, C-III; E
Lp(a)	TG, 5%; chol, 60%	Liver	B-100; Apo(a)

[a]Remainder of particle is composed of phospholipid and protein.
Chol, cholesterol; HDL, high-density lipoprotein; IDL, intermediate-density lipoprotein; LDL, low-density lipoprotein; Lp(a), lipoprotein(a); TG, triglyceride; VLDL, very-low-density lipoprotein.

- Nearly 90% of patients with CHD have some form of dyslipidemia. Increased levels of LDL cholesterol (LDL-C), remnant lipoproteins, and Lp(a) and decreased levels of HDL cholesterol have all been associated with an increased risk of premature vascular disease.[39,40] In addition, dyslipidemia is highly prevalent in children with nonalcoholic fatty liver disease and may play a role in its pathophysiology.[41]
- **Clinical dyslipoproteinemias**
  - Most dyslipidemias are multifactorial in etiology and reflect the effects of genetic influences coupled with diet, inactivity, smoking, alcohol use, and comorbid conditions such as obesity and DM.
  - Differential diagnosis of the major lipid abnormalities is summarized in Table 3-10.
  - The major genetic dyslipoproteinemias are reviewed in Table 3-11.[42,43]
    - Familial hypercholesterolemia (FH) and familial combined hyperlipidemia are disorders that contribute significantly to premature CVD.
    - FH is an underdiagnosed, autosomal co-dominant condition with a prevalence of approximately 1 in 200 people that causes elevated LDL-C levels from birth.[43,44] It is associated with significantly increased risk of early CVD.[45]
    - Familial combined hyperlipidemia has a prevalence of 1%–2% and typically presents in adulthood, although obesity and high dietary fat and sugar intake have led to increased presentation in childhood and adolescence.[46]
- **Standards of care for hyperlipidemia**
  - LDL-C–lowering therapy, particularly with hydroxymethylglutaryl-coenzyme A (HMG-CoA) reductase inhibitors (commonly referred to as statins), lowers the risk of CHD-related death, morbidity, and revascularization procedures in patients ***with***

TABLE 3-10 Differential Diagnosis of Major Lipid Abnormalities

Lipid Abnormality	Primary Disorders	Secondary Disorders
Hypercholesterolemia	Polygenic, familial hypercholesterolemia, familial defective apo B-100; PCSK9 gain of function mutation	Hypothyroidism, nephrotic syndrome, anorexia nervosa
Hypertriglyceridemia	Lipoprotein lipase deficiency, apo C-II deficiency, apo A-V deficiency, familial hypertriglyceridemia, dysbetalipoproteinemia	Diabetes mellitus, obesity, metabolic syndrome, alcohol use, oral estrogen, renal failure, hypothyroidism, retinoic acid, lipodystrophies
Combined hyperlipidemia	Familial combined hyperlipidemia, dysbetalipoproteinemia	Diabetes mellitus, obesity, metabolic syndrome, nephrotic syndrome, hypothyroidism, lipodystrophies
Low HDL	Familial hypoalphalipoproteinemia, Tangier disease (ABCA1 deficiency), apoA1 mutations, lecithin–cholesterol acyltransferase deficiency	Diabetes mellitus, obesity, metabolic syndrome, hypertriglyceridemia, smoking, anabolic steroids

apo, apolipoprotein; HDL, high-density lipoprotein.

TABLE 3-11 Review of Major Genetic Dyslipoproteinemias

Type of Genetic Dyslipidemia	Typical Lipid Profile	Type of Inheritance Pattern	Phenotypic Features	Other Information
Familial hypercholesterolemia	• Increased LDL cholesterol (>190 mg/dL) • Homozygous form or compound heterozygous form (rare) can have LDL cholesterol >500 mg/dL	Autosomal dominant (prevalence of 1 in 200–250 for heterozygote form and 1 in 250,000 for homozygous form)	• Premature CAD • Tendon xanthomas • Premature arcus corneae (full arc before age 40) • Homozygous form: planar and tendon xanthomas and CAD in childhood and adolescence	Mutations of the LDL receptor, apolipoprotein B-100, and gain-of-function mutations of proprotein convertase/kexin subtype 9 (PCSK9) lead to impaired uptake and degradation of LDL
Familial combined hyperlipidemia	• High levels of VLDL, LDL, or both • LDL apo B-100 level >130 mg/dL	Autosomal dominant (prevalence of 1–2%)	• Premature CAD • Patients do not develop tendon xanthomas	Genetic and metabolic defects are not established
Familial dysbetalipoproteinemia	• Symmetric elevations of cholesterol and triglycerides (300–500 mg/dL) • Elevated VLDL-to-triglyceride ratio (>0.3)	Autosomal recessive	• Premature CAD • Tuberous or tuberoeruptive xanthomas • Planar xanthomas of the palmar creases are essentially pathognomonic	Mutation of ApoE gene Many homozygotes are normolipidemic, and emergence of hyperlipidemia often requires a secondary metabolic factor such as diabetes mellitus, hypothyroidism, or obesity

(Continued)

TABLE 3-11 Review of Major Genetic Dyslipoproteinemias (Continued)

Type of Genetic Dyslipidemia	Typical Lipid Profile	Type of Inheritance Pattern	Phenotypic Features	Other Information
Familial hypertriglyceridemia (can result in chylomicronemia syndrome)	• Most patients have triglyceride levels in the range of 150–500 mg/dL • Clinical manifestations may occur when triglyceride levels exceed 1500 mg/dL	• Familial hypertriglyceridemia is an autosomal dominant disorder caused by overproduction of VLDL triglycerides and manifests in adults	• Eruptive xanthomas • Lipemia retinalis • Pancreatitis • Hepatosplenomegaly	Patients may develop the chylomicronemia syndrome in the presence of secondary factors such as obesity, alcohol use, or diabetes
Familial hyperchylomicronemia	• Similar to familial hypertriglyceridemia	• Onset before puberty indicates deficiency of lipoprotein lipase or apo C-II, both autosomal recessive	• Similar to familial hypertriglyceridemia	Homozygosity for mutations in apoAV, LMF, and GHIHBP1 also found (rare)

CAD, coronary artery disease; GHIHBP1, glycosylphosphatidylinositol-anchored high-density lipoprotein–binding protein 1; LDL, low-density lipoprotein; VLDL, very-low-density lipoprotein.

(secondary prevention) ***or without*** (primary prevention) known CHD.[47-54] LDL-lowering therapy has proven beneficial even in patients at low risk for vascular disease.[55]

- Prevention of **ASCVD** is the primary goal of the 2018 ACC/AHA guidelines. These guidelines address risk assessment, lifestyle modifications, evaluation and treatment of obesity, and evaluation and management of blood cholesterol and aim for a more personalized and shared decision-making approach to risk management.[56]

Screening

- Screening for hypercholesterolemia should be done **in all adults age 20 years or older.**[56]
- Screening is best performed with a lipid profile (total cholesterol, LDL-C, HDL cholesterol, and triglycerides) obtained after a 12-hour fast.
- If a fasting lipid panel cannot be obtained, total and HDL cholesterol should be measured. Non-HDL cholesterol ≥220 mg/dL may indicate a genetic or secondary cause. A fasting lipid panel is required if non-HDL cholesterol is ≥220 mg/dL or triglycerides are ≥500 mg/dL.

- If the patient does not have an indication for LDL-lowering therapy, screening can be performed every 4–6 years between ages 40 and 75.[56]
- Patients hospitalized for an acute coronary syndrome or coronary revascularization should have a lipid panel obtained within 24 hours of admission if lipid levels are unknown.
- Individuals with hyperlipidemia should be evaluated for potential **secondary causes**, including hypothyroidism, DM, obstructive liver disease, chronic renal disease such as nephrotic syndrome, and medications such as estrogens, progestins, anabolic steroids/androgens, corticosteroids, cyclosporine, retinoids, atypical antipsychotics, and antiretrovirals (particularly protease inhibitors).

RISK ASSESSMENT

- The 2019 guidelines emphasize risk stratification based on predicted future risk, with further stratification using risk-enhancing factors to identify groups in whom the benefits of LDL-C–lowering therapy with HMG-CoA reductase inhibitors (statins) clearly outweigh the risks and to aim for certain goals in the reduction of LDL-C. A key observation is that the more LDL-C is reduced, the greater the subsequent risk reduction.[56] In all individuals, a heart healthy lifestyle should be encouraged as it reduces ASCVD risk at all ages.
- Areas in which treatment with statin therapy is recommended:
  - Patients with clinical ASCVD
  - Patients with LDL-C ≥190 mg/dL
  - Patients with DM age 40–75
  - Patients age 40–75 with a calculated ASCVD risk ≥7.5% if a discussion of treatment options favors statin therapy.
- For patients **without** clinical ASCVD or an LDL-C ≥190 mg/dL, the guidelines advise having a clinician–patient risk discussion before starting statin therapy. This includes calculating a patient's risk for ASCVD based on age, sex, ethnicity, total and HDL cholesterol, SBP (treated or untreated), presence of DM, and current smoking status in addition to the presence of risk-enhancing factors.[56]
- For patients with family history of early ASCVD and LDL-C ≥160 mg/dL statin therapy can be considered.[57]
- The ACC/AHA risk calculator is available at tools.acc.org/ASCVD-Risk-Estimator-Plus/.
  - For patients of ethnicities other than African American or non-Hispanic white, risk cannot be well assessed with the risk calculator. Use of the non-Hispanic white risk calculation is suggested, with the understanding that risk may be lower than calculated in East Asian Americans and Hispanic Americans and higher in American Indians and South Asians.
  - Ten-year risk should be calculated beginning at age 40 in patients without ASCVD or LDL-C ≥190 mg/dL.
  - Lifetime risk may be calculated in patients age 20–39 and patients age 40–59 with a 10-year risk <7.5% to inform decisions regarding lifestyle modification.

TREATMENT

- The 2019 guidelines recognize lifestyle factors, including diet and weight management as an important component of risk reduction for all patients.[56]
- Patients should be advised to adopt a diet that is high in fruits and vegetables, whole grains, fish, lean meat, low-fat dairy, legumes, and nuts, with lower intake of red meat, saturated and trans fats, sweets, and sugary beverages (Table 3-12). Saturated fat should comprise no more than 5%–6% of total calories.[58]

TABLE 3-12 Nutrient Composition of the Therapeutic Lifestyle Change Diet[58]

Nutrient	Recommended Intake
Saturated fat[a]	<5%–6% of total calories
Polyunsaturated fat	Up to 10% of total calories
Monounsaturated fat	Up to 20% of total calories
Total fat	25%–35% of total calories
Carbohydrate[b]	50%–60% of total calories
Fiber	20–30 g/d
Protein	Approximately 15% of total calories
Cholesterol	<200 mg/d
Total calories (energy)[c]	Balance energy intake and expenditure to maintain desirable body weight/prevent weight gain

[a]Trans fatty acids are another low-density lipoprotein–raising fat that should be kept at a low intake.
[b]Carbohydrates should be derived predominantly from foods rich in complex carbohydrates, including grains (especially whole grains), fruits, and vegetables.
[c]Daily energy expenditure should include at least moderate physical activity (contributing approximately 200 kcal/d).

- Efforts should be made to replace dietary saturated fat with polyunsaturated and monounsaturated fats, as this has been shown to lower LDL-C and triglycerides. Polyunsaturated fat intake has been shown to promote atherosclerosis regression.[59]
- Physical activity, including aerobic and resistance exercise, at least 150 minutes per week of accumulated moderate-intensity physical activity or 75 minutes per week of vigorous-intensity physical activity is recommended in all patients.[58]
- For all obese patients (body mass index ≥30) and for overweight patients (body mass index ≥25) who have additional risk factors, sustained weight loss of 3%–5% or greater reduces ASCVD risk.[59]
- Consultation with a registered dietitian nutritionist may be helpful to plan, start, and maintain a saturated fat–restricted and weight loss–promoting diet. Diets such as Mediterranean diet, DASH diet, and plant-based diet which have increased fruit, nut, vegetable, legume, and lean vegetable or animal protein (preferably fish) consumption, with the inherent soluble and insoluble vegetable fiber consistently been associated with decreased all-cause mortality.
- Prior to the start of treatment, there should be a risk discussion between the patient and the clinician. Topics for discussion include the following:
  - Potential for ASCVD risk reduction benefits
  - Potential for adverse effects and drug–drug interactions
  - Heart healthy lifestyle and management of other risk factors
  - Patient preferences
- **Clinical ASCVD**
  - Clinical ASCVD includes acute coronary syndromes, history of MI, stable angina, arterial revascularization (coronary or otherwise), stroke, transient ischemic attack, or atherosclerotic peripheral arterial disease.
  - Secondary prevention is an indication for high-intensity statin therapy, which has been shown to reduce events more than moderate-intensity statin therapy. Statin regimens are listed in Table 3-13. Goal is reduction of LDL-C by >50%.

TABLE 3-13 Statin Therapy Regimens by Intensity[56]

High Intensity (↓ LDL ≥50%)	Medium Intensity (↓ LDL 30%–49%)	Low Intensity (↓ LDL <30%)
Atorvastatin 40–80 mg	Atorvastatin 10–20 mg	Fluvastatin 20–40 mg
Rosuvastatin 20–40 mg	Fluvastatin 40 mg bid, 80 mg XL Lovastatin 40 mg Pitavastatin 1–4 mg Pravastatin 40–80 mg Rosuvastatin 5–10 mg Simvastatin 20–40 mg	Lovastatin 20 mg Pravastatin 10–20 mg Simvastatin 10 mg

LDL, low-density lipoprotein; ↓, decreased.

- ◦ If high-dose statin therapy is contraindicated or poorly tolerated or there are significant risks to high-intensity therapy (including age >75 years), the maximally tolerated statin therapy is an option.
- ◦ In very-high-risk ASCVD, use a LDL-C threshold of 70 mg/dL (1.8 mmol/L) to consider addition of nonstatins to statin therapy. If proprotein convertase subtilisin/kexin type 9 (PCSK9) inhibitor is considered, add ezetimibe to maximal statin before adding PCSK9 inhibitor. Very high-risk ASCVD includes a history of multiple major ASCVD events or one major ASCVD event and multiple high-risk conditions (major ASCVD events are recent ACS [past 12 months], history of MI, history of ischemic stroke, symptomatic peripheral arterial disease).
- ◦ High-risk conditions include age >65 years, heterozygous FH, history of prior coronary bypass surgery or percutaneous intervention outside the major ASCVD event, DM, hypertension, CKD (eGFR 15–59 mL/min/1.73 m^2), current smoking, persistently elevated LDL-C (>100 mg/dL) despite maximally tolerated statin therapy and ezetimibe, history of CHF.

- **LDL-C ≥190 mg/dL**
  - ◦ These individuals have elevated lifetime risk because of long-term exposure to very high LDL-C levels, and the risk calculator does not account for this.
  - ◦ LDL-C should be reduced with high-intensity statin therapy. If high-intensity therapy is not tolerated, maximum tolerated intensity should be used.
  - ◦ If LDL-C on statin therapy remains >100 mg/dL (>2.6 mmol/L), adding ezetimibe is reasonable.
  - ◦ If the LDL-C level on statin plus ezetimibe remains >100 mg/dL (>2.6 mmol/L) and the patient has multiple factors that increase subsequent risk of ASCVD event, a PCSK9 inhibitor may be considered, although the long-term safety (>3 years) is uncertain.
  - ◦ LDL apheresis is an optional therapy in patients with homozygous FH and those with severe heterozygous FH with insufficient response to medication. Lomitapide, a microsomal triglyceride transfer protein inhibitor, and mipomersen, an apolipoprotein B (apo B) antisense oligonucleotide, are medications indicated for the treatment of patients with homozygous FH.[43]
  - ◦ Because hyperlipidemia of this degree is often genetically determined, discuss screening of other family members (including children) to identify candidates for treatment. In addition, screen for and treat secondary causes of hyperlipidemia.[44]
- **Patients with diabetes, aged 40–75, LDL-C >70 mg/dL**
  - ◦ Moderate-intensity statin therapy is indicated regardless of estimated 10-year ASCVD risk.

- In patients with DM at higher risk, especially those with multiple risk factors or those aged 50–75, it is reasonable to use a high-intensity statin to reduce the LDL-C by >50%.
- It is reasonable to assess the 10-year ASCVD risk and in adults with DM2 who have multiple ASCVD risk factors; it is reasonable to prescribe high-intensity statin therapy with the aim to reduce LDL-C levels by 50% or more.
- Diabetes-specific risk enhancers: long duration (>10 years for DM2 or >20 years for DM1), albuminuria (>30 mcg of albumin/mg creatinine), eGFR <60 mL/min/1.73 m^2, retinopathy, neuropathy, ankle-brachial index (ABI) <0.9.
- In adults with DM and 10-year ASCVD risk of 20% or higher, it may be reasonable to add ezetimibe to maximally tolerated statin therapy to reduce LDL-C by 50% or more.
- In adults 20–39 years with DM that is of long duration (>10 years of DM2 or >20 years of DM1), albuminuria, eGFR <60 mL/min/1.73 m^2, retinopathy, neuropathy, or ABI (<0.9), it may be reasonable to initiate statin therapy.

- **Patients without diabetes, aged 40–75, LDL-C between 70 and 189 mg/dL**
  - Using the AHA/ACC risk calculator, calculate 10-year risk of an ASCVD event in these patients (categories: >20%, ≥7.5%–<20%, 5.0%–7.5%, and <5.0%).
  - A 10-year risk ≥7.5%–<20% is an indication for moderate-intensity statin if a discussion of options favors statin therapy. Risk-enhancing factors favor statin therapy.
  - Risk-enhancing factors include family history of premature ASCVD, persistently elevated LDL-C levels (>160 mg/dL), metabolic syndrome, chronic kidney disease, history of pre-eclampsia or premature menopause (<40 years), chronic inflammatory disorders (e.g., rheumatoid arthritis, psoriasis, or chronic HIV), high-risk ethnic groups (e.g., South Asian), persistent elevations of triglycerides >175 mg/dL, and, if measured in selected individuals, apo B >130 mg/dL, high-sensitivity C-reactive protein >2.0 mg/L, ABI <0.9, and lipoprotein (a) >50 mg/dL or 125 nmol/L.
  - If statins are indicated, reduce LDL-C levels by 30%, and if 10-year risk is >20%, reduce LDL-C levels by 50%.
  - In intermediate-risk adults in whom high-intensity statins are advisable to reach goal reduction, but not acceptable or tolerated, it is reasonable to add a nonstatin drug (ezetimibe or bile acid sequestrant) to moderate-intensity statin.
  - A 10-year risk of >20% favors initiating statin therapy.
  - A 10-year risk between 5.0% and 7.5% and risk-enhancing factors may favor moderate-intensity statin therapy.
- **Other patient populations**
  - If a 10-year ASCVD risk is >7.5%–19.9% and decision about statin therapy is uncertain, consider measuring coronary artery calcium (CAC) to help identify risk. If the CAC is zero, it is reasonable to withhold statin therapy and reassess in 5–10 years, as long as higher risk conditions are absent. If CAC score is 1–99, it is reasonable to initiate statin therapy for patients >55 years. If CAC score is >100 and/or greater than 75th percentile, it is reasonable to initiate statin therapy.
  - Patients with stage 3–5 CKD are high risk for ASCVD[60] and the use of LDL-lowering therapy is indicated in patients with nondialysis-dependent CKD.[61]
  - Use of statin therapy should be individualized for patients older than 75. In randomized controlled trials, patients older than 75 continued to have benefit from statin therapy, particularly for secondary prevention.[50,62] In addition, many ASCVD events occur in this age group, and patients without other comorbidities may benefit substantially from cardiovascular risk reduction.
  - In adults >75 years it may be reasonable to stop statin therapy when functional decline (physical or cognitive), multimorbidity, frailty, or reduced life expectancy limits the potential benefits of statin therapy.
  - In adults with advanced kidney disease that requires dialysis treatment who are currently on LDL-lowering therapy with a statin, it may be reasonable to continue the statin.

- In adults with advanced kidney disease who require dialysis treatment, initiation of a statin is not recommended.
- In patients with HF with reduced ejection fraction attributable to ischemic heart disease who have a reasonable life expectancy (3–5 years) and are not already on a statin because of ASCVD, clinicians may consider initiation of moderate-intensity statin therapy to reduce the occurrence of ASCVD events.[56]

- **Treatment beyond statin therapy**
  - When statins are insufficient for LDL-C reduction, further therapy with nonstatins may be indicated. This would generally include ezetimibe, bile acid sequestrants, and PCSK9 monoclonal antibodies.[63]
- **Hypertriglyceridemia**
  - Hypertriglyceridemia may be an **independent cardiovascular risk factor**.[42,64-66]
  - Hypertriglyceridemia is often observed in the metabolic syndrome,[66] and there are many potential etiologies for hypertriglyceridemia, including obesity, DM, renal insufficiency, genetic dyslipidemias, and therapy with oral estrogen, glucocorticoids, β-blockers, tamoxifen, cyclosporine, antiretrovirals, and retinoids.
  - The classification of serum triglyceride levels is as follows: normal: <150 mg/dL; borderline high: 150–199 mg/dL; high: 200–499 mg/dL; and very high: ≥500 mg/dL.[66] The Endocrine Society has added two further categories: severe: 1000–1999 mg/dL (greatly increases the risk of **pancreatitis**) and very severe: ≥2000 mg/dL.[46]
  - Treatment of hypertriglyceridemia depends on the degree of severity.
    - For patients with very high triglyceride levels, triglyceride reduction through a very low–fat diet (≤15% of calories), exercise, weight loss, and drugs (fibrates, ω-3 fatty acids) is the primary goal of therapy to prevent acute pancreatitis.
    - When patients have a lesser degree of hypertriglyceridemia, controlling the LDL-C level is the primary aim of initial therapy. Lifestyle changes are indicated to lower triglyceride levels.[46]
- **Low HDL cholesterol**
  - Low HDL cholesterol is an **independent ASCVD risk factor** that is identified as a non–LDL-C risk and is included as a component of the ACC/AHA scoring algorithm.[67]
  - Etiologies for low HDL cholesterol include genetic conditions, physical inactivity, obesity, insulin resistance, DM, hypertriglyceridemia, cigarette smoking, high-carbohydrate (>60% of calories) diets, and certain medications (β-blockers, anabolic steroids/androgens, progestins). Acquired low HDL can also occur with plasma cell dyscrasias due to interference of paraproteins with the assay.[68]
  - Because therapeutic interventions for low HDL cholesterol are of limited efficacy, the guidelines recommend considering low HDL cholesterol as a component of overall risk, rather than a specific therapeutic target.
  - There are no clinical trial data showing a benefit of pharmacologic methods of elevating HDL cholesterol.
- **Starting and monitoring therapy**
  - Before starting therapy, guidelines recommend checking alanine aminotransferase (ALT), hemoglobin A1C (if diabetes status is unknown), labs for secondary causes (if indicated), and creatine kinase (if indicated).
  - Evaluate for patient characteristics that increase the risk of adverse events from statins, including impaired hepatic and renal function, history of statin intolerance, history of muscle disorders, unexplained elevations of ALT >3× the upper limit of normal, drugs affecting statin metabolism, Asian ethnicity, and age >75 years.[56]
  - **A repeat fasting lipid panel** is indicated 4–12 weeks after starting therapy to assess adherence, with reassessment every 3–12 months as indicated.
  - In patients without the anticipated level of LDL-C reduction based on intensity of statin therapy (≥50% for high intensity, 30%–50% for moderate intensity), assess adherence

to therapy and lifestyle modifications, evaluate for intolerance, and consider secondary causes. After evaluation, if the therapeutic response is still insufficient on maximally tolerated statin therapy, it is reasonable to consider adding a nonstatin agent.[63]

- Creatine kinase can be checked 4 weeks after the initiation of therapy should not be routinely checked in patients on statin therapy but is reasonable to measure in patients with muscle symptoms.
- In 2012, the FDA stated that liver enzyme tests should be performed before starting statin therapy and only as clinically indicated thereafter. The FDA concluded that serious liver injury with statins is rare and unpredictable and that routine monitoring of liver enzymes does not appear to be effective in detecting or preventing serious liver injury. Elevations of liver transaminases 2–3× the upper limit of normal are dose-dependent, may decrease on repeat testing even with continuation of statin therapy, and are reversible with discontinuation of the drug.

Treatment of Elevated LDL Cholesterol

- **HMG-CoA reductase inhibitors (statins)**
  - Statins (see Table 3-13) are the treatment of choice for elevated LDL-C and usually lower levels by 30%–50% with moderate-intensity and ≥50% with high-intensity statin therapy.[56,69,70]
  - The lipid-lowering effect of statins appears within the first week of use and becomes stable after approximately 4 weeks of use.
  - Statin therapy is effective in both men and women.[71]
  - Common side effects (5%–10% of patients) include gastrointestinal upset (e.g., abdominal pain, diarrhea, bloating, constipation) and muscle pain or weakness, which can occur without creatine kinase elevations. Other potential side effects include malaise, fatigue, headache, and rash.[70,72-74]
  - Myalgias are the most common cause of statin discontinuation and are often dose-dependent. They occur more often with increasing age and number of medications and decreasing renal function and body size.[73-75]
    - Discontinue statins in patients who develop muscle symptoms until they can be evaluated. For severe symptoms, a creatine kinase level can be measured.[56]
    - For mild to moderate symptoms, evaluate for conditions increasing the risk of muscle symptoms, including renal or hepatic impairment, hypothyroidism, vitamin D deficiency, rheumatologic disorders, and primary muscle disorders. Statin-induced myalgias are likely to resolve within 2 months of discontinuing the drug.
    - If symptoms resolve, the same or lower dose of the statin can be reintroduced.
    - If symptoms recur, use a low dose of a different statin and increase as tolerated.
    - If the cause of symptoms is determined to be unrelated, restart the original statin.
  - Statins have been associated with an increased incidence of DM. However, the total benefit of statin use usually outweighs the potential adverse effects from an increase in blood sugar.[76]
  - In a recent review of the use of statins, there was no aggregated evidence that statins have any negative impact on cognitive function.[77]
  - Because some statins undergo metabolism by the cytochrome P450 enzyme system, taking these statins in combination with other drugs metabolized by this enzyme system increases the risk of **rhabdomyolysis**.[70,72,73] Among these drugs are fibrates (greater risk with gemfibrozil), itraconazole, ketoconazole, erythromycin, clarithromycin, cyclosporine, nefazodone, and protease inhibitors.[73]
  - Statins may also interact with large quantities of grapefruit juice to increase the risk of myopathy.

- Simvastatin can increase the levels of warfarin and digoxin and has significant dose-limiting interactions with amlodipine, amiodarone, dronedarone, verapamil, diltiazem, and ranolazine. Rosuvastatin may also increase warfarin levels.
- Because a number of drug interactions are possible depending on the statin and other medications being used, drug interaction programs and package inserts should be consulted.[78]
- The use of statins is contraindicated during pregnancy and lactation.

- **Bile acid sequestrant resins**
  - Currently available bile acid sequestrant resins include the following:
    - **Cholestyramine:** 4–24 g/d PO in divided doses before meals.
    - **Colestipol:** tablets, 2–16 g/d PO; granules, 5–30 g/d PO in divided doses before meals.
    - **Colesevelam:** 625 mg tablets, three tablets PO bid or six tablets PO daily (maximum of seven tablets daily) with food, or one packet of oral suspension daily.
  - Bile acid sequestrants typically lower LDL-C levels by 15%–30% and thereby lower the incidence of CHD.[70,79]
  - These agents should not be used as monotherapy in patients with triglyceride levels >250 mg/dL because they can raise triglyceride levels. They may be combined with nicotinic acid or statins.
  - Common side effects of resins include constipation, abdominal pain, bloating, nausea, and flatulence.
  - Bile acid sequestrants may decrease oral absorption of many other drugs, including warfarin, digoxin, thyroid hormone, thiazide diuretics, amiodarone, glipizide, and statins.
    - Colesevelam interacts with fewer drugs than do the older resins but can affect the absorption of thyroxine.
    - Other medications should be given at least 1 hour before or 4 hours after resins.
- **Nicotinic acid (niacin)**
  - Niacin can lower LDL-C levels by ≥15%, lower triglyceride levels by 20%–50%, and raise HDL cholesterol levels by up to 35%.[64,80] The use of niacin is limited by its side effect profile.
  - Crystalline niacin is given 1–3 g/d PO in two to three divided doses with meals. Extended-release niacin is dosed at night, with a starting dose of 500 mg PO, and the dose may be titrated monthly in 500 mg increments to a maximum of 2000 mg PO (administer dose with milk, applesauce, or crackers).
  - Common side effects of niacin include flushing, pruritus, headache, nausea, and bloating. Other potential side effects include elevation of liver transaminases, hyperuricemia, and hyperglycemia.
    - Flushing may be decreased with the use of aspirin 325 mg 30 minutes before the first few doses.
    - Hepatotoxicity associated with niacin is partially dose-dependent and appears to be more prevalent with some over-the-counter time-release preparations.
  - Avoid use of niacin in patients with gout, liver disease, active peptic ulcer disease, and uncontrolled DM.
    - Niacin can be used with care in patients with well-controlled DM (hemoglobin A1C level ≤7%).
    - Serum transaminases, glucose, and uric acid levels should be monitored every 6–8 weeks during dose titration and then every 4 months.
  - The use of niacin in patients with well-controlled LDL-C levels (with statins) has not been shown to be of benefit in clinical trials.[81,82] Niacin can be useful as an additional agent in patients with severely elevated LDL-C levels.
- **Ezetimibe**
  - Ezetimibe is currently the only available cholesterol-absorption inhibitor. It appears to act at the brush border of the small intestine and inhibits cholesterol absorption.

- Ezetimibe may provide an additional 25% mean reduction in LDL-C when combined with a statin and provides an approximately 18% decrease in LDL-C when used as monotherapy.[83-86]
- The recommended dosing is 10 mg PO once daily. No dosage adjustment is required for renal insufficiency and mild hepatic impairment or in elderly patients. It is not recommended for use in patients with moderate to severe hepatic impairment.
- Side effects are infrequent and include gastrointestinal symptoms (e.g., diarrhea, abdominal pain) and myalgias.
- In clinical trials, there was no excess of rhabdomyolysis or myopathy when compared with statin or placebo alone.
- Liver enzymes should be monitored when used in conjunction with fenofibrate but are not required in monotherapy or with a statin.
- A clinical outcome trial showed decreased reduction of cardiovascular events with the combination of simvastatin and ezetimibe compared with placebo in patients with chronic renal failure.[87] The IMPROVE-IT trial showed a reduction in cardiovascular end points when ezetimibe was added to simvastatin in high-risk patients with already low LDL levels.[88]
- Ezetimibe is useful in patients with FH who do not achieve adequate LDL-C reductions with statin therapy alone.[89]

- **PCSK9 inhibitors**
  - Monoclonal antibodies have been developed that lower LDL-C. They work by inhibiting the PCSK9 enzyme, which is involved in breaking down the LDL-C receptor. Their use increases the number of available cell surface LDL receptors and subsequently remove more LDL from circulation. Major studies have shown significant reduction in LDL-C when PCSK9 inhibitors were added to statin therapy.[90]
  - These agents have shown great ability in further reducing LDL-C in high-risk patients and are approved for use as adjuncts in patients with clinical ASCVD and heterozygous FH and as monotherapy for homozygous FH.
  - Two PCSK9 inhibitors are approved for clinical use, evolocumab and alirocumab. **Evolocumab** is dosed at 140 mg subcutaneously every 2 weeks or 420 mg sc every 4 weeks. **Alirocumab** is dosed at 75 or 150 mg every 2 weeks or 300 mg every 4 weeks.
- Evolocumab has been shown to decrease major cardiovascular events.[90] Data on the outcome trial with alirocumab are pending publication.

Other Therapies

- **Lomitapide**, an inhibitor of microsomal triglyceride transfer protein that transfers triglycerides to apo B during assembly of VLDL in the liver, is recommended for patients with homozygous FH.
- **Bempedoic acid**, an inhibitor of adenosine triphosphate citrate lyase, could lower levels of LDL-C and other atherogenic proteins alone or in combination with statin or ezetimibe.
- **Mipomersen**, an antisense oligonucleotide complementary to the coding region for human apo B mRNA, inhibits the production of apo B.
- **LDL apheresis** has been recommended for those with homozygous FH who do not have an adequate response to maximum tolerated drug therapy.

Cardiovascular risk categories and recommendations based on 2019 ESC/EAS guidelines for the management of dyslipidemias are summarized in Table 3-14.

Treatment of Hypertriglyceridemia

- **Nonpharmacologic treatment**
  Nonpharmacologic treatments are important in the therapy of hypertriglyceridemia. Approaches include the following:
  - Changing oral estrogen replacement to transdermal estrogen;

TABLE 3-14 Cardiovascular Risk Categories and Recommendations for LDL-C Based on 2019 ESC/EAS Guidelines for the Management of Dyslipidemias

Risk	Description	Recommendation	
		Target	Intervention
Very high risk	Documented ASCVD, either clinical or unequivocal on imaging Documented ASCVD—includes previous ACS, stable angina, coronary revascularization, stroke and TIA, and peripheral arterial disease Unequivocally documented ASCVD on imaging, such as significant plaque on coronary angiography or CT scan or on carotid ultrasound, known to be predictive of clinical events DM with target organ damage ≥3 major risk factors or early onset of T1DM of long duration (>20 years) Severe CKD (eGFR <30 mL/min/1.73 m²) Family history with ASCVD or with another major risk factor Apparently healthy people with calculated SCORE ≥10% for 10-year risk of fatal CVD	An LDL-C reduction of at least 50% from baseline and an LDL-C goal of <1.4 mmol/L (<55 mg/dL) are recommended LDL-C goal of <1.0 mmol/L (<40 mg/dL) may be considered for patients with ASCVD who experience a second vascular event within 2 years while taking maximally tolerated statin therapy	**Secondary prevention:** Lifestyle interventions recommended and pharmacological intervention considered for all patients with very high cardiovascular risk Pharmacological intervention recommended for patients with LDL-C >55 mg/dL **Primary prevention:** Lifestyle interventions recommended and pharmacological intervention considered for patients with LDL levels above target (>55 mg/dL) Pharmacological intervention recommended for patients with LDL-C >70 mg/dL
High risk	Markedly elevated single risk factors, in particular TC >8 mmol/L (>310 mg/dL), LDL-C >4.9 mmol/L (>190 mg/dL), or BP ≥ 180/110 mm Hg Patients with FH without other major risk factors	An LDL-C reduction of at least 50% from baseline and an LDL-C goal of <1.8 mmol/L (<70 mg/dL) are recommended	**Primary prevention:** Lifestyle interventions recommended and pharmacological intervention considered for patients with LDL levels above target (>70 mg/dL)

(Continued)

TABLE 3-14 Cardiovascular Risk Categories and Recommendations for LDL-C Based on 2019 ESC/EAS Guidelines for the Management of Dyslipidemias (Continued)

Risk	Description	Recommendation	
		Target	Intervention
	Patients with DM without target organ damage, with DM duration ≥10 years or another additional risk factor Moderate CKD (eGFR 30–59 mL/min/1.73 m²) Apparently healthy people with calculated SCORE ≥5% and <10% for 10-year risk of fatal CVD		Pharmacological intervention recommended for patients with LDL-C levels >100 mg/dL
Moderate risk	Young patients (T1DM <35 years; T2DM <50 years) with DM duration <10 years, without other risk factors Apparently healthy people with calculated SCORE ≥1% and <5% for 10-year risk of fatal CVD	An LDL-C goal of <2.6 mmol/L (<100 mg/dL) should be considered	**Primary prevention:** Lifestyle interventions recommended and pharmacological intervention considered for patients with LDL levels above target (>100 mg/dL) Pharmacological intervention recommended for patients with LDL-C levels ≥190 mg/dL
Low risk	Apparently healthy people with calculated SCORE <1% for 10-year risk of fatal CVD	An LDL-C goal <3.0 mmol/L (<116 mg/dL) may be considered	**Primary prevention:** Lifestyle interventions recommended and pharmacological intervention considered for patients with LDL levels above target (>116 mg/dL) Pharmacological intervention recommended for patients with LDL-C levels ≥190 mg/dL

Pharmacological therapy includes the following points:

- For patients with no current statin use: Add high-intensity LDL-lowering therapy.
- For patients on LDL-lowering treatment: Increase treatment intensity.

ASCVD, atherosclerotic cardiovascular disease; CKD, chronic kidney disease; DM, diabetes mellitus; SCORE, systematic coronary risk estimation.

- Decreasing alcohol intake;
- Encouraging weight loss and exercise;
- Controlling hyperglycemia in patients with DM;
- Avoiding simple sugars and very high–carbohydrate diets.[46,66]

- **Pharmacologic treatment**
  - Pharmacologic treatment of severe hypertriglyceridemia consists of fibric acid derivative (fibrates), niacin, or ω-3 fatty acids.
  - Patients with severe hypertriglyceridemia (>1000 mg/dL) should be treated with pharmacotherapy in addition to reduction of dietary fat, alcohol, and simple carbohydrates to decrease the risk of pancreatitis.
  - Statins may be effective for patients with mild to moderate hypertriglyceridemia and concomitant LDL-C elevation.[46,66,91]
  - **Fibric acid derivatives**
    - Currently available fibric acid derivatives include the following:
      - **Gemfibrozil:** 600 mg PO bid before meals
      - **Fenofibrate:** available in several forms, dosage typically 48–145 mg/d PO
    - Fibrates generally lower triglyceride levels by 30%–50% and increase HDL cholesterol levels by 10%–35%. They can lower LDL-C levels by 5%–25% in patients with normal triglyceride levels but may actually increase LDL-C levels in patients with elevated triglyceride levels.[91,92]
    - Common side effects include dyspepsia, abdominal pain, cholelithiasis, rash, and pruritus.
    - Fibrates may potentiate the effects of warfarin.[70] Gemfibrozil given in conjunction with statins may increase the risk of rhabdomyolysis.[73,93-95]
  - **ω-3 Fatty acids**
    - High doses of ω-3 fatty acids from fish oil can lower triglyceride levels.[96,97]
    - The active ingredients are eicosapentaenoic acid (EPA) and docosahexaenoic acid (DHA).
    - To lower triglyceride levels, 1–6 g of ω-3 fatty acids, either EPA alone or with DHA, is needed daily.
    - Main side effects are burping, bloating, and diarrhea.
    - Prescription forms of ω-3 fatty acids are available and are indicated for triglyceride levels >500 mg/dL. One preparation contains EPA and DHA; four tablets contain about 3.6 g of ω-3 acid ethyl esters and can lower triglyceride levels by 30%–40%. Other preparations contain only EPA or contain unesterified EPA and DHA.
    - In practice, ω-3 fatty acids are being used as an adjunct to statins or other drugs in patients with moderately elevated triglyceride levels.
    - Large cardiovascular outcomes trials with ω-3 fatty acids are in progress.
    - In addition, EPA and DHA may help preserve physical function in CAD patients.[98]
    - The combination of ω-3 fatty acids plus a statin has the advantage of avoiding the risk of myopathy seen with statin–fibrate combinations.[99,100]

Treatment of Low HDL Cholesterol

- Low HDL cholesterol often occurs in the setting of hypertriglyceridemia and metabolic syndrome. Management of accompanying high LDL-C, hypertriglyceridemia, and the metabolic syndrome may result in improvement of HDL cholesterol.[101]
- Nonpharmacologic therapies are the mainstay of treatment, including the following:
  - Smoking cessation
  - Exercise
  - Weight loss
- In addition, medications known to lower HDL levels, such as β-blockers (except carvedilol), progestins, and androgenic compounds, should be avoided.
- No clinical outcomes trials have shown a clear benefit to pharmacologic treatment for raising HDL cholesterol.

Summary

- An estimated 1.4 billion people worldwide have high blood pressure, but just 14% have it under control.
- Use an average threshold of 140/90 mm Hg for office diagnosis of hypertension, but 135/85 mm Hg for home and 130/80 mm Hg for 24-hour ambulatory monitoring.
- Initial assessment in a patient who is hypertensive should be evaluated for cardiovascular risk and any hypertension-mediated organ damage.
- Secondary causes should be considered in patients 30 years or younger, especially without comorbidities, and any patient with resistant hypertension, sudden deterioration in control, severe BP elevations, or clinical signs of a cause for the secondary hypertension.
- LDL-C levels may be miscalculated in non-fasting measurements in groups who have high triglyceride (TG) levels. Hence, fasting or the direct measurement of LDL-C is recommended for individuals with high TG levels.
- The causality of LDL-C is well established; therefore, it is the primary target of therapy in all new guidelines (to keep LDL-C below 70 mg/dL).

Scan the QR code to access chapter references.

4 Ischemic Heart Disease

Nathan L. Frogge, Philip M. Barger, Marc A. Sintek, and G. G. Akshay Prabhu

Coronary Heart Disease and Stable Angina

GENERAL PRINCIPLES

Definition

- Coronary artery disease (CAD) refers to the luminal narrowing of a coronary artery, usually due to atherosclerosis. CAD is the leading contributor to ischemic heart disease (IHD). IHD includes angina pectoris, myocardial infarction (MI), and silent myocardial ischemia.
- Cardiovascular disease (CVD) includes IHD, cardiomyopathy, heart failure (HF), arrhythmia, hypertension, cerebrovascular accident (CVA), diseases of the aorta, peripheral vascular disease (PVD), valvular heart disease, and congenital heart disease.
- Stable angina is defined as angina symptoms or angina equivalent symptoms that are reproduced by consistent levels of activity and relieved by rest.
- American Heart Association/American College of Cardiology (AHA/ACC) guidelines provide a more thorough overview of stable IHD.[1,2]

Epidemiology

- In the United States, IHD is the cause of one of every six deaths.[3]
- South Asians make up to 25% of the global population, but over 50% of the world's cardiovascular deaths occur in patients of South Asian origin. South Asians have a threefold to fivefold increased risk of MI.
- South Asians also present with more severe disease and at an earlier age than Caucasians.
- Bainey and Jugdutt* proposed an algorithm to actively screen for CAD among South Asians and advocated that the Framingham score be multiplied by 1.4 to accurately assess the cardiovascular risk.
- Death due to CVD continues to decline in large part because of adherence to current guidelines. The spectrum of IHD is described in Figure 4-1.

Etiology

CAD most commonly results from luminal accumulation of atheromatous plaque.

Other causes of obstructive CAD include congenital coronary anomalies, myocardial bridging, vasculitis, and prior radiation therapy.

Pathophysiology

- Stable angina results from progressive luminal obstruction of angiographically visible epicardial coronary arteries or, less commonly, obstruction of the microvasculature, which results in a mismatch between myocardial oxygen supply and demand.
- Atherosclerosis is an inflammatory process, initiated by lipid deposition in the arterial intima layer followed by recruitment of inflammatory cells and proliferation of arterial smooth muscle cells to form an atheroma.

---

*Bainey KR, Jugdutt BI. Increased burden of coronary artery disease in South-Asians living in North America. Need for an aggressive management algorithm. *Atherosclerosis*. 2009 May;204(1):1–10.

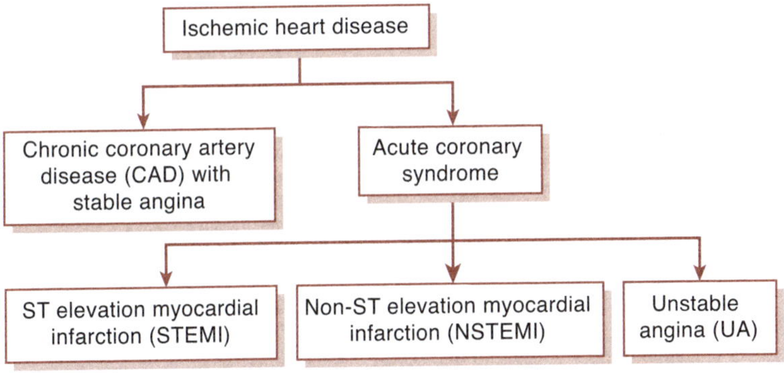

Figure 4-1 Spectrum of ischemic heart disease.

- The coronary lesions responsible for stable angina differ from the vulnerable plaques associated with acute MI. The stable angina lesion is fixed and is less prone to fissuring, hence producing symptoms that are more predictable.[4]
- All coronary lesions are eccentric and do not uniformly alter the inner circumference of the artery.
- Epicardial coronary lesions causing less than 40% luminal narrowing generally do not significantly impair coronary flow.
- Moderate angiographic lesions (40%–70% obstruction) may interfere with flow and are routinely underestimated on coronary angiograms given the eccentricity of CAD.

Risk Factors

- Of IHD events, >90% can be attributed to elevations in at least one major risk factor.[5]
- Nontraditional versus traditional CVD risk factors are listed in Figure 4-2.
- Note: diabetes is considered an IHD risk equivalent
- Low-density lipoprotein [LDL], high-density lipoprotein [HDL], triglycerides; direct LDL for non-fasting samples or very high triglycerides.
- Note: smoking cessation restores the risk of IHD to that of a non-smoker within approximately 15 years.[6]
- Family History - Defined as first-degree male relative with IHD before age 55 or female relative before age 65.
- Genome-wide association studies (GWAS) have identified several genetic variants associated with increased MI risk. For instance, polymorphisms within genes encoding components of the renin-angiotensin-aldosterone system (RAAS) and lipid metabolism pathways have been linked to MI susceptibility.
- Measures for obesity, particularly central obesity; body mass index goal is between 18.5 and 24.9 kg/m^2; and waist circumference goal is <40 inches for men and <35 inches for women.

Nonatherosclerotic Causes of Acute Coronary Syndrome

- The prevalence of nonobstructive coronary artery disease, defined clinically as luminal stenosis <50%, in patients presenting with MI is estimated to be as high as 30% in women and 11% in men. Important causes include the following:
  - **Spontaneous coronary artery dissection** (SCAD): Accounts for up to 35% of ACS in women aged <50 years, and has a true prevalence as high as 4% of all cases of ACS. Systemic conditions associated with SCAD include fibromuscular dysplasia, peripartum status, extreme emotion or exercise, and connective tissue diseases, such as Marfan syndrome, Ehlers–Danlos syndrome, and Loeys–Dietz syndrome.

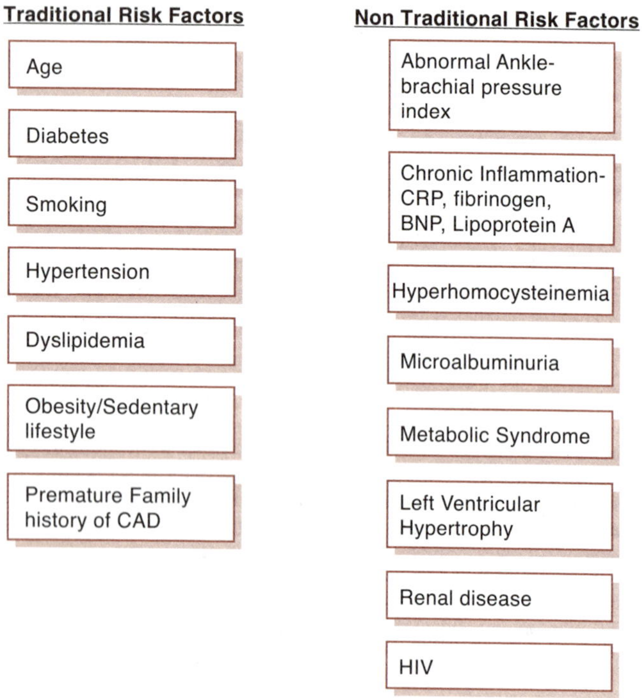

Figure 4-2 Risk factors of cardiovascular diseases.

- **Coronary artery embolism:** direct, paradoxical, or iatrogenic.
- **Coronary vasospasm** at the epicardial or microvascular level.
- **Coronary artery bridging:** A portion of myocardial muscle overlying a segment of an epicardial coronary artery is defined as a myocardial bridge.
- **Stress-induced cardiomyopathy**/Takotsubo syndrome (TTS).

• As of 2013, AHA/ACC guidelines recommend assessing 10-year atherosclerotic cardiovascular disease (ASCVD) risk for patients aged 40–79 years using new race and age-specific pooled cohort equations.[7]
  - The ASCVD risk calculator is available online (http://tools.cardiosource.org/ASCVD-Risk-Estimator/).
  - If there remains uncertainty about lower risk estimates, high-sensitivity C-reactive protein (≥2 mg/dL), coronary artery calcium score (≥300 Agatston units or ≥75th percentile), or ankle–brachial index (<0.9) may be obtained to revise risk estimates upward.
  - Traditional risk factors noted above should be assessed in patients younger than age 40 and every 4–6 years after 40; 10-year ASCVD risk should be calculated every 4–6 years in patients 40–79 years of age.
  - Lifetime risk can be assessed using the ASCVD risk calculator and may be helpful in the setting of counseling patients about lifestyle modifications.

Prevention

Primary prevention: See Chapter 3, Preventive Cardiology

DIAGNOSIS

Clinical Presentation

History

- **Typical angina** has three features: (1) substernal chest discomfort with a characteristic quality and duration that is (2) provoked by stress or exertion and (3) relieved by rest or nitroglycerin.
  - **Atypical angina** has two of these three characteristics.
  - **Noncardiac chest pain** meets one or none of these characteristics.
- Chronic stable angina is reproducibly precipitated in a predictable manner by exertion or emotional stress and relieved within 5–10 minutes by sublingual nitroglycerin or rest.
- The severity of angina may be quantified using the Canadian Cardiovascular Society (CCS) classification system (Table 4-1).
- Associated symptoms may include dyspnea, diaphoresis, nausea, vomiting, dizziness, jaw pain, and left arm pain.
- Female patients and those with diabetes or chronic kidney disease (CKD) may have minimal or atypical symptoms that serve as anginal equivalents. Such symptoms include dyspnea (most common), epigastric pain, and nausea.
- The clinician's assessment of the pretest probability of IHD is the important driver for further diagnostic testing in patients without known CAD and is largely ascertained from the clinical history. ACC/AHA recommends using the Diamond/Forrester score for calculating pretest probability for this purpose (Table 4-2). This score may, however, overestimate the pretest probability as it does not take into account other risk factors. Another score called the CAD consortium score which takes into account the coronary risk factors, more reliably assists the clinician in pretest assessment of the patient.* Patients with a low pretest probability (5–10%) of CAD are unlikely to benefit from further diagnostic testing aimed at detecting CAD.

Physical Examination

- Clinical examination should include measurement of BP, heart rate, and arterial pulses.
- Examination findings of a mitral regurgitation (MR) murmur or aortic stenosis murmur can alert the clinician to additional CVD that may be contributing to symptoms of angina.
- Stigmata of hyperlipidemia such as corneal arcus and xanthelasmas should be noted.
- Signs of HF, such as an S_3 gallop, inspiratory crackles on lung examination, elevated jugular venous pulsation, and peripheral edema, are also high-risk examination findings.

TABLE 4-1 Canadian Cardiovascular Society (CCS) Classification System

Class	Definition
CCS 1	Angina with strenuous or prolonged activity
CCS 2	Angina with moderate activity (walking greater than two level blocks or one flight of stairs)
CCS 3	Angina with mild activity (walking less than two level blocks or one flight of stairs)
CCS 4	Angina that occurs with any activity or at rest

Data from Sangareddi V, Chockalingam A, Gnanavelu G, Subramaniam T, Jagannathan V, Elangovan S. Canadian Cardiovascular Society classification of effort angina: an angiographic correlation. *Coron Artery Dis.* 2004;15(2):111-114.
Anginal symptoms may include typical chest discomfort or anginal equivalents.

* https://qxmd.com/calculate/calculator_287/pre-test-probability-of-cad-cad-consortium

TABLE 4-2 Pretest Probability of Coronary Artery Disease by Age, Gender, and Symptoms

Age (y)	Asymptomatic		Nonanginal Chest Pain		Atypical/Probable Angina Pectoris		Typical/Definite Angina Pectoris	
Gender	**Women**	**Men**	**Women**	**Men**	**Women**	**Men**	**Women**	**Men**
30–39	<5	<5	2	4	12	34	26	76
40–49	<5	<10	3	13	22	51	55	87
50–59	<5	<10	7	20	31	65	73	93
60–69	<5	<5	14	27	51	72	86	94
	Very Low <5%		**Low <10%**		**Intermediate 10%–80%**		**High >80%**	

Data from Gibbons RJ, Balady GJ, Timothy Bricker J. et al. (Committee Members) ACC/AHA 2002 guideline update for exercise testing: summary article: a report of the American College of Cardiology/American Heart Association task force on practice guidelines (Committee to update the 1997 exercise testing guidelines). *Circulation.* 2002;106(14):1883–1892.

- Vascular examination should include palpitation of radial, femoral, popliteal, posterior tibial, and dorsalis pedis pulses bilaterally to compare differences. Auscultation with the bell of the stethoscope should be performed to evaluate for femoral or carotid bruits.
- Pain that is reproducible on physical examination suggests a musculoskeletal cause of chest pain but does not exclude the presence of CAD.

Differential Diagnosis

- A wide range of disorders may manifest with chest discomfort and may include both cardiovascular and noncardiovascular etiologies (Table 4-3).
- A careful history focused on cardiac risk factors, physical examination, and initial laboratory evaluation usually narrows the differential diagnosis.
- In patients with established IHD, always look for exacerbating factors that contribute to ischemia.
- Any process that reduces myocardial oxygen supply or increases demand can cause or exacerbate angina (Table 4-4).

Diagnostic Testing

- **General diagnostic testing**
    - A resting ECG can be helpful in determining the presence of prior infarcts or conduction system disease and may alert the clinician to the possibility of CAD in patients with chest pain.
    - Chest radiography can be used to evaluate for cardiomegaly, HF, or vascular disease (pulmonary and aortic) that can be important in the management of patients with chest pain or IHD.
    - A transthoracic echocardiogram (TTE) can be useful in determining the presence of left ventricular (LV) dysfunction or valvular heart disease that may affect the management and diagnosis of IHD. TTE can also be used to assess for resting wall motion abnormalities that may be the result of prior MI.
    - Evidence of vascular disease or prior MI on the diagnostic testing modalities noted above should raise the pretest probability of IHD in patients presenting with chest pain.
- **Stress testing overview**
    - All stress testing requires (1) a cardiovascular stress and (2) a way of evaluating cardiac changes consistent with ischemia. The latter is always done with continuous ECG; however, it can be done either with or without an imaging modality.

TABLE 4-3 Differential Diagnosis of Chest Pain Excluding Epicardial Atherosclerosis

Diagnosis	Comments
Cardiovascular	
Aortic stenosis	Anginal episodes can occur with severe aortic stenosis.
HCM	Subendocardial ischemia may occur with exercise and/or exertion.
Prinzmetal angina	Coronary vasospasm that may be elicited by exertion or emotional stress.
Pericarditis	Pleuritic chest pain associated with pericardial inflammation from infectious or autoimmune disease.
Aortic dissection	May mimic anginal pain and/or involve the coronary arteries.
Cocaine use	Results in coronary vasospasm and/or thrombus formation.
Other	
Anemia	Marked anemia can result in a myocardial O_2 supply–demand mismatch.
Thyrotoxicosis	Increase in myocardial demand may result in an O_2 supply–demand mismatch.
Esophageal disease	GERD and esophageal spasm can mimic angina (responsive to NTG).
Biliary colic	Gallstones can usually be visualized on abdominal sonography.
Respiratory diseases	Pneumonia with pleuritic pain, pulmonary embolism, pulmonary hypertension.
Musculoskeletal	Costochondritis, cervical radiculopathy.

GERD, gastroesophageal reflux disease; HCM, hypertrophic cardiomyopathy; NTG, nitroglycerin.

- The stress and imaging methods are chosen by the clinician to meet the diagnostic needs of the patient.
- Many stress testing modalities provide not only detection of ischemia/CAD but also prognostic information based on the burden of ischemia.
- Table 4-5 provides an overview of the sensitivity and specificity for each stress and imaging modality along with advantages and disadvantages for the clinician to consider.

- **Stress testing indications**
  - See the ACCF 2013 Multimodality Appropriate Use Criteria for the Detection and Risk Assessment of Stable Ischemic Heart Disease for a comprehensive list of the indications for stress testing.[8]
  - The following are some of the more common indications:
    - Patients without known CAD:
      - Patients with anginal symptoms who are intermediate risk
      - Asymptomatic intermediate-risk patients who plan on beginning a vigorous exercise program or working in a high-risk occupation (e.g., airline pilot)
      - Atypical symptoms in patients with a high risk of IHD (i.e., diabetes or vascular disease patients)
    - Patients with known CAD:
      - Post-MI risk stratification (see section on ST-segment elevation MI)
      - Preoperative risk assessment if it will change management before surgery
      - Recurrent anginal symptoms despite medical therapy or revascularization

TABLE 4-4 Conditions That May Provoke or Exacerbate Ischemia/Angina Independent of Worsening Atherosclerosis

Increased Oxygen Demand	Decreased Oxygen Supply
Noncardiac	
Hyperthermia	Anemia
Hyperthyroidism	Sickle cell disease
Sympathomimetic toxicity (i.e., cocaine use)	Hypoxemia
Hypertension	*Pneumonia*
Anxiety	*Asthma exacerbation*
	Chronic obstructive pulmonary disease
	Pulmonary hypertension
	Pulmonary fibrosis
	Obstructive sleep apnea
	Pulmonary embolus
	Sympathomimetic toxicity (i.e., cocaine use, pheochromocytoma)
	Hyperviscosity
	Polycythemia
	Leukemia
	Thrombocytosis
	Hypergammaglobulinemia
Cardiac	
Hypertrophic cardiomyopathy	Aortic stenosis
Aortic stenosis	Elevated left ventricular end-diastolic pressure
Dilated cardiomyopathy	Hypertrophic cardiomyopathy
Tachycardia	Microvascular disease
Ventricular	
Supraventricular	

Data from AHA/ACC Guidelines on Stable Ischemic Heart Disease; Fihn SD, Gardin JM, Abrams J, et al. 2012 ACCF/AHA/ACP/AATS/PCNA/SCAI/STS guideline for the diagnosis and management of patients with stable ischemic heart disease: a report of the American College of Cardiology Foundation/American Heart Association task force on practice guidelines, and the American College of Physicians, American Association for Thoracic Surgery, Preventive Cardiovascular Nurses Association, Society for Cardiovascular Angiography and Interventions, and Society of Thoracic Surgeons. *J Am Coll Cardiol.* 2012;60(24):e44–e164; Fihn SD, Blankenship JC, Alexander KP, et al. 2014 ACC/AHA/AATS/PCNA/SCAI/STS focused update of the guideline for the diagnosis and management of patients with stable ischemic heart disease: a report of the American College of Cardiology/American Heart Association task force on practice guidelines, and the American Association for Thoracic Surgery, Preventive Cardiovascular Nurses Association, Society for Cardiovascular Angiography and Interventions, and Society of Thoracic Surgeons. *J Am Coll Cardiol.* 2014;64(18):1929–1949.

- **Contraindications to stress testing**
  - Acute MI within 2 days
  - Unstable angina (UA) not previously stabilized by medical therapy
  - Cardiac arrhythmias causing symptoms or hemodynamic compromise
  - Symptomatic severe aortic stenosis
  - Symptomatic HF
  - Acute pulmonary embolus, myocarditis, pericarditis, or aortic dissection

TABLE 4-5 Diagnostic Accuracy of Common Stress Testing Modalities in Patients Without Known Ischemic Heart Disease

Test Type	Sensitivity	Specificity	Advantages	Disadvantages
ECG				
Exercise	61%	70%–77%	• Easy to perform • Inexpensive	• Less diagnostic accuracy, especially in women • No viability assessment
Pharmacologic	—	—		
Echocardiography				
Exercise	70%–85%	77%–89%	• Gather other important information on diastolic function, valvular disorders, and pulmonary pressures • Can assess viability with pharmacologic stress	• Limited by image quality • Diagnostic accuracy reduced with resting wall motion abnormalities
Pharmacologic (dobutamine)	85%–90%	79%–90%		
Nuclear Perfusion Imaging				
Exercise	82%–88%	70%–88%	• More sensitive for small areas of ischemia/infarct • Very accurate ejection fraction assessment • Easy to compare to prior studies	• Significant radiation • May underestimate severe balanced ischemia • No other valve or other structural information • Viability may require separate testing
Pharmacologic (adenosine, regadenoson, or dobutamine)	82%–91%	75%–90%		
Cardiac MRI				
Exercise	—	—	• Excellent assessment of viability • Anatomic detail of heart and great vessels is outstanding	• Expensive • Requires closed MRI • Exercise option not typically available
Pharmacologic[a]	91%	81%		

All diagnostic accuracies unadjusted for referral bias.[1,2]

[a]Vasodilator stress only; dobutamine has sensitivity of 83% and specificity of 86%.

- **Stress Modalities**
  - **Exercise stress testing**
    - The stress modality of choice for evaluating most patients of intermediate risk for CAD (see Table 4-2).
    - Bruce protocol: Consists of 3-minute stages of increasing treadmill speed and incline. BP, heart rate, and ECG are monitored throughout the study and the recovery period.
    - The ECG portion of the study is considered positive if:
      - New ST-segment depressions of >1 mm in multiple contiguous leads
      - Hypotensive response to exercise
      - Sustained ventricular arrhythmias are precipitated by exercise
    - The Duke Treadmill Score provides prognostic information for patients presenting with chronic angina (Table 4-6).
    - When exercise testing is combined with imaging (e.g., echocardiography), and the test is normal at the target heart rate for age, the risk of infarction or death from CVD is <1% annually in patients with no prior history of IHD.
    - In patients who cannot exercise and require pharmacologic testing, the annual risk of infarction or death in a normal study doubles (i.e., 2% per year). This underscores the inability to perform physical activity as a marker of increased cardiovascular risk.
  - Pharmacologic stress testing
    - In patients who are unable to exercise, pharmacologic stress testing may be preferable.
    - Pharmacologic stress testing is preferred in patients with left bundle branch block (LBBB) or a paced rhythm on ECG. This is due to the increased incidence of false-positive stress tests seen with either exercise or dobutamine infusion.
    - Dipyridamole, adenosine, and regadenoson are vasodilators commonly used in conjunction with myocardial perfusion scintigraphy.
    - Technically, these agents do not impose a physiologic stress. Relative ischemia across a coronary vascular bed is elucidated as healthy vessels dilate more than diseased vessels with fixed obstruction. This in turn leads to relative changes in perfusion that are reflected in the post-vasodilator images.
    - Dobutamine is a positive inotrope commonly used with echocardiographic stress tests and may be augmented with atropine to achieve target heart rate for age.
- **Stress testing with imaging**
  Recommended for patients with the following baseline ECG abnormalities:
  - Pre-excitation (Wolf–Parkinson–White syndrome)
  - LVH
  - LBBB or paced rhythm
  - Intraventricular conduction delay
  - Resting ST-segment or T-wave changes

TABLE 4-6 Exercise Stress Testing: Duke Treadmill Score

Duke Treadmill Score (DTS) = Minutes exercised – [5 × maximum ST-segment deviation] – [4 × angina score]. Angina score: 0 = none, 1 = not test limiting, 2 = test limiting

DTS		
5	Annual mortality 0.25%	Low-risk study
−10 to 4	Annual mortality 1.25%	Intermediate-risk study
<−10	Annual mortality >5%	High-risk study

In general, β-blockers, other nodal blocking agents, and nitrates should be discontinued before stress testing.[82]

 - Patients unable to exercise or who do not have an interpretable ECG at rest or with exercise
 - May be considered in patients with high pretest probability of IHD who have not met the threshold of invasive angiography
- **Imaging Modalities**
 - **Myocardial perfusion imaging (MPI):** Both PET (positron emission tomography) and SPECT (single-photon emission tomography) use tracers that emit radiation detected by a camera in conjunction with exercise or pharmacologic stress. PET has better contrast and spatial resolution than SPECT, but PET is much more expensive and less widely available. Perfusion imaging compares rest perfusion to stress perfusion images to discern areas of ischemia or infarct. It can be limited by body habitus, breast attenuation, and the quality of the acquisition and processing of images. Severe CAD may cause balanced reduction in perfusion and an underestimation of ischemic burden.
 - **Echocardiographic imaging:** Exercise or dobutamine stress testing can be performed with echocardiography to aid in the diagnosis of CAD. Echocardiography adds to the sensitivity and specificity of the test by revealing areas with wall motion abnormalities. The technical quality of this study can be limited by imaging quality (i.e., obesity).
 - **Magnetic resonance perfusion imaging:** MRI sequences obtained with contrast and vasodilator stress testing (and very rarely exercise testing) provides viability assessment without additional testing, as well as evaluation for other causes of myocardial dysfunction that may mimic IHD (i.e., sarcoidosis or infiltrative cardiomyopathies). It can not be performed in certain patients with implanted cardiac devices (i.e., defibrillators and pacemakers).

Diagnostic Procedures

- **Coronary angiography**
 - The gold standard for evaluating epicardial coronary anatomy because it quantifies the presence and severity of atherosclerotic lesions, which has prognostic value.
 - Coronary angiography is invasive and associated with a small risk of death, MI, CVA, bleeding, arrhythmia, and vascular complications. Therefore, it is reserved for patients whose risk–benefit ratio favors an invasive approach such as:
   - ST-segment elevation MI (STEMI) patients
   - Most UA/non–ST-segment elevation MI (NSTEMI) patients
   - Symptomatic patients with high-risk stress tests who are expected to benefit from revascularization
   - Class III and IV angina despite medical therapy (see Table 4-1)
   - Survivors of sudden cardiac death or those with serious ventricular arrhythmias
   - Signs or symptoms of HF or decreased LV function
   - Angina that is inadequately controlled with medical therapy for the patient's lifestyle
   - Previous coronary artery bypass grafting (CABG) or percutaneous coronary intervention (PCI)
   - Suspected/known left main (≥50% stenosis) or severe three-vessel CAD
   - To diagnose CAD in patients with angina who have not undergone stress testing because of a high pretest probability of having CAD (see Table 4-2)
 - It can be both diagnostic and therapeutic if PCI is needed.
 - It can be used to evaluate patients who are suspected of having a nonatherosclerotic cause of ischemia (e.g., coronary anomaly, coronary dissection, radiation vasculopathy).
 - Intravascular ultrasound can be used to directly visualize plaque burden and plaque anatomy.
 - Functional significance of intermediate stenotic lesions (50%–70% narrowing) can further be assessed by fractional flow reserve (FFR) or instantaneous wave-free ratio (iFR)

  - Both FFR and iFR are calculated by determining the ratio of pressure distal to the coronary obstruction to that of the aortic pressure (flow) using slightly different methods.
  - An FFR ≤0.8 or iFR ≤0.89 is considered flow limiting, and PCI decreases the need for urgent revascularization for UA or MI, as well as risk of recurrent MI.[9]
  - Whether PCI in stable IHD improves cardiovascular outcomes or symptoms compared to medical therapy is controversial.[10]
- Measurement of LV filling pressures (diastolic function) and aortic and mitral valve gradients, assessment of regional wall motion and LV function, and assessment for certain aortopathies can be accomplished by placing a catheter in the LV cavity or aorta directly and making the appropriate pressure measurements and/or injection of contrast.

- **Contrast-induced nephropathy** (CIN) occurs after 24–48 hours in up to 5% of patients undergoing coronary angiography. In most patients, creatinine returns to baseline within 7 days. The following are considerations in the prevention of CIN:
  - The volume of contrast media used should be minimized.
  - All patients should receive some CIN prophylactic therapy: oral hydration, IV hydration, held IV diuretics, and statin therapy have proven benefit.
  - We recommend a 3 mL/kg bolus of normal saline at least 6 hours before the procedure with a 1-mg/kg continuous infusion rate until start of procedure.
  - *N*-Acetyl-L-cysteine has no advantage over simple hydration for prevention of CIN.
  - National Cardiovascular Data Registry Acute Kidney Injury (NCDR AKI) Risk Model is a robust risk stratification tool for acute kidney injury and the need for hemodialysis after cardiac catheterization (Table 4-7).[11]
- **Coronary CT Angiography**
  - A noninvasive technique used to establish a diagnosis of CAD. Like cardiac angiography, it exposes the patient to both radiation and contrast material.
  - Uses arterial phase contrast CT images to evaluate coronary stenosis. Where available, a proprietary software package can calculate intracoronary hemodynamics akin to FFR.
  - CT has a high negative predictive value; it is better suited to rule out diseases for symptomatic patients with a low pretest probability for CAD, such as a patient with repeated emergency room admissions for chest pain or patients with equivocal stress test results.
  - Trials such as PROMISE and SCOT-HEART indicate no advantage to CT over functional stress testing (e.g., MPI) for prediction of major adverse cardiovascular events among patients with an intermediate risk of IHD.[12,13]
  - May aid in the identification of congenital anomalies of the coronary arteries.
  - Because of diminished study quality, it is not useful in patients with extensive coronary calcification (e.g., elderly or advanced CKD), coronary stents, or small-caliber vessels.

TREATMENT

- The major goal of treatment is to reduce symptoms.
- An absolute reduction in incidence of MI or cardiac death in patients with stable IHD is accomplished mainly through medical therapy and not revascularization.
- A combination of lifestyle modification, medical therapy, and coronary revascularization can be used. A recommended strategy for the evaluation and management of the patient with stable angina can be found in Figure 4-3.
- Medical treatment is aimed at improving myocardial oxygen supply, reducing myocardial oxygen demand, controlling exacerbating factors (e.g., anemia), and limiting the development of further atherosclerotic disease.
- Medical treatment often is sufficient to control anginal symptoms in chronic stable angina.

TABLE 4-7 NCDR AKI Risk Model: Risk of AKI and AKI Resulting in HD in Patients Undergoing PCI

	Risk Conversion					
Points	**AKI**	**AKI+HD**	**Points Total**	**Risk AKI (%)**	**Points Total**	**Risk HD (%)**
Variables			0	1.9	≤6	<1
			5	2.6	7	1.5
Age ≤50	0		10	3.6	8	2.6
50–59	2		15	4.9	9	4.4
60–69	4		20	6.7	10	7.6
70–79	6		25	9.2	11	12.6
80–89	8		30	12.4	12	20.3
>90	10		35	16.5	13	31.0
Heart failure within 2 wk	11	2	40	21.7		
GFR ≤30	18	5	45	27.9		
GFR 31–44	8	3	50	35.1		
GFR 45–59	3	1	55	43		
Diabetes mellitus	7	1	>60	51.4		
Any prior heart failure	4	–				
Any prior cerebrovascular disease/stoke	4	–				
Anemia (Hgb <10 g/dL)	10	–				
NSTEMI/UA presentation	6	1				
STEMI presentation	15	2				
Shock before procedure	16	–				
Cardiac arrest before procedure	8	3				
IABP use	11	–				

Points are determined by the points column and total points are converted to risk in the risk conversion column.

AKI, acute kidney injury; GFR, glomerular filtration rate; HD, hemodialysis; Hgb, hemoglobin; IABP, intra-aortic balloon counterpulsation; NCDR, National Cardiovascular Data Registry; NSTEMI, non–ST-segment elevation myocardial infarction; PCI, percutaneous coronary intervention; STEMI, ST-segment elevation myocardial infarction; UA, unstable angina.

GFR calculated using the Modification of Diet in Renal Disease (MDRD) formula; AKI defined as at least a ≥0.3 mg/dL increase or ≥1.5-fold relative increase in creatinine after procedure or initiation of dialysis (HD) after procedure. Patients were excluded if on dialysis at the time of the procedure.

Medications

- **Anti-ischemic therapy**
  - **β-Adrenergic antagonists** (Table 4-8) control anginal symptoms by decreasing heart rate and myocardial work, leading to reduced myocardial oxygen demand.
    - β-Blockers with intrinsic sympathomimetic activity should be avoided.
    - Dosage can be adjusted to result in a resting heart rate of 50–60 bpm.

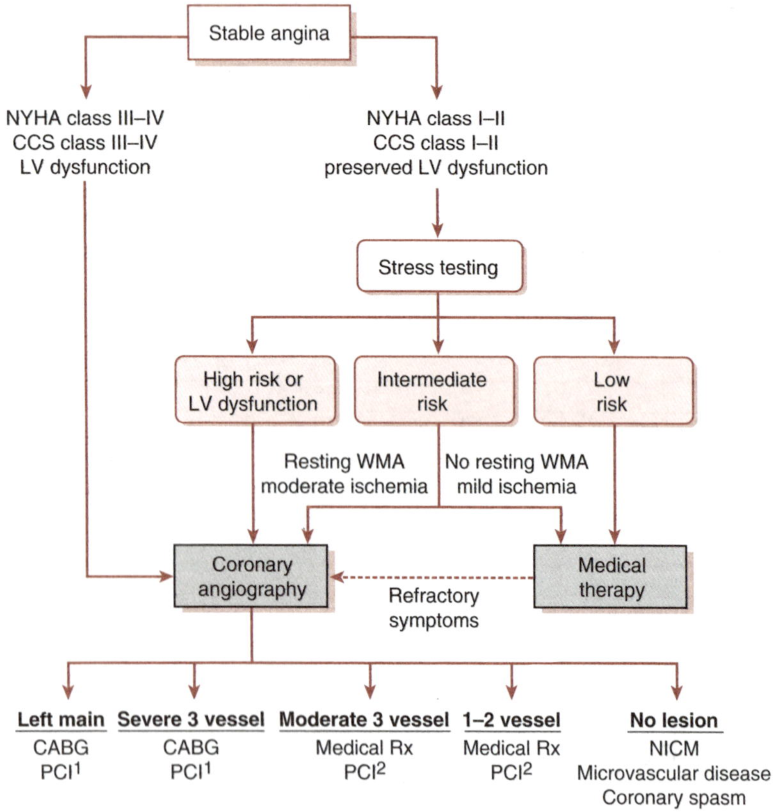

Figure 4-3 Approach to the evaluation and management of the patient with stable angina. Patients with clinical heart failure, severe limiting angina, and those with left ventricle (LV) dysfunction should undergo coronary angiography to define underlying coronary artery disease. Patients without these features may undergo further risk stratification with stress testing. Following stress testing, patients may undergo either coronary angiography or empiric medical therapy depending on their risk profile. Patients initially treated with medical therapy who have refractory symptoms should undergo angiography.[1] CABG is generally preferred because of known survival advantage over medical therapy alone; however, if the coronary lesions are not complex, PCI may offer similar results to CABG but with a higher need for future revascularizations.[2] PCI should be reserved for patients who have high-grade lesions, have severe ischemia, and are refractory to medical therapy. CABG, coronary artery bypass grafting; CCS, Canadian Cardiovascular Society Classification (angina); NICM, nonischemic cardiomyopathy; NYHA, New York Heart Association; PCI, percutaneous coronary intervention; WMA, wall motion abnormality.

  - Use with caution or avoid in patients with active bronchospasm, atrioventricular (AV) block, resting bradycardia, or poorly compensated heart failure (HF).
- **Calcium channel blockers** can be used either in conjunction with or in lieu of β-blockers in the presence of contraindications or adverse effects as a second-line agent (Table 4-9).
  - Calcium antagonists are often used in conjunction with β-blockers if the latter are not fully effective at relieving anginal symptoms. Both long-acting dihydropyridines and nondihydropyridine agents can be used.
  - Calcium channel blockers are effective agents for the treatment of coronary vasospasm.

TABLE 4-8 β-Blockers Commonly Used for Ischemic Heart Disease

Drug	β-Receptor Selectivity	Dose
Propranolol	β_1 and β_2	20–80 mg bid
Metoprolol	β_1	50–200 mg bid
Atenolol	β_1	50–200 mg daily
Nebivolol	β_1	5–40 mg daily
Nadolol	β_1 and β_2	40–80 mg daily
Timolol	β_1 and β_2	10–30 mg tid
Acebutolol[a]	β_1	200–600 mg bid
Bisoprolol	β_1	10–20 mg daily
Esmolol (IV)	β_1	50–300 μg/kg per minute
Labetalol	Combined α, β_1, β_2	200–600 mg bid
Pindolol[a]	β_1 and β_2	2.5–7.5 mg tid
Carvedilol	Combined α, β_1, β_2	3.125–25 mg bid

[a]β-blockers with intrinsic sympathomimetic activity.

TABLE 4-9 Calcium Channel Blockers Commonly Used for Ischemic Heart Disease

Drug	Duration of Action	Usual Dosage
Dihydropyridines		
Nifedipine	Long	30–180 mg/d
Amlodipine	Long	5–10 mg/d
Felodipine (SR)	Long	5–10 mg/d
Isradipine	Medium	2.5–10 mg/d
Nicardipine	Short	20–40 mg tid
Nondihydropyridines		
Diltiazem		
Immediate release	Short	30–90 mg qid
Slow release	Long	120–360 mg/d
Verapamil		
Immediate release	Short	80–160 mg tid
Slow release	Long	120–480 mg/d

  - Nondihydropyridine agents (verapamil/diltiazem) should be avoided in patients with systolic dysfunction because of their negative inotropic effects.
- **Nitrates,** either long-acting formulations for chronic use or sublingual/topical preparations for acute anginal symptoms, are more often used as adjunctive antianginal agents (Table 4-10).
  - Sublingual preparations should be used at the first indication of angina or prophylactically before engaging in activities that are known to precipitate angina. Patients should seek prompt medical attention if angina occurs at rest or fails to respond to the third sublingual dose.
  - Nitrate tolerance resulting in reduced therapeutic response may occur with all nitrate preparations. The institution of a nitrate-free period of 10–12 hours (usually at night) can enhance treatment efficacy.

TABLE 4-10 Nitrate Preparations Commonly Used for Ischemic Heart Disease

Preparation	Dosage	Onset (min)	Duration
Sublingual nitroglycerin	0.3–0.6 mg PRN	2–5	10–30 min
Aerosol nitroglycerin	0.4 mg PRN	2–5	10–30 min
Oral isosorbide dinitrate	5–40 mg tid	30–60	4–6 h
Oral isosorbide mononitrate	10–20 mg bid	30–60	6–8 h
Oral isosorbide mononitrate SR	30–120 mg daily	30–60	12–18 h
2% Nitroglycerin ointment	0.5–2.0 in. tid	20–60	3–8 h
Transdermal nitroglycerin patches	5–15 mg daily	>60	12 h
Intravenous nitroglycerin	10–200 μg/min	<2	During infusion

[a]In-hospital mortality of patients in 1965–1967 with no reperfusion therapy (n = 250).[83]
JDV, jugular venous distention; SBP, systolic blood pressure.

- For patients with CAD, nitrates have not shown a mortality benefit.
- Nitrates are contraindicated (even in patients with acute coronary syndrome [ACS]) for use in patients who are on phoshodiesterase-5 inhibitors due to risk of severe hypotension. A washout period of 24 hours for sildenafil and vardenafil and 48 hours for tadalafil is required before nitrate use.

◦ **Ranolazine** is indicated for angina refractory to standard medical therapy and has shown benefit in improving symptoms and quality of life. Ranolazine interacts with simvastatin metabolism and should not be used together.

- **Secondary prevention medications**
  - **Acetylsalicylic acid (ASA)** (75–162 mg/d) reduces cardiovascular events, including repeat revascularization, MI, and cardiac death, by approximately 33%.[14,15]
  - ASA 81 mg appears to be sufficient for most patients (primary or secondary prevention for both IHD and CVA).
  - ASA desensitization may be performed in patients with ASA allergy.
  - **Clopidogrel** (75 mg/d) can be used in those allergic/intolerant of ASA.
  - **Angiotensin-converting enzyme inhibitors (ACE Inhibitors) and angiotensin receptor blockers (ARBs)** have cardiovascular protective effects that reduce the recurrence of ischemic events.
    - ACE inhibitor therapy, or ARBs in those intolerant to ACE inhibitors, should be used in all patients with an LV ejection fraction (LVEF) <40%, hypertension, diabetes, or CKD.
    - It is reasonable to use ACE inhibitor in all stable angina patients.
  - **Statins** have a marked effect in secondary prevention, and all patients with IHD who can tolerate therapy should be on a high-potency statin (see Chapter 3, Preventive Cardiology).
    - In secondary prevention of coronary heart disease, statins have the most evidence demonstrating a robust mortality benefit.
    - **Proprotein convertase subtilisin/kexin type 9 (PCSK9) inhibitors** confer a mortality benefit to patients with IHD whose LDL levels remain >70 mg/dL despite high-intensity statins. Currently, expense and insurance coverage limit the use of this class of medications.[16]
    - **Ezetimibe** also improves cardiovascular outcomes among patients with IHD whose LDL remains >100 mg/dL despite high intensity statin therapy.[17] The adenosine citrate lyase inhibitor, bempedoic acid, may be considered as an add-on therapy to statins plus a second-line agent like ezetemibe or pcsk9 inhibitors, for patients who do not meet target or have contraindications to these drugs.
  - **Influenza vaccination** is recommended for all patients with IHD.

Newer Therapies

- **Inhibition of fatty acid oxidation**: During periods of stress, the heart uses more fatty acids as fuel, which is less oxygen efficient. Inhibition of fatty acid oxidation shifts the equilibrium toward increased use of glucose, improving the efficient use of oxygen.
    - **Trimetazidine**: 20 mg three times daily. Associated with greater improvements in time to onset of angina, and the mean weekly number of anginal episodes.
    - **Perhexiline:** Its use markedly declined after reports of hepatotoxicity and peripheral neuropathy.
- **Nicorandil**: 20 mg twice per day. It is a potassium channel activator. It is an arterial and venous dilator, and improves coronary blood flow due to potassium channel opening and nitrate effect. Since ATP-dependent potassium channels play a role in ischemic preconditioning, nicorandil may also mimic a natural process of ischemic preconditioning, protecting the heart from subsequent ischemic attacks.
- **Allopurinol**: The drug significantly improves endothelium-dependent vasodilation and completely abolishes oxidative stress. Further evaluation of allopurinol is necessary before it can be recommended as an antianginal agent.
- **Ivabradine**: Not recommended in patients with stable angina who do not have clinical heart failure.
- **Fasudil**: An inhibitor of Rho kinase that is involved in the vascular smooth muscle contractile response, is of benefit in patients with stable and microvascular angina (angina with normal coronary arteries). We do not recommend its use to treat angina.
- **Therapeutic angiogenesis for management of refractory angina**
    - **Indications**
        - Patients with angina that is refractory to medical therapy
        - Patients with angina who are not candidates for traditional revascularization (PCI) or CABG because of the inability to achieve complete revascularization or the high risk of CABG
    - The goal of therapeutic angiogenesis is the induction of new coronary arterial vessels that can effectively provide blood supply to the area of myocardium subtended by diseased or occluded native coronary arteries.
    - A number of angiogenic growth factors stimulate blood vessel growth including fibroblast growth factors (FGFs), vascular endothelial growth factors (VEGFs), and platelet-derived growth factor (PDGF) and many of these are under investigation.

Revascularization

- In general, medical therapy with at least two classes of antianginal agents should be attempted before medical therapy is considered a failure and coronary revascularization pursued in stable angina (Figure 4-4).
- Relief of angina symptoms is the most common objective of all revascularization procedures for stable angina.
- The indication for all revascularization procedures should consider the acuity of presentation, the extent of ischemia, and the ability to achieve full revascularization. The selection of revascularization should be tailored to the individual patient and, in complex cases, include the use of a multidisciplinary heart team.
- The choice between PCI and CABG surgery is dependent on the coronary anatomy, medical comorbidities, and patient preference.
    - In general, patients with complex and diffuse disease or diabetes do better with CABG, whereas PCI in select patients with the proper coronary anatomy can provide comparable results as CABG.[18]
    - Owing to the more invasive nature of CABG, patient comorbidities often necessitate PCI for revascularization.

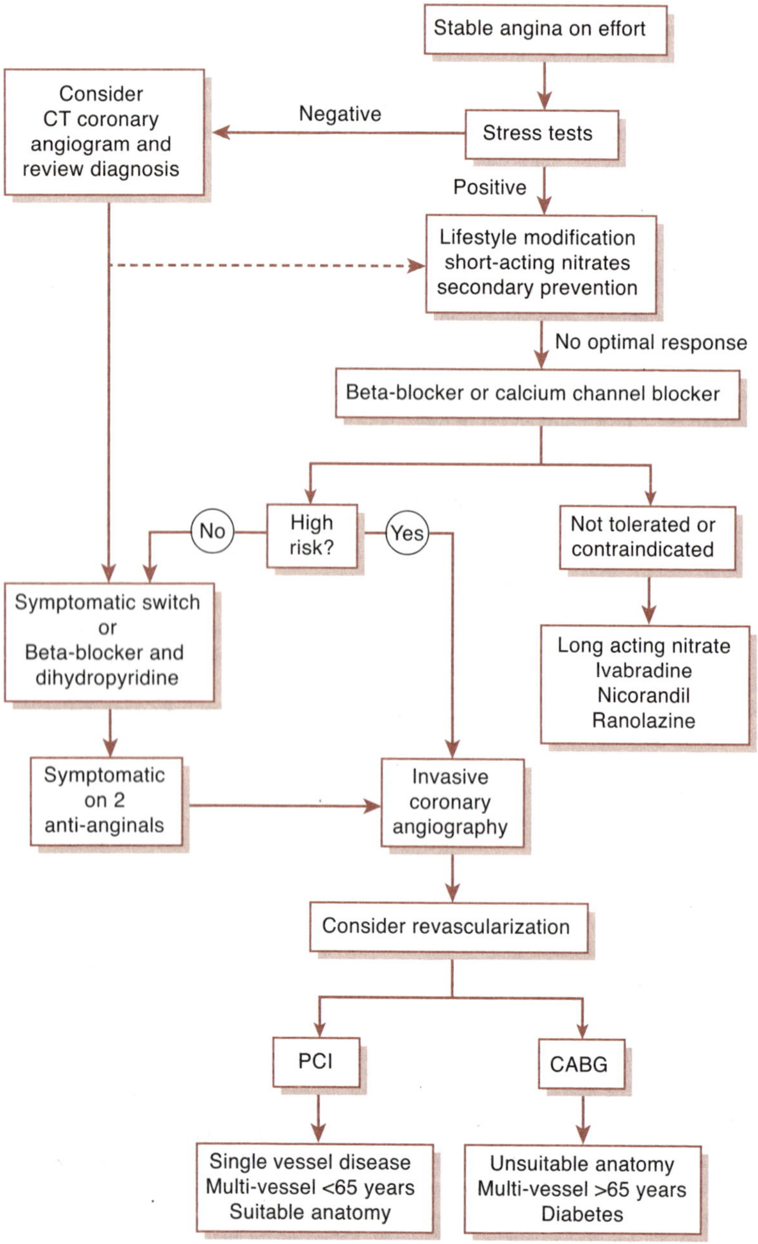

Figure 4-4 Scheme for the investigation and management of stable angina.

  - The Syntax Score is a validated angiographic model that can aid the clinician in determining outcomes after PCI or CABG. In general, patients with a low or intermediate Syntax Score do as well or better with PCI compared to CABG (available at http://www.syntaxscore.com/).[19]
  - The Society of Thoracic Surgeons (STS) score can help determine the risk of mortality and morbidity associated with CABG and should be determined for all patients when considering surgical revascularization (available at http://riskcalc.sts.org/).
- Revascularization is shown to **improve survival** in the following circumstances as compared to medical therapy:
  - CABG for >50% left main CAD that has not been grafted (unprotected). PCI is a reasonable alternative for patients with left main disease if the patient is a poor surgical candidate (STS score >5) and has a favorable morphology for PCI (low Syntax Score). PCI, in the right clinical context, can offer rates of MI, CVA, or death similar to CABG.[20]
  - CABG for three-vessel disease or two-vessel disease that includes the proximal left anterior descending (LAD) artery.
  - CABG for patients with two-vessel disease not including the LAD artery if there is extensive ischemia (>20% myocardium at risk) or in patients with isolated proximal LAD artery disease when an internal mammary artery revascularization is performed.
  - CABG, as compared to PCI or medical therapy, in patients with multivessel disease and diabetes, if a left internal mammary artery to the LAD artery can be placed. PCI *may* offer similar survival outcomes in diabetics with multivessel disease and a low Syntax Score (<22) but does have a higher need for repeat revascularization.[21,22]
  - PCI or CABG in patients who have survived sudden cardiac death due to ischemic ventricular tachycardia (VT).
  - PCI or CABG in patients with ACS.
- Owing to the morbidity of a repeat CABG, PCI is often used to improve symptoms in patients with recurrent angina after CABG.
- The use of internal mammary artery grafts is associated with 90% graft patency at 10 years, compared with 40%–50% for saphenous vein grafts. The long-term patency of a radial artery graft is 80% at 5 years. After 10 years of follow-up, 50% of patients develop recurrent angina or other adverse cardiac events related to late vein graft failure or progression of native CAD.
- The risks of elective PCI include <1% mortality, a 2%–5% rate of nonfatal MI, and <1% need for emergent CABG for an unsuccessful procedure. Patients undergoing PCI have shorter hospitalizations but require more frequent repeat revascularization procedures compared to CABG.
- Elderly patients represent a unique population when considering revascularization due to comorbidities, frailty, the physiology of aging as it relates to drug metabolism and cardiopulmonary function, and concern over polypharmacy. In general, this population has been underrepresented in most trials but still derives benefit from revascularization to relieve symptoms. Frailty should be heavily considered when considering a procedure or counseling about the benefits of revascularization.
- It is reasonable to revascularize selected patients with severe LV dysfunction (EF <35%), as evidenced by the long-term mortality benefit seen with CABG in the STICHES trial.[23]
- Viability testing (nuclear perfusion imaging or MRI) may provide some assistance to the clinician when trying to determine the possible benefit of revascularization in patients with prior MI or severe LV dysfunction, but it is still largely unproven.

PATIENT EDUCATION

- Compliance with medications, diet, and exercise should be stressed to patients. All patients should be encouraged to participate in cardiac rehab as well as meet with a registered dietician.
- Patients with known CAD should present for evaluation if any change in chest pain pattern, frequency, or intensity develops.
- Patients should also be reevaluated if they report the presence of any HF symptoms.

MONITORING/FOLLOW-UP

- Close patient follow-up is a critical component of the treatment of CAD because lifestyle modification and secondary risk factor reduction require serial reassessment and interventions.
- All patients should be aggressively treated for the traditional risk factors mentioned above.
- Relatively minor changes in anginal symptoms can be safely treated with titration and/or addition of antianginal medications.
- Significant changes in anginal complaints (frequency, severity, or time to onset with activity) should be evaluated by either stress testing (usually in conjunction with an imaging modality) or cardiac angiography as warranted.
- Cardiac rehabilitation or an exercise program should be offered or instituted.

Unstable Angina and Non–ST-Segment Elevation Myocardial Infarction

GENERAL PRINCIPLES

Definition

- NSTEMI and UA are closely related conditions whose pathogenesis and clinical presentations are similar but differ in severity.
- If coronary flow is not severe enough or the occlusion does not persist long enough to cause myocardial necrosis (as indicated by positive cardiac biomarkers), the syndrome is labelled UA.
- NSTEMI is defined by an elevation of cardiac biomarkers and the absence of ST-segment elevation on the ECG.
- NSTEMI, like STEMI, can lead to cardiogenic shock.
- AHA/ACC guidelines provide a more thorough overview of NSTEMI/UA.[24]

Epidemiology

- The annual incidence of acute coronary syndrome (ACS) is >780,000 events, with 70% being NSTEMI/UA.
- Among patients with ACS, approximately 60% have UA and 40% have MI (one-third of MIs present with an acute STEMI).
- At 1 year, patients with UA/NSTEMI are at considerable risk for death (~6%), recurrent MI (~11%), and need for revascularization (~50%–60%). It is important to note that although the short-term mortality of STEMI is greater than that of NSTEMI, the long-term mortality is similar.[24]
- Patients with NSTEMI/UA tend to have more comorbidities, both cardiac and noncardiac, than STEMI patients.
- Women with NSTEMI/UA have worse short-term and long-term outcomes and more complications compared to men. Much of this has been attributed to delays in

recognition of symptoms and underutilization of guideline-directed medical therapy and invasive management.[25]

Etiology and Pathophysiology

- Myocardial ischemia results from decreased myocardial oxygen supply and/or increased demand. In the majority of cases, NSTEMI is due to a sudden decrease in blood supply via partial occlusion of the affected vessel. In some cases, markedly increased myocardial oxygen demand may lead to NSTEMI (demand ischemia), as seen in severe anemia, hypertensive crisis, acute decompensated HF, surgery, or any other significant physiologic stressor.
- UA/NSTEMI most often represents severe coronary artery narrowing or acute atherosclerotic plaque rupture/erosion and superimposed thrombus formation. Alternatively, it may also be due to progressive mechanical obstruction from advancing atherosclerotic disease, in-stent restenosis, or bypass graft disease.
- Plaque rupture may be triggered by local and/or systemic inflammation as well as shear stress. Rupture allows exposure of lipid-rich subendothelial components to circulating platelets and inflammatory cells, serving as a potent substrate for thrombus formation. A thin fibrous cap (thin-cap fibroatheroma) is felt to be more vulnerable to rupture and is most frequently represented as only moderate stenosis on angiography.
- Less common causes include dynamic obstruction of the coronary artery due to vasospasm (Prinzmetal angina, cocaine), coronary artery dissection (more common in women), coronary vasculitis, and embolus.
- **Myocardial infarction with nonobstructive coronary arteries (MINOCA) and ischemia and no obstructive coronary artery disease (INOCA)**: Encompasses a heterogeneous group of issues, including plaque rupture without severe obstruction, but with resultant vasospasm, microscopic thromboembolism, or thrombosis with spontaneous thrombolysis. These diagnoses come into consideration only after cardiac catheterization (and perhaps infrequently after coronary CT) since they require objective evidence of nonobstructive CAD.

DIAGNOSIS

Clinical Presentation

History

- ACS symptoms include all the qualities of typical angina except the episodes are more severe, of longer duration, and may occur at rest.
- The three principal presentations for UA are **rest angina** (angina occurring at rest and prolonged, usually >20 minutes), **new-onset angina**, and **progressive angina** (previously diagnosed angina that has become more frequent, lasts longer, or occurs with less exertion). New-onset and progressive angina should occur with at least mild to moderate activity, CCS class III severity.
    - Female sex, diabetes, HF, end-stage kidney disease, and older age are traits that have been associated with a greater likelihood of atypical ACS symptoms. However, the most common presentation in these populations is still typical anginal chest pain.
    - Jaw, neck, arm, back, or epigastric pain and/or dyspnea can be anginal equivalents.
    - Pleuritic pain, pain that radiates down the legs or originates in the mid/lower abdomen, pain that can be reproduced by extremity movement or palpation, and pain that lasts seconds in duration are unlikely to be related to ACS.

Physical Examination

- Physical examination should be directed at identifying hemodynamic instability, pulmonary congestion, and other causes of acute chest discomfort.

TABLE 4-11 Hemodynamic Classification of Patients with Acute Myocardial Infarction

Based Clinical Examination (Killip's)			
Class I	**Class II**	**Class III**	**Class IV**
Rales and S_3 absent	Crackles, S_3 gallop, elevated jugular venous pressure	Frank pulmonary edema	Shock SBP <90 mm Hg
Mortality—6%	*Mortality—17%*	*Mortality—38%*	*Mortality—81%*
Based on Invasive Monitoring			
Subset I	**Subset II**	**Subset III**	**Subset IV**
Normal hemodynamics	Pulmonary congestion	Peripheral hypoperfusion	Pulmonary congestion and peripheral hypoperfusion
PCWP <18	PCWP >18	PCWP <18	PCWP >18
CI >2.2	CI >2.2	CI <2.2	CI <2.2

CI, cardiac index; PCWP, pulmonary capillary wedge pressure.

- Objective evidence of HF including peripheral hypoperfusion, heart murmur (particularly MR murmur), elevated jugular venous pulsation, pulmonary edema, hypotension, and peripheral edema worsens the prognosis.
- Killip classification can be useful to risk stratify and identify patients with features of cardiogenic shock (Table 4-11).
- Examination may also give clues to other causes of ischemia such as thyrotoxicosis or aortic dissection (see Table 4-4).

Diagnostic Testing

Electrocardiography

- Before or immediately on arrival to the emergency department, a baseline ECG should be obtained in all patients with suspected ACS. A normal tracing does not exclude the presence of disease.
- The presence of Q waves, ST-segment changes, or T-wave inversions is suggestive of CAD.
- Isolated Q waves in lead III only are a normal finding.
- Serial ECGs should be obtained to assess for dynamic ischemic changes.
- Comparison to prior ECGs is important when evaluating an ECG for dynamic changes.
- The posterior circulation (i.e., circumflex coronary artery distribution) is poorly assessed with standard ECG lead placement and should always be considered when evaluating patients with ACS. Posterior placed leads or urgent echocardiography may more accurately assess the presence of ischemia when the suspicion is high.
- Approximately 50% of patients with UA/NSTEMI have significant ECG abnormalities, including transient ST-segment elevations, ST depressions, and T-wave inversions.[24]
    - ST-segment depression in two contiguous leads is a sensitive indicator of myocardial ischemia, especially if dynamic and associated with symptoms.
        - The threshold value for abnormal J-point depression should be 0.5 mm in leads V_2 and V_3 and 1 mm in all other leads.
        - ST-segment depression in multiple leads plus ST-segment elevation in aVR and/or V_1 suggests ischemia due to multivessel or left main disease.

- Biphasic or deeply inverted T waves (>5 mm) with QT prolongation in leads V_2 to V_4 in the setting of stuttering chest pain within the past 24 hours suggests a critical lesion in the LAD artery distribution (Wellens Syndrome).[26]
- Nonspecific ST-segment changes or T-wave inversions (those that do not meet voltage criteria) are nondiagnostic and unhelpful in the management of acute ischemia but are associated with a higher risk for future cardiac events.

Laboratories

- A complete blood count, basic metabolic panel, fasting glucose, and lipid profile should be obtained in all patients with suspected CAD. Other conditions may be found to be contributing to ischemia (e.g., anemia) or mimicking ischemia (e.g., hyperkalemia-related ECG changes) or may alter management (e.g., severe thrombocytopenia).
- Cardiac biomarkers (Figure 4-5) are essential in the diagnosis of UA/NSTEMI and should be obtained in all patients who present with chest discomfort suggestive of ACS.
- **Troponin** is the recommended biomarker for assessment of myocardial necrosis.
  - Troponin T and I assays are highly specific and sensitive markers of myocardial necrosis. Serum troponin levels are usually undetectable in normal individuals, and any elevation is considered abnormal.
  - In patients with troponin below the detectable limit of the assay within 6 hours of the onset of pain, a second sample should be drawn 8–12 hours after symptom onset.
  - MI size and prognosis are directly proportional to the magnitude of increase in troponin.[27,28]
- Creatine kinase (CK)-MB is no longer a recommended marker for the initial diagnosis of NSTEMI. It lacks specificity because it is present in both skeletal and cardiac muscle cells.
  - CK-MB may be a useful assay for detecting postinfarct ischemia because a fall and subsequent rise in enzyme levels suggests reinfarction if accompanied by recurrent ischemic symptoms or ECG changes.
- Brain natriuretic peptide (BNP) can be a useful biomarker of myocardial stress in patients with ACS, and elevations are associated with worse outcomes. Severe elevations of BNP in the setting of ACS in patients without known HF should raise concern for a large infarction and urgent angiography.[29]
- Another promising biomarker is the heart-type fatty acid-binding protein (H-FABP), which is released into the bloodstream rapidly after myocardial injury. Combining high-sensitivity cTn and H-FABP measurements may enhance the diagnostic accuracy of MI, facilitating rapid triage, and treatment.

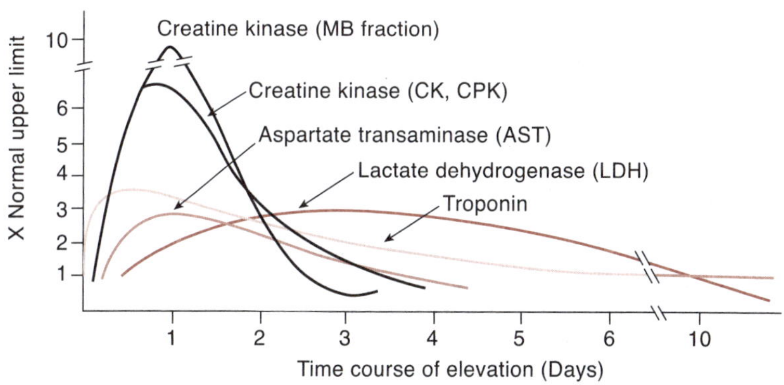

Figure 4-5 Cardiac biomarkers.

TREATMENT

- Acute treatment aims to reduce the symptoms of chest pain and risks of recurrent MI or death.
- Risk stratification can be helpful in determining the appropriate testing, pharmacologic interventions, and timing or need for coronary angiography.
  - Risk of death or MI progression is elevated with the following **high-risk ACS characteristics**, which should prompt **urgent coronary angiography** (<2 **hours**) with the intent to revascularize:
    - Recurrent/accelerating angina despite adequate medical therapy
    - Signs or symptoms of new HF, pulmonary edema, or shock (high Killip Classification)
    - New or worsening MR
    - New LBBB
    - VT
  - Several clinical tools can estimate a patient's risk of recurrent MI and cardiac mortality, such as the Thrombolysis in Myocardial Infarction (TIMI) and Global Registry of Acute Coronary Events (GRACE) risk scores. The TIMI risk score can be used to determine the risk of death or nonfatal MI up to 1 year after an ACS event (Figure 4-6).
- In the stabilized patient, two treatment strategies are available: the **ischemia-driven approach** (formerly termed *conservative*) versus the **routine invasive approach** (*early* defined as <24 hours of presentation or *delayed* >24 hours).
  - The planned approach should always be individualized to the patient (Figure 4-7). All patients should receive aggressive antithrombotic, antiplatelet, and ischemic medical therapy no matter the final revascularization strategy. Table 4-12 summarizes the selection approach.
  - In ACS, as opposed to stable IHD, a routine invasive approach with possible PCI has been shown to **reduce the incidence of recurrent MI, hospitalizations, and death.** In general, patients with ACS should undergo a routine invasive strategy unless it is clear that the risk outweighs the possible benefit in a given patient.
  - In the **ischemia-driven approach**, if the patient does not develop high-risk ACS features, has normal subsequent cardiac biomarkers, has no dynamic ECG changes, and responds to medical therapy, a noninvasive stress test should be obtained for further risk stratification.
    - Patients should be angina-free for at least 12 hours before stress testing.
    - If a patient with positive cardiac biomarkers is selected for noninvasive testing, a submaximal or pharmacologic stress test 72 hours after the peak value may be performed.
    - Coronary angiography is reserved for patients who develop high-risk ACS features, have a high-risk stress test, develop angina at low levels of stress, or are noted to have an LVEF <40%.
  - In the **routine invasive strategy**, the patient is planned for a coronary angiography with the intent to revascularize. An early (<24 hours from presentation) invasive approach is recommended for patients with high-risk scores or other high-risk features (see Table 4-12).
  - All patients with NSTEMI for whom an invasive evaluation is planned must receive P2Y12 inhibitor; ticagrelor or prasugrel is preferred over clopidogrel.
  - Refractory chest pain, hemodynamic instability, or serious ventricular arrhythmias are indications for an urgent/emergent invasive strategy similar to STEMI; this is not to be confused with a routine invasive strategy.
  - An early invasive strategy is also warranted in low- or intermediate-risk patients with repeated ACS presentations despite appropriate therapy.

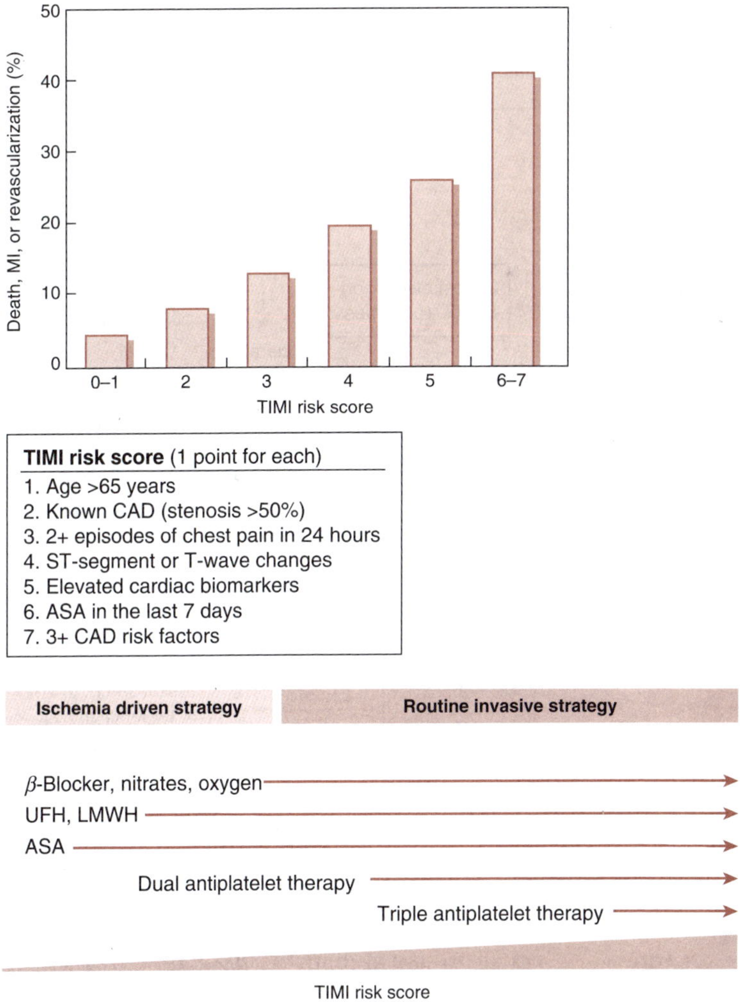

Figure 4-6 Fourteen-day rates of death, MI, or urgent revascularization from the TIMI 11B and ESSENCE trials based on increasing TIMI risk score. Coronary artery disease (CAD) risk factors include family history of CAD, diabetes, hypertension, hyperlipidemia, and tobacco use. ASA, aspirin; LMWH, low–molecular-weight heparin; MI, myocardial infarction; TIMI, Thrombolysis in Myocardial Infarction; UFH, unfractionated heparin.[76]

- A routine invasive strategy is not recommended for the following:
  - Patients with severe comorbid illnesses such as advanced CKD, end-stage liver or lung disease, or metastatic/uncontrolled cancer whereby the benefits of the procedure are likely outweighed by the risk from the routine invasive procedure.
  - Acute chest pain with a low likelihood of ACS and negative biomarkers, especially in women.

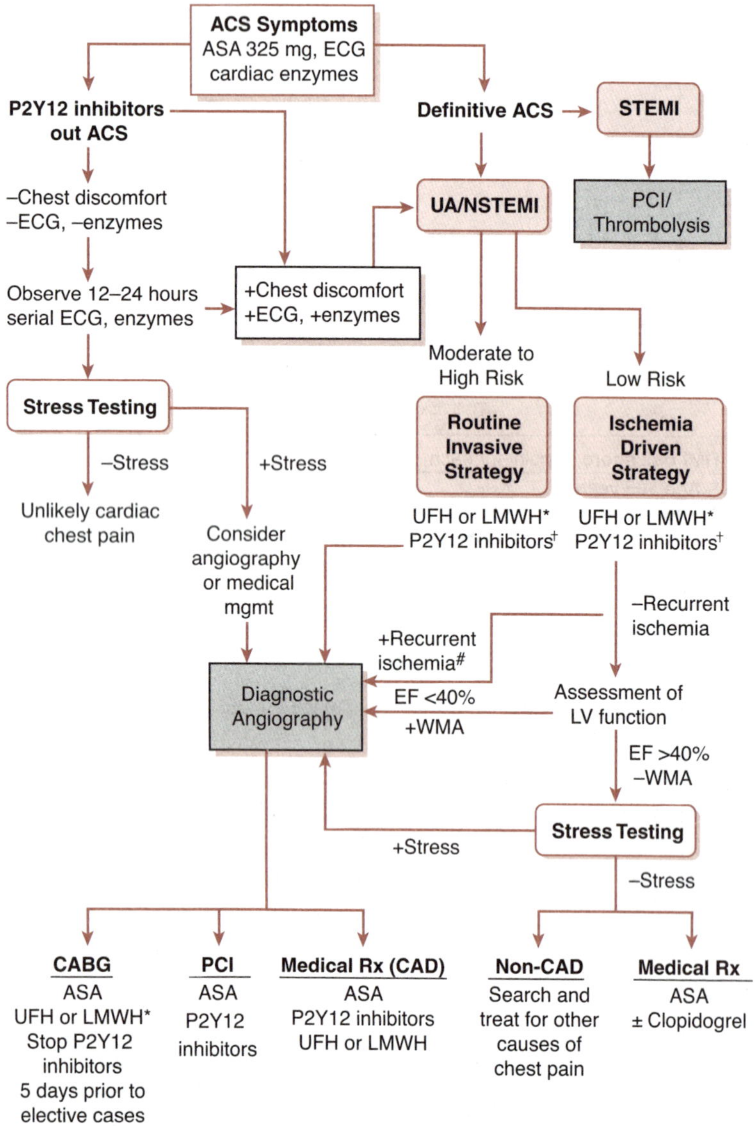

Figure 4-7 Diagnostic and therapeutic approach to patients presenting with acute coronary syndrome (ACS) focusing on antiplatelet and antithrombotic therapy.
*Bivalirudin is an appropriate alternative to UFH and LMWH, or at time of PCI, patients on UFH may be switched to bivalirudin. †Choose either P2Y12 inhibitors, ticagrelor, or prasugrel as the second antiplatelet agent. #Indicators of recurrent ischemia include worsening chest pain, increasing cardiac biomarkers, heart failure signs/symptoms, arrhythmia (VT/VF), and dynamic ECG changes.
ASA, aspirin; CABG, coronary artery bypass grafting; CAD, coronary artery disease; EF, ejection fraction; glycoprotein IIb/IIIa inhibitor; LMWH, low–molecular-weight heparin; NSTEMI, non–ST-segment elevation myocardial infarction; PCI, percutaneous coronary intervention; Rx, treatment; STEMI, ST-segment elevation myocardial infarction; UA, unstable angina; UFH, unfractionated heparin; VT/VF, ventricular tachycardia/ventricular fibrillation; WMA, wall motion abnormality.[24,77]

TABLE 4-12	Appropriate Selection of Routine Invasive Versus Ischemia-Driven Revascularization Strategy in Patients With NSTEMI/UA
Immediate/urgent invasive (within 2 h)	Refractory angina Worsening signs or symptoms of heart failure or mitral regurgitation Hemodynamic instability or shock Sustained VT or VF
Ischemia-driven	Low-risk score (TIMI ≤1 or GRACE <109) Low-risk biomarker-negative female patients Patient or clinician preference in the absence of high-risk features
Early invasive (within 24 h)	None of the above but a high-risk score (TIMI ≥3 or GRACE >140) Rapid rate of rise in biomarkers New or presumably new ST depressions
Delayed invasive (24–72 h)	None of the above but presence of diabetes Renal insufficiency (GFR <60) LV ejection fraction <40% Early postinfarction angina Prior PCI within 6 mo Prior CABG TIMI score ≥2 or GRACE score 109–140 and no indication for early invasive strategy

CABG, coronary artery bypass graft; GFR, glomerular filtration rate; GRACE, Global Registry of Acute Coronary Events; LV, left ventricular; NSTEMI, non–ST-segment elevation myocardial infarction; PCI, percutaneous coronary intervention; TIMI, Thrombolysis in Myocardial Infarction; UA, unstable angina; VF, ventricular fibrillation; VT, ventricular tachycardia.

Medications

- Patients presenting with UA/NSTEMI should receive medications that reduce myocardial ischemia through reduction in myocardial oxygen demand, improvement in coronary perfusion, and prevention of further thrombus formation.
- This approach should include antiplatelet, anticoagulant, and antianginal medications.
- Supplemental oxygen should be provided if the patient is hypoxemic (<90%) or having difficulty in breathing. Routine use of oxygen is not needed and possibly harmful.[30,31]
- **Antiplatelet therapy**
  - Table 4-13 summarizes available agents and dosing recommendations for use in ACS.
  - Early dual antiplatelet therapy (DAPT) with aspirin plus a $P2Y_{12}$ inhibitor is strongly recommended for patients with NSTEMI/UA without a contraindication (e.g., uncontrolled severe bleeding, recent neuraxial surgery or trauma, recent hemorrhagic stroke, or intra-cranial or spinal metastases).
  - DAPT should ideally be continued for 12 months from the index ACS event, regardless of whether revascularization is performed or not. See the 2016 2016 ACC/AHA Guideline Focused Update on Duration of Dual Antiplatelet Therapy in Patients With Coronary Artery Disease for specific recommendations tailored to stent type, bleeding risk, and other considerations.[32]
  - **Aspirin** blocks platelet aggregation within minutes.

TABLE 4-13 Antiplatelet Agents in UA/NSTEMI

Medication	Dosage	Comments
Aspirin (ASA)	162–325 mg initial, then 75–100 mg	In patients taking ticagrelor, the maintenance dose of ASA *should not* exceed 100 mg.
Clopidogrel	300–600 mg loading dose, 75 mg daily	In combination with ASA, clopidogrel (300–600 mg loading dose, then 75 mg/d) decreased the composite end point of cardiovascular death, MI, or stroke by 18%–30% in patients with UA/NSTEMI.[33]
Ticagrelor	180 mg loading dose, then 90 mg bid	Ticagrelor reduced incidence of vascular death, MI, or CVA (9.8% vs. 11.0%) but with higher major bleeding not related to CABG (4.5% vs. 3.8%) as compared to clopidogrel.[35]
Prasugrel	60 mg loading dose, 10 mg daily	Prasugrel has increased antiplatelet potency compared to clopidogrel. Prasugrel reduced the incidence of cardiovascular death, MI, and stroke (9.9% vs. 12.1%) at the expense of increased major (2.4% vs. 1.1%) and fatal bleeding (0.4% vs. 0.1%), compared to clopidogrel.[34]
Cangrelor	30 mcg/kg IV bolus, then 4 mcg/kg per minute	Currently FDA approved only for patients undergoing PCI. Expense and modest evidence of benefit compared to other $P2Y_{12}$ inhibitors limit use.
Eptifibatide	180 μg/kg IV bolus, 2 μg/kg per minute[a]	Eptifibatide reduces the risk of death or MI in patients with ACS undergoing either invasive or noninvasive therapy in combination with ASA and heparin.[84,85] Compared to abciximab and tirofiban, eptifibatide has the most consistent effects on platelet inhibition with shortest on-time and drug half-life.[90]
Tirofiban	0.4 μg/kg IV bolus, 0.1 μg/kg per minute[a]	Tirofiban reduces the risk of death or MI in patients with ACS undergoing either invasive or noninvasive therapy in combination with ASA and heparin.[24]
Abciximab	0.25 mg/kg IV bolus, 10 μg/min[b]	Abciximab reduces the risk of death or MI in patients with ACS undergoing coronary intervention. It should not be used in patients in whom percutaneous intervention is not planned.[24] Platelet inhibition may be reversed by platelet transfusion.

[a]Infusion doses should be decreased by 50% in patients with a GFR <30 mL/min and avoided in patients on HD.
[b]Abciximab may be used in patients with ESRD because it is not cleared by the kidney.
ACS, acute coronary syndrome; CABG, coronary artery bypass grafting; CVA, cerebrovascular accident; ESRD, end-stage renal disease; FDA, the Food and Drug Administration; GFR, glomerular filtration rate; HD, hemodialysis; MI, myocardial infarction; NSTEMI, non–ST-segment elevation myocardial infarction; UA, unstable angina.

- A chewable 162–325-mg dose of ASA should be administered immediately at symptom onset or at first medical contact, unless a contraindication exists. This should be followed by ASA 81 mg daily indefinitely.
- If an ASA allergy is present, clopidogrel may be substituted. An allergy consultation should be obtained for possible desensitization, preferably before the need for a coronary stent.
- After PCI, ASA 81 mg is the current recommended dose in the setting of DAPT.
- *If ticagrelor is chosen as platelet $P2Y_{12}$ inhibitor, the discharge dose of aspirin should not be greater than 100 mg/day.*

◦ **Clopidogrel** is a prodrug whose metabolite blocks the $P2Y_{12}$ receptor and inhibits platelet activation and aggregation by blocking the adenosine diphosphate receptor site on platelets.
- The addition of clopidogrel to ASA reduced cardiovascular mortality and recurrent MI both acutely and at 11 months of follow-up.[33]
- A loading dose of 600 mg should always be given in naïve patients.
- In patients unable to take oral medications or unable to absorb oral medications because of ileus, rectal administration is unproven but has been reported. Alternatively, parenteral agents (e.g., cangrelor or eptifibatide), may be considered.
- It can be used as part of the protocol in both the ischemia-driven and routinely invasive strategies.

◦ **Prasugrel** is also a prodrug that blocks the $P2Y_{12}$ adenosine receptor; its conversion to its active metabolite occurs faster and to a greater extent than clopidogrel.
- It results in faster, greater, and more uniform platelet inhibition compared to clopidogrel at the expense of higher risk of bleeding.[34]
- It decreases risk of CVD death, MI, CVA, and acute stent thrombosis as compared to clopidogrel in ACS patients, including STEMI patients.
- It should be used with caution or avoided in patients older than 75 years and who weigh less than 60 kg. It is contraindicated in those with prior stroke or transient ischemic attack.
- It is used **only in the invasive approach of ACS** and only after coronary anatomy is known and PCI is planned. There is no benefit over clopidogrel when tested before the initiation of PCI.

◦ **Ticagrelor** is not a prodrug and blocks the $P2Y_{12}$ adenosine receptor directly.
- It reduces the risk of death, MI, CVA, and stent thrombosis as compared to clopidogrel in ACS patients, including STEMI patients.[35]
- After the loading dose of ASA, the maintenance dose of ASA must be <100 mg.
- It can be used as part of the protocol in both the ischemia-driven and early invasive strategies.
- Barring any contraindication, ticagrelor is the preferred $P2Y_{12}$ inhibitor of choice because of the mortality advantage over medications in this class.
- The relative contraindications include baseline bradycardia, severe reactive airways disease, and prior hemorrhagic stroke.

◦ **Cangrelor** is a parenteral, direct, and reversible inhibitor of the $P2Y_{12}$ adenosine receptor.
- It has a uniquely rapid onset (<2 minutes), potency (>90% platelet inhibition), and short duration of action after cessation (normal platelet function after 1 hour).
- It reduces the risk of death, MI, urgent revascularization, or stent thrombosis among patients undergoing PCI.[36]
- The FDA approved it only for patients undergoing PCI and is currently very expensive. Thus, it is not yet recommended for routine use in either ischemia-guided or invasive strategy. Thus, we recommend consulting a cardiologist before the use of cangrelor.
- It is sometimes used as a bridging strategy in patients who have had recent PCI and require surgery where DAPT is prohibited. This approach is of unproven benefit.

- **Glycoprotein IIb/IIIa (GPIIb/IIIa) antagonists** (abciximab, eptifibatide, or tirofiban) block the interaction between platelets and fibrinogen, thus targeting the final common pathway for platelet aggregation.
  - GPIIb/IIIa inhibitors play a limited role in ACS management with the introduction of more potent oral antiplatelet agents.
  - The routine use of GPIIb/IIIa antagonists on initial presentation, before angiography, in patients undergoing the invasive approach *should be avoided* because of increased risk of major bleeding and a lack of improvement in outcomes.
  - GPIIb/IIIa agents may be considered in scenarios of worsening ischemia despite DAPT, complex PCI, or bridging strategy in patients with an indication for DAPT (e.g., recent PCI) but require surgery.
  - Thrombocytopenia, which can be severe, is an uncommon complication of these agents and should prompt discontinuation.
- **Other concerns with antiplatelet agents**
  - Timing of CABG
    - Owing to the increased risk of bleeding, it is currently recommended that clopidogrel be withheld for at least 5 days before CABG, prasugrel 7 days prior, ticagrelor 5 days prior, and cangrelor 1–6 hours prior.
    - Cangrelor or GPIIb/IIIa antagonists can be used as an alternative to clopidogrel, ticagrelor, and prasugrel in appropriate patients with UA/NSTEMI who are known to require surgical revascularization.
    - In general, **DAPT should not be withheld during the initial management of ACS (i.e., before angiography) out of concern for the potential need for surgical revascularization.** There is a larger risk of withholding beneficial therapy to patients in this setting than causing harm by delaying surgical revascularization.
  - Proton pump inhibitors (PPIs)
    - PPIs should be used in patients on DAPT with a prior history of gastrointestinal bleeding or increased risk of bleeding (e.g., elderly, known ulcers or *Helicobacter pylori* infection, or coprescribed warfarin, steroids, or NSAIDs).[37]
    - Pharmacologic studies have raised concerns about the potential of PPIs to blunt the efficacy of clopidogrel. However, in a prospective randomized trial, no apparent cardiovascular interaction was noted between PPIs and clopidogrel.[36]
  - Triple Therapy
    - Many patients requiring DAPT after PCI have a pre-existing indication for oral anticoagulation (OAC), such as atrial fibrillation or recent venous thromboembolism.
    - The use of DAPT and OAC (triple therapy) leads to higher bleeding risk, but recent trials suggest that triple therapy may not significantly reduce ischemic events any more than single antiplatelet therapy (SAPT; e.g., aspirin or clopidogrel) plus OAC.[38,39]
    - The most recent guidelines have not yet made specific recommendations, but they generally support tailoring selection of triple therapy (DAPT plus OAC) or SAPT plus OAC to the patient by comparing the risk of bleeding to the risk of ischemic events.[32]
    - In patients with an average risk of bleeding and average risk of ischemic events, we recommend triple therapy (e.g., aspirin, clopidogrel, and warfarin) for 4 weeks followed by SAPT plus OAC (e.g., clopidogrel and warfarin) for at least 1 year.
    - In patients with either high risk of bleeding or high risk of ischemic events, we recommend consultation with a cardiologist to tailor therapy.

- **Anticoagulant therapy**
  - See Table 4-14 for recommended use and dosing in ACS.
  - Anticoagulation accompanied by DAPT is required for all UA/NSTEMI patients, whether along the early invasive or conservative pathway.

TABLE 4-14 Anticoagulant Medications

Medication	Dosage	Comments
Heparin (UFH)	60 units/kg IV bolus (maximum dose: 4000 units), 12–14 units/kg per hour	Heparin therapy, when used in conjunction with ASA, has been shown to reduce the early rate of death or MI by up to 60%.[86] The aPTT should be adjusted to maintain a value of 1.5–2.0 times control.
Enoxaparin (LMWH)	1 mg/kg SC bid[a]	LMWH is at least as efficacious as UFH and may further reduce the rate of death, MI, or recurrent angina.[87] LMWH may increase the rate of bleeding and cannot be reversed in the setting of refractory bleeding.[40] LMWH does not require monitoring for clinical effect.
Fondaparinux	2.5 mg SC daily	Fondaparinux has efficacy similar to that of LMWH with possibly reduced bleeding rates.[88]
Bivalirudin[b]	0.75 mg/kg IV bolus, 1.75 mg/kg per hour	When used in conjunction with ASA and clopidogrel, bivalirudin is at least as effective as the combination of ASA, UFH, clopidogrel, and GPIIb/IIIa antagonists with decreased bleeding rates.[42] May increase risk for stent thrombosis. Monitoring is required with a goal aPTT of 1.5–2.5 times control.

[a]LMWH should be given at reduced dose (50%) in patients with a serum creatinine >2 mg/dL or GFR <30 mL/min.
[b]Bivalirudin requires dosage adjustment in patients with a GFR less than 30 mL/min or those on hemodialysis.
aPTT, activated partial thromboplastin time; ASA, aspirin; GFR, glomerular filtration rate; GP, glycoprotein; LMWH, low-molecular-weight heparin; MI, myocardial infarction; UFH, unfractionated heparin.

- **Unfractionated heparin** (UFH) works by binding antithrombin III, which catalyzes the inactivation of thrombin and other clotting factors.
    - Most commonly used and easily monitored but also most inconsistent in its anticoagulation and metabolism.
    - Heparin-induced thrombocytopenia (HIT) is a concern with prior use.
    - Easily reversed in the event of a severe hemorrhagic complication.
    - Always requires aggressive bolus dosing and anticoagulation monitoring in the setting of ACS.
    - Is a recommended anticoagulant to be used in the setting of ACS.
- **Low–molecular-weight heparin** (LMWH) inhibits mostly factor Xa but also affects thrombin activity and offers an ease of administration (weight-based, twice-daily subcutaneous dose). The risk of HIT is lower but not absent.
    - As compared to UFH, LMWH has a more predictable anticoagulant effect.
    - It has a similar efficacy as UFH but is associated with a higher risk of postprocedural bleeding.[40]
    - LMWH must be adjusted for renal dysfunction and should be avoided in patients with severe impairments.

- Enoxaparin 0.3 mg/kg IV should be administered at the time of PCI in patients who have received less than two therapeutic doses or if the last dose was received more than 8 hours before PCI.
- **Fondaparinux** is a synthetic polysaccharide that selectively inhibits factor Xa and can be subcutaneously administered on a daily routine.
  - It is associated with an increased risk of thrombosis during PCI and should not be used without additional antithrombin anticoagulation; as such, it is not recommended for the routine management of ACS.
  - In patients not undergoing invasive management, fondaparinux may significantly reduce bleeding and improve outcomes compared to LMWH.[41]
- **Bivalirudin** is a direct thrombin inhibitor given as a continuous IV infusion and requires partial thromboplastin time (PTT) monitoring when used for >4 hours.
  - It does not cause HIT and is used in the treatment of patients who develop HIT or patients with ACS who have history of HIT.
  - Bivalirudin can be given in conjunction with ASA and clopidogrel in patients presenting with UA/NSTEMI who will undergo a routine invasive strategy.
  - Bivalirudin alone compared to UFH/LMWH + GPIIb/IIIa inhibitor was associated with less bleeding.[42]
  - Recent evidence has shown that in ACS without significant GPIIb/IIIa inhibitor use, bivalirudin is associated with increased risk of stent thrombosis and target lesion revascularization.[43]
  - Caution should be taken with routine use of bivalirudin in ACS unless there is a high risk of bleeding.

- **Anti-ischemic therapy** (please also refer to Treatment section of stable angina)
  - **Nitroglycerin**
    - Treatment can be initiated at the time of presentation with sublingual nitroglycerin. **NOTE:** 40% of patients with chest pain *not* due to CAD will get relief with nitroglycerin (see Table 4-10).[44]
    - Patients with ongoing ischemic symptoms or those who require additional agents to control significant hypertension can be treated with IV nitroglycerin until pain relief, hypertension control, or both are achieved.
    - Rule out right ventricular (RV) infarct before administration of nitrates because this can precipitate profound hypotension.
  - **β-Adrenergic blockers (BBs)** (please also refer to the Treatment section for stable angina)
    - Oral therapy should be started early in the absence of contraindications.
    - Treatment with an IV preparation should be reserved for treatment of arrhythmia, ongoing chest pain, or advanced hypertension rather than routine use.
    - Routine use of IV BBs is associated with increased risk of cardiogenic shock and should be avoided.
    - Contraindications to BB therapy include advanced AV block, active bronchospasm, decompensated HF, cardiogenic shock, hypotension, and bradycardia.
  - **Morphine** 2–4 mg IV may be used as an adjunct to BB, nitrates, and calcium channel blockers. Care must be taken on not to mask further clinical evaluation by heavy use of narcotic medications.
- **Adjunctive medical therapy**
  - **ACE inhibitors** (refer to Treatment section for stable angina) are effective antihypertensive agents and have been shown to reduce mortality in patients with CAD and LV systolic dysfunction. ACE inhibitors should be used in patients with LV dysfunction (EF <40%), hypertension, or diabetes presenting with ACS. **ARBs** are appropriate in patients who cannot tolerate ACEIs.

- **Aldosterone antagonists** should be added, if there are no contraindications (potassium >5 mEq/L or creatinine clearance [CrCl] <30 mL/min), after initiation of ACE inhibitors in patients with diabetes or an LVEF <40%.
- **3-Hydroxy-3-methylglutaryl–coenzyme A (HMG-CoA) reductase inhibitors (statins)** are potent lipid-lowering agents that reduce the incidence of ischemia, MI, and death in patients with CAD. High-intensity statins should be routinely administered within 24 hours of presentation in patients presenting with ACS. A lipid profile should be obtained in all patients.
  - Statin therapy reduces adverse outcomes through lipid lowering and potentially through pleiotropic effects (anti-inflammatory/atherosclerotic plaque–stabilizing effects).
  - Aggressive statin therapy reduces the risk of recurrent ischemia, MI, and death in patients presenting with ACS.[45]
  - A reduction in adverse CVD outcomes following early initiation of a high-dose statin with achievement of an LDL <70 mg/dL can be seen as early as 30 days following initial presentation with ACS.[46] Aggressive LDL lowering also reduces the incidence of periprocedural MI following PCI.[47]
  - Patients who cannot achieve LDL <70 mg/dL after the use of a high-intensity statin should be evaluated for adjunctive PCSK9 inhibitors or ezetimibe.[16,17] (Please refer to "Treatment" section for stable angina)
- **NSAIDs** are associated with an increased risk of death, MI, myocardial rupture, hypertension, and HF in large meta-analyses.[48] Adverse outcomes have been observed for both nonselective and cyclooxygenase-2 (COX-2) selective agents. NSAIDs should be discontinued in patients presenting with UA/NSTEMI.
- **Blood glucose** should not be tightly controlled in diabetic patients who have suffered ACS because it may increase mortality. Goal is <180 mg/dL while avoiding hypoglycemia at all costs.
- **Marine omega-3 fatty acid:** High-dose icosapent ethyl is associated with reduction in CV events when used with other measures of secondary prevention.

Revascularization

- PCI
  - Please see "Revascularization" section under Stable Angina for invasive management strategies.
- CABG
  - The indications for PCI versus CABG in patients with UA/NSTEMI are similar to those for individuals with chronic stable angina (please see section on "Revascularization" under Stable Angina).
  - The urgency of revascularization should weigh heavily in the decision for CABG; patients in cardiogenic shock may benefit from PCI and mechanical support compared to emergency cardiac surgery.
  - NSTEMI in the setting of critical left main CAD should prompt urgent surgical revascularization and consideration of intra-aortic balloon pump (IABP) for stabilization before the induction of anesthesia.

MONITORING/FOLLOW-UP

The highest rate of progression to MI or development of recurrent MI is in the first 2 months after presentation with the index episode. Beyond that time, most patients have a clinical course similar to those with chronic stable angina.

- Patients should be discharged on dual antiplatelet, BB, and statin therapy.

- Most patients should be discharged on ACE inhibitors.
- Patients should be evaluated for the need of aldosterone antagonists.
- Screening for life stressors and depression should be carried out. Refer for depression treatment as needed.
- Smoking cessation and risk factor modification should be stressed.
- Referral to cardiac rehabilitation should also be pursued.

ST-Segment Elevation Myocardial Infarction

GENERAL PRINCIPLES

Definition

- STEMI is defined as a clinical syndrome of myocardial ischemia in association with persistent ECG ST elevations (see "Diagnostic Testing" section).
- STEMI is a medical emergency.
- Compared to UA/NSTEMI, STEMI is associated with a higher in-hospital and 30-day morbidity and mortality. Left untreated, the mortality rate of STEMI can exceed 30%, and the presence of mechanical complications (papillary muscle rupture, ventricular septal defect [VSD], and free wall rupture) increases the mortality rate to 90%.
- Ventricular fibrillation (VF) accounts for approximately 50% of mortality and often occurs within the first hour from symptom onset.
- Keys to treatment of STEMI include rapid recognition and diagnosis, coordinated mobilization of health-care resources, and prompt reperfusion therapy.
- Mortality is directly related to total ischemia time.
- AHA/ACC guidelines provide a more thorough overview of STEMI.[49]

Epidemiology

- STEMI accounts for approximately 25%–30% of ACS cases annually, and the incidence has been declining.
- Over the last several decades, there has been a dramatic improvement in short-term mortality to the current rate of 6%–10%.
- Approximately 30% of STEMI presentations occur in women, but outcomes and complications continue to be worse compared with male counterparts.

Types of MI

- **Type 1:** Spontaneous MI with ischemia due to a primary coronary event, for example, plaque erosion/rupture, fissuring, or dissection
- **Type 2:** Myocardial oxygen demand supply mismatch, that is, secondary to ischemia due to increased oxygen demand or decreased supply (e.g., coronary spasm, coronary embolism, anemia, arrhythmias, hypertension, or hypotension)
- **Type 3:** Diagnosis of MI resulting in sudden cardiac death
- **Type 4:** (a) PCI related MI (b) Stent thrombosis
- **Type 5:** MI after CABG—post-CABG

Pathophysiology

- STEMI is caused by acute, total occlusion of an epicardial coronary artery, most often due to atherosclerotic plaque rupture/erosion and subsequent thrombus formation.
- As compared to NSTEMI/UA, thrombotic occlusion is complete such that there is total transmural ischemia/infarct in the distribution of the large occluded artery.

DIAGNOSIS

Clinical Presentation

History

- Chest pain from STEMI resembles angina but lasts longer, is more intense, and is not relieved by rest or sublingual nitroglycerin. Chest discomfort may be accompanied by dyspnea, diaphoresis, palpitations, nausea, vomiting, fatigue, and/or syncope.
- Severe tearing chest pain or focal neurologic deficits should raise concern for aortic dissection. Aortic dissection can mimic ACS; in addition, dissections of the ascending aorta may involve the right coronary artery (RCA) and cause ST elevations on the ECG.
- It is imperative to determine the time of symptom onset because this is critical in determining the appropriate means of reperfusion.
- STEMI may have an atypical presentation particularly in female, elderly, and postoperative patients, as well as those with diabetes and chronic or end-stage kidney disease. Such patients may experience atypical or no chest pain and may instead present with confusion, dyspnea, unexplained hypotension, or HF.
- STEMI should always be considered as an etiology when any patient is hemodynamically compromised (i.e., postoperative, delirium, or shock).
- The initial history by the clinician should always include an inquiry about prior cardiac procedures or surgery. Prior PCI or CABG can have profound implications for acute revascularization management.
- The clinician should assess for absolute and relative contraindications to thrombolytic therapy (see the following text) and potential issues complicating primary PCI (IV contrast allergy, PVD/peripheral revascularization, renal dysfunction, central nervous system disease, pregnancy, bleeding diathesis, or severe comorbidity).
- An inquiry about recent cocaine use should be done. In this setting, aggressive medical therapy with nitroglycerin, coronary vasodilators, and benzodiazepines should be administered before reperfusion therapy is considered.

Physical Examination

Physical examination should be directed at identifying hemodynamic instability, pulmonary congestion, mechanical complications of MI, and other causes of acute chest discomfort.

- The Killip classification (Table 4-11) can be a useful guide when evaluating patients with ACS. The Forrester classification uses hemodynamic data to risk stratify patients and is less frequently used.
- The identification of a new systolic murmur may suggest the presence of ischemic MR or a VSD.
- A limited neurologic examination to detect baseline cognitive and motor deficits and a vascular examination (lower extremity pulses and bruits) will aid in determining candidacy and planning for reperfusion treatment.
- Cardiogenic shock due to right ventricular MI (RVMI) may be clinically suspected by the presence of hypotension, elevated jugular venous pressure, and absence of pulmonary congestion.
- Bilateral arm BPs should be obtained to assess for the presence of aortic dissection.

DIAGNOSTIC TESTING

Electrocardiography

The ECG is paramount to the diagnosis of STEMI and should be obtained within 10 minutes of presentation. If the diagnosis of STEMI is in doubt, serial ECGs may help elucidate the diagnosis. Classic findings include:

- Peaked upright T waves are the first ECG manifestation of myocardial injury.
- ST elevations correlate with the territory of injured myocardium (Table 4-15).

TABLE 4-15 Electrocardiogram-Based Anatomic Distribution

ST Elevation	Myocardial Territory	Coronary Artery
V_1–V_6 or LBBB	Anterior and septal walls	Proximal LAD or left main
V_1–V_2	Septum	Proximal LAD or septal branch
V_2–V_4	Anterior wall	LAD
V_5–V_6	Lateral wall	LCX
II, III, aVF	Inferior wall	RCA or LCX
I, aVL	High lateral wall	Diagonal or proximal LCX

LAD, left anterior descending artery; LBBB, left bundle branch block; LCX, left circumflex artery; RCA, right coronary artery.

- **Diagnostic ECG criteria for STEMI**[50]
  - When ST elevations reach threshold values in two or more anatomically contiguous leads, a diagnosis of STEMI can be made.
  - In men >40 years of age, the threshold value for abnormal ST-segment elevation at the J point is ≥2 mm in leads V_2 and V_3 and >1 mm in all other leads. In men <40 years of age, the threshold value for abnormal ST-segment elevation at the J point in leads V_2 and V_3 is >2.5 mm.
  - In women, the threshold value of abnormal ST-segment elevation at the J point is >1.5 mm in leads V_2 and V_3 and >1 mm in all other leads.
  - In right-sided leads (V_3R and V_4R), the threshold for abnormal ST elevation at the J point is 0.5 mm, except in males <30 years in whom it is 1 mm. Right-sided leads should be obtained in all patients with evidence of inferior wall ischemia to rule out RV ischemia. RV infarction can occur with proximal RCA lesions.
  - In posterior leads (V_7, V_8, and V_9), the threshold for abnormal ST elevation at the J point is 0.5 mm.
    - All patients with ST-segment depression in leads V_1 to V_3, inferior wall ST elevation, or tall R waves in V_1 to V_3 should have posterior leads placed to diagnose a posterior wall MI. Posterior STEMIs are usually due to occlusion of the circumflex artery and are often misdiagnosed as UA/NSTEMI. R waves in V_1 or V_2 represent Q waves of the posterior territory (Figure 4-8).
    - Ischemia of the circumflex artery may also be electrocardiographically silent.

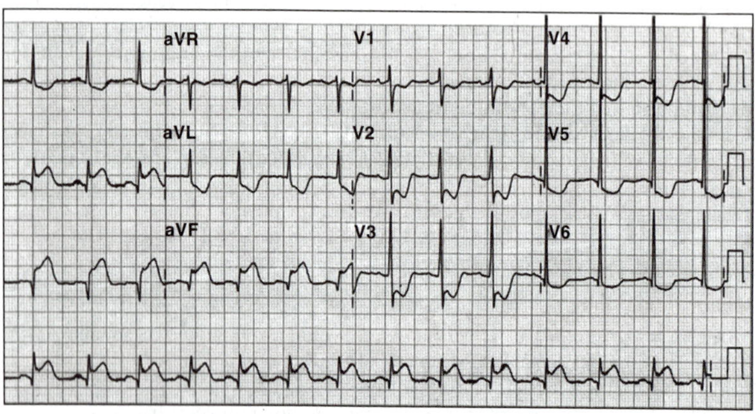

Figure 4-8 ECG changes in acute inferior wall and posterior wall MI.

- The presence of reciprocal ST-segment depression opposite of the infarct territory increases the specificity for acute MI.
- New LBBB suggests a large anterior wall MI with a worse prognosis.
- ECG criteria for STEMI in patients with preexisting LBBB or RV pacing can be found in Table 4-16. Above criteria do not apply.
- **ECG changes that mimic MI.** ST-segment elevation and Q waves may result from numerous etiologies other than acute MI, including prior MI with aneurysm formation, aortic dissection, LV hypertrophy, pericarditis, myocarditis, or pulmonary embolism, or they may be a normal finding (Table 4-17). It is critical to obtain prior ECGs to clarify the diagnosis.
- **Q waves.** Development of new pathologic Q waves is considered diagnostic for transmural MI but may occur in patients with prolonged ischemia or poor collateral supply. The presence of Q waves only is not an indication for acute reperfusion therapy; however, it is very helpful to have an old ECG to compare to determine chronicity.

  Diagnostic criteria include:

  - In leads V_2 and V_3, a pathologic Q wave is ≥0.02 second or a QS complex in V_2 or V_3. An isolated Q wave in lead V_1 or lead III is normal.

TABLE 4-16 Criteria for ST-Segment Elevation for Prior LBBB or RV-Paced Rhythm

ECG Change
ST-segment elevation >1 mm in the presence of a positive QRS complex (concordant with the QRS)
ST-segment elevation >5 mm in the presence of a negative QRS complex (disconcordant with the QRS)
ST-segment depression >1 mm in V_1–V_3

Sgarbossa's (GUSTO) criteria: *Am J Cardiol.* 1996;77:423; *N Engl J Med.* 1996;334:481; *Pacing Clin Electrophysiol.* 2001;24:1289.
LBBB, left bundle branch block; RV, right ventricular.

TABLE 4-17 Differential Diagnosis of ST-Segment Elevation on ECG Excluding STEMI

Cardiac Etiologies	Other Etiologies
Prior MI with aneurysm formation	Pulmonary embolism
Aortic dissection with coronary involvement	Hyperkalemia
Pericarditis	
Myocarditis	
LV hypertrophy or aortic stenosis (with strain)[a]	
Hypertrophic cardiomyopathy	
Coronary vasospasm (cocaine, Prinzmetal angina)	
Early repolarization (normal variant)	
Brugada syndrome	

[a]Strain may occur in numerous settings including systemic hypertension, hypotension, tachycardia, exercise, and sepsis.
LV, left ventricular; MI, myocardial infarction; STEMI, ST-segment elevation myocardial infarction.

- In leads other than V_1 through V_3, presence of a Q wave ≥0.03 second and ≥0.1 mV deep or a QS complex in any two contiguous leads suggests prior MI.
- R wave ≥0.04 second in V_1 and V_2 and R/S ratio ≥1 with a positive T wave suggest prior posterior MI (in the absence of RV hypertrophy or right bundle branch block).
- Changes in MI are described in Table 4-18.

TABLE 4-18 Sequential ECG Changes in STEMI

Time	Changes
Baseline	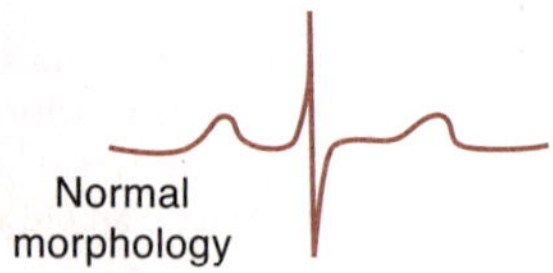
Lasts for a few minutes	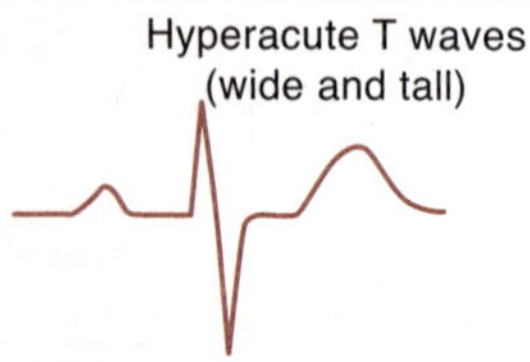
Minutes–hours infarction	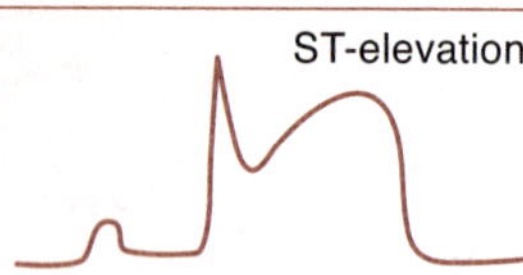
Hours–days fibrosis	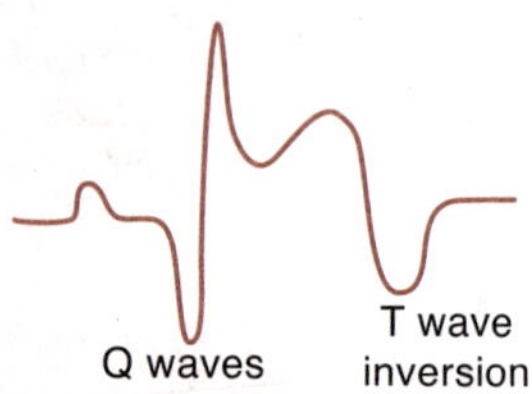
Days–weeks	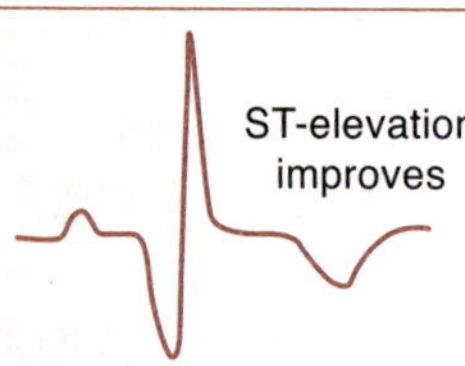
Years–decades	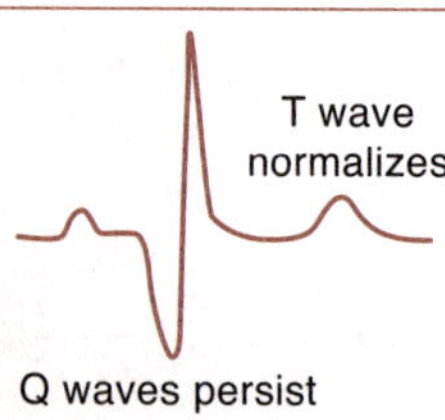

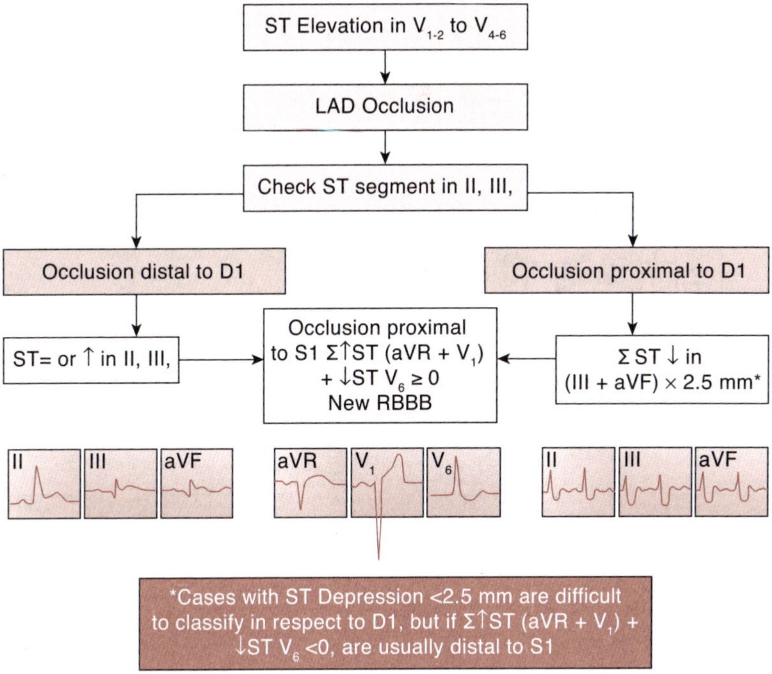

Figure 4-9 Localization of culprit vessel in anterior wall MI. D1, first diagonal branch; LAD, left anterior descending artery; RBBB, right bundle branch block.

Localization of culprit vessel in anterior wall MI and inferior wall MI has been described in Figures 4-9 and 4-10.

Laboratories and Imaging

- STEMI diagnosis and initiation of treatment are done in a patient who reports prolonged chest discomfort or anginal equivalent with qualifying ECG findings. Attempting to wait for results of cardiac biomarkers will add unnecessary delay.
- Blood samples should be sent for cardiac biomarkers (troponin), complete blood cell count, coagulation studies (aPTT, prothrombin time, international normalized ratio), creatinine, electrolytes including magnesium, and type and screen. A lipid profile should be obtained in all patients with STEMI for secondary prevention (note, however, that lipid levels may be falsely lowered during the acute phase of MI).
- Initial cardiac biomarkers (including troponin assays) may be normal, depending on the time in relation to symptom onset.
- CK-MB can be used to confirm that myocardial injury has reoccurred within the previous 48 hours because troponin levels may remain elevated for up to 2 weeks after MI.
- The risk of subsequent cardiac death is directly proportional to the increase in cardiac-specific troponins. The method of measuring biomarkers until the peak level has been attained can be used to determine the infarct size.
- Routine use of cardiac noninvasive imaging is not recommended for the initial diagnosis of STEMI. When the diagnosis is in question, a TTE can be performed to document regional wall motion abnormalities. If not adequately evaluated by TTE, a transesophageal

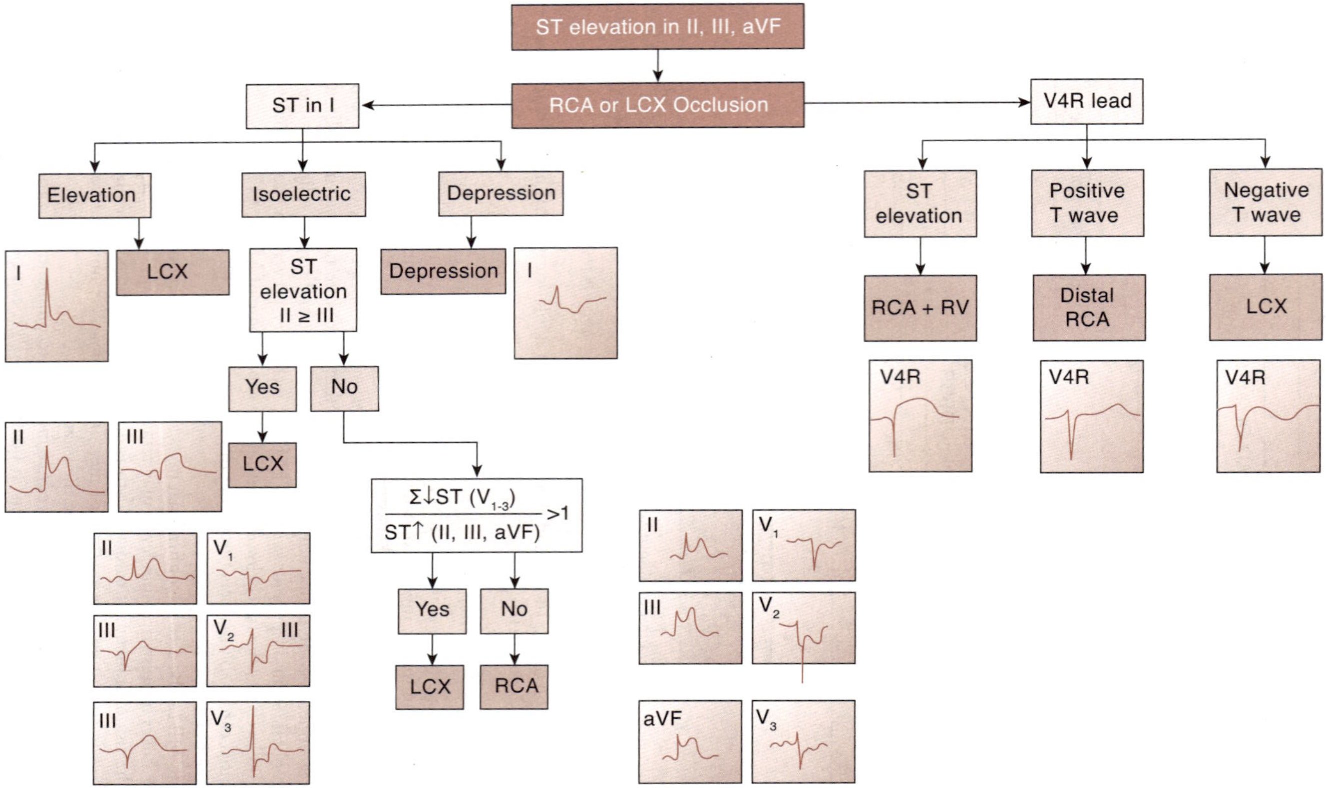

Figure 4-10 Localization of culprit vessel in inferior wall MI. LCX, left circumflex artery; RCA, right coronary artery; RV, right ventricle.

echocardiogram (TEE) can be obtained to assess for acute complications of MI and presence of aortic dissection.

- A portable chest radiograph is useful to assess for pulmonary edema and evaluate for other causes of chest pain including aortic dissection. Importantly, a normal mediastinal width does not exclude aortic dissection, especially if clinically suspected.

TREATMENT

- Prompt treatment should be initiated as soon as the diagnosis is suspected, as mortality and risk of subsequent HF are directly related to ischemia time (Figure 4-11).
- All medical centers should have in place and use an AHA/ACC guideline–based STEMI protocol. Centers that are not primary PCI capable should have protocols in place to

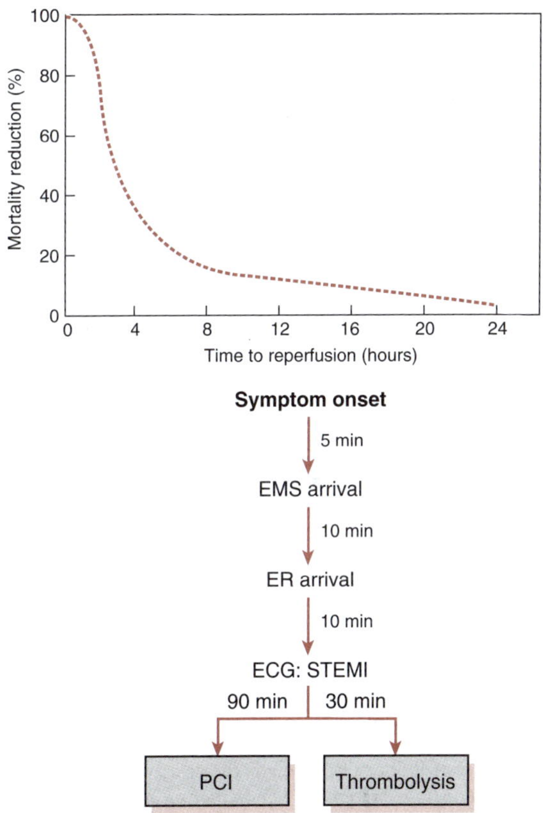

Figure 4-11 The benefit of coronary reperfusion is inversely related to ischemia time. **Top.** Graphic representation of mortality benefit of coronary reperfusion as a function of ischemia time.[78] **Bottom.** Recommended timeline of events following chest pain onset according to AHA/ACC guidelines.[49,79] AHA/ACC, American Heart Association/American College of Cardiology; ECG, electrocardiogram; EMS, emergency medical service; ER, emergency room; PCI, percutaneous coronary intervention; STEMI, ST-segment elevation myocardial infarction.

meet accepted time-to-therapy guidelines, with either rapid transfer to a PCI-capable facility or administration of thrombolytics with subsequent transfer to a PCI center.

- **In the emergency department**, an acute MI protocol should be activated that includes a targeted clinical examination and a 12-lead ECG completed within 10 minutes of arrival.
- The goal of immediate management in patients with STEMI is to identify candidates for reperfusion therapy and to immediately initiate that process. Other priorities include relief of ischemic pain, as well as recognition and treatment of hypotension, pulmonary edema, and arrhythmia.
  - Supplemental oxygen should be administered if saturations are <90%. If necessary, institution of mechanical ventilation decreases the work of breathing and reduces myocardial oxygen demand.
  - Two peripheral IV catheters should be inserted on arrival.
  - Serial ECGs should be obtained for patients who do not have ST-segment elevation on the initial ECG but experience ongoing chest discomfort as they may have an evolving STEMI. Telemetry should be placed to monitor for arrhythmias.

Medications

Upstream medical therapy should include administration of ASA, a second antiplatelet agent, an anticoagulant, and agents that reduce myocardial ischemia (Table 4-19).

- **ASA** 162–325 mg should be given orally (chewed) or rectally immediately to *all* patients with suspected acute MI; 325 mg is preferred for those who are ASA naïve. After PCI, the subsequent dose of ASA is 81 mg/d indefinitely.[51]
- **$P2Y_{12}$ inhibitor** loading dose should be given to all STEMI patients, as part of DAPT, as soon as possible after presentation. Cost and bleeding risk can be taken into consideration when choosing which agent. (Please refer to the "Antiplatelet" section under UA/NSTEMI (p 23) for background information and dosing on agents listed in the following text.)
- If the patient is going for PCI, **one** of the following should be added to ASA and anticoagulant:
  - **Ticagrelor** 180 mg loading dose, then 90 mg bid (Note: maintenance ASA must be <100 mg daily) for a minimum of 12 months. It is the preferred $P2Y_{12}$ inhibitor for ACS because of its mortality advantage over others in this class.
  - **Clopidogrel** 600 mg loading dose, then 75 mg daily for 12 months.
  - **Prasugrel** 60 mg loading dose, then 10 mg daily for minimum of 12 months (contraindicated in patients with prior CVA and avoided in those >75 years and with weight <60 kg). **Prasugrel should only be given after diagnostic angiography** (or within an hour of PCI) given a higher incidence of bleeding compared to clopidogrel.[52]
- If the patient is to receive fibrinolytic therapy, along with ASA and an anticoagulant, patients should receive: Clopidogrel 300 mg loading dose if given during the first 24 hours of therapy; if started 24 hours after administration of fibrinolytics, a 600-mg loading dose is preferred. Maintenance is 75 mg/d.
- Patients older than 75 years should not be given the loading dose. **GPIIb/IIIa inhibitors** do not have a routine role in the initial presentation of STEMI patients or as part of adjunctive therapy with thrombolytics.
- **Anticoagulant therapy** should be initiated on presentation in all patients with STEMI regardless of the choice of PCI or thrombolytic therapy. *Please also refer to the medication section under UA/NSTEMI for background information on agents listed in the following text.*
  - **Anticoagulant choice for patients who will receive primary PCI:**
    - **UFH** is often preferred during PCI by many operators because of the availability and real-time therapeutic monitoring with activating clotting times (ACTs) in the catheterization laboratory. Additional bolus doses of UFH are given at PCI, with the dose and ACT goal dependent on whether a GPIIb/IIIa antagonist has been given.

TABLE 4-19 Upstream Medical Therapy

Medication	Dosage	Comments
Aspirin (ASA)	162–325 mg	Non–enteric-coated formulations (chewed or crushed) given orally or rectally facilitate rapid drug absorption and platelet inhibition.
Clopidogrel	600 mg loading dose, 75–150 mg/d	600 mg loading dose followed by 150 mg maintenance dose for 7 d may reduce the incidence of stent thrombosis and MI compared to the standard 300 mg loading dose and 75 mg maintenance dose. Caution should be taken in the elderly because clinical trials validating clopidogrel use in STEMI either did not include elderly patients or did not use a loading dose.
Prasugrel	60 mg loading dose, 10 mg/d	Compared to clopidogrel, prasugrel is a quicker acting and more potent antiplatelet agent with improved efficacy but significantly increases CABG bleeding rates. Prasugrel should not be used in patients >75 yrs old, <60 kg, or with a history of stroke/TIA.
Ticagrelor	180 mg loading, then 90 mg bid	ASA dose should not exceed 100 mg. Ticagrelor has shown mortality benefit over clopidogrel at the expense of higher bleeding rates.
Cangrelor	30 μg/kg IV bolus, then 4 μg/kg per minute	Currently FDA approved only for patients undergoing PCI. Expense and modest evidence of benefit compared to other $P2Y_{12}$ inhibitors limit use.
Unfractionated heparin (UFH)	60 units/kg IV bolus, 12 units/kg per hour	UFH should be given to all patients undergoing PCI and those receiving thrombolytics with the exception of streptokinase. The maximum IV bolus is 4000 units.
Enoxaparin (LMWH)	30 mg IV bolus, 1 mg/kg SC bid	Patients >75 yrs old should not be given a loading dose and receive 0.75 mg/kg SC bid. An additional loading dose of 0.3 mg/kg should be given if the last dose of LMWH was >8 h before PCI. The use of LMWH is only validated in thrombolysis and rescue PCI.
Bivalirudin	0.75 mg/kg IV bolus, 1.75 mg/kg per hour	Bivalirudin has been validated in patients undergoing PCI and has not been studied in conjunction with thrombolysis. Patients who received a heparin bolus before bivalirudin had a lower incidence of stent thrombosis than those who only received bivalirudin.

(Continued)

TABLE 4-19 Upstream Medical Therapy (Continued)

Medication	Dosage	Comments
Fondaparinux	2.5 mg IV bolus, 2.5 mg SC daily	Shown to be superior to UFH when used during thrombolysis with decreased bleeding rates. Fondaparinux increases the risk of catheter thrombosis when used during PCI.[88]
Nitroglycerin	0.4 mg SL or aerosol infusion; 10–200 μg/min IV	Sublingual or aerosol nitroglycerin can be given every 5 min for a total of three doses in the absence of hypotension. IV nitroglycerin can be used for uncontrolled chest discomfort.
Metoprolol	25 mg PO qid, uptitrate as needed	β-Blockers should be avoided in patients with evidence of heart failure, hemodynamic instability, marked first-degree AV block, advanced heart block, and bronchospasm.

AV, atrioventricular; CABG, coronary artery bypass graft; FDA, the Food and Drug Administration; LMWH, low-molecular-weight heparin; MI, myocardial infarction; PCI, percutaneous coronary intervention; SL, sublingual; STEMI, ST-segment elevation myocardial infarction; TIA, transient ischemic attack.

- **Enoxaparin** use in STEMI patients as an anticoagulant for PCI is unclear, and we generally do not recommend it. An additional IV dose may be needed at PCI depending on the timing of the last dose and total number of doses given.
- **Bivalirudin** can be given to patients already treated with ASA and clopidogrel on presentation.
  - Bivalirudin is an acceptable alternative to the use of combined heparin and GPIIb/IIIa inhibitor during PCI with lower bleeding rates but higher rate of stent thrombosis.[42,43,53,54]
  - It is the agent of choice in patients with known HIT.
  - It can be given with or without prior treatment with UFH. If the patient is being treated with UFH, discontinue UFH for 30 minutes before starting bivalirudin.
  - Dose is 0.75 mg/kg bolus and then 1.75 mg/kg per hour infusion.

- **Patients who will receive fibrinolytic therapy should be started on either:**
  - **UFH** with monitoring to ensure the activated PTT is twice the upper limit of normal. UFH should be continued for at least 48 hours after fibrinolysis. If angiography with intent to perform PCI is anticipated to occur early after fibrinolysis, then UFH may be preferable.
  - **Enoxaparin,** if the serum creatinine is <2.5 mg/dL in men or 2.0 mg/dL in women, an initial 30-mg IV bolus is given followed 15 minutes later with 1 mg/kg SC bid. Give for the entirety of the index hospitalization but not to exceed 8 days.
  - **Bivalirudin** can be used for HIT-positive patients but has not been studied extensively in STEMI patients or patient with fibrinolysis.

- **Anti-ischemic therapy** (also refer to the Medications section under UA/NSTEMI for background information on agents listed here).
  - **Nitroglycerin** should be administered to patients with ischemic chest pain, to aid in control of hypertension, or as part of the management of HF. Nitroglycerin should either be avoided or used with caution in patients with:
    - Hypotension (systolic BP [SBP] <90 mm Hg)
    - RV infarct

    - Heart rate >100 bpm or <50 bpm
    - Documented use of phosphodiesterase inhibitors (e.g., sildenafil) in previous 48 hours
  - **Morphine** (2–4 mg IV) can be used for refractory chest pain that is not responsive to nitroglycerin. Adequate analgesia decreases levels of circulating catecholamines and reduces myocardial oxygen consumption.
  - **BBs** improve myocardial ischemia, limit infarct size, and reduce major adverse cardiac events including mortality, recurrent ischemia, and malignant arrhythmias.
    - Oral BBs should be started in all patients with STEMI within the first 24 hours who do not have signs of new HF, evidence of cardiogenic shock (Killip class II or greater), age older than 70 years, SBP <120 mm Hg, pulse >110 or <60 bpm, or advanced heart block.[55]
    - IV BBs can increase mortality in patients with STEMI and should be reserved for management of arrhythmias or acute treatment of accelerated hypertension in patients without the earlier mentioned features. Sinus tachycardia in the setting of a STEMI may be a compensatory response to maintain cardiac output and should not prompt IV BB use.
    - **Serum electrolyte monitoring**: AHA guidelines recommend maintaining potassium concentration above 4.0 mEq/L and serum magnesium above 2.0 mEq/L.
    - **Treatment of arrhythmias**: Sinus bradycardia can occur especially with inferior wall MI. If the patient is symptomatic, atropine is indicated.
    - AV nodal conduction abnormalities can occur in anterior wall STEMI; symptomatic patients may require temporary pacing.
    - There is no recommendation for either hematopoietic stem cell therapy or colchicine for patients with acute MI.

Acute Coronary Reperfusion

- The majority of patients who suffer an acute STEMI have thrombotic occlusion of a coronary artery. Early restoration of coronary perfusion limits infarct size, preserves LV function, and reduces mortality.
- All other therapies are secondary and should not delay the timely goal of achieving coronary reperfusion.
- Unless spontaneous resolution of ischemia occurs (as determined by resolution of chest discomfort and normalization of ST elevation), the choice of reperfusion strategy includes thrombolysis, primary PCI, or emergent CABG (Figure 4-12).
  - Normalization of the ECG and symptoms should not preclude the patient being referred for urgent diagnostic angiography. Morphine may mask ongoing ischemic symptoms.
  - Note: Ongoing symptoms are not criteria for treatment of STEMI in the first 12 hours of symptom onset. Patients who arrive within 12 hours of their symptoms, despite symptom resolution, but with continued ECG changes of STEMI are still candidates for immediate reperfusion (either primary PCI or fibrinolytics). We recommend angiography with intent for PCI/CABG in such a circumstance.
- The choice of reperfusion therapy should be considered of secondary importance to the overall goal of achieving reperfusion in a timely manner.
  - **Primary PCI**
    - Primary PCI is the preferred reperfusion strategy when available within 90 minutes of first medical contact. Compared to fibrinolytic therapy, PCI offers superior vessel patency and perfusion (TIMI 3 flow) with less reinfarction, less risk of intracranial hemorrhage, and improved survival regardless of lesion location or patient age. STEMI patients with symptom onset <12 hours prior have a better prognosis and outcome after PCI. PCI should still be routinely offered to patients with STEMI who have ongoing symptoms that began 12–24 hours before presentation.

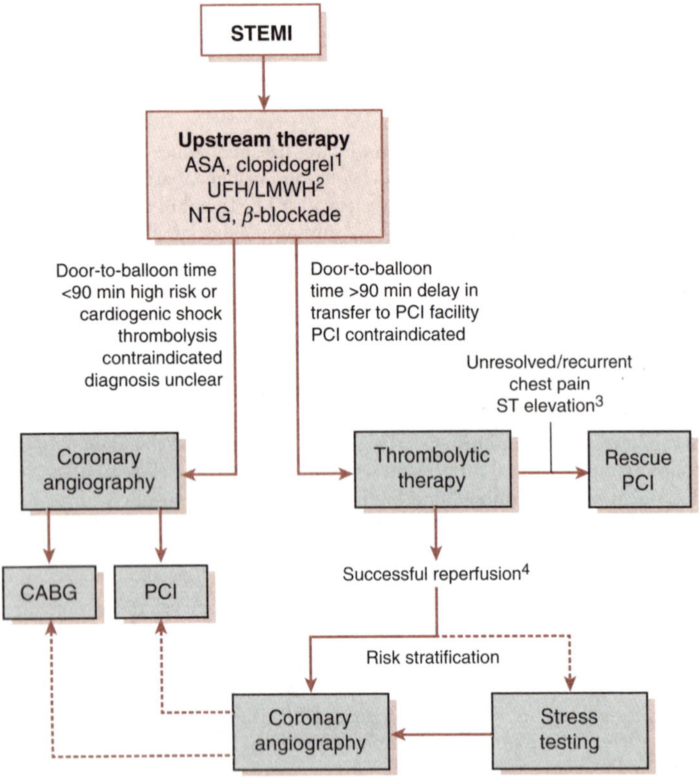

Figure 4-12 Strategies for coronary reperfusion and risk assessment.[1] If fibrinolytics are to be given, use clopidogrel only. If primary PCI is planned, give ticagrelor, prasugrel, or clopidogrel.[2] UFH may be used with either PCI or thrombolytic therapy, whereas bivalirudin has only been studied with PCI and LMWH has only been validated for fibrinolytic therapy and rescue PCI. In patients who are to receive fibrinolysis, LMWH and fondaparinux are preferred to UFH.[3] Patients who do not experience chest pain relief, have recurrent chest pain, have unstable arrhythmias, develop heart failure, or have ST-segment elevations that do not normalize 60–90 minutes following fibrinolysis should undergo rescue PCI.[4] Signs of successful reperfusion include chest pain relief, 50% reduction in ST-segment elevation, and idioventricular rhythm. ASA, aspirin; CABG, coronary artery bypass graft; LMWH, low–molecular-weight heparin; NTG, nitroglycerin; PCI, percutaneous coronary intervention; STEMI, ST-segment elevation myocardial infarction; UFH, unfractionated heparin.

- PCI may also be considered, although evidence of benefit is limited, in patients who are now asymptomatic but had symptoms in the previous 12- to 24-hour period.
- Asymptomatic patients who are hemodynamically and electrically stable without evidence of ischemia and whose symptoms began more than 24 hours prior should not be offered PCI of a totally occluded infarct artery.[56]
- **PCI** is always preferred over fibrinolysis in the following situations:
  - Patients who present with severe HF or cardiogenic shock should receive primary PCI (even if transfer to a PCI center may cause delays beyond current time goals for reperfusion). Patients with Killip class III/IV or TIMI risk score ≥5 represent high-risk groups where PCI is preferred despite a potential time delay.[49,57]

    - Have a contraindication to fibrinolytic therapy.
    - Have had recent PCI or prior CABG.
    - PCI is generally preferred to fibrinolysis in patients with symptom onset >12 hours prior.[58,59]
  - Coronary stenting is superior to balloon angioplasty alone and reduces the rates of target vessel revascularization.
  - Drug-eluting stents further reduce the need for target vessel revascularization without increasing the incidence of stent thrombosis.
  - If the infarct-related artery is successfully treated and patients have lesions in non–infarct-related arteries that are amenable to PCI, there may be a benefit for death or recurrent nonfatal MI to undergo revascularization at the time of STEMI.[60]
  - Patients in shock should have significant lesions in non–infarct-related arteries intervened on if feasible.
  - Transradial approach in STEMI reduces bleeding and may have a mortality benefit compared to transfemoral access.
  - Facilitated PCI, a strategy of reduced dose of GPIIb/IIIa inhibitors and/or fibrinolytic agent just before PCI, should not be routinely used because it does not improve efficacy and significantly increases bleeding rates.
- **Fibrinolytic therapy**
  - Fibrinolytic therapy has the main advantages of widespread availability and ease of delivery. The primary disadvantage of fibrinolytic therapy is the risk of intracranial hemorrhage, uncertainty of whether normal coronary flow has been restored, and risk of reocclusion of the infarct-related artery.
  - Fibrinolysis is indicated when primary PCI is not available in a timely fashion (i.e., delay >120 minutes or time-to-transfer >120 minutes). Transfer to a PCI-capable facility should occur regardless of whether fibrinolytics are given or not.
  - Fibrinolytic therapy is indicated for use if given within 12 hours of the symptom onset with qualifying ECG changes of ST elevation, new LBBB, or true posterior MI. When given, it should be administered within 30 minutes of initial patient contact. Fibrinolytic therapy is most successful when given in the first 3 hours of symptom onset, after which the benefit tapers.
  - Patients presenting to a hospital without PCI capability should be transferred for primary PCI, rather than being given fibrinolytics, if time from first medical contact to PCI will not be >120 minutes. This seems particularly relevant to patients arriving 3–12 hours from symptom onset.
  - In patients transferred for PCI, primary PCI significantly lowered the incidence of death, MI, or stroke compared to on-site thrombolysis.[61,62]
  - All patients should be transferred to a PCI-capable facility after fibrinolysis (early routine angiography); this should occur urgently if patients are in shock or have failed reperfusion.
  - Available thrombolytic agents include the fibrin-selective agents such as **alteplase (recombinant tissue plasminogen activator [rt-PA])**, **reteplase** (r-PA), and **tenecteplase** (TNK-tPA). **Streptokinase** is the only nonselective agent in use. Further details and dosing information can be found in Table 4-20.
    - TNK-tPA is the current agent of choice because of similar efficacy, lower risk of bleeding, and convenient single bolus administration as compared to rt-PA. Streptokinase is the cheapest and still widely used worldwide.
    - Fibrin-selective agents should be used in combination with anticoagulant therapy, ASA, and clopidogrel (see earlier). GPIIb/IIIa inhibitors should not be used in conjunction. Prasugrel and ticagrelor have not been studied for use with fibrinolytics.

TABLE 4-20 Fibrinolytic Agents

Medication	Dosage	Comments
Streptokinase (SK)	1.5 million units IV over 60 min	Produces a generalized fibrinolytic state (not clot specific). SK reduces mortality following STEMI: 18% relative risk reduction and 2% absolute risk reduction.[49] Allergic reactions including skin rashes, fever, and anaphylaxis may be seen in 1%–2% of patients. Isolated hypotension occurs in 10% of patients and usually responds to volume expansion. Because of the development of antibodies, patients who were previously treated with SK should be given an alternate thrombolytic agent.
Recombinant tissue plasminogen activator (rt-PA)	15 mg IV bolus 0.75 mg/kg over 30 min (maximum 50 mg) 0.50 mg/kg over 60 min (maximum 35 mg)	Fibrin-selective agent with improved clot specificity compared to SK. Does not cause allergic reactions or hypotension. Mortality benefit compared to SK at the expense of an increased risk of intracranial hemorrhage.[49]
Reteplase (r-PA)	Two 10-unit IV boluses administered 30 min apart	Fibrin-selective agent with a longer half-life but reduced clot specificity compared to rt-PA. Mortality benefit equivalent to that of rt-PA.[49,89]
Tenecteplase (TNK-tPA)	0.50 mg/kg IV bolus (total dose 30–50 mg)	Genetically engineered variant of rt-PA with slower plasma clearance, improved fibrin specificity, and higher resistance to PAI-1. Mortality benefit equivalent to that of rt-PA with reduced bleeding rates.[49] Monitoring is required with a goal aPTT of 1.5–2.5 times control.

aPTT, activated partial thromboplastin time; PAI-1, plasminogen activator inhibitor-1; STEMI, ST-segment elevation myocardial infarction.

- Fibrinolytic therapy is contraindicated:
  - In patients with ECG evidence of ST-segment depressions (unless posterior MI suspected).
  - In those who are asymptomatic with initial symptoms occurring >24 hours prior (*this is in contrast to patients who are asymptomatic with symptom onset <12 hours prior; see earlier*).
  - In patients with other contraindications to fibrinolysis (Table 4-21).
  - In patients with presence of five or more risk factors for intracranial hemorrhage.
- Any patient who experiences a sudden change in neurologic status should undergo urgent head CT, and all anticoagulant and thrombolytic therapies should be discontinued. Neurological and neurosurgical consultation should be obtained immediately.

TABLE 4-21 Contraindications to Thrombolytic Therapy

Absolute Contraindications	Relative Contraindications
History of intracranial hemorrhage or hemorrhagic stroke	Prior ischemic stroke >3 mo ago
Ischemic stroke within 3 mo	Allergy or previous use of streptokinase (>5 d ago)[a]
Known structural cerebrovascular lesion (AVMs, aneurysms, tumor)	Recent internal bleeding (2–4 wk)
Closed head injury within 3 mo	Prolonged/traumatic CPR more than 10 min
Aortic dissection	Major surgery within 3 wk
Severe uncontrolled hypertension (SBP >180 mm Hg, DBP >110 mm Hg)	Active peptic ulcer disease
Active bleeding or bleeding diathesis	Noncompressible vascular punctures
Acute pericarditis	History of intraocular bleeding
	Pregnancy
	Uncontrolled hypertension
	Use of oral anticoagulants

[a]Thrombolytics other than streptokinase may be used.
AVM, arteriovenous malformation; CPR, cardiopulmonary resuscitation; DBP, diastolic blood pressure; SBP, systolic blood pressure.

- Major bleeding complications that require blood transfusion occur in approximately 10% of patients.
- **Post fibrinolysis care**
  - All patients should receive appropriate DAPT and at least 48 hours of anticoagulation after fibrinolysis.
  - Routine coronary angiography within 24 hours of thrombolysis has reduced adverse cardiac events compared to rescue PCI.[63]
  - Immediate transfer for angiography (3–24 hours after fibrinolysis) at a PCI-capable facility is also proven to be beneficial.[64]
  - Evidence for successful fibrinolysis includes:
    - Relief of chest pain or angina symptoms
    - >50% reduction in ST-segment elevations at 90 minutes
    - Reperfusion arrhythmia (i.e., accelerated idioventricular rhythm) up to 2 hours after completion of infusion
- **Emergency CABG** is a high-risk procedure that should be considered only if the patient has severe left main disease or refractory ischemia in the setting of failed PCI or coronary anatomy that is not amenable to PCI. Emergency surgery should also be considered for patients with acute mechanical complications of MI including papillary muscle rupture, severe ischemic MR, VSD, ventricular aneurysm formation in the setting of intractable ventricular arrhythmias, or ventricular free wall rupture.

Peri-Infarct Management

- **The coronary care unit** (CCU) was the first major advance in the modern era of treatment of acute MI. All patients with STEMI should be observed in a specialized CCU or intensive care unit setting for at least 24 hours after STEMI.
- Bed rest is appropriate intermediate care for the first 24 hours after presentation with an acute MI. After 24 hours, clinically stable patients can progressively advance their activity as tolerated.
- Patients should have continuous telemetry monitoring to detect for recurrent ischemia and arrhythmias.

- Daily evaluation should include assessment for recurrent chest discomfort, new HF symptoms, and routine ECGs. Physical examination should focus on new murmurs and any evidence of HF.
- A baseline echocardiogram should be obtained to document EF, wall motion abnormalities, valvular lesions, and presence of ventricular thrombus.
- **Cardiac pacing** may be required in the setting of an acute MI. Rhythm disturbance may be transient in nature, in which case temporary pacing is sufficient until a stable rhythm returns (see the following text). As compared to inferior wall MIs where AV block is transient and stable, AV block with anterior wall MIs can be unstable with wide QRS escape rhythms with 80% mortality and usually requires temporary and then permanent pacemakers.

Post–ST-Segment Elevation Myocardial Infarction Medical Therapy

- See also Medications section for UA/NSTEMI.
- **ASA** should be continued indefinitely. Dose of 81 mg/d has been shown to be effective after PCI; however, the range of 75–162 mg/d has also been endorsed.
- **Clopidogrel** (75 mg/d), **prasugrel** (10 mg/d), or **ticagrelor** (90 mg bid) should be given for a minimum of 12 months regardless of whether a bare metal stent (BMS) or drug-eluting stent (DES) was used (*this is in contrast to non-ACS patients who receive a BMS and the minimum duration of therapy is 1 month*).
- **BBs** confer a mortality benefit following acute MI. Treatment should begin as soon as possible (preferably within the first 24 hours) and continue indefinitely unless contraindicated.
- **ACE inhibitors** provide a reduction in short-term mortality, incidence of HF, and recurrent MI when initiated within the first 24 hours of an acute MI.[65,66]
  - Patients with EF <40%, large anterior MI, and prior MI derive the most benefit from ACE inhibitor therapy.
  - Contraindications include hypotension, history of angioedema with use, pregnancy, acute renal failure, and hyperkalemia.
  - ARBs can be used in patients who are intolerant of ACE inhibitors.
- **HMG-CoA reductase inhibitors** should be started in all patients in the absence of contraindications. Several trials have shown the benefit of early and aggressive use of high-dose statins following acute MI. The goal is at least 50% reduction in LDL or LDL <70 mg/dL. Patients unable to achieve LDL <70 mg/dL despite a high-intensity should be evaluated for adjunctive therapy with a PCSK9 inhibitor or ezetimibe.[16,17]
- **Aldosterone receptor antagonists (spironolactone and eplerenone)** have shown benefit in post-MI patients with LVEF <40% and in diabetics. Caution should be taken in patients with hyperkalemia and renal insufficiency.[67,68]
- **Warfarin** should not be routinely prescribed to patients with apical hypokinesis in the setting of an anterior MI in the absence of LV thrombus or other indications for anticoagulation. Such therapy is associated with increased bleeding and death. The actual risk of developing LV thrombus is low because many patients will have recovery of hypokinesis.[69]

SPECIAL CONSIDERATIONS

Management of STEMI with Active or High Risk of Bleeding

Bleeding is a well-known complication of any acute coronary syndrome (ACS), including STEMI, and can independently increase the risk of stroke, recurrent MI, or death. Fibrinolysis should be avoided if significant bleeding is a concern. However, if fibrinolysis is deemed necessary, tenecteplase may present a preferable option due to its weight-based dosing, which contributes to a potentially safer bleeding risk profile compared to alteplase. When considering PCI, radial access should be prioritized whenever possible. Regarding anticoagulation during PCI, bivalirudin offers advantages in terms of reduced major bleeding when compared to a combination of heparin and a glycoprotein IIb/IIIa inhibitor. Finally, stent selection should be tailored to the patient's bleeding risk, with a preference for bare metal stents favored over drug-eluting stents in patients with high-bleeding risk.

Risk Assessment

- Asymptomatic patients who present >24 hours after symptom onset, patients who receive medical therapy alone, and patients who receive an incomplete revascularization should undergo further risk assessment. Patients may be evaluated using either noninvasive stress testing or an invasive (coronary angiography) strategy.
- **Stress testing** can be used to determine prognosis, residual ischemia, and functional capacity. Patients who are successfully revascularized do not need stress testing before discharge unless needed for referral to cardiac rehabilitation.
  - A submaximal exercise stress test can be performed as early as 2–3 days following MI in stable patients who have had no further ischemic signs/symptoms or signs of HF.
  - Alternatively, stress testing can be performed after hospital discharge (2–6 weeks) for low-risk patients and for patients starting cardiac rehabilitation.
  - Coronary angiography should be performed in patients with limiting angina, significant ischemic burden, and poor functional capacity.
- Patients treated medically or with fibrinolytics who experience complications of MI, including recurrent angina/ischemia, HF, significant ventricular arrhythmia, or a mechanical complication of the MI, should proceed directly to coronary angiography to define their anatomy and offer an appropriate revascularization strategy.

Special Clinical Situations

- **RVMI** is seen in patients with an acute inferior MI secondary to complete occlusion of the proximal RCA. RV function is very preload dependent, and frequently, hypotension responds to fluid resuscitation.
  - The clinical triad of hypotension, elevated jugular venous pressure, and clear lung fields in the setting of STEMI should prompt an evaluation for RV infarct or massive pulmonary embolism.
  - One-mm ST elevations in the V_1 or V_4R leads are the most sensitive marker of RV involvement.
  - LV filling pressures are typically normal or decreased, the right atrial pressures are elevated (>10 mm Hg), and the cardiac index is depressed. In some patients, elevated right atrial pressures may not be evident until IV fluids are administered.
  - Initial therapy is IV fluids. If hypotension persists, inotropic support with dobutamine and/or IABP may be necessary. Right-sided mechanical support devices are available when pharmacologic support fails.
  - Invasive hemodynamic monitoring is critical in the persistently hypotensive patient because it guides volume status and the need for inotropic and mechanical support.
  - In patients with heart block and AV dyssynchrony, sequential AV pacing has a marked beneficial effect.
- **Restenosis and stent thrombosis** are disease entities unique to patients who have previously undergone PCI.
  - **Restenosis** is a result of neointimal hyperplasia and occurs more frequently in patients with BMS placement, diabetics, long areas of prior stenting, and stenting in small arteries. Restenosis presents most frequently as stable progressive angina and is not affected by the discontinuation of DAPT.
  - **Stent thrombosis** is the thrombotic occlusion of a previously placed coronary stent and presents as ACS or sudden cardiac death. Stent thrombosis is associated with a high mortality rate and poor prognosis.[70,71]

        - Acute stent thrombosis occurs within 24 hours and is due to mechanical procedural complications as well as inadequate anticoagulation and antiplatelet therapies.
        - Subacute stent thrombosis (24 hours to 30 days) is a consequence of inadequate platelet inhibition and mechanical stent complications. Cessation of $P2Y_{12}$ inhibitor therapy during this time yields a 30- to 100-fold risk of stent thrombosis.
        - Late (30 days to 1 year) stent thrombosis and very late stent thrombosis occurs principally with DESs.
        - Neoatherosclerosis is atherosclerotic plaque unique to prior PCI, occurs in previously placed stents, and can predispose a patient to angina or plaque rupture with subsequent ACS.
- **Ischemic MR** is a poor prognostic indicator following MI. Papillary muscle rupture is associated with inferior and posterior infarcts. The anterior papillary muscle has a dual blood supply and is less vulnerable to rupture. The mechanism of chronic MR after STEMI includes papillary muscle dysfunction or leaflet tethering due to posterior wall akinesis.
    - Acute MR from papillary muscle rupture is a severe complication of MI associated with high mortality (see below).
    - Progressive MR following MI may develop as a result of LV chamber dilation, apical remodeling, or posterior wall dyskinesis. These changes lead to leaflet tethering or mitral annular dilation.
    - Echocardiography is the diagnostic modality of choice.
    - Transient ischemic MR occurs secondary to papillary muscle ischemia and results in transient severe MR and pulmonary edema. It can be hard to detect on examining or imaging when ischemia is not induced.
    - Initial treatment of MR involves aggressive afterload reduction and revascularization. *Stable* patients should receive a trial of medical therapy and undergo surgery only if they fail to improve.
- **STEMI** in the setting of recent **cocaine use** presents a unique and challenging management situation.[72] ST elevation can result from myocardial ischemia due to coronary vasospasm, in situ thrombus formation, and/or increased myocardial oxygen demand. The common pathophysiology is excessive stimulation of α- and β-adrenergic receptors. Chest pain due to cocaine use usually occurs within 3 hours but may be seen several days following use.
    - Oxygen, ASA, and heparin (UFH or LMWH) should be administered to all patients with cocaine-associated STEMI.
    - Nitrates should be used preferentially to treat vasospasm. Additionally, benzodiazepines may confer additional relief by decreasing sympathetic tone.
    - BBs are contraindicated; both selective and nonselective BBs should be avoided.
    - Phentolamine (α-adrenergic antagonist) and calcium channel blockers may reverse coronary vasospasm and are recommended as second-line agents.
    - The use of reperfusion therapy is controversial and should be reserved for those patients whose symptoms persist despite initial medical therapy.
        - Primary PCI is the preferred approach for the patient with persistent symptoms and ECG changes despite aggressive medical therapy. It is important to note that coronary angiography and intervention carry a significant risk of worsening vasospasm.
        - Fibrinolytic therapy should be reserved for patients who are clearly having a STEMI and who cannot undergo PCI.

COMPLICATIONS

Myocardial damage predisposes the patient to several potential adverse consequences and complications that should be considered if the patient experiences new clinical signs and/or symptoms. These include recurrent chest pain, cardiac arrhythmias, cardiogenic shock, and mechanical complications of MI (Figure 4-13).

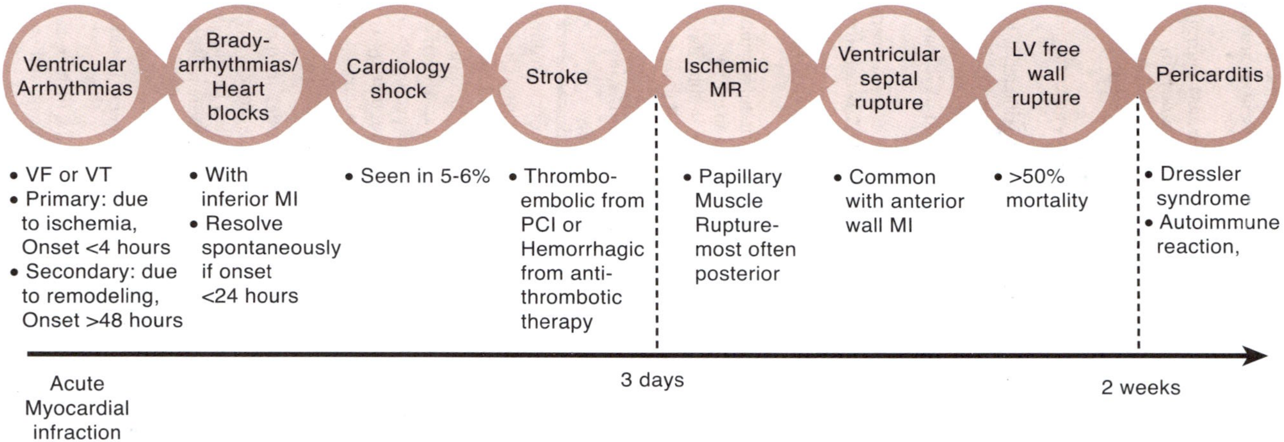

Figure 4-13 Time sequence of complication of MI.

- **Recurrent chest pain** may be due to ischemia in the territory of the original infarction, pericarditis, myocardial rupture, or pulmonary embolism.
  - Recurrent angina is experienced by 20%–30% of patients after MI who receive fibrinolytic therapy and up to 10% of patients in the early time period following percutaneous revascularization. These symptoms may represent recurrence of ischemia or infarct extension.
    - Assessment of the patient may include evaluation for new murmurs or friction rubs, ECG to assess for new ischemic changes, cardiac biomarkers (troponin and CK-MB), echocardiography, and repeat coronary angiography if indicated.
    - Patients with recurrent chest pain should continue to receive ASA, $P2Y_{12}$ inhibition, anticoagulants, nitroglycerin, and BB therapy.
    - If recurrent angina is refractory to medical treatment, urgent repeat coronary angiography and intervention should be considered.
  - **Acute pericarditis** occurs 24–96 hours after MI in approximately 10%–15% of patients. The associated chest pain is often pleuritic and may be relieved in the upright position. A friction rub may be noted on clinical examination, and the ECG may show diffuse ST-segment elevation and PR-segment depression. Lead aVR may have PR elevation. Treatment is directed at pain management.
    - High-dose ASA (up to 650 mg qid maximum) is generally considered a first-line agent. NSAIDs such as ibuprofen may be used if ASA is not effective but should be avoided early after acute MI.
    - Colchicine along with ASA may also be beneficial for recurrent symptoms and may also be superior to each agent alone.
    - Glucocorticoids (prednisone 1 mg/kg daily) may be useful if symptoms are severe and refractory to initial therapy. Steroids should be used sparingly because they may lead to an increased risk of recurrence of pericarditis. Use should also be deferred until at least 4 weeks after acute MI because of their adverse impact on infarct healing and risk of ventricular aneurysm.
    - Heparin should be avoided in the setting of pericarditis with or without pericardial effusion because it may lead to pericardial hemorrhage.
  - **Dressler syndrome** is thought to be an autoimmune process characterized by malaise, fever, pericardial pain, leukocytosis, elevated erythrocyte sedimentation rate, and often a pericardial effusion. In contrast to acute pericarditis, Dressler syndrome occurs 1–8 weeks after MI. Treatment is identical to acute pericarditis.
- **Arrhythmias.** Cardiac rhythm abnormalities are common following MI and may include conduction block, atrial arrhythmias, and ventricular arrhythmias. Arrhythmias that result in hemodynamic compromise require prompt, aggressive intervention. If the arrhythmia precipitates refractory angina or HF, urgent therapy is warranted. For all rhythm disturbances, exacerbating conditions should be addressed, including electrolyte imbalances, hypoxia, acidosis, and adverse drug effects. Details on specific arrhythmias can be found in Table 4-22.
  - **Atropine** should be attempted for all bradyarrhythmias in the setting of STEMI. Bradycardia is a common complication of intense vagal input to the AV node as a result of baroreceptor activation in the myocardium (also called Bezold–Jarisch reflex).
  - **Transcutaneous and transvenous pacing.** Conduction system disease that progresses to complete heart block or results in symptomatic bradycardia can be effectively treated with cardiac pacing. A transcutaneous pacing device can be used under emergent circumstances; however, a temporary transvenous system should be used for longer duration therapy.
    - Absolute indications for temporary transvenous pacing include asystole, symptomatic bradycardia, recurrent sinus pauses, complete heart block, and incessant polymorphic VT.

TABLE 4-22 Arrhythmias Complicating Myocardial Infarction

Arrhythmia	Treatment	Comments
Intraventricular conduction delays	None	The left anterior fascicle is most commonly affected because of isolated coronary blood supply. Bifascicular and trifascicular block may progress to complete heart block and other rhythm disturbances.
Sinus bradycardia	None Atropine 0.5 mg Temporary pacing[a]	Sinus bradycardia is common in patients with RCA infarcts. In the absence of hypotension or significant ventricular ectopy, observation is indicated.
AV block	Temporary pacing[a]	First-degree AV block usually does not require specific treatment. Mobitz I second-degree block occurs more often with inferior MI. The block is usually within the His bundle and does not require treatment unless symptomatic bradycardia is present. Mobitz II second-degree AV block originates below the His bundle and is more commonly associated with anterior MI. Because of the significant risk of progression to complete heart block, patients should be observed in the CCU and treated with temporary pacing if symptomatic. Third-degree AV block complicates large anterior and RV infarcts. In patients with anterior MI, third-degree heart block often occurs 12–24 h after initial presentation and may appear suddenly. Temporary pacing is recommended because of the risk of progression to ventricular asystole.
Sinus tachycardia	None[b]	Sinus tachycardia is common in patients with acute MI and is often due to enhanced sympathetic activity resulting from pain, anxiety, hypovolemia, anxiety, heart failure, or fever. Persistent sinus tachycardia suggests poor underlying ventricular function and is associated with excess mortality.
Atrial fibrillation and flutter	β-Blockers Anticoagulation Cardioversion	Atrial fibrillation and flutter are observed in up to 20% of patients with acute MI. Because atrial fibrillation and atrial flutter are usually transient in the acute MI period, long-term anticoagulation is often not necessary after documentation of stable sinus rhythm.

(Continued)

TABLE 4-22 **Arrhythmias Complicating Myocardial Infarction (Continued)**

Arrhythmia	Treatment	Comments
Accelerated junctional rhythm	None	Accelerated junctional rhythm occurs in conjunction with inferior MI. The rhythm is usually benign and warrants treatment only if hypotension is present.
Ventricular premature depolarizations (VPDs)	β-Blockers if symptomatic[c]	VPDs are common in the course of an acute MI. Prophylactic treatment with lidocaine or other antiarrhythmics has been associated with increased overall mortality and is not recommended.[91]
Accelerated idioventricular rhythm (AIVR)	None	Commonly seen within 48 h of successful reperfusion and is not associated with an increased incidence of adverse outcomes. If hemodynamically unstable, sinus activity may be restored with atropine or temporary atrial pacing.
Ventricular tachycardia (VT)	Cardioversion for sustained VT Lidocaine or amiodarone for 24–48 h[d]	Nonsustained ventricular tachycardia (NSVT, <30 s) is common in the first 24 h after MI and is only associated with increased mortality when occurring late in the post-MI course. Sustained VT (>30 s) during the first 48 h after acute MI is associated with increased in-hospital mortality.
Ventricular fibrillation (VF)	Unsynchronized cardioversion Lidocaine or amiodarone for 24–48 h[d]	VF occurs in up to 5% of patients in the early post-MI period and is life threatening.

[a]Atropine and temporary pacing should only be used for symptomatic or hemodynamically unstable patients.

[b]The use of β-blockers in the setting of sinus tachycardia and poor left ventricular function may result in decompensated heart failure.

[c]β-Blockers should be used with caution in the setting of bradycardia and frequent VPDs as they may increase the risk of polymorphic VT.

[d]Lidocaine should be used as a 1 mg/kg bolus followed by a 1–2 mg/kg per hour infusion. Amiodarone should be given as a 150–300 mg bolus followed by an infusion of 1 mg/kg per hour for 6 hours and then 0.5 mg/kg per hour for 18 hours.

AV, atrioventricular; CCU, coronary care unit; MI, myocardial infarction; RCA, right coronary artery; RV, right ventricular.

- Temporary transvenous pacing may also be warranted for new trifascicular block, new Mobitz II block, and patients with LBBB who require a pulmonary artery catheter, given the risk of developing complete heart block.

◦ **Implantable cardioverter-defibrillators (ICDs)** should not routinely be implanted in patients with reduced LV function following MI or those with VT/VF in the setting of ischemia or immediately following reperfusion (<48 hours).

    - Routine insertion of ICDs into patients with reduced LV function immediately following MI does not improve outcomes.[73]
    - In contrast, patients who continue to have depressed LV function (EF <35% and New York Heart Association [NYHA] class II or III or EF <30% regardless of NYHA class) >40 days following MI benefit from ICD therapy.[74,75]
    - In patients with LVEF <35% less than 40 days post MI, consideration of a wearable cardioverter defibrillation (e.g., Zoll LifeVest) as a bridge to re-evaluation for recovery of EF is reasonable. The clinical data for this are currently late-breaking.
    - ICD therapy is also indicated for patients with recurrent episodes of sustained VT or VF after >48 hours following coronary reperfusion.
- **Cardiogenic shock** is an infrequent, but serious, complication of MI and is defined as hypotension in the setting of inadequate ventricular function to meet the metabolic needs of the peripheral tissue. Risk factors include prior MI, older age, diabetes, and anterior infarction. Organ hypoperfusion may manifest as progressive renal failure, dyspnea, diaphoresis, or mental status changes. Hemodynamic monitoring reveals elevated filling pressures (wedge pressure >20 mm Hg), depressed cardiac index (<2.5 L/kg per minute), and hypotension.
  - Patients with cardiogenic shock in the setting of MI have a mortality rate in excess of 50%. Such patients require invasive hemodynamic monitoring and advanced therapeutic modalities including inotropic and mechanical support.
  - **Dobutamine and milrinone** are the most frequently used medications for inotropic support. They both possess vasodilatory properties (i.e., afterload reducing) and are arrhythmogenic. Milrinone should be avoided in the setting of renal insufficiency.
  - **Dopamine** can be used as both a vasopressor and inotrope but increases the risk of atrial arrhythmias in patients with shock and is not a preferred first-line agent.
  - **Norepinephrine and phenylephrine** may be required to maintain systemic BP. The use of any vasoconstrictive agents in the setting of cardiogenic shock should prompt an evaluation for mechanical circulatory support.
  - **Epinephrine** is a potent vasopressor and inotrope and is frequently used as an adjunct to other medical therapies. There may be some preferential benefit to RV function, and thus, epinephrine may be used for shock secondary to RV infarct or severe RV dysfunction.
  - **Mechanical circulatory support** includes both temporary and durable support devices. Temporary support devices include IABP, Impella catheter, or extracorporeal membrane oxygenation. Temporary support is offered as bridge to recovery or as bridge to decision about long-term durable mechanical support such as an LV assist device (see Chapter 5, Heart Failure and Cardiomyopathy). The choice of temporary support device is not always clear and should be made by a team familiar with the management of cardiogenic shock.
  - All patients with cardiogenic shock should undergo echocardiography to evaluate for mechanical complications of MI (see the following text).
  - **LV thrombus** occurs most often in setting of anterior MI and should be treated with anticoagulation. Warfarin is the recommended long-term anticoagulation agent; direct oral anticoagulants (e.g., rivaroxaban) have not yet been studied. Patients should receive warfarin for 3–6 months unless other indications warrant its continued use.
- **Mechanical complications**
  - **Aneurysm.** After MI, the affected area of the myocardium may undergo infarct expansion and thinning, forming an aneurysm. The wall motion may become dyskinetic, making the endocardial surface susceptible to mural thrombus formation.
    - LV aneurysm is suggested by persistent ST elevation on the ECG and may be diagnosed by imaging studies including ventriculography, echocardiography, and MRI.

- Anticoagulation is warranted to lower the risk of embolic events, especially if a mural thrombus is present.
- Surgical intervention may be appropriate if the aneurysm results in HF or ventricular arrhythmias that are not satisfactorily managed with medical therapy.

◦ **Ventricular pseudoaneurysm.** Incomplete rupture of the myocardial free wall can result in formation of a ventricular pseudoaneurysm. In this case, blood escapes through the myocardial wall and is contained within the visceral pericardium. In the post-CABG patient, hemorrhage from frank ventricular rupture may be contained within the fibrotic pericardial space producing a pseudoaneurysm.
- Echocardiography (TTE with contrast or TEE) is the preferred diagnostic test to assess for a pseudoaneurysm, often allowing differentiation from a true aneurysm.
- Prompt surgical intervention for pseudoaneurysms is advised because of the high incidence of myocardial rupture.

◦ **Free wall rupture** represents a rare but catastrophic complication of STEMI in the modern early-reperfusion era (Table 4-23). Rupture typically occurs within the first week after MI and presents with sudden hemodynamic collapse. This complication can occur after anterior or inferior MI and is more commonly seen in hypertensive women with their first large transmural MI, in patients receiving late therapy with fibrinolytics, and in patients given NSAIDs or glucocorticoids.
- Echocardiography may identify patients with particularly thinned ventricular walls at risk for rupture.
- Emergent surgical correction is necessary.
- Despite optimal intervention, mortality of free wall rupture remains >90%.

◦ **Papillary muscle rupture** (please also refer to earlier MR section) is a rare complication after MI and is associated with abrupt clinical deterioration. The posterior medial papillary muscle is most commonly affected because of its isolated vascular supply, but anterolateral papillary muscle rupture has been reported. Of note, papillary muscle rupture may be seen in the setting of a relatively small acute MI or even NSTEMI.
- The diagnostic test of choice is echocardiography with Doppler imaging and/or TEE because physical examination reveals a murmur in only ~50% of cases.
- Initial medical therapy should include aggressive afterload reduction. Patients with refractory HF and those with hemodynamic instability may require inotropic support with dobutamine and/or IABP. Surgical repair is indicated in the majority of patients.

◦ **Ventricular septal rupture** is most commonly associated with anterior MI occurring 3–5 days after MI. The perforation may follow a direct course between the ventricles or a serpiginous route through the septal wall (Table 4-23).
- Diagnosis can be made by echocardiography with Doppler imaging and often requires TEE.
- Diagnosis should be suspected in the postinfarct patient who develops HF symptoms and a new holosystolic murmur.
- Stabilization with afterload reduction, inotropic support, and/or IABP may be necessary for hemodynamically unstable patients until definitive therapy with surgical repair can be performed.
- In hemodynamically stable patients, surgery is best deferred for at least a week to improve patient outcome. Left untreated, mortality approaches 90%.
- Percutaneous device closure in the cardiac catheterization laboratory can be performed in select patients with an unacceptable surgical risk.

MONITORING/FOLLOW-UP

Routine office visits 1 month after discharge and every 3–12 months thereafter are suggested for patients presenting with an acute MI.

TABLE 4-23 Characteristics of Ventricular Septal Rupture, Rupture of Ventricular Free Wall, and Papillary Muscle Rupture

	Incidence	Time Course	Clinical Manifestations	Physical Manifestations
Ventricular septal rupture	1%–3% without reperfusion therapy 3.9% in those with cardiogenic shock 0.2%–0.34% with fibrinolytic therapy	Bimodal peaks—within 24 h or 3–5 d Seen between 1 and 14 d	Chest pain Dyspnea Hypotension	Harsh holosystolic murmur with thrill S3, accentuated S2 Pulmonary edema RV and LV failure Cardiogenic shock
Rupture of ventricular free wall	1%, fibrinolysis does not reduce risk Primary PCI reduces risk	Bimodal peaks—within 24 h or 3–5 d Seen between 1 and 14 d	Anginal, pleuritic pericardial chest pain Syncope Hypotension Restlessness Sudden death	Jugular venous distention (29%) Pulsus paradoxus (47%) Electromechanical dissociation Cardiogenic shock
Papillary muscle rupture	1%, posteromedial muscle rupture more than anteromedial	Bimodal peaks—within 24 h or 3–5 d Seen between 1 and 14 d	Abrupt-onset dyspnea Pulmonary edema Hypotension	Soft murmur, no thrill, variable signs of RV overload Severe pulmonary edema Cardiogenic shock

- Patients should be instructed to seek more frequent or urgent follow-up evaluation if they experience any noticeable changes in their clinical status.
- Specific plans for long-term follow-up care should be individualized based on clinical status, anatomy, prior interventions, and change in symptoms.
- All patients should be referred for cardiac rehabilitation.

Summary

- A distinction between stable ischemic heart disease and acute coronary syndrome (ACS) is essential where a more acute presentation with troponin elevation (i.e., myocardial infarction) or high-risk chest pain without troponin elevation (i.e., high-risk, UA) is required for the diagnosis.
- Long-term -blocker therapy is not recommended to improve outcomes in patients with chronic coronary disease in the absence of myocardial infarction in the past year, left ventricular ejection fraction ≤50%, or another primary indication for β-blocker therapy.

- Shorter durations of dual antiplatelet therapy are safe and effective in many circumstances, particularly when the risk of bleeding is high, and the ischemic risk is low to moderate.
- For patients with significant left main disease, surgical revascularization is indicated to improve survival relative to that likely to be achieved with medical therapy.
- Radial artery access is recommended in patients undergoing percutaneous intervention who have acute coronary syndrome or stable ischemic heart disease to reduce bleeding and vascular complications compared with a femoral approach.
- Patients with diabetes who have triple-vessel disease should undergo surgical revascularization; percutaneous coronary intervention may be considered if they are poor candidates for surgery.

Scan the QR code to access chapter references.

5 Heart Failure and Cardiomyopathy

Xiaowen Wang, Shane J. LaRue, Justin M. Vader, and Vivek S. Dandin

HEART FAILURE

General Principles

DEFINITION

Heart failure (HF) is a **clinical syndrome** in which either structural or functional abnormalities of the heart impair its ability to fill with or eject blood, resulting in dyspnea, fatigue, and fluid retention.[1] HF is a progressive disorder and is associated with extremely high morbidity and mortality.

CLASSIFICATION

- HF may be due to abnormalities in myocardial contraction (systolic dysfunction), relaxation and filling (diastolic dysfunction), or both.
- Left ventricular (LV) ejection fraction (EF) is used to subdivide HF patients into groups for therapeutic and prognostic purposes. These groups are
  - EF ≤40%: HF with reduced EF (HFrEF).
  - Previous LVEF <40% and a follow-up measurement of LVEF >40%: HFimpEF (HF with improved EF)
  - EF 40%–50%: HF with borderline EF (EF 41%–49% mildly reduced EF) (HFmrEF).
  - EF ≥50%: HF with preserved EF (HFpEF).
- HF is classified in terms of natural history by American College of Cardiology/American Heart Association (ACC/AHA) HF stage and in terms of symptom status by New York Heart Association (NYHA) Functional Class (Tables 5-1 and 5-2).

EPIDEMIOLOGY

- In the United States, over 6.5 million adults over 20 years of age are living with HF and this number is expected to exceed 8 million by 2030.[2]
- In Asia, prevalence rate ranges from 1.26% to 6.7%, varying among different countries and ethnicities.
- Looking specifically at individual countries and areas within Asia, the enormity of the problem becomes clear. For example, in China alone, approximately 4.2 million people have HF, whereas in India, prevalence estimates vary widely between 1.3 and 23 million, and in Southeast Asia, 9 million people are estimated to have HF.
- Approximately 1 million new cases of HF are diagnosed each year.
- HF accounts for approximately 1 million hospitalizations per year.
- Estimated 1- and 5-year mortality rates are 22% and 42.3%, respectively.[3]
- In Asia, patients are younger at HF onset with more severe symptoms, longer hospital stay, and higher mortality rates as compared to their Western counterparts.

TABLE 5-1 American College of Cardiology/American Heart Association Guidelines of Evaluation and Management of Chronic Heart Failure in Adults

Stage	Description	Treatment
A	No structural heart disease and no symptoms but risk factors: CAD, HTN, DM, cardio toxins, familial cardiomyopathy	Lifestyle modification—diet, exercise, smoking cessation; treat hyperlipidemia and use ACE inhibitor for HTN
B	No signs and symptoms of HF and evidence of one of the following: • Structural heart disease • Evidence of raised filling pressures • Patients with risk factors (raised BNP/persistently elevated cardiac troponin)	Lifestyle modifications, ACE inhibitor, β-adrenergic blockers
C	Structural heart disease and HF symptoms	Lifestyle modifications, ACE inhibitor, β-adrenergic blockers, diuretics, digoxin
D	Refractory HF symptoms to maximal medical management	Therapy listed under A, B, and C, and mechanical assist device, heart transplantation, continuous IV inotropic infusion, hospice care in selected patients

Adapted from HuntSA, AbrahamWT, ChinMH, et al. ACC/AHA guidelines for the evaluation and management of chronic heart failure in the adult: executive summary. *J Am Coll Cardiol.* 2005;46:1116.

ACE, angiotensin-converting enzyme; CAD, coronary artery disease; DM, diabetes mellitus; HF, heart failure; HTN, hypertension; LV, left ventricular; MI, myocardial infarction.

TABLE 5-2 New York Heart Association (NYHA) Functional Classification

NYHA Class	Symptoms
I (Mild)	No symptoms or limitation while performing ordinary physical activity (walking, climbing stairs, etc.).
II (Mild)	Mild symptoms (mild shortness of breath, palpitations, fatigue, and/or angina) and slight limitation during ordinary physical activity.
III (Moderate)	Marked limitation in activity because of symptoms, even during less than ordinary activity (walking short distances [20–100 m]). Comfortable only at rest.
IV (Severe)	Severe limitations with symptoms even while at rest. Mostly bedbound patients.

ETIOLOGY

- Coronary artery disease (CAD) is the most frequent cause of HF in the United States and also worldwide. Other risk factors with high population attributable risk include tobacco use, hypertension, diabetes, and obesity.[2]

- Other causes include valvular heart disease, toxin induced (alcohol, cocaine, chemotherapy), myocarditis (infectious or autoimmune), familial cardiomyopathy, infiltrative disease (amyloidosis, sarcoidosis, hemochromatosis), peripartum cardiomyopathy (PPCM), hypertrophic cardiomyopathy (HCM), constrictive pericardial disease, high-output states (i.e., arteriovenous malformation or fistula), generalized myopathy (Duchenne or Becker muscular dystrophy), tachycardia-induced cardiomyopathy, ventricular noncompaction cardiomyopathy, endomyocardial fibrosis (EMF), stress-induced cardiomyopathy, and idiopathic cardiomyopathy.
- HF exacerbations may be precipitated by dietary and medication noncompliance; however, myocardial ischemia, hypertension (accelerated hypertension), arrhythmias (particularly atrial fibrillation), infection, volume overload, alcohol/toxins, thyroid disease, drugs (NSAIDs, calcium channel blockers, doxorubicin), and pulmonary embolism are also potential triggers.

PATHOPHYSIOLOGY

- HF begins with an initial insult leading to myocardial injury.
- Regardless of etiology, the myocardial injury leads to a pathologic remodeling, which manifests as an increase in LV volume (dilatation) and/or mass (hypertrophy).
- Compensatory adaptations initially maintain cardiac output; specifically, there is activation of the renin–angiotensin–aldosterone system (RAAS) and vasopressin (antidiuretic hormone), which leads to increased sodium retention and peripheral vasoconstriction. The sympathetic nervous system is also activated, with increased levels of circulating catecholamines, resulting in increased myocardial contractility. Over time, these neurohormonal pathways result in direct cellular toxicity, fibrosis, arrhythmias, and pump failure.
- Cardiac dysfunction and pathologic remodeling alter the ventricular pressure–volume relationship, leading to an increase in chamber pressures, resulting in pulmonary and systemic venous congestion.

Diagnosis

CLINICAL PRESENTATION

History

- Affected patients most commonly present with symptoms of HF, including the following:
  - Dyspnea (on exertion and/or at rest)
  - Fatigue
  - Exercise intolerance
  - Orthopnea, paroxysmal nocturnal dyspnea
  - Bendopnea (dyspnea when leaning forward)
  - Systemic or pulmonary venous congestion (lower extremity swelling or cough/wheezing)
  - Presyncope, palpitations, and angina may also be present
- Other possible presentations include incidental detection of asymptomatic cardiomegaly or symptoms related to coexisting arrhythmia, conduction disturbance, thromboembolic complications, or sudden death.
- Clinical manifestations of HF vary depending on the severity and rapidity of cardiac decompensation, underlying etiology, age, and comorbidities of the patient.
- Extreme decompensation may present as cardiogenic shock (resulting from both low arterial and high venous pressures), characterized by hypoperfusion of vital organs, leading to renal failure—cardiorenal syndrome—(decreased urine output), mental status changes (confusion and lethargy), or "shock liver" (elevated liver function tests).

Physical Examination

- The goal of the physical examination in HF is to estimate intracardiac pressures, ventricular compliance, cardiac output, and end-organ perfusion.
- Elevated right-sided pressures result in lower extremity edema, jugular venous distension (JVD), basal crepitations, S3 gallop, sustained abdominojugular reflux, pleural and pericardial effusions, hepatic congestion, and ascites.
  - JVD is the most specific and reliable physical examination indicator of right-sided volume overload and is representative of left-sided filling pressures except in cases of disproportionate right heart dysfunction (e.g., pulmonary hypertension, severe tricuspid regurgitation, and pericardial disease).
  - JVD is best visualized with oblique light and the patient at 45 degrees. Venous pulsations are differentiated from carotid pulsation by their biphasic nature, respiratory variability, and compressibility.
  - Abdominojugular reflux suggests an impaired ability of the right ventricle to handle augmented preload and may be due to constriction or pulmonary hypertension in addition to myocardial disease.
- Elevated left-sided pressures may result in pulmonary rales, but rales are absent in the majority of HF patients with elevated left-sided filling pressures.
- In the setting of systolic dysfunction, a third (S_3) or fourth (S_4) heart sound as well as the holosystolic murmurs of tricuspid or mitral regurgitation (MR) may be present; carotid upstrokes may also be diminished.
- Low cardiac output is suggested by a proportional pulse pressure (pulse pressure/diastolic blood pressure) ≤25%, diminished carotid upstroke, and cool extremities.
- Useful framework in the bedside evaluation of patients with acute heart failure was developed by Stevenson and colleagues, which focuses on the adequacy of perfusion ("cold" vs. "warm") and congestion at rest ("wet" vs. "dry") (Figure 5-1).

Acute Decompensated Heart Failure

Acute decompensated heart failure (ADHF) is the most common form of heart failure that accounts for nearly 80% of hospitalizations. The causes are as follows:

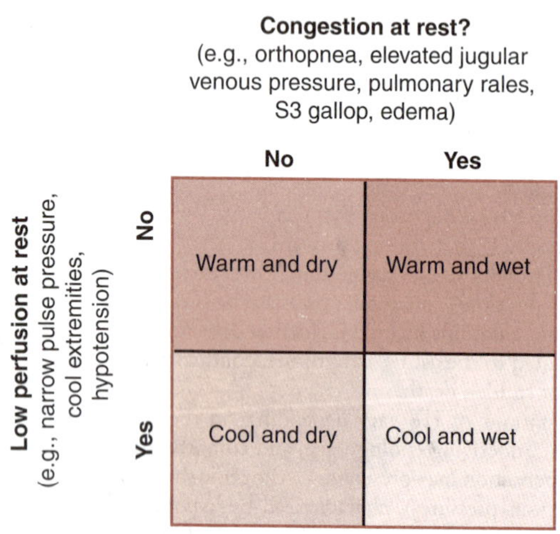

Figure 5-1 Types of clinical presentation of heart failure.

- Nonadherence to medication or dietary restrictions
- Arrhythmias
- Uncontrolled hypertension
- Infections
- Acute coronary syndrome/ischemia
- Alcohol intoxication or excess
- Thyrotoxicosis
- Pregnancy
- Other iatrogenic conditions, such as postoperative fluid replacement or administration of steroids or nonsteroidal anti-inflammatory drugs
- New-onset anemia or renal dysfunction

DIAGNOSTIC TESTING

Laboratories

- Initial laboratory studies should include complete blood count (CBC), urinalysis, serum electrolytes, blood urea nitrogen (BUN), creatinine, calcium, magnesium, glucose, liver function tests, lipid profile, and thyroid function tests.
- B-type natriuretic peptide (BNP) and the biologically inactive cleavage product N-terminal prohormone BNP (NT-proBNP) are released by myocytes in response to stretch, volume overload, and increased filling pressures. Elevated BNP/NT-proBNP is present in patients with asymptomatic LV dysfunction as well as symptomatic HF.
- BNP and NT-proBNP levels have been shown to correlate with HF severity and to predict survival.[4,5] A serum BNP >400 pg/mL is consistent with HF; however, specificity is reduced in patients with renal dysfunction. A serum BNP level <100 pg/mL has a good negative predictive value to exclude HF in patients presenting with dyspnea.[6] Age-specific cut points have also been identified, for example, NT-proBNP levels of 450, 900, and 1800 pg/mL optimally identified acute HF for patients age <50, 50–75, and >75, respectively.[5]
- High-sensitivity troponin tests are used to diagnose acute myocardial infarction with acute heart failure.
- Additional laboratory testing in a patient with new-onset HF without CAD may include diagnostic tests for HIV, hepatitis, and hemochromatosis. When clinically suspected, serum tests for rheumatologic diseases (antinuclear antibody [ANA], antineutrophil cytoplasmic antibody [ANCA], etc.), amyloidosis (serum protein electrophoresis [SPEP], urine protein electrophoresis [UPEP]), or pheochromocytoma (catecholamines) should be considered.[7]

Electrocardiography

An ECG should be performed to look for evidence of ischemia (ST-T wave abnormalities), hypertrophy (increased voltage), infiltration (reduced voltage), previous myocardial infarction (MI) (Q waves), conduction block (PR interval), interventricular conduction delays (QRS), and arrhythmias (supraventricular and ventricular).

Imaging

- Chest radiography should be performed to evaluate the presence of pulmonary edema or cardiomegaly and rule out other etiologies of dyspnea (e.g., pneumonia, pneumothorax). Although chest radiograph findings of cephalization and interstitial edema are highly specific for identifying patients presenting with acute HF (specificity of 98% and 99%, respectively), they have limited sensitivity (41% and 27%, respectively).[8]
- An echocardiogram should be performed to assess right ventricular (RV) and LV systolic and diastolic function, valvular structure and function, and chamber size and to exclude cardiac tamponade.

- LV function may also be evaluated using radionuclide ventriculography (i.e., multigated acquisition [MUGA] scan) or cardiac catheterization with ventriculography and invasive hemodynamics.
- Coronary angiogram with ventriculography is useful in diagnosing acute stress cardiomyopathy with ST elevation and normal epicardial coronaries.
- Cardiac MRI may also be useful in assessing ventricular function and evaluating the presence of intracardiac shunting, valvular heart disease, infiltrative cardiomyopathy, myocarditis, and previous MI.

Diagnostic Procedures

- Coronary angiography should be performed in patients with angina or evidence of ischemia by ECG or stress testing, unless the patient is not a candidate for revascularization.[7]
- Stress nuclear imaging or echocardiography may be an acceptable alternative for assessing ischemia in patients presenting with HF who have known CAD and no angina, unless they are ineligible for revascularization.[7]
- Right heart catheterization with placement of a pulmonary artery catheter may help guide therapy in patients with hypotension and evidence of shock.
- Cardiopulmonary exercise testing with measurement of peak oxygen consumption (VO_2) is useful in assessing functional capacity and in identifying candidates for heart transplantation.[9]
- Endomyocardial biopsy should be considered when seeking a specific diagnosis that would influence therapy, specifically in patients with rapidly progressive and unexplained cardiomyopathy, those in whom active myocarditis, especially giant cell myocarditis, is considered, and those with possible infiltrative processes such as cardiac amyloidosis and sarcoidosis.[10]

Treatment of Heart Failure

PHARMACOTHERAPY

- In general, pharmacologic therapy in chronic HF is aimed at blocking the neurohormonal pathways that contribute to cardiac remodeling and the progression of HF, while reducing symptoms, hospitalizations, and mortality.
- The cornerstone of medical therapy for HF includes RAAS blockade, β-adrenergic blockade, vasodilators, and diuretic therapy for volume overload.
- Pharmacotherapy is determined by the presence of a preserved or reduced LVEF. Several pharmacotherapies for HFrEF have been demonstrated to reduce death and hospitalization and improve quality of life in HF. No pharmacotherapy has been unequivocally demonstrated to improve mortality in patients with HFpEF.

Chronic Medical Therapy With Reduced Ejection Fraction (HFrEF)

- **β-Adrenergic receptor antagonists (β-blockers)** (Table 5-3). β-Blockers are a critical component of HF therapy and work by blocking the toxic effects of chronic adrenergic stimulation on the heart.
    - Large randomized trials have documented the beneficial effects of β-blockers on functional status, disease progression, and survival in patients with NYHA class II–IV symptoms.
    - Improvement in LVEF, exercise tolerance, and functional class are common after the institution of a β-blocker.[11]
    - Typically, 2–3 months of therapy is required to observe significant effects on LV function, but reduction of cardiac arrhythmia and incidence of sudden cardiac death (SCD) may occur much earlier.[12]

- β-Blockers should be instituted at a low dose and titrated with careful attention to blood pressure and heart rate. Some patients experience volume retention and worsening HF symptoms that typically respond to transient increases in diuretic therapy.
- The survival benefit of β-blockers is proportional to the heart rate reduction achieved.[13]
- Individual β-blockers have unique properties, and the beneficial effect of β-blockers may not be a class effect. Therefore, one of the three β-blockers with proven benefit on mortality in large clinical trials should be used[1]:
  - Carvedilol[14,15]
  - Metoprolol succinate[16]
  - Bisoprolol[17]
- **Angiotensin-converting enzyme (ACE) inhibitors** (see Table 5-3) attenuate vasoconstriction, vital organ hypoperfusion, hyponatremia, hypokalemia, and fluid retention attributable to compensatory activation of the renin–angiotensin system. They are the first choice for antagonism of the RAAS.

TABLE 5-3 Drugs Commonly Used for Treatment of Heart Failure

Drug	Initial Dose	Target
Angiotensin-Converting Enzyme Inhibitors		
Captopril	6.25–12.5 mg tid	50 mg tid
Enalapril	2.5 mg bid	10 mg bid
Fosinopril	5–10 mg daily; can use bid	20 mg daily
Lisinopril	2.5–5.0 mg daily; can use bid	10–20 mg bid
Quinapril	2.5–5.0 mg bid	10 mg bid
Ramipril	1.25–2.5 mg bid	5 mg bid
Trandolapril	0.5–1.0 mg daily	4 mg daily
Angiotensin Receptor Blockers		
Valsartan	40 mg bid	160 mg bid
Losartan	25 mg daily; can use bid	25–100 mg daily
Irbesartan	75–150 mg daily	75–300 mg daily
Candesartan[a]	2–16 mg daily	2–32 mg daily
Olmesartan	20 mg daily	20–40 mg daily
Angiotensin Receptor-Neprilysin Inhibitor		
Entresto (Sacubitril/Valsartan)	24/26 mg bid	97/103 mg bid
IKf Channel Inhibitor		
Ivabradine	5 mg bid	7.5 mg bid
Thiazide Diuretics		
HCTZ	25–50 mg daily	25–50 mg daily
Metolazone	2.5–5.0 mg daily or bid	10–20 mg total daily
Loop Diuretics		
Bumetanide	0.5–1.0 mg daily or bid	10 mg total daily (maximum)

(Continued)

TABLE 5-3 Drugs Commonly Used for Treatment of Heart Failure (Continued)

Drug	Initial Dose	Target
Furosemide	20–40 mg daily or bid	400 mg total daily (maximum)
Torsemide	10–20 mg daily or bid	200 mg total daily (maximum)
Aldosterone Antagonists		
Eplerenone	25 mg daily	50 mg daily
Spironolactone	12.5–25.0 mg daily	25 mg daily
β-Blockers		
Bisoprolol	1.25 mg daily	10 mg daily
Carvedilol	3.125 mg bid	25–50 mg bid
Metoprolol succinate	12.5–25.0 mg daily	200 mg daily
Digoxin	0.125–0.25 mg daily	0.125–0.25 mg daily

[a]Valsartan and candesartan are the only US Food and Drug Administration–approved angiotensin II receptor blockers in the treatment of heart failure.
HCTZ, hydrochlorothiazide.

- Multiple large clinical trials have clearly demonstrated that ACE inhibitors improve symptoms and survival in patients with LV systolic dysfunction.[1]
- ACE inhibitors may also prevent the development of HF in patients with asymptomatic LV dysfunction and in those at high risk of developing structural heart disease or HF symptoms (e.g., patients with CAD, diabetes mellitus, hypertension).
- Currently, no consensus has been reached regarding the optimal dosing of ACE inhibitors in HF, although higher doses have been shown to reduce morbidity without improving overall survival.[18]
- Absence of an initial beneficial response to treatment with an ACE inhibitor does not preclude long-term benefit.
- Most ACE inhibitors are excreted by the kidneys, necessitating careful dose titration in patients with renal insufficiency. ACE inhibitors should be used cautiously in the presence of renal dysfunction and use should be avoided in patients with bilateral renal artery stenosis. Renal function and potassium levels should be monitored with dose adjustment and periodically with chronic use.
- A rise in serum creatinine up to 30% above baseline may be seen when initiating an ACE inhibitor and should not result in reflexive discontinuation of therapy.[19]
- Additional adverse effects may include cough, rash, angioedema, dysgeusia, increase in serum creatinine, proteinuria, hyperkalemia, and leukopenia.
- Oral potassium supplements, potassium salt substitutes, and potassium-sparing diuretics should be used with caution during treatment with an ACE inhibitor.
- Agranulocytosis and angioedema are more common with captopril than with other ACE inhibitors, particularly in patients with associated collagen vascular disease or serum creatinine >1.5 mg/dL.
- **ACE inhibitors are contraindicated in pregnancy. Enalapril and captopril may be safely used by breastfeeding mothers.**

- **Angiotensin II receptor blockers (ARBs)** (see Table 5-3) inhibit the renin–angiotensin system via specific blockade of the angiotensin II receptor.
  - ARBs reduce morbidity and mortality associated with HF in patients who are not receiving an ACE inhibitor[20-22] and therefore should be instituted when ACE inhibitors are not tolerated.[1]

  - In contrast to ACE inhibitors, ARBs do not increase bradykinin levels and therefore are not associated with cough.
  - Renal precautions and monitoring for ARB use are similar to ACE inhibitor use.
  - Use of ARBs is contraindicated in patients taking ACE inhibitors and aldosterone antagonists due to a high risk for hyperkalemia.
  - **ARBs are contraindicated in pregnancy and breastfeeding.**
- **Sacubitril/valsartan (Entresto™)** is a combination of the ARB valsartan and the neprilysin inhibitor sacubitril.
  - Neprilysin is a neutral endopeptidase involved in the degradation of vasoactive peptides including the natriuretic peptides, bradykinin, and adrenomedullin. Inhibition of neprilysin increases the availability of these peptides, which exert favorable effects in HF.
  - Sacubitril/valsartan was shown to be *superior* to enalapril in reducing death and rehospitalization among NYHA class II–IV patients with HFrEF who were stably tolerant of ACE inhibitor or ARB therapy.[23,24]
  - Sacubitril/valsartan is approved for use in patients with HFrEF and NYHA class II–IV symptoms who are already tolerant to ACE inhibitors or ARBs.
  - Forthcoming clinical trials will determine its role as initial therapy for HFrEF and in treatment of NYHA class IV HF.
  - Rates of angioedema are increased with sacubitril/valsartan compared with ACE inhibitors.
- **Mineralocorticoid receptor antagonists (MRAs)** attenuate aldosterone-mediated sodium retention, vascular reactivity, oxidant stress, inflammation, and fibrosis.
  - **Spironolactone** is a nonselective aldosterone receptor antagonist that has been shown to improve survival and decrease hospitalizations in NYHA class III–IV patients with low EF.[25]
  - **Eplerenone** is a selective aldosterone receptor antagonist without the estrogenic side effects of spironolactone. It has proven beneficial in patients with HF following MI[26] and in less symptomatic HF patients (NYHA class II) with reduced EF.[27]
  - MRAs are recommended for use in patients with NYHA class II–IV HF and acceptable renal function (serum creatinine is <2.5 mg/dL in men or <2.0 mg/dL in women, and potassium is <5.0 mEq/L) (see Table 5-3).
  - Life-threatening hyperkalemia may occur with the use of these agents. Serum potassium must be monitored closely after initiation; concomitant use of ACE inhibitors and NSAIDs and the presence of renal insufficiency increase the risk of hyperkalemia.
  - Gynecomastia may develop in 10%–20% of men treated with spironolactone; eplerenone should be used in this case.
- **SGLT2 inhibitors:** These medications inhibit sodium glucose cotransporter 2 in the proximal renal tubule, thereby decreasing glucose reabsorption by the kidney. SGLT2i are recommended for patients with symptomatic chronic HFrEF to reduce hospitalizations for HF and cardiovascular mortality, irrespective of the presence of type 2 diabetes in patients.
  - Dapagliflozin (10 mg once daily) and empagliflozin (10 mg once daily)
  - Adverse effects may include fatigue, hypoglycemia, increased urine output, elevated hematocrit levels, and mycotic genital or urinary tract infections.
- **Vasodilator therapy** alters preload and afterload conditions to improve cardiac output.
  - **Hydralazine** acts directly on arterial smooth muscle to produce vasodilation and to reduce afterload.
  - **Nitrates** are predominantly venodilators and help relieve symptoms of venous and pulmonary congestion. They also reduce myocardial ischemia by decreasing ventricular filling pressures and by directly dilating coronary arteries.
  - **A combination of hydralazine and isosorbide dinitrate** (starting dose: 37.5/20 mg three times daily), when added to standard therapy with β-blockers and ACE inhibitors, has been shown to reduce mortality in African American patients.[28]
  - In the absence of ACE inhibitors, ARBs, aldosterone receptor antagonists, and β-blockers, the combination of nitrates and hydralazine improves survival in patients

with HFrEF[29] and should therefore be considered for use in all HFrEF patients unable to tolerate RAAS blockade.
  - Reflex tachycardia and increased myocardial oxygen consumption may occur in the setting of hydralazine use, requiring cautious use in patients with ischemic heart disease.
  - Nitrate therapy may precipitate hypotension in patients with reduced preload.
- **Ivabradine** is an inhibitor of the IK*f* channel involved in generating "pacemaker" currents in cardiac tissue.
  - Use of ivabradine in outpatients with HFrEF was shown to reduce HF hospitalization and HF death,[30] and it is indicated for the reduction of HF hospitalization in patients with EF <35%, stable HF symptoms, and sinus rhythm with a resting heart rate ≥70 bpm who are already taking β-blockers at the highest tolerated dose.[24]
- **Digitalis glycosides** increase myocardial contractility and may attenuate the neurohormonal activation associated with HF.
  - Digoxin has been shown to decrease rates of HF hospitalizations without improving overall mortality.[31]
  - Digoxin has a **narrow therapeutic index**, and serum levels should be followed closely, particularly in patients with unstable renal function.
  - The usual daily dose is 0.125–0.25 mg and should be decreased in patients with renal insufficiency.
  - Clinical benefits may not be related to serum levels. Although serum digoxin levels of 0.8–2.0 ng/mL are considered therapeutic, toxicity can occur in this range.
  - Women and patients with higher serum digoxin levels (1.2–2.0 ng/mL) have an increased mortality risk.[32,33]
  - Discontinuation of digoxin in patients who are stable on a regimen of digoxin, diuretics, and an ACE inhibitor may result in clinical deterioration.[34]
  - Drug interactions with digoxin are common and may lead to toxicity. Agents that may increase levels include erythromycin, tetracycline, quinidine, verapamil, flecainide, and amiodarone. Electrolyte abnormalities (particularly hypokalemia), hypoxemia, hypothyroidism, renal insufficiency, and volume depletion may also exacerbate toxicity.
  - Digoxin is not dialyzable, and toxicity is only treatable by the administration of digoxin immune Fab.
  - Vericiguat is a soluble guanylyl cyclase stimulator recommended for use in selected high-risk patients with HFrEF who are already on Goal Directed Medical Therapy. It helps reduce HF hospitalizations and cardiovascular death.
  - In patients with HF class II to IV symptoms, omega-3 polyunsatuated fatty acids (PUFA) supplementation may be considered a reasonable adjunctive therapy to reduce mortality and cardiovascular hospitalizations.
- **α-Adrenergic receptor antagonists** have not been shown to improve survival in HF, and hypertensive patients treated with doxazosin as first-line therapy are at increased risk of developing HF.[35]
- **Calcium channel blockers** have no favorable effects on mortality in HFrEF.
  - Dihydropyridine calcium channel blockers such as amlodipine may be used in hypertensive HF patients already on maximal guideline-directed medical therapy; however, these agents do not improve mortality.[36,37]
  - Nondihydropyridine calcium channel blockers should be avoided in HFrEF because their negative inotropic effects may potentiate worsening HF.
- **Diuretic therapy** (see Table 5-3), in conjunction with restriction of dietary sodium and fluids, often leads to clinical improvement in patients with symptomatic HF. Frequent assessment of the patient's weight and careful observation of fluid intake and output are essential during initiation and maintenance of therapy. Frequent complications of therapy include hypokalemia, hyponatremia, hypomagnesemia, volume contraction alkalosis, intravascular volume depletion, and hypotension. Serum electrolytes, BUN, and creatinine levels should be followed after institution of diuretic therapy.

Hypokalemia may be life threatening in patients who are receiving digoxin or in those who have severe LV dysfunction that predisposes them to ventricular arrhythmias. Potassium supplementation or a potassium-sparing diuretic should be considered in addition to careful monitoring of serum potassium levels.

- **Potassium-sparing diuretics (amiloride)** do not exert a potent diuretic effect when used alone.
- **Thiazide diuretics (hydrochlorothiazide, chlorthalidone)** can be used as initial agents in patients with normal renal function in whom only a mild diuresis is desired. **Metolazone**, unlike other oral thiazides, exerts its action at the proximal and distal tubule and may be useful in combination with a loop diuretic in patients with a low glomerular filtration rate.
- **Loop diuretics (furosemide, torsemide, bumetanide, ethacrynic acid)** should be used in patients who require significant diuresis and in those with markedly decreased renal function.
  - Furosemide reduces preload acutely by causing direct venodilation when administered intravenously, making it useful for managing severe HF or acute pulmonary edema.[38]
  - Use of loop diuretics may be complicated by hyperuricemia, hypocalcemia, ototoxicity, rash, and vasculitis. Furosemide, torsemide, and bumetanide are sulfa derivatives and may rarely cause drug reactions in sulfa-sensitive patients; ethacrynic acid can be used in such patients.
  - Dose equivalence of oral loop diuretics is approximately 50 mg ethacrynic acid = 40 mg furosemide = 20 mg torsemide = 1 mg bumetanide.

Medical therapy of HFmrEF are as follows:

(1) Diuretics; (2a) SGLT2i; (2b) ACEi, ARB, ARNi; (2b) MRA; (2b) Evidence-based beta blockers for HFrEF (Figure 5-2).

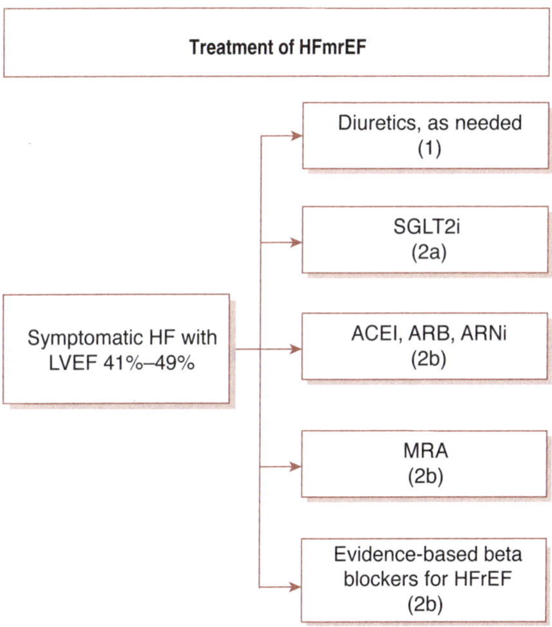

Figure 5-2 Treatment of HFmrEF.

Chronic medical therapy with preserved ejection fraction (HFpEF):

(1) Diuretics; (2b) SGLT2i; (2b) ARNi; (2b) MRA; (2b) ARB

- No pharmacotherapy has been definitively shown to improve mortality in HFpEF.
- Control of blood pressure is recommended.
  - The use of ACE inhibitors, ARBs, spironolactone, and β-blockers is reasonable. Use of these particular agents may be associated with a small reduction in HF hospitalization rates.[22]
  - **Spironolactone** reduced HF hospitalization in patients with HFpEF in a large randomized trial, but mortality was not reduced.[39]
- Treatment of atrial fibrillation through rate or rhythm control in accordance with practice guidelines is recommended.
- Treatment of coronary disease and angina through pharmacotherapy and/or revascularization in accordance with practice guidelines is recommended.

Parenteral Agents

- **Parenteral vasodilators** should be reserved for patients with severe HF not responding to oral medications. Intravenous (IV) vasodilator therapy may be guided by central hemodynamic monitoring (pulmonary artery catheterization) to assess efficacy and avoid hemodynamic instability. Parenteral agents should be started at low doses, titrated to the desired hemodynamic effect, and discontinued slowly to avoid rebound vasoconstriction.
- **Nitroglycerin** is a potent vasodilator with effects on venous and, to a lesser extent, arterial vascular beds. It relieves pulmonary and systemic venous congestion and is an effective coronary vasodilator. Nitroglycerin is the preferred vasodilator for treatment of HF in the setting of acute MI or unstable angina.
- **Sodium nitroprusside** is a direct arterial vasodilator with less potent venodilatory properties. Its predominant effect is to reduce afterload, and it is particularly effective in patients with HF who are hypertensive or who have severe aortic or mitral valvular regurgitation. Nitroprusside should be used cautiously in patients with myocardial ischemia because of a potential reduction in regional myocardial blood flow (**coronary steal**).
  - The initial dose of **0.25 μg/kg/min** can be titrated (**maximum dose of 10 μg/kg/min**) to the desired hemodynamic effect or until hypotension develops.
  - The half-life of nitroprusside is 1–3 minutes, and its metabolism results in the release of cyanide, which is metabolized by the liver to thiocyanate and is then excreted via the kidney.
  - Toxic levels of thiocyanate (>10 mg/dL) may develop in patients with renal insufficiency. Thiocyanate toxicity may manifest as nausea, paresthesias, mental status changes, abdominal pain, and seizures.
  - **Methemoglobinemia** is a rare complication of treatment with nitroprusside.
- **Recombinant BNP (nesiritide)** is an arterial and venous vasodilator.
  - IV infusion of nesiritide reduces right atrial and LV end-diastolic pressures and systemic vascular resistance and results in an increase in cardiac output.
  - It is administered as a 2-μg/kg IV bolus, followed by a continuous IV infusion starting at 0.01 μg/kg/min.
  - Nesiritide is approved for use in acute HF exacerbations and relieves HF symptoms early after its administration.[40] It does not have an effect on survival or rehospitalization in patients with HF.[41]
  - Hypotension is the most common side effect of nesiritide, and its use should be avoided in patients with systemic hypotension (systolic blood pressure <90 mm Hg) or evidence of cardiogenic shock. Episodes of hypotension should be managed with discontinuation of nesiritide and cautious volume expansion or vasopressor support if necessary.

- **Inotropic agents**
  - **Sympathomimetic agents** are potent drugs reserved for the treatment of severe HF. Beneficial and adverse effects are mediated by stimulation of myocardial β-adrenergic receptors. The most important adverse effects are related to the arrhythmogenic nature of these agents and the potential for exacerbation of myocardial ischemia. Treatment should be guided by careful hemodynamic and ECG monitoring. Patients with refractory chronic HF may benefit symptomatically from continuous ambulatory administration of IV inotropes as palliative therapy or as a bridge to mechanical ventricular support or cardiac transplantation. However, this strategy may increase the risk of life-threatening arrhythmias or indwelling catheter–related infections.[1]
  - **Norepinephrine**, rather than **dopamine** (Table 5-4), should be used for stabilization of the hypotensive HF patient. Although a large randomized trial found no mortality difference between dopamine and norepinephrine in a cohort of undifferentiated shock patients, there were more adverse events (primarily arrhythmic) in the dopamine group, and subgroup analysis of those with cardiogenic shock (n = 280) showed an increased rate of death at 28 days in the dopamine group.[42]
  - **Dobutamine** (see Table 5-4) is a synthetic analog of dopamine with predominantly β_1-adrenoreceptor activity. It increases cardiac output, lowers cardiac filling pressures, and generally has a neutral effect on systemic blood pressure. Dobutamine tolerance has been described, and several studies have demonstrated increased mortality in patients treated with continuous dobutamine. Dobutamine has no significant role in the treatment of HF resulting from diastolic dysfunction or a high-output state.
  - **Epinephrine** (see Table 5-4) may be considered in patients with refractory cardiogenic shock; however, its use has been associated with increased mortality. Escalation of therapy to include epinephrine should prompt consideration of mechanical circulatory support.

TABLE 5-4 Inotropic Agents[a]

Drug	Dose	Mechanism	Effects/Side Effects
Dopamine	1–3 μg/kg/min	Dopaminergic receptors	Splanchnic vasodilation
	2–8 μg/kg/min	β_1-Receptor agonist	+Inotropic
	7–10 μg/kg/min	α-Receptor agonist	↑ SVR
Dobutamine	2.5–15.0 μg/kg/min	β_1- > β_2- > α-Receptor agonist	+Inotropic, ↓ SVR, tachycardia
Epinephrine	0.05–1 μg/kg/min; titrate to desired mean arterial pressure. May adjust dose every 10–15 min by 0.05–0.2 μg/kg/min to achieve desired blood pressure goal	$\beta_1 > \alpha_1$ Low doses = β High doses = α	+Inotropic, ↓ SVR
Milrinone[b]	50-μg/kg bolus IV over 10 min, 0.375–0.75 μg/kg/min	↑ cAMP	+Inotropic, ↓ SVR

[a]Increased risk of atrial and ventricular tachyarrhythmias.
[b]Needs dose adjustment for creatinine clearance.
cAMP, cyclic adenosine monophosphate; SVR, systemic vascular resistance; ↑, increased; ↓, decreased.

- **Phosphodiesterase inhibitors** increase myocardial contractility and produce vasodilation by increasing intracellular cyclic adenosine monophosphate (cAMP). **Milrinone** is indicated for treatment of refractory HF. Hypotension may develop in patients who receive vasodilator therapy or have intravascular volume contraction, or both. Milrinone may improve hemodynamics in patients who are treated concurrently with dobutamine or dopamine. Data suggest that in-hospital short-term milrinone administration in addition to standard medical therapy does not reduce the length of hospitalization or the 60-day mortality or rehospitalization rate when compared with placebo.[43]

Antiarrhythmic Therapy

- Suppression of asymptomatic ventricular premature beats or nonsustained ventricular tachycardia (NSVT) using antiarrhythmic drugs in patients with HF does not improve survival and may increase mortality as a result of the proarrhythmic effects of the drugs.[44-46]
- For patients with atrial fibrillation (AF) as a suspected cause of new-onset HF, a rhythm control strategy should be pursued. For patients with preexisting HF who develop AF, despite evidence suggesting improved symptom status in patients treated with rhythm control, the use of antiarrhythmic drug therapy for the maintenance of sinus rhythm has not been shown to improve mortality.[47]
- Agents recommended for the maintenance of sinus rhythm in HF with reduced LVEF include dofetilide and amiodarone. Sotalol may also be considered in patients with mildly depressed LVEF. These agents require close monitoring of the QT interval.
- In patients with severe LV systolic dysfunction and HF, dronedarone should not be used.[48]
- Catheter ablation for atrial fibrillation in patients with HF as compared with medical therapy was associated with a lower rate of mortality in one randomized trial, but guideline consensus for use has not been formalized.[49]

Anticoagulant and Antiplatelet Therapy

- Although patients with HF are at relatively greater risk for thromboembolic events, the absolute risk is modest, and routine anticoagulation is not recommended in HF patients in the absence of AF, prior thromboembolism, or a prior cardioembolic source.
- In patients with AF, use of the CHADS2 or CHADS2-VASc risk score is recommended for determining when to use anticoagulant therapies.
- The novel anticoagulants dabigatran, rivaroxaban, and apixaban have been shown to be effective in HF patients with nonvalvular AF.
- There are insufficient data to support the routine use of aspirin in patients with HF who do not have coronary disease or atherosclerosis. Furthermore, certain data suggest that aspirin use may reduce the beneficial effects of ACE inhibitors.[50]

NONPHARMACOLOGIC THERAPIES FOR HEART FAILURE

Coronary revascularization reduces ischemia and may improve systolic function in some patients with CAD.

- Surgical or percutaneous revascularization is recommended in HF patients with angina and suitable anatomy (class I recommendation) and may be considered in patients without angina who have suitable anatomy, whether in the presence of viable myocardium (class IIa recommendation) or nonviable myocardium (class IIb recommendation).[1]
- In a large randomized trial of HF patients with CAD and LVEF <35% comparing medical therapy to medical therapy plus coronary artery bypass graft surgery (CABG), there was no difference in the primary outcome of death from any cause (hazard ratio [HR] with CABG, 0.86; 95% confidence interval [CI], 0.72–1.04; *P* = .12). A prespecified secondary analysis of death from cardiovascular causes favored CABG over medical therapy alone (HR with CABG, 0.81; 95% CI, 0.66–1.00; *P* = .05).[51]

At longer follow-up intervals of up to 10 years, the rates of death from any cause and death from cardiovascular causes were significantly lower in patients who underwent CABG in addition to medical therapy than those receiving medical therapy alone.[52]

- **Cardiac resynchronization therapy (CRT) or biventricular pacing** (see Chapter 7, Cardiac Arrhythmias) can improve quality of life and reduce the risk of death in certain patients with an EF of ≤35%, NYHA class II–IV HF, and conduction abnormalities (left bundle branch block [LBBB] and atrioventricular delay).[53,54]
  - CRT can also be useful (class IIA recommendation) in the following situations[1]:
    - LVEF ≤35%, sinus rhythm, a non-LBBB pattern with a QRS ≥150 ms, and NYHA class III/ambulatory class IV symptoms on GDMT.
    - LVEF ≤35%, sinus rhythm, LBBB with a QRS 120–149 ms, and NYHA class II, III, or ambulatory IV symptoms on GDMT.
    - AF and LVEF ≤35% on GDMT if the patient requires ventricular pacing and atrioventricular nodal ablation or rate control allows near 100% ventricular pacing with CRT.
    - Patients on GDMT who have LVEF ≤35% and are undergoing new or replacement device implantation with anticipated frequent ventricular pacing (>40% of the time).
    - Factors most strongly favoring response to CRT include female sex, QRS duration ≥150 ms, LBBB, body mass index <30 kg/m^2, nonischemic cardiomyopathy, and a small left atrium.[55]
  - **Implantable cardioverter-defibrillator (ICD)** placement for primary prevention of sudden cardiac death (SCD) is recommended for selected HF patients with a persistently reduced LVEF ≤35%.
    - SCD occurs six to nine times more often in patients with HF compared with the general population and is the leading cause of death in ambulatory HF patients.
    - Multiple large randomized trials have demonstrated a survival benefit of 1%–1.5% per year in patients with both ischemic and nonischemic cardiomyopathy.[1,53]
    - Patients should receive at least 3–6 months of optimal GDMT prior to reassessment of EF and implantation of an ICD.
    - Following an acute MI or revascularization, EF should be assessed after 40 days of GDMT prior to ICD implantation.
    - ICD therapy should be reserved for patients expected to otherwise live >1 year with good functional capacity. ICD therapy should not be used in end-stage HF patients who are not candidates for transplantation or durable mechanical circulatory support.
- An **intra-aortic balloon pump (IABP)** can be considered for temporary hemodynamic support in patients who have failed pharmacologic therapies and have transient myocardial dysfunction or are awaiting a definitive procedure such as a LV assist device (LVAD) or transplantation. Severe aortoiliac atherosclerosis and moderate to severe aortic valve insufficiency are contraindications to IABP placement.
- **Percutaneous LVADs** provide short-term hemodynamic support for patients in cardiogenic shock. These devices have been shown to provide superior hemodynamic effects compared with IABP. However, use of percutaneous LVADs compared with IABP did not improve 30-day survival in critically ill patients.[56]
- **CardioMEMS™** is an implantable hemodynamic monitoring system delivered into the pulmonary artery that can be used to monitor patient's ambulatory pulmonary artery pressures and allow clinicians to adjust medications accordingly. It has been shown to reduce hospitalization in patients with NYHA class III HF, irrespective of LV EF.[57]

SURGICAL MANAGEMENT

- **Surgical or nonsurgical replacement or repair** of the mitral valve in the setting of a reduced LVEF and severe MR is discussed elsewhere (see Chapter 6, Pericardial and Valvular Heart Disease).

- **Ventricular assist devices (VADs)** are surgically implanted devices that draw blood from the left ventricle, energize flow through a motor unit, and deliver the energized blood to the aorta, resulting in augmented cardiac output and lower intracardiac filling pressures. These devices may be temporary (CentriMag, percutaneous LVADs) or durable (HeartWare, HeartMate II, HeartMate III).
  - Temporary support is indicated for patients with severe HF after cardiac surgery or individuals with intractable cardiogenic shock after acute MI.
  - Durable support is indicated as a "bridge to transplantation" for patients awaiting heart transplantation or as "destination" therapy for select patients ineligible for transplant with refractory end-stage HF and HF-related life expectancy with therapy of <2 years.[1,58]
  - Currently available devices vary with regard to degree of mechanical hemolysis, intensity of anticoagulation required, and difficulty of implantation.
  - Patients should be monitored closely for complications related to LVAD therapy, such as bleeding (especially gastrointestinal bleed and intracranial hemorrhage), stroke, hemolysis, and infection (driveline infection, LVAD pocket infection, bacteremia, endocarditis).
  - Newer magnetic levitation technology offers less pump thrombosis and disabling stroke.[59,60]
  - The decision to institute mechanical circulatory support must be made in consultation with an HF cardiologist and a cardiac surgeon who have experience with this technology.
- **Cardiac transplantation** is an option for selected patients with severe end-stage HF that has become refractory to aggressive medical therapy and for whom no other conventional treatment options are available.
  - Only approximately 2200–3200 heart transplants are performed each year in the United States.[2]
  - Candidates considered for transplantation should generally be <65 years old (although selected older patients may also benefit), have advanced HF (NYHA class III–IV), have a strong psychosocial support system, have exhausted all other therapeutic options, and be free of irreversible extracardiac organ dysfunction that would limit functional recovery or predispose them to posttransplant complications.[61]
  - Survival rates after heart transplant are approximately 90%, 70%, and 50% at 1, 5, and 10 years, respectively. Annual statistics can be found on the United Network for Organ Sharing website (www.unos.org).
  - Functional capacity and quality of life improve significantly after transplantation, although VO_2 does not reach levels of age- and gender-matched controls, improving by approximately 40% at 2 years.[62]
  - **Posttransplant complications** may include acute or chronic rejection, typical and atypical infections, and adverse effects of immunosuppressive agents. Surgical complications and acute rejection are the major causes of death in the first posttransplant year. Cardiac allograft vasculopathy and malignancy are the leading causes of death after the first posttransplant year.

LIFESTYLE/RISK MODIFICATION

- Dietary counseling for sodium and fluid restriction should be provided. Daily intake of approximately 2 g of sodium per day is reasonable. Excessive restriction (<1.5 g/d of sodium) may be harmful.
- Smoking cessation should be strongly encouraged.
- Abstinence from alcohol is recommended in symptomatic HF patients with low EF.
- Exercise training is recommended in stable HF patients as an adjunct to pharmacologic treatment. Exercise training in patients with HF has been shown to improve exercise capacity (peak VO_2 max as well as 6-minute walk time), improve quality of life, and decrease neurohormonal activation.[63,64] Treatment programs should be individualized

and include a warm-up period, 20–30 minutes of exercise at the desired intensity, and a cool-down period.[65]

- Weight loss should be recommended in obese HF patients.

Special Considerations

- **Fluid and free water restriction** (<1.5 L/d) is especially important in the setting of hyponatremia (serum sodium <130 mEq/L) and volume overload.
- **Minimization of medications** with deleterious effects in HF should be emphasized.
    - **Negative inotropes** (e.g., verapamil, diltiazem) should be avoided in patients with impaired ventricular contractility, as should over-the-counter β stimulants (e.g., compounds containing ephedra, pseudoephedrine hydrochloride).
    - **NSAIDs**, which antagonize the effect of ACE inhibitors and diuretic therapy, should be avoided if possible.
- **Administration of supplemental oxygen** may relieve dyspnea, improve oxygen delivery, reduce the work of breathing, and limit pulmonary vasoconstriction in patients with hypoxemia but is not routinely recommended in patients without hypoxemia.
- **Sleep apnea** has a prevalence rate as high as 48% in the HF population. Treatment with nocturnal positive airway pressure improves symptoms and EF.[66,67] However, treatment of *central* sleep apnea with adaptive servo-ventilation was associated with increased mortality.[68] Treatment of *obstructive* sleep apnea may be warranted.
- **Dialysis or ultrafiltration** may be beneficial in patients with severe HF and renal dysfunction who cannot respond adequately to fluid and sodium restriction and diuretics.[69] Ultrafiltration is not superior to a scaled diuretic regimen in patients with acute HF and cardiorenal syndrome and is associated with higher rate of adverse events.[70] Other mechanical methods of fluid removal such as therapeutic thoracentesis and paracentesis may provide temporary symptomatic relief of dyspnea. Care must be taken to avoid rapid fluid removal and hypotension.
- **End-of-life considerations** may be necessary in patients with advanced HF who are refractory to therapy. Discussions regarding the disease course, treatment options, survival, functional status, and advance directives should be addressed early in the treatment of the patient with HF. For those with end-stage disease (stage D, NYHA class IV) with multiple hospitalizations and severe decline in their functional status and quality of life, hospice and palliative care should be considered.[71] Table 5-5 lists the predictors of poor outcome in chronic heart failure.

TABLE 5-5 Outcome Predictors in Chronic Heart Failure

- High NYHA functional class
- Reduced left ventricular ejection fraction
- Low peak oxygen consumption with maximal exercise (percentage predicted value)
- Third heart sound
- Increased pulmonary artery capillary wedge pressure
- Reduced cardiac index
- Diabetes mellitus
- Hyponatremia
- Raised plasma catecholamine and natriuretic peptide concentrations

Acute Heart Failure and Cardiogenic Pulmonary Edema

GENERAL PRINCIPLES

Cardiogenic pulmonary edema (CPE) occurs when the pulmonary capillary pressure exceeds the forces that maintain fluid within the vascular space (serum oncotic pressure and interstitial hydrostatic pressure).

- Increased pulmonary capillary pressure may be caused by LV failure of any cause, obstruction to transmitral flow (e.g., mitral stenosis [MS], atrial myxoma), or rarely, pulmonary veno-occlusive disease.
- Alveolar flooding and impairment of gas exchange follow accumulation of fluid in the pulmonary interstitium.

DIAGNOSIS

Clinical Presentation

- Clinical manifestations of CPE may occur rapidly and include dyspnea, anxiety, cough, and restlessness.
- The patient may expectorate pink frothy fluid.
- Physical signs of decreased peripheral perfusion, pulmonary congestion, hypoxemia, use of accessory respiratory muscles, and wheezing are often present.

Diagnostic Testing

- Radiographic abnormalities include cardiomegaly, interstitial and perihilar vascular engorgement, Kerley B lines, and pleural effusions.
- The radiographic abnormalities may follow the development of symptoms by several hours, and their resolution may be out of phase with clinical improvement.

TREATMENT

- Placing the patient in a sitting position improves pulmonary function.
- Bed rest, pain control, and relief of anxiety can decrease cardiac workload.
- **Supplemental oxygen** should be administered initially to raise the arterial oxygen tension to >60 mm Hg.
- **Mechanical ventilation** is indicated if oxygenation is inadequate or hypercapnia occurs. Noninvasive positive-pressure ventilation is preferred and may have particularly favorable effects in the setting of pulmonary edema.[72]
- **Precipitating factors** should be identified and corrected because resolution of pulmonary edema can often be accomplished with correction of the underlying process. The most common precipitants are
  - Severe hypertension
  - MI or myocardial ischemia (particularly if associated with MR)
  - Acute valvular regurgitation
  - New-onset tachyarrhythmias or bradyarrhythmias
  - Volume overload in the setting of severe LV dysfunction

Medications

- **Furosemide** is a venodilator that decreases pulmonary congestion within minutes of IV administration, well before its diuretic action begins. An initial dose of 20–80 mg IV should be given over several minutes and can be increased based on response to a maximum of 200 mg in subsequent doses.

- **Nitroglycerin** is a venodilator that can potentiate the effect of furosemide. IV administration is preferable to oral and transdermal forms because it can be rapidly titrated.
- **Nitroprusside** is an effective adjunct in the treatment of acute CPE and is useful when CPE is brought on by acute valvular regurgitation or hypertension (see Chapter 6, Pericardial and Valvular Heart Disease). Pulmonary and systemic arterial catheterization should be considered to guide titration of nitroprusside therapy.
- **Inotropic agents**, such as dobutamine or milrinone, may be helpful after initial treatment of CPE in patients with concomitant hypotension or shock.
- **Recombinant BNP (nesiritide)** is administered as an IV bolus followed by an IV infusion. Nesiritide reduces intracardiac filling pressures by producing vasodilation and indirectly increases the cardiac output. In conjunction with furosemide, nesiritide produces natriuresis and diuresis.
- **Morphine sulfate** reduces anxiety and dilates pulmonary and systemic veins; 2–4 mg can be given intravenously over several minutes and can be repeated every 10–25 minutes until an effect is seen.

SPECIAL CONSIDERATIONS

Right heart catheterization (e.g., Swan-Ganz catheter) may be helpful in cases where a prompt response to therapy does not occur by allowing differentiation between cardiogenic and noncardiogenic causes of pulmonary edema via measurement of central hemodynamics and cardiac output. It may then be used to guide subsequent therapy. The *routine* use of right heart catheterization in acute HF patients is not beneficial.[73]

Heart Failure with Preserved Ejection Fraction

GENERAL PRINCIPLES

Definition

- HFpEF, also called **diastolic HF**, refers to the clinical syndrome of HF in the presence of preserved systolic function (LVEF >50%).
- Diastolic dysfunction refers to an abnormality in the mechanical function of the heart during the relaxation phase of the cardiac cycle, resulting in elevated filling pressures and impairment of ventricular filling.

Epidemiology

- Almost half of the patients admitted to the hospital with HF have a normal or near-normal EF.[2]
- HFpEF is most prevalent in older women, most of whom have hypertension and/or diabetes mellitus. Many of these patients also have CAD and/or AF.

Etiology

- The vast majority of patients with HFpEF have hypertension and LV hypertrophy.
- Myocardial disorders associated with HFpEF include restrictive cardiomyopathy (RCM), obstructive and nonobstructive HCM, infiltrative cardiomyopathies, and constrictive pericarditis.

Pathophysiology

- Reduced ventricular compliance and elastance play a major role in the pathophysiology of HFpEF.

- Factors contributing to the clinical HFpEF syndrome include abnormal sodium handling by the kidneys, atrial dysfunction, autonomic dysfunction, increased arterial stiffness, pulmonary hypertension, sarcopenia, obesity, deconditioning, and other comorbidities.

DIAGNOSIS

- Differentiating between HFpEF and HFrEF cannot be reliably accomplished without assessment of LVEF, preferably with two-dimensional echocardiography.
- Diagnosis is based on echocardiographic criteria and Doppler findings of normal LVEF, impaired diastolic relaxation, and elevated filling pressures. More sensitive echocardiographic parameters of systolic function, such as LV strain, may be abnormal in patients with HFpEF.

TREATMENT

No pharmacologic therapy has been shown in a randomized controlled trial to reduce mortality in HFpEF patients. Subgroup analysis indicates a possible modest benefit with respect to morbidity from the use of aldosterone receptor antagonists, ACE inhibitors/ARBs, and β-blockers. Practice guidelines for HFpEF emphasize blood pressure control, heart rate control or restoration of sinus rhythm in symptomatic patients, judicious diuretic use, and treatment of ischemic heart disease (Figure 5-3).

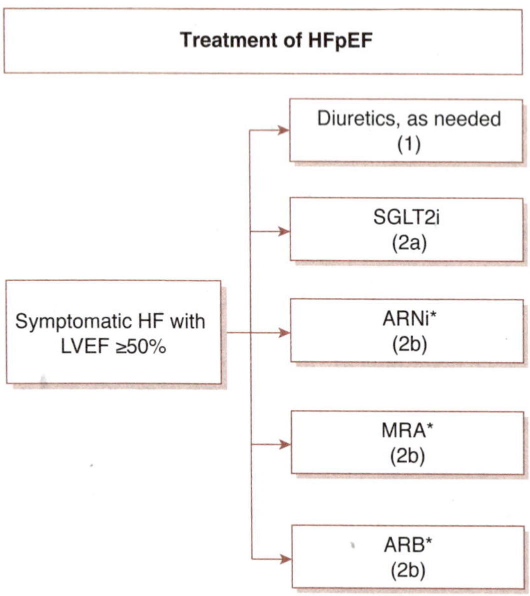

Figure 5-3 Treatment of HFpEF.

CARDIOMYOPATHY

Dilated Cardiomyopathy

GENERAL PRINCIPLES

Definition

Dilated cardiomyopathy (DCM) is a disease of heart muscle characterized by dilation of the cardiac chambers and reduction in ventricular contractile function.

Epidemiology

DCM is the most common form of cardiomyopathy and is responsible for approximately 10,000 deaths and 46,000 hospitalizations each year. The lifetime incidence of DCM is about 30 cases per 100,000 persons.

Pathophysiology

- DCM may be secondary to progression of any process that affects the myocardium, and dilation is directly related to neurohormonal activation. Familial DCM accounts for up to 50% of cases and is likely underestimated.[2,74]
- Dilation of the cardiac chambers and varying degrees of hypertrophy are anatomic hallmarks. Tricuspid and mitral regurgitation are common because of the effect of chamber dilation on the valvular apparatus.
- **Atrial and ventricular arrhythmias** are present in as many as one-half of these patients and contribute to the high incidence of sudden death in this population.

DIAGNOSIS

Clinical Presentation

- Symptomatic HF (dyspnea, volume overload) is often present.
- A portion of patients with clinical disease may be asymptomatic.
- The ECG is usually abnormal, but changes are typically nonspecific.

Diagnostic Testing

Imaging

- Diagnosis of DCM can be confirmed with echocardiography, CMR, or radionuclide ventriculography.
- Two-dimensional and Doppler echocardiography is helpful in differentiating this condition from HCM or RCM, pericardial disease, and valvular disorders.

Diagnostic Procedures

Coronary angiography (conventional or CT) is useful to rule out atherosclerosis and ischemic cardiomyopathy.

Endomyocardial biopsy provides little information that affects treatment of patients with DCMs and is not routinely recommended.[1,75] Settings where endomyocardial biopsy for DCM is recommended include the following:

- New-onset HF of <2 weeks in duration with normal-sized or dilated left ventricle and hemodynamic compromise.
- New-onset HF of 2 weeks to 3 months in duration associated with a dilated left ventricle and new ventricular arrhythmias, high-grade atrioventricular block (type II second-degree or third-degree), and failure to respond to usual care.

- Clinical scenarios that may result in the diagnosis of a treatable form of acute myocarditis, such as giant cell myocarditis or eosinophilic myocarditis.

TREATMENT

Medications

- The medical management of symptomatic patients is identical to that for HFrEF from other causes. This consists of controlling total body sodium and volume and pharmacotherapy including β-blockers, ACE inhibitors or ARBs, aldosterone antagonists, and vasodilator therapy.
- Immunizations against influenza and pneumococcal pneumonia are recommended.
- Immunosuppressive therapy with agents such as prednisone, azathioprine, and cyclosporine for biopsy-proven myocarditis has been advocated by some, but efficacy has not been established, with the possible exception of the very rare patient with giant cell myocarditis.[1,76]

Other Nonpharmacologic Therapies

Nonpharmacologic therapies for DCM are identical to those for HFrEF in general and, when indicated by practice guidelines, include ICD implantation, CRT, and temporary mechanical circulatory support.

Surgical Management

- Cardiac transplantation should be considered for selected patients with HF due to DCM that is refractory to medical therapy.
- LVAD placement may be necessary for stabilization of patients in whom cardiac transplantation is an option or in select patients who are not eligible for transplantation.

Hypertrophic Cardiomyopathy

GENERAL PRINCIPLES

Definition

HCM can be defined broadly as the presence of increased LV wall thickness that is not solely explained by abnormal loading conditions.[77] More specifically, HCM is a genetically determined disease wherein sarcomere mutations lead to LV hypertrophy associated with nondilated ventricular chambers in the absence of another disease that would be capable of causing the magnitude of hypertrophy present in a given individual.[78]

Epidemiology

- HCM is the most commonly inherited heart defect, occurring in 1 out of 500 individuals.
- Approximately 500,000 people have HCM in the United States, although many are unaware. An estimated 36% of young athletes who die suddenly have probable or definite HCM, making it the leading cause of SCD in young people in the United States, including trained athletes.[1]

Pathophysiology

- HCM results from a mutation in a gene encoding one of the proteins involved in essential myocardial sarcomere functions, such as structural or contractile proteins, calcium handling proteins, or mitochondrial proteins.
    - There are currently at least 50 HCM susceptibility genes that lead to autosomal dominant transmission with variable phenotypic expression and penetrance.[2,79,80]

 - The most common mutations involve myosin binding protein C *(MYBPC3)* and myosin heavy chain 7 *(MYH7)*.
 - Over 50% of clinically affected patients have an identified mutation.[81]
- The histopathologic change in HCM consists of hypertrophied myocytes arranged in a disorganized manner with interstitial fibrosis.
- These changes lead grossly to myocardial hypertrophy that is typically predominant in the ventricular septum (asymmetric septal hypertrophy) but may involve any and all ventricular segments. HCM can be classified clinically according to the presence or absence of LV outflow tract (LVOT) obstruction. When present, it is termed **hypertrophic obstructive cardiomyopathy** (HOCM).
- LVOT obstruction may occur at rest but is enhanced by factors that increase LV contractility (exercise), decrease ventricular volume (e.g., Valsalva maneuver, volume depletion, large meal), or decrease afterload (vasodilators).
- Delayed ventricular diastolic relaxation and decreased compliance are common and, along with MR, may lead to pulmonary congestion.
- Myocardial ischemia is common, secondary to a myocardial oxygen supply–demand mismatch.
- **Systolic anterior motion** (SAM) of the anterior leaflet of the mitral valve is often associated with MR and likely determines the severity of LVOT obstruction.

DIAGNOSIS

HCM is usually diagnosed by maximal LV wall thickness ≥15 mm in the absence of another disease that could account for the degree of hypertrophy, often accompanied by supporting information (family history of HCM or sudden death, SAM, genetic testing).

Clinical Presentation

- Presentation varies but may include exertional dyspnea, angina, fatigue, dizziness, syncope, palpitations, or sudden death.
- Sudden death is most common in children and young adults between the ages of 10 and 35 years and often occurs during or immediately after periods of strenuous exertion.

Physical Examination

- **Coarse systolic outflow murmur localized along the left sternal border:** Diminished intensity with increased preload (squatting) or afterload (handgrip) and increased intensity with a decrease in preload (Valsalva maneuver, standing), and with any decrease in afterload (vasodilator administration)
- **Bisferiens (double peak per cardiac cycle) carotid pulse (in the presence of obstruction):** A double/triple apical impulse due to forceful left atrial contraction against a highly noncompliant left ventricle, normal S1 and split S2, S3 due to decompensated heart failure, and prominent "a wave" of jugular venous pressure

Diagnostic Testing

Electrocardiography

The ECG of HCM is usually abnormal and invariably so in symptomatic patients with LVOT obstruction. The most common abnormalities are ST-segment and T-wave abnormalities, followed by evidence of LV hypertrophy.[82] The ECG in apical-variant HCM is characterized by large, inverted T waves across the precordial leads. ECG findings include prominent Q waves in the inferior (II, III, and aVF) and lateral (I, aVL, and V4–V6) leads, left atrial or biatrial enlargement, left-axis deviation, and deeply inverted T waves. The combination of left ventricular hypertrophy (LVH) with right atrial enlargement is str deviation, and deeply inverted T waves. *The combination of left ventricular hypertrophy (LVH) with right atrial enlargement is strongly suggestive of HCM* (Figure 5-4).

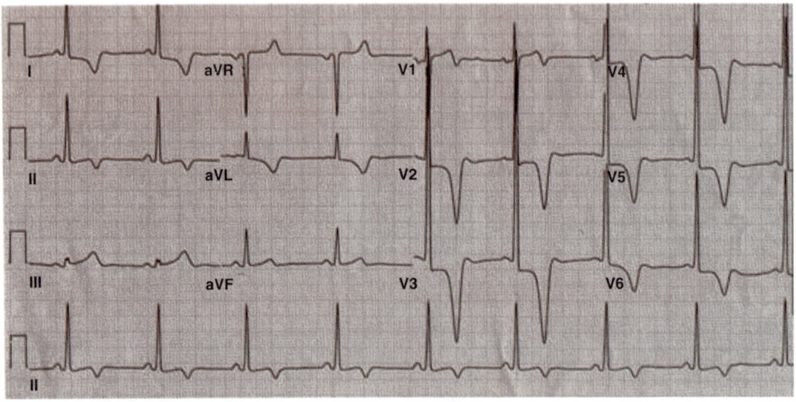

Figure 5-4 ECG showing left ventricular hypertrophy and deep T wave inversions suggestive of HOCM.

Imaging

- Two-dimensional echocardiography and Doppler flow studies can establish the presence of a significant LV outflow gradient at rest or with provocation.
- Additional risk stratification should be pursued with 24- to 48-hour Holter monitoring and exercise testing.
- Cardiac MRI is indicated in patients with suspected HCM in whom the diagnosis cannot be confirmed with echocardiography.
- Invasive hemodynamic assessment using cardiac catheterization is reserved for patients with suspected HCM and one or more of the following situations:
  - Persons in whom the additional diagnosis of RCM or constrictive pericarditis is being considered
  - Persons in whom invasive coronary angiography is being performed for the evaluation of obstructive coronary disease
  - Persons in whom a suspicion for LVOT obstruction is present but the clinical and imaging data are discrepant
  - Persons in whom endomyocardial biopsy is indicated to exclude nonsarcomeric disease (e.g., Fabry disease, amyloidosis, Danon disease)
  - Pre-cardiac transplantation evaluation

Genetic Testing

Genetic testing for HCM is commercially available. Roughly 50% of patients with HCM have a known pathogenic mutation. Genetic testing can be used to aid in diagnosis of HCM when the clinical presentation is unclear. Genetic testing is reasonable in an index patient to facilitate family screening to determine at-risk first-degree relatives.[78]

TREATMENT

- Management is directed toward relief of symptoms and prevention of sudden death.
- Infective endocarditis prophylaxis remains controversial, and prophylactic antibiotics are no longer recommended by guidelines.[77]
- Treatment in asymptomatic individuals is controversial, and no conclusive evidence has been found that medical therapy is beneficial.
- All individuals with HCM should avoid strenuous physical activity, including most competitive sports. Activity-specific recommendations are available.[83]

Medications

- β-Blockers are generally the first-line agent to reduce symptoms of HCM by reducing myocardial contractility and heart rate.
- Nondihydropyridine calcium channel antagonists (verapamil and diltiazem) may improve the symptoms of HCM by reducing myocardial contractility and heart rate. Therapy should be initiated at low doses, with careful titration in patients with outflow obstruction. The dose should be increased gradually over several days to weeks if symptoms persist. Dihydropyridines should be avoided in patients with LVOT obstruction as a result of their vasodilatory properties.
- Disopyramide, a negative inotropic agent that results in lowering of the LVOT gradient, may be added for HCM patients who remain symptomatic despite the use of β-blockers and calcium channel blockers (alone or in combination). Use requires monitoring of the QT interval, and concomitant use of other antiarrhythmic drugs should be avoided.
- Diuretics may improve pulmonary congestive symptoms in patients with elevated pulmonary venous pressures. These agents should be used cautiously in patients with LVOT obstruction because excessive preload reduction worsens the obstruction.
- Nitrates and vasodilators should be avoided because of the risk of increasing the LVOT gradient.
- **Atrial and ventricular arrhythmias** occur commonly in patients with HCM. Supraventricular tachyarrhythmias are tolerated poorly and should be treated aggressively. Cardioversion is indicated if hemodynamic compromise develops.
  - **Digoxin is relatively contraindicated** because of its positive inotropic properties and potential for exacerbating ventricular outflow obstruction.
  - AF should be converted to sinus rhythm when possible, and anticoagulation is recommended if paroxysmal or chronic AF develops.
  - **Diltiazem, verapamil, or β-blockers** can be used to control the ventricular response before cardioversion. Procainamide, disopyramide, or amiodarone (see Chapter 7, Cardiac Arrhythmias) may be effective in the chronic suppression of AF.
  - ICD implantation is recommended for patients with HCM and prior cardiac arrest, ventricular fibrillation, or hemodynamically significant ventricular tachycardia.
  - ICD placement is reasonable in high-risk patients such as those with the following:
    - Recent unexplained syncope
    - LV hypertrophy with a maximal wall thickness >30 mm
    - History of sudden death presumably caused by HCM in one or more first-degree relatives
    - Multiple episodes of NSVT on Holter recordings (especially in patients <30 years old)
    - Hypotensive response to exercise
  - Symptomatic ventricular arrhythmias should be treated as outlined in Chapter 7, Cardiac Arrhythmias.

Nonpharmacologic Therapies for HCM

Dual-chamber pacing (see Chapter 7, Cardiac Arrhythmias) improves symptoms in some patients with HCM. Alteration of the ventricular activation sequence via RV pacing may minimize LVOT obstruction secondary to asymmetric septal hypertrophy. Only 10% of patients with HCM meet the criteria for pacemaker implantation, and the effect on decreasing the LVOT gradient is only 25%. A subset of patients with HCM may derive symptomatic benefit from dual-chamber pacing without an effect on survival.[84]

Surgical Management

- Septal reduction therapy (surgical myectomy or catheter-based alcohol septal ablation) provides symptom relief without proven survival benefit in the treatment of medication-refractory HCM symptoms.

- Septal myectomy is the most commonly performed surgical intervention in HCM. In experienced centers, it is associated with symptom improvement in 95% of patients with <1% operative mortality.[85] Concomitant mitral valve intervention (mitral valve repair or replacement) is rarely required in experienced centers because MR generally responds well to septal reduction.
- Alcohol septal ablation, a catheter-based alternative to surgical myectomy, also provides relief of obstruction and symptomatic benefit with low procedural mortality, although it can be associated with heart block, requiring pacemaker placement in up to 20% of patients.[86]
- Cardiac transplantation should be considered for patients with refractory end-stage HCM with symptomatic HF.

PATIENT EDUCATION

Genetic counseling and family screening are recommended for first-degree relatives of patients with HCM because it is transmitted as an autosomal dominant trait.

SPECIAL CONSIDERATIONS

- Apical nonobstructive cardiac hypertrophy (**Yamaguchi syndrome**) is a relatively rare form of HCM.
- Typical features of apical HCM include giant T-wave negativity on the electrocardiogram, especially in the left precordial leads, and a "spade-like" configuration of the LV cavity at end-diastole on left ventriculography.
- In Japan, where it was first described, it constitutes 15%–25% of all cases of hypertrophic cardiomyopathies and is seen more commonly in men.

Restrictive Cardiomyopathy

GENERAL PRINCIPLES

Definition

- RCM is characterized by a rigid heart with poor ventricular filling but generally a nondilated LV and normal LVEF. Right HF symptoms often predominate.
- RCM may be primary, including conditions such as idiopathic RCM, EMF, and Löeffler endocarditis, or secondary to either infiltrative conditions (amyloidosis, sarcoidosis, hypereosinophilic syndrome) or storage diseases (Fabry disease, hemochromatosis, and Hurler disease). Other causes include scleroderma, Anderson–Fabry disease, Danon disease, and drug induced—anthracycline, methysergide, ergot.
- Constrictive pericarditis may present similarly to RCM but is a disease wherein the pericardium limits diastolic filling. Constriction carries a different prognosis and therapy, and the distinction between constriction and RCM is essential.

Pathophysiology

- In amyloidosis, misfolded protein (amyloid) deposits in the cardiac interstitium, interrupting the normal myocardial contractile units and causing restriction. Most commonly, the misfolded protein is either immunoglobulin light chain (AL) or transthyretin (TTR).
- In sarcoidosis, granulomatous infiltration of the myocardium is often subclinical and more commonly presents with arrhythmias or conduction system disease; however, in up to 5% of sarcoidosis cases, restriction is manifested.
- In hemochromatosis, excess iron is deposited in the cardiomyocyte sarcoplasm, ultimately overcoming antioxidant capacity and resulting in lipid peroxidation and membrane permeability. Injury occurs initially in the epicardium and then later in the myocardium and endocardium, with systolic function initially preserved.

- Fabry disease, an X-linked genetic disorder, is characterized by deficient activity of the lysosomal enzyme α-galactosidase A, resulting in lysosomal accumulation of globotriaosylceramide in tissues, with more than half of patients manifesting cardiomyopathy, typically with LV hypertrophy and RCM.
- EMF predominantly involves right ventricle affecting primarily children and adolescents in tropical countries of sub-Saharan Africa, Latin America, and South Asia. It is the most common cause of RCM worldwide. Most commonly, it involves right ventricle inflow tract along with AV subvalvular apparatus. Pulmonary valves and arteries are spared. Pathological specimens seldom show eosinophils and inflammation.
- Endocardial fibroelastosis is a pathological entity rather than precise disease representing endocardial reaction to several cardiac diseases. It is mostly described in children with hypoplastic left heart syndrome.
- Carcinoid heart disease (Hedinger syndrome) is a rare disorder that occurs due to vasoactive amines reaching right side of the heart producing progressive fibrotic plaque and thickening along the tricuspid and pulmonary valves.

DIAGNOSIS

Diagnostic Testing

Electrocardiography

The classic ECG finding in amyloidosis is low voltage (despite echocardiographically evident ventricular thickening) with poor R-wave progression and pseudoinfarction pattern in inferior and septal leads. In sarcoidosis, conduction disease is often present with varying degrees of heart blocks.

Imaging

- In RCM, echocardiography with Doppler analysis often demonstrates thickened myocardium with normal or abnormal systolic function, abnormal diastolic filling patterns, and evidence of elevated intracardiac pressure. Compared with constrictive pericarditis, respiratory variation is less marked and tissue Doppler velocities are reduced.
- Cardiac MRI, position emission tomography (PET), and CT are emerging as useful diagnostic tools for patients with cardiac sarcoidosis because granulomas, inflammation, and edema may be seen, which appear to improve with therapy.[87,88]
- Cardiac MRI is useful in the diagnosis of amyloidosis. In addition, bone-seeking radiotracers have strong avidity for TTR-variant amyloid and nuclear imaging with tracers such as 99mTc-pyrophosphate is highly sensitive and specific for TTR-cardiac amyloidosis. A granular, speckled appearance of the ventricular myocardium combined with clinical suspicion and other laboratory findings is suggestive of cardiac amyloidosis.

Diagnostic Procedures

- On cardiac catheterization, elevated and equalized RV and LV filling pressures are seen with a classic "dip-and-plateau" pattern in the RV and LV pressure tracing. Although pericardial constriction may produce similar findings, absence of ventricular interdependence identifies RCM as opposed to constriction.[89]
- RV endomyocardial biopsy should be considered in patients in whom a diagnosis is not established or where characterization of a protein species will alter therapy, as in cardiac amyloidosis.

TREATMENT

- Specific therapy aimed at amelioration of the underlying cause should be initiated.
- In patients with AL cardiac amyloidosis, chemotherapy to reduce AL production should be pursued in conjunction with a hematologist.

- In patients with TTR amyloidosis, emerging therapies to deplete TTR (combination of doxycycline and taurodeoxycholic acid) or stabilize abnormal TTR (Diflunisal and Tafamidis) are under investigation. In patients with a defined TTR gene mutation, dual liver-heart transplantation may be considered.
- Cardiac hemochromatosis may respond to reduction of total body iron stores via phlebotomy or chelation therapy with deferoxamine.[90]
- Cardiac sarcoidosis may respond to glucocorticoid therapy or other immunomodulatory therapies.
- Fabry disease may be treated with recombinant α-galactosidase A enzyme replacement therapy.[91,92]
- In those with syncope and/or ventricular arrhythmias, placement of an ICD is indicated. Patients with high-grade conduction disease warrant pacemaker placement.
- No pharmacotherapy is known to be effective at reversing the progression of cardiac amyloidosis.
- Digoxin should be avoided in patients with AL cardiac amyloidosis because digoxin is bound extracellularly by amyloid fibrils and may cause hypersensitivity and toxicity.[93] β-Blockers should be avoided in patients with cardiac amyloidosis.

Table 5-6 lists the differences between RCM and constrictive pericarditis.

TABLE 5-6 Differences Between Restrictive Cardiomyopathy and Constrictive Pericarditis

Clinical and Investigation Features	Restrictive Cardiomyopathy	Constrictive Pericarditis
History	Systemic disease (e.g., sarcoidosis, hemochromatosis)	Prior history of pericarditis or conditions affecting the pericardium
Physical examination	±Kussmaul sign, S_3 and S_4 gallop, murmurs of mitral and tricuspid regurgitation	Pericardial knock
Chest X-ray	Atrial dilatation	Pericardial calcification
ECG	Low QRS voltages (mainly amyloidosis), conduction disturbances, nonspecific ST abnormalities	Nonspecific ST and T abnormalities, low QRS voltage (<50%)
2D echocardiography	±Wall and valvular thickening, sparkling myocardium	±Pericardial thickening, respiratory ventricular septal shift
Doppler echocardiography	Decreased variation in mitral and/or tricuspid inflow E velocity, increased hepatic vein inspiratory diastolic flow reversal, presence of mitral and tricuspid regurgitation	Increased variation in mitral and/or tricuspid inflow E velocity, hepatic vein expiratory diastolic reversal ratio ≥0.79, medial e′/lateral e′ ≥0.91

(Continued)

TABLE 5-6 Differences Between Restrictive Cardiomyopathy and Constrictive Pericarditis (Continued)

Clinical and Investigation Features	Restrictive Cardiomyopathy	Constrictive Pericarditis
Catheterization hemodynamics	LVEDP–RVEDP ≥5 mm Hg RVSP ≥55 mm Hg RVEDP/RVSP ≤0.33	LVEDP–RVEDP <5 mm Hg RVSP <55 mm Hg RVEDP/RVSP >0.33 Inspiratory decrease in RAP <5 mm Hg Systolic area index >1.1 Left ventricular height of rapid filling wave >7 mm Hg
CT	Normal pericardium	Thickened/calcified pericardium
MRI	Measurement of iron overload, various types of LGE	Thickened pericardium
Biopsy	May reveal underlying cause	Normal myocardium

LGE, late gadolinium enhancement; LVEDP, left ventricular end-diastolic pressure; RAP, right atrial pressure; RVEDP, right ventricular end-diastolic pressure; RVSP, right ventricular systolic pressure.

Peripartum Cardiomyopathy

GENERAL PRINCIPLES

Definition

- PPCM is defined as nonischemic LV systolic dysfunction diagnosed in the last month of pregnancy up to 5 months postpartum.
- The incidence of PPCM is 1 in 1000–4000 pregnancies in the United States,[94] with the highest incidence in Nigeria (1 in 100 deliveries) and the least in Japan (1 in 20,000).

Etiology

- The etiology of PPCM remains unclear. There is evidence to support **viral triggers**, including coxsackievirus, parvovirus B19, adenovirus, and herpesvirus, which may replicate unchecked in the reduced immunologic state brought on by pregnancy.[95,96]
- **Fetal microchimerism**, wherein fetal cells escape into the maternal circulation and induce an autoimmune myocarditis, has also been suggested as a cause.[97]
- The most accepted hypothesis in the development of PPCM is cleavage product of **prolactin.**[98] Other vasculo-hormonal pathways have also been suggested to post a toxic challenge to the heart and lead to PPCM.[94]

Risk Factors

Risk factors that predispose a woman to PPCM include advanced maternal age, multiparity, multiple pregnancies, preeclampsia, and gestational hypertension. There is a higher risk in African American women, but this may be confounded by the higher prevalence of hypertension in this population.

DIAGNOSIS

Clinical Presentation

- Majority develop PPCM in the first month after the delivery.
- Clinically, women with PPCM present with the signs and symptoms of HF.
- Because dyspnea on exertion and lower extremity edema are common in late pregnancy, PPCM may be difficult to recognize. Cough, orthopnea, and paroxysmal nocturnal dyspnea are warning signs that PPCM may be present, as is the presence of a displaced apical impulse and a new MR murmur on examination.
- Most commonly, patients present with NYHA class III and IV HF, although mild cases and sudden cardiac arrest also occur.
- Minority of patients develop cardiogenic shock, severe arrhythmias and thromboembolic complications.

Diagnostic Testing

Electrocardiography

On ECG, LV hypertrophy is often present, as are nonspecific ST-T–wave abnormalities. Normal ECG does not rule out PPCM.

Imaging

Diagnosis requires an echocardiogram with a newly depressed EF and/or LV dilatation. It may also show features suggestive of functional MR or TR, RV dilation, pulmonary hypertension, and rarely intracardiac apical thrombus; cardiac MRI is rarely indicated if ECHO is inconclusive. *Differential diagnosis*: PPCM is the diagnosis of exclusion. Careful attention should be given to rule out preexisting heart disease (cardiomyopathies and valvular heart disease). Severe preeclampsia can cause diastolic heart failure.

TREATMENT

Medications

- The mainstay of treatment is afterload and preload reduction with special modifications to ensure fetal safety. Most medications are compatible with breastfeeding.
- **ACE inhibitors** are used in the postpartum patient, whereas hydralazine is used in the patient who is still pregnant.
- **β-Blockers** are used to reduce tachycardia, arrhythmia, and risk of SCD and are relatively safe, although β_1-selective blockers are preferred (metoprolol tartrate) because they avoid peripheral vasodilation and uterine relaxation.
- **Digoxin** is also safe during pregnancy and may be used to augment contractility and for rate control, although levels need to be closely monitored.
- **Diuretics** are used for preload reduction and symptom relief and are also safe.
- In those with thromboembolism, **heparin** is required, followed by **warfarin** after delivery.
- Anticoagulation is also required in patients with LVEF <35% even without any thromboembolic features.
- Patients with PPCM treated with bromocriptine 2.5 mg twice daily for 2 weeks and once daily for 6 weeks show significant improvement of LV systolic function.*

OUTCOME/PROGNOSIS

- The prognosis in PPCM is better than that seen in other forms of nonischemic cardiomyopathy.
- The extent of ventricular recovery at 6 months after delivery can predict overall recovery, although continued improvement has been seen up to 2–3 years after diagnosis.

---

*Melinda BD, Zolt A, Dennis MM, et al. Peripartum cardiomyopathy. *J Am Coll Cardiol.* 2020;75:207–221.

- Subsequent pregnancies in patients with PPCM may be associated with significant deterioration in LV function and can even result in death. Family planning counseling is essential after the diagnosis of PPCM is made, and women who do not recover their LV function should be encouraged to consider foregoing future pregnancy.

Stress Cardiomyopathy

GENERAL PRINCIPLES

- Stress cardiomyopathy is a clinical syndrome characterized by an acute and transient (< 21 days) LV systolic (and diastolic) dysfunction often related to an emotional or physical stressful event, most often identified in the preceding days (1–5 days).
- It was first described in Japan in 1990, and is also called **Takotsubo cardiomyopathy**, broken heart syndrome, and apical ballooning syndrome.
- Prevalence is currently estimated at 1%–2% of patients with suspected acute coronary syndrome.
- Exact pathophysiology is unknown and the most accepted hypothesis is that norepinephrine and neuropeptide Y (NPY) are stored in the presynaptic terminations of the postganglionic sympathetic system. The spillover of norepinephrine and NPY, from presynaptic terminations at myocardial level following intense stress, may induce a direct toxic effect and epicardial and microvascular dysfunction.
- Risk factors include female sex, menopausal, psychiatric illness, diabetes mellitus, obstructive airway disease, and substance abuse disorder.
- Stress cardiomyopathy can be classified accordingly in to either primary form (main reason for care seeking) or secondary form (found during evaluation of other illnesses).
- Anatomical variants of stress cardiomyopathy are as follows:
  - **Apical ballooning (typical) 75%–80%:** Associated with LV outflow tract obstruction and/or apical thrombus formation with variable prognosis
  - **Midventricular 10%–20%:** Present with severe LV dysfunction, and acute heart failure syndrome is common
  - **Basal or inverted 5%:** Less severe hemodynamic compromise
  - **Biventricular <0.5%:** Present with severe hemodynamic compromise and cardiogenic shock
  - **Focal dysfunction:** Rare with benign course and more commonly associated with chest pain

DIAGNOSIS

Clinical Presentation

- Clinical presentation of a typical patient with stress cardiomyopathy includes a postmenopausal woman who presents with acute or subacute onset of chest pain (>75%) and/or shortness of breath (approximately 50%), often with dizziness (>25%), and occasional syncope (5%–10%).
- In majority of the cases, the patient has experienced an emotional or physical stress that he/she may not share with the healthcare provider unless asked.
- Physical examination reveals features of acute decompensated left-sided heart failure and a systolic murmur when there is accompanying LVOT obstruction.

Diagnostic Testing

Diagnosis is based on regional wall motion abnormalities (RWMA) beyond territory supplied by single coronary artery with reversible in due course and associated with physical/emotional stress.

- The InterTAK International Registry Group developed pretest probability scoring system for diagnosis of Takotsubo cardiomyopathy which includes five clinical and two ECG variables.

- Diagnostic score (0–100) ≥50 favors Takotsubo cardiomyopathy and ≤31 favors acute coronary syndrome (specificity of >95%).
- Electrocardiogram is abnormal in >95% of patients with ischemic ST segment and T-wave changes. T-wave inversions are usually deep and wide associated with prolonged QTc likely occurring after 24–48 hours of the precipitating factor.
- Cardiac biomarkers are elevated in most of the cases.
- Coronary angiography is mostly normal or suggests mild coronary artery disease (which is unlikely to be cause of acute event).
- LV ventriculography should be done unless contraindicated (suspected apical thrombosis), especially in midventricular variant which is difficult to visualize.
- Cardiac magnetic resonance (CMR) allows visualization of myocardial edema, inflammation, and scarring with the use of delayed gadolinium enhancement (DGE).
- Coronary computed tomography angiography has been proposed as a noninvasive imaging modality alternative to invasive angiography to exclude coronary culprit lesions in selected stable patients, and a convincing clinical and echocardiographic picture of stress cardiomyopathy.

TREATMENT

- Management is mainly a supportive therapy and prevention of complications until recovery. Treatment of heart failure with or without cardiogenic shock is as per the guideline-directed heart failure management.
- Anticoagulation is considered for apical thrombus (for up to 3 months) or large area of akinesis (until LVEF improves).
- Recurrence is seen in 2%–4% of the patients and in-hospital mortality is seen in up to 5% of the patients.
- Recovery of LVEF is seen from 48 hours up to 6 weeks.

Left Ventricular Noncompaction Cardiomyopathy

GENERAL PRINCIPLES

- Left ventricular noncompaction cardiomyopathy (LVNC) is defined by three markers: prominent LV trabeculae, deep intertrabecular recesses, and the thin compacted layer.
- It is classified as a genetic cardiomyopathy by the AHA, and an unclassified cardiomyopathy by the ESC and WHO. It occurs as familial and nonfamilial forms and can manifest as an isolated form or in association with other genetic or congenital defect, e.g., Barth syndrome.
- Nonsporadic acquired forms are seen in athletes, pregnant women, persons with chronic kidney disease, persons with sickle cell anemia, etc.

Diagnostic Testing

Clinical spectrum extends from normal LV function to LV dysfunction and remodeling.

Echocardiography is the first choice of noninvasive imaging tool with predefined criteria by experts review as follows:

- Greater than three prominent trabeculae along the left ventricular endocardial border, which are visible in end-diastole
- Trabeculations form the noncompacted part of the two-layer myocardial structure, best visible at end-systole
- Ratio of > 2:1 noncompacted to compacted (NC/C) layer at end-systole
- Perfusion of the intertrabecular spaces from the ventricular cavity is present at end-diastole

Limitation of Echocardiography: difficulty in visualization of apex in LVNC.

CMR is performed in patients with evidence or suspicion of LVNC. In clinical practice, NC/C ratio >2.3 is diagnostic of LVNC (Peterson criteria).

TREATMENT

Symptomatic patients with LV systolic dysfunction and arrhythmias are treated according to the guideline-directed management. Oral anticoagulation is considered to prevent mural thrombosis.

Myocarditis

GENERAL PRINCIPLES

- It is an inflammatory disease of myocardium caused by different infectious and noninfectious triggers.
- Defined by the WHO, myocarditis is diagnosed by established histological (Dallas criteria), immunological, and immunohistochemical criteria. It often results from common viral infections and postviral immune-mediated responses.
- The most common viruses associated are coxsackie, enterovirus, adenovirus, HHV-6, parvovirus, EBV, CMV, HIV, and HCV. Other infectious causes include leptospirosis, diphtheria, *Staphylococcus*, *Streptococcus*, *Borrelia*, *Ehrlichia*, *babesiosis*, *T. cruzi*, helminths, and some fungi.
- Noninfectious causes include alcohol, drugs (doxorubicin, anticonvulsants, antibiotics, and antipsychotics), radiation, toxins (hydrocarbons and arsenic), autoimmune (sarcoid and lupus), and idiopathic.
- It is an important cause of dilated cardiomyopathy worldwide.

DIAGNOSIS

Clinical Manifestations

- Acute myocarditis
  - Acute coronary syndrome–like with acute chest pain in the absence of angiographic evidence of CAD
  - New onset or worsening HF in the absence of CAD and known causes of HF
  - Life-threatening condition (cardiogenic shock with severe LV dysfunction, arrhythmias) in the absence of CAD and known causes of HF
- Subacute/chronic myocarditis
  - Few patients with myocarditis present with an insidious onset of illness, i.e., developing over more than 3 months.
- Chronic active myocarditis
  - Presenting with frequent clinical and histologic relapses
  - Development of ventricular systolic dysfunction associated with chronic inflammatory changes
  - Mild to moderate fibrosis on endomyocardial biopsy
- Chronic persistent myocarditis
  - Presenting with a less distinct onset of illness characterized by a persistent histologic infiltrate, often with foci of myocyte necrosis
  - No ventricular systolic dysfunction despite persistent chest pain or palpitation

Diagnostic Workup

- Invasive diagnostic testing, such as endomyocardial biopsy, and specific therapies, such as immunosuppression, should be reserved for patients presenting with major clinical syndromes (severe heart failure and/or life-threatening arrhythmias) that are refractory to conventional therapies.
- Cardiac biomarkers (troponin I/T, BNP, and NT-proBNP) are elevated.
- Electrocardiography shows diffuse and saddle-shaped ST-segment elevation, bradyarrhythmia or advanced AV conduction defects, and low-voltage complexes.
- Echocardiography varies from normal to transient wall motion anomalies, transient mild ventricular dysfunction, pericardial effusion to (in severe cases) global impairment of LV with severe biventricular dysfunction without major remodeling, and wall motion abnormalities not relating to coronary artery distribution.
- CMR has become a primary tool for accurate distinction between myocarditis and acute coronary syndromes (subepicardial vs. subendocardial/transmural LGE distribution).
- Coronary angiography/CT-CAG and endomyocardial biopsy are indicated in the presence of severe clinical syndromes refractory to medical therapy.

TREATMENT

- Treatment of myocarditis includes supportive heart failure therapy and treatment of arrhythmias. Potential options for patients with refractory HF despite optimum medical therapy include mechanical circulatory support (e.g., ventricular assist devices) and cardiac transplantation.
- Immunosuppressive therapy is suggested for specific autoreactive disorders (giant cell myocarditis, cardiac sarcoidosis, eosinophilic myocarditis, and myocarditis associated with inflammatory connective tissue disorders).

Summary

- Heart failure is a complex clinical syndrome with symptoms and signs that result from any structural or functional impairment of ventricular filling or ejection of blood.
- Treatment of each stage aims to modify risk factors (stage A), treat risk and structural heart disease to prevent HF (stage B), and reduce symptoms, morbidity, and mortality (stages C and D).
- HFimpEF (HF with improved EF) is defined as previous LVEF $\leq$40% and a follow-up measurement of LVEF $>$40%.
- A critical component of the history and physical examination is to assess for clinical congestion (ie, those signs and symptoms resulting from elevated cardiac-filling pressures).
- Guideline-directed medical therapy (GDMT) for heart failure (HF) with reduced ejection fraction (HFrEF) now includes 4 medication classes that include sodium-glucose cotransporter-2 inhibitors (SGLT2i) ARNi, ACEi, ARB, MRA, and beta blockers.

Scan the QR code to access chapter references.

6 Pericardial and Valvular Heart Disease

Brittany M. Dixon, Nishath Quader, Ashwini M. V. and Anjali Sahni

PERICARDIAL DISEASE

Acute Pericarditis

ETIOLOGY

- Viral (coxsackie A and B, echovirus, HIV), neoplastic, autoimmune, tuberculous, bacterial (nontuberculous), uremia, postcardiac surgery, idiopathic, trauma, postmyocardial infarction (Dressler syndrome), drugs (procainamide, hydralazine), dissecting aortic aneurysm, and connective tissue disorder (RA, SLE).

Pathophysiology

- The pericardium is a fibrous sac surrounding the heart consisting of two layers: a thin visceral layer attached to the pericardium and a thicker parietal layer.
- The pericardial space is normally filled with 15–50 mL of fluid, and the two layers slide smoothly against each other, allowing for normal expansion and contraction of the heart.
- Pericarditis occurs when these layers are inflamed.

DIAGNOSIS

History

- The clinical presentation of acute pericarditis can vary depending on the underlying etiology.
- Chest pain: typically, sudden onset, anterior chest, sharp and pleuritic; improved by sitting up and leaning forward, made worse by inspiration and lying flat.

Physical Examination

- Pericardial friction rub: highly specific for acute pericarditis. Described as a "scratchy, grating, or squeaking sound," heard best with the diaphragm of the stethoscope.

Diagnostic Testing

- **Electrocardiogram** (**ECG**): diffuse ST-segment elevation (usually in more than one coronary artery distribution) and PR depression (Figure 6-1). The ECG differences between acute pericarditis and acute ST-segment elevation myocardial infarction (STEMI) have been highlighted in Table 6-1.
- **Chest X-ray** (**CXR**): typically normal.
- **Transthoracic echocardiogram** (**TTE**): may observe an associated pericardial effusion.
- Other tests: complete blood count, C-reactive protein (CRP), erythrocyte sedimentation rate (ESR), blood cultures (if suspect infection).

TREATMENT

- Treat the underlying cause whenever possible.
- Bed rest and avoid physical activity.

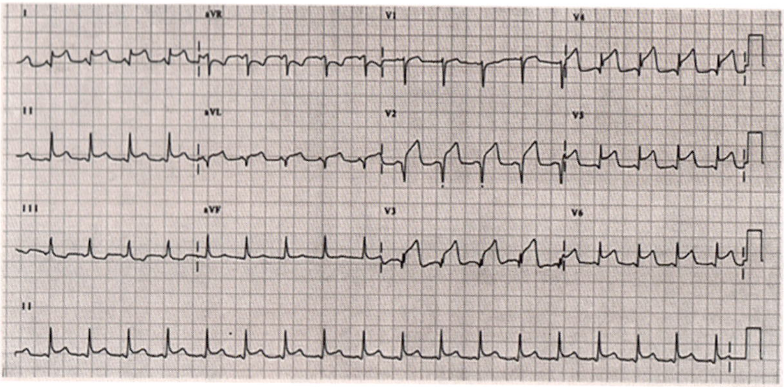

Figure 6-1 ECG showing PR-segment elevation in aVR, ST elevation in V2–V6, I, aVL, and depression in aVR suggestive of acute pericarditis.

TABLE 6-1 Differences in ECG Changes between Acute Pericarditis and Acute ST-elevation MI

ECG Changes	Acute Pericarditis	Acute ST-Elevation MI
Shape of ST segment	Concave upward	Convex upward
Reciprocal ST-segment changes	Absent	Present
Location of ST-segment changes	Diffuse (except aVR and V1)	Follows a vascular territory
Depression of PR segment	Present	Absent
Concomitant presence of ST and T changes	Absent (T-wave inversion occurs after ST segments have normalized)	Present

- **NSAIDs:**
  - Aspirin in the dose of 600 mg 4 hourly is the drug of choice for patients with a recent myocardial infarction.
  - Ibuprofen 300–800 mg, three times daily may also be used.
  - Indomethacin is a more potent anti-inflammatory drug and can be given in the dose of 25 mg, three times daily.
- **Colchicine:** 0.5 mg twice a day when added to conventional anti-inflammatory therapy, significantly reduces symptoms, recurrence rates, and hospitalizations (COPE trial).[1]
- **Glucocorticoids:** reserved for cases refractory to standard therapy or in the setting of uremia, connective tissue disease, or immune-mediated pericarditis.

Constrictive Pericarditis

Constrictive pericarditis is often difficult to distinguish from restrictive cardiomyopathies (RCMs). Multiple imaging modalities, invasive hemodynamic tests, history, and physical examination are often needed to confirm the diagnosis.

ETIOLOGY

Idiopathic, viral pericarditis (chronic or recurrent), postcardiotomy, chest irradiation, autoimmune connective tissue disorders, end-stage renal disease, uremia, malignancy (e.g., breast, lung, lymphoma), and tuberculosis (more common in endemic countries).

Pathophysiology

- In the setting of chronic inflammation, the pericardial layers become thickened, scarred, and calcified.
- The pericardial space is obliterated, and the pericardium becomes noncompliant. This impairs ventricular filling and leads to an equalization of pressures in all four chambers and subsequent heart failure symptoms.

DIAGNOSIS

History

- The clinical presentation of constrictive pericarditis is insidious, with gradual development of fatigue, exercise intolerance, and venous congestion.

Physical Examination

- Features of right-sided heart failure: lower extremity edema, hepatomegaly, ascites, elevated jugular venous pressure (JVP).
- Other characteristic signs:
  - **Kussmaul sign:** paradoxical increase in JVP with inspiration or lack of appropriate decrease in JVP with inspiration.
  - **Pericardial knock:** early, loud, high-pitched S_3.

Constriction versus Restriction

Both constrictive and restrictive diseases may share similar clinical features. However, it is important to distinguish the two physiologies. Constrictive pericarditis is a potentially reversible condition, whereas restrictive disease has fewer therapeutic options. The differences between constrictive pericarditis and restrictive cardiomyopathy are shown in Table 6-2.

TABLE 6-2 Constrictive Pericarditis vs Restrictive Cardiomyopathy

	Constrictive Pericarditis	Restrictive Cardiomyopathy
Ventricular interdependence	Present	Absent
Echocardiography	Preserved (or increased) tissue Doppler velocities	Decreased tissue Doppler velocities
Septal motion	Septal bounce (exaggerated septal motion)	Normal septal motion
Pulmonary hypertension	Mild or absent	Present
B-type natriuretic peptide	Mildly elevated	Significantly elevated
JVP	Prominent “x” and “y” descents (“square root sign”)	Blunted “x” descent

Diagnostic Testing

- **TTE:**
  - First-line diagnostic test.
  - Ventricular systolic function can be deceptively "normal."
  - Features suggestive of constrictive pericarditis include the following:
    - Increased pericardial thickness/tethering of the pericardium to the myocardium.
    - Dilated, incompressible inferior vena cava (IVC).
    - Septal bounce.
    - Inspiratory variation in mitral flow velocity curves.
    - Expiratory diastolic flow reversal in hepatic veins.
    - Preserved (or increased) tissue Doppler velocities of the mitral annulus.
    - Blunted superior vena cava flow.
- **Cardiac catheterization:** allows for simultaneous measurement of right ventricular and left ventricular pressures.
- **Cardiac CT and MRI**
  - Provide excellent visualization of pericardial anatomy (thickness and calcification).
  - An MRI and gated CT can show evidence of ventricular interdependence (septal bounce).
  - Can provide other anatomic information that may be helpful in making the diagnosis of constriction (i.e., engorgement of IVC and hepatic veins) and its etiology (i.e., lymph nodes, tumors).

TREATMENT

- Limited role for medical therapy: diuretics, low-sodium diet.
- Patients with constriction often have a resting sinus tachycardia. Because of limited stroke volume (SV), they are more dependent on heart rate for adequate cardiac output (CO). Avoid efforts to slow down the heart rate.
- **Surgical pericardiectomy is the only definitive treatment for constrictive pericarditis.** Operative mortality is 5%–15%; more advanced heart failure symptoms confer higher operative risk.

Cardiac Tamponade

Cardiac tamponade is a **clinical diagnosis** and is considered a medical emergency. Imaging is used to confirm the presence of a pericardial effusion; however, it should not be solely relied on to make the diagnosis of tamponade.

ETIOLOGY

Procedural complications, infection, neoplasms, or idiopathic pericarditis, postcardiotomy, autoimmune connective tissue disorders, uremia, trauma, radiation, myocardial infarction (subacute), drugs (hydralazine, procainamide, isoniazid, phenytoin, minoxidil), hypothyroidism.

Pathophysiology

- Fluid accumulation in the pericardial space increases pericardial pressure. The pressure depends on the amount of fluid, the rate of accumulation, and the compliance of the pericardium.
- Tamponade develops when the pressure in the pericardial space is sufficiently high to interfere with adequate cardiac filling, resulting in a decrease in cardiac output.

DIAGNOSIS

History

- The diagnosis of cardiac tamponade should be suspected in patients with **elevated JVP, hypotension, and distant heart sounds** (**Beck's triad**).
- Symptoms can include dyspnea, fatigue, anxiety, presyncope, chest discomfort, abdominal fullness, and lethargy.

Physical Examination

- **Pulsus paradoxus** refers to an abnormally large decrease in systolic blood pressure, SV, and pulse wave amplitude with inspiration.
- A normal fall in pressure is less than 10 mm Hg. **A decrease in systolic pressure >10 mm Hg is one of the physical examination findings in tamponade.**
- Patients are also frequently tachycardic and hypotensive.

Diagnostic Testing

- **Remember, cardiac tamponade is a clinical diagnosis that can be made based on history, physical examination, and vital signs (blood pressure, pulsus paradoxus) alone.**
- **ECG:** low voltage (more likely with larger pericardial effusions), sinus tachycardia, electrical alternans (specific but not sensitive).
- **TTE:**
  - First-line diagnostic test to evaluate the hemodynamic significance of pericardial effusion.
  - Features suggestive of a hemodynamically significant pericardial effusion:
    - Dilated, incompressible IVC.
    - Significant respiratory variation of tricuspid and mitral inflow velocities (>25% mitral, >40% tricuspid).
    - Early diastolic collapse of the right ventricle and systolic collapse of the right atrium.

TREATMENT

- Limited role for medical therapy to treat cardiac tamponade. **Goal is to maintain adequate filling pressures** with IV fluids. Avoid diuretics, nitrates, and any other preload-reducing medications. Avoid efforts to slow down sinus tachycardia: it compensates for a reduced SV to try to maintain adequate cardiac output.
- **Percutaneous pericardiocentesis** with echocardiographic guidance can be a relatively safe and effective way to drain the pericardial fluid; the approach should be guided by location of the fluid and is usually easiest when the effusion is in anterior location.
- Creation of a **pericardial window** is preferred for recurring effusions, loculated effusions, or those not safely accessible percutaneously.

VALVULAR HEART DISEASE

The 2014 and updated 2017 and 2020 American Heart Association/American College of Cardiology (AHA/ACC) Guidelines describe different stages in the progression of valvular heart disease (VHD).[2,3]

- **Stage A (at risk):** patients with risk factors for development of VHD.
- **Stage B (progressive):** patients with progressive VHD (mild to moderate severity and asymptomatic).
- **Stage C (asymptomatic severe):** asymptomatic patients who meet criteria for severe VHD.
  - C1: asymptomatic patients with a compensated left and right ventricle.
  - C2: asymptomatic patients with decompensation of the left or right ventricle.
- **Stage D (symptomatic severe):** patients who have developed symptoms as a result of VHD.

Acute Rheumatic Fever

ETIOLOGY

Rheumatic fever is an acute, poststreptococcal, immune-mediated, multisystem inflammatory disease, occurring as a sequela to group A streptococcal pharyngitis after a latent period of 2–6 weeks.

Serotype M-type 5 is commonly implicated in rheumatic fever.

Pathophysiology

- **Molecular mimicry:** The antibodies produced against antigenic components of the *Streptococcus* cross-react with human tissues (heart, joint) because of the antigenic similarity. Carditis manifests as pancarditis involving all three layers of the heart such as endocardium, myocardium, and pericardium. Valvular damage is the hallmark of rheumatic fever.
- **Streptococcal superantigens:** Superantigens are glycoproteins that bridge class II MHC molecules to specific T-cell receptors, simulating activation of CD4+ T cells.
- **Host factors:** In India, HLA-DR3 is associated more frequently with rheumatic fever.

DIAGNOSIS

History

- History of streptococcal pharyngitis in the past 2–3 weeks.
- Migrating polyarthritis: acute, painful, migratory, asymmetric, fleeting, and flitting arthritis usually involving large joints.
- Chest pain.

Physical Examination

- Migrating polyarthritis: involved joints show signs of inflammation. Pain and swelling develops quickly and subsides within 5–7 days, without leaving any residual deformity.
- Tachycardia disproportionate to fever and features of congestive heart failure.
- Apical soft mid-diastolic murmur, also known as a Carey Coombs murmur: due to valvulitis with nodules on the mitral valve leaflets.
- Pericardial friction rub.
- Subcutaneous nodules: small, painless, and mobile nodules along the extensor surface.
- Erythema marginatum: red macules with serpiginous spreading edge and central clearing, mostly found on the trunk and limbs.
- Rheumatic chorea: chorea, muscle weakness, and emotional instability.

Diagnostic Testing

Diagnosis of acute rheumatic fever is based on modified Jones criteria (Table 6-3).

Other investigations include the following:

- Raised ESR and CRP.
- Raised streptococcal antibody levels: ASO, anti-DNase B, and antihyaluronidase.
- Isolation of group A streptococci by throat swab culture.
- ECG: prolongation of the PR interval and T-wave inversion.
- ECHO: to assess cardiac function, valvular abnormalities, and pericardial effusion.

TABLE 6-3 Diagnostic Criteria for Rheumatic Fever—Modified 2015 Jones Criteria

Major Criteria	
Low-Risk Population	**High-Risk Population**
Carditis (clinical or subclinical) Arthritis—only polyarthritis Chorea Erythema marginatum Subcutaneous nodules	Carditis (clinical or subclinical) Arthritis—monoarthritis or polyarthritis Polyarthralgia Chorea Erythema marginatum Subcutaneous nodules
Minor Criteria	
Low-Risk Population	**High-Risk Population**
Polyarthralgia Hyperpyrexia (≥38.5°C) ESR ≥60 mm/h and/or CRP ≥3.0 mg/dL Prolonged PR interval (after taking into account the differences related to age; if there is no carditis as a major criterion)	Monoarthralgia Hyperpyrexia (≥38.0°C) ESR ≥30 mm/h and/or CRP ≥3.0 mg/dL Prolonged PR interval (after taking into account the differences related to age; if there is no carditis as a major criterion)

CRP, C-reactive protein; ESR, erythrocyte sedimentation rate.
The diagnosis of RF in the whole population with evidence of antecedent group A β-hemolytic streptococcal infection requires a confirmation of two major criteria or one major and two minor criteria—the first episode of the disease.

TREATMENT

Supportive Measures

- Treatment of congestive cardiac failure: digitalis and diuretics.
- Treatment of chorea.
- Rest to joints and supportive splinting.

Primary Prevention: Eradication of Streptococci

- Benzathine Penicillin 1.2 million units single-dose intramuscular (IM), or oral penicillin V.

Anti-Inflammatory Agents

- Aspirin is given in doses of 75–100 mg/kg body weight/day divided into four doses for 6 weeks.
- Corticosteroids are indicated in patients with carditis or severe arthritis. Prednisolone 1.0–2.0 mg/kg/day is given in divided doses for 4 weeks and then tapered off.

Secondary Prevention of Rheumatic Fever: Prevention of Recurrent Attacks

- Penicillin G benzathine 1.2 million units IM every 3 weeks. The duration of prophylaxis is guided by the presence or absence of carditis and residual heart disease.

Infective Endocarditis

It is defined as an endovascular infection of cardiovascular structures by microbes.

PATHOPHYSIOLOGY

- Endocardial damage and formation of sterile thrombus.
- Adherence of the microorganisms to the sterile vegetations during transient bacteremia.
- Proliferation of microorganisms within vegetations.
- Formation of infective emboli: they may result in infarction or abscess.
- Septic emboli cause arteritis with weakness of arterial wall leading to mycotic aneurysms.

Predisposing Factors

- Congenital heart diseases: ventricular septal defect, tetralogy of Fallot, and idiopathic subaortic stenosis.
- Cardiac prosthetic valves.
- Parenteral narcotic drug abuse.
- Conditions with bacteremia: all dental procedures in which there is handling of gingival tissue or the periapical region of teeth or perforation of the oral mucosa; any invasive procedure of the respiratory tract involving respiratory mucosa.

CLASSIFICATION

- According to the clinical course: acute, subacute, and chronic.
- According to the causative organism: bacterial (commonly *Streptococcus*, *Staphylococcus aureus*), viral, rickettsial, or fungal.
- According to the nature of valve or device: native or prosthetic.
- According to the side affected: left-sided or right-sided infective endocarditis.

DIAGNOSIS

History

- Fever, fatigue, loss of appetite, and loss of weight.

Physical Examination

- Clubbing.
- Splenomegaly.
- Evidence of new valve lesion (regurgitant)/murmurs or change of murmur.
- Cutaneous manifestations: purpura and petechiae and subungual splinter hemorrhages.
- Janeway lesions: erythematous, nontender nodules on palms or soles.
- Osler nodes: tender, small, painful, swollen, and purplish/erythematous subcutaneous papules/nodules in pulp of distal fingers due to hypersensitive angiitis.
- Roth spots: circular retinal hemorrhages with white or pale center spots composed of fibrin.
- Focal segmental glomerulonephritis: hematuria.

Diagnostic Testing (Table 6-4)

Investigations

- Blood cultures: at least three sets of blood cultures should be taken from different venipuncture sites over 24 hours before commencing the therapy.
- ECG: to detect complications such as conduction abnormalities.

TABLE 6-4 2023 Duke-International Society for Cardiovascular Infectious Diseases Infective Endocarditis (IE)

I. Major Criteria

A. Microbiologic Major Criteria

i. Positive blood cultures
   a. Microorganisms that commonly cause IE isolated from 2 or more separate blood culture sets (typical).
   or
   b. Microorganisms that occasionally or rarely cause IE isolated from 3 or more separate blood culture sets (nontypical).

ii. Positive laboratory tests
   a. Positive polymerase chain reaction (PCR) or other nucleic acid-based techniques for *Coxiella burnetii, Bartonella* species, or *Tropheryma whipplei* from blood.
   or
   b. *Coxiella burnetii* antiphase I immunoglobulin G (IgG) antibody titer >1:800 or isolated from a single blood culture.
   or
   c. Indirect immunofluorescence assays (IFA) for detection of IgM and IgG antibodies to *Bartonella henselae* or *Bartonella quintana* with immunoglobulin G (IgG) titer ≥1:800.

B. Imaging Major Criteria

i. Echocardiography and cardiac computed tomography (CT) imaging
   a. Echocardiography and/or cardiac CT showing vegetation, valvular/leaflet perforation, valvular/leaflet aneurysm, abscess, pseudoaneurysm, or intracardiac fistula.
   or
   b. Significant new valvular regurgitation on echocardiography as compared with previous imaging. Worsening or changing of preexisting regurgitation is not sufficient.
   or
   c. New partial dehiscence of prosthetic valve as compared with previous imaging.

ii. Positron emission computed tomography with 18F-fluorodeoxyglucose ([18[F] FDG PET/CT imaging)

Abnormal metabolic activity involving a native or prosthetic valve, ascending aortic graft (with concomitant evidence of valve involvement), intracardiac device leads, or other prosthetic material.

C. Surgical major criteria

Evidence of IE documented by direct inspection during heart surgery neither major imaging criteria nor subsequent histologic or microbiologic confirmation

II. Minor Criteria

A. Predisposition
   i. Previous history of IE
   ii. Prosthetic valve
   iii. Previous valve repair
   iv. Congenital heart disease
   v. More than mild regurgitation or stenosis of any etiology

(*Continued*)

TABLE 6-4 2023 Duke-International Society for Cardiovascular Infectious Diseases Infective Endocarditis (IE) (Continued)

vi. Endovascular intracardiac implantable electronic device (CIED)
vii. Hypertrophic obstructive cardiomyopathy
viii. Injection drug use

B. Fever documented temperature greater than 38.0°C (100.4°F)

C. Vascular phenomena clinical or radiological evidence of arterial emboli, septic pulmonary infarcts, cerebral or splenic abscess, mycotic aneurysm, intracranial hemorrhage, conjunctival hemorrhages, Janeway lesions, and purulent purpura.

D. Immunologic phenomena positive rheumatoid factor, Osler nodes, Roth spots, or immune complex-mediated glomerulonephritis.

E. Microbiologic evidence, falling short of a major criterion
Positive blood cultures for a microorganism consistent with IE but not meeting the requirements for major criterion.
or
Positive culture, PCR, or other nucleic acid-based test (amplicon or shotgun sequencing, in situ hybridization) for an organism consistent with IE from a sterile body site other than cardiac tissue, cardiac prosthesis, or arterial embolus; or a single finding of a skin bacterium by PCR on a valve or wire without additional clinical or microbiological supporting evidence.

F. Imaging criteria
Abnormal metabolic activity as detected by (18F) FDG PET/CT within 3 months of implantation of prosthetic valve, ascending aortic graft (with concomitant evidence of valve involvement), intracardiac device leads, or other prosthetic material.

G. Physical examination criteria
New valvular regurgitation identified on auscultation if echocardiography is not available. Worsening or changing of preexisting murmur not sufficient.

I. Definite Endocarditis

A. Pathologic Criteria

i. Microorganisms identified in the context of clinical signs of active endocarditis in a vegetation; from cardiac tissue; from an explanted prosthetic valve or sewing ring; from an ascending aortic graft (with concomitant evidence of valve involvement); from an endovascular intracardiac implantable electronic device (CIED); or from an arterial embolus.
or
ii. Active endocarditis (may be acute or subacute/chronic) identified in or on a vegetation; from cardiac tissue; from an explanted prosthetic valve or sewing ring; from an ascending aortic graft (with concomitant evidence of valve involvement); from a CIED; or from an arterial embolus.

B. Clinical Criteria

i. 2 major criteria
or
ii. 1 major criterion and 3 minor criteria
or
iii. 5 minor criteria

II. Possible Endocarditis

i. 1 major criterion and 1 minor criterion
or
ii. 3 minor criteria

(*Continued*)

TABLE 6-4 2023 Duke-International Society for Cardiovascular Infectious Diseases Infective Endocarditis (IE) (Continued)

III. Rejected Endocarditis

i. Firm alternate diagnosis explaining signs/symptoms.
or
ii. Lack of recurrence despite antibiotic therapy for less than 4 days.
or
iii. No pathologic or macroscopic evidence of IE at surgery or autopsy, with antibiotic therapy for less than 4 days.
or
iv. One does not meet criteria for possible IE, as above.

- Echocardiography: to identify the presence and size of vegetations, and assess valve damage, abscess formation, and cardiac function.
- Complete blood counts: may show normocytic normochromic anemia and increased WBC counts.
- Urea and creatinine: may be increased due to glomerulonephritis.
- Liver biochemistry: serum alkaline phosphatase may be increased.
- Increased ESR and CRP.
- Urine: proteinuria and hematuria.

TREATMENT

- Penicillins are fundamental to the therapy of bacterial endocarditis.
- Empirical treatment: no suspicion of staphylococci—benzylpenicillin 1.2 g IV 4 hourly for 4–6 weeks plus gentamicin 80 mg IV 12 hourly for 2–6 weeks.
- Suspected staphylococcal endocarditis: Vancomycin 30 mg/kg/day (not to exceed 2 g/day) IV 12 hourly for 6 weeks plus gentamicin 80–120 mg IV 8 hourly for 1–2 weeks. In prosthetic valve endocarditis, add rifampicin.
- Progressive cardiac failure due to valvular damage, abscess formation, and large and mobile vegetations are indications for surgery.

PROPHYLAXIS

- Indications for antibiotic regimen for prophylaxis of endocarditis are as follows:
  - Prosthetic heart valves.
  - Prior bacterial endocarditis.
  - Complex cyanotic congenital heart disease.
  - Surgically constructed systemic-pulmonary shunts.
  - Repaired shunts within 6 months.
  - Valvulopathy after cardiac transplantation.
- Standard regimen: amoxycillin 2.0 g PO 1 hour before procedure.
- Inability to take oral medication: ampicillin 2.0 g IV or IM 30 minutes before procedure.
- Other alternatives: clarithromycin, cephalexin or cefadroxil, and clindamycin.

Mitral Stenosis

- Mitral stenosis (MS) is characterized by incomplete opening of the mitral valve during diastole, which limits antegrade flow and yields a sustained diastolic pressure gradient between the left atrium (LA) and the left ventricle (LV).

ETIOLOGY

- **Rheumatic MS**
  - Because of the increased use of antibiotics, the incidence of rheumatic heart disease as a cause of MS has decreased.
  - Two-thirds of patients with rheumatic MS are female; may be associated with mitral regurgitation (MR).
  - Rheumatic fever can cause fibrosis, thickening, and calcification, leading to fusion of the commissures, leaflets, chordae, and/or papillary muscles.
- **Other causes of MS:** substantial mitral annular calcification (calcific MS), systemic lupus erythematosus (SLE), rheumatoid arthritis, congenital, oversewn or small mitral annuloplasty ring; "functional MS" may occur with obstruction of the LA outflow because of tumor (particularly myxoma), LA thrombus, or endocarditis with a large vegetation.

Pathophysiology

- Increased transvalvular flow or decreased diastolic filling time may lead to worsening symptoms of MS. This occurs with pregnancy, exercise, hyperthyroidism, atrial fibrillation (AF) with rapid ventricular response, and fever.
- MS causes increased pressure in the LA, which then dilates as a compensatory mechanism. This causes the LA to dilate and fibrose, which then leads to atrial arrhythmias and thrombus formation.
- A sustained increase in pulmonary venous pressures is transmitted backward to cause pulmonary hypertension (PH) and with time, increased pulmonary vascular resistance and right ventricular pressure overload and dysfunction.

DIAGNOSIS

History

- After a prolonged asymptomatic period, patients may report any of the following: dyspnea, decreased functional capacity, orthopnea, paroxysmal nocturnal dyspnea, fatigue, palpitations, systemic embolism, hemoptysis, chest pain.

Physical Examination

- Mitral facies.
- Pulse: low volume; rhythm is irregularly irregular and varying volume in AF.
- Apex beat is not shifted and is tapping in character.
- Diastolic thrill at apex.
- Loud first heart sound.
- Opening snap (OS) caused by sudden tensing of the valve leaflets; the A_2-OS interval varies inversely with the severity of stenosis (shorter interval = more severe stenosis)
- Mid-diastolic rumble: low-pitched, rumbling, mid-diastolic murmur, best heard with the bell of the stethoscope held lightly at the apex with the patient lying on the left lateral position, breath held in expiration; the severity of stenosis is related to the duration of the murmur, not intensity.
- Signs of right-sided heart failure and PH (palpable P2, left parasternal heave, epigastric pulsations of RV type).
- Murmur of pulmonary regurgitation (Graham Steell murmur).

Diagnostic Testing

- **ECG:** left atrial enlargement (LAE), AF, right ventricular hypertrophy.
- **CXR:** straightening of left heart border (mitralization of heart), evidence of pulmonary venous and arterial hypertension, calcification of the mitral valve and/or annulus.

- TTE:
  - Assess valve leaflets and subvalvular apparatus.
  - Determine mitral valve area (MVA) and mean transmitral gradient.
  - Estimate pulmonary artery systolic pressure and evaluate right ventricular size and function.
- **Transesophageal echocardiogram** (TEE): evaluate MV morphology and hemodynamics in patients with MS for whom TTE was suboptimal. Also used to rule out left atrial thrombus.
- **Exercise stress testing:** indicated when symptoms are out of proportion to severity indicated by TTE. Can get assessment of exercise capacity, mean transmitral gradient with exercise, and increase in PA pressures with exercise.
- **Cardiac catheterization**
  - Rarely indicated; however, it can be performed when clinical and echocardiography assessment are discordant; however, to obtain an accurate assessment, direct left atrial hemodynamics via transseptal puncture is required.
  - Reasonable in patients with MS to assess the cause of severe PH when out of proportion to the severity of MS as determined by noninvasive testing.

TREATMENT

Medical Management

- Diuretics, β-blockers, and low-salt diet for heart failure symptoms.
- AF occurs in 30%–40% of patients with severe MS.
  - Therapy is mostly aimed at rate control and prevention of thromboembolism.
  - **AHA/ACC Guidelines—Class I indications for anticoagulation** for prevention of systemic embolization in patients with MS regardless of CHADS2VASC score.[2,3]

Percutaneous Mitral Balloon Commissurotomy

- Balloon inflation separates the leaflets, yielding an increased valve area.
- Indicated only in rheumatic MS where there is thickening of the leaflets and annulus is mostly spared.
- It compares favorably with surgical mitral commissurotomy (open or closed) and is the procedure of choice in experienced centers in patients without contraindications (such as moderate or more MR and left atrial appendage thrombus).
- **Recommendations for percutaneous mitral balloon commissurotomy**[2,3]:
  - Symptomatic patients with severe MS (valve area $\leq$1.5 cm^2) (stage D) and favorable valve anatomy in the absence of contraindications (i.e., LA clot or moderate to severe MR) (Class I)
  - Asymptomatic patients with very severe MS (valve area $\leq$1.0 cm^2) (stage C) and favorable valve anatomy in the absence of contraindication (Class IIa)
  - Asymptomatic patients with severe MS (stage C) and favorable valve anatomy in the absence of a LA clot or moderate to severe MR who have new-onset AF (Class IIb)
  - Symptomatic patients with MVA <1.5 cm^2 with hemodynamically significant MS during exercise (Class IIb)
  - Severely symptomatic patients with severe MS (MVA <1.5 cm^2) (stage D) who have suboptimal valve anatomy and are not surgical candidates or high-risk surgical candidates (Class IIb)

Surgical Management

Recommendations for mitral valve surgery[2,3]:

- Severely symptomatic patients with severe MS (valve area <1.5 cm^2; stage D) who are not high risk for surgery and who are not candidates for or failed previous percutaneous mitral balloon commissurotomy (Class I).

- Concomitant MV surgery is indicated for patients with severe MS (valve area <1.5 cm^2; stage C or D) undergoing other cardiac surgery (Class I).

Complications of Mitral Stenosis

- Atrial fibrillation: most common complication. AF worsens symptoms of MS.
- Systemic embolization.
- Pulmonary hypertension and right heart failure.
- Pulmonary edema.
- Ortner syndrome: paralysis of left recurrent laryngeal nerve due to compression between the enlarged tense pulmonary artery and the aorta at ligamentum arteriosum. It produces hoarseness of voice.
- Hemoptysis.
- Cardiac cirrhosis.
- Pulmonary hemosiderosis.
- Dysphagia due to compression of esophagus.
- Infective endocarditis (rare).

Mitral Valve Prolapse

Mitral valve prolapse (MVP) is an abnormal movement of one or both of the mitral valve leaflets ≥2 mm beyond annular plane into the left atrium during systole with or without MR.

PATHOPHYSIOLOGY

- It is caused by congenital anomalies or degenerative myxomatous changes that are associated with excessive or redundant mitral leaflet tissue, for example, Marfan syndrome and cystic medial necrosis.
- Familial: autosomal dominant mode of inheritance.
- Prolapse of the cusp occurs in systole → tensing of the chordae → pulling of papillary muscles which sometimes may interfere with blood supply.

DIAGNOSIS

History

- Most patients are asymptomatic.
- Atypical chest pain, palpitation, syncope, and fatigue may be present.

Physical Examination

- Asthenic built, straight back/pectus excavatum.
- Midsystolic click: in mildest forms, the valve is competent but bulges back into the atrium during systole, causing a midsystolic click without any murmur.
- Late systolic murmur: when there is MR, the click is followed by a late systolic apical murmur.
- The length of the murmur increases as the regurgitation becomes more severe.
- The systolic murmur of MVP increases during standing and Valsalva maneuver, but decreases during squatting and isometric exercise.

Diagnostic Testing

- **ECG:** nonspecific ST-T changes or inverted T waves in leads II, III, and aVF.
- **Echocardiography:** used for confirmation of the diagnosis. Color Doppler is used to assess the degree of MR.

TREATMENT

- No need for infective endocarditis prophylaxis.
- Reassurance for patients without symptoms.

Medical Management

- **β-Blockers:** for atypical chest pain.
- **Antiarrhythmic drugs:** for the treatment of arrhythmias.
- **Transient ischemic attacks:** aspirin, dipyridamole, or anticoagulants.

Surgical Management

- Mitral valve repair or replacement in severe MR.

Aortic Stenosis

- **Aortic stenosis** (AS) is the most common cause of LV outflow tract obstruction.
- Other causes of obstruction occur above the valve (supravalvular) and below the valve (subvalvular), both fixed (i.e., subaortic membrane) and dynamic (i.e., hypertrophic cardiomyopathy with obstruction).
- **Aortic sclerosis** is thickening of the aortic valve leaflets that causes turbulent flow through the valve and a murmur but no significant gradient; over time, it can develop into AS.

ETIOLOGY

- **Calcific/degenerative**
  - Most common cause in the United States.
  - Trileaflet calcific AS usually presents in the seventh to ninth decades of life.
- **Bicuspid**
  - Occurs in 1%–2% of population (congenital lesion).
  - AS in this population occurs in much younger patients.
  - Can be associated with aortopathies (i.e., dissection, aneurysm).
- **Rheumatic**
  - More common cause worldwide; much less common in the United States.
  - Almost always accompanied by MV disease.
- **Radiation induced**

Pathophysiology

- The pathophysiology for calcific AS involves both the valve and the ventricular adaptation to the stenosis.
- Within the valve (trileaflet and bicuspid), there is growing evidence for an active biologic process that begins much like the formation of an atherosclerotic plaque and eventually leads to calcification (Figure 6-2).

DIAGNOSIS

History

- The classic triad of symptoms includes **angina, syncope, and heart failure.**
- Symptoms may be masked by a progressive decline in functional capacity as patients modify their activities to suit their symptoms.

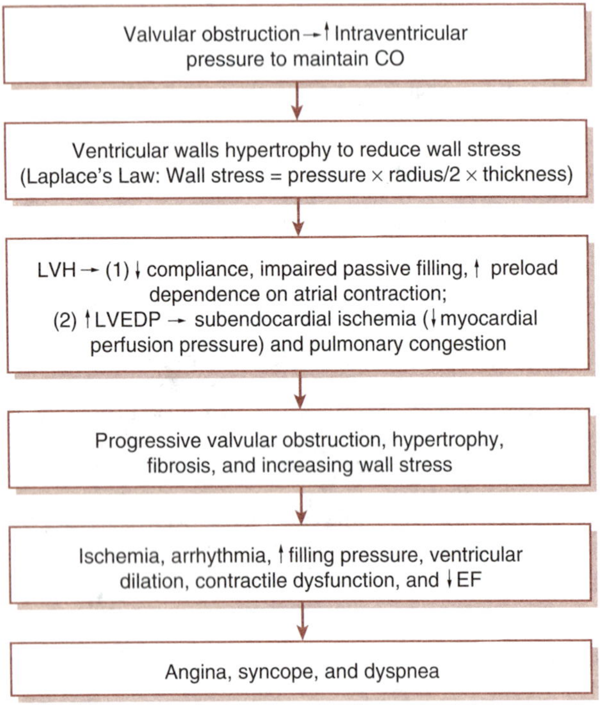

Figure 6-2 Pathophysiology of aortic stenosis. CO, cardiac output; EF, ejection fraction; LVEDP, left ventricular end-diastolic pressure; LVH, left ventricular hypertrophy.

Physical Examination

- Pulsus parvus et tardus: slow rising, late peaking, and low amplitude.
- Blood pressure: systolic decapitation (SBP <120 mm Hg).
- **Harsh systolic crescendo–decrescendo murmur** heard best at the right upper sternal border and radiating to both carotids; time to peak intensity correlates with severity (later peak = more severe).
- Diminished or absent A_2 (soft S_2) suggests severe AS.
- Gallavardin phenomenon is an AS murmur heard best at the apex (could be confused with MR).

Diagnostic Testing

- **ECG:** LAE, left ventricular hypertrophy (LVH).
- **CXR:** cardiomegaly, calcification of the aorta, and/or aortic valve.
- **TTE:**
  - Determine valve morphology (tricuspid vs. bicuspid), calculate valve area using continuity equation, and measure transvalvular mean and peak gradients.
  - **Severe AS:** peak jet velocity ≥4.0 m/s, mean gradient ≥40 mm Hg, valve area <1.0 cm^2.
- **TEE:** useful in select patients to better visualize valve morphology and determination of AS severity.

- **Dobutamine stress echocardiography**
  - Useful to assess the patient with a reduced stroke (reduced or preserved ejection fraction [EF]) and small calculated valve area but a low (<30–40 mm Hg) mean transvalvular gradient.
  - Can help distinguish truly severe AS from pseudo-severe AS.
- **Cardiac catheterization**
  - Hemodynamic assessment of severity of AS in patients for whom noninvasive tests are inconclusive or when there is discrepancy between noninvasive tests and clinical findings regarding AS severity.
  - **Gorlin equation:** used to calculate aortic valve area during invasive hemodynamic assessment; based on principle that aortic valve area is equal to systolic flow across valve divided by systolic pressure gradient times a constant.

TREATMENT

- **Severe symptomatic AS requires surgery or percutaneous intervention;** currently, there are no medical treatments proven to decrease mortality or to delay surgery.
- Hypertension should be treated in patients with AS to reduce afterload.
- Diuretics may alleviate shortness of breath in patients with symptomatic AS and evidence of volume overload.
- Severe AS with decompensated HF:
  - Several options may help bridge the patient to definitive surgery or percutaneous procedure: intra-aortic balloon pump (IABP) (contraindicated in patients with moderate to severe aortic regurgitation [AR]), sodium nitroprusside, balloon aortic valvuloplasty.
  - Each of the above measures provides some degree of afterload reduction, either at the level of the valve (valvuloplasty) or systemic vascular resistance (sodium nitroprusside), which can facilitate forward flow.

Percutaneous Interventions

Balloon aortic valvuloplasty has a limited role in the treatment of patients with severe AS; the improvement in valve area is modest, and the clinical improvement that it provides usually lasts weeks to months.[4-7]

- **Transcatheter aortic valve replacement (TAVR)**
  - Requires evaluation by a team of cardiologists and cardiac surgeons. TAVR procedure uses fluoroscopic and echocardiographic guidance to place a stented bioprosthetic valve within the stenotic valve. This can be performed via a transfemoral, transaortic, subclavian, transcaval, or transapical approach.
  - To date, clinical trials have demonstrated that in patients at prohibitive risk for surgery, TAVR reduces mortality compared with medical therapy[8]; for high-risk patients and intermediate-risk patients, TAVR and surgical valve replacement have similar outcomes.[9-11]
  - Ongoing studies are assessing the role of TAVR in expanded patient populations.
  - These less-invasive, catheter-based techniques for valve replacement are rapidly evolving and are being investigated in ongoing clinical trials and clinical registries.

Surgical Management

- Symptomatic with severe high-gradient AS (stage D1) (Class I)
- Asymptomatic with severe AS and left ventricular ejection fraction (LVEF) <50% (stage C2) (Class I).
- Patients with severe AS (stage C or D) undergoing other cardiac surgery (Class I)
- Asymptomatic patients with very severe AS (stage C1) and low surgical risk (Class IIa)
- Asymptomatic patients with severe AS (stage C1) and decreased exercise tolerance or fall in blood pressure on exercise testing (Class IIa).

PROGNOSIS

- AS is a progressive disease typically characterized by an asymptomatic phase until the valve area reaches a minimum threshold, generally <1.0 cm^2. In the absence of symptoms, patients with AS have a good prognosis with a risk of sudden death estimated to be approximately 1% per year.
- Once patients experience symptoms, their average survival is 2–3 years with a high risk of sudden death.

Mitral Regurgitation

- Prevention of MR is dependent on the integrated and proper function of the MV (annulus and leaflets), subvalvular apparatus (chordae tendineae and papillary muscles), LA, and LV; abnormal function or size of any one of these components can lead to MR.
- **Primary MR** refers to MR caused primarily by lesions to the valve leaflets and/or chordae tendineae (i.e., myxomatous degeneration, endocarditis, rheumatic).
- **Secondary MR,** or functional MR, refers to MR caused primarily by ventricular dysfunction usually with accompanying annular dilatation (i.e., dilated cardiomyopathy and ischemic MR).
- It is critical to define the mechanism of MR and the time course (acute vs. chronic) because these significantly impact clinical management.

ETIOLOGY

- **Primary MR**
  - **Degenerative** (overlap with MV prolapse syndrome).
    - Usually occurs as a primary condition (Barlow disease or fibroelastic deficiency) but has also been associated with heritable diseases affecting the connective tissue including Marfan syndrome, Ehlers-Danlos syndrome, osteogenesis imperfecta, etc.
    - Occurs in 1.0%–2.5% of the population in a female-to-male ratio of 2:1.
    - Myxomatous proliferation and cartilage formation can occur in the leaflets, chordae tendineae, and/or annulus.
  - **Rheumatic**
    - May be isolated MR or combined MR/MS.
    - Caused by thickening and/or calcification of the leaflets and chords.
  - **Infective endocarditis:** usually caused by destruction of the leaflet tissue (i.e., perforation).
- **Secondary MR**
  - **Dilated cardiomyopathy**
    - Annular dilatation from ventricular enlargement.
    - Papillary muscle displacement because of ventricular enlargement and remodeling prevents adequate leaflet coaptation.
  - **Ischemic**
    - Mechanism of MR usually involves one or both of the following: (1) annular dilatation from ventricular enlargement; (2) local LV remodeling with papillary muscle displacement (both the dilatation of the ventricle and the akinesis/dyskinesis of the wall to which the papillary muscle is attached can prevent adequate leaflet coaptation).
    - MR may develop acutely from papillary muscle rupture (see below).
- **Other causes of MR**
  - Congenital, infiltrative diseases (i.e., amyloid), SLE (Libman-Sacks endocarditis), hypertrophic obstructive cardiomyopathy, mitral annular calcification, paravalvular prosthetic leak, drug toxicity (e.g., Fen-phen).

- **Acute causes of MR**
  - Ruptured papillary muscle or ruptured chordae tendineae, usually in setting of acute MI. The posteromedial papillary muscle is more likely to rupture than the anterolateral papillary muscle; the anterolateral muscle has dual blood supply from both the left anterior descending artery and left circumflex artery.
  - Infective endocarditis.

Pathophysiology

- Acute MR. (Figure 6-3)
- Chronic MR. (Figure 6-4)

DIAGNOSIS

History

- **Acute MR:** most prominent symptom is relatively rapid onset of significant shortness of breath, which may lead quickly to respiratory failure.
- **Chronic MR**
  - Symptoms will depend on the etiology of MR and timing of presentation.
  - In primary MR (usually degenerative MR) that has gradually progressed, the patient may be asymptomatic even when the MR is severe. As compensatory mechanisms fail, patients may note dyspnea on exertion (may be because of PH and/or pulmonary edema), palpitations (from an atrial arrhythmia), fatigue, and volume overload.

Physical Examination

- **Acute MR**
  - Tachypnea with respiratory distress, tachycardia, hypotension.
  - Systolic murmur, usually at the apex (may not be holosystolic and may be absent).

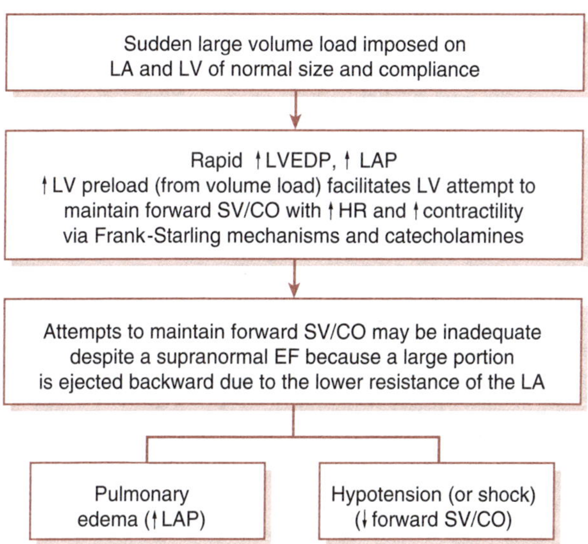

Figure 6-3 Acute mitral regurgitation. CO, cardiac output; EF, ejection fraction; HR, heart rate; LA, left atrium; LAP, left atrial pressure; LV, left ventricle; LVEDP, left ventricular end-diastolic pressure; SV, stroke volume.

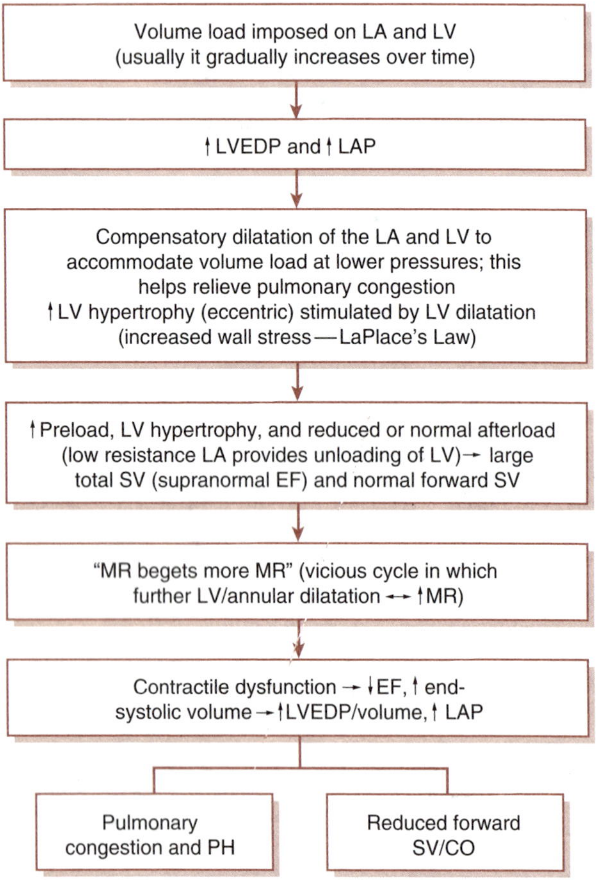

Figure 6-4 Chronic mitral regurgitation. CO, cardiac output; EF, ejection fraction; LA, left atrium; LAP, left atrial pressure; LV, left ventricle; LVEDP, left ventricular end-diastolic pressure; MR, mitral regurgitation; PH, pulmonary hypertension; SV, stroke volume.

- **Chronic MR**
  - Apical high-pitched, blowing holosystolic murmur that radiates widely over the precordium, into the axilla, and left interscapular area (if anterior leaflets involved as in rheumatic) or radiating to base (if posterior leaflets involved).
  - In MV prolapse, there is a mid-systolic click heard before the murmur.
  - S_2 may be widely split because of an early A_2.
  - Other signs of heart failure (lower extremity edema, increased JVP, rales, etc.).

Diagnostic Testing

- **ECG:** LAE, LVH, and AF.
- **CXR:** enlarged LA, pulmonary edema, enlarged pulmonary arteries, and cardiomegaly.
- **TTE:** assess etiology of MR, LA size and LV dimensions (dilated in chronic severe MR), EF (LV dysfunction is present if EF ≤55%), qualitative and quantitative measures of MR severity.

- TEE:
  - Provides better visualization of the valve to help define anatomy, presence of endocarditis (valvular vegetations), and feasibility of repair.
  - May help determine severity of MR when TTE is nondiagnostic, particularly in the setting of an eccentric jet.
- **Right heart catheterization**
  - Better characterize PH in patients with chronic severe MR and determine LA filling pressure in patients with unclear symptoms.
  - Giant "V" waves on pulmonary capillary wedge pressure tracing may suggest severe MR.
- **Left heart catheterization**
  - May influence therapeutic strategy in ischemic MR.
  - Evaluation of CAD in patients with risk factors undergoing MV surgery.
- **MRI/nuclear testing**
  - Assess EF in patients with severe MR but with an inadequate assessment of EF by echocardiography.
  - Assess quantitative measures of MR severity when echocardiography is nondiagnostic.
  - Viability assessment may play a role in considering therapeutic strategy in ischemic MR.

TREATMENT

Acute Mitral Regurgitation

- While awaiting surgery, aggressive afterload reduction with IV nitroprusside or an IABP can diminish the amount of MR and stabilize the patient by promoting forward flow and reducing pulmonary edema.
- These patients are usually tachycardic, but attempts to slow down their heart rate should be avoided because they are often heart rate dependent for an adequate forward CO.

Chronic Mitral Regurgitation

- **Chronic primary MR**
  - Medical therapy is reasonable in patients with chronic primary MR and LVEF less than 60% not undergoing surgery.
  - Angiotensin-converting enzyme (ACE) inhibitors and angiotensin receptor blocker have been shown to reduce the regurgitant fraction and aid with ventricular remodeling. β-Blockers have also been shown to reduce severity of MR in asymptomatic patients.
  - There is no benefit of vasodilator therapy in the asymptomatic patient with normal LV function and chronic severe MR.
- **Chronic secondary MR**
  - Treat symptoms related to LV dysfunction.
  - ACE inhibitors and β-blockers are indicated and have been shown to reduce mortality and the severity of MR.
  - Some patients may also qualify for cardiac resynchronization therapy, which can favorably remodel the LV and reduce the severity of MR.

Percutaneous Intervention

- The mitral clip pinches the leaflets together in an attempt to enhance coaptation (a percutaneous treatment analogous to the surgical Alfieri stitch), creating a double-orifice valve.
  - This procedure is performed via femoral venous access, and a transseptal puncture is used to position the delivery system in the LA.
  - Using fluoroscopy and TEE guidance, the clip is advanced and attempts are made to grasp the leaflet tips of the anterior and posterior MV leaflets and clip them together.

- Transcatheter mitral valve replacement is an emerging structural intervention and currently being investigated in a number of clinical trials. Currently, this technology is only reserved for degenerative MR.
- Recent data from the COAPT trial have shown benefit of transcatheter mitral valve repair in select heart failure patients with severe or moderate-to-severe secondary MR who remain symptomatic despite maximal guideline-directed medical therapy.[12,13]

Surgical Management

- **Primary MR**[2,3]
  - Symptomatic with chronic severe primary MR (stage D), regardless of the LV function (Class I).
  - Asymptomatic with chronic severe primary MR with EF <60% or LV end-systolic dimension ≥40 mm) (stage C2; Class I).
  - Chronic severe primary MR undergoing cardiac surgery for other indications (Class I).
  - Repair is recommended over replacement (Class I).
  - Asymptomatic patients with chronic severe primary MR (stage C1) in whom repair is highly likely (>95%) and operative mortality is low (<1%) or in the setting of new-onset AF or PH (Class IIa).
- **Secondary MR**[2,3]
  - Class IIa: chronic severe secondary MR undergoing cardiac surgery for other indications.
  - Class IIb: severely symptomatic patients (NYHA III/IV) with chronic severe secondary MR (stage D).
  - Note that the benefits of surgery are not well established for secondary MR.
- Patients with AF should be considered for a concomitant surgical maze procedure.

Aortic Regurgitation

- AR may result from pathology of the aortic valve, the aortic root, or both; it is important that both the aortic valve and the aortic root are evaluated to determine the appropriate management and treatment.
- AR usually progresses insidiously with a long asymptomatic period; when it occurs acutely, patients are often very sick and must be managed aggressively.

ETIOLOGY

- **More common**
  Bicuspid aortic valve, rheumatic disease, calcific degeneration, infective endocarditis, idiopathic dilatation of the aorta, myxomatous degeneration, systemic hypertension, dissection of the ascending aorta, and Marfan syndrome.
- **Less common**
  Traumatic injury to the aortic valve, collagen vascular diseases (ankylosing spondylitis, rheumatoid arthritis, reactive arthritis, giant cell aortitis, and Whipple disease), syphilitic aortitis, discrete subaortic stenosis, ventricular septal defect with prolapse of an aortic cusp.
- **Acute AR**
  Infective endocarditis, dissection of the ascending aorta, trauma.

Pathophysiology

- Acute AR (Figure 6-5)
- Chronic AR (Figure 6-6)

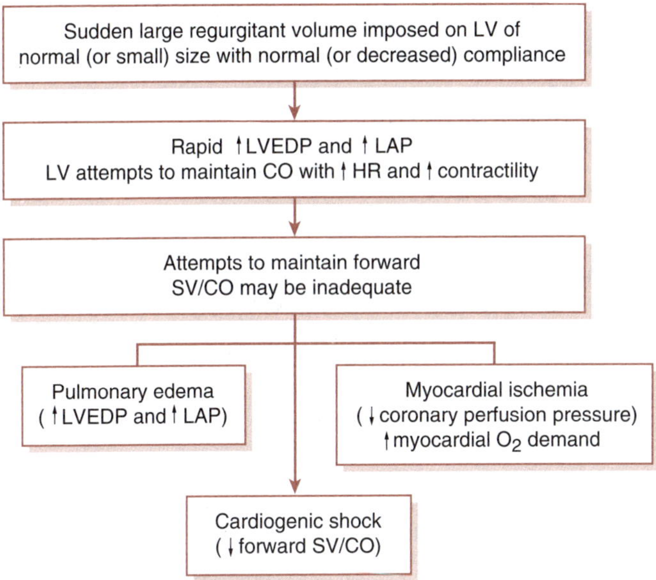

Figure 6-5 Acute aortic regurgitation. CO, cardiac output; HR, heart rate; LAP, left atrial pressure; LV, left ventricle; LVEDP, left ventricular end-diastolic pressure; SV, stroke volume.

DIAGNOSIS

History

- **Acute AR:** patients with acute AR may present with **symptoms of cardiogenic shock and severe dyspnea.** Other presenting symptoms may be related to the cause of acute AR.
- **Chronic AR:** symptoms depend on the presence of LV dysfunction and whether the patient is in the **compensated versus decompensated stage.** Compensated patients are typically asymptomatic, whereas those in the decompensated stage may note decreased exercise tolerance, dyspnea, fatigue, and/or angina.

Physical Examination

- Acute AR
  - Widened pulse pressure may be present, but it is often not present because forward SV (and therefore systolic blood pressure) is reduced.
  - May hear brief soft diastolic murmur or systolic flow murmur.
  - Look for evidence of aortic dissection, infective endocarditis, and characteristics associated with Marfan's disease.
- Chronic AR
  - LV heave; point of maximal impulse is laterally displaced.
  - Diastolic decrescendo murmur heard best at left sternal border leaning forward at end-expiration (**severity of AR correlates with duration, not intensity, of the murmur**).
  - Systolic flow murmur (mostly because of volume overload; concomitant AS may also be present).
  - **Widened pulse pressure** (often >100 mm Hg) with a low diastolic pressure; there are numerous eponyms for the characteristic signs related to a wide pulse pressure.

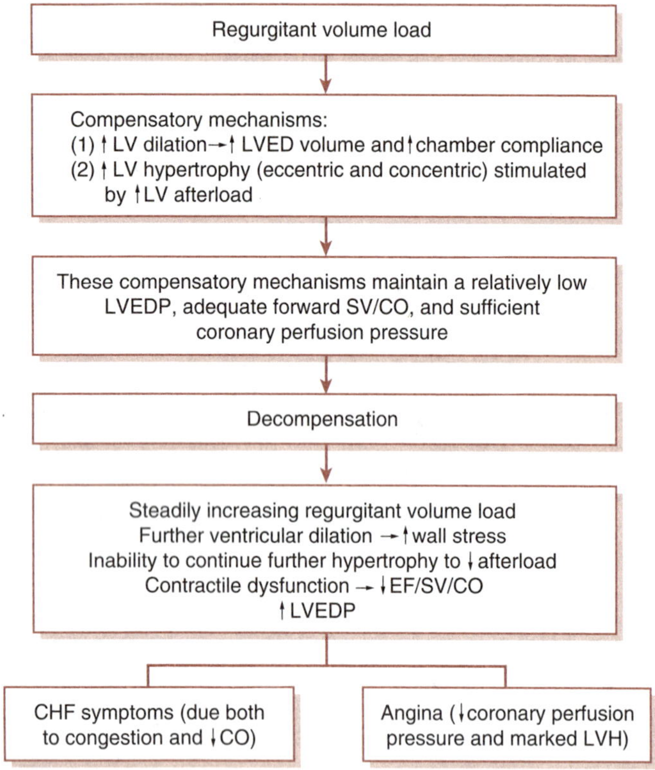

Figure 6-6 Chronic aortic regurgitation. CO, cardiac output; CHF, congestive heart failure; EF, ejection fraction; LV, left ventricle; LVED, left ventricular end-diastolic; LVEDP, left ventricular end-diastolic pressure; LVH, left ventricular hypertrophy; SV, stroke volume.

Diagnostic Testing

- **ECG:** tachycardia, LVH, and LAE (more common in chronic AR).
- **CXR:** pulmonary edema, widened mediastinum, and cardiomegaly.
- **TTE:**
  - Assess LV systolic function, LV dimensions at end systole and diastole, leaflet number and morphology, assessment of the severity of AR.
  - Look for evidence of endocarditis or aortic dissection; dimension of aortic root.
- **TEE:**
  - Clarify whether there is a bicuspid valve if unclear on TTE.
  - Better sensitivity and specificity for aortic dissection than TTE.
  - Clarify whether there is endocarditis with or without root abscess if unclear on TTE.
  - Better visualization of aortic valve in patients with a prosthetic aortic valve.
- **Cardiac catheterization:** assessment of LV pressure, LV function, and severity of AR (via aortic root angiography) is indicated in symptomatic patients in whom the severity of AR is unclear on noninvasive imaging or discordant with clinical findings.
- **MRI/CT**
  - Either of these may be the imaging modality of choice for evaluating aortic dimensions and/or for evaluation of aortic dissection.

- If echocardiography assessment of the severity of AR is inadequate, MRI is useful for assessing the severity of AR.

TREATMENT

- **The role of medical therapy in patients with AR is limited.**
- **Vasodilator therapy (i.e., nifedipine, ACE inhibitor, hydralazine)** is indicated to reduce systolic blood pressure in hypertensive patients with AR.
- Retrospective data suggest that β-blocker use may be associated with a survival benefit in patients with severe AR, but prospective studies are needed.
- When endocarditis is suspected or confirmed, appropriate antibiotic coverage is critical.

Surgical Management

- AHA/ACC recommendations for intervention[2,3]:
  - Symptomatic patients with severe AR (stage D) regardless of LV systolic function (Class I).
  - Asymptomatic patients with chronic severe AR and LV systolic dysfunction (EF ≤55%) (stage C2; Class I).
  - Patients with severe AR (stage C or D) undergoing cardiac surgery for other indications (Class I).
  - Asymptomatic patients with severe AR and normal LV systolic function (EF >55%) but with severe LV dilation (LV end-systolic dimension >50 mm) (stage C2; Class IIa).
- **Acute, severe AR is almost universally symptomatic and is treated surgically.**
- If the aortic root is dilated, it may be repaired or replaced at the time of aortic valve replacement (AVR). For patients with a bicuspid valve, Marfan syndrome, or a related genetically triggered aortopathy, surgery on the aorta should be considered at the time of AVR.

OUTCOME/PROGNOSIS

- Asymptomatic patients with normal LV systolic function (LVEF ≥50%): progression to symptoms and/or LV dysfunction approximately 6% per year.[14]
- Asymptomatic patients with LV dysfunction (LVEF <50%): progression to cardiac symptoms >25% per year.[14,15]
- Symptomatic patients: mortality rate approximately 9.4% per year.[14]

Tricuspid Valve Disease

Most often, tricuspid valve disease presents as functional regurgitation secondary to left-sided valvular disease or heart failure (mostly in the setting of PH). Structural causes of tricuspid valve disease are less common, and include rheumatic heart disease, endocarditis, carcinoid, papillary muscle dysfunction, trauma (biopsy), endomyocardial fibrosis, methysergide, and congenital anomalies (Ebstein).

CLINICAL FEATURES

- Signs and symptoms are often consistent with congestive heart failure and can include dyspnea on exertion, orthopnea, jugular venous distention, ascites, and peripheral edema.
- Advanced disease also can present with hemoptysis and paroxysmal nocturnal dyspnea.
- Physical examination reveals a pansystolic (TR) or presystolic (tricuspid stenosis [TS]) murmur in the fourth and fifth intercostal spaces at the left sternal border or epigastrium. Murmur increase with inspiration (Carvallo sign), exercise, leg raising, and hepatic compression.

- Jugular venous distension—prominent c-v wave (x-x′ disappears) with ear lobe pulsations - Lancisi sign. Y descent is sharp.
- Hepatojugular reflux, pulsatile liver, and signs of hepatic dysfunction may also be present.

DIAGNOSTICS

- Electrocardiographic features include right atrial volume overload and enlargement.
- Plain chest radiography may demonstrate cardiomegaly with right-sided chamber enlargement.
- Doppler and two-dimensional echocardiography confirm the diagnosis, revealing structural abnormalities and measuring pulmonary arterial pressures, degree of stenosis/regurgitation, and right ventricular dysfunction.
- Cardiac catheterization usually confirms elevated right atrial and ventricular end-diastolic pressures in TR. A diastolic pressure–atrioventricular pressure gradient that increases with respiration is found in patients with significant TS.
- Tricuspid endocarditis is typically diagnosed in the setting of major criteria that include valvular vegetations and pyrexia; positive blood cultures, septic pulmonary emboli, and a murmur constitute the minor criteria.

TREATMENT

- Tricuspid valve repair or replacement is indicated for TS and moderate-to-severe TR, usually associated with New York Heart Association class III or IV symptoms. TS is usually treated with commissurotomy.
- Surgical techniques for TR include bicuspidization, De Vega suture annuloplasty, Carpentier ring annuloplasty, and prosthetic valve replacement.

Prosthetic Heart Valves

- The choice of valve prosthesis depends on many factors including the patient, surgeon, cardiologist, and clinical scenario.
- With improvements in bioprosthetic valves, the recommendation for a mechanical valve in patients <65 years of age is no longer as firm, and bioprosthetic valve use has increased in younger patients.
- **Mechanical valves**
  - Ball-and-cage (Starr–Edwards): rarely, if ever, used today.
  - Bileaflet (i.e., St. Jude, Carbomedics): most commonly used.
  - Single tilting disk (i.e., Björk–Shiley, Medtronic Hall, Omnicarbon).
  - **Advantages of mechanical valve:** structurally stable, long-lasting, relatively hemodynamically efficient (particularly bileaflet).
  - **Disadvantages of mechanical valve:** need for anticoagulation/risk of bleeding, risk of thrombosis/embolism despite anticoagulation, severe hemodynamic compromise if disk thrombosis or immobility occurs (single tilting disk), risk of endocarditis, anticoagulation issues in women of child-bearing age.
- **Bioprosthetic valves**
  - Porcine aortic valve tissue (i.e., Hancock, Carpentier-Edwards).
  - Bovine pericardial tissue (i.e., Carpentier-Edwards Perimount).
  - **Advantages of bioprosthetic valve:** no need for anticoagulation, low thromboembolism risk, low risk of catastrophic valve failure.
  - **Disadvantages of bioprosthetic valve:** structural valve deterioration, risk of endocarditis, still a small risk (approximately 0.04%–0.34% per year in recent meta-analysis) of thromboembolism without anticoagulation.[16]
  - **Homograft (cadaveric):** rarely used; most commonly used to replace the pulmonic valve.

TREATMENT

- **Anticoagulation with a vitamin K antagonist and international normalized ratio (INR) monitoring is recommended in patients with a mechanical prosthetic valve** (Class I).[2,3]
  - Goal INR of 2.5 is recommended in patients with a mechanical AVR and no risk factors for thromboembolism. Goal INR 3.0 in patients with a mechanical AVR and additional risk factors for thromboembolic events (AF, previous thromboembolism, LV dysfunction, or hypercoagulable conditions) or an older generation mechanical AVR (such as ball-in-cage) (Class I).
  - Goal INR 3.0 in patients with a mechanical MV replacement (Class I).
  - Aspirin 75–100 mg daily is recommended in addition to anticoagulation with a vitamin K antagonist in patients with a mechanical valve prosthesis (Class I).
  - Aspirin 75–100 mg daily is reasonable in all patients with a bioprosthetic aortic valve or MV (Class IIa).
  - **Anticoagulant therapy with oral direct thrombin inhibitors or anti-Xa agents should not be used in patients with mechanical valve prostheses (Class III).**
- **Bridging therapy for prosthetic valves**[2,3]:
  - For patients with mechanical heart valves who are undergoing minor procedures (e.g., dental extractions or cataract removal), where bleeding is easily controlled, continuation of VKA anticoagulation with a therapeutic INR is recommended (Class 1).
  - For patients with a bileaflet mechanical AVR and no other risk factors for thromboembolism who are undergoing invasive procedures, temporary interruption of VKA anticoagulation without bridging agents while the INR is subtherapeutic is recommended (Class 2a).
  - For patients with a mechanical valve prosthesis receiving VKA therapy who require immediate/emergency noncardiac surgery or an invasive procedure, administration of 4-factor prothrombin complex concentrate (or its activated form) is reasonable (Class 2a).
  - For patients with bioprosthetic heart valves or annuloplasty rings who are receiving anticoagulation for AF, it is reasonable to consider the need for bridging anticoagulant therapy around the time of invasive procedures on the basis of the CHA2DS2-VASc score weighed against the risk of bleeding (Class 2a).
  - For patients who are undergoing invasive procedures and have (1) a mechanical AVR and any thromboembolic risk factor, (2) an older-generation mechanical AVR, or (3) a mechanical mitral valve replacement, bridging anticoagulation therapy during the preoperative time interval when the INR is subtherapeutic is reasonable on an individualized basis, with the risks of bleeding weighed against the benefits of thromboembolism prevention.

Infective Endocarditis in Native or Prosthetic Valves

- Patient at risk or with suspected endocarditis should receive antibiotic therapy after two sets of blood cultures (Class I).[2,3]
- These patients should be evaluated for need and timing of surgery: early surgery is recommended (Class I) for those with valve dysfunction causing heart failure, resistant organisms (fungi, staphylococcus), heart block/abscess, persistent infection.
- Surgery is also recommended for relapsing prosthetic valve (Class I).[2,3]
- Those with large mobile vegetations of the native valve and recurrent emboli can be evaluated for early surgery (Class II).[2,3]

Management of Pregnant Patients With Prosthetic Heart Valves (Figure 6-7)

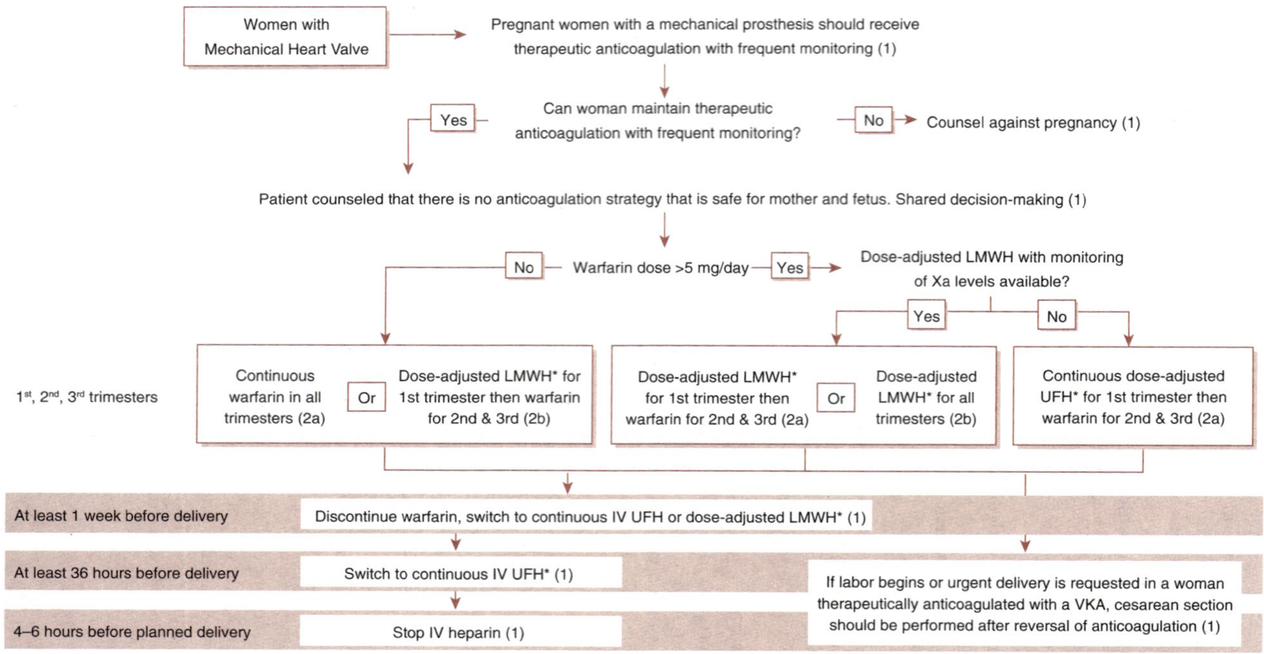

*Dose-adjusted LMWH should be given at least 2 times per day, with close monitoring of anti-Xa levels. Target to Xa level of 0.8 to 1.2 U/mL, 4 to 6 hours after dose. Trough levels may aid in maintaining patient in therapeutic range. Continuous UFH should be adjusted to aPTT 2 times control.

Abbreviations: aPTT indicates activated partial thromboplastin time; IV, intravenous; LMWH, low-molecular-weight heparin; UFH, unfractionated heparin; and VKA, vitamin K antagonist.

Figure 6-7 Anticoagulants management in pregnant patient with prosthetic valve. Otto CM, Nishimura RA, Bonow RO, Carabello BA, Erwin III JP, Gentile F, Jneid H, Krieger EV, Mack M, McLeod C, O'Gara PT. 2020 ACC/AHA guideline for the management of patients with valvular heart disease: executive summary: a report of the American College of Cardiology/American Heart Association Joint Committee on Clinical Practice Guidelines. Journal of the American College of Cardiology. 2021 Feb 2;77(4):450-500.

Summary

- Colchicine is recommended as a combined drug with NSAIDs to optimize the treatment and reduce the recurrence of pericarditis.
- Over the last two decades, there has been a resurgence of interest in RF/RHD possibly due to increasingly wide-spread availability of echocardiography.
- The revised Jones criteria addressed two significant features: (a) Distinguished criteria between low-risk and moderate-to-high risk populations based on ARF incidence or RHD prevalence; and (b) Recommending echocardiography of all suspected cases of ARF and incorporating subclinical carditis as evidenced by echocardiography as a major criteria.
- The highest risk of IE is observed in patients with previous history of IE, followed by patients with prosthetic valves.
- Embolic complications were detected in 25.3% of patients of IE, and cardiac conduction abnormalities were found in 11.5%.
- The POET trial has shown that after an initial phase of intravenous treatment, up to 20% patients could complete the treatment by oral antibiotic therapy.

Scan the QR code to access chapter references.

7 Cardiac Arrhythmias

Sandeep S. Sodhi, Daniel H. Cooper, Mitchell N. Faddis, Vidarshan Mathavan, and M. Harsha Sagar

TACHYARRHYTHMIAS

Approach to Tachyarrhythmias

GENERAL PRINCIPLES

- Tachyarrhythmias are encountered in both the inpatient and outpatient settings.
- Recognition and analysis of these rhythms in a stepwise manner will facilitate initiation of appropriate therapy.
- Clinical decision-making is guided by patient symptoms and signs of hemodynamic stability.

Definition

Cardiac rhythms whose ventricular rate exceeds **100 beats per minute** (bpm).

Classification

Tachyarrhythmias are broadly classified into the following based on the width of the QRS complex on the ECG.

- Narrow-complex tachyarrhythmia (QRS <120 ms): Arrhythmia originates within the atria (supraventricular tachycardia [SVT]) and rapidly activates the ventricles via the His-Purkinje system.
- Wide-complex tachyarrhythmia (QRS ≥120 ms): Arrhythmia originates within the ventricles and does not depend on the His-Purkinje system (ventricular tachycardia [VT]) or originates in the atria and travels to the ventricles either via an abnormal His-Purkinje system (SVT with aberrancy) or through an accessory pathway.

Etiology

Mechanism (Figure 7-1) is divided into disorders of **impulse conduction** and **impulse formation**:

- **Disorders of impulse conduction:** Reentry is the most common mechanism of tachyarrhythmias. A reentrant mechanism can occur when differential refractory periods and conduction velocities allow for propagation of an activation wavefront in a unidirectional manner around a zone of scar or refractory cardiac tissue. Reentry of the activation wavefront around a myocardial circuit sustains the arrhythmia (e.g., VT).
- **Disorders of impulse formation: Enhanced automaticity** (e.g., accelerated junctional and accelerated idioventricular rhythm) **and triggered activity** (e.g., long QT syndrome [LQTS] and digitalis toxicity) are other less common mechanisms of tachyarrhythmias.

DIAGNOSIS

Clinical Presentation

- Tachyarrhythmias often produce symptoms that lead to patient presentation at an outpatient or acute care setting.
- Tachyarrhythmias can be associated with systemic illnesses in patients being evaluated in the emergency department or being treated in the inpatient setting.

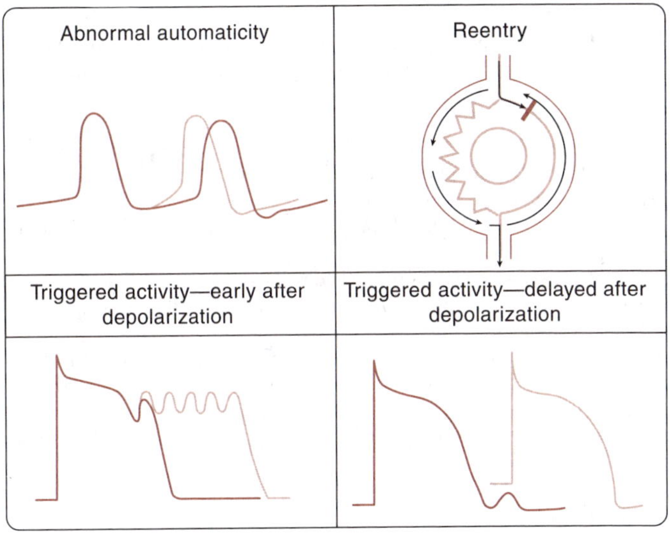

Figure 7-1 Mechanism of arrhythmogenicity.

History

- Symptoms generally guide clinical decision-making.
- **Dyspnea, angina, lightheadedness or syncope, and decreased level of consciousness** are severe symptoms that mandate urgent treatment.
- Baseline symptoms that reflect **poor left ventricular (LV) function**, such as dyspnea on exertion (DOE), orthopnea, paroxysmal nocturnal dyspnea (PND), and lower extremity swelling, are critical to identify.
- **Palpitations** are a common symptom of tachyarrhythmias. The pattern of onset and termination is useful to suggest the presence of a primary arrhythmia.
  - Sudden onset and termination of palpitations is highly suggestive of a reentrant tachyarrhythmia.
  - Termination of palpitations with breath holding or the Valsalva maneuver is suggestive of a supraventricular tachyarrhythmia.
- History or presence of **organic heart disease** (i.e., ischemic, nonischemic, or valvular cardiomyopathy) or **endocrinopathy** (i.e., thyroid disease, pheochromocytoma) should be determined.
- History of **familial or congenital causes of arrhythmias** such as hypertrophic cardiomyopathy (HCM), LQTS, or other congenital cardiac conditions should be ascertained as well.
  - **Hypertrophic obstructive cardiomyopathy** (HOCM) is associated with atrial arrhythmias (atrial fibrillation [AF] in 20%–25%), as well as malignant ventricular arrhythmias.
  - **Mitral valve prolapse** (MVP) is associated with supraventricular and ventricular arrhythmias.
  - **Repaired congenital heart disease,** such as surgically corrected tetralogy of Fallot (TOF) and d-transposition of the great arteries (d-TGA) with Mustard or Senning baffles, are substrates for ventricular and supraventricular tachyarrhythmias, respectively.
- **Medication and ingestion history** (including over-the-counter drugs, herbal supplements, and illicit substances) should be carefully taken to assess a possible causal link.

Physical Examination

- Assessment of clinical stability or instability—achieved by evaluating vital signs, mental status, and peripheral perfusion—is critical in guiding initial decision-making.
- If clinically stable, physical examination should be focused on determining underlying cardiovascular abnormalities that may make certain rhythms more or less likely.
- Findings of **congestive heart failure (CHF)**, including elevated jugular venous pressure (JVP), pulmonary rales, peripheral edema, and S_3 gallop, make the diagnosis of malignant ventricular arrhythmias more likely.
- If an arrhythmia is sustained, special considerations during physical examination include the following:
  - **Palpation of the pulse** to assess for rate and regularity.
    - If the rhythm is irregular and the rate is approximately 150 bpm, suspect atrial flutter (AFL) with 2:1 block.
    - If the pulse is irregular with no pattern, suspect atrial fibrillation (AF).
    - An irregular pulse with a discernible pattern (group beating) suggests the presence of second-degree heart block.
  - **Presence of "Cannon" A waves:** Revealed on inspection of JVP; reflect atrial contraction against a closed tricuspid valve.
    - If irregular, may be suggestive of underlying atrioventricular (AV) dissociation and possible presence of VT.
    - If regular in a 1:1 ratio with peripheral pulse, then suggestive of an AV nodal reentrant tachycardia (AVNRT), AV reentrant tachycardia (AVRT), or a junctional tachycardia (JT), all leading to retrograde atrial activation occurring simultaneously with ventricular contraction.

Diagnostic Testing

Laboratories

Serum electrolytes, complete blood count (CBC), thyroid function tests, serum concentration of digoxin (if applicable), and urine toxicology screen should be considered for all patients.

Electrocardiography

- **12-lead ECG, in the presence of the rhythm abnormality and in normal sinus rhythm,** is the most useful initial diagnostic test.
- If the patient is clinically stable, obtain a 12-lead ECG and a **continuous rhythm strip** with leads that best demonstrate atrial activation (e.g., V_1, II, III, aVF).
- Examine the ECG for evidence of conduction abnormalities, such as preexcitation or bundle branch block, or signs of structural heart disease such as prior myocardial infarction (MI).
- Comparison of the ECG obtained during arrhythmia with that at baseline can highlight subtle features of the QRS deflection that indicate the superposition of atrial and ventricular depolarization.
- Rhythm strip is useful to document response to interventions (e.g., vagal maneuvers, antiarrhythmic drug therapy, or electrical cardioversion).

Imaging

Chest radiography (CXR) and **transthoracic echocardiogram** (TTE) can help provide evidence of structural heart disease that may make ventricular arrhythmias more likely.

Diagnostic Testing

- Continuous ambulatory ECG monitoring
  - To aid in outpatient diagnosis of tachyarrhythmias.
  - 24- or 48-hour Holter monitor; useful for documenting symptomatic transient arrhythmias that occur with sufficient frequency.

- Recording mode useful for assessment of patient's heart rate response to daily activities or antiarrhythmic drug treatment.
- Correlation between patient-reported symptoms in a time-marked diary and heart rhythm recordings is the key to determining if symptoms are attributable to an arrhythmia.

- Event recorders
  - Weeks to months of ambulatory monitoring; useful for documenting symptomatic transient arrhythmias that occur infrequently.
  - A "loop recorder" is worn by the patient and continuously records the cardiac rhythm. When activated by the patient or via an autodetection feature, a rhythm strip is saved with several minutes of preceding data.
  - An **implantable loop recorder** (ILR) is a subcutaneous monitoring device used to provide an automated or patient-activated recording of significant arrhythmic events that occur very infrequently (over many months) or for patients who are unable to activate external recorders.
- Exercise ECG
  Useful for studying exercise-induced arrhythmias or to assess the sinus node response to exercise.
- Inpatient telemetry monitoring
  Mainstay of surveillance monitoring during the course of hospitalization for cardiac arrhythmia patients who are seriously ill or are having life-threatening arrhythmias.
- Electrophysiology study (EPS)
  - Invasive catheter-based procedure used to study a patient's susceptibility to arrhythmias or to investigate the mechanism of a known arrhythmia.
  - EPS is also combined with catheter ablation for curative treatment of many arrhythmia mechanisms.
  - The efficacy of EPS to induce and study arrhythmias is highest for reentrant mechanisms.

TREATMENT

Please refer to the treatment of individual tachyarrhythmias for hemodynamically unstable patients and advanced cardiac life support (ACLS) algorithm for tachycardias in Appendix C.

Supraventricular Tachyarrhythmias

GENERAL PRINCIPLES

- **Supraventricular tachyarrhythmias** (SVT) are often recurrent, rarely persistent, and frequently a cause of visits to emergency departments and primary care physician offices.
- The evaluation of patients with SVT should always begin with prompt assessment of hemodynamic stability and clinical status.
- The diagnostic and therapeutic discussion that follows is aimed at the hemodynamically stable patient. If a patient is deemed clinically unstable based on clinical signs and symptoms, one should immediately proceed to cardioversion per ACLS guidelines.

Definition

- Tachyarrhythmias that require atrial or AV nodal tissue or both for their initiation and maintenance are termed SVT.
- The QRS complex in most SVTs is narrow (QRS <120 ms). However, SVTs can present as a wide-complex tachycardia (QRS ≥120 ms) if they are aberrantly conducted or in an accessory pathway–mediated tachycardia.

Classification

- SVT is initially classified by ECG in an effort to understand the likely underlying arrhythmia mechanism.
- A diagnostic approach, based on the ECG, is summarized in Figure 7-2.
- Narrow QRS complex tachyarrhythmias can be divided into those arrhythmias requiring only atrial tissue for initiation and maintenance (atrial tachycardia [AT], AF, and AFL) versus those that require the AV junction for perpetuation (JT, AVNRT, and AVRT).
- **Paroxysmal SVT** specifically refers to intermittent SVT other than AF, AFL, and multifocal AT (MAT).

Epidemiology

- The estimated prevalence of paroxysmal SVT in the normal population is 2.25/1000, with an incidence of 35/100,000 person-years.[1]
- In the absence of structural heart disease, SVT most commonly presents between the ages of 12 and 30.[1]
- Women are twice as likely to develop SVT as men.[1]

DIAGNOSIS

- A general understanding of the prevalence of various arrhythmia mechanisms is useful to guide evaluation of an individual patient.
- **AF** is the most common narrow-complex tachycardia seen in the inpatient setting. **AFL** can often accompany AF and is diagnosed one-tenth as often as AF, but first time AFL is diagnosed twice as often as the paroxysmal SVTs. The other atrial tachyarrhythmias are far less common.
- In one case series, **AVNRT** was reported as the most common diagnosis of the paroxysmal SVTs (60%), followed by AVRT (30%).[2]
- Mechanism of paroxysmal SVT is significantly influenced by gender and age.
  - Irrespective of gender, AVRT tends to present at a younger age (most commonly in the first two decades of life), whereas AVNRT and AT tend to present more commonly later in life.

Clinical Presentation

The clinical presentation for SVT is similar to tachyarrhythmias in general and has been previously outlined in this section.

Differential Diagnosis

- **Atrial fibrillation (AF)**
  The most common sustained tachyarrhythmia is discussed as a separate topic later in this section.
- **Atrial flutter (AFL)**
  - The overall incidence of AFL in the United States is 88 per 100,000 person-years. Adjusted for age, the incidence in men is more than 2.5 times that of women.[3]
  - AFL usually presents as a **regular rhythm** but can be **irregularly irregular** when associated with variable AV block (2:1 to 4:1 to 3:1, etc.) (Table 7-1).
  - **Mechanism:** Type of macroreentrant atrial tachycardia circuit usually within the right atrium around the perimeter of the tricuspid valve. This form of AFL is called "typical" AFL. Atrial rate is 250–350 bpm with conduction to ventricle that is usually not 1:1, but most often 2:1. **(An SVT with regular ventricular rate of 150 bpm should raise suspicion for AFL.)**
  - Chronic AFL commonly coexists with AF and is associated with the same risk factors (obesity, hypertension, diabetes mellitus, and obstructive sleep apnea).

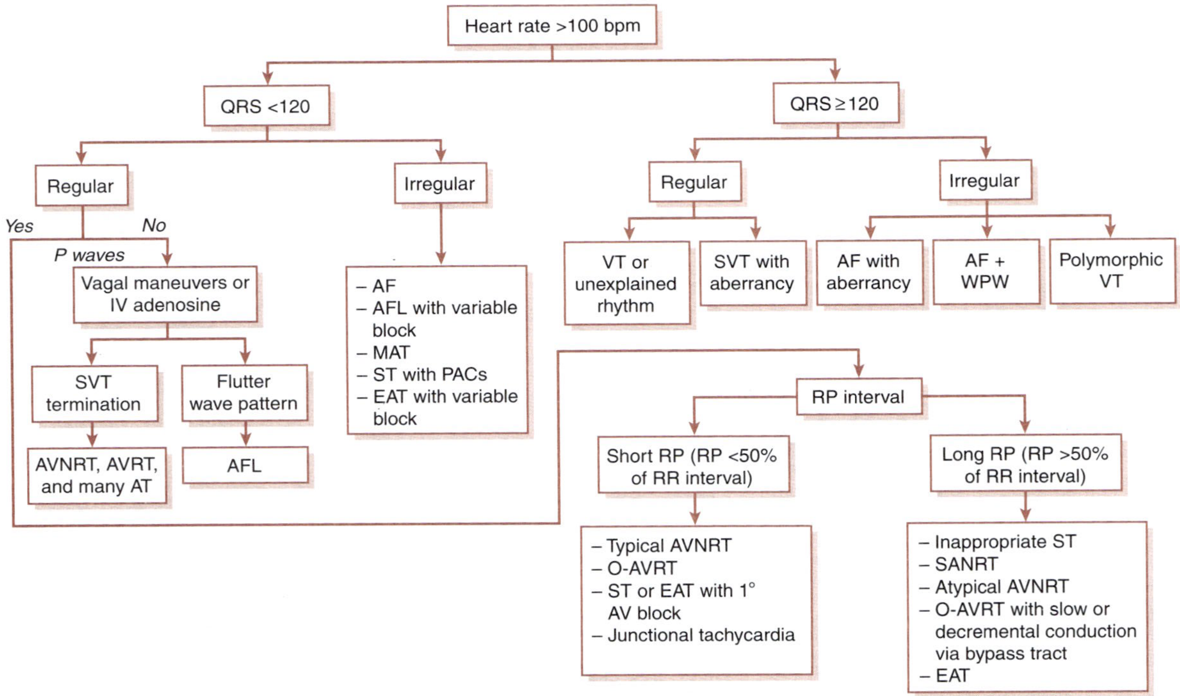

Figure 7-2 Diagnostic approach to tachyarrhythmias. AF, atrial fibrillation; AFL, atrial flutter; AT, atrial tachycardia; AV, atrioventricular; AVNRT, atrioventricular nodal reentrant tachycardia; AVRT, atrioventricular reentrant tachycardia; EAT, ectopic atrial tachycardia; MAT, multifocal atrial tachycardia; O-AVRT, orthodromic AVRT; PAC, premature atrial complex; SANRT, sinoatrial nodal reentrant tachycardia; ST, sinus tachycardia; SVT, supraventricular tachyarrhythmia; VT, ventricular tachycardia; WPW, Wolff-Parkinson-White.

TABLE 7-1 ECG Features of Atrial Flutter

Narrow complex tachycardia
Regular atrial activity at approximately 300 bpm
Flutter or sawtooth waves pattern, best in leads II, III, aVF. Flutter waves in V_1 may look like P waves
Loss of isoelectric baseline
Fixed AV blocks—ventricular rate is a fraction of the atrial rate

2:1 block—150 bpm

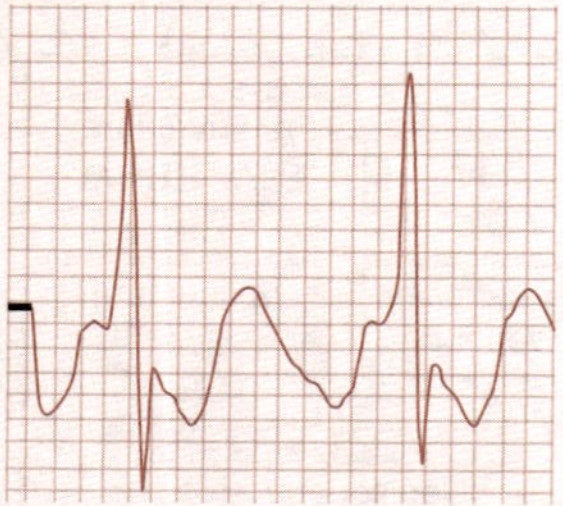

3:1 block—100 bpm

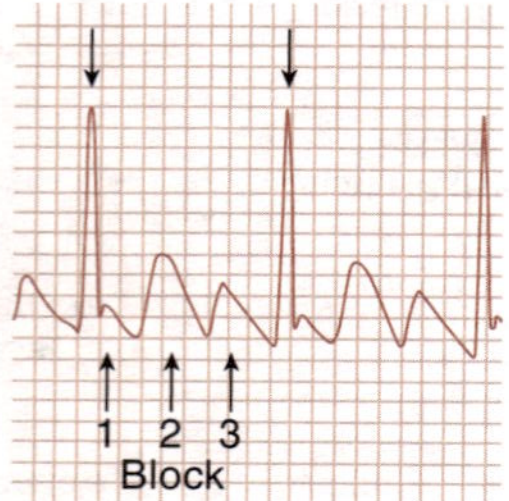

4:1 block—75 bpm

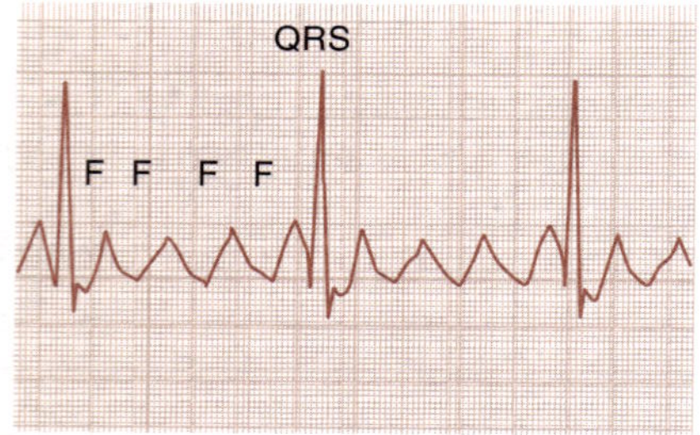

Variable AV blocks—ventricular response is irregular and may mimic AF

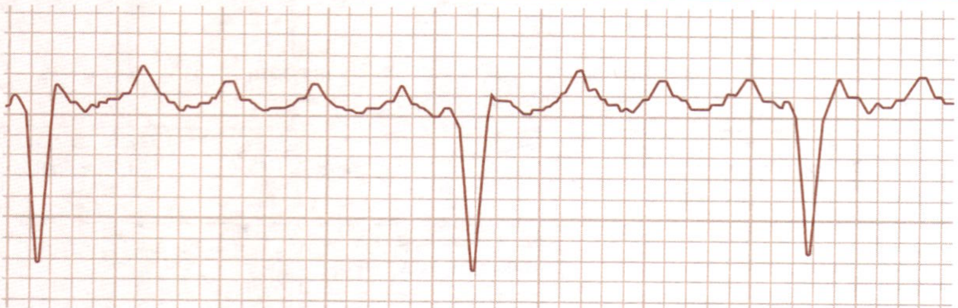

- **ECG:** In typical AFL, a "saw tooth" pattern best visualized in leads II, III, and aVF with negative deflections in V_1 (Table 7-1).

- **Multifocal atrial tachycardia (MAT) (Figure 7-3)**
  - **Irregularly irregular** SVT generally seen in elderly hospitalized patients with multiple comorbidities.
  - MAT is most often associated with chronic obstructive pulmonary disease (COPD) and CHF but may also be associated with glucose intolerance, hypokalemia, hypomagnesemia, drugs (e.g., theophylline), and chronic renal failure.
  - **ECG:** SVT with at least **three distinct P-wave morphologies**, generally best visualized in leads II, III, and V_1.
- **Sinus tachycardia (ST) (Figure 7-4)**
  - ST is the most common mechanism of **long RP tachycardia.**
  - Usually, ST is a normal physiologic response to hyperadrenergic states (fever, pain, hypovolemia, anemia, hypoxia, etc.) but can also be induced by illicit (cocaine, amphetamines, methamphetamine) and prescription drugs (theophylline, atropine, β-adrenergic agonists).
  - **Inappropriate ST** refers to persistently elevated sinus rate in the absence of an identifiable physical, pathologic, or pharmacologic influence.
- The cause of the increased automaticity, however, remains elusive. Theories suggest hypersensitivity to catecholamines, disturbance in the autonomic nervous system, etc.
- Inappropriate sinus tachycardia may be diagnosed only when all other causes of sinus tachycardia have been ruled out.
- No clear evidence points to any increased mortality in inappropriate sinus tachycardia. This is somewhat unexpected given that tachycardia is a well-known risk factor for cardiomyopathy (tachycardia-induced cardiomyopathy).
- Maximum discharge rate in the sinoatrial node is estimated by:
  - Women: 206 – age × 0.88
  - Men: 208 – age × 0.7
  - Coronary heart disease on beta-blockers: 164 – age × 0.7
- **Ectopic atrial tachycardia (EAT)**
  - EAT with variable block can present as an **irregularly irregular** rhythm and can be distinguished from AFL by an **atrial rate of 150–200 bpm.**

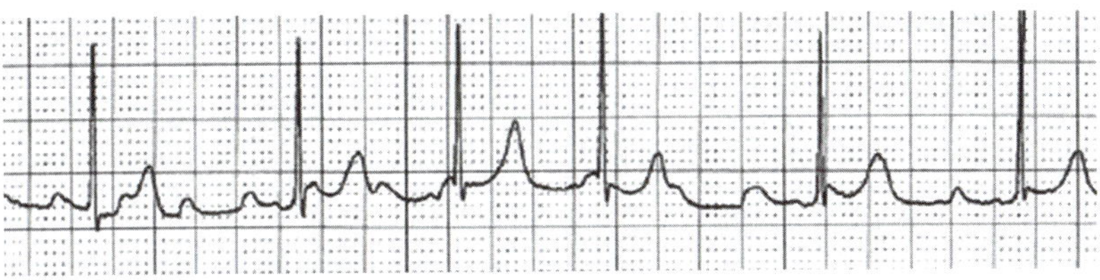

Figure 7-3 ECG showing multifocal atrial tachycardia.

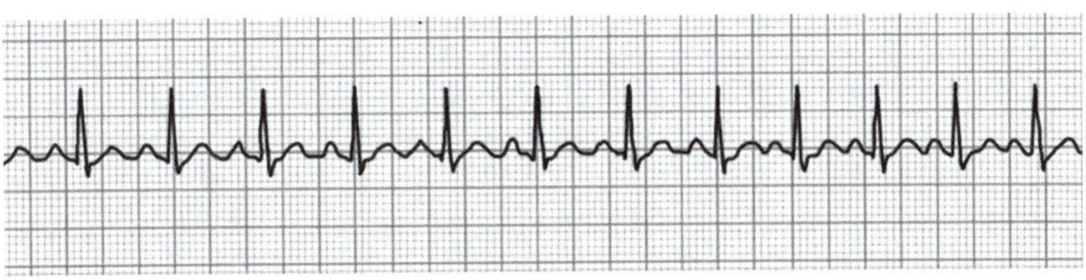

Figure 7-4 ECG showing sinus tachycardia.

- EAT with variable block is associated with **digoxin toxicity.**
- EAT is characterized by a regular atrial activation pattern with a P-wave morphology originating outside of the sinus node complex resulting in a **long RP tachycardia.**
- **Mechanism:** Enhanced automaticity, triggered activity, and possibly microreentry.

- **Atrioventricular node reentrant tachycardia** (AVNRT)
  - This reentrant rhythm requires functional dissociation of the AV node into two pathways with antegrade conduction down a "slow" AV nodal pathway and retrograde conduction up a "fast" AV nodal pathway. AVNRT can occur at any age, with a predilection for **middle age** and **female gender**. AVNRT is not correlated with structural heart disease.
  - **Typical AVNRT (Figure** 7-5 **and Table** 7-2) is a major cause of short RP tachycardia.
    - **ECG appearance has characteristic "absent P waves"** because atrial activation is coincident with the QRS complex. Commonly, atrial activation can occur at the terminal portion of the QRS to create a pseudo-r' (V_1) or pseudo-s' (II) compared with the sinus rhythm QRS.
- **Atypical AVNRT**
  - Less common; antegrade conduction proceeds down a fast AV nodal pathway with retrograde conduction up a slow AV nodal pathway, leading to a **long RP tachycardia.**
  - **ECG:** The retrograde P wave is inscribed well after the QRS complex in the second half of the RR interval (Table 7-2).
- **Atrioventricular reentrant tachycardia** (AVRT)
  - **Orthodromic AVRT** (O-AVRT) is the most common AVRT, accounting for about 95% of all AVRT.
    - Accessory pathway–mediated reentrant rhythm with antegrade conduction to the ventricle down the AV node and retrograde conduction to the atrium up an accessory or "bypass" tract (bundle of Kent), leading to a **short RP tachycardia.**
    - **ECG:** Retrograde P waves are frequently seen after the QRS complex and are usually distinguishable from the QRS (i.e., separated by >70 ms) (Figure 7-6).
    - O-AVRT is the most common mechanism of SVT in patients with Wolff-Parkinson-White (WPW) syndrome who have preexcitation (defined by short PR and a delta wave on upstroke of QRS) present on sinus rhythm ECG. Algorithm for localizing the site of the accessory pathway is described in Figure 7-7.
    - O-AVRT can occur without preexcitation when conduction through the bypass tract occurs only during tachycardia in a retrograde fashion ("concealed pathway").

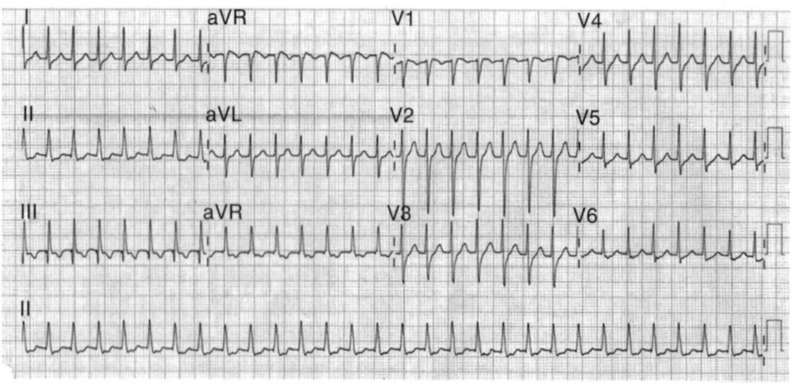

Figure 7-5 ECG showing typical AVNRT.

TABLE 7-2 ECG Features of Typical and Atypical AVNRT

Typical AVNRT (slow–fast): 90% of all cases	
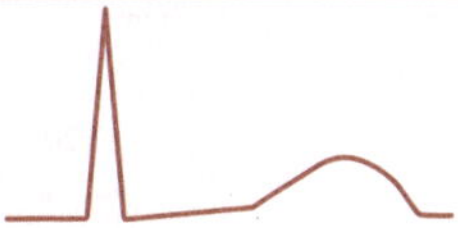	In most cases, the P wave is hidden in the QRS complex
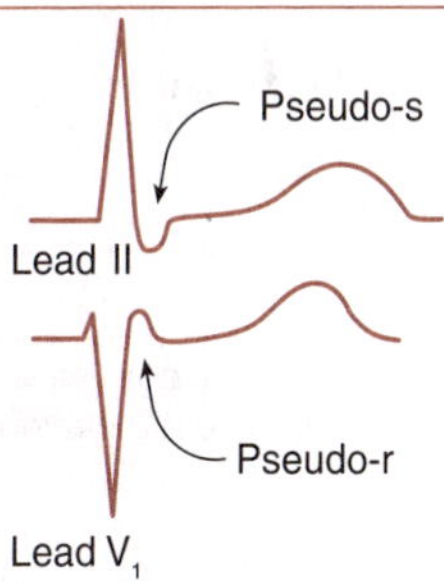	The P wave is sometimes seen after the QRS complex. It will present itself as "pseudo-s" in lead II and "pseudo-r" in lead V_1
Atypical AVNRT (fast–slow): 10% of all cases	
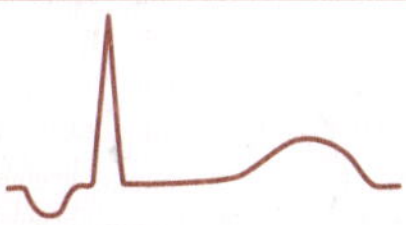	P wave before QRS complex
Very atypical AVNRT (slow–slow): <1% of all cases	
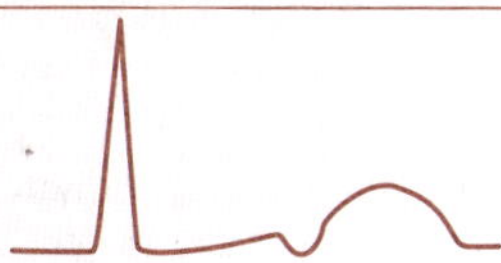	P waves on the ST-T segment

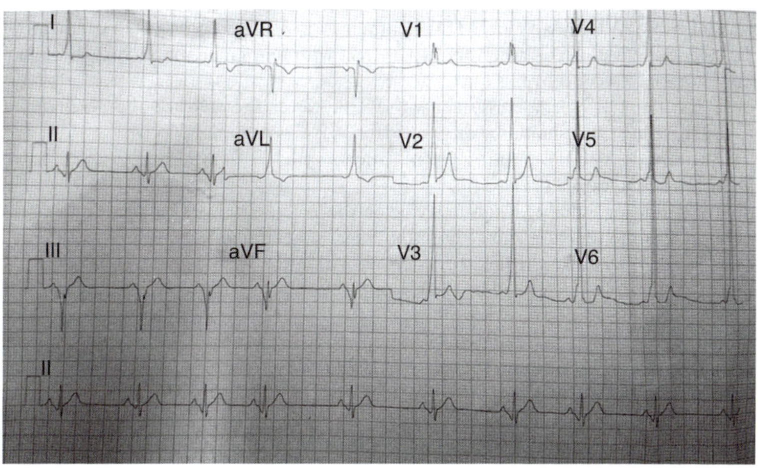

Figure 7-6 ECG of Wolff-Parkinson-White (WPW) syndrome (left posteroseptal pathway).

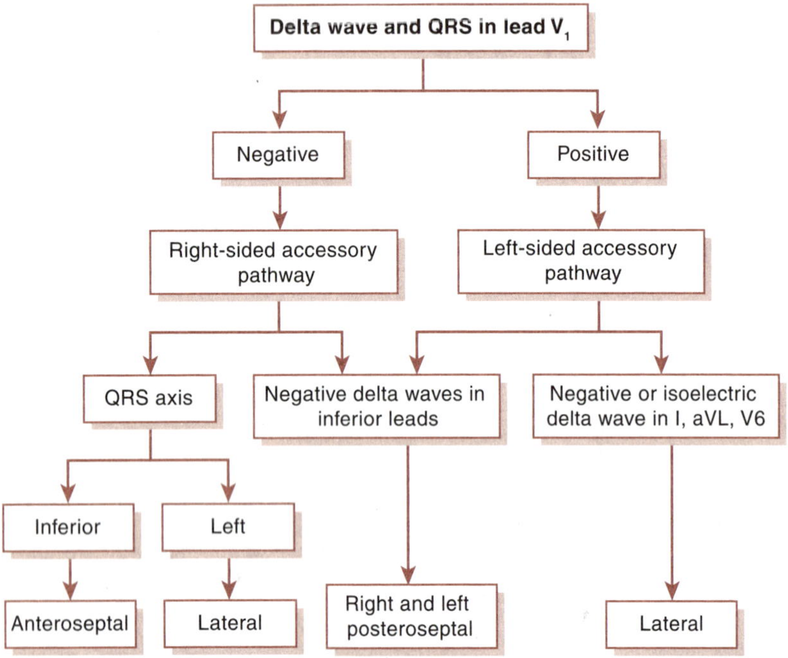

Figure 7-7 Algorithm for localizing the site of the accessory pathway in WPW syndrome.

- Less commonly, retrograde conduction through the accessory pathway to the atrium proceeds slowly enough for atrial activation to occur in the second half of the RR interval, leading to a **long RP tachycardia.** The associated incessant tachycardia can cause tachycardia-induced cardiomyopathy.

- **Antidromic AVRT (A-AVRT):** This reentrant form of SVT occurs when conduction to the ventricle is down an accessory bypass tract with retrograde conduction through the AV node or a second bypass tract.
  - **ECG:** The QRS seems consistent with VT; however, the presence of preexcitation on the baseline QRS should be diagnostic for WPW syndrome.
  - Antidromic AVRT is seen in <5% of patients with WPW syndrome.

- **Junctional tachycardia** (JT)
  - This is due to enhanced automaticity of the AV junction. The electrical impulses conduct to the ventricle and atrium simultaneously, similar to typical AVNRT, so that retrograde P waves are frequently concealed within the QRS complex. Common junctional rhythms are described in Table 7-3.
  - Uncommon in adults.
  - Common in young children, particularly after cardiac surgery.
- **Sinoatrial nodal reentrant tachycardia** (SANRT)
  - Reentrant circuit is localized at least partially within the sinoatrial node.
  - Abrupt onset and termination, triggered by a premature atrial complex.
  - **ECG:** P-wave morphology and axis are identical to the native sinus P wave during normal sinus rhythm.

TABLE 7-3 Junctional Rhythms

Classification by Rate		
Junctional Escape Rhythm	**Accelerated Junctional Rhythm**	**Junctional Tachycardia**
40–60 bpm 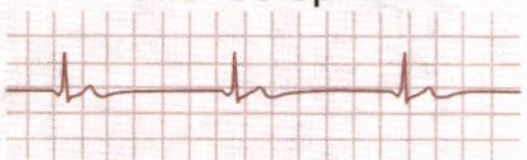	60–100 bpm 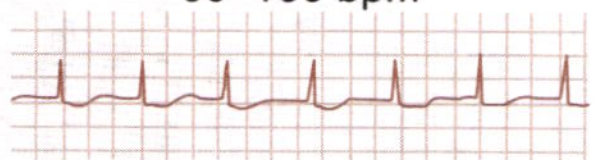	>100 bpm 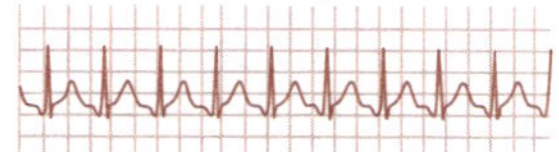

Classification by Etiology	
Automatic Junctional Rhythm	**Reentrant Junctional Rhythm**
Due to enhanced automaticity in AV nodal cells 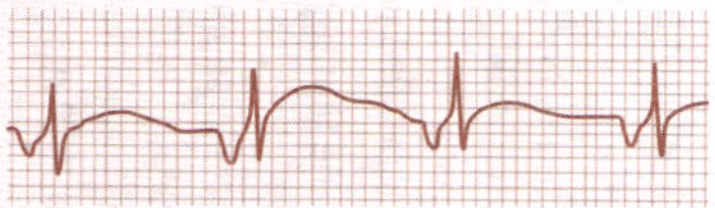	Due to reentrant loop involving AV node 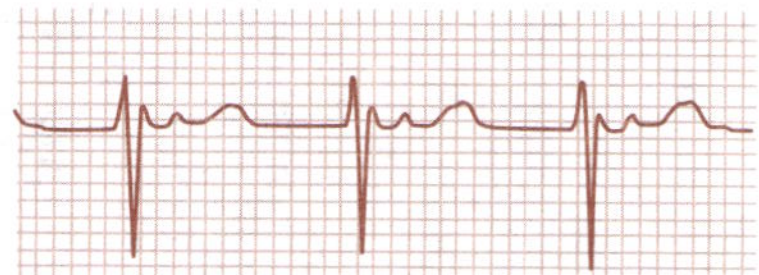

TREATMENT

- Please refer to Table 7-4 for general therapeutic approach to common SVTs (Figures 7-8 and 7-9).
- Acute treatment of symptomatic SVT should follow the **ACLS protocol** as outlined in Appendix C.

TABLE 7-4 Treatment of Common Supraventricular Tachyarrhythmias[4]

Treatment Strategies	
Atrial flutter (AFL)	Anticoagulation similar to AF; risk of thromboembolic complications is similar. Rate control with same agents as AF. If highly symptomatic or rate control difficult, electrical or chemical cardioversion is appropriate. If pacemaker present, overdrive atrial pacing can achieve cardioversion. Catheter ablation of typical right AFL with long-term success above 90% and rare complications.
Multifocal atrial tachycardia (MAT)	Therapy targeted at treatment of underlying pathophysiologic process. Antiarrhythmic, if symptomatic rapid ventricular response. Individualize β-adrenergic blockers vs. calcium channel blocker therapy. DC cardioversion is not effective.
Sinus tachycardia (ST)	Therapy targeted at treatment of underlying pathophysiologic process.
Ectopic atrial tachycardia (EAT)	**Acute therapy:** Identify and treat precipitating factors like digoxin toxicity; if hemodynamically stable, then β-blockers and calcium channel blockers. In rare cases, amiodarone, flecainide, or sotalol. **Chronic therapy:** Rate control with β-adrenergic blockers and calcium channel blockers. If unsuccessful, options include catheter ablation (86% success rate), flecainide, propafenone, sotalol, or amiodarone.
AV nodal reentrant tachycardia (AVNRT)	Catheter ablation highly successful (96%) but has to be individualized to each patient. If medical therapy more desirable—β-adrenergic blockers, calcium channel blockers, and digoxin; then consider propafenone, flecainide, etc.
Orthodromic AV reentrant tachycardia (O-AVRT)	**Acute therapy:** Vagal maneuvers, adenosine, calcium channel blockers. If ineffective, then procainamide or β-blockers. **Chronic suppressive therapy:** Catheter ablation highly successful (95%) but has to be individualized to each patient. If medical therapy more desirable for prevention, flecainide and procainamide are indicated.
Antidromic AV reentrant tachycardia (A-AVRT)	**Acute therapy:** Avoid adenosine or other AV node–specific blocking agents. Consider ibutilide, procainamide, or flecainide. **Chronic suppressive therapy:** Accessory pathway catheter ablation is preferred and successful (95%). If medical therapy desired, consider flecainide and propafenone.

AF, atrial fibrillation; AV, atrioventricular; DC, direct current.

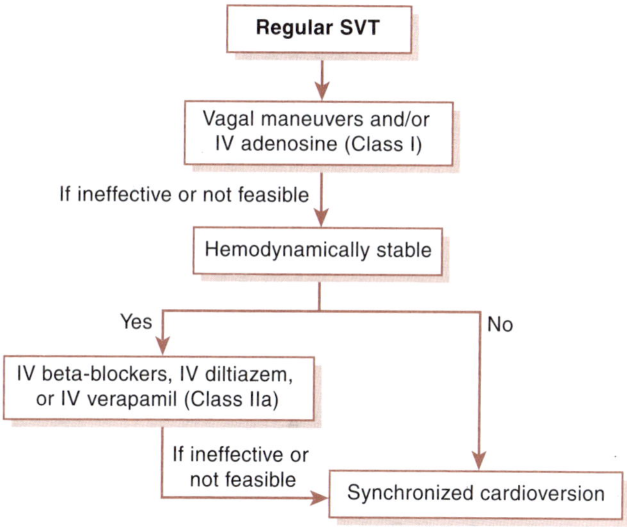

Figure 7-8 Algorithm for management of SVT.

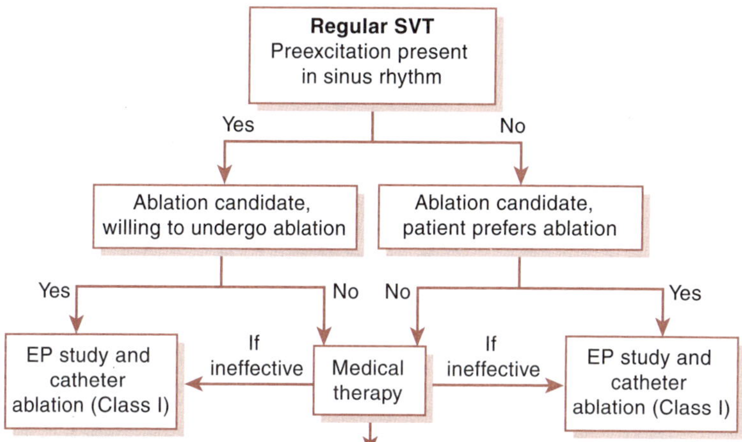

Drug Options			
Class I	**Class IIa**	**Class IIb**	**Class IIb**
Beta-blockers, diltiazem, or verapamil (in the absence of preexcitation)	Flecainide or propafenone (in the absence of SHD)	Amiodarone, dofetilide, or sotalol	Digoxin (in the absence of preexcitation)

Figure 7-9 Algorithm for management of SVT. SHD, structural heart disease.

- Chronic treatment is guided by the severity of associated symptoms, as well as the frequency and duration of recurrent events.[4]
- Many SVTs can be terminated by **AV nodal blocking agents or vagal techniques** (Table 7-5), whereas AF, AFL, and some atrial tachycardias will persist despite a slowing of the ventricular rate because of partial AV nodal blockade.

TABLE 7-5 Common Vagal Maneuvers and Adenosine

	Patient Preparation[a]	Mechanism	Dose/Duration/Details	Toxicity	Contraindication	Potentiators/ Antagonists	Common Side Effects
Valsalva	Describe the procedure.	Vagal stimulation during relaxation phase.	Exhale forcefully against a closed airway for several seconds followed by relaxation.	Well tolerated.	Patient unable to follow commands.	–	–
Carotid sinus massage	Check for carotid bruits and history of CVA; then place in recumbent position with neck extended.	Vagal stimulation.	First, apply enough pressure to simply feel carotid pulse with index and middle fingers. If no effect, then use rotating motion for 3–5 s.	Well tolerated. Risk of embolizing carotid plaque. **Never massage both carotids.**	Recent TIA or stroke or ipsilateral significant carotid artery stenosis or carotid artery bruit.	–	–
Adenosine	Explain the potential side effects to the patient.	AV nodal blocking agent. Short acting (serum half-life 4–8 min).	Initial: 6 mg IV rapid bolus via antecubital vein, followed by 10–30 mL saline flush. If desired or effect not achieved, can repeat 12 mg followed by 12 mg after 1- to 2-min intervals. Central venous line: 3 mg IV initial dose.	Precipitate prolonged asystole in patients with sick sinus syndrome or second- or third-degree AV block.	Significant bronchospasm.	Potentiators: Dipyridamole and carbamazepine. **Effect pronounced in heart transplant recipients.** Antagonists: Caffeine and theophylline.	Facial flushing, palpitations, chest pain, hypotension, exacerbation of bronchospasm.

Atrioventricular nodal reentrant tachycardia, atrioventricular reentrant tachycardia, and many atrial tachycardias will terminate with vagal maneuvers or adenosine, and in atrial flutter, the appearance of flutter waveform will help diagnosis.

Water immersion, eyeball pressure, coughing, gagging, deep breathing, etc., are other alternative vagal maneuvers.

[a]Patients should be under continuous ECG monitoring for each of these procedures. To enhance diagnostic value of rhythm strip, use leads V_1 and II (atrial activity).

AV, atrioventricular; CVA, cerebrovascular accident; TIA, transient ischemic attack.

- **Radiofrequency ablation (RFA):** Definitive cure with high success rates ranging from 80%–100% for many SVTs including AVNRT, accessory bypass tract–mediated tachycardias, focal atrial tachycardia, and AFL. Complication risk is generally <3% for ablation of common SVTs. This risk includes major bleeding, cardiac perforation or tamponade, stroke, pulmonary embolism, and complete heart block requiring permanent pacemaker (PPM) implantation.[4]
- There is limited evidence—but no large randomized trials with long-term follow-up—suggesting that catheter ablation improves quality of life and is more cost-effective than chronic antiarrhythmic drug therapy for long-term management of SVT.[5]

Atrial Fibrillation

GENERAL PRINCIPLES

The medical management of **AF** requires careful consideration of three issues: **rate control, rhythm control, and prevention of thromboembolic events.**

Definition

- Atrial tachyarrhythmia characterized by chaotic activation of the atria with loss of normal atrial mechanical function.
- AF has a pattern on 12-lead ECG characterized by the absence of consistent P waves. Instead, rapid, low-amplitude oscillations or fibrillatory waves are noted in the baseline of leads that best demonstrate atrial activation (V_1, II, III, aVF).
- The ventricular response to AF is characteristically irregular and, often, rapid in the presence of intact AV conduction.
- AF is the most common sustained cardiac arrhythmia encountered in clinical practice.

Classification

AF has been classified (Figure 7-10) into the following forms based on clinical presentation: first occurrence, paroxysmal, persistent, and permanent.

- **First occurrence** may be symptomatic or asymptomatic. The spontaneous conversion rate is high, measured at >60% in hospitalized patients.
  - Stage 1: At risk for AF presence of modifiable and nonmodifiable risk factors
  - Stage 2: Pre-AF (evidence of structural or electrical findings predisposing to AF)
  - Stage 3A: Paroxysmal AF (intermittent, lasting up to 7 days and usually <48 hours in duration)
  - Stage 3B: Persistent AF (continuous and sustained for over 7 days and requires intervention)
  - Stage 3C: Long-standing persistent AF (continuous AF lasting >12 months)
  - Stage 3D: Successful AF ablation (free from AF after ablation or surgical intervention)
  - Stage 4: Permanent AF (no further attempts at rhythm control). Early rhythm control is associated with a greater likelihood of maintaining sinus rhythm in the long term and minimizing AF burden and reducing the progression of the disease

Epidemiology

- AF is the most common sustained tachyarrhythmia for which patients seek treatment and the most likely etiology for an irregularly irregular rhythm discovered on an inpatient ECG. The estimated global prevalence was 50 million patients in 2020.[6] AF is typically a disease of the elderly, affecting >10% of those >75 years old.

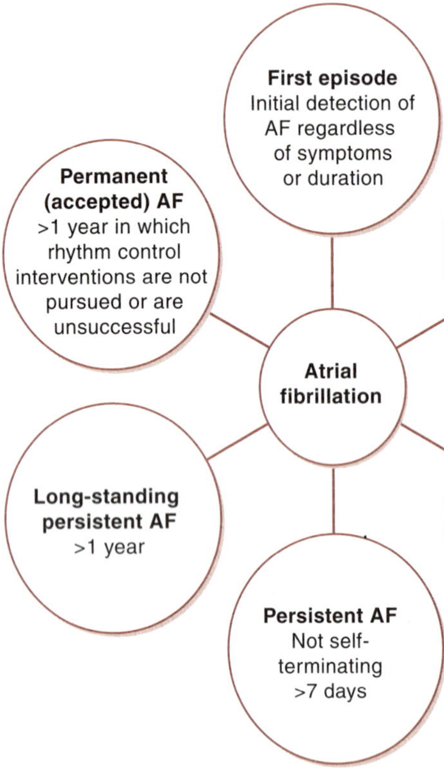

Figure 7-10 Classification of atrial fibrillation.

- Independent risk factors for AF include advanced age, male gender, and the comorbid presence of diabetes mellitus and cardiovascular diseases such as CHF, valvular heart disease, hypertension (HTN), and previous myocardial infarction (MI).[7] Age less than 65, obesity and obstructive sleep apnea (OSA) are important risk factors for new-onset AF.[8]
- Following cardiothoracic surgery, AF occurs in 20%–50% of patients.[9]

Pathophysiology

- The precise mechanisms giving rise to AF are not completely understood.
- Initiation of AF is commonly because of rapid, repetitive firing of an ectopic focus within the pulmonary veins with fibrillatory conduction to the bodies of the atria.
- Maintenance of persistent AF likely requires multiple reentrant circuits varying in location and timing to explain the self-perpetuating characteristic of AF (Table 7-6).
- Structural and electrical remodeling of the left atrium associated with cardiovascular disease promotes ectopic activity and heterogeneous conduction patterns that provide the substrate for AF. AF, when present, also promotes structural and electrical remodeling in the atria that stabilizes the rhythm.

TABLE 7-6 Mechanism of Atrial Fibrillation

Focal Activation	Multiple Wavelets
AF originates from an area of focal activity which may be triggered due to increased automaticity, or from micro-reentry. Usually in the pulmonary veins	Multiple wandering small wavelets are formed, and the fibrillation is maintained by reentry circuits formed by some wavelets. This is potentiated in the presence of a dilated left atria due to the larger surface facilitating continuous waveform propagation

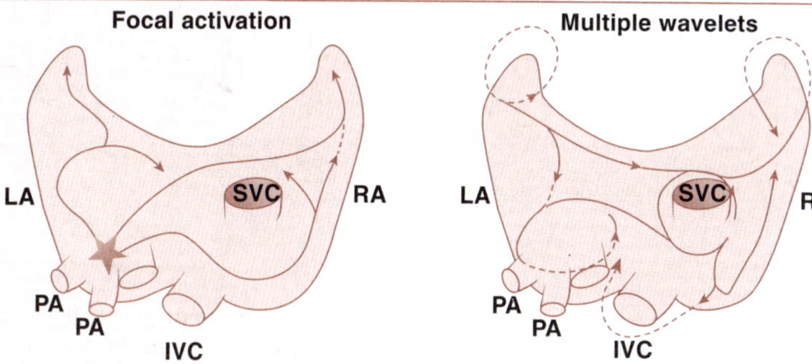

- Inflammation and fibrosis may play a major role in initiation and maintenance of AF. Inflammatory markers, such as interleukin-6 and C-reactive protein, are increased in AF and correlate with the duration of AF, success of cardioversion, and thrombogenesis.

Prevention

- Currently, there is a lack of prospective clinical trials that examine the value of primary prevention of non–postoperative AF through treatment of associated conditions or risk factor modification.
- Some analysis suggests that statins may reduce recurrent AF by 61%, independent of their lipid-lowering effect.[10]
- Angiotensin-converting enzyme inhibitors (**ACE-I**) and angiotensin receptor blockers (**ARB**) have been shown to prevent atrial remodeling in animals via suppression of the renin–angiotensin system. A meta-analysis of patients with CHF and HTN treated with either ACE-I or ARB demonstrated a reduction in new-onset AF by 20%–30%.[11]
- A number of pharmacologic and nonpharmacologic strategies have been evaluated to prevent postoperative AF. Perioperative continuation of **β-adrenergic antagonists has** been shown to reduce postoperative AF rates. **Amiodarone, sotalol, magnesium, and omega-3 fatty acids** used in the perioperative period have also demonstrated a reduction in postoperative AF.[12]
- Lifestyle and risk factor modification serve as essential pillars of AF management to prevent onset, progression, and associated adverse outcomes. For patients with AF, guidelines recommend:
  1. Weight loss in those with body mass index >27 kg/m^2
  2. Moderate-to-vigorous exercise training to a target of 210 minutes per week
  3. Tobacco cessation
  4. Minimization or elimination of alcohol consumption
  5. Optimal blood pressure control
  6. Screening for sleep-disordered breathing

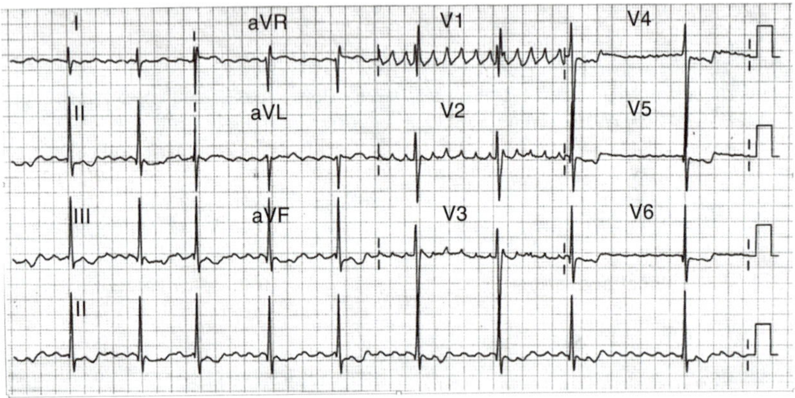

Figure 7-11 ECG showing atrial fibrillation.

DIAGNOSIS

- AF is diagnosed by 12-lead ECG with a stereotypical pattern of an irregularly fluctuating baseline with an irregular, and often rapid, ventricular rate (>100 bpm) (Figure 7-11).
- AF should be distinguished from other tachycardia mechanisms with an irregular ventricular response such as MAT and AFL with variable conduction.

Clinical Presentation

- Symptoms associated with AF can range from nonexistent to nonspecific (fatigue) to severe (acute pulmonary edema, palpitations, angina, syncope).
- Symptoms are usually secondary to the rapid ventricular response to AF rather than the loss of atrial systole. However, patients with significant ventricular systolic or diastolic dysfunction can have symptoms directly attributable to the loss of atrial systole.
- Prolonged episodes of tachycardia because of AF may lead to a **tachycardia-induced cardiomyopathy**.

TREATMENT

- Medical management of AF is directed at three therapeutic goals: **rate control, prevention of thromboembolic events, and rhythm control** through maintenance of sinus rhythm.
- Previous studies have shown that there is no mortality benefit to a strategy aimed at maintaining sinus rhythm.[13] Therefore, rate control and management of thromboembolic risk are the preferred strategy in asymptomatic and minimally symptomatic patients. Rhythm control is reserved for patients who remain symptomatic despite reasonable efforts at pharmacologic rate control.

Medications

- Medical management begins with consideration of appropriate antithrombotic therapy. Warfarin has been shown to be consistently superior to aspirin (ASA) or ASA in combination with clopidogrel for prevention of thromboembolus.
- Direct oral anticoagulants (DOAC) dabigatran, rivaroxaban, apixaban, and edoxaban have been directly compared with warfarin in randomized prospective trials and have

been shown to be either noninferior or superior to warfarin in preventing stroke in AF patients.

- Rate control of the ventricular response to AF is achieved with medications that limit conduction through the AV node such as **non-dihydropyridine calcium channel blockers** (verapamil, diltiazem, etc.), **β-adrenergic antagonists, and digoxin.**
- Rhythm control through maintenance of sinus rhythm can be attempted with selected antiarrhythmic drugs. Pharmacologic control with antiarrhythmic drugs is more effective at preventing recurrence of AF than chemical cardioversion (Table 7-7).

First Line

- **Prevention of stroke and systemic emboli** is a central tenet of AF management guided by individual risk assessment in each patient. Systemic anticoagulation with Coumadin or a DOAC will attenuate the risk of stroke or systemic emboli associated with AF; however, the use of any one of these agents requires a careful risk–benefit analysis to identify patients who are at sufficient risk for thromboembolic events to outweigh the increased risk of hemorrhagic complications.
  - The **CHA_2DS_2-VASc score (Table 7-8)** is a validated risk stratification tool used in nonvalvular AF to predict stroke or systemic embolus risk based on the presence of the following risk factors: CHF, HTN, age >65 or >75 years, diabetes mellitus, female gender, prior stroke or transient ischemic attack (TIA), and history of vascular disease Table 7-9).[14]
  - Antithrombotic therapy can be omitted in patients with a **CHA_2DS_2-VASc score = 0.**
  - In patients with a **CHA_2DS_2-VASc score of 1, no antithrombotic therapy or treatment with an oral anticoagulant or ASA may be considered.**
  - Systemic anticoagulation with warfarin or DOAC is recommended for patients with a CHA_2DS_2-VASc risk of ≥2 and no contraindications for anticoagulation.
  - Measurement of renal function is critical to assess the safety and dosing of certain DOACs in patients with a **CHA_2DS_2-VASc score of ≥2 and chronic kidney disease.**
  - The role of antithrombotic therapy leading up to and after restoration of sinus rhythm is discussed later in the context of cardioversion.
  - The second aspect with regard to thromboprophylaxis is to assess bleeding risk. The HAS-BLED score (Table 7-10) is the recommended score in the ESC and Canadian guidelines for this purpose. A high HAS-BLED score (≥3) is indicative of the need for regular clinical review and follow-up, but should not be used per se as a reason for stopping oral anticoagulation.
- **Rate control** of AF can be achieved with drugs that prolong conduction through the AV node. These include the non-dihydropyridine calcium channel blockers (diltiazem, verapamil), β-adrenergic blockers, and digoxin. Refer to Table 7-7 for loading and dosing recommendations.
  - **Digoxin** can be useful in controlling the resting ventricular rate in AF in the setting of LV dysfunction and CHF when other agents fail. Its utility in other clinical settings is limited by reduced efficacy of rate control during exertion and significant concerns of toxicity.
    - **Digitalis toxicity** is characterized by symptoms of **nausea, abdominal pain, vision changes, confusion, and delirium.** Patients with renal dysfunction are at high risk for digitalis toxicity as are patients on agents known to increase digoxin levels (e.g., verapamil, diltiazem, erythromycin, cyclosporine). **Paroxysmal atrial tachycardia with varying degrees of AV block and bidirectional VT** is the most commonly seen arrhythmias in association with digitalis toxicity. Treatment is supportive—withholding the drug, inserting a temporary pacemaker for prolonged AV block, and administering **IV phenytoin for bidirectional VT.**

TABLE 7-7 Pharmacologic Agents Used for Heart Rate Control in Atrial Fibrillation[9]

Drug	Loading Dose	Onset of Action	Maintenance Dose	Major Side Effects	Recommendation
Without Evidence of Accessory Pathway					
Esmolol[a]	IV: 500 μg/kg over 1 min, followed by 50 μg/kg for 4 min	IV: 2–10 min	IV: Up to 200 μg/kg/min continuous infusion	↓BP, ↓HR, HB, HF, bronchospasm	I
Metoprolol[a]	IV: 2.5–5 mg over 2 min, repeat doses every 5 min as needed up to 15 mg	IV: 20 min		↓BP, ↓HR, HB, HF, bronchospasm	I
	PO: 50–100 mg (in single or divided doses depending upon formulation)	PO: Within 1 h	PO: Up to 400 mg daily		
Propranolol[a]	IV: 1 mg over 1 min, repeat every 2 min as needed up to 3 doses			↓BP, ↓HR, HB, HF, bronchospasm	I
	PO: 10–30 mg every 6-8 h	PO: 1–2 h	PO: 10–40 mg tid or qid		
Diltiazem	IV: 0.25 mg/kg over 2 min, followed by 0.35 mg/kg over 2 min if needed	IV: 3 min	IV: 5–10 mg/h, up to 15 mg/h	↓BP, HB, HF	I
	PO: 120 mg daily (in single or divided doses depending upon formulation)	PO: 30–60 min (for immediate release formulation)	PO: 120–360 mg daily		
Verapamil	IV: 0.075–0.15 mg/kg over 2 min, followed by 10 mg bolus after 15–30 min if needed	IV: 3–5 min	IV: 5 mg/h	↓BP, HB, HF	I
	PO: 180–480 mg daily (in single or divided doses depending upon formulation)	PO: 1–2 h (for immediate release formulation)	PO: Up to 480 mg daily		

(Continued)

TABLE 7-7 Pharmacologic Agents Used for Heart Rate Control in Atrial Fibrillation[8] (Continued)

Amiodarone	IV: 150 mg over 10 min, followed by 1 mg/min for 6 h, followed by 0.5 mg/min for 18 hPO: 600–800 mg daily in divided doses for total load of 10 g over 2–4 wk	2 d–3 wk for antiarrhythmic effects of IV and PO	PO: 200 mg once daily, can be decreased to 100 mg in elderly and patients with low BMI	↓BP, HB, ↓HR, warfarin interaction; see text for description of dermatologic, thyroid, pulmonary, corneal, and liver side effects	Acute setting: IIa (IV) Nonacute/chronic: IIb (PO)
With Evidence of Accessory Pathway[c]					
Amiodarone	IV: 150 mg over 10 min, followed by 1 mg/min for 6 h, followed by 0.5 mg/min for 18 h	2 d–3 wk	PO: 200 mg once daily	See above	IIa
With Heart Failure and Without Accessory Pathway					
Digoxin	IV: 0.25–0.5 mg over several min, repeat 0.25 mg doses every 6 h to maximum dose of 1.5 mg in 24 h; dose may need to be reduced by 50% in patients with CKD/ESRD	IV: 5–60 min PO: 1–2 h	PO: 0.125–0.25 mg once daily; 0.0625 mg once daily for GFR of 10–50 mL/min; 0.0625 mg once every 48 h for GFR <10 mL/min	Digoxin toxicity, HB, ↓HR	I

[a]Only representative β-blockers are included in the table, but other similar agents could be used for this indication in appropriate doses.
[b]Onset is variable, and some effects occur earlier.
[c]Conversion to sinus rhythm and catheter ablation of the accessory pathway are generally recommended; pharmacologic therapy for rate control may be appropriate therapy in certain patients. See text for discussion of atrial fibrillation in setting of preexcitation/Wolff-Parkinson-White syndrome.
[d]Amiodarone can be useful to control the heart rate in patients with atrial fibrillation when other measures are unsuccessful or contraindicated.
BMI, body mass index; ↓BP, hypotension; CKD, chronic kidney disease; ESRD, end-stage renal disease; GFR, glomerular filtration rate; HB, heart block; HF, heart failure; ↓HR, bradycardia; NA, not applicable.

TABLE 7-8 CHA_2DS_2-VASc

Clinical Risk Factors for Stroke, Transient Ischemic Attack, and Systemic Thromboembolism	Condition	Points
C	**Congestive heart failure** Clinical features of heart failure or objective evidence of left ventricular systolic dysfunction (reduced left ventricular ejection fraction)	1
H	**Hypertension** Resting blood pressure above 140/90 mm Hg on more than two occasions or on antihypertensives	1
A_2	**Age ≥75 yrs**	2
D	**Diabetes mellitus** Fasting glucose >125 mg/dL (7 mmol/L) or on treatment with oral hypoglycemic agents and/or insulin	1
S_2	**Prior stroke or TIA or thromboembolism**	2
V	**Vascular disease** Peripheral artery disease, myocardial infarction, aortic plaque	1
A	**Age 65–74 yrs**	1
Sc	**Sex category (female)**	1
	Maximum score—9	

TABLE 7-9 Annual Stroke Risk in Patients With Nonvalvular Atrial Fibrillation Not Treated With Anticoagulation According to the CHA_2DS_2-VASc Score[14]

CHA_2DS_2-VASc Score	Stroke Risk (%)[a]
0	0
1	1.3
2	2.2
3	3.2
4	4.0
5	6.7
6	9.8
7	9.6
8	12.5
9	15.2

CHA_2DS_2-VASc, cardiac failure, hypertension, age 65–74 or age >74 (doubled), diabetes, female sex, stroke (doubled), and a history of vascular disease.

[a]The adjusted stroke rate was derived from multivariate analysis assuming no aspirin usage.

- **Nonpharmacologic rate control** of AF can be accomplished by AV nodal ablation in association with PPM implantation. This strategy should be reserved for patients deemed to be in permanent AF, who have failed pharmacologic rate control and in whom rhythm control is either ineffective or contraindicated.

TABLE 7-10 HAS-BLED Bleeding Risk Score

	Clinical Characteristic	Points
H	**Hypertension** Uncontrolled, >160 mm Hg systolic	1
A	**Abnormal renal function** Dialysis, transplant, Cr >2.26 mg/dL or >200 μmol/L **Abnormal liver function** Cirrhosis or bilirubin >2x normal or AST/ALT/AP >3x normal	1 1
S	**Stroke** Prior history of stroke	1
B	**Bleeding** Prior major bleeding or predisposition to bleeding	1
L	**Labile INR** Unstable/high INR, time in therapeutic range <60%	1
E	**Elderly** Age >65 yrs	1
D	**Prior alcohol or drug usage history** ≥8 drinks/wk **Medication usage predisposing to bleeding** Antiplatelet agents, NSAIDs	1 1
	Maximum score—9	
	0 point — 1.13 bleeds per 100 patient-years	
	1 point — 1.02 bleeds per 100 patient-years	
	2 points — 1.88 bleeds per 100 patient-years	
	3 points — 3.74 bleeds per 100 patient-years	
	4 points — 8.70 bleeds per 100 patient-years	
	5–9 points — Insufficient data	

Second Line

Pharmacologic rhythm control of AF is accomplished with antiarrhythmic drugs that modify impulse formation or propagation to prevent initiation of AF. **The risk of thromboembolus associated with a pharmacologic cardioversion should be considered before beginning antiarrhythmic drug therapy (Tables 7-10 and 7-11(A) and (B)).**

Guidelines for anticoagulation are discussed in the following text and Figure 7-12:

- **Pharmacologic cardioversion** should be done in the hospital setting with continuous ECG monitoring because of a small risk of life-threatening tachyarrhythmias or bradyarrhythmias. **Ibutilide** is the only drug that is approved by the US Food and Drug Administration for pharmacologic cardioversion. Clinical trials have shown a 45% conversion rate for AF and a 60% conversion rate for AFL. Ibutilide is associated with a 4%–8% risk for torsades de pointes (TdP), especially in the first 2–4 hours after administration of the drug. Because of this risk, patients must be monitored on telemetry with an external defibrillator immediately available during ibutilide infusion and for at least 4 hours after the infusion. The risk for TdP is higher in patients with cardiomyopathy and CHF. Ibutilide is given via an IV, at a dosage of 1 mg (0.01 mg/kg if patient is <60 kg), **infused slowly over 10 minutes.** Faster administration can promote TdP. The efficacy of antiarrhythmics to achieve pharmacologic conversion drops sharply when AF is >7 days in duration. For shorter duration AF episodes, dofetilide, sotalol, flecainide, and propafenone have some efficacy, whereas amiodarone has limited efficacy to achieve pharmacologic cardioversion.

TABLE 7-11(A) Commonly Used Antiarrhythmic Drugs in Atrial Fibrillation

Drug	Channels Blocked	Cardiovascular Toxicity	Other Adverse Effects
Amiodarone	IKr, INa, ICaL, IKur, Ito, IKACh, If, β-AR, α-AR	Sinus Bradycardia	Thyroid- hypothyroidism, Hyperthyroidism Pulmonary- Chronic Interstitial Infiltrates, Acute hypersensitivity pneumonitis Hepatitis Blue-grey skin discoloration Photosensitivity Nausea, Ataxia, Tremor Alopecia
Dronedarone	IKr, INa, ICaL, IKur, Ito, IKACh, If, β-AR, α-AR	Bradycardia	Anorexia Nausea Hepatotoxicity
Flecainide	INa	AFl with 1:1 conduction Ventricular tachycardia May unmask Brugada-type ST elevation	Dizziness Headache Visual blurring
Propafenone	INa, β-AR	AFl with 1:1 conduction Ventricular tachycardia May unmask Brugada type ST elevation	Metallic taste Dizziness Visual blurring
Sotalol	IKr, β-AR	Bradycardia, Torsades de pointes	Bronchospasm
Dofetilide	IKr	Torsades de pointes	None
Disopyramide	INa, IKr, Acetylcholine	Exacerbation of congestive heart failure Torsades de pointes	Anticholinergic effects- dry mouth, urinary retention, blurry vision

AFl, atrial flutter; IKr, rapidly activating delayed rectifier potassium current; INa, sodium current; ICaL, L-type calcium current; IKur, ultra-rapidly activating delayed rectifier potassium current; Ito, transient outward potassium current; IKACh, acetylcholine-activated inward rectifier potassium current; If, funny current; AR, adrenoreceptor.

- **Maintenance of sinus rhythm** with antiarrhythmic agents is associated with a small risk for life-threatening proarrhythmia. As a result, antiarrhythmic therapy should be reserved for patients who have highly symptomatic AF despite adequate rate control. Commonly used antiarrhythmic agents, their major route of elimination, and dosing regimens are listed in Table 7-11(A) and (B). The most effective agents for maintenance of sinus rhythm are flecainide, propafenone, sotalol, dofetilide, amiodarone, and dronedarone.
  - **Flecainide and propafenone** can be considered for maintenance of sinus rhythm in patients with **structurally normal hearts.** In patients with structural heart disease,

TABLE 7-11(B) Commonly Used Antiarrhythmic Drugs

Class	Drug	Route of Administration (Elimination)	Initial/Loading Dose	Maintenance Dose
Ia	Procainamide	IV (R, H) PO (R, H)	15–18 mg/kg at 20 mg/min 50 mg/kg/24 h, Max: 5 g/24 h	1–4 mg/min IR: 250–500 mg q3–6h SR: 500 mg q6h Procanbid: 1000–2500 mg q12h
	Quinidine	PO (H)	Sulfate, 200–400 mg q6h; gluconate, 324–972 mg q8–12h	NA
	Disopyramide	PO (H, R)	300–400 mg	IR: 100–200 mg q6h SR: 200–400 mg q12h
Ib	Lidocaine	IV (H)	1 mg/kg over 2 min (may repeat × 2 up to 3 mg/kg total)	1–4 mg/min
	Mexiletine	PO (H)	400 mg one-time dose	200–300 mg q8h
Ic	Flecainide	PO (H, R)	50 mg q12h	Increase by 50–100 mg/d every 4 d to max 400 mg/d
	Propafenone	PO (H)	IR: 150 mg q8h ER: 225 mg q12h	IR: Increase at 3- to 4-day intervals up to 300 mg q8h; ER: May increase at 5-day intervals, up to 425 mg q12h
III	Sotalol	PO (R)	80 mg q12h	May increase every 3 d up to 240–320 mg/d in two to three divided doses
	Dofetilide	PO (R, H)	CrCl (mL/min): Dose (μg bid): >60: 500 40–60: 250 20–39: 125 <20: Contraindicated	Dose adjusted based on QTc 2–3 h after inpatient doses 1 through 5 Chronic therapy requires calculation of QTc and CrCl every 3 mo with adjustment as necessary
	Ibutilide	IV (H)	1 mg (0.01 mg/kg if patient <60 kg) over 10 min; can repeat if no response 10 min after initial infusion	NA

(Continued)

TABLE 7-11(B) Commonly Used Antiarrhythmic Drugs (Continued)

Class	Drug	Route of Administration (Elimination)	Initial/Loading Dose	Maintenance Dose
	Amiodarone	IV (H) PO (H)	IV: 150 mg over 10 min PO: 800 mg/d for 1 wk, then 600 mg/d for 1 wk, then 400 mg/d for 1 wk	1 mg/min × 6 h, then 0.5 mg/min 100–400 mg PO daily

[a]Either common or life-threatening adverse effects of these medications are listed. This is not a comprehensive list of all possible adverse effects.

AMI, acute myocardial infarction; ANA, antinuclear antibodies; ↓BP, hypotension; CNS, central nervous system; CHF, congestive heart failure; CrCl, creatinine clearance; ER, extended release; GI, gastrointestinal; H, hepatic; HA, headache; HB, heart block; HF, heart failure; ↓HR, bradycardia; IR, immediate release; NA, not applicable; NAPA, *N*-acetylprocainamide; R, renal; SLE, systemic lupus erythematosus; SR, sustained release; TdP, torsades de pointes; VT, ventricular tachycardia.

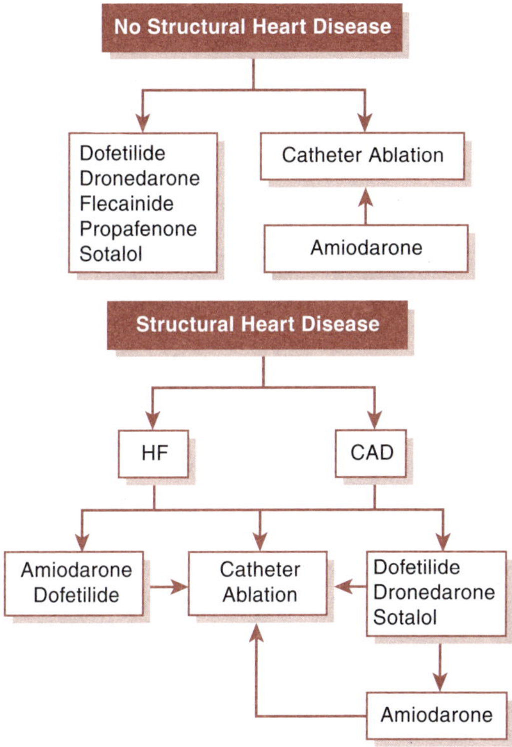

Figure 7-12 Algorithm for rhythm control in atrial fibrillation.

these agents are associated with an increased mortality rate.[15] Both agents are potent negative inotropes that can provoke or exacerbate heart failure. Both agents prolong the QRS duration as an early manifestation of toxicity. Toxicity increases with heart rate because of preferential blockade of active sodium channels. This property is described as **positive-use dependence.** Exercise ECG can be used to give additional information about dose safety at higher heart rates. Flecainide should be used with caution without concomitant dosing with an AV nodal blocker because a paradoxical increase in the ventricular rate may occur because of drug-induced conversion of AF to AFL. Propafenone is less prone to this phenomenon because of intrinsic β-adrenergic antagonism.

- **Sotalol** is useful for the maintenance of sinus rhythm. Sotalol is a mixture of stereoisomers (DL-); D-sotalol is a potassium channel blocker, whereas L-sotalol is a β-antagonist. Side effects of the drug reflect both mechanisms of action. In addition to QT interval prolongation leading to TdP, DL-sotalol may result in sinus bradycardia or AV conduction abnormalities. Sotalol should not be used in patients with decompensated CHF (because of the negative inotropic effect) or with a prolonged QT interval. Initiation of sotalol should be performed in an inpatient monitored setting.
- **Dofetilide** is useful for the maintenance of sinus rhythm. Dofetilide is a pure potassium channel blocker. Initiation of dofetilide should be done in an inpatient monitored setting.

- QT prolongation with sotalol or dofetilide is intensified by bradycardia, a characteristic known as "**reverse-use dependence.**" The main risk of dofetilide is TdP. Dofetilide is contraindicated in patients with a baseline corrected QT interval (QT_c) >440 ms or >500 ms in patients with a baseline bundle branch block. Initial dosing of dofetilide is based on the creatinine clearance. A 12-lead ECG should be obtained before the first dose of dofetilide and 1–2 hours after each dose. If the QT_c interval after the first dose is prolonged by 15% of the baseline or exceeds 500 ms, a 50% dosage reduction is indicated. If the QT_c exceeds 500 ms after the second dose, dofetilide must be discontinued. Several medications block the renal secretion of dofetilide (verapamil, cimetidine, prochlorperazine, trimethoprim, megestrol, ketoconazole) and are contraindicated with dofetilide. The advantages of dofetilide are that it is not associated with increased CHF or mortality in patients with LV dysfunction and it does not cause sinus node dysfunction or conduction abnormalities.[16]

○ **Dronedarone** is the newest antiarrhythmic agent approved for treatment of AF. Like amiodarone—from which it was derived—dronedarone shares properties with Vaughan Williams classes I–IV antiarrhythmic drugs. Dronedarone has been shown to be more effective than placebo at maintaining sinus rhythm after cardioversion but less effective than amiodarone at maintenance of sinus rhythm. The incidence of proarrhythmia is low with dronedarone, as is the incidence of organ toxicity. A trend toward increased mortality has been shown in patients with advanced heart failure symptoms; as such, it is contraindicated in this patient group. Dronedarone is metabolized in the liver and should not be used in patients with significant hepatic dysfunction. Dronedarone can be used in patients with significant renal dysfunction because clearance is predominantly in the GI tract.

○ **Amiodarone** is arguably the most effective antiarrhythmic agent for maintenance of sinus rhythm. **Because of the extensive toxicity profile of amiodarone, it should not be considered as a first-line agent for rhythm control of AF in patients in whom an alternative antiarrhythmic can safely be used.** IV amiodarone has a low efficacy for acute conversion of AF, although conversion after several days of IV amiodarone has been observed. Given its common use and relatively high incidence of side effects, a more detailed discussion of these effects is required.

- Adverse effects of oral amiodarone are partially dose dependent and may occur in up to 75% of patients treated at high doses for 5 years. At lower doses (200–300 mg/d), adverse effects that require discontinuation occur in approximately 5%–10% of patients per year.
- **Pulmonary toxicity** occurs in 1%–15% of treated patients but appears less likely in those who receive <300 mg/d.[17] Patients characteristically have a dry cough and dyspnea associated with pulmonary infiltrates and rales. The process appears to be reversible if detected early, but undetected cases may result in a mortality rate of up to 10% among those affected. A CXR and pulmonary function tests should be obtained at baseline and every 12 months or when patients report symptoms of dyspnea. The presence of interstitial infiltrates on the chest radiograph and a decreased diffusing capacity raise concern of amiodarone pulmonary toxicity.
- **Photosensitivity** is a common adverse reaction, and in some patients, a violaceous skin discoloration develops in sun-exposed areas. The blue-gray discoloration may not resolve completely with discontinuation of therapy.
- **Thyroid dysfunction** is a common adverse effect. Hypothyroidism and hyperthyroidism have both been reported, with an incidence of 2%–5% per year. Thyroid-stimulating hormone should be obtained at baseline and monitored every 6 months. If hypothyroidism develops, concurrent treatment with levothyroxine may allow continued amiodarone use.

- **Corneal microdeposits**, detectable on slit-lamp examination, develop in virtually all patients. These deposits rarely interfere with vision and are not an indication for discontinuation of the drug. Optic neuritis, leading to blindness, is rare but has been reported in association with amiodarone.
- The most common **ECG changes** are lengthened PR intervals and bradycardia; however, high-grade AV block may occur in patients who have preexisting conduction abnormalities. Amiodarone may prolong QT intervals, although usually not extensively, and **TdP is rare**. Other agents that prolong the QT interval, however, should be avoided in patients who are taking amiodarone.
- **Liver dysfunction** usually manifests in an asymptomatic and transient rise in hepatic transaminases. If the increase exceeds three times normal or doubles in a patient with an elevated baseline level, amiodarone should be discontinued or the dose should be reduced. Aspartate transaminase (AST) and alanine transaminase (ALT) should be monitored every 6 months in patients who are receiving amiodarone.
- **Drug interactions.** Amiodarone may raise the blood levels of warfarin and digoxin; therefore, these drugs should be reduced routinely by one-half when amiodarone is initiated, and levels should be followed closely.

Nonpharmacologic Therapies

- Nonpharmacologic methods of rhythm control include electrical cardioversion or ablation via catheter or surgical techniques that block the initiation and maintenance of AF.
- **Direct current cardioversion** (DCCV) is the safest and most effective method of acutely restoring sinus rhythm. Prior to cardioversion, consideration of thromboembolic risk and anticoagulation is critical, when possible, to minimize thromboembolic events triggered by the cardioversion process. AF with a rapid ventricular response in the setting of ongoing myocardial ischemia, MI, hypotension, or respiratory distress should receive prompt cardioversion regardless of the anticoagulation status.
  - If the duration of AF is documented to be **<48 hours**, cardioversion may proceed without anticoagulation. If AF has persisted for **>48 hours** (or for an unknown duration), patients should be therapeutically anticoagulated for at least 3 weeks before cardioversion (in an elective situation), and anticoagulation should be continued in the same therapeutic range following successful cardioversion for a minimum of 4 weeks.
  - An alternative to anticoagulation for 3 weeks before cardioversion is to perform a **transesophageal echocardiogram** (TEE) to rule out left atrial appendage thrombus before cardioversion. This method is safe and has the advantage of a shorter time to cardioversion than 3 weeks of anticoagulation. Therapeutic anticoagulation is indicated after the cardioversion for a minimum of 4 weeks.[18]
  - When practical, periprocedural sedation should be accomplished with midazolam (1–2 mg IV q2min to a maximum of 5 mg), methohexital (25–75 mg IV), etomidate (0.2–0.6 mg/kg IV), or propofol (initial dose, 5 mg/kg/h IV).
  - Proper synchronization of the DC shock to the QRS is critical to avoid induction of VT by a cardioversion shock delivered during a vulnerable period of the ventricle.
  - For cardioversion of atrial arrhythmias, the anterior patch electrode should be positioned just right of the sternum at the level of the third or fourth intercostal space, with the second electrode positioned just below the left scapula posteriorly. **Care should be taken to position patch electrodes at least 6 cm from PPM or implantable-cardioverter defibrillator (ICD) generators.** If electrode paddles are used, firm pressure and conductive gel should be applied to minimize contact impedance. Direct contact with the patient or the bed should be avoided. Atropine (1 mg IV) should be readily available to treat prolonged pauses. Reports of serious arrhythmias, such as VT, ventricular fibrillation (VF), or asystole are rare and are more likely in the setting of improperly synchronized cardioversions, digitalis toxicity, or concomitant antiarrhythmic drug therapy.

- **Catheter ablation of AF** has been shown to be highly effective in younger patients with structurally normal hearts and a paroxysmal pattern of AF.
  - Success rates in this patient category are in the range of 70%–80% over a 12–18 month follow-up period. Success rates are diminished in patients with structural heart disease, advanced age, and persistent AF. A significant fraction of patients require more than one ablation procedure to achieve long-term successful elimination of AF.[9]
  - The goal of the catheter ablation procedure in paroxysmal AF patients is to achieve electrical isolation of the pulmonary veins. In patients with persistent AF, this goal is frequently combined with substrate modification strategies whereby regions of the atria are targeted for ablation to block reentry or the presence of focal drivers of AF.
  - Because of potential procedural complications and modest success, patients generally undergo at least one trial of an antiarrhythmic drug for maintenance of sinus rhythm. If this trial is ineffective or poorly tolerated, catheter ablation can be considered.
  - Alternatively, select patients—particularly those with paroxysmal atrial fibrillation—may choose to forgo a trial of an antiarrhythmic drug in favor of catheter ablation as a primary rhythm control strategy.[9]
- Left atrial appendage occlusion (LAAO) devices:
  - In patients with CHA2DS2-VASc score ≥2 and a contraindication to long-term OAC, percutaneous LAAO (pLAAO) is reasonable (Class 2a). Patients with a moderate to high risk of stroke and a high risk of major bleeding while on OAC, pLAAO may represent a reasonable alternative to OAC (Class 2b).[19]
  - For patients with symptomatic but infrequent, acute, and nondestabilizing episodes, the use of an antiarrhythmics only at the time of an episode that can quickly restore sinus rhythm, generally as an out-patient, without the burden of a daily drug regimen, may be better. This is called "pill-in-the-pocket" therapy.[20] The drugs used are 300 mg of flecainide or 600 mg of propafenone.
  - "Pill-in-the-pocket" anticoagulation is a novel paradigm where patients initiate oral anticoagulation only in response to a documented episode of atrial fibrillation. The safety and efficacy of this strategy will be tested in the pivotal REACT-AF trial.

Surgical Management

Surgical techniques for cure of AF have been evaluated since the 1980s. Of these techniques, the Cox-maze procedure has the highest demonstrated efficacy and the most substantial published follow-up data documenting sustained efficacy. Taking into account patients with persistent AF and structural heart disease, success rates approach 90%. Because of its highly invasive nature, surgical treatment is usually reserved for patients who have failed a catheter ablation strategy or who have planned concomitant cardiac surgery.[9]

Ventricular Tachyarrhythmias

GENERAL PRINCIPLES

- Ventricular tachyarrhythmias should be initially approached with the assumption that they will have a malignant course until proven otherwise.
- Characterization of the arrhythmia involves consideration of hemodynamic stability, duration and ECG morphology of the tachycardia, and presence or lack of underlying structural heart disease.
- Ultimately, this characterization will aid in determining the patient's risk for **sudden cardiac arrest** (SCA) and the need for therapeutic intervention and/or device implantation.

Definition (Table 7-12)

- Ventricular arrhythmias are the major cause of **sudden cardiac death** (SCD). SCD is defined as unexpected death that generally occurs within 1 hour of the onset of symptoms in a person without any prior condition that would appear fatal. In the United States, approximately 350,000 cases of SCD occur annually. Among patients with aborted SCD, ischemic heart disease is the most common associated cardiac structural abnormality. Most cardiac arrest survivors do not have evidence of an acute MI; however, >75% have evidence of previous infarcts. Nonischemic cardiomyopathy (NICM) is also associated with an elevated risk for SCD.[21]

TABLE 7-12 Ventricular Arrhythmias

Arrhythmias	Comments
Premature ventricular complexes	Spontaneous ventricular depolarization of supraventricular impulse. Usually benign but can cause tachycardia-induced cardiomyopathy and heart failure or precipitate ventricular tachycardia or ventricular fibrillation
Nonsustained ventricular tachycardia	≥consecutive ventricular depolarizations at a rate >100 bpm and ≥30 sec
Sustained ventricular tachycardia	Repetitive ventricular depolarizations at a rate >100 for >30 sec or requiring termination <30 sec owing to hemodynamic instability
Monomorphic ventricular tachycardia	Single stable QRS morphology from beat-to-beat cycle length variation and QRS alternans may be seen Heart rate can be <100 if on antiarrhythmic therapy LBBB-like pattern—predominantly negative QRS polarity in V_1 (QS, rS, qrS) RBBB-like pattern—predominantly positive QRS polarity in V_1 (rs-R', qR, R-R, R, R-S)
Polymorphic ventricular tachycardia	Continuously changing QRS morphology (without a constant QRS morphology for >5 complexes) No clear isoelectric baseline between QRS complexes with different morphologies in multiple simultaneously recorded leads Indicates a variable sequence of ventricular activation and/or no single site of origin
Torsades de pointes	Polymorphic VT associated with a long QT interval. Twisting of the peaks of the QRS complexes around the isoelectric line Seen in drug-induced and in congenital long QT syndrome
Bidirectional ventricular tachycardia	Beat-to-beat alternation of QRS frontal plane axis Associated with catecholaminergic VT and digitalis toxicity
Ventricular flutter	Regular, rapid (300 bpm with a cycle length variability usually <30 msec) monomorphic ventricular arrhythmia without any isoelectric interval between successful QRS complexes
Ventricular fibrillation	Rapid (≥300 bpm), grossly irregular ventricular rhythm with marked variability in QRS cycle length, morphology, and amplitude

Etiology

- **VT associated with structural heart disease**
  - Most ventricular arrhythmias are associated with structural heart disease, typically related to active ischemia or prior infarct.
    - Scar and the peri-infarct area provide the substrate for reentry that produces SMVT.
    - PMVT and VF are commonly associated with ischemia and are the presumed cause of most out-of-hospital SCD.
  - NICM typically involves progressive dilation and fibrosis of the ventricular myocardium, providing an arrhythmogenic substrate.
  - Infiltrative cardiomyopathies (secondary to sarcoidosis, hemochromatosis, amyloidosis, etc.) affect a smaller patient population that is at significant risk for ventricular arrhythmias and whose management is less clearly defined.
  - Adults with prior repair of congenital heart disease are commonly afflicted with both VT and SVT.
  - Arrhythmogenic right ventricular dysplasia (ARVD) or cardiomyopathy (ARVC) is marked by fibrofatty replacement of the RV (and sometimes LV) myocardium that gives rise to left bundle branch block (LBBB) morphology VT and is associated with sudden death, particularly in young athletes.
  - Bundle branch reentry VT is a form of ventricular tachyarrhythmia that uses the His-Purkinje system in a reentrant circuit and is typically associated with cardiomyopathy and an abnormal conduction system.
- **VT in the absence of structural heart disease**
  - Inherited ion channelopathies, such as those seen in Brugada syndrome and LQTS, can lead to PMVT and sudden death in patients without evidence of structural heart disease on imaging.
  - Catecholaminergic PMVT involves inherited, exercise-induced VT that is related to irregular calcium processing.
  - **Idiopathic VT** is a diagnosis of exclusion that requires the documented absence of structural heart disease, genetic disorders, and reversible etiologies (i.e., ischemia, metabolic abnormalities). Most idiopathic VTs originate from the RV outflow tract (RVOT) and are amenable to ablation. Less commonly, LV outflow tract (LVOT) VT or fascicular VT (using anterior and posterior divisions of the left bundle branch) may be discovered on EPS.

DIAGNOSIS

Clinical Presentation

- The evaluation of wide-complex tachyarrhythmias (WCTs) should always begin with prompt assessment of vital signs and clinical symptoms. If the arrhythmia is poorly tolerated, postpone further detailed evaluation and proceed to acute management per ACLS guidelines. If the patient is clinically stable, the rhythm should be carefully analyzed to distinguish VT from SVT. A common mistake is the assumption that hemodynamic stability supports the diagnosis of SVT over VT.
- VT represents the vast majority of WCT seen in the inpatient setting with reported prevalence around 80%. Eliciting certain historical points of emphasis and closely assessing ECG properties of the arrhythmia can help to further delineate the mechanism of the underlying rhythm disturbance. Begin with the following questions:
  - Does the patient have a history of structural heart disease?
    - Patients with structural heart disease are much more likely to have VT rather than SVT as the etiology of a WCT. In one analysis, 98% of patients with WCT who had prior MI proved to have VT.[22]
  - Does the patient have an implanted device (PPM or ICD) or a wide QRS at baseline?

- The presence of either a pacemaker or an ICD should raise suspicion for a device-mediated WCT.
- **Device-mediated WCT** can be because of ventricular pacing at a rapid rate either caused by device tracking of an atrial tachyarrhythmia or alternatively by an "endless loop tachycardia" from tracking of retrograde atrial impulses created by the preceding ventricular paced beat. In either case, the tachycardia rate is a clue to the mechanism because it is typically equal to the programmed upper rate limit (URL) of the device. A commonly programmed URL is 120 bpm. A tachycardia rate above the URL effectively excludes a device-mediated WCT.
- The presence of an implantable device can be confirmed by inspection of the chest wall (usually left chest for right-handed patients), CXR, or the appearance of pacing spikes on ECG or telemetry.
- Patients with known right bundle branch block (RBBB), LBBB, or intraventricular conduction delay (IVCD) at baseline presenting with WCT will have a QRS morphology identical to baseline in the presence of SVT. In contrast, some patients with a narrow QRS at baseline will manifest a WCT due to SVT when a rate-related bundle branch block is present (SVT with aberrancy).

◦ What are the patient's home medications?
- The patient's home medication list should be carefully reviewed for any drugs with proarrhythmic side effects, especially those that can prolong the baseline QT interval. These medicines include many of the class I and III antiarrhythmics, certain antibiotics and antipsychotics, etc.
- The use of medications that can potentially lead to electrolyte derangements, such as loop and potassium-sparing diuretics, ACE-I, ARB, should be discussed with the patient. Practitioners should also consider digoxin toxicity, if applicable, in the setting of any arrhythmia.

Differential Diagnosis

- WCT may be because of either SVT with aberrant conduction or VT. Differentiation between these rhythm abnormalities is of utmost importance. **The pharmacologic agents used in the management of SVT (i.e., adenosine, β-blockers, calcium channel blockers) may cause hemodynamic instability if used in the setting of VT.** Therefore, all WCTs are considered to be ventricular in origin until proven otherwise.
- Other less common mechanisms of WCT include **A-AVRT, hyperkalemia-induced arrhythmia, or pacemaker-induced tachycardia.**
- **Telemetry artifact** because of poor lead contact or repetitive patient motion (tremor, shivering, brushing teeth, chest physical therapy, etc.) can mimic VT or VF.

Diagnostic Testing

Laboratories

- Basic laboratory studies should include CBC, complete metabolic panel (CMP), magnesium level, and serial troponins.
- Additional labs based on clinical suspicion should also be obtained during initial workup.

Electrocardiography

- **Differentiation of SVT with aberrancy from VT** (Figures 7-13 and 7-14) based on ECG analysis is critical for the determination of appropriate acute and chronic therapy. Features that are diagnostic of VT are **AV dissociation, capture or fusion beats**, an absence of RS morphology in all precordial leads (V_1–V_6), and **LBBB morphology with right axis deviation.** In the absence of these features, examination of an RS complex in a precordial lead for an RS interval >100 ms is consistent with VT (Figure 7-15).

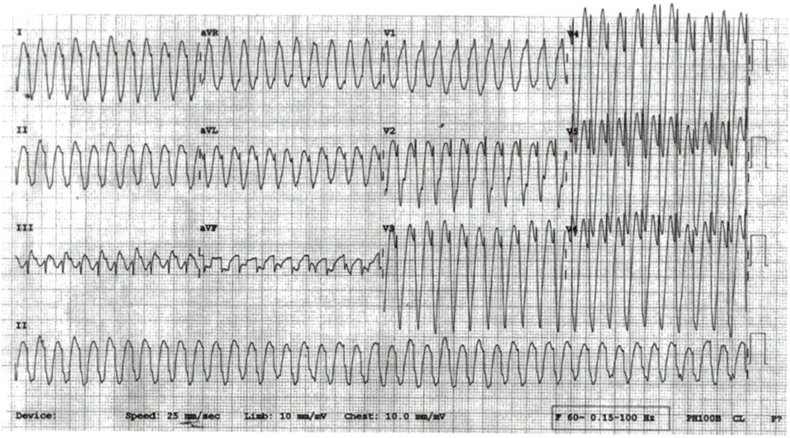

Figure 7-13 ECG of ventricular tachycardia.

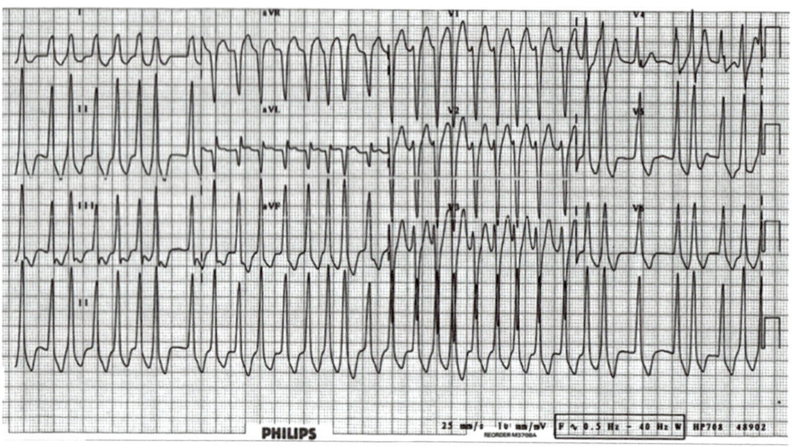

Figure 7-14 ECG showing irregular wide complex tachycardia—WPW with AF.

- In addition, characteristic QRS morphologies that are suggestive of VT may be sought, as shown in Figure 7-16.
- **ECG pearls**
  - **Brugada syndrome ECG patterns** (Table 7-13 and Figure 7-17)
  - **Arrhythmogenic RV dysplasia (ARVD)**
    - Normal sinus rhythm (NSR) ECG at baseline with presence of an **epsilon wave** (late potential just after QRS) and/or T wave inversions in the right precordial leads are diagnostic criteria for ARVD.
    - VT in ARVD generally arises from an RV origin and is therefore likely to have a LBBB configuration; patients may present with NSVT or PMVT

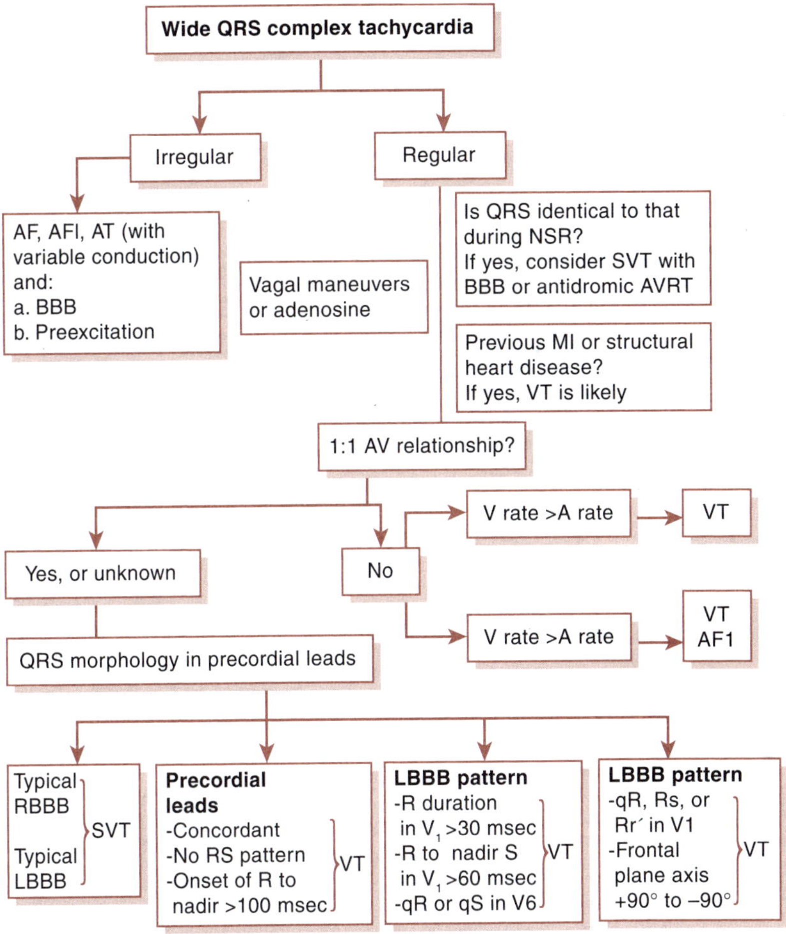

Figure 7-15 Algorithm of approach to wide complex tachycardia.

- **Bundle branch reentrant VT**
  - Baseline ECG often shows IVCD
  - In VT the ECG typically presents with a LBBB morphology with the electrical impulse traveling "down" the right bundle and "up" the left bundle)
- **Fascicular VT**
  ECG in VT shows an RBBB morphology with superior axis
- **Long QT syndrome (LQTS)** (Table 7-14)
  - Abnormal prolongation of the QT interval on ECG at baseline (ideally measured in leads II and V_5 or V_6).
  - $QT_c \geq 450$ ms in men and 460 ms in women.
  - ECG in VT often shows TdP degenerating into VF.

• **Outflow tract VT** ECG characteristically has an inferior axis with an LBBB morphology. R/S transition in the precordial leads can aid in localization: early transition (V_1 or V_2)

suggests an LV outflow tract origin, whereas later transition (V_4 or after) is suggestive of an RV outflow tract origin.

Imaging

- The presence or absence of structural heart disease should be initially evaluated by TTE.
- Further imaging (cardiac MRI, noninvasive stress test, coronary angiogram, etc.) should be obtained based on suspected etiology.

TREATMENT

- **Differentiation of SVT with aberrancy from VT** based on analysis of the surface ECG is critical in the determination of appropriate acute and chronic treatment.
  - For acute therapy of SVT, IV medications such as adenosine, calcium channel blockers, or β-blockers are used (see Treatment of Supraventricular Tachyarrhythmias earlier in

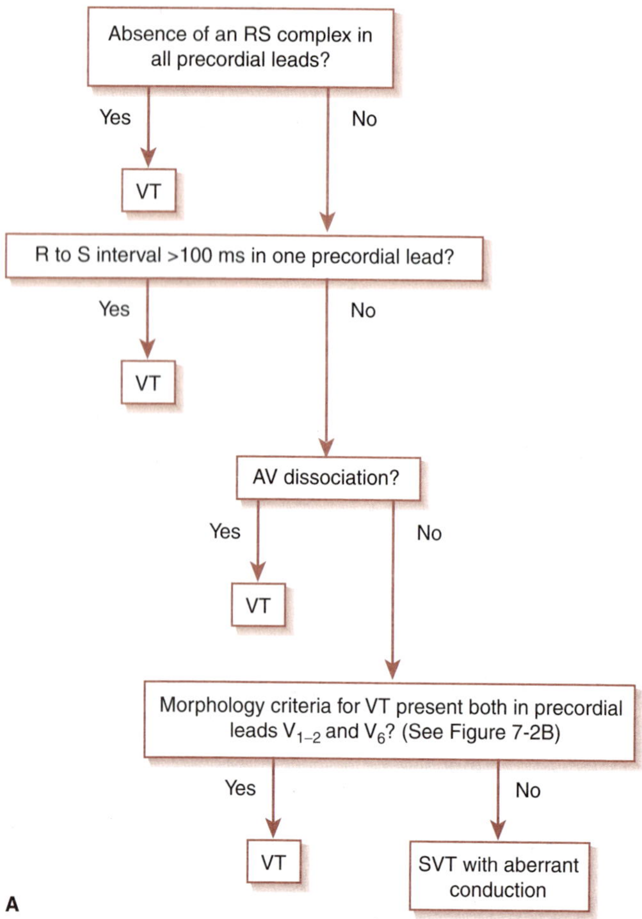

Figure 7-16 (*Continued*)

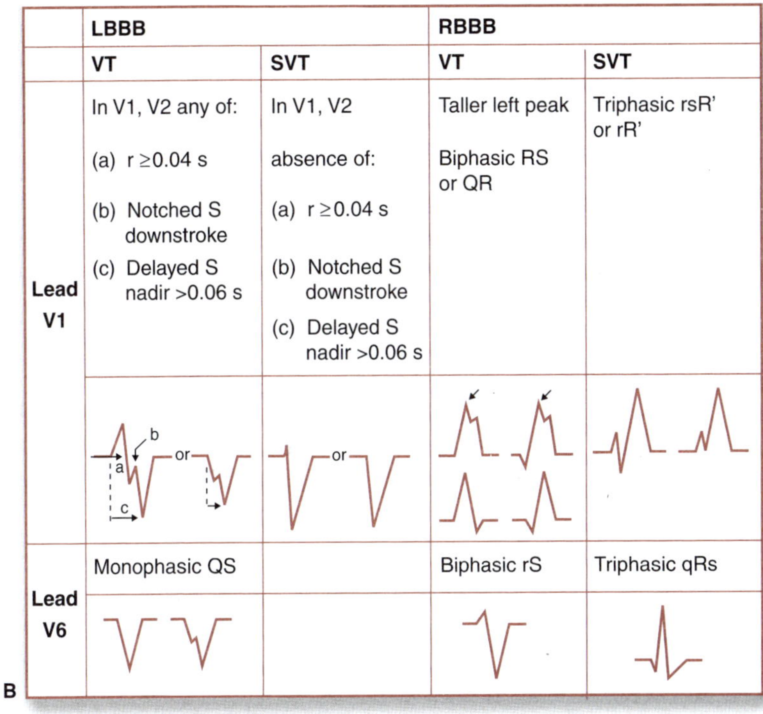

Figure 7-16 (*Continued*) A and B, Brugada criteria for distinguishing ventricular tachycardia from supraventricular tachycardia with aberrancy in wide-complex tachycardias. LBBB, left bundle branch block; RBBB, right bundle branch block; SVT, supraventricular tachyarrhythmia; VT, ventricular tachycardia. (Reprinted from Sharma S, Smith T. Advanced electrocardiography. In: Cuculich PS, Kates AM, eds. The Washington Manual of Cardiology Subspecialty Consult. 3rd ed. Philadelphia, PA: Lippincott, Williams and Wilkins; 2014 with permission.)

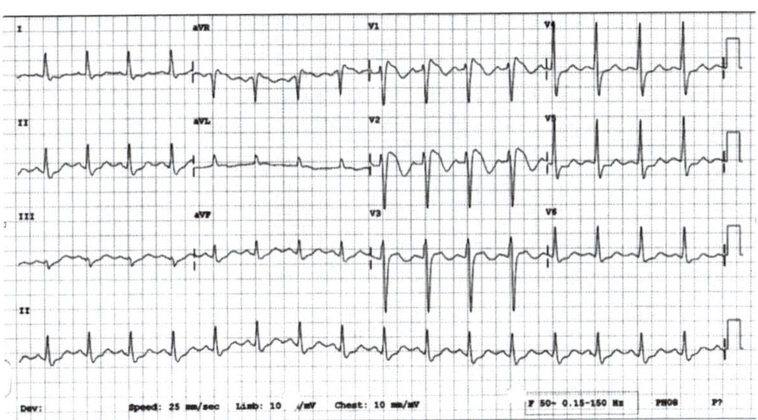

Figure 7-17 ECG showing Brugada syndrome.

TABLE 7-13 ECG Types of Brugada Syndrome

ECG Pattern	Type 0	Type 1	Type 2	Type 3
ST segments in V1-3	J-wave amplitude or ST-segment elevation ≥2 mm (0.2 mV) at its peak followed by absent or shallow negative T wave (<1 mm), with little or no isoelectric separation	J-wave amplitude or ST-segment elevation ≥2 mm (0.2 mV) at its peak followed by a negative T wave (<1 mm), with little or no isoelectric separation	High take-off ST-segment elevation, but the J-wave amplitude (≥2 mm) gives rise to a gradually descending ST-segment elevation (remaining ≥1 mm above baseline), followed by a positive or biphasic T wave that results in a saddleback configuration	J-wave amplitude ≥2 mm, but right precordial ST-segment elevation < 1 mm
ST segment configuration	Coved	Coved	Saddleback	Saddleback or coved or both
ECG	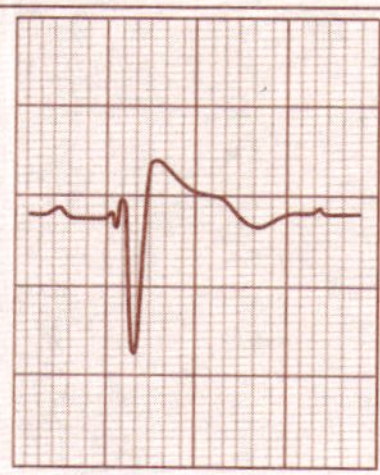	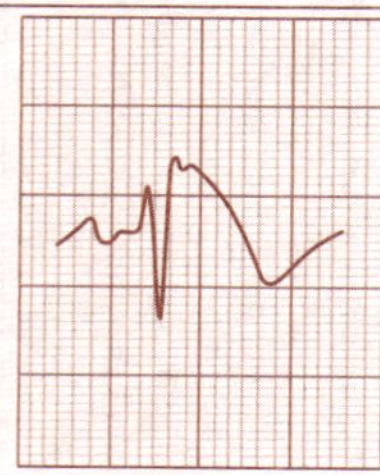	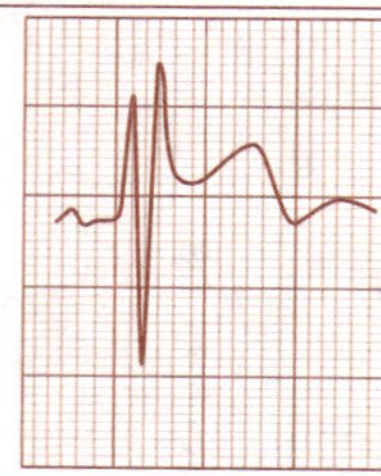	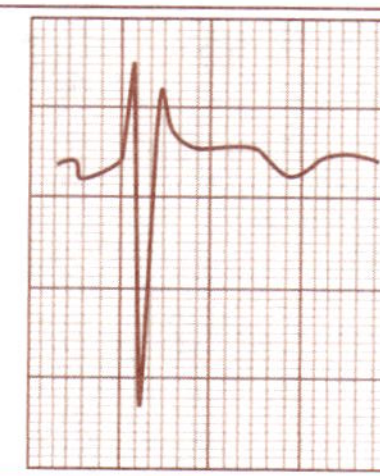

TABLE 7-14 Diagnostic Criteria for Long QT Syndrome

Clinical history	Syncope		1
	Congenital deafness		0.5
ECG features	QTc interval	>480 msec	3
		460–479 msec	2
		<460 msec	1
	Torsades de pointes		2
	T-wave alternans		1
	Notched T wave in three leads		1
	Low heart rate for age		0.5
Family history	Family history of definite long QT syndrome		1
	Unexplained sudden cardiac death in younger than 30 yrs among immediate family members		0.5

Definite LOTS is defined by an LQTS score >4:

- ≤1.0 point: low probability of LQTS
- 1.5–3.0 points: intermediate probability of LQTS
- ≥3.5 points: high probability of LQTS

this chapter). However, calcium channel blockers and β-blockers can produce hemodynamic instability in patients with VT.

- Immediate unsynchronized DCCV is the primary therapy for pulseless VT and VF.

Nonpharmacologic Therapies

- **ICDs** provide automatic recognition and treatment of ventricular arrhythmias. ICD implantation improves survival in patients resuscitated from ventricular arrhythmias (secondary prevention of SCD) and in individuals without prior symptoms who are at high risk for SCD (primary prevention of SCD).
  - **Secondary prevention of SCD** with ICD implantation is indicated for most patients who survive SCD outside of the peri-MI setting. The superiority of ICD therapy to chronic antiarrhythmic drug therapy has been demonstrated.[23]
  - **Primary prevention of SCD** with ICD implantation is indicated for patients who are at high risk of SCD. The efficacy of ICD implantation for primary prevention of SCD in the setting of cardiomyopathy has been established in multiple prospective clinical trials.[24–27] Most patients with an LV ejection fraction of <35% for more than 3 months on optimal medical therapy for cardiomyopathy meet indications for prophylactic ICD implantation.
  - **Other indications for ICD placement**
    - Phenotypes associated with **HCM, ARVD, congenital LQTS, or Brugada syndrome have a higher risk of SCD**. ICD implantation is indicated if patients with one of these syndromes have had a resuscitated cardiac arrest or documented ventricular arrhythmia. Prophylactic ICD implantation is based on disease-specific risk factors.
    - Patients who are awaiting cardiac transplantation are at high risk for SCD, especially if they are receiving an intravenous inotrope. Prophylactic ICD implantation is reasonable to protect against SCD prior to transplantation.
    - ICDs are **contraindicated** in patients who have incessant VT, recent MI <40 days or revascularization <3 months in the case of primary prevention, significant psychiatric illnesses, or life expectancy of <12–24 months.
- **Radiofrequency ablation (RFA) of VT** is most successfully performed in patients with hemodynamically stable forms of idiopathic VT that are not associated with structural

heart disease. Long-term cure rates in these patients are similar to those achieved for catheter ablation of SVT. In the presence of structural heart disease, catheter ablation has a lower efficacy and a higher morbidity but is an important treatment option, particularly in drug-refractory, symptomatic VT leading to ICD therapy.

- **Idiopathic VT** is usually associated with a structurally normal heart, but tachycardia-mediated cardiomyopathy can result if left untreated.
  - **Outflow tract VT** often presents as repetitive, nonsustained bursts of VT that originate most commonly from the RVOT and less commonly from the LVOT near the coronary cusps or aortomitral continuity (AMC). These can be responsive to β-adrenergic blockers, diltiazem, verapamil, and/or adenosine.
  - Idiopathic VT is thought to be benign in the absence of structural heart disease. Therefore, ICD implantation is not appropriate. Idiopathic VT is amenable to treatment with RFA or drug therapy.
- **VT associated with ischemic heart disease** can also be treated by catheter ablation targeting the scar-based substrate. Emergent catheter ablation in the setting of frequent hemodynamically unstable VT requiring defibrillation (VT storm) can be life-saving. Ablation has been shown to reduce ICD therapy and to improve quality of life.
- **Ablation of VT** in NICM is also a reasonable management option, particularly in drug-refractory patients. However, VT circuits may be intramyocardial or epicardial, and as a result, success rates are typically lower than those associated with ischemic VT. In such cases, referral to a center that routinely performs both endocardial and epicardial ablations should be considered.

Medications

- VT or VF that is resistant to external defibrillation requires the addition of IV antiarrhythmic agents.
  - IV lidocaine is frequently used; however, IV amiodarone appears to be more effective in increasing survival of VF when used in conjunction with defibrillation.[28]
  - After successful defibrillation, continuous IV infusion of effective antiarrhythmic therapy should be maintained until any reversible causes have been corrected.
- Chronic antiarrhythmic drug therapy is indicated for the treatment of recurrent symptomatic ventricular tachyarrhythmias. In the setting of hemodynamically unstable ventricular arrhythmias treated with an ICD, antiarrhythmic drug therapy is often necessary to prevent frequent device shocks.

Acute Drug Therapy

- **Amiodarone** is safe and well tolerated for the acute management of ventricular arrhythmias. Amiodarone has complex pharmacokinetics and is associated with significant toxicities arising from chronic therapy.[29]
  - After loading, amiodarone prevents the recurrence of sustained VT or VF in up to 60% of patients. A therapeutic latency of more than 5 days exists before beneficial antiarrhythmic effects are observed with oral dosing, and full suppression of arrhythmias may not occur for 4–6 weeks after therapy is initiated. Unfortunately, recurrence of ventricular arrhythmias during long-term follow-up is common.
- **Lidocaine** is a **class Ib** agent available only in IV form with efficacy in the management of sustained and recurrent VT/VF. The prophylactic use of lidocaine for suppression of premature ventricular contractions and nonsustained VT in the otherwise uncomplicated post-MI setting should be avoided.
  - Toxicities of lidocaine include central nervous system (CNS) effects (convulsions, confusion, stupor, and, rarely, respiratory arrest), all of which resolve with discontinuation of therapy.
  - Serum levels should be followed during prolonged use.

- **Class II** agents, the β-adrenergic antagonists, are the only class of antiarrhythmic agents to have consistently shown improved survival in post-MI patients.
  - β-Adrenergic blockers reduce postinfarction total mortality by 25%–40% and SCD by 32%–50%.[30–34]
  - After acute therapy of VT/VF and stabilization, β-adrenergic blockers should be initiated and titrated as blood pressure and heart rate allow.

Chronic Drug Therapy

- **Sotalol** is a **class III** agent indicated for the chronic treatment of VT/VF. Sotalol prevents the recurrence of sustained VT and VF in 70% of patients but must be used with caution in individuals with CHF.[35]
- **Class I** agents in general have not been shown to reduce mortality in patients with VT/VF. In fact, the class Ic agents, **flecainide** and **propafenone**, are associated with increased mortality in patients with ventricular arrhythmias after MI.[36] **Mexiletine** is similar to lidocaine (also an Ib agent) but is available in oral form. **Mexiletine is most often used in combination with either amiodarone or sotalol for chronic treatment of refractory ventricular arrhythmias.** CNS toxicity includes tremor, dizziness, and blurred vision. Higher levels may result in dysarthria, diplopia, nystagmus, and an impaired level of consciousness. Nausea and vomiting are common.
- **Phenytoin** can be used in the treatment of **digitalis-induced ventricular arrhythmias.** It may have a limited role in the treatment of ventricular arrhythmias associated with congenital LQTS and those with structural heart disease.

SPECIAL CONSIDERATIONS

- **Class IV** agents have no role in the chronic management of VT associated with structural heart disease.
- Primary therapy for VF that occurs secondary to ischemia in the setting of an MI is complete revascularization. In the absence of complete revascularization, the patient remains at high risk for recurrent VT/VF.
- In the case of **TdP associated with LQTS**, acute therapy is immediate defibrillation.
- Bolus administration of magnesium sulfate in 1- to 2-g increments up to 4–6 g IV is effective.
- In cases of acquired long QT, identification and treatment of the underlying condition should be undertaken, if possible.
- Elimination of long–short triggering sequences and shortening of the QT interval can be achieved by increasing the heart rate to the range of 90–120 bpm by either IV isoproterenol infusion (initial rate at 1–2 μg/min) or temporary transvenous pacing.

BRADYARRHYTHMIAS

GENERAL PRINCIPLES

- Bradyarrhythmias are commonly encountered rhythms in the inpatient setting that result in a ventricular rate of <60 bpm.
- **Anatomy of the conduction system (Figure 7-18)**
  - **The sinoatrial (SA) node** is a collection of specialized pacemaker cells located in the high right atrium. Under normal conditions, it initiates a wave of depolarization that spreads inferiorly and leftward via atrial myocardium and intranodal tracts, producing atrial systole.

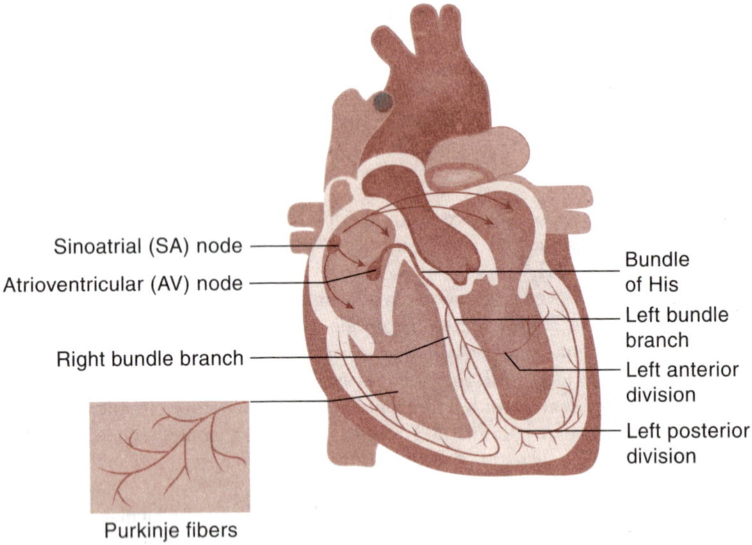

Figure 7-18 Conduction system of the heart.

- The wave of depolarization then reaches another grouping of specialized cells, the atrioventricular (**AV**) **node**, located in the lower right atrial side of the interatrial septum. Normally, the AV node should serve as the lone electrical connection between the atria and ventricles.
- From the AV node, the wave of depolarization travels down the **His bundle**, located in the membranous septum, and into the **right and left bundle branches** before reaching the **Purkinje fibers** that depolarize the remaining ventricular myocardium.

ETIOLOGY

Common causes of bradycardia are listed in Table 7-15.

DIAGNOSIS

Clinical Presentation

- When evaluating a suspected bradyarrhythmia, one should efficiently use the history, physical examination, and available data to address stability, symptoms, reversibility, site of dysfunction, and need for temporary as well as permanent pacing.
- If the patient is demonstrating signs of poor perfusion (hypotension, confusion, decreased consciousness, cyanosis, etc.), immediate management per ACLS protocol should be initiated. The clinical manifestations of bradyarrhythmias are variable, ranging from asymptomatic to nonspecific (lightheadedness, fatigue, weakness, exercise intolerance) to overt (syncope).
- Emphasis should be placed on delineating **whether the presenting symptoms have a direct temporal relationship to underlying bradycardia.** Other historical points of emphasis include the following:

TABLE 7-15 Causes of Bradycardia[47]

Causes of Bradycardia
Intrinsic
Congenital disease (may present later in life)
Idiopathic degeneration (aging)
Infarction or ischemia
Cardiomyopathy
Infiltrative disease: sarcoidosis, amyloidosis, hemochromatosis
Collagen vascular diseases: systemic lupus erythematosus, rheumatoid arthritis, scleroderma
Surgical trauma: valve surgery, transplantation
Infectious disease: endocarditis, Lyme disease, Chagas disease
Extrinsic
Autonomically mediated
Neurocardiogenic syncope
Carotid sinus hypersensitivity
Increased vagal tone: coughing, vomiting, micturition, defecation, intubation
Drugs: β-blockers, calcium channel blockers, digoxin, antiarrhythmic agents
Hypothyroidism
Hypothermia
Neurologic disorders: increased intracranial pressure
Electrolyte imbalances: hyperkalemia, hypermagnesemia
Hypercarbia/obstructive sleep apnea
Sepsis

- Ischemic heart disease, particularly involving the right-sided circulation, can precipitate a number of bradyarrhythmias. Therefore, signs and symptoms of acute coronary syndrome should always be thoroughly investigated.
- **Precipitating circumstances** (micturition, coughing, defecation, noxious smells) surrounding episodes may help identify a neurocardiogenic etiology of bradycardia.
- **Tachyarrhythmias,** particularly in patients with underlying sinus node dysfunction, can be followed by long pauses because of sinus node suppression during tachycardia. These are commonly referred to as conversion pauses.
- History of structural heart disease, hypothyroidism, obstructive sleep apnea, collagen vascular disease, infections (bacteremia, endocarditis, Lyme, Chagas), infiltrative diseases (amyloid, hemochromatosis, and sarcoid), neuromuscular diseases, and prior cardiac surgery (valve replacement, congenital repair) should be elicited.
- **Medications** should be reviewed with emphasis on those that affect the SA and AV nodes (i.e., calcium channel blockers, β-adrenergic blockers, digoxin).

- After hemodynamic stability is confirmed, a more thorough examination with particular emphasis on the cardiovascular examination and any findings consistent with the above comorbidities is appropriate (Figure 7-19).

Diagnostic Testing

Laboratories

Laboratory studies should include serum electrolytes and thyroid function tests in most patients. Digoxin levels and serial troponins should be drawn when clinically appropriate.

Electrocardiography

- The **12-lead ECG** is the cornerstone for diagnosis in any workup where arrhythmia is suspected.

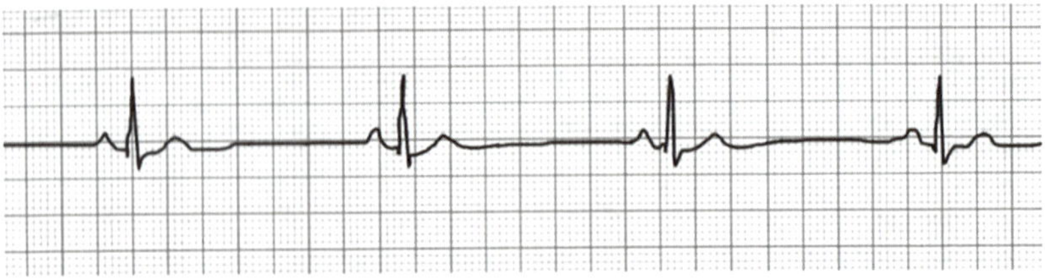

Figure 7-19 ECG showing sinus bradycardia.

- Rhythm strips from leads that provide the best view of atrial activity (II, III, aVF, or V_1) should be examined closely.
- Emphasis should be placed on identifying evidence of **SA node dysfunction** (P-wave intervals) or **AV conduction abnormalities** (PR interval).

Special Considerations

- Often, episodes of bradycardia are transient and episodic; therefore, a baseline ECG may not be sufficient to capture the bradycardia. Some form of continuous monitoring is often required.
  - In the inpatient setting, **continuous central telemetry monitoring** can be used.
  - If further workup is done as an outpatient, **24- to 72-hour Holter monitoring** can be used if the episodes occur somewhat frequently. If infrequent, **an event recorder** or **ILR** should be considered.
  - It is vital to correlate symptoms with the rhythm disturbances discovered via continuous monitoring. Therefore, the importance of accurate symptom diaries in the ambulatory setting should be emphasized to patients.
- To evaluate the sinus node's response to exertion (chronotropic competence), walking the patient in the hallway or up a flight of stairs under appropriate supervision is easy and inexpensive. A formal **exercise ECG** can be ordered if necessary.
- An **EPS** can also be used to assess sinus node function and AV conduction, but it is rarely necessary if the rhythm is already discovered via noninvasive modalities.

Differential Diagnosis

- **Sinus node dysfunction,** or sick sinus syndrome, represents the most common reason for pacemaker implantation in the United States. Manifestations of sick sinus syndrome include the following
  - **Sinus bradycardia (Figure 7-19)** defined as a regular rhythm with QRS complexes preceded by "sinus" P waves at a rate <60 bpm. Young patients and athletes often have resting sinus bradycardia that is well tolerated. Nocturnal heart rates are lower in all patients, but the elderly tend to have higher resting heart rates and sinus bradycardia is a far less common normal variant
  - **Sinus arrest** and **sinus pauses** (Figure 7-20) refer to failure of the sinus node to depolarize, which manifest as periods of atrial asystole (no P waves). This may be accompanied by ventricular asystole or escape beats from junctional tissue or ventricular myocardium. Pauses of 2–3 seconds can be found in healthy, asymptomatic people, especially during sleep. Pauses >3 seconds, particularly during daytime hours, raise concern for significant sinus node dysfunction.
  - **Sinus exit block** represents the appropriate firing of the sinus node, but the wave of depolarization fails to traverse past the perinodal tissue. It is indistinguishable from sinus arrest on surface ECGs except that the R-R interval will be a multiple of the R-R preceding the bradycardia.

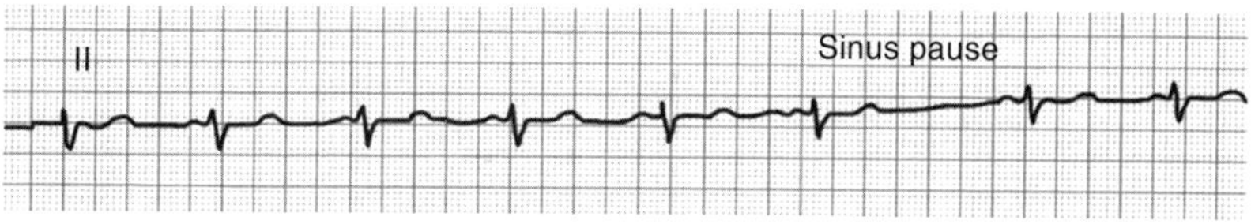

Figure 7-20 ECG showing sinus pause.

- ◦ **Tachy-brady syndrome** occurs when tachyarrhythmias alternate with bradyarrhythmias. This can be seen in conjunction with a number of types of SVT but is most commonly noted in patients with paroxysmal AF
- ◦ **Chronotropic incompetence** is the inability to increase the heart rate appropriately in response to metabolic need. This is usually determined by exercising the patient.
- **AV conduction disturbances**
  - ◦ AV conduction can be **diverted** (fascicular or bundle branch blocks); **delayed** (first-degree AV block); **occasionally interrupted** (second-degree AV block); **frequently, but not always, interrupted** (advanced or high-degree AV block); or **completely absent** (third-degree AV block). Assignment of the bradyarrhythmia under investigation to one of these categories allows one to better determine prognosis and, therefore, guide therapy.
  - ◦ **First-degree AV block** describes a conduction delay that results in a PR interval >200 ms on the surface ECG (Figure 7-21).
  - ◦ **Second-degree AV block** is present when there are periodic interruptions (i.e., "dropped beats") in AV conduction. Distinction between Mobitz I and II is important because the entities possess differing natural rates of progression to complete heart block.
    - ▪ **Mobitz type I block (Wenckebach) (Figure 7-22)** is represented by a progressive delay in AV conduction with successive atrial impulses until an impulse fails to conduct. On surface ECG, classic Wenckebach block manifests as the following:
      - ▫ Progressive prolongation of the PR interval of each successive beat before the dropped beat.
      - ▫ Shortening of each subsequent RR interval before the dropped beat.
      - ▫ A regularly irregular grouping of QRS complexes (group beating).
      - ▫ Type I block is usually within the AV node and portends a more benign natural history with progression to complete heart block unlikely.
    - ▪ **Mobitz type II block** carries a less favorable long-term prognosis and is characterized by abrupt AV conduction block without evidence of progressive conduction delay (Figure 7-23).

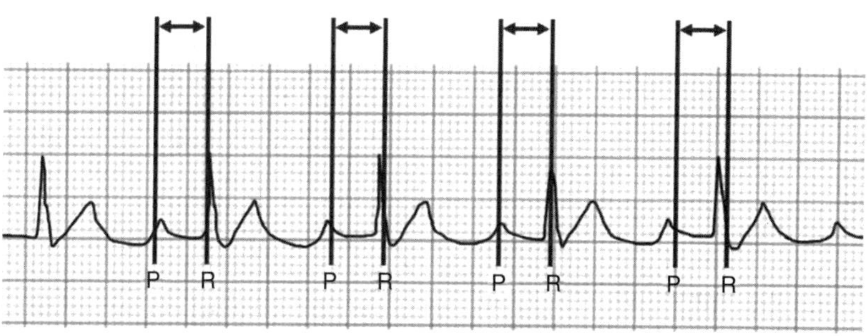

Figure 7-21 ECG showing first-degree heart block.

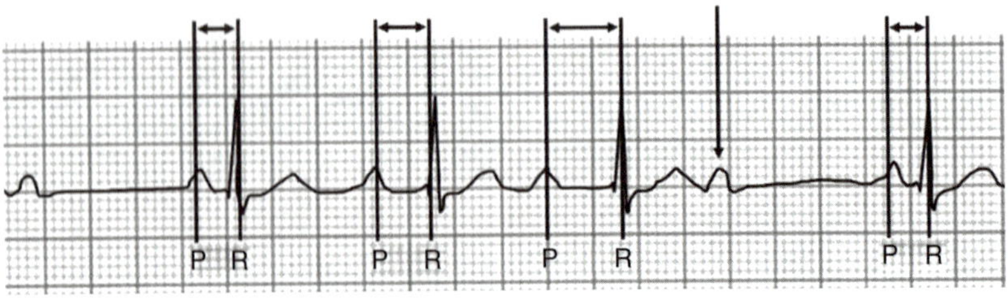

Figure 7-22 ECG showing Mobitz type I block.

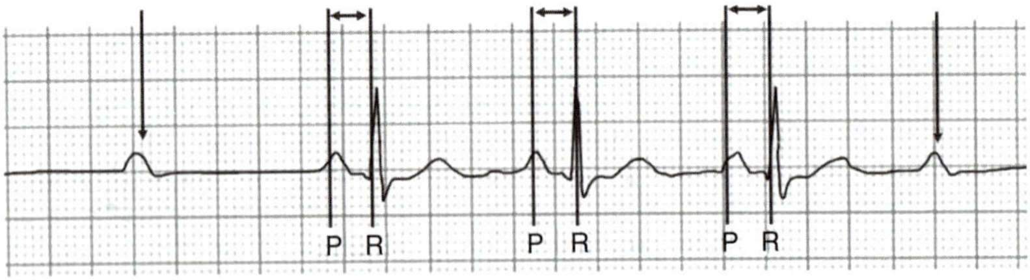

Figure 7-23 ECG showing Mobitz type II block.

- On ECG, the PR intervals remained unchanged preceding the nonconducted P wave.
- The presence of type II block, particularly if a bundle branch block is present, often antedates progression to complete heart block.

- The presence of **AV 2:1 block** makes the differentiation between Mobitz type I or II mechanisms difficult. Diagnostic clues to the site of block include the following:
  - Concomitant first-degree AV block, periodic AV Wenckebach, or improved conduction (1:1) with enhanced sinus rates or sympathetic input suggests a more proximal interruption of conduction (i.e., Mobitz type I mechanism).
  - Concomitant bundle branch block, fascicular block, or worsened conduction (3:1, 4:1, etc.) with enhanced sympathetic input localizes the site of block more distally (Mobitz type II mechanism).
  - Site of block in 2:1 AV block is discussed in Table 7-16.
- **Third-degree (complete) AV block** is present when all atrial impulses fail to conduct to the ventricles. There is complete dissociation between the atria and ventricles ("A >V" rates). This should be distinguished from dissociation with competition at the AV node ("V >A" rates) (Figure 7-24).
- **Advanced or high-degree AV block** is present when more than one consecutive atrial depolarization fails to conduct to the ventricles (i.e., 3:1 block or greater). On ECG,

TABLE 7-16 Site of Block in 2:1 AV Block

His-Purkinje System	AV Node
PR fixed despite varying RP interval	Type 1 Wenckebach pattern preceding 2:1 Block
Wide QRS complex	Narrow QRS complex
Pulse rate <160	Pulse rate >300
No improvement of block on atropine administration	Improvement of block on exercise and atropine administration

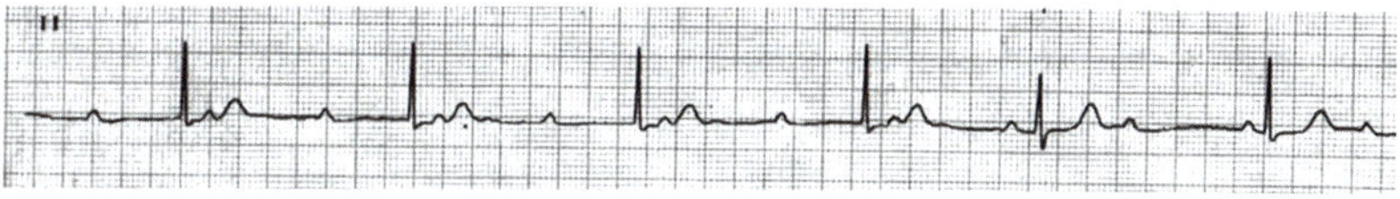

Figure 7-24 ECG showing third-degree (complete) AV block.

consecutive P waves will be seen without associated QRS complexes. However, there will be demonstrable P:QRS conduction somewhere on the record to avoid a "third-degree" designation

Imaging

- The presence or absence of structural heart disease should be initially evaluated by TTE.
- Further imaging should be obtained based on suspected etiology.

TREATMENT

Pharmacologic Therapy

- Bradyarrhythmias that lead to significant symptoms and hemodynamic instability should be managed emergently as outlined in ACLS guidelines (see Appendix C).
- **Atropine,** an anticholinergic agent given in doses of 0.5–2.0 mg IV, is the cornerstone pharmacologic agent for emergent bradycardia treatment.
  - Dysfunction localized more proximally in the conduction system (i.e., symptomatic sinus bradycardia, first-degree AV block, Mobitz I second-degree AV block) tends to be responsive to atropine.
  - Distal disease is not responsive and can be worsened by atropine.
  - Reversible causes of bradyarrhythmias should be identified, and any agents (digoxin, calcium channel blockers, β-adrenergic blockers) that caused or exacerbated the underlying dysrhythmia should be withheld.

Nonpharmacologic Therapies

- For bradyarrhythmias that have irreversible etiologies or that are secondary to medically necessary pharmacologic therapy, pacemaker therapy should be considered.
  - Temporary pacing is indicated for symptomatic second-degree or third-degree heart block caused by transient drug intoxication or electrolyte imbalance and complete heart block or Mobitz II second-degree AV block in the setting of an acute MI.
  - Sinus bradycardia, AF with a slow ventricular response, or Mobitz I second-degree AV block should be treated with temporary pacing only if significant symptoms or hemodynamic instability is present.
  - Temporary pacing is achieved preferably via insertion of a transvenous pacemaker. Transthoracic external pacing can be used, although the lack of reliability of capture and patient discomfort make this a second-line modality.
- Once hemodynamic stability has been established, attention turns to the indications for PPM placement.
  - In symptomatic patients, the key determinants include **potential reversibility of causative factors** and **temporal correlation of symptoms to the arrhythmia.**
  - In asymptomatic patients, the key determinant is based on whether the **discovered conduction abnormality has a natural history of progression to higher degrees of heart block** that portends a poor prognosis.

- **Permanent pacing**
  - Permanent pacing involves the placement of anchored, intracardiac pacing leads for the purpose of maintaining a heart rate sufficient to avoid symptoms and hemodynamic instability. Current devices, through maintenance of AV synchrony and rate-adaptive programming, more closely mimic normal physiologic heart rate behavior.
    - Class I and IIa indications for permanent pacing are listed in Figure 7-3.
    - Pacemakers are designed to provide an electrical stimulus to the heart whenever the rate drops below a preprogrammed **lower rate limit**. Therefore, the ECG appearance of a PPM varies depending on the heart rate and state of AV conduction.
    - The pacing spikes produced by modern pacemakers are low amplitude, sharp, and immediately preceding the generated P wave or QRS complex indicating capture of the chamber. Figure 7-25 illustrates some common ECG appearances of normally and abnormally functioning pacemakers.

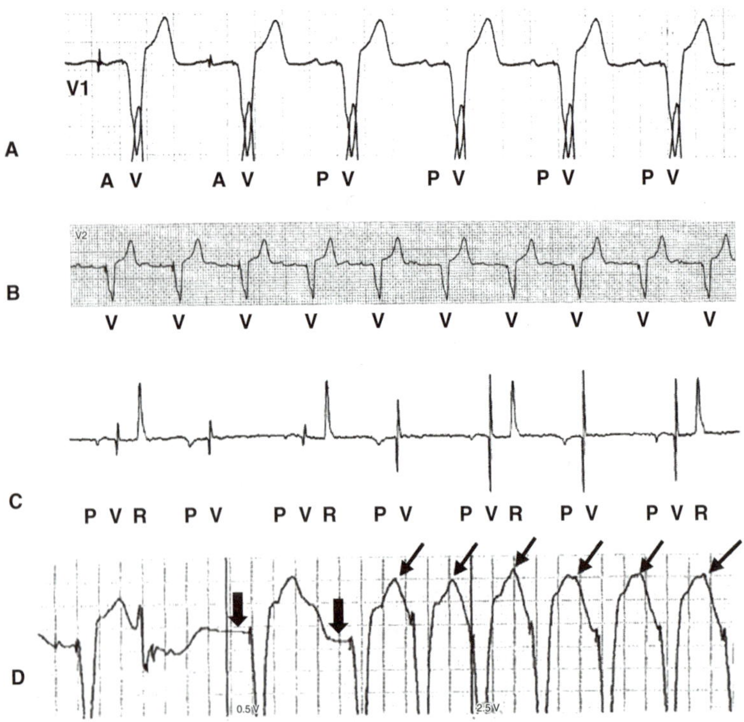

Figure 7-25 Pacemaker rhythms. A, Normal dual-chamber (DDD) pacing. First two complexes are atrioventricular (AV) sequential pacing, followed by sinus with atrial sensing and ventricular pacing. B, Normal single-chamber (VVI) pacing. The underlying rhythm is atrial fibrillation (no distinct P waves), with ventricular pacing at 60 bpm. C, Pacemaker malfunction. The underlying rhythm is sinus (P) at 80 bpm with 2:1 heart block and first-degree AV block (long PR). Ventricular pacing spikes are seen (V) after each P wave, demonstrating appropriate sensing and tracking of the P waves; however, there is failure to capture. D, Pacemaker-mediated tachycardia. A, paced atrial events; V, paced ventricular events; P, sensed atrial events; R, sensed ventricular events. (Reprinted from Fansler D, Chen J. Bradyarrhythmias and permanent pacemakers. In: Cuculich PS, Kates AM, eds. The Washington Manual Cardiology Subspecialty Consult. 3rd ed. Philadelphia, PA: Lippincott, Williams and Wilkins; 2014 with permission.)

- The pacemaker generator is commonly placed subcutaneously in the pectoral region on the side of the nondominant arm. The electronic lead(s) is/are placed in the cardiac chamber(s) via central veins. Complications of placement include **pneumothorax, device infection, bleeding, and, rarely, cardiac perforation with tamponade.**
  - Before implantation, the patient must be free of any active infections, and anticoagulation issues must be carefully considered. Hematomas in the pacemaker pocket develop most commonly in patients who are receiving IV heparin or subcutaneous low-molecular-weight heparin. In severe cases, surgical evacuation is required.
  - Following implantation, **posteroanterior (PA) and lateral CXR** are obtained to confirm appropriate lead placement. The pacemaker is interrogated at appropriate intervals—typically, before discharge, 2–6 weeks following implantation, and every 6–12 months thereafter.
- **Pacing modes** are classified by a sequence of three to five letters. Most pacemakers are referred to by the three-letter code alone (Table 7-17).
  - **Position I denotes the chamber that is paced:** A for atria, V for ventricle, or D for dual (A + V).
  - **Position II refers to the chamber that is sensed:** A for atria, V for ventricle, D for dual (A + V), or O for none.
  - **Position III denotes the type of response the pacemaker will have to a sensed signal:** I for inhibition, T for triggering, D for dual (I + T), or O for none.
  - **Position IV is used to signify the presence of rate-adaptive pacing (R)** in response to increased metabolic need.
- The most common pacing systems used today include VVI, DDD, or AAI.
  - AAI systems should be used only for sinus node dysfunction in the absence of any AV conduction abnormalities.
  - The presence of AV nodal or His-Purkinje disease makes a dual-chamber device (i.e., DDD) more appropriate.
  - Patients in permanent AF warrant a single ventricular lead with VVI programming.
- Modern-day pacemakers also have the capability of **mode switching.** This is useful in patients with DDD pacers who have concurrent paroxysmal tachyarrhythmias. When these patients develop an atrial arrhythmia faster than a programmed mode switch rate, the device will change to a mode (i.e., VVI) that does not track atrial signals. It will return to DDD when the tachyarrhythmia resolves.
- Although infrequent, **pacemaker malfunction** is a potentially life-threatening situation, particularly for patients who are pacemaker dependent. The workup of suspected malfunction should begin with a 12-lead ECG.
  - If no pacing activity is seen, one can place a magnet over the pacemaker to assess for output failure and ability to capture. **Application of the magnet switches the pacemaker to an asynchronous pacing mode.** For example, VVI mode becomes VOO

TABLE 7-17 Pacing Modes

I	II	III	IV	V
Chamber(s) paced	Chamber(s) sensed	Response to sensing	Rate modulation	Multisite pacing
O: none	O: none	O: none	O: none	O: none
A: atrium	A: atrium	T: triggered	R: rate modulation	A: atrium
V: ventricle	V: ventricle	I: inhabited		V: ventricle
D: dual (A + V)	D: dual (A + V)	D: dual (T + I)		D: dual (A + V)

(ventricular asynchronous pacing) and DDD mode becomes DOO (asynchronous AV pacing).
    - If malfunction is obvious or if the ECG is unrevealing and malfunction is still suspected, then a formal interrogation of the device should be performed. **Patients are given a card to carry on implantation that will identify the make and model of the device to facilitate this evaluation.**
    - **Two view CXR** should also be obtained to assess for evidence of overt lead abnormalities (dislodgement, fracture, migration, etc.).
  - General categories of pacemaker malfunction include failure to pace (output failure), failure to capture, failure to sense (undersensing), and pacemaker-mediated dysrhythmias.

Syncope

GENERAL PRINCIPLES

Syncope is a common clinical problem. A primary goal of evaluation is to determine whether the patient is at increased risk of death.

Definition

Sudden, self-limited loss of consciousness and postural tone caused by transient global cerebral hypoperfusion, followed by spontaneous, complete, and prompt recovery.

Classification

Syncope can be classified into four major categories based on etiology[37]:

- **Neurocardiogenic** (most common): vasovagal, carotid sinus hypersensitivity, and situational
- **Orthostatic hypotension:** hypovolemia, medication-induced (iatrogenic), and autonomic dysfunction
- **Cardiovascular:**
  - **Arrhythmogenic:** sinus node dysfunction, AV block, pacemaker malfunction, VT/VF, SVT (rare)
  - **Mechanical:** HCM, valvular stenosis, aortic dissection, myxomas, pulmonary embolism, pulmonary HTN, acute MI, subclavian steal, etc.
- **Miscellaneous** (not true syncope): seizures, stroke/TIA, hypoglycemia, hypoxia, psychogenic, etc.
  - Atherosclerotic cerebral artery disease is a rare cause of true syncope; the exception is severe obstructive four-vessel cerebrovascular disease (expect focal neurologic findings prior to syncope).

Epidemiology

- Studies report prevalence rates as high as 41%, with recurrent syncope occurring in 13.5%.
- Common in the general population: 6% of medical admissions and 3% of emergency room visits.[38]
- Incidence is similar among men and women; one of the largest epidemiologic studies revealed an 11% incidence during an average follow-up of 17 years, with a sharp rise after age 70.[38]

Pathophysiology

- The two components of **neurocardiogenic syncope** are described as **cardioinhibitory**, in which bradycardia or asystole results from increased vagal outflow to the heart, and

vasodepression, where peripheral vasodilation results from sympathetic withdrawal to peripheral arteries. Most patients have a combination of both components as the mechanism of their syncope.

- Specific stimuli (e.g., micturition, defecation, coughing, swallowing) may evoke a neurocardiogenic mechanism, leading to **situational syncope**.

Risk Factors

- **Cardiovascular disease**, history of **stroke or TIA**, and **HTN have been shown to predispose patients to syncope.**[37]
- Low body mass index (BMI), increased alcohol intake, and diabetes are also associated with syncope.[37–39]
- Causes of syncope could be cardiac, vascular, or unknown (Table 7-18).

DIAGNOSIS

- A syncopal event may be the presenting result of an otherwise unsuspected, potentially lethal cardiac condition, Therefore, a careful evaluation of the patient with syncope is warranted.
- A meticulous history and physical examination are vital to an accurate diagnosis of the etiology of syncope. In 40% of episodes, the mechanism of syncope remains unexplained.[40,41]

TABLE 7-18 Causes of Syncope

<table>
<tr><th>Vascular</th><th colspan="2">Cardiac</th></tr>
<tr><td>Anatomic
Vascular steal syndromes</td><td colspan="2" rowspan="2">Anatomic
Obstructive cardiac valve disease
Aortic dissection
Pericardial tamponade
Hypertrophic obstructive cardiomyopathy
Myocardial infarction
Pulmonary embolism
Pulmonary hypertension
Atrial myxoma</td></tr>
<tr><td>Orthostatic
Autonomic insufficiency
Idiopathic
Volume depletion
Drugs
Alcohol induced</td></tr>
<tr><td rowspan="2">Reflex Mediated
Carotid sinus hypersensitivity
Glossopharyngeal syncope
Neurally mediated vasovagal
Situational (cough, acute hemorrhage, defecation, laugh, micturition, sneeze, swallow, postprandial)</td><td colspan="2">Arrhythmias</td></tr>
<tr><td>Bradyarrhythmias
Atrioventricular blocks, sinus node dysfunction, bradycardia</td><td>Tachyarrhythmias
Supraventricular tachycardias—atrial fibrillation, AVNRT, WPW
Ventricular tachycardias—structural heart disease, inherited syndromes (ARVD, HCM, Brugada syndrome, long QT syndrome), drug-induced proarrhythmias</td></tr>
<tr><td colspan="3">Syncope of Unknown Origin</td></tr>
</table>

Clinical Presentation

History

- Special attention should be focused on the **symptoms** that **precede and follow** the syncopal episode, **eyewitness** accounts during the event, the **time course** of loss and resumption of consciousness (abrupt vs. gradual), and the patient's **medical history**.
- A characteristic prodrome of nausea, diaphoresis, visual changes, or flushing suggests neurocardiogenic syncope.
  - Identification of a particular emotional or situational trigger and postepisode fatigue are also clues to a neurocardiogenic/situational cause of syncope.
- Alternatively, an unusual sensory prodrome, incontinence, or a decreased level of consciousness that gradually clears suggests a seizure as a likely diagnosis.
- With transient ventricular arrhythmias, an abrupt loss of consciousness with a rapid recovery may occur.
- Syncope with exertion is a matter of concern for structural heart disease, pulmonary HTN, and/or CAD.

Physical Examination

- **Cardiovascular** and **neurologic** examinations should be the primary focus of initial evaluation (Table 7-19).
- Orthostatic vital signs can aid in the diagnosis of orthostatic hypotension. All patients should have blood pressure checked in both arms.
- Cardiac examination findings may help detect valvular heart disease, LV dysfunction, pulmonary HTN, etc.
- Neurologic findings are often absent but, if present, may point to a neurologic etiology of the syncopal event.
- Carotid sinus massage for 5–10 seconds with reproduction of symptoms and consequent ventricular pause >3 seconds is considered positive for carotid sinus hypersensitivity. It is critical to take proper precautions of telemetry monitoring, availability of bradycardia treatments, and avoidance of the maneuver in patients with known or suspected carotid disease.

Diagnostic Testing

- The presence of known **structural heart disease, abnormal ECG, age >65 years, focal neurologic findings, and severe orthostatic hypotension** suggest a potentially more ominous etiology of a syncopal event. Therefore, these patients should be admitted for further workup to avoid delay and adverse outcomes.
- After the history and physical examination, the ECG is the most important diagnostic tool in the evaluation of the syncopal patient. It will be abnormal in 50% of cases but alone will yield a diagnosis in only 5% of these patients.
- If the patient has no history of heart disease or baseline ECG abnormalities, **tilt-table testing** has been used to evaluate a patient's hemodynamic response during transition from supine to an upright state to precipitate a neurocardiogenic response. In an unselected population, the predictive value of this test is low.
- Refer to Figures 7-26 and 7-27 for the diagnostic approach to syncope.

TREATMENT

- In general, therapy is tailored to the underlying etiology of syncope with goals of preventing recurrence and reducing risk of injury or death.

TABLE 7-19 Differentiation of Syncope

	Demographic, Clinical Setting	Premonitory Symptoms	Observation During the Event	Residual Symptoms
Neurally mediated hypotension	Females >males Age <55 yrs >2 episodes Standing, warm room Emotional-upset mood	Longer-duration palpitations (>5 sec), blurred vision, nausea, warmth, diaphoresis, light-headedness	Pallor diaphoresis, dilated pupils, slow pulse, low BP, incontinence, Brief clonic movements	Common, prolonged fatigue in >90% oriented
Arrhythmias	Males >females Age >55 yrs <3 episodes During erect or supine Family history of sudden cardiac death	Shorter-duration (<6 sec) palpitations may be present	Blue, not pale Incontinence may óccur Brief tonic–clonic movements may occur	Uncommon unless prolonged unconsciousness, oriented
Seizures	Age <45 yrs Any setting	Sudden onset or brief aura	Blue face, no pallor Frothing at mouth Lasts >5 min Tongue bite Horizontal eye deviation Elevated pulse and BP Incontinence Tonic–clonic movements	Common, aching muscles, disoriented, fatigue, headache, slow recovery
Psychogenic	Females >males Age <40 yrs Many episodes (multiple in 1 d) Occurs in the presence of others No identifiable trigger	Usually absent	Normal color, Not diaphoretic Eyes closed Normal pulse, BP Prolonged for a few minutes commonly	Uncommon, oriented

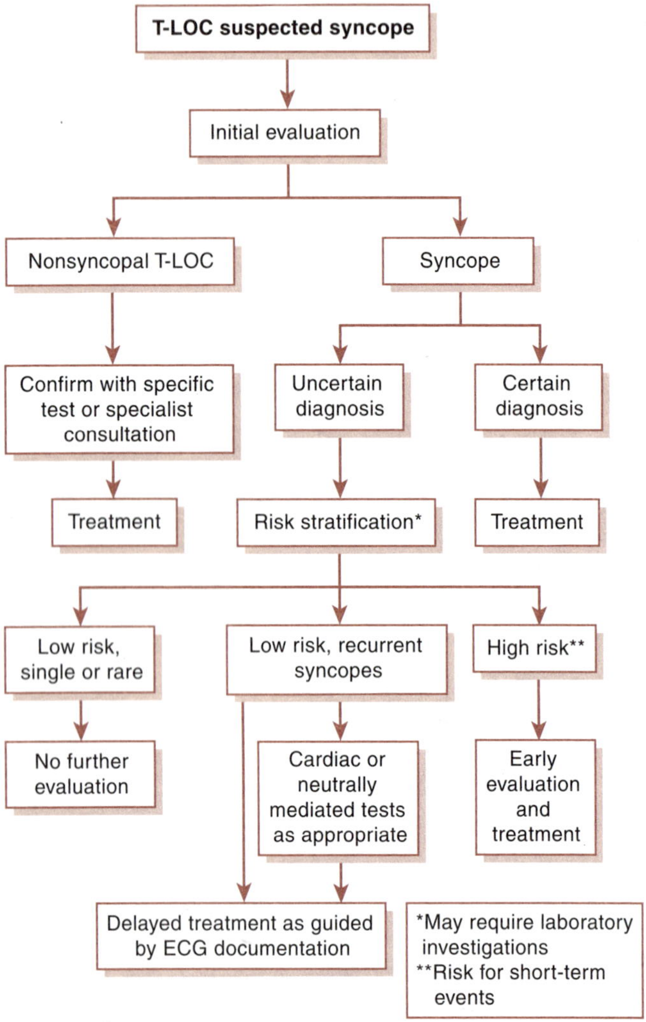

Figure 7-26 Algorithmic approach to transient loss of consciousness—T-LOC.

- **Neurocardiogenic syncope**
  - **Counsel** patients to take steps to avoid injury by being aware of prodromal symptoms and maintaining a **horizontal position** at those times.
  - Avoid known precipitants and maintain adequate **hydration.**
  - Employ **isometric muscle contraction** during prodrome to abort a syncopal episode.
  - Evidence suggests that β-adrenergic blockers are probably unhelpful; **selective serotonin reuptake inhibitor** (SSRI) **antidepressants** and **fludrocortisone** have a debatable effect; **midodrine** (initiated at 5 mg PO tid and can be increased to 15 mg tid) is probably helpful in the treatment of neurocardiogenic syncope.[42–44]

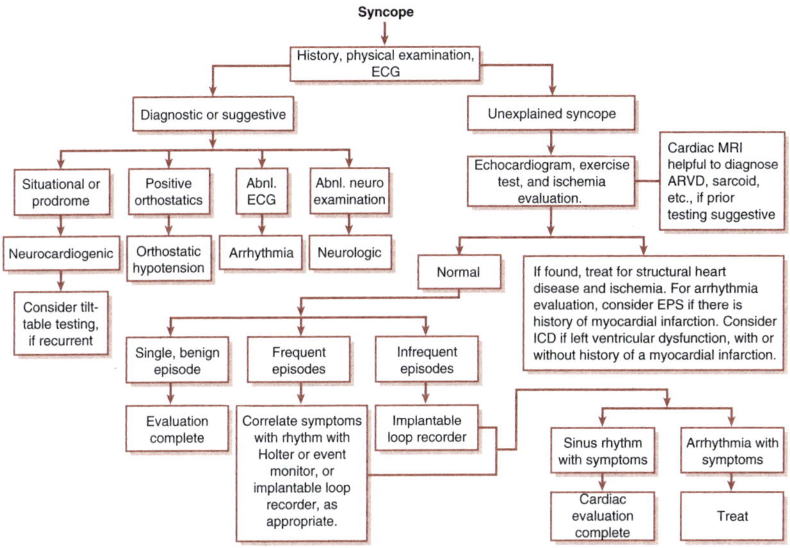

Figure 7-27 Algorithm for the evaluation of syncope. ARVD, arrhythmogenic right ventricular dysplasia; EPS, electrophysiology study; ICD, implantable cardioverter-defibrillator. (Reprinted from Strickberger SA, Benson DW, BiaggioniI, et al. AHA/ACCF scientific statement on the evaluation of syncope from the American Heart Association Councils on Clinical Cardiology, Cardiovascular Nursing, Cardiovascular Disease in the Young, and Stroke, and the Quality of Care and Outcomes Research Interdisciplinary Working Group; and the American College of Cardiology Foundation in Collaboration with the Heart Rhythm Society. *J Am Coll Cardiol.* 2006;47(2):473-484 with permission from Elsevier.)

  - In general, **PPMs** have no proven benefit in the management of neurocardiogenic syncope.[45] However, permanent dual-chamber pacemakers with a hysteresis function (high-rate pacing in response to a detected sudden drop in heart rate) have been shown to be useful in highly selected patients with recurrent neurocardiogenic syncope with a prominent cardioinhibitory component.[45,46]
  - **Cardiac pacing** for **carotid sinus hypersensitivity** is appropriate in syncopal patients.
  - In general, neurocardiogenic syncope is not associated with increased risk of mortality.
- **Orthostatic hypotension**
  - **Adequate hydration** and elimination of offending drugs.
  - Salt supplementation, compressive stockings, and counseling on gradual position changes.
  - Midodrine and fludrocortisone can help by increasing systolic BP and expanding plasma volume, respectively.
- **Cardiovascular (arrhythmia or mechanical)**
  - Treatment of **underlying disorder** (valve replacement, antiarrhythmic agent, coronary revascularization, etc.)
  - **Cardiac pacing** for sinus node dysfunction or high-degree AV block
  - Discontinuation of QT-prolonging drugs
  - Catheter **ablation** procedures in select patients with syncope associated with SVT
- **ICD** for documented VT without correctable cause and for syncope in presence of significant LV dysfunction even in absence of documented arrhythmia.

Summary

- Comprehensive phenotyping is recommended for most patients with arrythmias, encompassing noninvasive cardiac functional testing, multimodality imaging, and genetic testing in select circumstances.
- AF is the most common arrhythmia in the world and accounts for significant morbidity and mortality.
- The CHA2DS2-VASc score is considered the most validated score for predicting stroke risk in AF.
- Catheter ablation is increasingly being considered a feasible first-line alternative to medical therapy.
- Invasive electrophysiology study (EPS) provides both diagnostic insights, through the mode of induction and discrimination between the type of VA, as well as risk stratification.
- The use of an ICD remains a cornerstone in the prevention of SCD.

Scan the QR code to access chapter references.

8 Critical Care

James G. Krings, Marin H. Kollef, Mahesha Padyana, and Sunil Karanth

Respiratory Failure

GENERAL PRINCIPLES

Definitions

- **Hypoxemic (type 1) respiratory failure:** Occurs when normal gas exchange is seriously impaired, causing hypoxemia (arterial oxygen tension [PaO_2] <60 mm Hg or arterial oxygen saturation [SaO_2] <90%). Usually associated with tachypnea and hypocapnia; however, progression can lead to hypercapnia as well.

  Acute respiratory distress syndrome (ARDS) is an important form of hypoxemic respiratory failure caused by acute lung injury. The common end result is disruption of the alveolocapillary membrane, leading to increased vascular permeability and accumulation of inflammatory cells and protein-rich fluid within the alveolar space.
  - The ARDS Definition Task Force defined ARDS as follows[1]:
    - Onset within 1 week of a known clinical insult or new or worsening respiratory symptoms;
    - Bilateral opacities not fully explained by effusions, lobar/lung collapse, or nodules;
    - Respiratory failure not fully explained by cardiac failure or volume overload; and
    - Impaired oxygenation with low PaO_2 to a fraction of inspired oxygen (FiO_2) ratio ($PaO_2/FiO_2 \leq 300$ mm Hg)
  - The severity of ARDS is stratified based on PaO_2/FiO_2:
    - Mild: 200 <$PaO_2/FiO_2 \leq 300$ mm Hg with positive end-expiratory pressure (PEEP) or continuous positive airway pressure (CPAP) ≥5 cm H_2O
    - Moderate: 100 <$PaO_2/FiO_2 \leq 200$ mm Hg with PEEP ≥5 cm H_2O
    - Severe: $PaO_2/FiO_2 \leq 100$ mm Hg with PEEP ≥5 cm H_2O

  Recently, with the widespread adoption of high-flow nasal cannula (HFNC)/noninvasive ventilation (NIV), an SpO_2/FiO_2 ratio less than 315 with HFNC requiring >30 L/min has been proposed as an alternate diagnosis of ARDS. Matthay et al., in the global definition of ARDS, have recommended ultrasound instead of chest radiography for identifying bilateral loss of lung aeration (multiple B lines and/or consolidation) in resource-limited settings.[2]
- **Hypercapnic (type 2) respiratory failure:** Occurs with acute elevation of carbon dioxide (arterial carbon dioxide tension ([$PaCO_2$] >45 mm Hg), producing a respiratory acidosis (pH <7.35).
- **Postoperative (type 3) respiratory failure:** Occurs when patients develop atelectasis from pain or the use of sedatives postoperatively. In reality, this is a subset of type 1 or 2 respiratory failure; however, as this is so common, it is often classified as its own type of respiratory failure.
- **Respiratory failure from shock (type 4):** Respiratory failure where the metabolic demands of the patient are too high for the respiratory system to compensate for (e.g., from sepsis or fever). Patients are often intubated in the process of resuscitation to off-load the respiratory system and decrease oxygen consumption.
- **Mixed respiratory failure:** Most commonly, respiratory failure is due to multiple pathophysiologic processes that can lead to both hypercarbia and hypoxemia. Types of respiratory failure and pathophysiological mechanisms have been summarized in Tables 8-1 and 8-2.

TABLE 8-1 Classification of Acute Respiratory Failure Based on Mechanisms of Hypoxia

	Type I—Hypoxemic Respiratory Failure, *Lung Failure*	Type II—Hypercapnic Respiratory Failure, *Pump Failure*	Type III—Postoperative Respiratory Failure	Type IV—Respiratory Failure From Shock
Definition	• PaO_2 <60 mm Hg • Acute: Develops in minutes to hours • Chronic: Develops over several days or longer	• Hypercapnic respiratory failure: $PaCO_2$ >45 mm Hg • Acute: Develops in minutes to hours • Chronic: Develops over several days or longer	Occurs when patients develop atelectasis from pain or the use of sedatives postoperatively	Respiratory failure where the metabolic demands of the patient are too high for the respiratory system to compensate for
Mechanism	• Decreased FiO_2 • V/Q mismatch • Shunting • Diffusion limitation	Hypoventilation due to either increased dead space or reduced minute ventilation	• Shunting • Hypoventilation • V/Q mismatch	Hypoperfusion or inadequate oxygenation of peripheral tissues
Location of pathological process	• Inhaled air composition • Alveolar–capillary unit • Oxygen-carrying capacity of blood	• Airway • Neuromuscular system • Chest wall	Alveolar–capillary unit collapse with regional hypoventilation	• Cardiovascular system • Peripheral tissues
Common clinical causes	• Cardiogenic pulmonary edema • ARDS • Pneumonia • ILD • Pulmonary embolism • Atelectasis • Alveolar hemorrhage • Carbon monoxide poisoning • Anatomic shunts	• COPD • CNS depression (intoxication) • CNS trauma or injury • Neuromuscular disorders • Skeletal disorders • Obesity hypoventilation syndrome	• Thoracic or upper abdominal surgery or trauma • Inadequate postoperative analgesia • Pleural tumor or inflammation • Trapped lung • Subdiaphragmatic tumor or inflammation • Obesity	• Septic shock • Hypovolemic shock • Cardiogenic shock • Hypermetabolic states

ARDS, acute respiratory distress syndrome; CNS, central nervous system; COPD, chronic obstructive pulmonary disease; FiO_2, fraction of inspired oxygen; ILD, interstitial lung disease; $PaCO_2$, arterial carbon dioxide tension; V/Q ventilation–perfusion.

TABLE 8-2 Pathophysiological Mechanisms Causing Hypoxia

Mechanism	Description	Alveolar Partial Pressure of Oxygen (PaO_2)	Alveolar–Arterial Oxygen Difference ('A–a gap')	PaO_2 Response to Increased Inspired Oxygen (FiO_2)	Other Comments
Decreased FiO_2 For example, high-altitude travel	Occurs owing to a low partial pressure of inspired oxygen	Reduced	Normal	Improves	-
V/Q mismatch For example, emphysema, pneumonia, pulmonary edema, pulmonary embolism	Occurs when perfusion does not compensate for a change in ventilation or vice versa	Reduced locally	Increased	Improves	Note: Supplemental oxygen paradoxically worsens V/Q mismatching in emphysema via reversing hypoxic vasoconstriction of pulmonary capillaries supplying poorly ventilated alveoli
Shunt See Table 8-3 for different causes of shunt	Occurs when mixed venous blood bypasses lung units and enters systemic arterial circulation without receiving oxygenation	Reduced locally	Increased	Minimal	Congenital (e.g., intracardiac shunt) or acquired (e.g., atelectasis, hepatopulmonary syndrome)
Diffusion limitation For example, pulmonary fibrosis	Occurs owing to abnormalities of the interstitium wherein the time it takes for gas equilibration is longer than the red blood cell transit time through the pulmonary capillaries	Normal	Increased	Improves	
Hypoventilation (See type 2 respiratory failure)	Occurs owing to a decrease in minute ventilation that results in an increase in $PaCO_2$ and displacement of oxygen	Reduced	Normal	Improves	

FiO_2, fraction of inspired oxygen; $PaCO_2$, arterial carbon dioxide tension.

Pathophysiology

- **Hypoxemic respiratory failure (type 1):** Usually is the result of the lung's reduced ability to deliver oxygen across the alveolocapillary membrane. The severity of gas exchange impairment is determined by calculating the P(A–a) O_2 gradient (A-a gradient) using the alveolar gas equation:

$$PaO_2 = FiO_2\left(P_{ATM} - P_{H_2O}\right) - \frac{PaCO_2}{R}$$

where FiO_2 = the fraction of inspired oxygen, P_{ATM} = atmospheric pressure, P_{H_2O} = water vapor pressure, and R = the respiratory quotient. Hypoxemia is caused by one of the following five mechanisms:
  - **Ventilation/perfusion (V/Q) mismatch:** Occurs when perfusion does not compensate for a change in ventilation or vice versa (e.g., emphysema, pneumonia, pulmonary edema, pulmonary embolism). V/Q mismatch leads to an elevated A-a gradient. Administration of supplemental oxygen increases PaO_2 (of note, supplemental oxygen paradoxically worsens V/Q mismatching in emphysema via reversing hypoxic vasoconstriction of pulmonary capillaries supplying poorly ventilated alveoli).
  - **Shunt:** Occurs when mixed venous blood bypasses lung units and enters systemic arterial circulation without receiving oxygenation. Shunts can be congenital (e.g., intracardiac shunt) or acquired (atelectasis, hepatopulmonary syndrome). Shunt leads to an elevated A-a gradient. In pure shunt, administration of supplemental oxygen does not increase PaO_2. See Table 8-3 for different causes of shunt.

TABLE 8-3 Causes of Shunt

Cause	Examples
Pulmonary Shunts	
Pus	Pneumonia
Water	• Cardiogenic pulmonary edema ○ Acute myocardial infarction ○ Systolic or diastolic left ventricular failure ○ Mitral regurgitation or stenosis • Noncardiogenic pulmonary edema ○ Primary acute respiratory distress syndrome ▪ Aspiration ▪ Inhalational injury ▪ Near drowning ○ Secondary acute respiratory distress syndrome ▪ Sepsis ▪ Pancreatitis ▪ Reperfusion injury ○ Upper airway obstruction pulmonary edema ○ Neurogenic pulmonary edema ○ High-altitude pulmonary edema ○ Transfusion-associated lung injury (TRALI)
Blood	Diffuse alveolar hemorrhage
Atelectasis	• Pleural effusion with atelectasis • Mucous plugging with lobar collapse
Cardiac shunts	• Patent foramen ovale • Atrial septal defect • Ventricular septal defect
Vascular shunts	Arteriovenous malformation

- ◦ **Diffusion abnormality:** Occurs owing to abnormalities of the interstitium wherein the time it takes for gas equilibration is longer than the red blood cell transit time through the pulmonary capillaries (e.g., pulmonary fibrosis). Diffusion abnormalities lead to an elevated A-a gradient. Administration of supplemental oxygen increases PaO_2.
- ◦ **Hypoventilation:** Occurs owing to a decrease in minute ventilation that results in an increase in $PaCO_2$ (see causes of hypercapnia below) and displacement of oxygen. The A-a gradient is normal. Primary treatment is directed at correcting the cause of hypoventilation. Administration of supplemental oxygen increases PaO_2.
- ◦ **Low inspired oxygen:** Occurs owing to a low partial pressure of inspired oxygen (e.g., high-altitude travel). A-a gradient is normal. Administration of supplemental oxygen increases PaO_2.

- **Hypercapnic respiratory failure (type 2):** Primarily occurs owing to ventilatory failure, resulting in an elevated $PaCO_2$ >45 mm Hg:

$$PaCO_2 = \frac{\dot{V}CO_2}{\dot{V}_A} = \frac{\dot{V}CO_2}{\dot{V}_E - \dot{V}_D}$$

where CO_2 = CO_2 production, V_A = alveolar ventilation, V_E = expired total ventilation, and V_D = dead space ventilation. The cause of hypercapnia is generally failure of one of the following components of the respiratory system:

- ◦ Disorders of the central nervous system: An impaired respiratory drive causes a decreased respiratory rate ("won't breathe"); e.g., opiate overdose, central apnea/hypoventilation, metabolic alkalosis, central nervous system (CNS) infection.
- ◦ Disorders of anterior horn cells, peripheral nervous system, or muscles: Neuromuscular failure or muscle weakness causes decreased tidal volume ("can't breathe"); e.g., Guillain–Barré syndrome, myasthenia gravis, amyotrophic lateral sclerosis, muscular dystrophies, myopathies.
- ◦ Disorders of the thoracic cavity: Anatomic abnormality causes decreased tidal volume; e.g., kyphoscoliosis, morbid obesity, pleural effusions.
- ◦ Disorders of the airway or lung parenchyma: Lung pathology causes increased dead space; e.g., asthma, chronic obstructive pulmonary disease (COPD).
- ◦ Hypermetabolic states can cause increased CO_2 production and lead to hypercapnia; e.g., sepsis, seizure, thyrotoxicosis, serotonin syndrome.

Presentation

- Hypoxemia presents with tachycardia/bradycardia, tachypnea, hypertension/hypotension, cyanosis, anxiety, diaphoresis, altered mental status, confusion, seizures, coma, and lactic acidosis.
- Hypercapnia manifests with somnolence, lethargy, restlessness, slurred speech, headache, asterixis, papilledema, coma, and diaphoresis.

Noninvasive Oxygen Therapy

GENERAL PRINCIPLES

- **Nasal cannulas:** Most commonly used, but the exact FiO_2 delivered is unknown because it is influenced by peak inspiratory flow demand. Each additional liter of flow increases FiO_2 by approximately 4% (e.g., 2 L/min delivers ~28%). Flow rates should generally be limited to ≤6 L/min. An oxygen reservoir device can increase oxygen delivery.
- **Simple facemask:** Delivers oxygen at FiO_2 of 35%–55% using flows of 5–12 L/min (lower flow rates should be avoided to prevent breathing in expired CO_2).

- **Venturi masks:** Allow the precise administration of oxygen via a Venturi facemask. Usual FiO_2 values delivered are 24%, 28%, 31%, 35%, 40%, and 50%. The oxygen flow exceeds the patient's peak expiratory flow. Hence, the patient is unlikely to breath in air from the room.
- **Nonrebreathing masks:** Use a reservoir bag to achieve higher oxygen concentrations (up to 80%). Flow rates are generally at least 8–15 L/min. A one-way valve prevents exhaled gases from entering the reservoir bag, maximizing the FiO_2 that is inspired.
- **Heated humidified high-flow nasal cannula (HFNC):** Delivers heated and humidified oxygen at high flows and concentrations such that it flushes out a significant amount of nonoxygenated air from the upper airway. The system can be titrated up to 60 L/min and 100% FiO_2 and may provide a small amount of PEEP at high flow rates.
  - The use of HFNC devices has increased recently, with some studies showing encouraging benefits. In one open-label trial, patients with hypoxemic nonhypercapnic respiratory failure were randomly assigned to HFNC versus standard oxygen therapy or noninvasive positive-pressure ventilation (NPPV). Intubation rates were similar between groups; however, there was a significant improvement in a 90-day mortality in patients who received HFNC as compared with other modalities.[3]
  - The role of HFNC following extubation is discussed in the mechanical ventilation section below. Figure 8-1 outlines the various breathing/ventilation strategies available.
- **NPPV:** Delivers respiratory support with positive airway pressure via a sealed facemask, nasal mask, or helmet device. NPPV includes continuous positive airway pressure (CPAP) and bilevel positive airway pressure (BiPAP) ventilation. NPPV can be delivered by home devices or ventilators.
  - CPAP: Delivers continuous positive airway pressure throughout the respiratory cycle and prevents alveolar collapse during expiration. CPAP is often used in the treatment of obstructive sleep apnea and pulmonary edema. Initially, 5 cm H_2O of pressure should be applied, and if hypoxemia persists, the level should be increased by 3–5 cm H_2O up to a level of 10–15 cm H_2O.
  - BiPAP: Delivers two different airway pressures during inspiration and expiration to decrease the work of breathing. BiPAP is often used for COPD exacerbations, weaning,

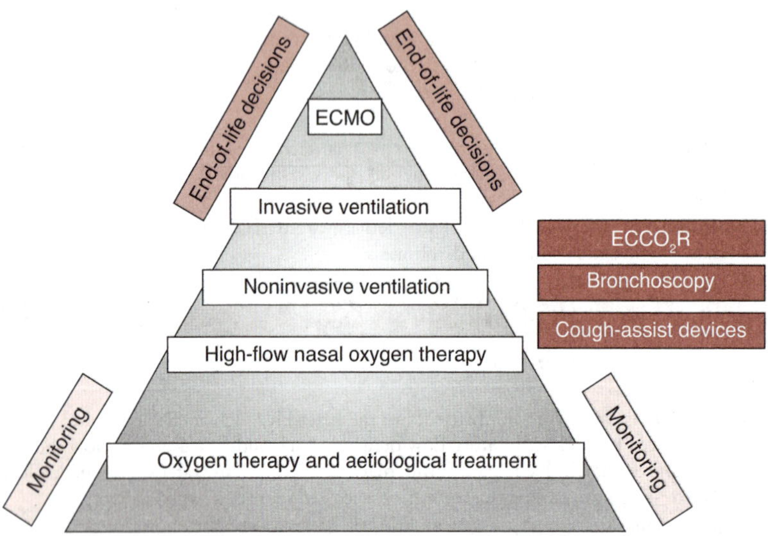

Figure 8-1 Outline on breathing/ventilation strategies.

and neuromuscular weakness. An inspiratory pressure of 5–10 cm H_2O and an expiratory pressure of 5 cm H_2O are reasonable starting points. Ventilation is determined by the difference between inspiratory and expiratory pressures (i.e., "drive pressure"), and inspiratory pressures can be uptitrated to achieve adequate tidal volumes and minute ventilation.

- Benefits of NPPV: NPPV decreases the need for mechanical ventilation in appropriately selected patients.[4] The benefits of NPPV are particularly strong in patients with neuromuscular disease, COPD, pulmonary edema, and postoperative respiratory insufficiency.[5] A recent single-center trial found that NPPV delivered via a transparent helmet device covering the entire head reduced the need for intubation and improved survival in patients with ARDS.[6]
- Potential harms of NPPV: NPPV is generally safe but can cause skin damage, eye irritation, claustrophobia, and aerophagia and be difficult to tolerate for some patients. Use should be limited to patients who are conscious, are cooperative, able to protect their airway, and are hemodynamically stable.[7] **NPPV use should be limited to those with an anticipated short duration of respiratory failure. Close monitoring is required during its use.**

Contraindications for noninvasive ventilation

- The need for emergent intubation (e.g., cardiac or respiratory arrest, severe respiratory distress, and unstable cardiac arrhythmia).
- Inability to cooperate, protect airway, or clear secretions (e.g., patients at high risk or aspiration).
- Nonrespiratory organ failure that is acutely life-threatening.
- Severe encephalopathy (e.g., GCS <10).
- Severe upper gastrointestinal bleeding.
- Hemodynamic instability.
- Facial or neurological surgery, trauma, or deformity.
- Significant airway obstruction (e.g., laryngeal mass or tracheal tumor).

Airway Management and Endotracheal Intubation

GENERAL PRINCIPLES

Airway Management Before Intubation

- **Head and jaw positioning:** First, the oropharynx should be inspected and all foreign bodies should be removed. If the patient is unresponsive, the head tilt–chin lift maneuver should be performed (see Airway Emergencies in Chapter 26, Medical Emergencies). If neck immobilization is required, jaw thrust should be performed.
- **Oral and nasopharyngeal airways:** Airway adjunct devices can be used to maintain a patent airway. Initially inserted with the concave curve of the airway facing toward the roof of the mouth, the oral airway then is turned 180 degrees as it is inserted so that the concave curve of the airway follows the natural curve of the tongue. Careful monitoring of airway patency is required, as malpositioning can push the tongue posteriorly and result in oropharyngeal obstruction. Nasopharyngeal airways are made of soft plastic and passed easily down one of the nasal passages to the posterior pharynx after topical nasal lubrication and anesthesia with viscous lidocaine jelly.
- **Bag-valve-mask ventilation:** Ineffective respiratory efforts can be augmented with simple bag-valve-mask ventilation. Proper fitting and positioning of the mask using the "EC" hand position—thumb and index finger forming a "C" around the mask and the remaining fingers forming an "E" to support the jaw—ensure a tight seal around the mouth and nose. Used in conjunction with proper positioning and airway adjuncts, e.g., oral airway. If possible, two hands should be used to optimize seal while a second clinician ventilates the patient.
- **Laryngeal mask airway (LMA):** The LMA is a supraglottic airway device shaped like an endotracheal tube connected to an elliptical mask. It is designed to be inserted over the

tongue and seated in the hypopharynx, covering the supraglottic structures and relatively isolating the trachea. It is a temporary airway and should not be used for prolonged ventilatory support. LMAs can be lifesaving in establishing an airway when endotracheal intubation cannot be easily achieved.

Endotracheal Intubation

- **Indications:** Refractory hypoxemic respiratory failure, hypercapnic respiratory failure, airway protection (e.g., intoxication, head trauma), upper airway obstruction (e.g., angioedema, tumor), severe metabolic acidosis or shock (e.g., type 4 respiratory failure, severe diabetic ketoacidosis), and the need for hyperventilation as a treatment for increased intracranial pressure.
- **Before endotracheal tube intubation** is attempted.
- **Prepare**
  - Assure that monitoring equipment is working (including pulse oximetry, telemetry, and blood pressure monitoring) and that the patient has adequate working intravenous (IV) access.
  - Assure that all necessary equipment is at the bedside, including a working suction equipment, endotracheal tube (with stylet, lubricant, and balloon tested), 10 mL syringe to fill endotracheal tube balloon, oral or nasopharyngeal airway, bag-valve-mask connected to 15 L/min oxygen, direct or video laryngoscope, end-tidal CO_2 monitor, medications for intubation, and a tape or endotracheal holder.
  - Have the plan articulated and the equipment at the bedside (e.g., tracheal tube introducer and supraglottic device) in case of a difficult airway.
- Evaluate head and neck **positioning.**
  - Oral, pharyngeal, and tracheal axes should be aligned by flexing the neck and extending the head, achieving the "sniffing" position. Obese patients may require a shoulder roll or ramp.
- **Preoxygenation**
  - Administration of 100% oxygen, for 3 minutes of normal tidal volume breathing in a normal healthy adult, establishes an adequate oxygen reservoir to permit 6–8 minutes of safe apnea before oxygen desaturation to less than 90% occurs. **Preoxygenation can be done by using bag-valve-mask device with a reservoir bag, HFNC, or NIV.** The All India Difficult Airway Association (AIDAA) guidelines in 2016 recommended the use of **HFNC oxygen from preoxygenation till the end of intubation.**
- **Pretreatment, paralysis,** and induction
  - The selected agents for intubation including neuromuscular blocking agents, opiates, and anxiolytics should be chosen based on their respective advantages and disadvantages in the given clinical situation. Commonly used agents for intubation are listed in Table 8-4.
  - If patient not in extremis/cardiac arrest, a verbal time-out should be performed.
- Techniques
  - Direct laryngoscopic orotracheal intubation: Most commonly used, requiring only a direct laryngoscope and light source. Procedure available in Table 8-6 and can be found in video form on the *New England Journal of Medicine* website.[8]
  - Video laryngoscopic orotracheal intubation: Allows for direct visual confirmation of intubation by a second observer via video monitoring and is particularly beneficial in more difficult airways.
  - Advanced techniques for specialists include blind nasotracheal intubation and flexible fiber optically guided orotracheal or nasotracheal intubation.
- **Postintubation management**
- Verification of correct endotracheal tube location and positioning: Proper tube location must be ensured by
  - Fiber optic inspection of the airways through the endotracheal tube; *or*
  - Direct visualization of the endotracheal tube passing through the vocal cords; *and*
  - Use of an end-tidal CO_2 monitor; *and*
  - CXR

TABLE 8-4 Drugs to Facilitate Endotracheal Intubation

Drug	Action	Dose (IV)	Onset	Duration	Comment
Propofol	Sedation, amnesia	Unstable: 0.5 mg/kg Stable: 1–1.5 mg/kg	30–60 s	5–10 min	Causes hypotension and bradycardia; beneficial in seizures
Midazolam	Sedation, amnesia	0.02–0.08 mg/kg (generally 1–5 mg in adult)	30–60 s	15–30 min	Causes hypotension; beneficial in seizures
Fentanyl	Analgesia	~2 μg/kg	15 s	30–60 min	Causes hypotension; used at lower doses as an adjunctive agent
Etomidate	Sedation	Unstable: 0.15 mg/kg Stable: 0.3 mg/kg	15–45 s	3–12 min	Hemodynamically neutral; inhibits cortisol synthesis; decreases seizure threshold
Ketamine	Sedation, amnesia, analgesia	1–3 mg/kg	30 s	5–10 min	Increases HR and BP; bronchodilator; may elevate ICP
Succinylcholine	Paralytic	1–1.5 mg/kg	30–60 s	5–15 min	Contraindicated in hyperkalemia, history of malignant hypothermia, myopathy
Rocuronium	Paralytic	1 mg/kg	45–60 s	30–45 min	Caution if difficult intubation or bag-valve-mask ventilation anticipated

BP, blood pressure; HR, heart rate; ICP, intracranial pressure.

  - Clinical evaluation of the patient (i.e., listening for bilateral breath sounds over the chest and the absence of ventilation over the stomach) and radiographic evaluation alone are unreliable for establishing correct endotracheal tube location.
  - The tip of the endotracheal tube should be 3–5 cm above the carina, depending on head and neck position.
- After successful intubation
  - Tracheal tube cuff pressures: Should be monitored at regular intervals and maintained below capillary filling pressure (25 mm Hg) to prevent ischemic mucosal injury.
  - Sedation: Anxiolytics and opiates are frequently used to facilitate endotracheal intubation and mechanical ventilation. Commonly used agents are listed in Table 8-5.

TABLE 8-5 Commonly Used Sedation Medications in the Intensive Care Unit

Drug	Dose (IV)	Time to Arousal	Comment
Propofol	20–100 μg/kg/min	10–15 min	Causes hypotension, may cause hypertriglyceridemia or propofol-related infusion syndrome, beneficial in bronchospasm
Midazolam	1–10 mg/h	1–2 h	Arousal time can be prolonged; active metabolite accumulates in renal failure; associated with delirium
Fentanyl	25–200 μg/h	15 s	Can cause chest wall rigidity and serotonin syndrome at higher doses
Ketamine	0.5–3 mg/kg/h	5–10 min	May cause hypertension and tachycardia; may experience reemergence hallucinations, beneficial in bronchospasm.
Dexmedetomidine	0.1–1.5 mg/kg/h	6–10 min	Does not cause respiratory depression, can cause hypotension and bradycardia

- **Complications:** Improper endotracheal tube location or positioning is the most important immediate complication to be recognized and corrected.
  - Esophageal intubation should be suspected if no end-tidal CO_2 is detected after three to five breaths, hypoxemia persists or develops, there is a lack of breath sounds, or abdominal distention or regurgitation of stomach contents occurs.
  - Mainstem intubation should be suspected if peak airway pressures are elevated or there are unilateral breath sounds.
  - Other complications include dislodgment of teeth and upper airway trauma.

Surgical Airways

- **Indications** for surgical airways in critical care
  - Life-threatening upper airway obstruction (e.g., epiglottitis, angioedema, facial burns, laryngeal/vocal cord edema) preventing bag-valve-mask ventilation and endotracheal intubation.
  - Need for prolonged respiratory support.
- **Needle cricothyrotomy:** Indicated in emergency settings when the patient cannot be ventilated noninvasively, standard endotracheal intubation is unsuccessful, and a surgical airway cannot be immediately performed. The steps of the procedure are listed in Table 8-6.
- **Cricothyrotomy:** Indicated in emergency settings when the patient cannot be ventilated noninvasively and standard endotracheal intubation is unsuccessful. The steps of the procedure are listed in Table 8-6.
- **Tracheostomy:** Predominantly performed owing to need for prolonged respiratory support.
  - The optimal time to perform a tracheostomy in a patient requiring prolonged respiratory support is somewhat controversial. A recent randomized controlled trial did not demonstrate any benefit in regard to occurrence of ventilator-associated pneumonia (VAP) or long-term outcomes for those who received an early tracheostomy (after 6–8 days of intubation) compared with late tracheostomy (after 12–14 days of intubation).[9]

TABLE 8-6 Procedure for Endotracheal Intubation, Needle Cricothyroidotomy, and Cricothyrotomy

Endotracheal Intubation Using Direct Laryngoscopy		
Equipment	Oxygen tubing, bag-valve-mask device, suction and tubing, oral airway, laryngoscope, laryngoscope blades, endotracheal tube with stylet, syringe, end-tidal carbon dioxide colorimeter	
Technique	Step 1	Place the patient in the "sniffing" position, with neck flexed and head extended; obese patients will require shoulder roll or ramp.
	Step 2	Preoxygenate the patient with 100% oxygen through the bag-valve-mask device until saturations are maintained at >95% for 3–5 min and suction oral secretions as necessary.
	Step 3	During preoxygenation, ensure that all equipment necessary is present and functional: check the endotracheal tube cuff with inflation and deflation and that the light of the laryngoscope is functional.
	Step 4	Administer intravenous (IV) sedation; once the patient is appropriately sedated, open the mouth with the right hand and insert the laryngoscope blade into the right side of mouth with the left hand, sweeping the tongue to the left.
	Step 5	Advance the blade to the base of the tongue and then lift vertically to visualize the vocal cords; **do not tilt the laryngoscope**.
	Step 6	If vocal cords are visible, insert the endotracheal tube with the stylet with the right hand; once the cuff is past the vocal cords, remove stylet. **Do not attempt intubation if the vocal cords are not visible.**
	Step 7	Advance the endotracheal tube until it is at 21 cm at the gum/teeth for women and 22 cm for men and inflate the cuff.
	Step 8	**Check tube location** with end-tidal carbon dioxide by using portable capnograph, auscultation over the chest and abdomen, AND chest radiograph.
Needle Cricothyroidotomy		
Equipment	Large bore IV catheter with needle stylet, 3-mL Luer lock syringe with plunger removed, 7-mm inner diameter endotracheal tube adapter	
Technique	Step 1	Extend the neck and identify the cricothyroid membrane, located inferior to the thyroid cartilage and superior to the thyroid gland.
	Step 2	Stabilize the thyroid cartilage with the nondominant hand and using the dominant hand, introduce the IV catheter with the needle stylet at a 45-degree angle through the cricothyroid membrane into the trachea, aspirating air to confirm location.
	Step 3	Advance the catheter to the hub and remove the needle stylet.
	Step 4	Attach the Luer lock syringe to the catheter and then the endotracheal tube adapter to the syringe to allow for bag-valve ventilation.

(Continued)

TABLE 8-6	Procedure for Endotracheal Intubation, Needle Cricothyroidotomy, and Cricothyrotomy (Continued)	
Cricothyrotomy		
Equipment	Scalpel, Kelly forceps, 6-mm inner diameter or smaller endotracheal tube	
Technique	Step 1	Extend the neck and identify the cricothyroid membrane, located inferior to the thyroid cartilage and superior to the thyroid gland.
	Step 2	Stabilize the thyroid cartilage with the nondominant hand and using the dominant hand, make a 1-cm horizontal incision just above the superior border of the cricoid.
	Step 3	Using the Kelly forceps, dissect until the cricothyroid membrane is visualized and then make a vertical incision through the midline of the membrane, being careful to not pass the blade too deeply.
	Step 4	Widen the incision with Kelly forceps until the endotracheal tube can be inserted and then inflate the cuff.

Generally, tracheostomy should be considered if prolonged ventilatory support is anticipated after 10–14 days of endotracheal intubation.

- **Complications:** Tracheostomy sites require at least 72 hours to mature, and tube dislodgment before maturation can lead to serious and life-threatening complications.
  - A tracheostomy tube that has been dislodged before stoma maturation **should not be reinserted** owing to the risk of creating a false tract.
  - **Standard endotracheal intubation** should be performed if a tracheostomy tube is dislodged before stoma maturation.
  - **Tracheoinnominate artery fistulas** are an uncommon but life-threatening complication of a tracheostomy that occurs when an abnormal tract develops between the innominate artery and trachea, leading to hemorrhage. This complication most commonly occurs 7–14 days after the tracheostomy but can occur up to 6 weeks after the procedure. Immediate management includes overinflation of the tracheostomy tube cuff, digital compression of the stoma, and surgical exploration.[10]

Mechanical Ventilation

GENERAL PRINCIPLES

Indications of mechanical ventilation with the underlying physiological mechanism are listed in Table 8-7.

Basic modes of ventilation: One can determine how the ventilator initiates a breath (triggering), how the breath is delivered, how patient-initiated breaths are supported, and when to terminate the breath to allow expiration (cycling).

- **Initiation of a breath:** Triggering of a ventilator occurs after a period of time has elapsed (time triggered) or when the patient has generated sufficient negative airway pressure or inspiratory flow exceeding a predetermined threshold (patient triggered).
- **Modes of ventilation**
  - **Assist-control (AC) ventilation:** Ventilator delivers a fully supported breath whether time or patient triggered. Primary mode of ventilation is used in respiratory failure.
  - **Synchronized intermittent mandatory ventilation (SIMV):** Ventilator delivers a fully supported breath when time triggered. However, when the breath is patient triggered, the ventilator delivers a pressure-supported breath (at a level set by the clinician).

TABLE 8-7 Potential Indications for Mechanical Ventilation

Physiologic Mechanism	Clinical Parameters to be Observed	Normal Range	Values Indicating Need for Mechanical Ventilation
Hypoxemia	$P(A\text{–}a)O_2$ gradient (mm Hg)	25–65	>350
	PaO_2/FiO_2 ratio	425–475	<300
	SaO_2	98%	<90% despite supplemental oxygen
Hypercarbia	$PaCO_2$	35–45 mm Hg	Acute increase from patient's baseline pH <7.20 Mental status decline
Oxygen delivery/oxygen consumption imbalance	Elevated lactate	≤2.2 mg/dL	≥4 mg/dL despite adequate resuscitation
	Decreased mixed venous oxygen saturation	70%	<70% despite adequate acute resuscitation
Increased work of breathing	Minute ventilation	5–10 L/min	>15–20 L/min
	Dead space	0.15–0.30	≥0.5 (acute)
Inspiratory muscle weakness	Negative inspiratory pressure	80–100 cm H_2O	<20–30
	Vital capacity	60–75 mL/kg	<15–20
Acute decompensated heart failure	Jugular venous distention Pulmonary edema Decreased EF		Clinical judgment combined with the listed factors
Inadequate lung expansion	Tidal volume (mL/kg)	5–8	<4–5
	Vital capacity (mL/kg)	60–75	<10–15
	Respiratory rate (breaths/min)	12–20	≥35

The size of the patient-triggered breath depends on lung compliance and patient's effort. This mode is commonly used in surgical patients.

- **Pressure support ventilation (PSV):** Spontaneous mode of ventilation without a set respiratory rate. Delivers a clinician-determined inspiratory pressure during patient-triggered breathing. **No respiratory rate is set, so there is no guaranteed minute ventilation.**

• **Type of breath delivered**

- **Volume control (VC):** Ventilator delivers a clinician-determined tidal volume (V_T) for each breath regardless of whether the breath was time or patient triggered. When predetermined V_T is delivered, airflow is terminated and exhalation occurs.
- **Pressure control (PC):** Delivers a practitioner-determined inspiratory pressure for each breath. When inspiratory time has elapsed, inspiratory pressure is terminated and exhalation occurs. The tidal volume varies based on lung compliance. **PC ventilation does not deliver a guaranteed V_T or minute ventilation and may lead to hypoventilation.** However, PC may improve patient synchrony and comfort while on the ventilator.
- Overview of features of selected modes of mechanical ventilation is listed in Table 8-8.

• **Basic ventilator terminology and management:** Flow-time and pressure-time tracings are demonstrated in Figure 8-2.

TABLE 8-8 Overview of Features of Selected Modes of Mechanical Ventilation

Ventilator Mode	Trigger	Control	Cycling	Inspiratory Flow (See Figure 8-1)	Advantages	Disadvantages
Continuous mandatory ventilation	Time	Flow or pressure	Volume or time	Selected or decelerating	Rests muscles of respiration	Requires use of heavy sedation/ neuromuscular blockade
Volume control/ assist control (VC/AC)	Patient or time	Flow	Volume	Square, decelerating, or sinusoidal	• Reduced work of breathing • Guarantees delivery of set tidal volume (unless peak pressure limit alarm is exceeded)	• Potential adverse hemodynamic effects • May lead to inappropriate hyperventilation and excessive inspiration pressures
Pressure control (PC)/AC	Patient or time	Pressure	Time	Decelerating	• Delivers set inspiratory pressure for each breath • Allows limitation of peak inspiratory pressures	• Same as for assist volume control • Potential hyperventilation or hypoventilation with lung resistance/compliance changes

(Continued)

TABLE 8-8 Overview of Features of Selected Modes of Mechanical Ventilation (Continued)

Synchronized intermittent mandatory ventilation	Patient or time	Pressure for patient breaths	Flow for spontaneous breaths	Decelerating for spontaneous breath	Less interference with normal cardiovascular function	• Increased work of breathing compared with AC • Patient may find it difficult to adjust to two different types of ventilator breaths
		Flow (VC) or pressure (PC) for ventilator breaths	Volume or time for ventilator breaths	Square (VC), decelerating (VC or PC), sinusoidal for spontaneous breaths	• Patient comfort Improved patient-ventilator interaction Decreased work of breathing	• Apnea alarm is only backup Variable patient tolerance
Stand-alone pressure-support ventilation	Patient	None	Flow	Decelerating	Rests muscles of respiration	Requires use of heavy sedation/neuromuscular blockade

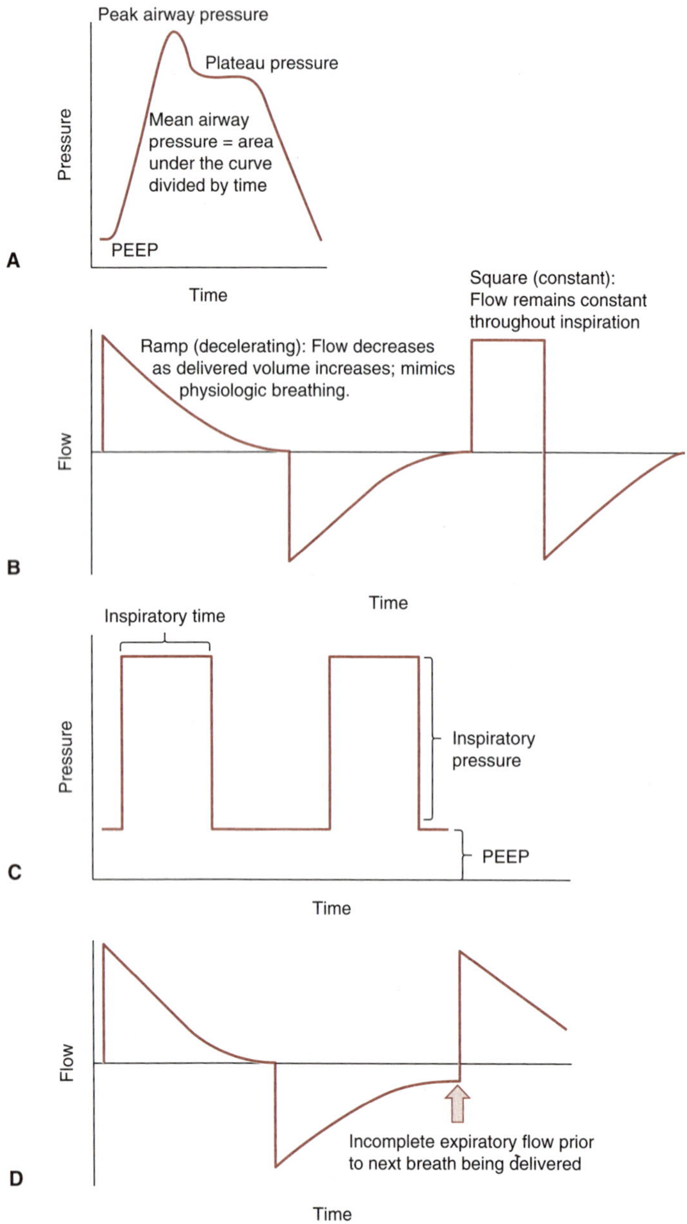

Figure 8-2 Flow-time and pressure-time tracings. A, Pressure-time curve for one breath. B, Flow-time curve for volume control ventilation. Pressure varies throughout inspiratory time, depending on lung compliance. C, Pressure-time curve for pressure control ventilation. Flow varies throughout inspiratory time, depending on lung compliance. D, Pressure-time curve demonstrating auto-positive end-expiratory pressure (auto-PEEP).

◦ **Minute ventilation:** Defined as the product of V_T and respiratory rate ($V_T \times RR$). Normally between 5 and 10 L/min in resting adults, but may be much higher in high metabolic states, e.g., septic shock.
◦ **Peak airway pressure:** Composed of pressures necessary to overcome inspiratory airflow resistance, chest wall recoil resistance, and alveolar opening resistance. Does not reflect alveolar pressure.
◦ **Mean airway pressure:** Mean pressures applied during the inspiratory cycle. Approximates alveolar pressure until overdistention occurs.
◦ **Plateau pressure:** Reflects alveolar pressure. Checked by performing an end-inspiratory hold maneuver to allow pressures through the tracheobronchial tree to equilibrate.

Ventilator Settings

- **Initial ventilator settings:** Typical initial ventilator settings are summarized in Table 8-9.
- **Advanced modes of ventilation:** Advanced modes should generally only be used after discussion with higher level practitioners (Table 8-10).
  ◦ **Pressure-regulated VC ventilation:** Ventilator determines after each breath if inspiratory pressure was sufficient to achieve targeted V_T; if insufficient or excessive, then ventilator will adjust inspiratory pressure to achieve desired V_T.
  ◦ **Inverse-ratio ventilation (IRV):** A pressure-controlled method of ventilation most commonly used in ARDS. Inspiratory time exceeds expiratory time to improve oxygenation at the expense of ventilation; patients are permitted to become hypercapnic to pH 7.20. If obstructive lung disease is present, then this can cause auto-PEEP and excessive hypercapnia.
  ◦ **Airway pressure release ventilation (APRV):** An extreme version of IRV; inspiratory pressure (P_{high}) applied for a prolonged period of time (T_{high}) with a short expiratory time (T_{low}, or release time)—usually <1 s—to allow for ventilation. Like IRV, patients are permitted to be hypercapnic to pH 7.20.

TABLE 8-9 Typical Initial Ventilator Settings

Parameter	Settings	Comments
Mode	A/C	Use A/C mode for patients not breathing spontaneously and for starting assisted ventilation
Respiratory rate	8–12 bpm	• For patients without spontaneous breathing efforts, set rate to achieve a desired $PaCO_2$ guided by ABGs • For spontaneously breathing patients in A/C or SIMV mode, set rate 2–3 bpm below spontaneous rate • Set initial rate higher than 8–12 bpm if lung disease is present—for example, asthma and COPD, depending on the disease
Tidal volume	6-8 mL/kg IBW	For patients with ARDS or at risk for ARDS, low tidal volumes (i.e., 6 mL predicted body weight [PBW]) are recommended
FiO_2	1.0	• Start at 1.0 and taper as guided by PaO_2 or SaO_2 • Maintain SaO_2 >87% or PaO_2 >55 mm Hg • Hyperoxia after intubation may actually worsen patient survival
PEEP	5–10	Higher values are frequently used in the treatment of ARDS

(Continued)

TABLE 8-9 Typical Initial Ventilator Settings (Continued)

Parameter	Settings	Comments
Inspiratory flow rate	60 L/min or greater	Higher flow rates increase expiration time, which may be important in obstructive lung disease to prevent auto-PEEP (ventilator delivers a breath before the patient has been able to fully expire)
I:E ratio	1:2	Usually a derived and not a preset parameter

Male IBW = 50 kg + 2.3 kg/in × (height [in] – 60) (imperial),
50 kg + 1.1 kg/cm × (height [cm] – 152.4) (metric).
Female IBW = 45.5 kg + 2.3 kg/in × (height [in] – 60) (imperial),
45.5 kg + 1.1 kg/cm × (height [cm] – 152.4) (metric).

ABG, arterial blood gas; bpm, beats per minute; FiO_2, fraction of inspired oxygen; IBW, ideal body weight; $PaCO_2$, arterial carbon dioxide tension; PEEP, positive end-expiratory pressure; SaO_2, arterial oxygen saturation.

TABLE 8-10 Advanced Modes of Ventilation

Mode	Description
Pressure-regulated VC ventilation	Ventilator determines after each breath whether inspiratory pressure was sufficient to achieve targeted V_T; if insufficient or excessive, then ventilator will adjust inspiratory pressure to achieve the desired V_T
Inverse ratio ventilation	• A pressure-controlled method of ventilation most commonly used in ARDS • Inspiratory time exceeds expiratory time to improve oxygenation at the expense of ventilation; patients are permitted to become hypercapnic to pH 7.20 • If obstructive lung disease is present, it can cause auto-PEEP and excessive hypercapnia
Airway pressure release ventilation	• An extreme version of IRV; inspiratory pressure (P_{high}) applied for a prolonged period of time (T_{high}) with a short expiratory time (T_{low}, or release time)—usually • It is used as an alternative modality in ARDS patients
High-frequency oscillation ventilation	• Generates very small tidal volumes with respiratory rates > 100/min • Has been used in patients with ARDS
Proportional assist ventilation	• Continuous spontaneous ventilation in which pressure generated is proportional to patient's inspiratory effort (volume and flow) • It enhances patient-ventilator synchrony
Neurally adjusted ventilatory assist ventilation	• Continuous spontaneous ventilation in which pressure generated is proportional to the electrical activity of the diaphragm • It enhances patient-ventilator synchrony
Adaptive support ventilation	• Combines dual-control, breath-to-breath, time-cycled (mandatory), and flow-cycled (spontaneous) breaths into a single mode • Ventilator chooses ventilator parameter based on clinician input of IBW and percent minute volume to meet minute ventilation target while minimizing WOB • Breaths may be triggered by patient or ventilator

ARDS, acute respiratory distress syndrome; IBW, ideal body weight; PEEP, positive end-expiratory pressure; V_T, tidal volume; WOB, work of breathing.

MECHANICAL VENTILATION PRINCIPLES FOR PATIENTS WITH ARDS

- Owing to severe hypoxia associated with ARDS, oxygenation and prevention of barotrauma may have to be prioritized over ventilation, resulting in hypercapnia.
  - Hypercapnia resulting in a pH of 7.20–7.35 often is tolerated to sufficiently oxygenate the patient ("**permissive hypercapnia**").
  - The plateau pressure should be checked and the tidal volume should be decreased down to 4 mL/kg of IBW as pH allows to achieve a plateau pressure ≤30 cm H_2O.
  - There is growing evidence that driving pressure (ratio of V_T/respiratory system compliance) is a key variable to optimize when ventilating patients with ARDS. The driving pressure can be calculated as the plateau pressure minus the PEEP and should be kept below 14 cm H_2O when possible.[11,13,14]
  - Ventilation management in special situations is summarized in Table 8-11.

TABLE 8-11 Ventilatory Management in Specific Situations

Clinical Condition	Initial Ventilator Setting	Monitoring
ARDS	• Mode: A/C VC • Low V_T: 4–8 mL/kg IBW • Pplat: <30 cm H_2O • RR: up to 35/min • FiO_2: 1 (initially) • PEEP is set according to FiO_2/PEEP combinations to achieve oxygenation goals	• Avoid $PEEP_i$ • SpO_2 goal 88%–95% • PaO_2 goal 55–80 mm Hg • pH goal 7.30–7.45 • Permissive hypercapnia may be needed • Patient-ventilator synchrony • Hemodynamic status
COPD	• NIPPV should be considered in COPD patients prior to invasive ventilation • Mode: A/C VC or PC • Low V_T: 6–8 mL/kg IBW • Pplat: <30 cm H_2O • RR: 8–12/min • FiO_2: ≤0.5 (or to meet SpO_2 goal) • PEEP: ≤5 cm H_2O or as needed to offset PEEP (80% of $PEEP_i$) • T_i: 0.6–1.25 sec • Peak flow: ≥80 L/min (decelerating flow) in VC	• Avoid $PEEP_i$ • SpO_2 goal >88% • Avoid hyperventilation • $PaCO_2$ goal is patient's baseline in COPD • Permissive hypercapnia may initially be required in asthmatic patients • Patient-ventilator synchrony • Hemodynamic status • Airway pressure assessment and flow-volume patterns can be used to monitor bronchodilator effectiveness
Asthma	• Mode: A/C VC or PC • Low V_T: 6–8 mL/kg IBW • Pplat: <30 cm H_2O • RR: 10–15/min • FiO_2: ≤0.5 (or to meet SpO_2 goal) • PEEP: 0–≤5 cm H_2O or as needed to offset PEEP (80% of PEEP)	• Avoid $PEEP_i$ • SpO_2 goal >90% • Permissive hypercapnia may initially be required in asthmatic patients • Patient-ventilator synchrony • Hemodynamics • Use of helium–oxygen mixtures should be considered

(Continued)

TABLE 8-11 Ventilatory Management in Specific Situations (Continued)

Clinical Condition	Initial Ventilator Setting	Monitoring
	• T_i: 0.6–1.25 sec • Peak flow: 60 L/min (constant flow) or 80–100 L/min (decelerating flow) in VC	• Airway pressure assessment and flow-volume patterns can be used to monitor bronchodilator effectiveness
Chronic restrictive disease	• Mode: A/C VC or PC • Low V_T: 4–8 mL/kg IBW • Pplat: <30 cm H_2O • RR: 15–30/min • FiO_2: ≤0.5 • PEEP: 5 cm H_2O • T_i: <1 sec • Peak flow: ≥60 L/min in VC	• SpO_2 goal 88%–95% • PaO_2 goal 55–80 mm Hg • Patient-ventilator synchrony • Hemodynamic status
Neuromuscular disease	• NIPPV should be considered early • Mode: A/C VC or PC • Low V_T: 6-8 mL/kg IBW • Pplat: <30 cm H_2O • RR: 10–15/min • FiO_2: ≤0.5 (or to meet SpO_2 goal) • PEEP: 5 cm H_2O • T_i: 1 sec	• Spontaneous V_T and RR • Vital capacity • Intubate if <10 mL/kg • Wean if = 10 mL/kg • Extubate if >15 mL/kg post-SBT • PImax ◦ Intubate if <–20 cm H_2O ◦ Wean if = –20 cm H_2O ◦ Extubate if >–30 cm H_2O post-SBT
Head trauma	• Mode: A/C VC or PC • Low V_T: 6–8 mL/kg IBW • Pplat: <30 cm H_2O • RR: 15–20/min • FiO_2: ≤0.5 (or to meet SpO_2 goal) • PEEP: 5 cm H_2O • T_i: 1 sec	• Monitor ICP or signs of raised ICP • Avoid hypoxia or hypercapnia; can raise ICP • PaO_2 goal 70–100 mm Hg • $PaCO_2$ goal 35–40 mm Hg • $ETCO_2$ 30–35 • Ensure PEEP level does not raise ICP • Avoid PEEP

A/C, assist/control; COPD, chronic obstructive pulmonary disease; $ETCO_2$, end-tidal carbon dioxide; IBW, ideal body weight; ICP, intracranial pressure; NIPPV, noninvasive positive-pressure ventilation; $PaCO_2$, arterial carbon dioxide tension; PC, pressure control; Pplat, plateau pressure; PEEP, positive end-expiratory pressure; RR, respiratory rate; SBT, spontaneous breathing trial; VC, volume-cycled.

ADJUNCTS TO MECHANICAL VENTILATION

General Principles

- **Nitric oxide (NO):** Improves oxygenation by preferential vasodilation of capillary beds of ventilated lung.
  - NO may have some benefit in patients with pulmonary hypertension who are severely hypoxemic.

  - The use of NO in patients without pulmonary hypertension is limited. Studies have suggested that its usage does not improve mortality in patients with ARDS regardless of the degree of hypoxia.[15]
- **Inhaled prostacyclins:** Similar to NO, theoretically, inhalation of prostacyclins—a class of vasodilators—improves oxygenation by preferential vasodilation of the capillary beds of ventilated lung.
  - Studies have shown that inhaled prostaglandins improve oxygenation and pulmonary artery pressure in patients with ARDS.[16] However, no studies have been performed to investigate whether mortality benefit exists.
  - Have antiplatelet effects, so theoretical concern for worsening diffuse alveolar hemorrhage.
- **Helium-oxygen mixture (Heliox):** Used in asthma and severe bronchospasm. Usually, a mixture of 70%–80% helium and 20%–30% oxygen. Theoretically decreases airway resistance owing to its low density leading to improvement in the ratio of laminar to turbulent flow and decreasing work of breathing. Studies have suggested some benefit in patients with severe asthma exacerbations.[17]

CONSIDERATIONS IN ACUTE RESPIRATORY DISTRESS SYNDROME

- **Fluids:** Conservative fluid management (pulmonary capillary wedge pressure <8, central venous pressure [CVP] <4) in an ARDS patient is associated with shorter mechanical ventilation time.[18]
- **Steroids:** Data exist that the use of glucocorticoids later in the course of ARDS (≥14 days) is not beneficial and may be harmful. The use of glucocorticoids earlier in the course of ARDS is less clear, but there is no good evidence of benefit and steroids are often avoided owing to their detrimental side effects, particularly with paralytics.[19]
- **Paralysis:** Decreases oxygen consumption from accessory inspiratory muscle use and is frequently used in ARDS.
  - A randomized controlled multicenter trial showed that early neuromuscular blockade with cisatracurium was associated with an improvement in a 90-day mortality and fewer ventilator days in patients with PaO_2/FiO_2 <120 mm Hg.[20]
- **Prone positioning:** Improves oxygenation in patients with ARDS by reducing V/Q mismatching and improving shunting by decreasing the amount of atelectatic lung.
  - Early application of prone positioning is associated with improved mortality in patients with ARDS with a PaO_2/FiO_2 <150 mm Hg ARDS.[21]
  - Patients should receive neuromuscular blockade to tolerate proning.
  - Absolute contraindications to proning include spinal instability or unstable fractures. Use of vasopressors, renal replacement therapy, or obesity are not contraindications to proning, but obesity can make proning challenging.
  - Patients should remain proned for at least 16 consecutive hours at a time for benefit and to limit the frequency of turns.
  - A video demonstration of proning can be found on the *New England Journal of Medicine* website.[21]

EXTRACORPOREAL MEMBRANE OXYGENATION IN ADULTS

Introduction

- Extracorporeal membrane oxygenation (ECMO) is a type of mechanical cardiopulmonary support that is used to support patients with cardiac failure or both cardiac and respiratory failure, despite optimal conventional care, by removing blood from the venous system, oxygenating it, and returning it to either the venous (venous–venous [VV] ECMO) or the arterial (venoarterial [VA] ECMO) system.
  - **Venovenous ECMO:** Used to support patients with respiratory failure.

- ◦ **VA ECMO:** Used to support patients with cardiac failure or both cardiac and respiratory failure.

INDICATIONS

- Acute severe heart or lung failure with high mortality risk despite optimal conventional therapy.
- Hypoxic respiratory failure, with a partial pressure of arterial oxygen (PaO_2)/FiO_2 <150 mm Hg with FiO_2 >0.9 and Murray score of 2–3.
- ARDS.
- Severe cardiac failure of any cause.
- Primary allograft failure following heart or lung transplantation.
- As a bridge to either cardiac or lung transplantation or placement of a ventricular assist device.

CONTRAINDICATIONS

- Most contraindications are relative.
  - ◦ Conditions incompatible with normal life if the patient recovers.
  - ◦ Pre-existing conditions which affect the quality of life (CNS status, end-stage malignancy, and risk of systemic bleeding with anticoagulation).

Complications

- Bleeding due to anticoagulants used is seen in around 50% of patients and can be life-threatening.
- Systemic thromboembolism may be present due to clots formed in the circuit.
- Heparin-induced thrombocytopenia, cannula-related problems, and neurological dysfunction have also been reported.
- Infection risk at the cannula insertion site or systemic infections range from 7% to 20%.

Extracorporeal Carbon Dioxide Removal ($ECCO_2R$)

- It removes carbon dioxide via external, gas-permeable membrane lung without providing significant oxygenation. It is used in patients with unavoidable hypercapnia, such as during lung-protective ventilation with low tidal volumes. This has been reported to reduce markers of inflammation and ventilator-induced lung injury in patients with ARDS.

COMMON COMPLICATIONS OF MECHANICAL VENTILATION

- **Airway malpositioning and occlusion:** See Airway Management and Tracheal Intubation section.
- **Troubleshooting ventilator alarms:** See Figure 8-3.
- **Hypoxia in ventilated patients:** Causes and management (mnemonic **DOPES**) are summarized in Table 8-12.
- **Auto-PEEP:** Occurs when inspiration is initiated before complete exhalation is complete. May be detected on physical examination by wheezing that does not terminate before the next breath. Demonstrated on ventilator flow-time loop by flow not returning to baseline before delivery of next breath (see Figure 8-2). Excessive auto-PEEP can lead to cardiac decompensation owing to tension pneumothorax-like physiology. Treated by adjusting ventilator settings to prolong the expiratory time and treating any reversible airway obstruction. In the acute setting, the patient may need to be disconnected from the ventilator to allow for full exhalation.
- **Barotrauma/volutrauma:** Occurs when excessive PEEP, inspiratory pressures, or tidal volumes are applied, resulting in alveolar rupture and dissection of air along interstitial tissues causing pneumothorax, pneumomediastinum, pneumopericardium, or pneumoperitoneum. If undetected, can result in life-threatening cardiac decompensation.

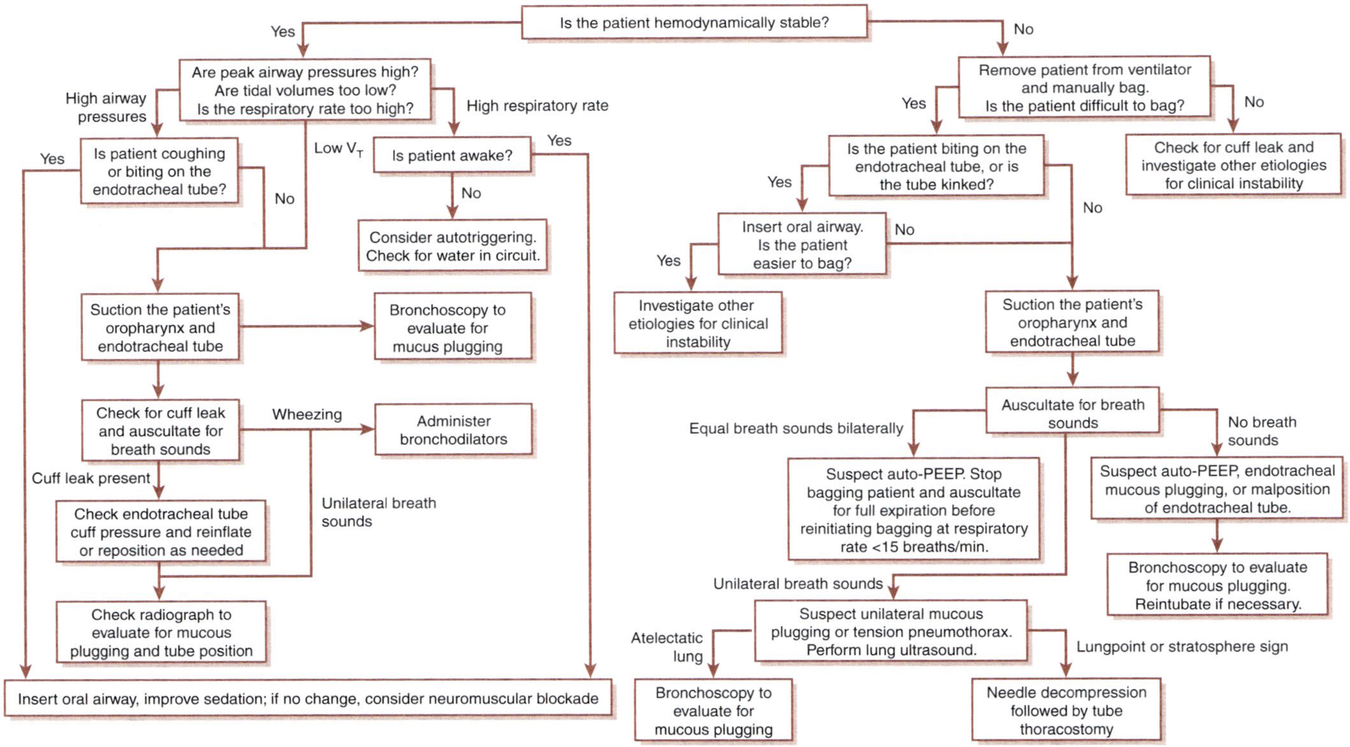

Figure 8-3 Troubleshooting ventilator alarms: what to do when the patient is hypoxic. *Auto-PEEP*, auto-positive end-expiratory pressure.

TABLE 8-12	Hypoxia in Ventilated Patients—Causes and Management (Mnemonic DOPES)	
Displacement/ disconnection	• Displacement of endotracheal tube • Disconnection from the ventilator	• Confirm with $ETCO_2$, bilateral breath sounds • Bag until recovery and reconnection to ventilator
Obstruction	• Mucus plug • Patient biting the tube	• Deep suctioning bronchoscopy, aggressive chest physiotherapy • Sedation/bite block
Pathology	• Pneumothorax • Pulmonary embolism • Pulmonary edema	• Get CXR, chest tube insertion • ECHO/CT angio, thrombolysis • Increase PEEP and FiO_2/ consider diuretics
Equipment	Technical problem	Respiratory therapist to look in
Stacked breaths	In obstructive airway diseases, new breath may be delivered even before patient exhales	Change settings to allow prolonged expiration, decrease respiratory rate

- **Ventilator-associated pneumonia (VAP):** Defined as pneumonia in a patient who has been intubated for >48 hours.
  - VAP is generally identified by a new infiltrate on CXR in addition to ≥2 of the following criteria: fever, leukocytosis, worsening oxygenation, and purulent secretions.
  - When VAP is suspected, microbiologic specimens should be obtained via tracheal aspirate or bronchoscopy with bronchoalveolar lavage.
  - Treatment with broad-spectrum empiric antibiotics based on the local prevalence of pathogens and antibiotic sensitivities should be initiated if there is high clinical suspicion for VAP. If an organism has been identified, the antibiotic choice should be tailored to the specific pathogen.
  - The antibiotic duration for VAP is generally 7 days, as longer durations are not more effective and may increase the risk of antibiotic resistance.[22–25]
- **Stress-induced peptic ulcer disease:** Critically ill patients are at an increased risk of developing upper gastrointestinal (GI) bleeding, which can be prevented by the appropriate use of pharmacologic prophylaxis.
  - The primary indications for stress ulcer prophylaxis are the presence of a significant coagulopathy (platelets <50k, international normalized ratio >1.5, or partial thromboplastin time >2 upper limits of normal) or the use of mechanical ventilation for >48 hours. The other indications for prophylaxis include a history of an upper GI bleed in the last year, presence of brain or spinal cord injury, or any 2 of the following: occult bleeding for ≥6 days, use of high-dose steroids (>250 mg of hydrocortisone), sepsis, or an intensive care unit (ICU) stay >1 week.
  - A histamine-2 receptor antagonist or proton pump inhibitor can be used for prophylaxis with some controversy on what agent is preferred.
  - The use of ulcer prophylaxis may increase the risk of nosocomial infections, but benefits are likely greater than risks in the above patients.
- **Oxygen toxicity:** Breathing high FiO_2 can lead to excessive free radical generation and result in lung injury.
  - Reducing FiO_2 to the lowest tolerable oxygen saturation (O_2 saturation of 90% or PaO_2 of 65 mm Hg) is advisable. There is evidence that tolerating hyperoxia after intubation may worsen patient survival.[12]

LIBERATION FROM MECHANICAL VENTILATION

- **Parameters demonstrating readiness to wean:** Daily assessment of readiness for extubation should be done once the underlying disease process begins to resolve and minimal ventilator support is required. The following criteria should generally be met before extubation:
  - Minimal ventilator support: FiO_2 ≤40%, PEEP 5 cm H_2O to maintain SpO_2 >90%.
  - Arterial blood gas: pH and $PaCO_2$ should be at the patient's baseline, particularly important for patients with chronic CO_2 retention.
  - Ventilation requirement: Minute ventilation should be <10 L/min and respiratory rate <30 breaths/min.
  - Mental status: Patient should be awake, alert, and cooperative.
  - Secretions: Secretions should be thin, scant in amount, and easily suctioned; patient should not require suctioning more frequently than every 4 hours before extubation.
  - Strength: Patient should have strong cough and be able to lift head off the bed and hold it in flexion for >5 s.
  - Breathing trial: Patient should be able to generate spontaneous V_T >5 mL/kg IBW.
  - **Rapid shallow breathing index (RSBI): RSBI should be ≤105.** Defined as a ratio of respiratory rate to V_T in liters (f/V_T). RSBI >105 accurately predicts weaning failure, but RSBI ≤105 is less accurate at predicting weaning success.[26]
  - **Patency of airway:** In patients with concern for laryngeal edema (e.g., angioedema, traumatic intubation), cuff leak should be checked before extubation. **Absence of cuff leak should generally preclude extubation**, and patients should be treated with IV corticosteroids for 12–24 hours before extubation.[27]
- **Weaning strategies: Sedation interruption and breathing trials for 30–120 minutes should be done daily** and is the most important predictor of timely liberation from mechanical ventilation.[28] Weaning strategies include the following:
  - **PSV:** No time-triggered breaths, but patient remains connected to the ventilator. PEEP is usually at 5 cm H_2O, with low levels of pressure support (5–10 cm H_2O) during spontaneous breathing.
  - **T-piece/spontaneous breathing trial:** Patient is removed from the ventilator but remains intubated. Endotracheal tube is connected to a heated, humidified circuit with minimal or no supplemental oxygen. End-tidal CO_2 monitoring may be used for additional safety.
  - **SIMV:** Used most frequently in surgical and neurosurgical patients. Set respiratory rate is gradually decreased over hours to days until patient is primarily breathing spontaneously.
  - SIMV has the poorest weaning outcomes of all techniques. However, neither T-piece nor PSV has proven to be more predictive of successful extubation.[29]
- **Management following extubation:** Patients need to be closely monitored following extubation. Good airway clearance and oxygenation decrease the risk of reintubation.
  - **Extubation to NPPV:** In patients with COPD who are intubated for acute respiratory failure, extubation to NPPV is associated with a reduction in mortality and healthcare–associated pneumonia.[30] Similar benefit has not been demonstrated in other etiologies of respiratory failure.
  - **Extubation to HFNC:** The use of HFNC may also have a beneficial role in the prevention of postextubation respiratory failure in select low-risk patients. When patients were randomly assigned to HFNC versus conventional oxygen therapy after extubation, patients who received HFNC were less likely to be intubated within 72 hours.[31] Other studies have shown HFNC to be noninferior when compared with NPPV in preventing reintubation.[32,33]

- **Failure to wean:** Defined as inability to liberate from mechanical ventilation 48–72 hours after resolution of underlying disease process. Factors that should be considered include the following:
  - Endotracheal tubes with smaller inner diameter increase airway resistance and may make breathing trials more difficult.
  - Use of neuromuscular blockade is associated with prolonged weakness, particularly when used with corticosteroids.[34]
  - Acid–base disturbances may make liberation from mechanical ventilation difficult.
  - Non-anion gap metabolic acidosis causes compensatory increase in minute ventilation (respiratory alkalosis) to normalize pH, which can lead to tachypnea and respiratory fatigue upon extubation.
  - Metabolic alkalosis causes blunting of ventilatory drive and decrease in minute ventilation (respiratory acidosis) to maintain normal pH, which can lead to hypercapnia upon extubation.

Shock

GENERAL PRINCIPLES

- A process in which blood flow and oxygen delivery to tissues are deranged, leading to tissue hypoxia and resultant compromise of cellular metabolic activity and organ function.
- Main goal of therapy is rapid cardiovascular resuscitation to reestablish tissue perfusion.
- Definitive treatment requires reversal of underlying processes.

Classifications

Hemodynamic patterns associated with the different shock states are listed in Table 8-13.

- **Distributive:** Shock caused by massive vasodilation and impaired distribution of blood flow, resulting in tissue hypoxia. Usually associated with hyperdynamic cardiac function, unless cardiac function is somehow impaired (see later discussion of cardiogenic shock).
  - **Primary etiologies** are septic shock and anaphylactic shock. Septic shock is most commonly seen in medical ICUs and will be further discussed in the next section. Anaphylaxis is discussed in Chapter 11, Allergy and Immunology.
  - **Hemodynamic parameters** will generally demonstrate increased cardiac output (CO), decreased systemic vascular resistance (SVR) due to vasodilation, and elevated central venous oxygen saturation ($ScvO_2$) due to ineffective oxygen extraction by tissue.

TABLE 8-13 Hemodynamic Patterns Associated With Specific Shock States

Type of Shock	CI	SVR	PVR	SvO_2	RAP	RVP	PAP	PAOP
Cardiogenic	↓	↑	N	↓	↑	↑	↑	↑
Hypovolemic	↓	↑	N	↓	↓	↓	↓	↓
Distributive	N–↑	↓	N	N–↑	N–↓	N–↓	N–↓	N–↓
Obstructive[a]	↓	↑–N	↑	N–↓	↑	↑	↑	N–↓

[a]Equalization of RAP, PAOP, diastolic PAP, and diastolic RVP establishes a diagnosis of cardiac tamponade.

CI, cardiac index; N, normal; PAOP, pulmonary artery occlusion pressure; PAP, pulmonary artery pressure; PVR, pulmonary vascular resistance; RAP, right atrial pressure; RVP, right ventricular pressure; SvO_2, mixed venous oxygen saturation; SVR, systemic vascular resistance.

- Primary goals of therapy
  - Volume resuscitation: Owing to massive peripheral vasodilation, patients have a functionally decreased oxygen-carrying capacity, requiring volume resuscitation. IV crystalloid fluids are primarily used.
  - Treatment of underlying infection: Inadequate initial antimicrobial therapy is an independent risk factor for in-hospital mortality in patients with septic shock, so timely, effective antimicrobial therapy is a cornerstone of treatment.
  - Removal of the offending agent in anaphylactic shock.
  - Cardiovascular support with vasoactive agents (e.g., norepinephrine). Vasoactive agents will be discussed in more detail in a later section.

- **Hypovolemic:** Shock caused by a decrease in effective intravascular volume and decreased oxygen-carrying capacity.
  - **Primary etiologies** are hemorrhagic (e.g., trauma, gastrointestinal bleeding) or fluid depletion (e.g., diarrhea, vomiting).
  - **Hemodynamic parameters** will generally demonstrate a decreased CO, increased SVR, and decreased $ScvO_2$ due to increased oxygen extraction by peripheral tissue.
  - Primary goals of therapy
    - Volume resuscitation: IV blood product and crystalloid are used for resuscitation of hemorrhagic and fluid depletion shock, respectively, with goal mean arterial pressure (MAP) of 60–65 mm Hg. Recent studies indicate that over-resuscitation may be detrimental in hemorrhagic shock and patients without significant comorbidities may tolerate lower hemoglobin levels (7 g/dL) than previously believed.
    - Definitive treatment of underlying etiology of volume loss: For hemorrhagic shock, surgical intervention may be necessary for definitive treatment.
- **Obstructive:** Shock caused by obstruction of the heart or great vessels, resulting in decreased left ventricular filling and cardiovascular collapse.
  - **Primary etiologies** are pulmonary embolism, cardiac tamponade, and tension pneumothorax.
  - **Hemodynamic parameters** will generally demonstrate decreased CO, normal to increased SVR, and normal to decreased $ScvO_2$.
  - Primary goals of therapy
    - Supportive: Although patients are preload dependent, excessive fluid administration can lead to right ventricular overload, thereby worsening shock.
    - In a carefully selected group of patients, thrombolytic therapy may be beneficial in patients with pulmonary emboli.
- **Cardiogenic:** Shock caused by left ventricular systolic failure, resulting in decreased CO and subsequent insufficient oxygen distribution.
  - **Primary etiologies** are myocardial infarction, acute mitral regurgitation, and myocarditis.
  - **Hemodynamic parameters** will demonstrate decreased CO, increased SVR, and decreased $ScvO_2$.
  - Primary goals of therapy
    - Mitigation of pulmonary edema: NPPV or endotracheal intubation with mechanical ventilation reduces afterload, thereby encouraging forward flow. Additionally, the application of positive pressure to the alveolar space causes pulmonary edema fluid to move to the interstitial space.
    - Careful fluid management: Adequate preload to optimize ventricular function is important, but volume overload will worsen respiratory status, so careful fluid management is necessary.
    - Definitive therapy for underlying cardiac disease: In the event of myocardial infarction, percutaneous revascularization should be performed in a timely fashion.
    - Supportive: Inotropic agents such as dobutamine may be used to augment CO. Other inotropes are discussed in Pharmacologic Therapies. Mechanical circulatory assist

devices, including left ventricular assist devices and intra-aortic balloon pumps, may be necessary in patients who do not respond to medical therapy.

Septic Shock

- **Definition of sepsis:** Sepsis is defined as a life-threatening organ dysfunction caused by dysregulation of the host response to an infection.
  - Sepsis was previously identified based on the presence of at least two systemic inflammatory response syndrome (SIRS) criteria:
    - Tachypnea: Respiratory rate >20 breaths/min or $PaCO_2$ <32 mm Hg
    - White blood cell count <4000 cells/μL or >12,000 cells/μL
    - Tachycardia: Pulse >90 bpm
    - Hypo- or hyperthermia: Temperature >38°C or <36°C
  - The new sepsis guidelines now identify organ dysregulation in sepsis as an increase in the Sequential Organ Failure Assessment (SOFA) score of ≥2.[35]
  - Septic shock is a subset of sepsis identified by persistent hypotension requiring vasopressors to maintain a mean arterial blood pressure ≥65 mm after adequate volume resuscitation. Mortality in these patients is ~40%.
- **Management of septic shock:** Management of septic shock involves early aggressive volume resuscitation and attempting to achieve hemodynamic stability quickly.[36]
- **Hour-1 bundle: Initial resuscitation for sepsis and septic shock.**
  - Measure lactate level. Remeasure lactate if initial lactate elevated (> 2 mmol/L).
  - Obtain blood cultures before administering antibiotics.
  - Administer broad-spectrum antibiotics.
  - Begin rapid administration of 30 mL/kg crystalloid for hypotension or lactate ≥ 4 mmol/L.
  - Apply vasopressors if hypotensive during or after fluid resuscitation to maintain a mean arterial pressure ≥ 65 mm Hg.
- **Volume resuscitation:** Patients should initially receive **at least 30 mL/kg IBW IV crystalloid fluid** within the first hour of presentation, with additional volume administered if the patient remains volume responsive. Parameters to determine volume responsiveness (discussed in Hemodynamic Measurements section) should be closely monitored during volume resuscitation to prevent volume overload.
  - Some recent studies have found that balanced crystalloids (i.e., lactated Ringer solution) may be associated with lower rates of renal dysfunction and even improved mortality when used as compared with normal saline.[37]
- Resuscitation goals include the following:
  - Mean arterial pressure >65 mm Hg.
  - Urine output >0.5 mL/kg/h.
  - Mixed venous oxygen saturation >65%.
  - Target resuscitation to normalize lactate in patients with elevated lactate levels. Lactate clearance is associated with improved mortality in septic patients.
  - **Cardiovascular support:** Vasoactive medications may be necessary if volume resuscitation is insufficient to maintain MAP ≥65 mm Hg. **Norepinephrine has become the first-line agent** after it was demonstrated that dopamine had more adverse events.[38] Vasopressin is frequently used as a second-line agent. Mechanisms of action and other agents are discussed in Pharmacologic Therapies.
  - **Timely, effective antimicrobial administration:** Delays in starting appropriate antimicrobials are associated with increased mortality in numerous studies.[39]
  - **Source control:** If a specific anatomical source of infection is identified (e.g., necrotizing soft tissue infection), intervention for source control should be performed as soon as reasonably possible.[40]

- **Early goal-directed therapy:** Protocol for management of the **first 6 hours** of sepsis was proposed by Rivers et al. in 2001.[36] Widely adapted in practice before recent multicenter, prospective, randomized controlled trials called its effectiveness into question[41,42]; studies limited by practice changes in control group.
- **Lactate clearance:** Lactate clearance is associated with improved mortality in septic patients.[43] Most recent Surviving Sepsis Guidelines recommend targeting resuscitation to normalize lactate in patients with elevated lactate levels.[44]
- **Procalcitonin (PCT):** PCT is a biomarker that may aid in diagnosing sepsis, assessing treatment response, and determining antibiotic duration. An elevated PCT >0.5 ng/mL is suggestive of a bacterial infection while a PCT <0.1 ng/mL makes bacterial infection less likely.[45] Some studies have shown that use of PCT may reduce the unnecessary usage of antibiotics.[46] However, caution must be used, as a low PCT does not exclude the possibility of a severe bacterial infection.

Pharmacologic Therapies

Vasoconstrictive and Inotropic Agents

- **Norepinephrine:** Causes potent vasoconstriction via α_1- and β_1-adrenergic activity. Preferred agent in septic shock.
- **Vasopressin:** Causes vasoconstriction via three different G-peptide receptors. Primarily used as an adjunct to norepinephrine. Weak evidence that it may have mortality benefit over norepinephrine in less severe septic shock (defined as requiring treatment with norepinephrine 5–14 µg/min to maintain MAP ≥65 mm Hg).[47]
- **Epinephrine:** Has inotropic and vasoconstrictive properties in a dose-dependent fashion owing to α_1- and β-adrenergic activity. At low doses (≤0.05 µg/kg/min), it increases CO and slightly reduces SVR owing to predominant β activity. At higher doses (>0.05 µg/kg/min), vasoconstriction predominates owing to increased α_1 activity. Preferred agent for anaphylactic shock.
- **Phenylephrine:** Selective α_1-receptor agonist causing vasoconstriction of larger arterioles. Few studies supporting its use in septic shock. May be administered via peripheral IV catheters if central venous access has not yet been established.
- **Angiotensin II:** Recent studies have investigated angiotensin II which engages the renin–angiotensin–aldosterone system. These studies showed that angiotensin II increased blood pressure in patients with vasodilatory shock.[48]
- **Dobutamine:** Inotropic agent that reduces afterload and increases stroke volume and heart rate via β_1-agonist activity. Good agent for cardiogenic shock but increases risk of cardiac arrhythmias.
- **Dopamine:** Has inotropic, vasodilatory, and vasoconstrictive properties in a dose-dependent fashion due to action on peripheral α_1-receptors, cardiac β_1-receptors, and renal and splanchnic dopaminergic receptors. At doses <5 µg/kg/min, primarily behaves as a vasodilator, increasing renal blood flow. At doses of 5–10 µg/kg/min, behaves as an inotrope. At doses >10 µg/kg/min, behaves as a vasopressor. Is associated with a higher rate of cardiac arrhythmias than norepinephrine.[38]
- **Milrinone:** Phosphodiesterase III inhibitor that has positive inotropic effect, causing an increase in CO. Also causes systemic vasodilation, which improves afterload but may cause hypotension.

Adjunctive Therapies

- **Corticosteroids:** Relative adrenal insufficiency may contribute to refractory hypotension during septic shock. Data do not support the use of corticosteroids in mild septic shock. However, corticosteroids should be considered on an individual basis in patients with more severe shock, particularly in patients chronically on steroids. Generally, hydrocortisone 200–300 mg daily divided on a q6–8h basis is given.[49,50]

- **Sodium bicarbonate:** No evidence supports the use of bicarbonate therapy in lactic acidemia from sepsis with a pH ≥7.15. Effect of bicarbonate on hemodynamics and vasopressor requirements with more severe acidemia is unknown, but bicarbonate is often recommended in patients with severe lactic acidemia (pH <7.1) who are hemodynamically unstable.
- **Methylene blue:** Selective guanylate cyclase inhibitor, thereby mitigating nitric oxide–mediated vasodilation. Observational studies have demonstrated beneficial effects on hemodynamic parameters, but effects on morbidity and mortality are unknown.[51]

Hemodynamic Measurements and Critical Care Ultrasound

Although CVP, MAP, and $SvO_2/ScvO_2$ are used as therapeutic end points in treating shock, there is evidence that these parameters do not reflect intravascular volume. There is a growing body of evidence that dynamic parameters, including pulse pressure variation and inferior vena cava (IVC) diameters, may better reflect intravascular volume, but it is unclear that the use of these lead to improved outcomes.

Hemodynamic Measurements

- **Static parameters**
  - **CVP:** An approximation of right atrial pressure and, therefore, preload. Should be measured from an internal jugular or subclavian venous catheter because readings from femoral catheters are influenced by intra-abdominal pressures and thus inaccurate. Poor relationship between CVP and blood volume,[52] but low values (<4 mm Hg) should generally lead to fluid resuscitation with careful monitoring.[53]
  - **$ScvO_2/SvO_2$:** $ScvO_2$ is a surrogate that is often used to reflect SvO_2, which is the percentage of oxygen bound to hemoglobin in blood returning to the right side of the heart. $ScvO_2$ is measured from an internal jugular or subclavian venous catheter, while a true SvO_2 must be measured with a pulmonary artery catheter (PAC). Normal values are 65%–75%. A high value often represents decreased oxygen consumption (commonly seen in mitochondrial dysfunction with sepsis), whereas low values indicate inadequate oxygen delivery (often due to low CO states such as cardiogenic shock).
  - **PACs:** A PAC catheter provides direct measurements of pressures in the right atrium, right ventricle, and pulmonary artery, as well as a pulmonary capillary wedge pressure. Previously commonly used in the management of septic shock and ARDS but did not affect mortality or morbidity.[54] CO can be measured from a PAC via thermodilution or Fick principle:
    - Thermodilution: An injectate of a known volume and temperature is injected into the PAC, and the cooled blood traverses a thermistor at the distal end of the catheter. The CO is inversely proportional to the duration of transit of cooled blood (i.e., the longer the transit time, the lower the CO).
    - Fick principle: CO is the quotient of oxygen consumption and the arteriovenous oxygen difference. To calculate CO, arterial and mixed venous blood are drawn to determine the arteriovenous oxygen difference, and oxygen consumption is determined by respiratory gas analysis or indirect calorimetry.
- **Dynamic parameters**
  - **Esophageal Doppler:** A Doppler probe is placed into the esophagus and rotated to measure blood flow through the descending aorta. The system can be used to calculate CO and stroke volume. Correlates well with CO as measured by PAC.[55] Predicts volume responsiveness in critically ill ventilated patients without spontaneous breathing.[56]
  - **Pulse pressure variation (ΔPp):** Requires arterial line placement. Calculated as the difference between maximal and minimal systolic blood pressures measured over one respiratory cycle divided by the mean of those values. ΔPp of 13% was an accurate predictor of fluid responsiveness in mechanically ventilated patients without spontaneous breathing.[57]

- **IVC distensibility index (dIVC):** Calculated as the difference between maximal and minimal IVC diameter measured over one respiratory cycle divided by the minimal IVC diameter. dIVC of 18% discriminated between volume responders and nonresponders with 90% sensitivity and specificity in mechanically ventilated patients without spontaneous breathing in one study,[58] but more recent studies have shown this method to be a poor predictor of fluid responsiveness.[59]
- **Thoracic bioreactance:** A noninvasive device is applied to the chest and measures bioreactance across the thorax using sensor pads placed on a patient's thorax surrounding their heart. Blood flow (which is predominately in the aorta in the thorax) causes phase shifts in impedance, which is detected by the sensors. From these measurements, stroke volume and CO can be estimated. There are conflicting data on the ability of thoracic bioreactance devices to reliably determine fluid responsiveness.[60,61]

Critical Care Ultrasound

The use of bedside ultrasonography has greatly expanded recently and is rapidly becoming the standard of care in ICUs. Courses in critical care ultrasonography are becoming more readily available and are necessary for complete proficiency. This section is intended to serve as an overview of basic concepts only. Critical care ultrasound should be used as an adjunct to other clinical data.

- **Basic concepts:** Air and calcified structures transmit sound waves poorly. Free-flowing fluids transmit sound waves well.
- **Basic definitions**
  - Echogenicity: The ability of an object to reflect sound waves.
  - Hyperechoic: Structures that reflect sound waves well; shows as white on ultrasound (e.g., bone, pleura, lung).
  - Hypoechoic: Containing structures that reflect sound waves poorly; shows as gray on ultrasound. Deeper structures are also more hypoechoic owing to attenuation with distance (e.g., lymph nodes, adipose tissue, muscle).
  - Anechoic: Containing structures that allow sound waves to pass through freely; shows as black on ultrasound. Examples include blood vessels, transudative pleural effusion.
- **Ultrasound to facilitate vascular access:** More detailed instructions are available in the *Washington Manual of Critical Care*, Section XIX. Use of ultrasound to guide central venous access results in increased success and reduced complication rates.
  - Location: Ultrasound guidance is most commonly used for internal jugular and femoral venous access.
  - Before starting the procedure: Both internal jugular and femoral veins should be scanned to evaluate for aberrant anatomy or venous thrombosis.
  - After applying the sterile field: The probe is positioned so that the needle is visualized for the entire duration of accessing the vessel.
  - During the procedure: Following insertion of the guidewire, the length of the vessel is scanned to ensure that the guidewire does not inadvertently enter any adjacent arteries.
  - After the procedure: Lung ultrasound can be used to rule out a pneumothorax.
- **Cardiac ultrasound:** Includes five standard views, reviewed below. Uses body transducer. Intended to facilitate assessment of volume responsiveness, global left and right ventricular systolic function, and valvular function.
  - Parasternal long axis view: Probe is placed adjacent to the sternum in the left third to fifth intercostal space with the orientation marker pointing toward the patient's right shoulder. The right ventricular outflow tract, left ventricular cavity, ascending aorta, mitral valve, and left atrium should be visualized. Assesses for pericardial effusion, left and right ventricular dysfunction, and valvular pathologies.
  - Parasternal short axis view: Probe remains adjacent to the sternum in the left third to fifth intercostal space, but orientation marker is rotated 90 degrees clockwise to point

at the patient's left shoulder. Cross-sectional view of the left and right ventricles at the level of the papillary muscles should be visualized. Assesses for pericardial effusion and left and right ventricular dysfunction.

- Apical four-chamber view: Probe is placed between the midclavicular and midaxillary lines of the left lateral chest between the fifth and seventh intercostal spaces, underneath the left nipple, with the orientation marker pointed at three o'clock. The left and right ventricles and atria, as well as the tricuspid and mitral valves, should be visualized. Assesses left and right ventricular size and function. See Figure 8-4.
- Subcostal long axis view: Probe is placed below the xiphoid process with the orientation marker pointed at three o'clock. The left and right ventricles and atria should be visualized. Assesses for pericardial effusion and left and right ventricular dysfunction. May be used for rapid assessment of cardiac function during performance of cardiopulmonary resuscitation.
- IVC longitudinal view: Probe remains below the xiphoid process, but orientation marker is rotated 90 degrees counterclockwise to point at 12 o'clock. IVC in the longitudinal axis should be visualized. Assesses IVC diameter during the respiratory cycle to determine volume responsiveness.

- **Thoracic ultrasound:** Includes four standard positions, performed bilaterally. Uses the body transducer on the abdominal setting to examine lung parenchyma; vascular transducer may be used for detailed examination of the pleura. Intended to facilitate the diagnosis of pleural effusion, pulmonary edema, pulmonary consolidation, and pneumothorax. Also used to guide a safe thoracentesis.
  - **Probe placement**: Bedside lung ultrasound in emergency (BLUE)s protocol, intended for immediate diagnosis of acute respiratory failure, defines four areas for investigation.[62] The orientation marker should be pointed toward the patient's head.
    - Upper BLUE point: Midclavicular line, second intercostal space
    - Lower BLUE point: Anterior axillary line, fourth or fifth intercostal space
    - Phrenic point: Midaxillary line, sixth or seventh intercostal space; location of the diaphragm
    - Posterolateral alveolar and/or pleural syndrome point: Posterior to the posterior axillary line, fourth or fifth intercostal space
  - **Anatomic landmarks and ultrasound appearance:** Knowledge of the normal sonographic appearance of thoracic anatomy is paramount to identifying key structures.

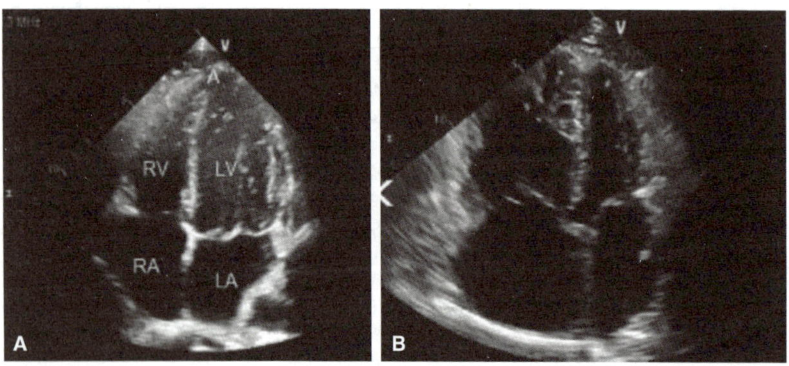

Figure 8-4 Cardiac ultrasound. Left (A): normal apical four-chamber view. A, apex; RV, right ventricle; RA, right atrium; LV, left ventricle; LA, left atrium. Right (B): demonstrates same view in a patient with right ventricular hypertrophy and dilation.

    - Chest wall: Hypoechoic, linear shadows of soft tissue density.
    - Ribs: Hyperechoic, curvilinear structures with a deep, hypoechoic, posterior acoustic shadow.
    - Pleura: Bright, hyperechoic, roughly horizontal line located approximately 0.5 cm below the rib shadows.
    - Diaphragm: Curvilinear, hyperechoic line that moves caudally with inspiration. In a seated patient, it is located caudad to the ninth rib.
    - Splenorenal and hepatorenal recesses: Should be confirmed before any procedure because its curvilinear appearance is similar to that of the diaphragm. Identified by visualization of the liver or spleen and the kidney caudally.
    - Lung: Air-filled lung appears hyperechoic due to the poor echogenicity of air. Atelectatic or consolidated lung appears hypoechoic relative to normal lung.
- **Sonographic artifacts and terminology:** A number of sonographic artifacts are caused by air–tissue interfaces, and presence or absence of these artifacts is indicative of disease.[63]
    - Pleural line: Brightly echogenic, roughly horizontal line; caused by parietopulmonary interface and indicating the lung surface.
    - A-lines: Brightly echogenic horizontal lines roughly parallel to the chest wall; caused by reverberations of the pleural line.
    - B-lines: Also called "comet tails"; a grouping within one intercostal space is called "lung rockets." Hyperechoic line arising perpendicularly from the pleural line that extends across the whole screen without fading, erasing A-lines; moves with lung slide. Caused by thickened interlobular septa or ground-glass areas; isolated B-lines are a normal variant. See Figure 8-5.
    - Lung slide: "Twinkling" movement of the pleural line that occurs with the respiratory cycle; caused by movement of the lung along the craniocaudal axis during respiration. In M-mode, lung slide is visualized as the "seashore sign," with the chest wall generating the "waves," the aerated lung forming the "sand," and the pleural line as the interface.
    - Lung pulse: Pulsation of the pleural line due to transmission of the heartbeat through noninflated lung.

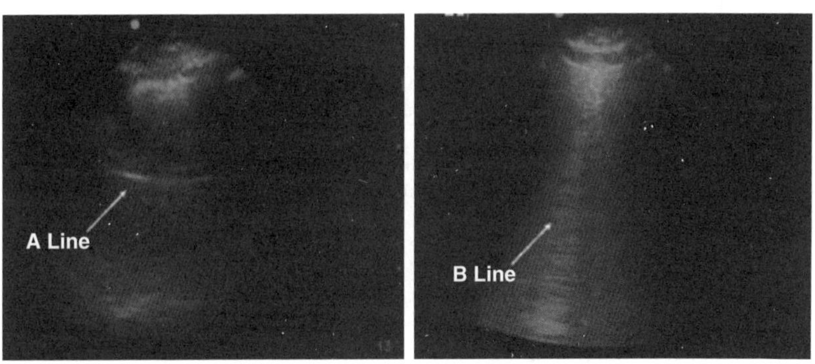

Figure 8-5 Lung ultrasound. A-lines demonstrated on left are equidistant horizontal lines created by reflections of the pleural line. B-lines demonstrated on the right are bright vertical lines that move with the pleura and extend to the bottom of the screen representing thickened fluid-filled interlobular septae.

- **Ultrasonography of lung pathology:**
  - Pleural effusion: A fluid collection bordered by the diaphragm, chest wall, and lung surface. Transudative effusions are typically anechoic; exudative effusions may have some echogenicity. If the effusion is loculated, septations—visualized as hyperechoic, weblike structures—may be seen. Atelectatic lung may be seen in the effusion.
    - Pneumothorax: Owing to air's poor echogenicity, diagnosis of pneumothorax on ultrasound is made by artifact analysis.
    - The presence of lung slide or lung pulse effectively rules out pneumothorax in the location being investigated.
    - Abolishment of lung slide has a characteristic stratosphere sign in M-mode, with loss of the "sand," but is neither sufficient nor specific for diagnosis of pneumothorax.
    - Lung point is pathognomonic for pneumothorax but has poor sensitivity. Occurs at the interface of the pneumothorax and aerated lung. Characterized by alternation between absent lung slide and present lung slide or B-lines in one location with respirations. In M-mode, it will transition between seashore sign and stratosphere sign.
  - Pneumonia: Can only be visualized when the consolidation abuts the pleura. A heterogeneous, hypoechoic area with irregular margins where aerated lung abuts the consolidated area. Air bronchograms should be seen to make the diagnosis of pneumonia.
  - Pulmonary edema: Presence of multiple B-lines within one intercostal space ("lung rockets") may indicate cardiogenic or noncardiogenic pulmonary edema. Corresponds to the Kerley B-lines seen on chest radiograph. Isolated B-lines are a normal variant.

- **Abdominal ultrasound:** Abdominal ultrasound in critical care is limited and intended to evaluate for intra-abdominal fluid and assess the urinary tract and abdominal aorta.
  - Evaluating for intra-abdominal fluid: Standard evaluation of the trauma patient who may have intra-abdominal bleeding includes the focused assessment with sonography for trauma (FAST) examination. The patient is in the supine position, and four views are obtained:
    - Hepatorenal space: The probe is placed on the right in the 10th or 11th intercostal space at the posterior axillary line with the orientation mark pointed cephalad.
    - Pelvis: The probe is placed in the suprapubic area with the orientation mark in the three o'clock position.
    - Perisplenic space: The probe is placed on the left in the 10th or 11th space at or slightly posterior to the posterior axillary line with the orientation mark pointed cephalad.
    - Pericardial space: The probe is placed in the subxiphoid position with the orientation marker in the three o'clock position.
- In the setting of trauma, an extended FAST (eFAST) examination is carried out, which involves assessing each hemithorax to rule out the presence of pneumothorax and hemothorax.
  - Paracentesis: Paracentesis should be performed under ultrasound guidance because there is evidence supporting a decrease in complications. More details can be found in the *Washington Manual for Critical Care*, Section XIX.
  - Assessment of the urinary tract: Bedside ultrasonography can identify bladder distention or hydronephrosis.
    - Bladder distention: The probe is placed in the suprapubic position with the orientation marker pointed cephalad for longitudinal dimensions and in the three o'clock position for transverse dimensions.
    - Hydronephrosis: The probe should be placed slightly caudad to the locations used for examination of the hepatorenal and perisplenic spaces in the FAST examination. Hydronephrosis is characterized by thinning of the renal cortex as the collecting system dilates.

    ◦ Assessment of the abdominal aorta: The goal is to visualize the entire abdominal aorta to ensure that its diameter from outer wall to outer wall is <3 cm. The examination begins caudad to the xiphoid process, with the probe perpendicular to the abdominal wall and the orientation marker in the three o'clock position.
- **Vascular diagnostic ultrasound:** Bedside ultrasonography may be performed to evaluate for deep vein thrombosis when clinically indicated. The target vein is visualized in the transverse plane. A vessel with normal blood flow should appear internally anechoic and should be easily compressible. Organized thrombus appears as a discrete, echogenic structure within the venous lumen. A very recently formed thrombus may be anechoic, but the vessel will be incompressible.

Summary

- The use of low-tidal-volume ventilation (LTVV), proposing a reduction in tidal volume from 10 to 6 mL/kg, is associated with improved clinical outcomes for mechanically ventilated patients.
- Treatment with an HFNC induces multiple effects, including increased oxygenation, lower respiratory rates, and reduced inspiratory effort, thus improving survival rates for patients with acute hypoxic respiratory failure.
- Antimicrobial therapy is the first pillar of sepsis/septic shock treatment.
- Vasopressors are required if a patient's MAP is <65 mm Hg despite fluid replacement.
- Balanced crystalloids are the fluid of choice in septic shock.

Scan the QR code to access chapter references.

9 Obstructive Lung Disease

Patrick R. Aguilar, Mario Castro, and Navyashree H. C.

Chronic Obstructive Pulmonary Disease

GENERAL PRINCIPLES

Definition

GOLD 2023 defines chronic obstructive pulmonary disease (COPD) as a heterogeneous lung condition characterized by chronic respiratory symptoms (dyspnea, cough, expectoration, and/or exacerbations) due to abnormalities of the airways (bronchitis, bronchiolitis) and/or alveoli (emphysema) that cause persistent, often progressive, airflow obstruction.[1]

The airflow obstruction in COPD is caused by emphysema and airway disease.

- Emphysema is defined pathologically as permanent enlargement of air spaces distal to the terminal bronchiole accompanied by destruction of the alveolar walls and absence of associated fibrosis.
- The airway disease in COPD occurs principally in small airways (i.e., those with an internal diameter of <2 mm). Located at a transitional zone between larger airways and lung interstitium, small airways may be affected in a wide variety of pathophysiological conditions.
- Chronic bronchitis is a common feature of COPD and is defined clinically as productive cough on most days for at least three consecutive months per year for at least two consecutive years, in the absence of other lung diseases that could account for this symptom. Individuals with chronic bronchitis but without airflow obstruction do not have COPD.

Epidemiology

- Although the prevalence of COPD is difficult to determine, it is estimated to affect approximately 15 million Americans.
- COPD and other chronic lower respiratory diseases represent the third leading cause of death in the United States.[2]
- In the United States, the age-adjusted mortality rate remains higher among Caucasians compared with African Americans, Hispanics, or Pacific Islanders, but rate differences between men and women have closed.
- Recent studies have found that the numbers of COPD-related cases, deaths, and DALYs increased globally from 1990 to 2019 by 86%, 30%, and 26%, respectively.
- COPD is the second leading cause of death and disability in South Asia, next only to cardiovascular diseases.
- COPD alone accounts for over 9.5% of the total deaths in India (GBD 2019 Report). Out of the chronic respiratory disease burden in India, COPD accounts for over 50% of the disease burden and 70% of the years of life lived with disability.[*]

Etiology

- Most cases of COPD are attributable to **cigarette smoking.** Although only a minority of cigarette smokers develop clinically significant COPD, a much higher proportion develop

[*] Salvi S, Ghorpade D. What is the true burden of chronic obstructive pulmonary disease in India and what are its implications at a national level? *Lung India.* 2021 Nov-Dec;38(6):503–505.

abnormal lung function.[3] However, never smokers develop airflow obstruction ~8% of the time which confirms other environmental and genetic influences in disease pathogenesis. Studies have shown that cigarette smoke (an exogenous source of reactive oxygen species) generates an imbalance of antioxidants in the body and an increase in the restriction of airflow, which together can result in a higher risk of COPD.

- **Environmental (e.g., wood-burning stoves) and occupational dusts, fumes, gases, and chemicals** are other etiologic agents of COPD. Household indoor air pollution is a major cause of fatal COPD in underdeveloped countries.[4] Women, spending more time indoors for cooking than men, are exposed to biomass fuel combustion products and are prone to develop COPD.
- The most relevant genetic risk factor for COPD identified are mutations in SERPINA1, leading to alpha-1 antitrypsin deficiency, a major circulating inhibitor of serine proteases. **α_1-Antitrypsin deficiency** is found in 1%–2% of COPD patients. Clinical characteristics of affected patients may include a minimal smoking history, early-onset COPD (e.g., younger than 45 years of age), a family history of lung disease, or lower lobe–predominant panacinar emphysema. Despite its relative rarity, some authorities recommend diagnostic testing for this condition in all patients with COPD.

Pathophysiology

- The pathogenesis of COPD involves inflammation, immune reactions, imbalance of proteinases and antiproteinases, turnover of extracellular matrix, oxidative stress, and apoptosis.
- Pathologic features include destruction of alveolar tissue and small airways, airway wall inflammation, edema and fibrosis, and intraluminal mucus.
- Pulmonary function changes include decreased maximal expiratory airflow, hyperinflation, air trapping, and alveolar gas exchange abnormalities.
- An increased incidence of osteoporosis, skeletal muscle dysfunction, and coronary artery disease (CAD) occur in COPD, perhaps indicating a systemic component of inflammation.[5]

Prevention

- **Abstinence from smoking is the most effective measure for preventing COPD.**
- In patients with COPD, smoking cessation may result in a reduction in the rate of lung function decline and improve survival.[6,7]
- Tobacco dependence warrants repeated treatment until patients stop smoking.[8] Most smokers fail initial attempts at smoking cessation, and relapse reflects the nature of the dependence and not the failure of the patient or the physician.
- A multimodality approach is recommended to optimize smoking quit rates.
  - Counseling on the preventable health risks of smoking, providing advice to stop smoking, and encouraging further attempts to stop smoking even after previous failures
  - Providing smoking cessation materials to patients
  - Prescribing pharmacotherapy (Table 9-1); providers should take every advantage to counsel and provide pharmacotherapy (including in the inpatient setting)
- Formal smoking cessation programs, often administered in a group setting, can be more effective than non–face-to-face methods.
- The US Department of Health and Human Services has developed a telephone-based support system (1-800-QUIT NOW) with an Internet analog (smokefree.gov).

DIAGNOSIS

Clinical Presentation

History

- Common symptoms are dyspnea on exertion, cough, sputum production, and wheezing.
- Typically, dyspnea on exertion progresses gradually over years.

TABLE 9-1 Pharmacotherapy for Smoking Cessation

Product	Dosing	Side Effects/Precautions
Nicotine Replacement Therapy[a]		
Transdermal patch[b]	7, 14, or 21 mg/24 h Usual regimen = 21 mg/d = 6 wk, 14 mg/d × 2 wk, 7 mg/d × 2 wk	Headache, insomnia, nightmares, nausea, dizziness, blurred vision (applies to all nicotine products)
Chewing gum, lozenges	2–4 mg q1–8h Gradually taper use	
Inhaler	10 mg/cartridge (4 mg delivered dose) 6–16 cartridges/d	
Nasal spray	0.5 mg/spray 1–2 sprays in each nostril q1h	
Nonnicotine Pharmacotherapy		
Bupropion ER (*Zyban*)	150 mg/d × 3 days, then bid × 7–12 wk Start 1 wk before quit date	Dizziness, headache, insomnia, nausea, xerostomia, hypertension, seizure Avoid monoamine oxidase inhibitors
Varenicline (*partial agonist selective for α4β2 nicotinic acetylcholine receptors*)	0.5 mg/d × 3 days, bid × 4 days, then 1 mg bid × 12–24 wk Start 1 wk before quit date	Nausea, vomiting, headache, insomnia, abnormal dreams Worsening of underlying psychiatric illness
Cytisine (partial agonist selective for α4β2 nicotinic acetylcholine receptors)	1 tablet (1.5 mg) every 2 h up to 6 tablets per day on day 1–3, later slowly tapering the number of tablets per day	Nausea, vomiting, clonic seizures, tachycardia, mydriasis, headache, fatigue, respiratory pump failure

[a]Combination therapy is often used. A long-acting product (e.g., patch) is used for basal nicotine replacement, with a short-acting product (e.g., inhaler) used for breakthrough cravings.
[b]If patient smokes less than a half pack per day, start at 14-mg dose.

- Significant nocturnal symptoms should lead to a search for comorbidities, such as gastroesophageal reflux, congestive heart failure, or sleep-disordered breathing.
- Clinicians should obtain a lifelong smoking history and quantify exposure to environmental and occupational risk factors.
- Careful assessment of severity of symptoms and frequency of COPD exacerbations is very important, as these will guide treatment choices.
- Some tools used to evaluate dyspnea and symptom severity in COPD include the COPD Assessment Tool (Table 9-2) and patient-oriented questionnaires such as the Modified (British) Medical Research Council questionnaire (Table 9-3).
- Weight loss often occurs in patients with end-stage COPD, but other etiologies, such as malignancy and depression, should be ruled out.

TABLE 9-2 Chronic Obstructive Pulmonary Disease Assessment Tool (CAT)

I never cough.	1	2	3	4	5	I cough all the time.
I have no phlegm or mucus in my chest.	1	2	3	4	5	My chest is completely full of mucus or phlegm.
My chest does not feel tight.	1	2	3	4	5	My chest feels tight.
When I walk up a hill or one flight of stairs, I am not breathless.	1	2	3	4	5	When I walk up a hill or one flight of stairs, I am very breathless.
I am not limited doing any activities at home.	1	2	3	4	5	I am limited doing activities at home.
I am confident leaving my home despite my lung condition.	1	2	3	4	5	I am not at all confident leaving my home because of my lung condition.
I sleep soundly.	1	2	3	4	5	I do not sleep soundly because of my lung condition.
I have lots of energy.	1	2	3	4	5	I have no energy at all.

Reproduced with permission from GlaxoSmithKline. GlaxoSmithKline is the copyright owner of the COPD Assessment Test (CAT).
Total score is sum of scores from individual question scales.

TABLE 9-3 Modified British Medical Research Council Questionnaire

0	I only get breathless with strenuous exercise.
1	I get short of breath when hurrying on level ground or walking up a slight hill.
2	On level ground, I walk slower than people of the same age because of breathlessness or have to stop for breath when walking at my own pace.
3	I stop for breath after walking about 100 yards or after a few minutes on level ground.
4	I am too breathless to leave the house or I am breathless when dressing.

Reprinted from Launois C, Barbe C, Bertin E, et al. The modified Medical Research Council scale for the assessment of dyspnea in daily living in obesity: a pilot study. *BMC Pulm* Med. 2012;12:61. © Launois et al.; licensee BioMed Central Ltd. 2012.

- Although dyspnea contributes predominantly to the morbidity of COPD, death in patients with COPD commonly results from cardiovascular disease, lung cancer, or non-lung cancers.[5,7]

Physical Examination

- Until significant reduction of lung function occurs (e.g., forced expiratory volume in 1 second [FEV_1] <50% predicted), physical signs of COPD are usually not present.
- Patients with severe COPD may exhibit prolonged (>6 seconds) breath sounds on a maximal forced exhalation, decreased breath sounds, use of accessory muscles of respiration, and hyperresonance to chest percussion. Expiratory wheezing may or may not be present.
- Signs of pulmonary hypertension (PH) and right-sided heart failure may be present.
- **Clubbing is not a feature of COPD**, so its presence should prompt an evaluation for other conditions, especially lung cancer.

COMORBIDITIES IN COPD (FIGURE 9-1)

- Muscle dysfunction and malnutrition in COPD: skeletal muscle weakness, general cachexia, and loss of fat-free mass.
- Cardiovascular disease: CAD, or congestive heart failure, secondary pulmonary hypertension, and ventricular dysfunction cor pulmonale.
- Normocytic anemia secondary to chronic inflammation and due to resistance to the effects of erythropoietin.
- Osteoporosis resulting in traumatic and nontraumatic fractures and vertebral compression fractures.
- Depression.
- Lung cancer: patients are three to four times more likely to develop lung cancer, with risk of small cell and squamous cell cancers being greater than that of adenocarcinomas.
- Diabetes (relative risk 1.5–1.8).
- Obstructive sleep apnea (OSA): ~20% of patients with OSA also have COPD, whereas ~10% of patients with COPD have OSA independent of disease.
- Others: stroke, cognitive decline, hypertension, GI bleed, CKD, and other cancers.

Differential Diagnosis

Airway tumors, asthma, bronchiectasis, chronic pulmonary thromboembolic disease, congestive heart failure, cystic fibrosis, constrictive bronchiolitis, diffuse panbronchiolitis, eosinophilic granuloma, ischemic heart disease, lymphangioleiomyomatosis, mycobacterial infection (tuberculous and nontuberculous), tracheobronchomalacia, and tracheal stenosis all must be considered as part of the differential in the workup of COPD.

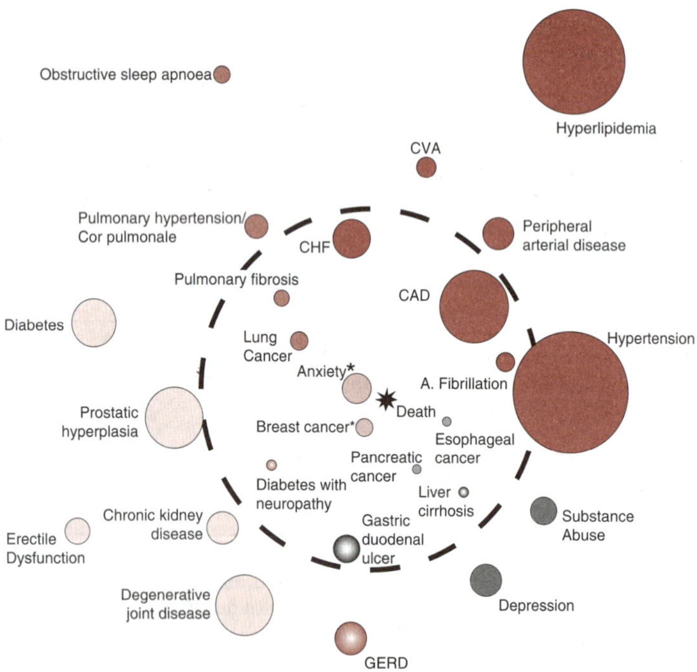

Figure 9-1 Comorbidities of COPD.

Diagnostic Testing

- Consider the diagnosis of COPD in any patient with chronic cough, dyspnea, or sputum production as well as any patient with a history of exposure to COPD risk factors, especially cigarette smoking.[1]
- **Pulmonary function testing**
  - A definite diagnosis of COPD requires the presence of expiratory airflow limitation on postbronchodilator spirometry, measured as the FEV_1/forced vital capacity (FVC) ratio, after 400 μg of albuterol/salbutamol. Although 0.7 is taken as the lower limit of normal for all adults, with advancing age, the ratio may decrease below 0.7 in individuals who are asymptomatic and have never smoked. Therefore, a reduced ratio should not be interpreted automatically as diagnostic of COPD. The FEV_1 is usually reduced.
  - The FEV_1 relative to the predicted normal defines the severity of expiratory airflow obstruction (Table 9-4) and is a predictor of mortality.
  - The FEV_1 is often used to assess the clinical course and response to therapy.
  - Spirometry may assist in the evaluation of worsened symptoms of unclear etiology.
  - The total lung capacity, functional residual capacity, and residual volume often increase to supernormal values in patients with COPD, indicating lung hyperinflation and air trapping.
  - The diffusing capacity for carbon monoxide may be reduced in patients with emphysema.
- Pre-COPD
  - This term is proposed to characterize individuals of any age who exhibit respiratory symptoms and/or other identifiable structural (e.g., emphysema) and/or functional abnormalities (e.g., hyperinflation, reduced lung diffusing capacity, or rapid FEV_1 decline) without airflow obstruction on post-bronchodilator spirometry (i.e., FEV_1/FVC >0.7)
- PRISm (preserved ratio impaired spirometry)
  - This term is proposed to describe individuals with FEV_1/FVC ≥0.7 and FEV_1 <80% of reference values after bronchodilation.

Laboratories

- A baseline arterial blood gas (ABG) is recommended for patients with severe COPD to assess for the presence and severity of hypoxemia and hypercapnia. Annual monitoring may be considered.
- Elevated venous bicarbonate may signify chronic hypercapnia.
- Polycythemia may reflect a physiologic response to chronic hypoxemia and inadequate supplemental oxygen use.

TABLE 9-4 Classification of Severity of Airflow Limitation in Chronic Obstructive Pulmonary Disease (Based on Postbronchodilator FEV_1)

In patients with FEV_1/FVC <0.70:		
GOLD 1	Mild	$FEV_1 \geq 80\%$ predicted
GOLD 2	Moderate	$50\% \leq FEV_1 < 80\%$ predicted
GOLD 3	Severe	$30\% \leq FEV_1 < 50\%$ predicted
GOLD 4	Very severe	$FEV_1 < 30\%$ predicted

Reprinted from the *Global Strategy for Diagnosis, Management, and Prevention of COPD;* 2018. © Global Initiative for Chronic Obstructive Lung Disease (GOLD), all rights reserved. Available from http://www.goldcopd.com.

FEV_1, forced expiratory volume in 1 second; FVC, forced vital capacity; GOLD, Global Initiative for Chronic Obstructive Lung Disease.

Imaging

- CXRs are not sensitive for determining the presence of COPD, but they are useful for evaluating alternative diagnoses.
- Features suggestive of emphysema include low-set flat diaphragm, translucent lung field, long and narrow heart (tubular heart), loss of peripheral vascular markings, and prominent pulmonary artery shadows at the hilum and bullae.
- Chest CT without contrast can detect emphysema and other conditions associated with tobacco smoking and COPD, especially lung cancer (see Comorbidities section). However, routine diagnostic chest CT adds little to management and is not required to exclude many alternative diagnoses, unless historical or examination findings suggest occult thromboembolic or interstitial lung disease.
- With increasing severity of COPD, patients often develop radiographic signs of thoracic hyperinflation, including flattening of the diaphragm, increased retrosternal/retrocardiac air spaces, and lung hyperlucency with diminished vascular markings. Bullae may be visible. In severe disease, chest CT is used to determine candidacy for lung volume reduction surgery (LVRS) (see Treatment: Surgical Therapy section).

TREATMENT

- Long-term management of patients with COPD aims to improve quality of life, decrease the frequency and severity of acute exacerbations, slow the progression of disease, and prolong survival.
- Of all chronic medical therapies, **smoking cessation and the correction of hypoxemia with supplemental oxygen have the best evidence for improving survival.**[7] Among surgical interventions, LVRS improves survival only in select patients.[9]
- COPD assessment should proceed in a personally tailored manner with recognition that spirometric severity, exacerbation frequency, and symptom burden may be inter-related but not entirely overlapping predictors of outcome (Table 9-5). Therapy should consider each factor and attempt to use best available evidence.
- Patients with clinical, historical, and spirometric evidence of an asthma overlap may be considered to have asthma-COPD overlap and should have treatment that addresses the predominant disease entity, e.g., if they have predominant asthma, treat as asthma; if predominant COPD, treat as COPD; and if features of both, start treatment as asthma pending further investigation.

TABLE 9-5 Refined ABCD Assessment Tool for Chronic Obstructive Lung Disease

Group	Description
A	0–1 exacerbations, no hospitalizations, minimal symptoms by mMRC or CAT
B	0–1 exacerbations, no hospitalizations, moderate to severe symptoms by mMRC or CAT
C	>2 exacerbations or >1 hospitalization, minimal symptoms by mMRC or CAT
D	>2 exacerbations or >1 hospitalization, moderate to severe symptoms by mMRC or CAT

Data from the *Global Strategy for Diagnosis, Management, and Prevention of COPD;* 2018. © Global Initiative for Chronic Obstructive Lung Disease (GOLD).
CAT, COPD Assessment Test; mMRC, Modified Medical Research Council Dyspnea Scale.
Initiative for Chronic Obstructive Lung Disease.

Gold Assessment Tool (Figure 9-2)

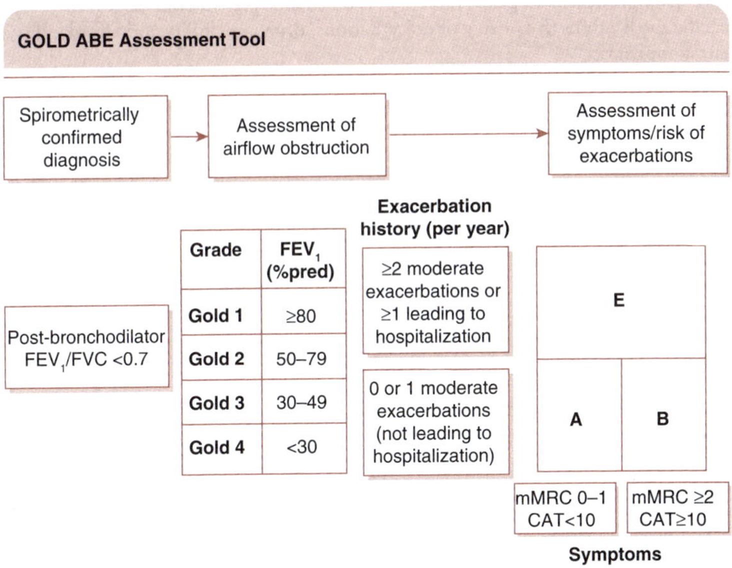

Figure 9-2 GOLD ABE assessment tool. Exacerbation history refers to exacerbations suffered the previous year. CAT, COPD assessment test; FEV$_1$, forced expiratory volume in 1 s; FVC, forced vital capacity; mMRC, modified Medical Research Council Dyspnea Questionnaire. *Source*: Global Initiative for Chronic Obstructive Lung Disease (GOLD), Global strategy for the diagnosis, management, and prevention of chronic obstructive lung disease (2023 Report). https://goldcopd.org/2023-gold-report-2/

Initial Pharmacological Treatment (Figure 9-3)

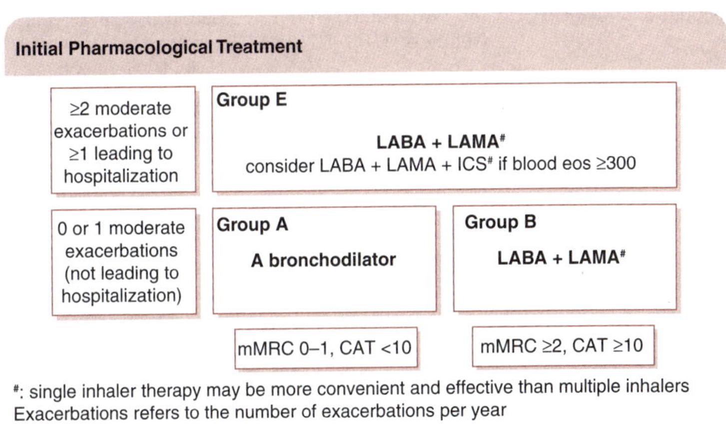

Figure 9-3 Initial pharmacological treatment. CAT, COPD assessment test; eos, eosinophils; ICS, inhaled corticosteroid; LABA, long-acting β2 receptor agonist; LAMA, long-acting anti-muscarinic antagonist; mMRC, modified Medical Research Council Dyspnea Questionnaire. *Source*: Global Initiative for Chronic Obstructive Lung Disease (GOLD), Global strategy for the diagnosis, management, and prevention of chronic obstructive lung disease (2023 Report). https://goldcopd.org/2023-gold-report-2/

Medications

A pharmacologic treatment plan (Table 9-6) is based on a patient's disease severity, response to specific medications, frequency of exacerbations, drug availability and affordability, and patient compliance.

- **Inhaled bronchodilators**
  - Inhaled bronchodilators are the foundation of COPD pharmacotherapy. They work mainly by relaxing airway smooth muscle tone. This results in a reduction in expiratory airflow obstruction.
  - Proper use of a metered-dose inhaler (MDI) results in equally effective drug delivery as use of a nebulizer in most patients. Health-care providers should routinely assess a patient's MDI technique and provide training.
  - Long-acting inhaled anticholinergic agents result in significant improvements in lung function, quality of life, and COPD exacerbations, although the rate of decline of FEV_1 is unaffected.[10]
  - Long-acting β-adrenergic agonists (LABAs) offer improvements that are at least similar to long-acting anticholinergic agents and inhaled corticosteroids (ICSs).[11]
- **ICSs**
  - The rationale for using ICSs stems from the central role of inflammation in the pathogenesis of COPD.

TABLE 9-6 Inhalational Pharmacotherapy for Stable Chronic Obstructive Pulmonary Disease[a]

Name	Dose	Side Effects[b]
Short-Acting β-Agonists		
Albuterol	MDI: two puffs q4–6h Nebulizer: 2.5 mg q6–8h	Palpitations, tremor, anxiety, nausea/vomiting, throat irritation, dyspepsia, tachycardia, arrhythmia, hypertension
Levalbuterol *(Xopenex)*	MDI: two puffs q4–6h Nebulizer: 0.63–1.25 mg q6–8h	Cardiovascular effects may be less common with levalbuterol
Long-Acting β-Agonists		
Salmeterol *(Serevent Diskus)*	DPI: one inhalation (50 μg) bid	Headache, upper respiratory tract infection, cough, palpitations, fatigue, diarrhea
Formoterol *(Foradil)*	DPI: one capsule (12 μg) bid	
Arformoterol *(Brovana)*	Nebulizer: 15 μg bid	
Indacaterol[c] *(Arcapta)*	DPI: one capsule (75 μg) daily	
Anticholinergics[d]		
Ipratropium *(Atrovent)*	MDI: two puffs q4–6h Nebulizer: 0.5 mg q6–8h	Xerostomia, cough, nausea/vomiting, diarrhea, urinary retention
Tiotropium *(Spiriva)*	DPI: one puff (18 μg) daily	
Aclidinium *(Tudorza)*	DPI: one puff (400 μg) bid	

(Continued)

TABLE 9-6 Inhalational Pharmacotherapy for Stable Chronic Obstructive Pulmonary Disease[a] (Continued)

Name	Dose	Side Effects[b]
Fixed Combination Medications		
Albuterol/Ipratropium *(Combivent Respimat, DuoNeb)*	Inhalational spray: one spray qid Nebulizer: one 3-mL vial qid (each vial contains 2.5 mg albuterol and 0.5 mg ipratropium)	As above for each individual medication class (anticholinergic, β-agonist)
Fluticasone/Salmeterol *(Advair)*	DPI: one puff bid Recommended dose is 250 μg fluticasone/50 μg salmeterol Reduced exacerbations seen with 500/50 μg dose	As above, plus lower respiratory tract infection (pneumonia) and oral candidiasis
Budesonide/Formoterol *(Symbicort)*	DPI: two puffs bid 160 μg budesonide/4 μg formoterol	
Umeclidinium/Vilanterol *(Anoro)*	DPI: one puff daily 62.5 μg umeclidinium/25 μg vilanterol	As above for each individual medication class

[a]Commonly used medications are listed. This table is not exhaustive.
[b]Only the most common side effects are listed.
[c]Indacaterol dosage approved in United States is lower than in other countries including Canada.
[d]Short-acting anticholinergic therapy (e.g., ipratropium) is usually discontinued with initiation of long-acting anticholinergic therapy (e.g., tiotropium), because minimal additional benefit is expected, side effects may increase, and use of two inhaled anticholinergic agents has had limited evaluation.
DPI, dry powder inhaler; MDI, metered-dose inhaler.

- ICSs may increase the FEV_1, reduce the frequency of COPD exacerbations, and improve quality of life. They do not slow the rate of decline of lung function over time.
- Adding ICS has little or no effect at a blood eosinophil count <100 cells·μL−1 whilst blood eosinophils ≥300 cells·μL−1 identify patients with a strong likelihood of treatment benefit.

- **Combination therapy:** The GOLD committee's ABE classification should be used to guide therapy. Patients who fall into group A should be offered an intermittent short-acting bronchodilator and assessed for effect before a long-acting agent is added. In contrast, for patients in Group B, a combination of dual long-acting bronchodilator combination (β2 adrenergic [LABA] + anti-muscarinic [LAMA] bronchodilators) is now recommended, as dual therapy is more effective than monotherapy with similar side effects. Similarly, for patients in Group E, LAMA + LABA is the recommended initial therapy, except for those patients with blood eosinophils ≥300 cells·μL1, for whom starting triple therapy (LABA + LAMA + inhaled corticosteroid [ICS]) can be considered.

Compared to single-agent therapy, a combination of medications may yield superior efficacy while reducing the potential for toxicity. Some examples follow:
  - The combination of an ICS and a LABA is effective in reducing the rate of COPD exacerbations, but this benefit must be balanced against an increased risk of pneumonia.[12]
  - Combination therapy with a LABA and a long-acting anticholinergic agent sustains improved lung function compared to either agent alone.[13]
  - Fixed-dose, long-acting combination therapies improve lung function better than either preparation alone, but data on symptom and exacerbation reduction are limited.[14]
  - Questions remain regarding the value of the incremental gains of adding long-acting anticholinergic therapy to LABA/ICS combinations, suggesting a stepwise approach with individualized therapy based on symptoms, side effects, and exacerbation frequency.[15]
  - Some studies have demonstrated good tolerance of ICS withdrawal in COPD patients treated with single dose–inhaled combinations of a LABA, anticholinergic, and ICS while others have demonstrated an improvement in exacerbation frequency with continuation of triple therapy.[16,17]
- **Macrolide antibiotics** (e.g., azithromycin 250 mg daily)
  - It may function as an anti-infective or direct anti-inflammatory in COPD.
  - In patients with previous exacerbations, the frequency of subsequent exacerbations decreased by 19%; however, improvement in clinical symptoms was modest.[18]
  - The benefit may be absent in current smokers and greater in older individuals (>65 years) and those with milder disease (FEV_1 >50%).
  - Hearing loss in the absence of tinnitus was reported, suggesting routine monitoring with audiometry should be considered with chronic therapy.
- **Phosphodiesterase-4 (PDE4) inhibitors** (e.g., roflumilast 500 μg daily)
  - The US Food and Drug Administration (FDA) approved for a relatively narrow indication of severe COPD (FEV_1 <50%) and chronic bronchitis with frequent exacerbations, demonstrating a 17% reduction in exacerbations.[19]
  - It appears to be safe when used as additional therapy to chronic bronchodilators.
  - It did not result in improvements in clinical symptoms possibly due to a higher frequency of side effects, particularly gastrointestinal, which limit the dose tolerated.
  - Limited long-term data and the possibility of weight loss and increased psychiatric symptoms suggest close monitoring is indicated.
- **Theophylline**
  - Theophylline is a xanthine derivative with bronchodilator properties. Patients not responding adequately to inhaled bronchodilator therapy may benefit from the addition of theophylline, but potential toxicities and lack of data regarding efficacy in patients already on long-acting inhaled combination therapies limit its use.
  - Patients with severe COPD may experience clinical deterioration with discontinuation of theophylline.
  - Theophylline clearance is increased in current smokers and reduced in the elderly and patients with liver disease or congestive heart failure.
- **Systemic corticosteroids** are not recommended for the long-term management of COPD owing to an unfavorable side effect profile and limited efficacy. However, they are sometimes used in patients with severe disease who are not responding to other therapies. If used, chronic oral steroid therapy should be administered at the minimum effective dose and discontinued as soon as is feasible. Routine bone mineral density assessment to prevent complications of osteoporosis should be incorporated.
- **IV α_1-antitrypsin (A1AT)** augmentation therapy may benefit select patients with severe A1AT deficiency and COPD.[20] Weekly infusion of 60 mg/kg is the standard treatment.
- For the treatment of stable COPD, antibiotics, mucolytics, antioxidants, immunoregulators, antitussives, vasodilators, respiratory stimulants, narcotics, and leukotriene inhibitors have not shown significant benefit.

Other Nonpharmacologic Therapies

- **Supplemental oxygen** has utility in patients with significant desaturation or those who have other comorbid lung disease.
  - A room-air resting ABG is the gold standard test for determining the need for supplemental oxygen. Pulse oximetry may be useful for routine checks after a baseline oxyhemoglobin saturation is assessed and compared for accuracy with the measured arterial oxyhemoglobin saturation (SaO_2).
  - A large randomized trial demonstrated that among patients with stable COPD and moderate resting or exertional desaturations, supplemental oxygen did not improve functional capacity, decrease hospitalizations, or reduce mortality.[21] Patients with comorbid fibrotic lung disease, those with significant PH, and those with more significant desaturation should continue to receive supplemental oxygen with a goal SpO_2 around 92%.
  - Supplemental oxygen requirements are typically greatest during exertion and least at rest while awake. Patients who require supplemental oxygen during exertion often need it during sleep as well. It is reasonable to initially estimate the amount of oxygen needed by setting the oxygen flow rate at 1 L/min greater than that required during rest while awake. Formal nocturnal oximetry should be performed to validate this dose. Patients with significant nocturnal desaturation or those who have symptoms of sleep apnea should undergo polysomnography.
- **Noninvasive ventilation** in combination with oxygen therapy has been shown to delay the median time to readmission or death in patients with persistent hypercapnia ($PaCO_2$ >53 mm Hg).[22]
- **Pulmonary rehabilitation** is a multidisciplinary intervention that improves symptoms and quality of life and reduces the frequency of exacerbations in patients with COPD. Components of a rehabilitation program include exercise training, nutritional counseling, and psychosocial support. Pulmonary rehabilitation should be considered for all patients with moderate to severe COPD.[23]
- **Vaccinations**
  - Annual influenza vaccination reduces the incidence of influenza-related acute respiratory illnesses in COPD patients.
  - Data supporting the use of pneumococcal vaccine in patients with COPD have been contradictory though a recent Cochrane review demonstrated a reduction in acute exacerbations.[24] Given the suggested benefits and the low likelihood of harm, pneumococcal vaccination (both PCV13 and PPSV23) should be part of the routine care of patients with COPD.
  - The WHO and CDC recommend SARS-CoV-2 vaccination for people with COPD (GOLD 2024).[46]

Surgical Therapy

- **Lung transplantation** for severe COPD can improve quality of life and functional capacity. The data are conflicting regarding survival, and a consistent survival benefit has not been demonstrated. Selection criteria for transplantation for COPD patients includes using estimates of survival likelihood without transplantation such as the BODE index (see Outcomes/Prognosis) as well as symptom burden and exacerbation frequency.
- **Surgical LVRS** may provide quality of life and survival benefits in a specific subset of patients with upper lobe–predominant emphysema and significantly reduced exercise capacity.[9] Further data are needed in defining the optimal patient population for bronchoscopic lung volume reduction.

SPECIAL CONSIDERATIONS

Interventions That Reduce the Frequency of COPD Exacerbations

Bronchodilators (LABAs, LAMAs, LABA + LAMA), corticosteroid-containing regimens (LABA + ICS, LABA + LAMA + ICS), anti-inflammatory (roflumilast), anti-infectives (vaccines, long-term macrolides), mucoregulators (N-acetylcysteine, carbocysteine, erdosteine), and others (smoking cessation, rehabilitation, LVRS, vitamin D, shielding measures such as mask wearing, minimizing social contact, and frequent handwashing).[46]

Acute Exacerbation of Chronic Obstructive Pulmonary Disease

- GOLD 2023 has adopted the recent consensus of the Rome proposal which defines ECOPD as: "an event characterized by dyspnea and/or cough and sputum that worsen over ≤14 days, which may be accompanied by tachypnea and/or tachycardia and is often associated with increased local and systemic inflammation caused by airway infection, pollution, or other insult to the airways."
- Patients with two or more exacerbations per year are classified as "**frequent exacerbators.**"
- Respiratory infections (viral and bacterial) and air pollution cause most exacerbations.[25]
- The differential diagnosis includes pneumothorax, pneumonia, pleural effusion, congestive heart failure, cardiac ischemia, and pulmonary embolism. These conditions may mimic and/or aggravate exacerbations and have to be treated if identified.
- In addition to the history and physical examination, assessment of a patient with a suspected COPD exacerbation should include oxyhemoglobin saturation, ABG, ECG, and CXR.
- Criteria for hospital admission include a significant increase in symptom severity, severe underlying COPD, significant comorbidities, failure to respond to initial medical management, diagnostic uncertainty, and insufficient home support.[1]
- Criteria for admission to an intensive care unit include the need for invasive mechanical ventilation, hemodynamic instability, severe dyspnea that does not adequately respond to therapy, mental status changes, and persistent or worsening hypoxemia, hypercapnia, or respiratory acidosis despite supplemental oxygen and noninvasive ventilation.[1]
- **Pharmacotherapy** (Table 9-7; Figure 9-4)
  - **Short-acting β-agonists (SABAs) are the first-line therapy for COPD exacerbations.** Short-acting anticholinergic agents can be added in the event of inadequate response to SABAs.
  - Many patients experiencing an acute exacerbation of COPD have difficulty performing optimal MDI technique. Therefore, numerous clinicians opt to deliver bronchodilators via nebulization.
  - Long-acting bronchodilators should be considered once stable.
  - Owing to the risk of serious side effects, clinicians typically avoid using methylxanthines (e.g., theophylline) for acute exacerbations. However, if a patient uses methylxanthines chronically, discontinuation during an exacerbation is discouraged because of the risk of decompensation.
  - **Systemic corticosteroids** produce improvement in hospital length of stay, lung function, and the incidence of relapse. They are recommended for all inpatients and most outpatients experiencing an exacerbation of COPD. A prednisone dose of 40 mg for 5 days is recommended over longer regimens.[27]
  - **Antibiotic therapy** is routinely administered but most often benefits patients with sputum purulence as well as patients with a need for mechanical ventilation. Duration of therapy should be 5–7 days.
- **Supplemental oxygen** should be administered with a target oxygen saturation of 88%–92%.
- **Thromboprophylactic measures** should be used given the increased risk of deep venous thrombosis in patients hospitalized for COPD exacerbation.[28]

TABLE 9-7 Pharmacotherapy for Acute Exacerbations of Chronic Obstructive Pulmonary Disease

Medication Name	Dose	
Albuterol	MDI: two to four puffs q1–4h Nebulizer: 2.5 mg q1–4h	
Ipratropium	MDI: two puffs q4h Nebulizer: 0.5 mg q4h	
Prednisone	40 mg/d × 5 days	
Antibiotics[a]		
Patient Characteristics	Pathogens to Consider	Antibiotic[b] (One of the Following)
No risk factors for poor outcome or drug-resistant pathogen[c]	*Haemophilus influenzae* *Streptococcus pneumoniae* *Moraxella catarrhalis*	Macrolide, second- or third-generation cephalosporin, doxycycline, trimethoprim/sulfamethoxazole
Risk factors present	As above, plus gram-negative rods, including *Pseudomonas*	Antipseudomonal fluoroquinolone or β-lactam

[a]Indicated for all inpatients and most outpatients. Dosing recommendation from Global Strategy for Diagnosis, Management, and Prevention of COPD, 2018, © Global Initiative for Chronic Obstructive Lung Disease (GOLD).[1]

[b]Treat for 3–7 days. If recent antibiotic exposure, select an agent from an alternative class. Take local resistance patterns into account.

[c]Risk factors: age >65 years, comorbid conditions (especially cardiac disease), forced expiratory volume in 1 second (FEV_1) <50%, more than three exacerbations/year, antibiotic therapy within the past 3 months.[26]

MDI, metered-dose inhaler.

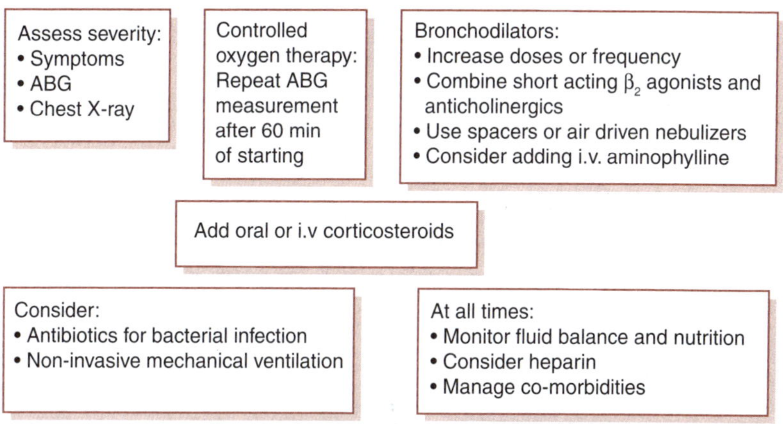

Figure 9-4 Stepwise management of acute exacerbation of COPD.*

*Rodriguez-Roisin R, Lloyd-Owen S, Wedzicha JA, et al. Exacerbations of COPD. Timely Topics in Medicine, Prous Science; 2003.

- **Noninvasive ventilation** (Table 9-8) should be considered the first mode of ventilator support as it reduces intubation rate, improves respiratory acidosis, decreases respiratory rate, and decreases hospital length of stay.[29]
- **Endotracheal intubation** and invasive mechanical ventilation are required in some patients (Table 9-9).
- Discharge criteria for patients with acute exacerbations of COPD include the need for inhaled bronchodilators less frequently than every 4 hours; clinical and ABG stability for at least 12–24 hours; the ability to eat, sleep, and ambulate fairly comfortably; adequate patient understanding of home therapy; and adequate home arrangements. Before discharging from the hospital, chronic therapy issues should be readdressed, including supplemental oxygen requirements, vaccinations, smoking cessation, assessment of inhaler technique, and pulmonary rehabilitation.

Management of Patients with COPD and Suspected or Proven Covid-19

Swab/saliva PCR, if new or worsening symptoms, consider CT for COVID pneumonia, assess for coinfection, and avoid bronchoscopy unless essential.

TABLE 9-8 Indications and Contraindications for Noninvasive Ventilation in Acute Exacerbations of Chronic Obstructive Pulmonary Disease

Indications	Contraindications
Moderate to severe dyspnea with evidence of increased work of breathing	Respiratory arrest Hemodynamic instability Altered mental status, inability to cooperate
Acute respiratory acidosis with pH ≤7.35 and/or $PaCO_2$ >45 mm Hg (6 kPa)	High risk of aspiration Viscous or copious secretions Recent facial or gastroesophageal surgery
Respiratory rate >25	Craniofacial trauma Fixed nasopharyngeal abnormalities Burns Extreme obesity

Data from the *Global Strategy for Diagnosis, Management, and Prevention of COPD;* 2018. © Global Initiative for Chronic Obstructive Lung Disease (GOLD).

TABLE 9-9 Indications for Invasive Mechanical Ventilation in Acute Exacerbations of Chronic Obstructive Pulmonary Disease

Failure to improve with or not a candidate for noninvasive ventilation (see Table 9-8
Severe dyspnea with evidence of increased work of breathing
Acute respiratory acidosis with pH <7.25 and/or $PaCO_2$ >60 mm Hg (8 kPa)
PaO_2 <40 mm Hg (5.3 kPa)
Respiratory rate >35
Coexisting conditions such as cardiovascular disease, metabolic abnormalities, sepsis, pneumonia, pulmonary embolism, pneumothorax, large pleural effusion

Data from the *Global Strategy for Diagnosis, Management, and Prevention of COPD;* 2018. © Global Initiative for Chronic Obstructive Lung Disease (GOLD).

Continue maintenance therapy unchanged, including ICS, and use antibiotics and oral steroids in line with recommendations for exacerbations. Use antivirals, corticosteroids, and immunomodulator therapy. Use HFNC or NIV for respiratory failure and mechanical ventilation if they fail. Maintain physical distance and wear a mask.

COMPLICATIONS OF COPD (TABLE 9-10)

- Annual low-dose CT screening of asymptomatic heavy smokers (age >55 years, >30 pack-year history) provides a 20% reduction in mortality from lung cancer. This must be balanced with the risk of invasive procedures from false-positive tests that were seen in approximately 40% of screened individuals.[30] In the largest screening trial, the majority of false-positive results could be resolved with repeat imaging.
- Many patients with mild and moderate (GOLD stage I/II) COPD will die of cardiovascular disease. Therefore, cardioselective β-blockers should be used when indicated.
- Osteoporosis, multimorbidity, frailty, and vitamin D deficiency are common in COPD and should be monitored and treated.

OUTCOME/PROGNOSIS

The **BODE index** is a composite of body mass index, airflow obstruction, dyspnea, and exercise tolerance that has been validated as a more accurate predictor of COPD mortality than FEV_1 alone.[31] It can be useful in predicting survival after LVRS. A reduced BODE score index postoperatively has been associated with reduced mortality.

Asthma

GENERAL PRINCIPLES

Definition

- Asthma is a heterogeneous airway disease characterized by chronic inflammation, hyperresponsiveness with exposure to a wide variety of stimuli, and variable airflow obstruction. As a consequence, patients have paroxysms of cough, dyspnea, chest tightness, and wheezing.
- **Asthma is a chronic disease with episodic acute exacerbations that are interspersed with periods of symptomatic variability.** Exacerbations are characterized by a progressive increase in asthma symptoms that can last minutes to hours. They are associated with viral infections, allergens, and occupational exposures, and occur when airway reactivity is increased and lung function becomes unstable.
- A clinical diagnosis of asthma should be suspected in the presence of recurrent/episodic wheezing, breathlessness, cough, and/or chest tightness with no alternative explanation for these symptoms.

TABLE 9-10 Complications of COPD

Acute	Chronic
Type 1 respiratory failure	Type 2 respiratory failure
Exacerbation	Cor pulmonale—right heart failure
Pneumonia	Polycythemia
Pneumothorax	Arrhythmias (atrial fibrillation, multifocal atrial tachycardia)
Pulmonary embolism	Lung cancer

Classification

- Asthma severity should be classified based on both level of impairment (symptoms, lung function, daily activities, and rescue medication use) and risk (exacerbations, lung function decline, and medication side effects).
- At the initial evaluation, this assessment will determine the level of severity in patients not on controller medications (Table 9-11). The level of severity is based on the most severe category in which any feature appears. On subsequent visits, or if the patient is on a controller medication, this assessment is based on the lowest step of therapy to maintain clinical control (Table 9-12). Control of asthma is based on the most severe impairment or risk category.
- During an exacerbation, the acute severity of the attack should be classified based on symptoms, signs, and objective measures of lung function (Table 9-13).
- Patients who have had two or more exacerbations requiring systemic corticosteroids in the past year may be considered in the same category as those who have persistent asthma, regardless of level of impairment.

Epidemiology

In the United States:

- Asthma is a highly prevalent problem, affecting 8.3% of American adults and children.[33]
- The prevalence of asthma is highest among black children, with 15.7% of that population carrying the diagnosis.
- The recent Global Burden of Disease (GBD, 1990–2019) estimated the total burden of asthma in India as 34.3 million, accounting for 13.09% of the global burden. Asthma accounted for 27.9% of disability-adjusted life years (DALYs) in the Indian population.[34]

Etiology

Possible factors for asthma development can be broadly divided into host, genetic, and environmental factors.

- There have been multiple genes, chromosomal regions, and epigenetic changes associated with the development of asthma. Racial and ethnic differences have also been reported in asthma and are likely the result of a complex interaction between genetic, socioeconomic, and environmental factors.
- There are multiple environmental factors that contribute to the development and persistence of asthma. Severe viral infections early in life, particularly respiratory syncytial virus and rhinovirus, are associated with the development of asthma in childhood and play a role in its pathogenesis.
- Childhood exposure and sensitization to a variety of allergens and irritants (e.g., cigarette smoke, mold, pet dander, dust mites, cockroaches) may play a role in the development of asthma, but the exact nature of this relationship is not yet fully elucidated. By contrast, early-life exposure to indoor allergens together with certain bacteria (microbiome) may be protective for urban children. The prevalence of asthma in children raised in a rural setting is reduced, although the reason for this is not fully known.

Pathophysiology

Asthma is characterized by airway obstruction, hyperinflation, and airflow limitation resulting from multiple processes:

- Acute and chronic airway inflammation characterized by infiltration of the airway wall, mucosa, and lumen by activated eosinophils, mast cells, macrophages, and T lymphocytes. Components of innate immunity including natural killer T cells, neutrophils, and innate lymphoid lymphocytes are also implicated.

TABLE 9-11 Classification of Asthma Severity on Initial Assessment[32]

Components of Severity		Classification of Asthma Severity ≥12 years of age			
			Persistent		
		Intermittent	Mild	Moderate	Severe
Impairment **Normal FEV_1/FVC:** **8–19 yr 85%** **20–39 yr 80%** **40–59 yr 75%** **60–80 yr 70%**	Symptoms	≤2 days/week	>2 days/week but not daily	Daily	Throughout the day
	Nighttime awakenings	≤2x/month	3–4x/month	>1x/week but not nightly	Often 7x/week
	Short-acting $beta_2$-agonist use for symptom control (not prevention of EIB)	≤2 days/week	>2 days/week but not daily, and not more than 1x on any day	Daily	Several times per day
	Interference with normal activity	None	Minor limitation	Some limitation	Extremely limited
	Lung function	• Normal FEV_1 between exacerbations • FEV_1 >80% predicted • FEV_1/FVC normal	• FEV_1 >80% predicted • FEV_1/FVC normal	• FEV_1 >60% but <80% predicted • FEV_1/FVC reduced 5%	• FEV_1 >60% predicted • FEV_1/FVC reduced >5%
Risk	**Exacerbations requiring oral systemic corticosteroids**	**0–1/year (see note)**	**≥2/year (see note)** →		
		← **Consider severity and interval since last exacerbation.** → **Frequency and severity may fluctuate over time for patients in any severity category.**			
		Relative annual risk of exacerbations may be related to FEV_1.			
Recommended Step for Initiating Treatment **(See Figure 4-5 for treatment steps.)**		**Step 1**	**Step 2**	**Step 3**	**Step 4 or 5**
				and consider a short course of oral systemic corticosteroids	
		In 2–6 weeks, evaluate level of asthma control that is achieved and adjust therapy accordingly.			

TABLE 9-12 Assessment of Asthma Control

	Well Controlled	Not Well Controlled	Very Poorly Controlled
Daytime symptoms	≤2 d/wk	>2 d/wk	Throughout the day
Nighttime symptoms	None	1–3×/wk	≥4×/wk
Activity limitations	None	Some	Extreme
Reliever medicine use	≤2×/wk	>2×/wk	Frequent
FEV_1 or PEF	≥80%	60%–80%	<60%
Validated questionnaire	ACT ≥20 ACQ <0.75	ACT 16–19 ACQ >1.5	ACT ≤15
Exacerbations	0–1/yr	≥2×/yr	≥2×/yr
Management	Maintain at lowest step possible Consider step down if well controlled for ≥3 mo	Step up one step	Step up one to two steps and consider short-course OCS
Follow-up	1–6 mo	2–6 wk	2 wk

Data from the *2020 GINA Report: Global Strategy for Asthma Management and Prevention.* Global Initiative for Asthma – GINA.

ACT, Asthma Control Test; ACQ, Asthma Control Questionnaire; FEV_1, forced expiratory volume in 1 second; OCS, oral corticosteroids PEF, peak expiratory flow.

TABLE 9-13 Classification of Asthma Exacerbation Severity

	Moderate	Severe	Impending Respiratory Arrest
FEV_1 or PEF predicted or personal best	40%–69%	<40%	<25% or unable to measure
Symptoms	DOE or SOB with talking	SOB at rest	Severe SOB
Exam	Expiratory wheeze Some accessory muscle use	Inspiratory and expiratory wheeze Increased accessory muscle use Chest retraction Agitation or confusion	Wheeze may become absent Accessory muscle use with paradoxical thoracoabdominal movement Depressed mental status
Vitals	RR <28/min HR <110 bpm O_2sat >91% RA No pulsus paradoxus	RR >28/min HR >110 bpm O_2sat <91% RA Pulsus paradoxus >25 mm Hg	Same as severe but could develop respiratory depression and/or bradycardia

(*Continued*)

TABLE 9-13	Classification of Asthma Exacerbation Severity (Continued)		
	Moderate	Severe	Impending Respiratory Arrest
$PaCO_2$	Normal to hypocapnia	>42 mm Hg	Hypercapnia is a late sign

Data from the *2020 GINA Report: Global Strategy for Asthma Management and Prevention.* DOE, dyspnea on exertion; FEV_1, forced expiratory volume in 1 second; HR, heart rate; O_2sat, oxygen saturation; PEF, peak expiratory flow; RA, room air; RR, respiratory rate; SOB, shortness of breath.

- Bronchial smooth muscle contraction resulting from mediators released by a variety of cell types including inflammatory, local neural, and epithelial cells.
- Epithelial damage manifested by denudation and desquamation of the epithelium leading to mucous plugs that obstruct the airway.
- Airway remodeling characterized by the following findings:
  - Subepithelial fibrosis, specifically thickening of the lamina reticularis from collagen deposition
  - Smooth muscle hypertrophy and hyperplasia
  - Goblet cell and submucosal gland hypertrophy and hyperplasia resulting in mucous hypersecretion
  - Airway angiogenesis
  - Airway wall thickening due to edema and cellular infiltration

Asthma Phenotypes

- **Type 2 Inflammation (Th2 high) asthma:** This is the most common type and includes 40%–70% of asthma patients. It is defined by sputum eosinophilia of ≥2% of leukocytes in a sample. Other ways to confirm the presence of type 2 inflammation are blood eosinophilia of 150/microliter and fractional exhaled nitric oxide (FeNO) 20 ppb. It has three distinct phenotypes, namely early onset allergic phenotype, late onset allergic phenotype, and aspirin-exacerbated respiratory disease (AERD) phenotype.
- **Non-Type 2 (Th2 low) asthma:** This can further be subdivided into 2 types:
  - Neutrophilic phenotype: Neutrophils of >40% of leukocytes in an induced sputum.
  - Pauci-granulocytic
- **Mixed type 2-high and type 2-low (granulocytic) asthma:** This type has features of both eosinophilic and neutrophilic inflammation, including their cytokines profile.

Risk Factors

A number of factors increase airway hyperresponsiveness and can cause an acute and chronic increase in the severity of the disease:

- Allergens such as dust mites, cockroaches, pollens, molds, and pet dander in susceptible patients.
- Viral upper respiratory tract infections.
- Many occupational allergens and irritants such as perfumes, cleaners, or detergents, even in small doses.
- Changes in weather (i.e., from warm to cold), strong emotional stimuli, and exercise.
- Indoor and outdoor pollutants, such as nitrogen dioxide (NO_2) and tobacco and wood smoke, can trigger acute bronchospasm and should be avoided by all patients.
- Obesity is associated with increased asthma severity.
- Medications such as β-blockers (including ophthalmic preparations), aspirin, and NSAIDs can cause the sudden onset of severe airway obstruction.

Prevention

- Strict compliance and appropriate follow-up can help prevent worsening of asthma control.
- Identification and avoidance of risk factors (allergens, irritants) that exacerbate symptoms play a key role in prevention.
- Recognition and management of comorbidities such as obesity, sinonasal diseases, gastroesophageal reflux disease (GERD), and psychiatric disorders are important.
- All patients with asthma should receive a yearly influenza vaccination.

Associated Conditions

- **Rhinosinusitis**, with or without nasal polyps, is frequently present and should be treated with intranasal or oral corticosteroids, saline rinses, and/or antihistamines. Antibiotics should be reserved for superimposed bacterial infections.
- **Vocal cord dysfunction (VCD)** can coexist with or masquerade severe, uncontrolled asthma. Diagnosis often requires provocation testing with laryngoscopy, otherwise the findings are often normal. Treatment consists of speech and, if needed, behavioral therapy.
- **Symptomatic GERD** can cause cough and wheezing in some patients and may benefit from treatment with H_2 blockers or proton pump inhibitors. Empiric treatment of GERD in asymptomatic patients with uncontrolled asthma is not an effective strategy.
- **Obesity** is increasingly being recognized as a comorbid condition as well as possibly playing a role in worsening asthma control. This may be related to altered lung mechanics, altered respiratory patterns, or an increase in systemic inflammation. Obese patients should be strongly encouraged to focus on weight loss through diet and exercise.
- Smoking prevalence in patients with asthma is the same as the general population. Although no convincing evidence links tobacco use with developing asthma, it may make patients less responsive to ICSs and more difficult to control. Tobacco cessation should be encouraged in all patients.
- OSA may make asthma more difficult to control and should be addressed with an overnight polysomnogram if suspected.

DIAGNOSIS

Clinical Presentation

History

- Recurring episodes of cough, dyspnea, chest tightness, and wheezing are suggestive of asthma. Symptoms are often worse at night or early morning, in the presence of potential triggers, and/or in a seasonal pattern.
- A personal or family history of atopy can increase the likelihood of asthma.
- Patients over 50 years old presenting for the first time, patients with >20 pack-years of smoking, and lack of response to asthma therapy are features that make asthma less likely as the sole cause of respiratory symptoms.

Physical Examination

- Auscultation of wheezing and a prolonged expiratory phase can be present on examination, but a normal chest examination does not exclude asthma.
- Signs of atopy, such as eczema, rhinitis, or nasal polyps, often coexist with asthma. The presence of nasal polyps should prompt questioning regarding the possibility of aspirin-exacerbated respiratory disease (AERD).
- During a suspected asthma exacerbation, a rapid assessment should be performed to identify patients who require immediate intervention (see Table 9-13).
    - Respiratory distress and/or peak expiratory flow (PEF) <25% of predicted.

- The presence or intensity of wheezing is an unreliable indicator of the severity of an attack.
- SC emphysema should alert the examiner to the presence of a pneumothorax or pneumomediastinum.

Diagnostic Criteria

- In general, the diagnosis is supported by the presence of symptoms consistent with asthma combined with demonstration of variable expiratory airflow obstruction.
- Adequate response to asthma treatment is a valid method to assist with making the diagnosis.

Differential Diagnosis

Other conditions may present with wheezing and must be considered, especially in patients who are not responsive to therapy (Table 9-14).

Diagnostic Testing

Laboratories

- Although laboratory analysis is not necessary for the diagnosis, a complete blood count with cellular differential should be obtained to assist with clinical phenotyping (i.e., to

TABLE 9-14 Conditions That Can Present as Refractory Asthma

Upper Airway Obstruction
Tumor
Epiglottitis
Vocal cord dysfunction
Obstructive sleep apnea
Lower Airway Disease
Allergic bronchopulmonary aspergillosis
Chronic obstructive pulmonary disease
Cystic fibrosis
α_1-Antitrypsin deficiency
Bronchiectasis
Bronchiolitis obliterans
Tracheomalacia
Endobronchial lesion
Foreign body
Herpetic tracheobronchitis
Adverse Drug Reaction
Aspirin
β-Adrenergic antagonist
Angiotensin-converting enzyme inhibitors
Inhaled pentamidine
Congestive heart failure
Gastroesophageal reflux
Sinusitis
Hypersensitivity pneumonitis
Eosinophilic granulomatosis with polyangiitis (Churg-Strauss)
Eosinophilic pneumonia
Hyperventilation with panic attacks
Dysfunctional breathlessness

identify those with predominant eosinophilia—absolute peripheral blood eosinophil level of $0.3 \times 10^9/mm^3$ or greater).

- During an exacerbation, monitor oxygen saturation. ABG measurement should be considered in patients in severe distress or with an FEV_1 of <40% of predicted values after initial treatment.
  - A PaO_2 <60 mm Hg is a sign of severe bronchoconstriction or of a complicating condition, such as pulmonary edema or pneumonia.
  - Initially, the $PaCO_2$ is low owing to an increase in respiratory rate. With a prolonged attack, the $PaCO_2$ may rise as a result of severe airway obstruction, increased dead space ventilation, and respiratory muscle fatigue. **A normal or increased $PaCO_2$ is a sign of impending respiratory failure and necessitates hospitalization.**

Allergy Tests

- Allergy skin tests or immunoassays for allergen-specific IgE are helpful to identify sensitization to specific inhalant allergens when allergen exposure is concerned as a trigger.
- Results of allergy tests must correlate with history and clinical presentation.

Exhaled Nitric Oxide

- Fractional concentration of exhaled nitric oxide (FeNO) may be used as a marker of eosinophilic airway inflammation in asthma.
- An FeNO level >50 parts per billion (ppb) is associated with a good response to ICSs. However, it is generally recommended not to use FeNO to guide asthma therapy.

Imaging

- Obtaining a CXR is not routinely required and is performed only if a complicating pulmonary process, such as pneumonia or pneumothorax, is suspected or to rule out other causes of respiratory symptoms in patients being evaluated for asthma.
- CT of the chest can be considered in patients with severe asthma refractory to treatment to evaluate for alternative diagnosis.

Diagnostic Procedures

- **Pulmonary function tests (PFTs)** are essential to the diagnosis of asthma. In patients with asthma, PFTs demonstrate an obstructive pattern—the hallmark of which is a decrease in expiratory flow rates.
  - A reduction in FEV_1 and a proportionally smaller reduction in the FVC occur. This produces a decreased FEV_1/FVC ratio (generally <0.7 or the lower limit of normal value). With mild obstructive disease that involves only the small airways, the FEV_1/FVC ratio may be normal, with the only abnormality being a decrease in airflow at midlung volumes (forced expiratory flow 25%–75%).
  - The clinical diagnosis of asthma is supported by an obstructive pattern that improves after bronchodilator therapy. **Improvement is defined as an increase in FEV_1 of >12% and 200 mL after two to four puffs of a short-acting bronchodilator.** Most patients will not demonstrate reversibility at each assessment.
  - In patients with chronic, severe asthma, the airflow obstruction may no longer be completely reversible. In these patients, the most effective way to establish the maximal degree of airway reversibility is to repeat PFTs after a course of oral corticosteroids (usually 40 mg/d for 10–14 days) and to use the same criteria as above for reversibility. The lack of demonstrable airway obstruction or reactivity does not rule out a diagnosis of asthma.
  - In cases in which spirometry is normal, the diagnosis can be made by showing heightened airway responsiveness to a **methacholine challenge**. A methacholine challenge is considered positive when a provocative concentration of 8 mg/mL or less causes a drop in FEV_1 of 20% (PC_{20}). If the patient is on ICS, a PC_{20} of 8–16 mg/mL is considered

borderline positive. A PC_{20} >16 mg/mL is considered a negative test. Repeat testing with the patient off of ICS may be necessary.

- An objective measurement of airflow obstruction is essential to the evaluation of an exacerbation. The severity of the exacerbation should be classified as:
  - Mild (PEF or FEV_1 >70% of predicted or personal best)
  - Moderate (PEF or FEV_1 40%–69%)
  - Severe (PEF or FEV_1 <40%)
  - Life-threatening/impending respiratory arrest (PEF or FEV_1 <25%)

TREATMENT

- Medical management involves chronic management and a plan for acute exacerbations, otherwise known as the **asthma action plan.** Most often, it includes the daily use of an anti-inflammatory, disease-modifying medication (long-term control medications) and as-needed use of a short-acting bronchodilator (quick-relief medications).
- The goals of daily management are to **avoid impairment** (lack of symptoms while maintaining normal activity and pulmonary function) and to **minimize risk** (preventing exacerbations, loss of lung function, and medication side effects). Successful management requires patient education, objective measurement of airflow obstruction, and a medication plan for daily use and for exacerbations.
- When initiating therapy for a patient not already on controller medicine, one should assess the patient's severity and assign the patient to the highest level in which any one feature has occurred over the previous 2–4 weeks (see Table 9-11).
- Assessment of control on subsequent visits is used to modify therapy when following patients already on controller medication (see Table 9-12).
- Address the following issues before stepping up the therapy when there is a poor response to controller medicine after 2–3 months of treatment.
  - Nonadherence to medications
  - Incorrect inhaler technique
  - Ongoing exposure to allergens and/or irritants
  - Comorbidities: obesity, sinonasal diseases, GERD, OSA, and depression
  - Alternative diagnoses (see Table 9-14)
- The goal of the stepwise approach is to gain control of symptoms as quickly as possible. At the same time, level of control varies over time and, consequently, medication requirements as well, so therapy should be reviewed regularly to check whether stepwise reduction is possible (Figure 9-5).
- **Management of an exacerbation** requiring hospital-based care should follow a treatment algorithm to triage patients based on response to treatment (Figure 9-6).
  - The response to initial treatment (three treatments with a short-acting bronchodilator every 20 minutes for 60–90 minutes) can be a better predictor of the need for hospitalization than the severity of an exacerbation.
  - Patients at high risk of asthma-related death (see Outcome/Prognosis section) should be advised to seek medical attention early in the course of an exacerbation.
- A low threshold for admission is appropriate for patients with recent hospitalization, a failure of aggressive outpatient management (with oral corticosteroids), or a previous life-threatening attack.
- Conditions that mimic asthma exacerbation include exacerbation of chronic obstructive pulmonary disease, acute heart failure, pulmonary thromboembolism, pneumothorax, hyperventilation (panic attacks/uremia), vocal cord dysfunction, and foreign body inhalation.

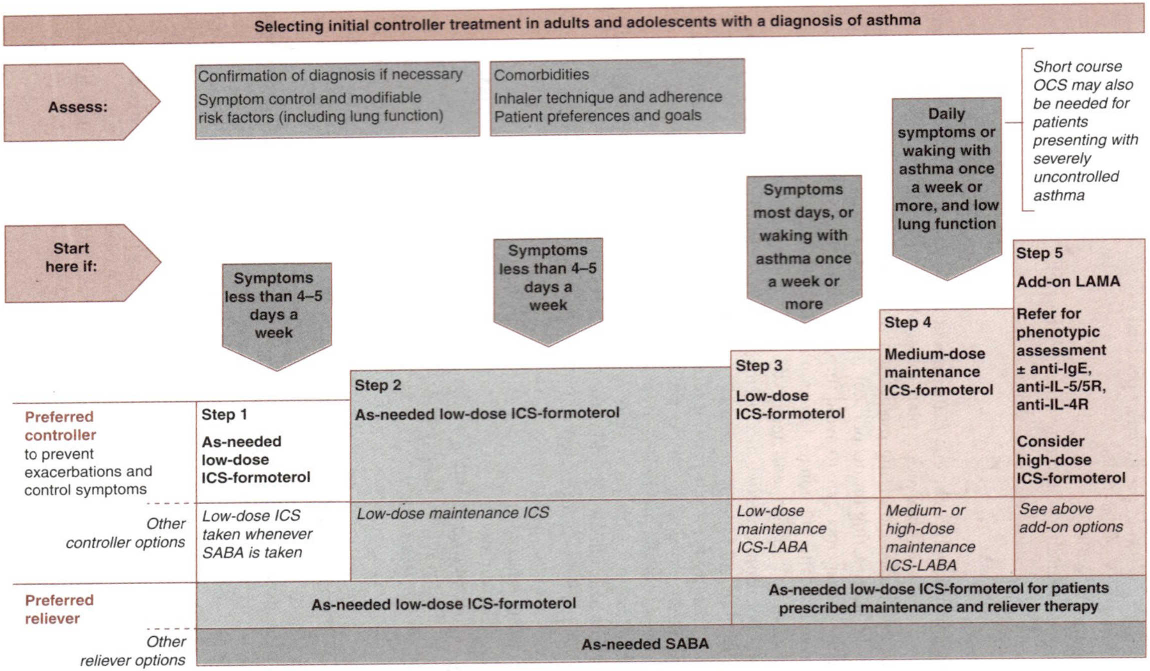

BDP = beclomethasone dipropionate; FEV_1 = forced expiratory volume in 1 second; HDM SLIT = house dust mite sublingual immunotherapy; ICS = inhaled corticosteroid; Ig = immunoglobulin; IL = interleukin; LABA = long-acting β_2-agonist; LAMA = long-acting muscarinic antagonist; LTRA = leukotriene receptor antagonist; OCS = oral corticosteroid; SABA = short-acting β_2-agonist.

GINA. Global Strategy for Asthma Management and Prevention. Updated 2021 (https://ginasthma.org/wp-content/uploads/2021/05/GINA-Main-Report-2021-V2-WMS.pdf). Accessed 7/25/21.

Figure 9-5 Management algorithm based on level of control.

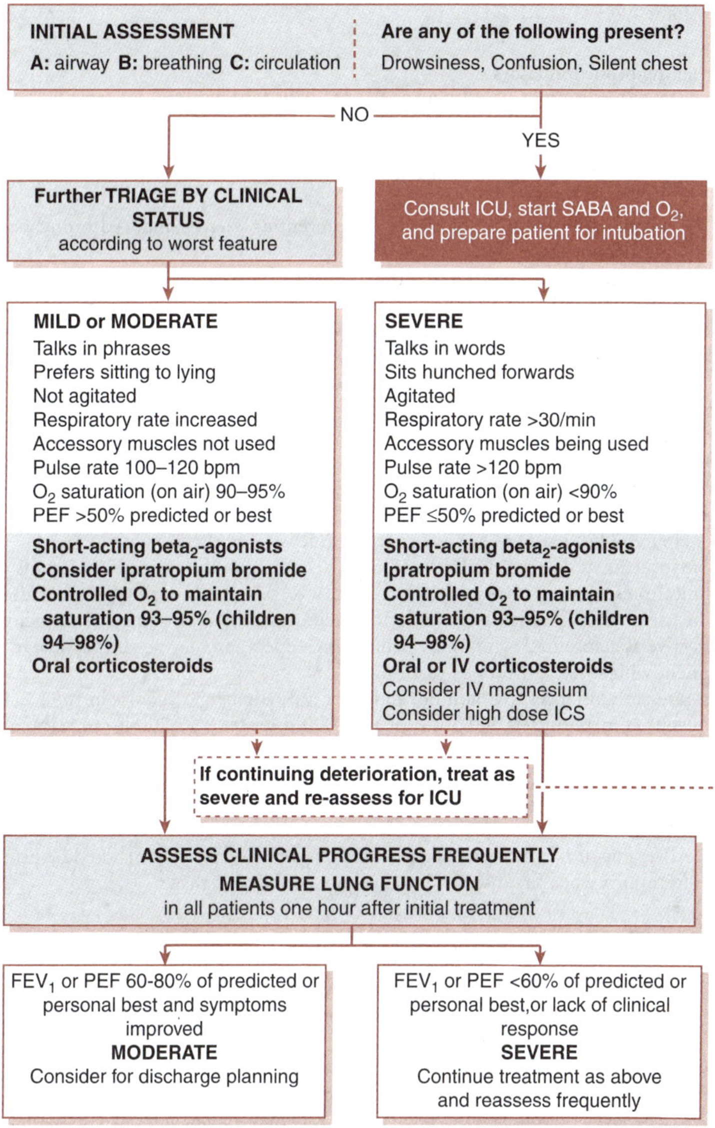

Figure 9-6 Treatment algorithm for asthma exacerbations in acute care facility. FEV_1, forced expiratory volume in 1 second; ICS, inhaled corticosteroids; ICU, intensive care unit; O_2, oxygen; PEF, peak expiratory flow. (From the *2018 GINA Report: Global Strategy for Asthma Management and Prevention.* Global Initiative for Asthma - GINA. Available from https://ginasthma.org/.)

Medications

First Line

- **Short-acting bronchodilators**
  - Quick-relief medications used on an as-needed basis for long-term management of all severities of asthma as well as for rapid treatment of exacerbations given via either MDI or nebulization.
  - For long-term management, a **SABA** used on an as-needed basis (e.g., albuterol, two puffs q6h) is appropriate.
  - SABA is considered the drug of choice for preventing exercise-induced bronchoconstriction (EIB).
  - During an exacerbation, reversal of airflow obstruction is achieved most effectively by frequent administration of an inhaled SABA.
    - For a **mild to moderate exacerbation**, initial treatment starts with two to six puffs of albuterol via MDI with a spacer or 2.5 mg via nebulizer and is repeated q20min until improvement is obtained or toxicity is noted.
    - For a **severe exacerbation**, albuterol 2.5–5 mg q20min with ipratropium bromide 0.5 mg q20min should be administered via nebulizer. Alternatively, albuterol 10–15 mg, administered continuously over an hour, may be more effective in severely obstructed adults. If used, telemetry monitoring is necessary.
    - Levalbuterol four to eight puffs or nebulized 1.25–2.5 mg q20min can be substituted for albuterol but has not been associated with fewer side effects in adults.
    - The subsequent dosing schedule is adjusted according to the patient's symptoms and clinical presentation. Often, patients require a SABA q2–4h during an acute attack. The use of an MDI with a spacer device under supervision of trained personnel is as effective as aerosolized solution by nebulizer. Cooperation may not be possible in the patient with severe airflow obstruction.
    - In rare circumstances, SC administration of a β_2-adrenergic agonist in the form of aqueous epinephrine (0.3–0.5 mL of a 1:1000 solution SC q20min) or terbutaline (0.25 mg SC q20min) for up to three doses can be used. Inhaled medications remain the preferred approach and SC therapy should only be provided in the absence of an effective inhaled option. Importantly, recent myocardial infarction or active angina are contraindications to SC therapy.
  - All SABAs now use hydrofluoroalkane (HFA) as a propellant. They should be primed with four puffs when first used and again if not used over 2 weeks.
- **ICSs**
  - ICSs are safe and effective for the treatment of persistent asthma. They are generally administered via a dry powder inhaler, MDI with a spacing device, or nebulized.
  - Dosing depends on assessment of severity and control (Table 9-15).
  - Once-daily dosing of ICS may be as effective as twice-daily dosing.
  - Systemic corticosteroid absorption can occur in patients who use high doses of ICS. Consequently, prolonged therapy with high-dose ICS should be reserved for patients with severe disease or for those who otherwise require oral corticosteroids.
  - Pharmacological inhibitors of cytochrome P450 may reduce steroid elimination in patients on ICS, thus increasing steroid side effects.
  - Attempts should be made to decrease the dose of ICS every 2–3 months to the lowest possible dose to maintain control.
- **LABAs**
  - Recommended for moderate and severe persistent asthma in patients not adequately controlled with ICS.
  - Salmeterol or the faster-acting formoterol added to ICS has consistently been shown to improve lung function, improve both day and nighttime symptoms, reduce exacerbations, and minimize the required dose of ICS.

TABLE 9-15 Comparative Daily Adult Dosages for Inhaled Corticosteroids

Drug	Low Dose	Medium Dose	High Dose
Beclomethasone HFA (40 or 80 µg/puff)	80–240 µg	>240–480 µg	>480 µg
Budesonide DPI (90, 180, or 200 µg/dose)	180–600 µg	>600–1200 µg	>1200 µg
Budesonide nebulized respules (250, 500, or 1000 µg/respules)	250–500 µg	>500–1000 µg	>1000 µg
Ciclesonide HFA (80 or 160 µg/puff)	160–320 µg	>320–640 µg	>640 µg
Fluticasone propionate HFA (44, 110, or 220 µg/puff)	88–264 µg	>264–440 µg	>440 µg
Fluticasone furoate (100, 220 µg/puff)	100–300 µg	>300–500 µg	>500 µg
Mometasone furoate DPI (110 or 220 µg/puff)	220 µg	440 µg	>440 µg
Combination Agents			
Budesonide/formoterol (MDI: 80/4.5 or 160/4.5 µg/puff)	Two puffs bid: 80/4.5 µg/puff	Two puffs bid: 80/4.5 to 160/4.5 µg/puff	Two puffs bid: 160/4.5 µg/puff
Fluticasone/salmeterol (MDI: 45/21, 115/21, or 230/21 µg/puff) (DPI: 100/50, 250/50, or 500/50 µg/dose)	One inhalation bid: 100/50 µg	One inhalation bid: 250/50 µg	One inhalation bid: 500/50 µg
Fluticasone/vilanterol (DPI: 100/25, 200/25 µg/puff)	One inhalation daily: 100/25 µg	One inhalation daily: 200/25 µg	One inhalation daily: 200/25 µg
Mometasone/formoterol (MDI: 100/5 or 200/5 µg/puff)	Two inhalations bid: 100/5 µg/puff	Two inhalations bid: 100/5 µg/puff to 200/5 µg/puff	Two inhalations bid: 200/5 µg/puff

Data from the *2018 GINA Report: Global Strategy for Asthma Management and Prevention*. Global Initiative for Asthma – GINA. https://ginasthma.org/2018-gina-report-global-strategy-for-asthma-management-and-prevention/. Updated 2018. Accessed September 13, 2018 and Asthma NAE and PP Third Expert Panel on the Diagnosis and Management of Asthma. *Expert Panel Report 3: Guidelines for the Diagnosis and Management of Asthma*. National Heart, Lung, and Blood Institute (US); 2007.
DPI, dry powder inhaler; MDI, metered-dose inhaler.

- LABAs should only be used in combination with ICS in patients with asthma (salmeterol/ fluticasone, budesonide/formoterol, or mometasone/formoterol).
- The benefits of adding LABAs are more substantial than those achieved by leukotriene modifiers (LTMs), theophylline, or increased doses of ICS.

- Maintenance and reliever therapy (MART) with the combination of formoterol and inhaled corticosteroids (ICS) has an established scientific rationale and demonstrated to reduce asthma exacerbations.
- Single inhaler triple therapy (SITT), comprising ICS, LABA, and LAMA, includes formulations such as fluticasone furoate/umeclidinium/vilanterol, beclomethasone dipropionate/formoterol/glycopyrronium, and mometasone furoate/glycopyrronium/indacaterol.

- **Systemic corticosteroids**
  - It may be necessary to gain control of disease quickly via either oral or IV route.
  - If chronic symptoms are severe and accompanied by nighttime awakening or PEF is <70% of predicted values, a short course of oral corticosteroid (prednisone 40–60 mg/d for 5–7 days) might be necessary.
  - Long-term therapy is occasionally necessary and should be started at low dose (≤10 mg/d prednisone or equivalent), and repeated attempts should be made to reduce the dose while patients are receiving high-dose ICS. Side effects associated with long-term therapy should be closely monitored. Osteoporosis prophylaxis may be necessary.
    - **During an exacerbation, systemic corticosteroids speed the resolution of exacerbations of asthma and should be administered promptly to all patients.**
    - The ideal dose of corticosteroid needed to speed recovery and limit symptoms is not well defined. A single or divided daily dose equivalent to prednisone 40–60 mg is usually adequate. Oral corticosteroid administration seems to be as effective as IV administration if given in equivalent doses.
    - IV methylprednisolone, 125 mg, given on initial presentation, decreases the rate of return to the emergency department (ED) for patients who are discharged.
    - For maximal therapeutic response, tapering of high-dose corticosteroids should not take place until objective evidence of clinical improvement is observed (usually 36–48 hours or when PEF >70%). Initially, patients are given a daily dose of oral prednisone, which is then reduced slowly.
    - A 7- to 14-day tapering dose of prednisone is usually successful in combination with an ICS instituted at the beginning of the tapering schedule. In patients with severe disease or with a history of respiratory failure, a slower dose reduction is appropriate.
    - Patients discharged from the ED should receive oral corticosteroids. A dose of prednisone, 40 mg/d for 5–7 days, can be substituted for a tapering schedule in selected patients. Either regimen should be accompanied by the initiation of an ICS or an increase in the previous dose of ICS.

Second Line

- **Leukotriene Modifiers**
  - **Montelukast** (10 mg PO daily) and **zafirlukast** (20 mg PO bid) are oral leukotriene receptor antagonists (LTRAs), and **zileuton** (extended-release 1200 mg bid) is an oral 5-Lipoxygenase inhibitor. The LTRAs are recommended as an alternative first-line medication for mild persistent asthma and as an add-on to ICS for more severe forms of asthma.
  - As add-on therapy to ICS, these agents have been shown to improve lung function, lead to improved quality of life, and lead to fewer exacerbations. However, compared with ICS plus LABA, they are not as effective in improving asthma outcomes.
  - A LTM should be considered for patients with aspirin-sensitive asthma, EIB, or concurrent allergic rhinitis, or individuals who cannot master the use of an inhaler.
- **Biologic therapy**

  Biologic therapy with monoclonal antibodies against IgE and interleukin (IL)-4, -5, and -13 in patients selected with the appropriate phenotype had been shown to be highly effective means of precision medicine in patients with severe persistent asthma not controlled on high doses of ICS plus long-acting bronchodilators:

- **Mepolizumab and Reslizumab** are humanized monoclonal antibodies against IL-5, which reduce eosinophilic inflammation and have been shown to significantly reduce the frequency of exacerbations and hospitalizations in patients with severe asthma and improve lung function.[35,36]
- **Benralizumab** is a monoclonal antibody directed against the α subunit of IL-5 that has been shown to significantly decrease exacerbations, improve lung function, and reduce systemic corticosteroid exposure and exacerbation frequency in patients with severe, steroid-dependent asthma.[37,38]
- **Dupilumab** is a human monoclonal antibody against IL-4 receptor α that blocks signaling for IL-4 and IL-13. Among patients with uncontrolled severe asthma, dupilumab was shown to decrease the rate of severe exacerbation rates, improve lung function, and improve asthma control.[39] This effect was most pronounced in patients with an eosinophil count greater than 300 cells/mm^3 or FeNO ≥25 ppb.
- **Omalizumab** is a monoclonal antibody against IgE that has been shown to reduce exacerbation rate, decrease emergency health-care utilization, and improve asthma-related quality of life in patients with moderate to severe persistent allergic asthma with a demonstrable sensitivity to a perennial aeroallergen and incomplete symptom control with ICS.[40]
- **Tezepelumab** binds to thymic stromal lymphopoietin (TSLP) and prevents it from activating immune cells such as dendritic cells, T cells, and mast cells, which can lead to a reduction in inflammation and its airway hyperresponsiveness has been approved for the treatment of severe asthma.

- **Long-acting muscarinic antagonists:** Tiotropium bromide as add-on therapy to ICS with or without LABA is associated with improved lung functions, fewer symptoms, and reduced exacerbations in patients with inadequately controlled asthma.[41]
- **Methylxanthines:** Theophylline has historical utility in the management of asthma but should be a last-line option given the wide variety of options with less toxicity. Doxofylline is a newer alternative to theophylline. It is postulated to cause lesser side effects due to lack of adenosine receptor antagonism and calcium channel receptor blocking ability.
- **IV magnesium sulfate:** During a severe exacerbation refractory to standard treatment over 1 hour, one dose of 2 g IV over 20 minutes in the ED should be considered. It has been shown to acutely improve lung function especially in those with severe, life-threatening exacerbations.
- **Inhaled heliox:** During a severe exacerbation refractory to standard treatment over 1 hour, heliox-driven albuterol nebulization in a mixture with oxygen (70:30) should be considered. It has been shown to acutely improve lung function, especially in those with severe, life-threatening exacerbations.[42]
- **Antibiotics:** Antibiotic therapy has not been shown to have any benefit when used to treat exacerbations. Antibiotics can only be recommended as needed for treatment of comorbid conditions, such as pneumonia or bacterial sinusitis.
- **Bronchial thermoplasty:** Bronchial thermoplasty is a novel therapy for severe asthma in which a specialized radiofrequency catheter is introduced through a bronchoscope to deliver thermal energy to smaller airways to reduce smooth muscle mass surrounding the airways. Although asthma symptoms worsen immediately after the procedure, long-term (at least 5 years) asthma-related quality of life and health-care utilization improve with bronchial thermoplasty.[43] Bronchial thermoplasty should be performed by experienced bronchoscopists in conjunction with an asthma specialist.

Other Nonpharmacologic Therapies

- **Supplemental oxygen** should be administered to the patient who is awaiting an assessment of arterial oxygen tension and should be continued to maintain an oxygen saturation >92% (95% in patients with coexisting cardiac disease or pregnancy).
- **Mechanical ventilation** may be required for respiratory failure.
  - General principles include use of a **large endotracheal tube (≥7.5 mm), prolonged expiratory time with high inspiratory flows, and low respiratory rate. Positive end-expiratory pressure (PEEP) should be patient-targeted and may need to be upwardly adjusted in some cases to avoid development of intrinsic PEEP.**
  - Ketamine and propofol may provide modest bronchodilatory effect in addition to sedation. After deep sedation, paralytics may have an advantage in decreasing muscular tone and minimizing patient–ventilator dyssynchrony.
  - Evidence is lacking to suggest modes of noninvasive ventilation are beneficial.
  - Although prospective data are lacking, Extracorporeal Life Support may be beneficial in cases of severe ventilatory failure associated with asthma exacerbations and offers the most benefit early in the course of disease.
- **Subcutaneous allergen immunotherapy** (SCIT) can be considered in allergic patients with mild to moderate disease with persistent symptoms despite adherence to allergen avoidance and medication. SCIT is relatively contraindicated in patients with severe or unstable asthma (chronic oral corticosteroid use or severe exacerbations requiring hospitalization or intubation in the previous 6 months). Sublingual immunotherapy (SLIT) and subcutaneous multiple allergen immunotherapy in polysensitized patients need more supporting evidence to corroborate their efficacy in practice.

Lifestyle/Risk Modification

Diet

There is no general diet that is known to improve asthma control. However, a small percentage of patients may have reproducible deterioration after exposure to dietary sulfites used to prevent discoloration in foods such as beer, wine, processed potatoes, and dried fruit, and therefore, these foods should be avoided in patients if they have had prior reactions to these foods.

Activity

Patients should be encouraged to lead an active lifestyle. If their asthma is well controlled, they should expect to be as physically active as they desire. If exercise is a trigger, patients should be advised to continue physical activity after prophylactic use of an LTM (montelukast 10 mg 2 hours before exercise) or an inhaled β_2-adrenergic agonist (two to four puffs 15–20 minutes before exposure).

SPECIAL CONSIDERATIONS

- During pregnancy, patients should have more frequent follow-up because the severity of asthma often changes and requires medication adjustment. **There is more potential risk to the fetus with poorly controlled asthma than with exposure to asthma medications, most of which are generally considered safe.**[44]
- Occupational asthma requires a detailed history of occupational exposure to a sensitizing agent, lack of asthma symptoms before exposure, and a documented relationship with symptoms and the workplace. Beyond standard asthma medical treatment, exposure avoidance is crucial.

COMPLICATIONS

Medication Side Effects

- **SABA:** Sympathomimetic symptoms (tremor, anxiety, tachycardia), decrease in serum potassium and magnesium, mild lactic acidosis, prolonged QT_c.
- ICS
  - Increased risk for systemic effects at high doses (equivalent >1000 µg/d of beclomethasone) including skin bruising, cataracts, elevated intraocular pressure, and accelerated loss of bone mass.
  - Pharyngeal and laryngeal effects are common, such as sore throat, hoarse voice, and oral candidiasis. **Patients should be instructed to rinse their mouth after each administration to reduce the possibility of thrush.** A change in the delivery method and/or use of a valved holding chamber/spacer may alleviate the other side effects.
- LABA
  - Fewer sympathomimetic-type side effects.
  - Associated with an increased risk of severe asthma exacerbations and asthma-related death when used without ICS based on the Salmeterol Multicenter Asthma Research Trial, which showed a very low but significant increase in asthma-related deaths in patients receiving salmeterol (0.01%–0.04%).[45]
  - Should only be used in combination with ICS. FDA recommends discontinuation of LABA once asthma control is achieved and maintained.
- LTM
  - Cases of newly diagnosed eosinophilic granulomatosis with polyangiitis (Churg-Strauss) after exposure to LTRA have been described, but it is unclear whether they are related to unmasking of a preexisting case with concurrent corticosteroid tapering or whether there is a causal relationship.
  - Zileuton can cause a reversible hepatitis, so it is recommended that hepatic function be monitored at initiation once a month during the first 3 months, every 3 months for the first year, and then periodically.
- **Biologic therapy:** All biologic therapies pose the risk of immunogenicity, hypersensitivity or rarely, anaphylaxis. For most therapies, 30 minutes of monitoring after drug administration should be routine. For omalizumab, 1 hour of monitoring should occur after the first dose and at least 30 minutes after each subsequent dose. Epinephrine should be available for self-administration in patients treated with omalizumab.
- **Methylxanthines**
  - Theophylline has a narrow therapeutic range with significant toxicities, such as arrhythmias and seizures, as well as many potential drug interactions, especially with antibiotics.
  - Serum concentrations of theophylline should be monitored on a regular basis, aiming for a peak level of 5–10 µg/mL; however, at the lower doses used for asthma, toxicity is much less likely.

PATIENT EDUCATION

- Patient education should focus on the chronic and inflammatory nature of asthma, with identification of factors that contribute to increased inflammation.
  - The consequences of ongoing exposure to chronic irritants or allergens and the rationale for therapy should be explained. Patients should be instructed to avoid factors that aggravate their disease, on how to manage their daily medications, and on how to recognize and deal with acute exacerbations (known as an asthma action plan).
  - Review the principles of asthma medications and skills of inhaler technique.
  - The use of a **written daily management plan** as part of the education strategy is recommended for all patients with persistent asthma.

- It is important for patients to recognize signs of poorly controlled disease.
  - These signs include an increased or daily need for bronchodilators, limitation of activity, waking at night because of asthma symptoms, and variability in the PEF.
  - Specific instructions about handling these symptoms, including criteria for seeking emergency care, should be provided.

MONITORING/FOLLOW-UP

- PEF monitoring provides an objective measurement of airflow obstruction and can be considered in patients with moderate to severe persistent asthma. However, symptom-based asthma action plans are equivalent to PEF-based plans in terms of overall self-management and control.
  The patient must be able to demonstrate correct use of the peak flow meter. The personal best PEF (the highest PEF obtained when the disease is under control) is identified, and the PEF is checked when symptoms escalate or in the setting of an asthma trigger. This should be incorporated into an asthma action plan, setting 80%–100% of personal best PEF as the "green" zone, 50%–80% as the "yellow" zone, and <50% as the "red" zone.
- Patients should learn to anticipate situations that cause increased symptoms. For most individuals, monitoring symptoms instead of PEF is sufficient (symptom-based asthma action plan).
- Questionnaires can also provide objective monitoring of asthma control. The Asthma Control Test and Asthma Control Questionnaire are useful instruments to rapidly assess patient-reported asthma control.

OUTCOME/PROGNOSIS

- Most patients with asthma can be effectively treated and achieve good control of their disease when following the stepwise treatment approach. Goals should include minimal use of reliever medication, freedom from troublesome symptoms, near-normal lung function, absence of serious attacks, and ability to lead a physically active life.
- Previous exacerbations that have required the use of oral corticosteroids or led to respiratory failure, as well as the use of more than two canisters per month of inhaled short-acting bronchodilator and seizures with asthma attacks, have been associated with severe and potentially fatal asthma.

DIFFERENCES BETWEEN BRONCHIAL ASTHMA AND COPD (TABLE 9-16)

TABLE 9-16 Comparison Between Asthma and COPD

	Asthma	COPD
Cause	Sensitive agent, usually with atopy	Noxious agent (mainly cigarette smoking), without atopy
Airway inflammation	CD4+ T lymphocytes and eosinophils	CD8+ T lymphocytes, macrophages, and neutrophils
Key mediators	Eotaxin, IL-4, IL-5,IL-13, NO^{+++}	IL-8, TNF-α, IL-1β, IL-6, NO^{+}
Oxidative stress	+	+++
Airflow limitation	Reversible	Not fully reversible

(Continued)

TABLE 9-16 Comparison Between Asthma and COPD (Continued)

	Asthma	COPD
Site of disease	Proximal airways	Peripheral airways, lung parenchyma, pulmonary vessels
Age	Usually child or young age	>45 years
Course	Variable, remissions, sometimes progressive	Progressive
Response to bronchodilators	Good	Bad
Response to corticosteroids	Good	Bad
Functional pulmonary testing		
Flow	=/-	-
BD response	+	-/+
Variability	+	-
BHR	++	+
DLCO	+	-
Hyperinflation	0/+	+(++)
Lung elasticity	0	-
Treatment		
Anti-inflammatory drugs	Corticosteroids Antileukotrienes Chromones	Corticosteroids
Bronchodilators	β-2 agonists Anticholinergics Anti-IgE	β-2 agonists Anticholinergics Theophylline
Mucoactive drugs	-	+
Antibiotics	-	+
Vaccines	-	+

BHR, bronchial hyperreactivity; DLCO, diffusing capacity of carbon monoxide.
Reproduced from Cukic V, Lovre V, Dragisic D, Ustamujic A. Asthma and Chronic Obstructive Pulmonary Disease (COPD) - Differences and Similarities. Mater Sociomed. 2012;24(2):100–105.

Other Considerations

ASTHMA CHRONIC OBSTRUCTIVE PULMONARY DISEASE OVERLAP SYNDROME

- Asthma COPD overlap syndrome (ACOS) comprises up to 15% of the patients with COPD.
- Three characteristic features that help us to identify them are as follows: enhanced bronchial and systemic eosinophilic inflammation, increased reversibility of airflow, and increased response to ICS compared with in patients with COPD alone.
- ACOS included six criteria:

Major

1. Persistent airflow limitation (postbronchodilator FEV1/FVC <0.70 or LLN) in individuals 40 years of age or older; LLN is preferred.
2. At least 10 pack-years of tobacco smoking
   OR equivalent indoor or outdoor air pollution exposure [e.g., biomass]
3. Documented history of asthma before 40 years of age
   OR
   BDR of >400 mL in FEV1

Minor

1. Documented history of atopy or allergic rhinitis
2. BDR of FEV1 ≥200 mL and 12% from baseline values on two or more visits
3. Peripheral blood eosinophil count of ≥300 cells μL

- The presence of two major criteria or one major plus two minor criteria defines ACOS.*

Exercise-Induced Asthma (EIA)

- EIB/EIA has been defined as a fall in FEV_1 of 10% or greater on an exercise challenge test (4–6 minutes of exercise at near-maximum targets with a total duration of exercise of 6–8 minutes).
- EIB can be prevented by using SABA or ICS/formoterol a few minutes before exercise. A warm-up period before exercise may also reduce EIB symptoms.

Aspirin-Induced Asthma (AIA)

- Aspirin-exacerbated respiratory disease is a special phenotype characterized by a triad of asthma, chronic rhinosinusitis with nasal polyposis, and respiratory reactions to aspirin. It occurs because of the inhibition of the enzyme cyclooxygenase-1 (COX-1) by aspirin and other NSAIDs.
- The diagnosis of AIA can be established by oral, nasal, or bronchial challenge testing with aspirin in patients with a suggestive history.
- COX-2 inhibitors can be safely used in patients with AIA.

Cough-Variant Asthma

- Patients with cough-variant asthma may exhibit chronic cough, often intensified at night, which can manifest as their sole symptom.

Brittle Asthma

- Type 1: Wide PEF variability (>40% diurnal variation for >50% of the time over a period of >3–6 months) despite intense therapy
- Type 2: Sudden severe attacks on a background of apparently well-controlled asthma

Summary

- The new definition of chronic obstructive pulmonary disease (COPD) appropriately emphasizes the heterogeneous nature of the disease.
- The previous ABCD Assessment Tool for initial assessment and initiation of pharmacological management of COPD has been changed to the ABE Assessment Tool.
- The preferred choice is a combination of a long-acting muscarinic antagonist (LAMA) and a long-acting beta-agonist (LABA) in the management of stable COPD.

---

* Sin DD, Miravitlles M, Mannino DM, et al. What is asthma–COPD overlap syndrome? Towards a consensus definition from a roundtable discussion. *Eur Respir J.* 2016;48:664–673.

- The latest guidelines from GINA recommend the use of inhaled corticosteroids (ICS) in combination with a long-acting β2-agonist (LABA) as reliever therapy for all asthma patients, regardless of their severity. Based on the severity of asthma symptoms, this treatment can also be used as maintenance therapy (MART).
- The fractional concentration of exhaled nitric oxide (FeNO) and sputum eosinophilia are useful biomarkers in asthma and are associated with steroid responsiveness.

Scan the QR code to access chapter references.

10 Pulmonary Diseases

Adrian Shifren, Tonya D. Russell, Chad Witt, Danish Ahmad, Adam Anderson, Shail Mehta, Yuka Furuya, Suchitra Pilli, Alexander Chen, Praveen Chenna, Murali Chakinala, and Isha Tiwari

Pulmonary Hypertension

GENERAL PRINCIPLES

Definition

Pulmonary hypertension (PH) is the sustained elevation of the mean pulmonary artery pressure (mPAP) to ≥25 mm Hg (at rest), pulmonary arterial wedge pressure ≤15 mm Hg, and pulmonary vascular resistance >240 dyn second/cm^5.

Classification

- PH is subcategorized into five major groups (Table 10-1)[1]:
  - Group I—**Pulmonary arterial hypertension (PAH)**
  - Group II—**PH due to left heart disease**
  - Group III—**PH due to lung diseases and/or hypoxemia**
  - Group IV—**Chronic thromboembolic pulmonary hypertension (CTEPH)**
  - Group V—**PH with unclear multifactorial mechanisms**
- **PAH represents a specific group of disorders with similar pathologies and clinical presentation, with a propensity for right heart failure in the absence of elevated left-sided pressures.**

Epidemiology

- PH is most often due to left heart disease (Group II) or parenchymal lung disease (Group III).
- **Idiopathic PAH (IPAH)** (Group I) is a rare disorder with an estimated prevalence of 6–9 cases per million compared to an overall PAH prevalence of 15–26 cases per million.[2,3] The average age of PAH patients in modern registries is approximately 50 years.[2–4] IPAH patients tend to be even younger, with a mean age of approximately 35 years.[5]
- Despite increased awareness, PAH continues to be diagnosed late in its course, with a reported delay of 27 months from symptom onset and the majority of patients in advanced World Health Organization (WHO) functional class III or IV.[2]
- IPAH and PAH associated with systemic sclerosis are the most common subtypes of PAH.[4,6]
- Incidence of **CTEPH** (Group IV) may be as high as 4% among survivors of acute pulmonary embolism.[7]
- South Asian population also had similar survival rates as compared to other national registries with the most common etiologies being attributed to congenital heart disease–associated PAH (35.8%), idiopathic PAH (29.7%), and then connective tissue disease–associated PAH (24.3%).*

Pathophysiology

- Complex origins of PAH include infectious/environmental insults or comorbid conditions that "trigger" the condition in individuals susceptible because of a genetic predisposition.

---

* Lim Y, Low TT, Chan SP, et al. Pulmonary arterial hypertension in a multi-ethnic Asian population: characteristics, survival and mortality predictors from a 14-year follow-up study. *Respirology*. 2019;24:162–170.

TABLE 10-1 Clinical Classification of Pulmonary Hypertension: Dana Point (2008) Classification System of Pulmonary Hypertension
I. **Pulmonary arterial hypertension (PAH)** Idiopathic PAH Heritable: *BMPR-II, ACVRL1, ENG, SMAD9, CAV1, KCNK3* *Unknown* Drug and toxin induced Associated with: *Connective tissue diseases* *HIV infection* *Portal hypertension* *Congenital heart diseases* *Schistosomiasis* Pulmonary veno-occlusive disease and/or pulmonary capillary hemangiomatosis Persistent pulmonary hypertension of the newborn
II. **Pulmonary hypertension due to left heart disease** Left ventricular systolic dysfunction Left ventricular diastolic dysfunction Valvular disease Congenital/acquired left heart inflow/outflow tract obstruction and congenital cardiomyopathies
III. **Pulmonary hypertension due to lung diseases and/or hypoxemia** Chronic obstructive lung disease Interstitial lung disease Other pulmonary diseases with mixed obstructive and restrictive pattern Sleep-disordered breathing Alveolar hypoventilation disorders Chronic exposure to high altitude Developmental lung diseases
IV. **Chronic thromboembolic pulmonary hypertension (CTEPH)**
V. **Pulmonary hypertension with unclear multifactorial mechanisms** Hematologic disorders: *chronic hemolytic anemia, myeloproliferative disorders, splenectomy* Systemic diseases: *sarcoidosis, pulmonary Langerhans cell histiocytosis, neurofibromatosis, lymphangioleiomyomatosis* Metabolic disorders: *glycogen storage disease, Gaucher disease, thyroid disorders* Others: *tumoral obstruction, fibrosing mediastinitis, chronic renal failure on hemodialysis*

ALK1 (ACVR1), activin-like receptor kinase-1; *BMPR-II*, bone morphogenetic protein receptor II; *CAV1*, caveolin-1; *ENG*, endoglin; *KCNK3*, potassium channel super family K member-3.

Reprinted from Simonneau G, Gatzoulis MA, Adatial, et al. Updated clinical classification of pulmonary hypertension. *J Am Coll Cardiol.* 2013;62:D34–D41; with permission from Elsevier.

- Mutations in the bone morphogenetic protein receptor II (*BMPR-II*) gene are an overwhelming cause of heritable PAH (HPAH).[8] Other susceptibility factors are speculated to exist but have not been identified.
- A total of 70% of familial PAH and 10%–40% of sporadic or anorexigen-associated cases are found to have mutations in *BMPR-II*.[9]

- PAH involves a complex interplay of factors resulting in progressive vascular remodeling with endothelial cell and smooth muscle proliferation, vasoconstriction, and in situ thrombosis at an arteriolar level. Vessel wall changes and luminal narrowing restrict the flow of blood and lead to higher than normal pressure as blood flows through the vessels, which is quantifiable by an elevated pulmonary vascular resistance (PVR).[10]
  - Elevated PVR results in increased afterload to the right ventricle (RV), which over time increases RV wall tension and work, ultimately impacting RV contractility.
  - Initially, cardiac output diminishes during strenuous exercise. As PH severity worsens, maximal cardiac output is achieved at progressively lower workloads; ultimately, resting cardiac output is reduced.
  - Unlike the left ventricle (LV), the RV has limited ability to hypertrophy and tolerates high afterload poorly, causing "vascular–ventricular uncoupling" and eventual RV failure, the most common cause of death.
  - In very advanced stages, pulmonary artery pressures decline as the failing RV cannot generate enough blood flow to maintain high pressures.
- Mechanisms of PH in Groups II–V vary and may include high post-capillary pressures, hypoxemia-mediated vasoconstriction and remodeling, parenchymal destruction, thromboembolic narrowing or occlusion of large arteries, compression of proximal vasculature, and hyperdynamic states leading to increased circulatory flow.

Prevention

Yearly screening transthoracic echocardiogram (TTE) is indicated for high-risk groups including individuals with known *BMPR-II* mutation, scleroderma spectrum of disease, portal hypertension undergoing liver transplantation evaluation, and congenital systemic-to-pulmonary shunts (e.g., ventricular septal defects, patent ductus arteriosus).

A more formal screening algorithm for early detection of PAH associated with scleroderma is available.[11]

DIAGNOSIS

Clinical Presentation

- **Symptoms** include **dyspnea** (most common), exercise intolerance, fatigue, palpitations, exertional dizziness, **syncope**, chest pain, lower extremity swelling, increased abdominal girth (ascites), and hoarseness (impingement of recurrent laryngeal nerve by enlarging pulmonary artery).
- Explore for underlying exposures (i.e., anorectic drugs, methamphetamines, chemotherapeutic agents)[1] or associated conditions (e.g., connective tissue diseases (CTDs), LV heart failure [congestive heart failure (CHF)], obstructive sleep apnea syndrome [OSAS], and venous thromboembolism [VTE]).
- Auscultatory signs of PH include **prominent second heart sound** (loud S_2) with loud P_2 component, RV S_3, tricuspid regurgitation, and pulmonary insufficiency murmurs.
- **Signs of right heart failure**
  - Elevated jugular venous pressure
  - Hepatomegaly
  - Pulsatile liver
  - Pedal edema
  - Ascites

- Physical examination should focus on identifying underlying conditions linked to PH: skin changes of scleroderma, stigmata of liver disease, clubbing (congenital heart disease), aortic/mitral murmurs, and abnormal breath sounds (parenchymal lung disease).

Diagnostic Testing

- **The purpose of diagnostic testing is to confirm clinical suspicion of PH, determine etiology of PH, and gauge severity of condition, which assist treatment planning.**
- **Acute illnesses** (e.g., pulmonary edema, pulmonary embolism, pneumonia, adult respiratory distress syndrome) can cause **mild PH** (pulmonary artery systolic pressure [PASP] <50 mm Hg) or aggravate preexisting PH.
- Evaluation of **chronic PH** becomes necessary if pulmonary artery pressures remain elevated after resolution of the acute process.
- If chronic PH is considered based on clinical suspicion or during the evaluation of a vulnerable population (see Prevention section), **TTE should be the initial test.**

TTE with Doppler and Agitated Saline Injection

- **Estimate PASP** by Doppler interrogation of tricuspid valve regurgitant jet. The absence of tricuspid regurgitation does not exclude elevated pulmonary artery pressure. Sensitivity for PH is 80%–100%, and correlation coefficient with invasive measurement is 0.6–0.9.[12] **Invasive measurement is recommended if suspicion remains despite a normal estimation by echocardiogram.**
- **Assess RV characteristics**, looking for pressure overload and dysfunction (e.g., RV hypertrophy and/or dilation, RV hypokinesis, displaced intraventricular septum, paradoxical septal motion, LV compression, and pericardial effusion from impaired pericardial drainage). Measures of RV function include tricuspid annular systolic excursion, systolic velocity of the free wall, RV index of myocardial performance, and free wall strain. TAPSE <1.8 cm is associated with worse survival.[13] Absence of any RV abnormalities makes moderate or severe PH unlikely.
- **Identify causes of PH** (e.g., LV systolic or **diastolic dysfunction**, left-sided valvular disease, left atrial structural anomalies, and congenital systemic-to-pulmonary shunts). Left atrial enlargement, elevated LV filling pressures, and diastolic dysfunction are important clues for LV diastolic heart disease that frequently leads to PH, especially in the elderly.[14]
- Transesophageal echocardiogram is indicated to exclude intracardiac shunts suspected by TTE, although majority of shunts are patent foramen ovale and do not require further evaluation.
- Additional studies, as outlined in the following text and in Figure 10-1, should be completed if PH is unexplained by TTE, if there is suspicion of lung disease or if PAH is still a consideration after echocardiography.[12,15]

Laboratories

- Evaluate for causative conditions and gauge degree of cardiac impairment.
  - Complete blood counts (CBCs)
  - Blood urea nitrogen, serum creatinine
  - Hepatic function tests
  - Brain natriuretic peptide (BNP) or N-terminal BNP
  - HIV serology
  - Antinuclear antibody (ANA), antitopoisomerase antibodies, anticentromere antibodies, extractable nuclear antigen antibody, and potentially other serologies of autoimmune disease
- Additional laboratory studies, based on initial findings, include thyroid function studies, hepatitis B and C serologies, hemoglobin electrophoresis, antiphospholipid antibody, and lupus anticoagulant.

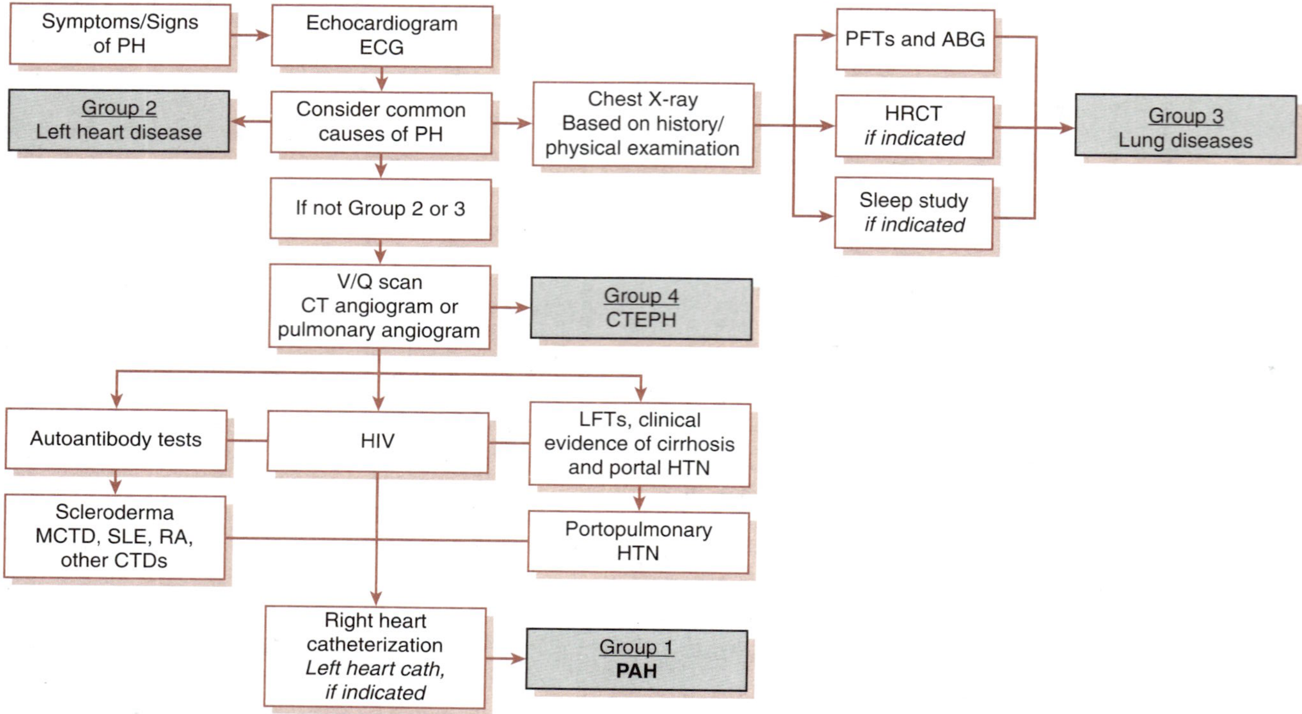

Figure 10-1 Algorithm for diagnostic workup of pulmonary hypertension. ABG, arterial blood gas; CTD, connective tissue disease; CTEPH, chronic thromboembolic pulmonary hypertension; HRCT, high-resolution CT; HTN, hypertension; LFT, liver function test; MCTD, mixed connective tissue disease, PAH, pulmonary arterial hypertension; PFT, pulmonary function test; PH, pulmonary hypertension; RA, rheumatoid arthritis; SLE, systemic lupus erythematosus; V/Q, ventilation-perfusion.

Electrocardiography

Signs of **right heart enlargement** include RV hypertrophy, right atrial enlargement, right bundle branch block, and RV strain pattern (S wave in lead I with Q wave and inverted T wave in lead III), but these findings have low sensitivity in milder PH.

Pulmonary Function Testing

- **Spirometry and lung volumes** to assess for obstructive (e.g., **chronic obstructive lung disease**) or restrictive (e.g., interstitial lung disease [ILD]) ventilatory abnormalities.
- **Diffusing capacity for carbon monoxide (DLCO)** is mildly reduced (in isolation) in PAH; but more severe reductions in DLCO (i.e., <40% predicted) is a clue for significant parenchymal lung disease or pulmonary veno-occlusive disease.
- **Arterial blood gas (ABG):** Elevated arterial partial pressure of carbon dioxide ($PaCO_2$) is an important clue for a hypoventilation syndrome or a severe obstructive ventilatory defect.
- **Six-minute walk (6MW) or simple exercise test**
  - Unexplained exercise-induced desaturation could indicate PH.
  - Distance walked correlates with WHO functional classification and provides intermediate prognosis.[16]
- **Nocturnal oximetry:** Nocturnal desaturations could indicate OSAS. PH patients with symptoms of sleep-disordered breathing should undergo **polysomnography** (PSG). Nocturnal desaturations are common in PAH, even in the absence of OSAS, and should be treated with nocturnal supplemental oxygen.[17]

Imaging

- General findings include enlarged central pulmonary arteries as well as RV enlargement with opacification of retrosternal space, seen best on lateral view.
- Clues to specific PH diagnosis include the following:
  - Decreased peripheral vascular markings or pruning (PAH)
  - Very large pulmonary vasculature throughout lung fields (pulmonary to systemic)
  - Regional oligemia of pulmonary vasculature (chronic thromboembolic disease)
  - Interstitial infiltrates (ILD)
  - Hyperinflated lungs (chronic obstructive lung disease)
- **Ventilation–perfusion (V/Q) lung scan**
  - Critical for excluding chronic thromboembolic disease but could also be abnormal in pulmonary veno-occlusive disease and fibrosing mediastinitis.
  - **Heterogeneous perfusion patterns** are associated with PAH.
  - Presence of one or more segmental mismatches raises concern for chronic thromboembolic disease and should be investigated with computed tomography (CT) or pulmonary angiography.[15]
- **Chest CT scan**
  - Angiogram confirms CTEPH if initial screening V/Q scan is suspicious, and also helps determine surgical feasibility; CT should not be used as screening tool for CTEPH.
  - Evaluates lung parenchyma and mediastinum.
  - High-resolution images to assess for interstitial or bronchiolar disease.
- **Pulmonary angiography** can be done safely in the setting of severe PH.
  - Confirms CTEPH.
  - Determines surgical feasibility.
- **Cardiac MRI**
  - Investigates cardiac anomalies leading to the development of PAH, especially if transesophageal echocardiogram is contraindicated.
  - Provides anatomic and functional information about the RV, including ventricular volumes, ejection fraction, and stroke volume index, which have prognostic value.

Diagnostic Procedures

- **Lung biopsy**
  Risk of surgery is usually prohibitive in the setting of severe PH or RV dysfunction but is rarely performed to diagnose variants such as PVOD or capillary hemangiomatosis.
- **Right heart catheterization: Essential investigation if PAH is suspected and treatment is being considered.**
  - **Confirm noninvasive estimate of PASP** because TTE can under- and overestimate PASP.[18]
  - **Measure cardiac output and mean right atrial pressure (RAP) to gauge severity of condition and predict future course.** Increased RAP is an indicator of RV dysfunction and has the greatest hemodynamic odds ratio for mortality.[5]
  - **Investigate etiologies of PH**, including left heart disease (by measuring pulmonary artery wedge pressure [PAWP] manually at end-expiration) or missed systemic-to-pulmonary shunts (by noting "step-ups" in oxygen saturations).
  - Exercise testing can elicit PH occurring during exercise or also confirm suspicion of diastolic heart failure, but exercise protocols and methods of measurement are not standardized and should be done at expert centers.
- **Acute vasodilator testing** is recommended as part of PAH evaluation, especially if IPAH, HPAH, or drug/toxin-induced PAH is likely.
  - Performed with a **short-acting vasodilator**, such as IV adenosine, IV epoprostenol, or inhaled nitric oxide. **Long-acting calcium channel blockers (CCBs) should not be used for initial vasodilator testing** because of risk of sustained systemic hypotension.[19]
  - **Not recommended in extreme right heart failure** (mean RAP >20 mm Hg).
  - Definition of a **responder** is **decline in mPAP of 10 mm Hg *and* concluding mPAP of 40 mm Hg with stable or improved cardiac output.**[19]
  - Responders should undergo a CCB trial with pulmonary artery catheter in place. If vasoresponsiveness is recapitulated, chronic CCB therapy can be prescribed (see Treatment section).
- **Left heart catheterization** should be done to directly measure **LV end-diastolic pressure** if PAWP cannot reliably exclude left heart disease, especially in patients older than 65 years.

TREATMENT

- Regardless of specific PH diagnosis, normoxemia should be maintained to avoid hypoxic vasoconstriction and further aggravation of pulmonary artery pressures. Supplemental oxygen to maintain adequate arterial saturations (>89%) 24 hours a day is recommended. However, normoxemia may not be possible with a significant right-to-left intracardiac shunt.
- **In-line filters** should be used to prevent paradoxical air emboli from IV catheters in PH patients with large right-to-left shunts.
- **Pneumovax and influenza vaccination** should be given to avoid respiratory tract infections.
- Patients with severe PH and RV dysfunction should **minimize behaviors** that can acutely decrease RV preload and/or increase RV afterload, which could cause circulatory collapse:
  - **Deep Valsalva** maneuvers can raise intrathoracic pressure and induce syncope through diminished central venous return (e.g., vigorous exercise, severe coughing paroxysm, straining during defecation, or micturition).
  - **High altitudes** (>5000 ft) because of low inspired concentration of oxygen.
  - **Cigarette smoking** because of nicotine's vasoactive effects.
  - **Pregnancy** because of hemodynamic alterations that further strain the heart.
  - Systemic **sympathomimetic** agents, such as decongestants and cocaine.
- **Management of PH depends on the specific category of PH.**
  - Patients with PH because of left heart disease should receive appropriate therapy for the underlying causative condition with the goal of minimizing post-capillary pressures.
  - Patients with underlying lung diseases should be treated appropriately for specific condition, e.g., bronchodilators for obstructive lung disease, immunomodulators or

antifibrotics for ILDs, noninvasive ventilation for OSAS or obesity hypoventilation syndrome, and supplemental oxygen if hypoxemic.
  - CTEPH is often treated by **pulmonary thromboendarterectomy or percutaneous balloon angioplasty (BPA)** at specialized centers and requires careful screening to determine resectability and expected hemodynamic response.[20,21] Patients with inoperable CTEPH can benefit from medical therapy (see Table 10-2).

Medications

- **PAH patients are candidates for vasomodulator/vasodilator** therapy (Figure 10-2 and Table 10-2).
  - There are four categories of PAH-specific therapies with unique mechanisms of action:
    - **Endothelin receptor antagonists** block endothelin-1 from binding to receptors on pulmonary artery smooth muscle cells, thus abrogating vasoconstriction and cellular hypertrophy/growth.
    - **Phosphodiesterase-5 inhibitors** block the enzyme that shuts down nitric oxide–mediated vasodilation and platelet inhibition.
    - **Soluble guanylate cyclase stimulator** activates the downstream signal of nitric oxide through stimulation soluble guanylate cyclase and induces vasodilation and platelet inhibition.
    - **Prostacyclin pathway activators, including prostacyclin analogues and prostacyclin receptor agonists,** induce vasodilation, inhibit cellular growth, and inhibit platelet aggregation.
  - Initial choice of PAH-specific therapy should be individualized based on the severity of the condition (see Figure 10-2). Risk assessment models have been developed:
  - **REVEAL includes numerous predictors of mortality**[22]:
    - PAH subtype: scleroderma, portopulmonary hypertension, familial PAH
    - Men older than 60 years
    - Renal insufficiency
    - BNP >180 pg/mL
    - PVR >32 Wood units
    - RAP >20 mm Hg
    - DLCO ≤32%
    - Pericardial effusion
    - Systolic blood pressure >110 mm Hg
    - Resting heart rate >92 bpm
    - New York Heart Association (NYHA) functional class IV
    - 6MW distance <165 m
  - **French Registry model** tallies the number of low-risk characteristics that an individual satisfies[23]: NYHA functional class I or II, 6MWD >440 m, RAP <8 mm Hg, cardiac index ≥2.5 L/min/m^2.
  - **Because of the complexity of some therapies, an individual's comorbid conditions, cognitive abilities, and psychosocial makeup must also be heavily factored.**
  - Combination therapy regimens, which include medications from more than one class of therapy, are generally the preferred approach even for newly diagnosed patients (see Figure 10-2).[24,25]
  - Because current therapies for PAH are palliative and not curative, patients require close follow-up as deterioration often occurs, requiring alternative/additional medical and possibly surgical intervention (see Figure 10-2). Although there is no consensus on follow-up strategy, regular functional (e.g., 6MW and WHO functional classification) and periodic cardiac (e.g., TTE, MRI, or right heart catheterization) assessments provide the most sound strategy.[25]
- **Diuretic therapy** (loop diuretic ± aldosterone antagonist ± thiazides)
  - Alleviates **right heart failure** and improves symptoms.

TABLE 10-2 Vasomodulator/Vasodilatory Therapy for Pulmonary Arterial Hypertension

Drug	Therapeutic Class	Route of Delivery	Dosing Range	Adverse Effects	Cautions
Nifedipine, amlodipine, diltiazem	Calcium channel blockers	PO	Varies by patient tolerance	Peripheral edema, hypotension, fatigue	**Use only in patients who are vaso-responsive during acute vasodilator challenge**; avoid if low cardiac output or decompensated right heart failure
Sildenafil, Tadalafil	Phosphodiesterase-5 inhibitor	PO	20 mg TID; 40 mg/d	Headache, hypotension, dyspepsia, myalgias, visual disturbances	Avoid using with **nitrates** or **protease inhibitors**
Riociguat	Soluble guanylate cyclase stimulator	PO	2.5 mg TID	Hypotension	Avoid using with **nitrates; approved for PAH and CTEPH that is inoperable or** persistent after endarterectomy
Bosentan	Endothelin receptor antagonist	PO	125 mg BID	Hepatotoxic, teratogen, peripheral edema	**Monthly liver function monitoring**; avoid using with glyburide and glipizide
Ambrisentan	Endothelin receptor antagonist	PO	5–10 mg/d	Teratogen, peripheral edema	Fluid retention, particularly in older patients
Macitentan	Endothelin receptor antagonist	PO	10 mg/d	Teratogen, peripheral edema	Monitor for anemia
Iloprost, Treprostinil	Prostacyclin analogue	IH	2.5–5 μg 6–8×/d; 9 or more breaths QID	Cough, flushing, headache, trismus	**Suboptimal adherence due to dosing frequency**; overnight drug holiday
Selexipag	Prostacyclin receptor agonist	PO	200–1600 mcg BID	Headache, jaw pain, diarrhea, extremity pain	Hyperthyroidism
Treprostinil	Prostacyclin analogue	SC, IV, or PO	Varies by patient tolerance	Headache, jaw pain, diarrhea, extremity pain	**With continuous parenteral use**, catheter-related complications (IV); **site pain/reaction (SC)**; GI distress with PO use
Epoprostenol	Prostacyclin analogue	IV	Varies by patient tolerance	Headache, jaw pain, diarrhea, extremity pain	**Continuous parenteral agent; very short half-life**; catheter-related complications (IV); **high-output state at higher doses**

CTEPH, chronic thromboembolic pulmonary hypertension; GI, gastrointestinal; PO, oral; IH, inhaled; SC, subcutaneous; IV, intravenous.

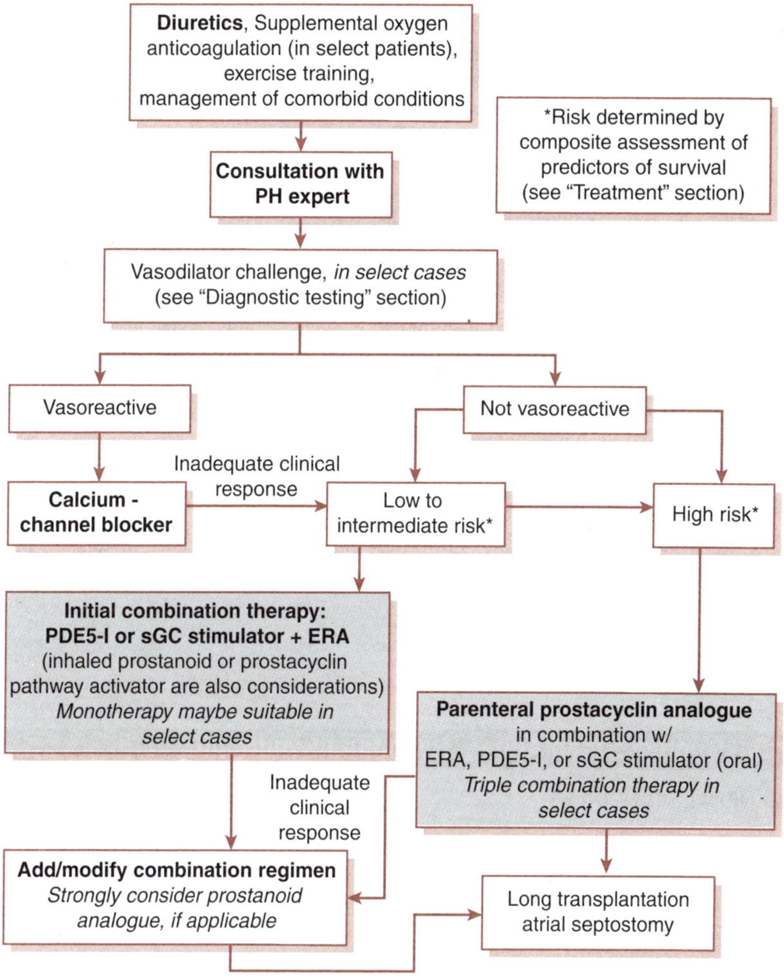

Figure 10-2 Algorithm for management of pulmonary arterial hypertension. ERA, endothelin receptor antagonist; PDE-5 I, phosphodiesterase-5 inhibitor; PH, pulmonary hypertension; sGC, soluble guanylate cyclase.

 - Overdiuresis may be poorly tolerated because of **preload dependency** of the RV and limited ability of the cardiac output to compensate for systemic hypotension.
- **Anticoagulation**
  - Chronic anticoagulation improves survival, primarily in IPAH.[26] Use of anticoagulation in other types of PAH is controversial.[27]
  - Warfarin is dosed to **target international normalized ratio of 1.5–2.5.**[19]
  - Anticoagulant therapy is not urgent and bridging therapy is unnecessary.
- **Inotropic agents**
  Dobutamine and milrinone are best suited for **short-term use** in extremely decompensated states.

Surgical Management

- **Lung transplantation or heart–lung transplantation**
  - Reserved for suitable patients with PAH who **remain in advanced functional class III–IV despite maximal medical therapy.**
  - The **lung allocation score** (LAS), derived from multiple clinical variables, provides a mechanism for prioritizing PAH patients beyond their imputed LAS. This improves the likelihood for patients with IPAH to receive transplants; however, mortality on the waiting list is high compared with other diagnoses.
  - Because the RV recovers after isolated lung transplantation, heart–lung transplantation is usually reserved for complex congenital heart defects that cannot be repaired.
- **Atrial septostomy**
  - Palliative right-to-left intracardiac shunt that is percutaneously created in cases of severe right heart failure (i.e., syncope, hepatic congestion, prerenal azotemia) refractory to medical therapy.
  - Despite arterial oxyhemoglobin desaturation and hypoxemia, oxygen delivery increases from improved LV filling and cardiac output.
- **Septal defect closure**
  - In select cases of intracardiac defects that still have significant left-to-right shunting, closure can be undertaken by **percutaneous or surgical** means.
  - Criteria for closure include net left-to-right shunt with flow ratio (pulmonary flow/systemic flow) ≥1.5, resistance ratio (PVR/systemic vascular resistance) ≤0.6,[28] and PVR >4.6 Wood units.[1]

Prognosis

The 1-, 3-, and 5-year survival rates in PAH are 85%, 70%, and 55%, respectively.[9,29]

Obstructive Sleep Apnea–Hypopnea Syndrome

GENERAL PRINCIPLES

Definition

Obstructive sleep apnea–hypopnea syndrome (OSAHS) is a disorder in which patients experience apneas or hypopneas because of upper airway narrowing. It is associated with excessive daytime somnolence.[30]

Classification

- **Apneas** represent complete cessation of airflow.
  - Obstructive events are associated with continued respiratory effort.
  - Central events are associated with no respiratory effort.
- **Hypopneas** represent diminished airflow associated with at least a 3%–4% oxygen desaturation.
- **Respiratory effort–related arousals (RERAs)** represent changes in airflow that lead to an arousal, but do not meet criteria for an apnea or hypopnea.
- **All respiratory events** must last **at least 10 seconds** to be counted.
- **Apnea–hypopnea index (AHI)** is the number of apneas and hypopneas per hour of sleep.
- **Respiratory disturbance index (RDI)** is the number of apneas, hypopneas, and RERAs per hour of sleep.
- **Respiratory event index (REI)** is the apneas + hypopneas/total recording time.

Epidemiology

- The prevalence of OSAHS in the general population is estimated to be about 4%, with men being twice as likely as women to be affected.[31]
- Obesity is a significant risk factor for obstructive sleep apnea (OSA).[31]
- Given the significant increase in the prevalence of obesity since the original epidemiological studies on OSA were performed, it is estimated that the current prevalence of moderate OSA as defined by an AHI ≥15 is 13% in men and 6% in women.[32]
  - OSAS affects approximately 2% of women and 4% of men living in the Western communities, whereas the average prevalence of OSA is around 7%, and OSAS prevalence is around 3.5% in Hong Kong. In India, the prevalence of OSA is 13.74% and that of OSAS is 3.57%.*

Etiology

- **Obstructive sleep apnea:** Narrowing of the upper airway because of excessive soft tissue or structural abnormalities
- **Central sleep apnea:** Disturbance of central control of respiration during sleep

Pathophysiology

OSA occurs because of narrowing of the upper airway, which results in diminished airflow or cessation of airflow leading to arousals that fragment sleep.

Risk Factors

Risk factors for OSA include obesity (BMI >30), large neck circumference (>17 in for men and >16 in for women), increased soft tissue of the posterior oropharynx (enlarged tonsils, adenoid hypertrophy, macroglossia, or elongated uvula), and abnormal jaw structure (micrognathia or retrognathia). Patients with comorbid conditions such as congestive heart failure, coronary artery disease, hypothyroidism, acromegaly, CKD, Parkinson disease, atrial fibrillation, difficult to control hypertension, and diabetes are also more likely to have OSA.[33]

Prevention

- Weight loss
- Avoiding sedatives such as hypnotic medications or alcohol

Associated Conditions

- **Cardiovascular disease**, including systemic hypertension, heart failure, arrhythmia, myocardial infarction, and stroke.[34] OSA has been established as an independent risk factor for hypertension.[35]
- **Increased risk of death in moderate to severe OSA**, mainly because of cardiovascular events.[36,37]
- Increased prevalence of **diabetes** has been noted in patients with OSAHS, independent of the effect of obesity.[38]
- There is approximately a 2.5-fold increased risk of **motor vehicle accidents** (MVA) in patients with OSA when compared with those without OSA. However, compliance with continuous positive airway pressure (CPAP) treatment can significantly reduce the risk of MVA in patients with OSA.[39]

---

* Mirrakhimov AE, Sooronbaev T, Mirrakhimov EM. Prevalence of obstructive sleep apnea in Asian adults: a systematic review of the literature. *BMC Pulm Med.* 2013;13:10.

DIAGNOSIS

Clinical Presentation

History

- **Habitual loud snoring** is the most common symptom of OSAHS, although not all people who snore have this syndrome. Patients with OSA may experience snore arousals along with a sensation of gasping or choking. Witnessed apneic periods, periods of silence followed by loud snoring, and restless or fitful sleep also suggest OSA.
- Excessive daytime sleepiness (**hypersomnolence**) is a classic symptom of OSAHS (Table 10-3). Patients may describe falling asleep while driving or having difficulty concentrating at work.
- Patients may also complain of personality changes, intellectual deterioration, morning headaches, nocturnal angina, loss of libido, and chronic fatigue.

Physical Examination

- All patients should have a thorough nose and throat examination to detect sources of upper airway obstruction that are surgically correctable (e.g., septal deviation, enlarged tonsils), especially if CPAP is poorly tolerated.
- Increased severity of OSA has been associated with a higher **Mallampati class** (Table 10-4).[40]
- STOP-Bang questionnaire, the Epworth Sleepiness Scale (ESS), the Berlin score, and the sleep apnea clinical score can be used as evaluation tools.

Diagnostic Criteria

A **PSG** demonstrating obstructive events with an RDI >5 is diagnostic of OSA. If the RDI is between 5 and 15, a patient may qualify for CPAP if there is a comorbid condition such

TABLE 10-3 Symptoms Associated With Obstructive Sleep Apnea–Hypopnea Syndrome

Excessive daytime sleepiness
Snoring
Nocturnal arousals
Nocturnal apneas
Nocturnal gasping, grunting, and choking
Nocturia
Enuresis
Awakening without feeling refreshed
Morning headaches
Impaired memory and concentration
Irritability and depression
Impotence

TABLE 10-4 Mallampati Airway Classification

Class	Visible Structures with Mouth Maximally Open and Tongue Protruded
I	Hard palate, soft palate, uvula, tonsillar pillars
II	Hard palate, soft palate, uvula
III	Hard palate, soft palate, base of uvula
IV	Hard palate

Adapted from Mallampati SR, Gatt SP, Gugino LD, et al. A clinical sign to predict difficult tracheal intubation: a prospective study. *Can Anaesth Soc J.* 1985;32:429–434.

as hypertension, coronary artery disease, depression, or hypersomnolence. If there are no comorbid conditions, then the RDI has to be >15 for a patient to qualify for CPAP.

Differential Diagnosis

- In addition to OSAHS and sleep-related hypoventilation, the differential diagnosis for daytime sleepiness includes sleep deprivation, periodic limb movement disorder, narcolepsy, nocturnal seizures, and medication side effects.
- Patients should also be evaluated for other medical conditions that may cause nighttime awakenings and dyspnea and thus mimic OSAHS, such as chronic lung disease (nocturnal asthma), congestive heart failure, and gastroesophageal reflux disease (GERD).

Diagnostic Testing

- The gold standard for the diagnosis of OSAHS is overnight PSG with direct observation by a qualified technician.[41] Sleep studies are typically performed in the outpatient setting.
- Typical indications for a sleep study include snoring with excessive daytime sleepiness, titration of optimal positive airway pressure therapy, and assessment of objective response to therapeutic interventions.
- PSG involves determination of sleep stages using electroencephalography, electromyography, and electro-oculography and assessment of respiratory airflow and effort, oxyhemoglobin saturation, cardiac electrical activity (e.g., ECG), and body position.
- Data are analyzed for sleep staging, the frequency of respiratory events, limb movements, and abnormal behaviors. Respiratory events are categorized as obstructive or central.
- Most sleep studies are performed as "split studies," where the first few hours of the study are diagnostic and the latter part of the study is used for CPAP titration if the AHI is consistent with moderate-to-severe OSA.
- Some patients only have significant events when lying in certain positions (usually supine) or during rapid eye movement sleep. These patients may require a complete overnight study for diagnosis and a second study for initiation of therapy.
- The American Academy of Sleep Medicine supports the use of unattended portable monitoring as an alternative to PSG for patients with a high pretest probability of moderate to severe OSA without significant comorbid medical conditions or other suspected sleep disorders. The portable device must record airflow, respiratory effort, and blood oxygenation. A sleep specialist should review the results. Portable devices can underestimate the severity of OSA because the number of events per hour is calculated using total recording time rather than total sleep time. If the portable sleep study is inconclusive, strong consideration should be given to performing an in-lab PSG.[41]

TREATMENT

The therapeutic approach to OSAHS depends on the severity of the disease, comorbid medical conditions, patient preference, and expected compliance. Treatment must be highly individualized, with special attention paid to correcting potentially reversible exacerbating factors.

Medications

- No pharmacologic agent has sufficient efficacy to warrant replacement of positive airway pressure as the primary therapeutic modality for OSAHS.
- Stimulant pharmacotherapy with **modafinil** or **armodafinil** may improve objective and subjective daytime sleepiness in patients with persistent symptoms despite adequate CPAP use.[42] Other drugs such as theophylline, acetazolamide, desipramine, oxybutynin, and atomoxetine have been tried.

- Medical treatment of conditions that may contribute to muscle hypotonia or weight gain, such as hypothyroidism, is of benefit.

Nonpharmacologic Therapies

- **Positive airway pressure**
- **Indications:**
  - Patients with an AHI >5 events per hour of sleep plus one or more clinical or physiologic sequelae attributable to OSA.
  - Patients with an AHI ≥15 events per hour of sleep, even in the absence of symptoms.
  - Patients with an increased number of RERAs (≥10 per hour) and excessive daytime sleepiness.
- **CPAP** delivers air via a face mask at a constant pressure throughout the respiratory cycle with the goal of pneumatically splinting open the upper airway, thus preventing collapse and airflow obstruction.
  - The PSG determines the positive airway pressure (expressed in cm H_2O) required to optimize airflow. The pressure setting is gradually increased until obstructive events, snoring, and oxygen desaturations are minimized.
  - The benefits of positive airway pressure include consolidated sleep and decreased daytime sleepiness. Hypertension, nocturia, peripheral edema, polycythemia, and PH may also improve. Additionally, CPAP is a highly cost-effective intervention[43] that appears to reduce the risk of cardiovascular events[44] and may also improve the metabolic syndrome associated with OSA.[45] Treatment of OSA results in a higher survival-free rate without recurrent atrial fibrillation after pulmonary vein isolation.[46]
- **Nasal CPAP (nCPAP) is the current treatment of choice for most patients with OSAHS.**
  - The compliance rate with nCPAP is approximately 50%.
    - Compliance can be improved with education, instruction, follow-up, adjustment of the mask for fit and comfort, humidification of the air to decrease dryness, and treatment of nasal or sinus symptoms.
    - Use of a full face mask (oronasal) has not been shown to improve compliance compared with the use of nCPAP.[47] However, full-face masks are frequently used in patients who "mouth breathe" or patients who require higher CPAP pressures because they will often experience air leak through the mouth when using nCPAP.
  - Autotitrating positive airway pressure machines use flow and pressure transducers to sense airflow patterns and then automatically adjust the pressure setting in response. Small studies have shown that autotitrating CPAP may be as effective as traditional CPAP and appears to be preferred by patients.[48,49]
- **Bilevel positive airway pressure** is typically used to treat OSA in the following settings: pressures >15–20 cm and H_2O are required, intolerance of CPAP, or concern for concomitant hypoventilation.
  - All noninvasive positive-pressure ventilation devices may induce dryness of the airway, nasal congestion, rhinorrhea, epistaxis, skin reactions to the mask, nasal bridge abrasions, and aerophagia. Some of these nasal symptoms may be treated with nasal saline, decongestants, and use of a humidifier.
- Some patients, such as those with coexisting chronic obstructive pulmonary disease, require supplemental oxygen to maintain adequate nocturnal oxygen saturations (SaO_2 ≥90%).
- **Oral appliances**
  - Used for mild OSAHS, with aim to increase airway size to improve airflow. These devices, such as the mandibular advancement device, can be fixed or adjustable, and most require customized fitting. Many devices have not been well studied.
  - Contraindications include temporomandibular joint disease, bruxism, full dentures, and inability to protrude the mandible.

- **Upper airway stimulation device**
  - A hypoglossal nerve stimulator to improve tongue protrusion is approved for use in patients with moderate to severe obstructive sleep apnea who cannot tolerate CPAP.
  - Although AHI and daytime sleepiness improved with this device, there was residual mild OSA.[50]

Surgical Management

- **Tracheostomy**
  - Tracheostomy is very effective in treating OSAHS but is rarely used since the advent of positive airway pressure therapy.
  - Tracheostomy should be reserved for patients with life-threatening disease (cor pulmonale, arrhythmias, or severe hypoxemia) or significant alveolar hypoventilation that cannot be controlled with other measures.
- **Uvulopalatopharyngoplasty (UPPP)**
  - UPPP is the most common surgical treatment of mild-to-moderate OSAHS in patients who do not respond to medical therapy.
  - UPPP enlarges the airway by removing tissue from the tonsils, tonsillar pillars, uvula, and posterior palate. UPPP may be complicated by change in voice, nasopharyngeal stenosis, foreign body sensation, velopharyngeal insufficiency with associated nasal regurgitation during swallowing, and CPAP tolerance problems.
  - The success rate of UPPP for treatment of OSAHS is only approximately 50%, when defined as a 50% reduction of the AHI, and improvements related to UPPP may diminish over time.[51] Thus, UPPP is considered a second-line treatment for patients with mild-to-moderate OSAHS who cannot successfully use CPAP and who have retropalatal obstruction.
- **Staged procedures**
  In experienced centers, other staged procedures for OSA can be performed, including mandibular osteotomy with genioglossus advancement, hyoid myotomy with suspension, and maxillomandibular advancement (MMA).[52] Significant reductions in AHI have been reported with MMA, but more research is needed.[53]

Lifestyle/Risk Modification

- Weight loss, both surgical and through reduced caloric intake, has been shown to reduce the severity of OSA by reduction in AHI.[54,55]
- OSAHS patients should avoid use of alcohol, tobacco, and sedatives.
- Clinicians should counsel patients with OSAHS regarding the increased risk of driving and operating dangerous equipment.
- Sleeping in a nonsupine position (lateral recumbent) can improve symptoms of OSA.

SPECIAL CONSIDERATIONS

Patients with a body mass index >40 kg/m^2 are at increased risk for concomitant sleep-related hypoventilation because of morbid obesity.

COMPLICATIONS

- Patients with OSAHS are at greater risk for perioperative complications because of intubation difficulty and/or impaired arousal secondary to the effects of anesthetics, narcotics, and sedatives.[56]
- The risk of death, hypertension, and poor neuropsychological functioning rises with increasing severity of OSA.

REFERRAL

Patients with risk factors and symptoms or sequelae of OSAHS should be referred to a sleep specialist and sleep laboratory for further evaluation.

Interstitial Lung Disease

GENERAL PRINCIPLES

Definition

ILDs are a heterogeneous group of disorders, pathologically characterized by infiltration of the lung interstitium with cells, fluid, and/or connective tissue.

Classification

- ILD of known etiology
  - Medication (e.g., bleomycin, amiodarone, nitrofurantoin, methotrexate)
  - CTD (e.g., rheumatoid arthritis, scleroderma, Sjögren syndrome, antisynthetase syndrome)
  - Pneumoconiosis (e.g., coal worker's pneumoconiosis, silicosis, asbestosis)
  - Radiation
  - Lymphangitic carcinomatosis
- Idiopathic interstitial pneumonias[57]
  - Major idiopathic interstitial pneumonias:
    - Idiopathic pulmonary fibrosis (IPF) (idiopathic usual interstitial pneumonia [UIP])
    - Idiopathic nonspecific interstitial pneumonia (NSIP)
    - Desquamative interstitial pneumonia (DIP)
    - Respiratory bronchiolitis interstitial lung disease (RB-ILD)
    - Cryptogenic organizing pneumonia (COP) (idiopathic organizing pneumonia)
    - Acute interstitial pneumonia
  - Rare idiopathic interstitial pneumonias:
    - Idiopathic lymphoid interstitial pneumonia (LIP)
    - Idiopathic pleuroparenchymal fibroelastosis (IPPFE)
  - Unclassifiable idiopathic interstitial pneumonia
- Granulomatous ILD
  - Sarcoidosis
  - Hypersensitivity pneumonitis (HP)
- Cystic lung disease
  - Lymphangioleiomyomatosis (LAM)
  - Pulmonary Langerhans cell histiocytosis (PLCH)
  - Genetic diseases (Birt–Hogg–Dubé, tuberous sclerosis)
  - Light chain deposition disease

DIAGNOSIS

Clinical Presentation

History

- Patients typically present with indolently progressive breathlessness with exertion or a persistent nonproductive cough. History often reveals years of gradually worsening symptoms, although a subset (acute interstitial pneumonia, acute eosinophilic pneumonia) may present acutely.
- Careful questioning should focus on symptoms of CTD.

- Exposures both at home and in the workplace should be evaluated. These may include exposures to medications, radiation, asbestos, fumes or dusts, birds (including down comforters and/or pillows), and molds.
- Smoking is associated with pulmonary Langerhans cell histiocytosis, desquamative interstitial pneumonitis, respiratory bronchiolitis-interstitial lung disease, and idiopathic pulmonary fibrosis.
- The patient should be asked about exposure to radiation and drugs.
- Clinical features of common ILDs are described in Table 10-5.

TABLE 10-5 Clinical and Radiologic Features of Interstitial Lung Diseases

	Clinical Features	HRCT Findings
UIP	• Insidious onset and progressive dyspnea • Dry cough • Poorly responsive to treatment, poor long-term survival • Variable course punctuated by intermittent exacerbations • Pattern can be associated with connective tissue disease • Older patients >50 years • Male predominance	• UIP on CT or biopsy forms the radiologic basis for diagnosing IPF in the absence of underlying cause • Subpleural, basal predominant reticulation / interstitial thickening • Honeycombing with/without traction bronchiectasis • Absence of ground glass, consolidation, micronodules, cysts or air-trapping • May have atypical distribution in familial cases
NSIP	• Associated with younger patients • More common in females • Commonly associated with collagen vascular diseases, including scleroderma, rheumatoid arthritis, and myositis • Response to therapy is variable depending on etiology	• Interstitial thickening, often with peripheral subpleural sparing • Ground-glass infiltrates • Traction bronchiectasis • In end-stage disease, may develop fibrotic changes and "bronchiolectasis" that resembles UIP
RB-ILD	• Associated with cigarette smoking • Generally responsive to smoking cessation	• Bronchiolocentric ground-glass nodules with an upper lobe predominance
DIP	• Associated with cigarette smoking and occupational exposures • Generally responsive to smoking cessation • May be treated with corticosteroids	• Peripheral ground-glass opacities or consolidation • May have small, well-defined cysts
AIP	• Rapidly progressive ILD with progressive hypoxemia and high mortality • Clinically (and histologically) similar to ARDS (may be considered "idiopathic ARDS")	• Ground-glass opacities admixed with consolidation in geographic pattern • Eventually progresses to fibrosis with architectural distortion and traction bronchiectasis

(Continued)

TABLE 10-5 Clinical and Radiologic Features of Interstitial Lung Diseases (Continued)

	Clinical Features	HRCT Findings
COP	• Subacute course, often presents as multiple outpatient treatment failures of bronchitis/pneumonia • Often associated with infections or drug exposures • Responsive to prolonged courses of corticosteroids • Often recurs if steroids are withdrawn too rapidly	• Multifocal ground-glass opacities and consolidations • Usually lower lobe predominant • Infiltrates may be migratory on serial imaging • May have "reverse halo" or atoll sign
CEP	• Presents as progressive dyspnea and cough • Patients may have a history of underlying asthma • Peripheral blood and BAL eosinophil counts usually elevated	• Peripheral consolidations described as the "reverse image of pulmonary edema" • Infiltrates may be migratory
Sarcoidosis	• Dyspnea, cough, and chest pain are common presenting symptoms • Systemic symptoms may be prominent • Approximately 1 in 20 cases are asymptomatic and incidentally detected on CXR • Almost any organ system may be affected	• Perilymphatic nodules • Patchy ground-glass opacities • Reticular infiltrates • Traction bronchiectasis • Progressive massive fibrosis • Hilar or mediastinal lymphadenopathy
Chronic HP	• Presents in a similar fashion to UIP/IPF • There may be a history of systemic symptoms (fever, myalgias) • Associated with environmental exposures (birds, molds, hot tubs) but these are identified in <50% of cases	• Reticular abnormality with an upper or mid-lung predominance • Micronodules • Mosaic attenuation/air trapping • Peribronchovascular predominance

AIP, acute interstitial pneumonia; ARDS, acute respiratory distress syndrome; BAL, bronchoalveolar lavage; CEP, chronic eosinophilic pneumonia; COP, cryptogenic organizing pneumonia; DIP, desquamative interstitial pneumonia; HP, hypersensitivity pneumonitis; HRCT, high-resolution CT; ILD, interstitial lung disease; IPF, idiopathic pulmonary fibrosis; NSIP, nonspecific interstitial pneumonia; RB-ILD, respiratory bronchiolitis interstitial lung disease; UIP, usual interstitial pneumonia.

Data from Kadoch MA, Cham MD, Beasley MB, et al. Idiopathic interstitial pneumonias: a radiology-pathology correlation based on the revised 2013 American Thoracic Society-European Respiratory Society classification system. *Curr Probl Diagn Radiol.* 2015;44:15–25; Raghu G, Collard HR, Egan JJ, et al. An official ATS/ERS/JRS/ALAT statement: idiopathic pulmonary fibrosis: evidence-based guidelines for diagnosis and management. *Am J Respir Crit Care Med.* 2011;183:788–824; Webb RW, Higgins CB. *Thoracic Imaging: Pulmonary and Cardiovascular Radiology.* New York: Lippincott Williams & Wilkins; 2005.

Physical Examination

Findings may include inspiratory velcro crackles and digital clubbing. Close attention should be paid to extrapulmonary findings that point toward CTDs. Examples include sclerodactyly, mechanic's hands, Raynaud phenomenon, dry mucous membranes, and dermatologic findings such as telangiectasias, rashes, or facial erythema. Cardiac examination may reveal signs of pulmonary hypertension and cor pulmonale.

Diagnostic Approach

Imaging

- Plain radiographs of the chest have variable appearance, with lung volume loss, interstitial thickening, and cystic changes being most common in ILD.
- If initial radiograph or clinical scenario is consistent with ILD, the patient should be referred for high-resolution CT (HRCT), which is the radiographic test of choice for patients with suspected ILD.
- The pattern of radiographic infiltrate is important in the differential diagnosis of ILD. Imaging patterns of common ILDs are described in Table 10-5. Notably, published guidelines exist for the definitive radiologic diagnosis of certain ILDs, specifically IPF/UIP.[58]

Pulmonary Function Testing

- Spirometry typically demonstrates a restrictive ventilatory defect characterized by a symmetric reduction in forced vital capacity (FVC) and forced expiratory volume in 1 second (FEV_1). Definitive diagnosis of a restrictive ventilatory defect requires documentation of a reduction in total lung capacity (TLC) to <80% of the patients predicted TLC.
- In certain ILDs (e.g., sarcoidosis, PLCH, LAM), bronchiolar involvement may result in airflow obstruction and an obstructive ventilatory defect, causing the FEV_1 to decrease disproportionately to the FVC resulting in an FEV_1:FVC ratio of <70%.
- In some cases, a mixed obstructive and restrictive defect may be seen. This circumstance may also exist in cases of ILD with comorbid emphysema.
- DLCO is often significantly decreased in patients with ILD.

Laboratory Analysis

- Patients with a diagnosis of ILD, especially those with evidence of CTD on history or clinical examination, should be evaluated with serologies.
- Identifying CTD can be difficult as it may manifest primarily with pulmonary symptoms. As an example, approximately 10%–20% of patients with rheumatoid arthritis may have lung disease as their initial clinical presentation.[59]
- ANA and rheumatoid factor (RF) should be tested in most patients, even patients with UIP on thoracic imaging. Cyclic citrullinated peptide should also be tested to evaluate for rheumatoid arthritis because RF may be insufficiently sensitive and has a low positive predictive value.
- Aldolase and creatinine kinase should be tested to evaluate for evidence of myositis. In cases where suspicion is high for myositis, panels of muscle-specific antibodies should also be obtained.
- In any patient with evidence of scleroderma such as telangiectasias, esophageal dysmotility, or sclerodactyly, antibodies against topoisomerase I (anti-Scl-70) should be obtained.

Diagnostic Procedures

- Bronchoalveolar lavage is controversial in the evaluation of ILD outside of excluding infection.
- Lung biopsy should be undertaken with the input of pulmonologists and thoracic surgeons with expertise in ILD.
  - Three types of lung biopsy are available: transbronchial forceps biopsy, cryobiopsy, and surgical biopsy.

- Generally, biopsy should be reserved for circumstances where the diagnosis is uncertain and clarification would result in a significantly altered approach to management.
- Transbronchial forceps lung biopsy has the highest yield in bronchocentric ILDs, such as sarcoidosis, in which small biopsy samples suffice for diagnosis.[60]
- Transbronchial forceps biopsies are insufficient at differentiating most idiopathic ILDs, and especially between UIP from NSIP, given inadequate sample size.
- Transbronchial cryobiopsy is a developing option that allows for larger tissue sampling without a surgical lung biopsy. Further studies are required to integrate this technique into the ILD diagnostic algorithm.[61]
- Surgical lung biopsy can be performed by video-assisted thoracoscopic surgery (VATS) or open thoracotomy. HRCT is used to target areas of active disease and avoid lung regions with end-stage fibrosis.
- Although many patients tolerate lung biopsy well, certain subgroups of patients are predisposed to complications, including decompensation of their ILD following lung biopsy.[62] Patients with IPF in particular may develop disease exacerbations following lung biopsy, resulting in disease progression and even death.

SPECIFIC INTERSTITIAL LUNG DISEASES

Idiopathic Pulmonary Fibrosis

- The incidence of IPF is estimated to be 4.6–16.3 cases per 100,000 population.
- Prevalence and incidence of IPF are higher in American population than in European and Asian population.[*,†]
- South Korean 2011-2012 incidence of IPF was 1.7/100,000.[‡]
- Japan from 2003 to 2007 indicated that the prevalence and cumulative incidence of IPF was 10.0 and 2.23 per 100,000 population, respectively, with 72.7% of cases involving males.[§]
- Males are more frequently affected than females.
- Mutations in telomerase RNA component (*TERC*), telomerase reverse transcriptase (*TERT*), pulmonary surfactant protein C (*SFTPC*), surfactant protein A2 (*SFTPA2*), and mucin 5B (*MUC5B*) have been identified in individuals and families with IPF.[63]
- Although the pathophysiology is incompletely understood, pulmonary epithelial cell injury and aberrant wound healing are thought to play a central role.
- Diagnosis is made by either a definite radiographic pattern for UIP on HRCT (Table 10-5, Figure 10-3) or UIP pattern on surgical lung biopsy in the absence of other known causes after thorough workup has been completed.[58]
- In the setting of a familial fibrotic lung disease, the CT pattern may be atypical, often lacking a basal predominance. Even histologically, strictly defined UIP is identified in less than half of familial fibrotic lung disease cases.[64]
- Disease-modifying treatment options are limited in IPF.
  - Increased risks of death and hospitalization have been associated with combined use of *N*-acetylcysteine, azathioprine, and prednisone.[65]

---

[*] Nalysnyk L, Cid-Ruzafa J, Rotella P, Esser D. Incidence and prevalence of idiopathic pulmonary fibrosis: review of the literature. *Eur Respir Rev*. 2012;21:355–361.

[†] Hutchinson JP, McKeever TM, Fogarty AW, Navaratnam V, Hubbard RB. Increasing global mortality from idiopathic pulmonary fibrosis in the twenty-first century. *Ann Am Thorac Soc*. 2014;11:1176–1185.

[‡] Sun C, Sun Y, Shen H, Yang C, Xu S. Idiopathic pulmonary fibrosis in East Asian. *Intractable Rare Dis Res*. 2017;6(2):80–86.

[§] Natsuizaka M, Chiba H, Kuronuma K, et al. Epidemiologic survey of Japanese patients with idiopathic pulmonary fibrosis and investigation of ethnic differences. *Am J Respir Crit Care Med*. 2014;190:773–779.

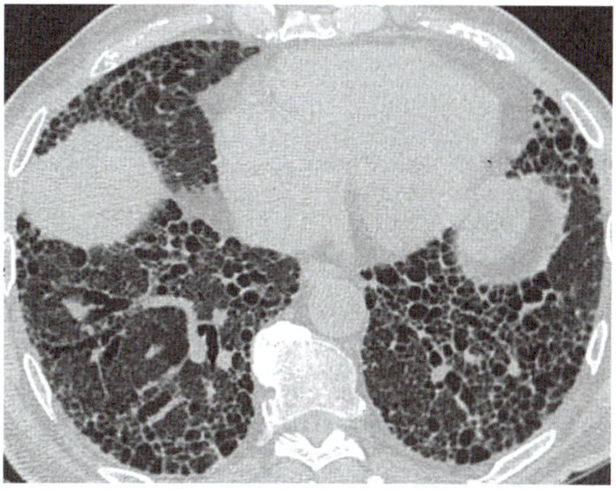

Figure 10-3 Usual interstitial pneumonitis. (Figure courtesy of Sanjeev Bhalla, Mallinckrodt Institute of Radiology.)

- Pirfenidone, an oral antifibrotic agent, and nintedanib, an oral tyrosine kinase inhibitor, have both been shown to slow down the rate of decline in lung function in patients with IPF.[66,67]
- **Pirfenidone** in a dose of 40 mg/kg/day inhibits transforming growth factor beta (TGF-β)-stimulated collagen synthesis.
- **Nintedanib**, a receptor blocker for multiple tyrosine kinases that mediate elaboration of fibrogenic growth factors at a dose of 150 mg twice daily, is seen to slow the rate of disease progression in IPF.

- Pulmonary rehabilitation has been associated with improvements in 6MW distance and quality of life in IPF.[68]
- Patients have a widely variable course, but those diagnosed with spirometrically mild, moderate, and severe disease have been reported to have median survivals of 55.6, 38.7, and 27.4 months, respectively.[69]
- Poor prognostic factors for IPF include a decline in FVC of >10% over 6 months, a decrease in 6MW distance of >150 m over 12 months, and a decrease in DLCO of >15% over 6 months.
- Acute exacerbations of IPF are characterized by acute worsening of dyspnea or oxygenation with no evidence of infection, pulmonary embolus, or heart failure.[58] Exacerbations are typically treated with high-dose corticosteroids, although their benefit has not been systematically proven. Patients often do not return to their pre-exacerbation baseline after IPF exacerbations and mortality rates are high.[70]
- Lung transplantation remains the ultimate therapy in patients with advanced IPF. Criteria for lung transplantation are listed in Table 10-6. Without lung transplantation, outcomes in IPF remain poor. Patients in the community should be referred to a tertiary center with a lung transplant program for consideration of lung transplantation at time of diagnosis of IPF.

Nonspecific Interstitial Pneumonia

- NSIP is rarely idiopathic; there is normally an identifiable etiology. Idiopathic NSIP is a diagnosis of exclusion. Careful history and physical examination should be performed to guide laboratory testing in the search for an underlying etiology.

TABLE 10-6 Criteria for Listing for Lung Transplantation in Idiopathic Pulmonary Fibrosis and Sarcoidosis

IPF
• SpO_2 <88% during a 6-min walk test • Walk distance <250 m on 6-min walk test • ≥50 m decline in walk distance on 6-min walk test over 6 mo of follow-up • ≥15% decline in DLCO over 6 mo of follow-up • ≥10% decline in FVC over 6 mo of follow-up • Pulmonary hypertension (right heart catheterization or echocardiogram) • Respiratory hospitalization secondary to decline or acute exacerbation of IPF
Sarcoidosis
NYHA functional class III or IV and any of the following: • Hypoxemia at rest • Pulmonary hypertension (right heart catheterization or echocardiogram) • Right atrial pressure >15 mm Hg

DLCO, diffusing capacity of the lung for carbon monoxide; FVC, forced vital capacity; HRCT, high-resolution CT; IPF, idiopathic pulmonary fibrosis; NYHA, New York Heart Association; SpO_2, oxyhemoglobin saturation by pulse oximetry; UIP, usual interstitial pneumonia.
Adapted from Orens
JB, Estenne M, Arcasoy S, et al. International guidelines for the selection of lung transplant candidates: 2006 update–a consensus report from the Pulmonary Scientific Council of the International Society for Heart and Lung Transplantation. *J Heart Lung Transplant.* 2006;25:745–755.

- Imaging (Figure 10-4) demonstrates ground-glass opacities with reticular infiltrates in a peripheral distribution. There is often sparing of the immediate subpleural space from infiltration. Traction bronchiectasis may progress to "bronchiolectasis" in advanced disease. This can appear radiographically similar to UIP.

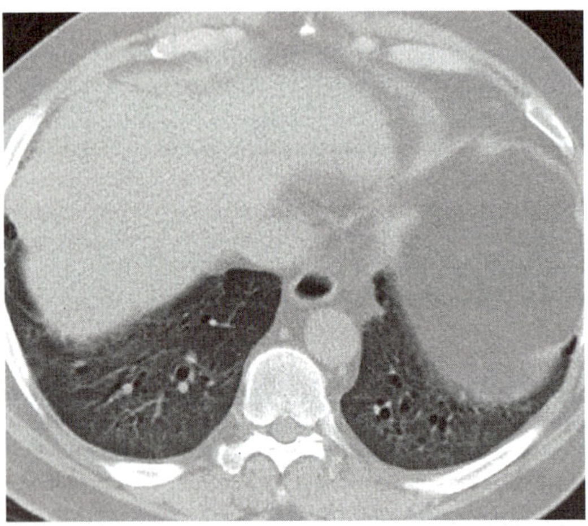

Figure 10-4 Nonspecific interstitial pneumonitis. (Figure courtesy of Sanjeev Bhalla, Mallinckrodt Institute of Radiology.)

- Patients with NSIP fare better than those with IPF.[71]
- Treatment of NSIP secondary to CTDs usually involves immunosuppression with steroids, in combination with agents such as mycophenolate, azathioprine, cyclophosphamide, or rituximab.
- Management of patients with CTD-related ILD should be undertaken in a multidisciplinary fashion with input from providers who are familiar and experienced with these conditions.
- The effects of treating idiopathic NSIP are not well known but are an area of active investigation. Treatment with mycophenolate mofetil in particular seems promising and has been associated with stable or improved pulmonary physiology.[72]

Hypersensitivity Pneumonitis

- HP is a complex syndrome caused by poorly understood immunologic processes directed against inhaled antigens.
- HP is characterized by acute, subacute, and chronic phases, with most patients presenting in the chronic phase.
- Symptoms of dyspnea and cough may manifest acutely or progress indolently over time.
- Unlike IPF, with which it is commonly confused, HP may manifest with systemic symptoms including fevers, chills, and myalgias in acute disease and anorexia, weight loss, and fatigue in chronic disease.
- Radiographically, HRCT demonstrates peribronchovascular nodularity with ground-glass opacities and evidence of air trapping. Findings will generally affect the upper lobes. In advanced disease, pulmonary fibrosis with architectural distortion may occur.[73]
- Innumerable antigenic stimuli have been associated with the development of HP. A careful exposure history should be taken and should include inquiry about exposure to birds or bird feathers (including down pillows and comforters), hot tubs (associated with aerosolized mycobacterial exposure), air humidifiers, molds, animal furs, epoxies, plant matter, industrial dusts, and chemicals.
- Specific antibody measurements can be sent to specialized labs when indicated, although positive serologies only support exposure to the antigens against which the antibodies are directed, and do not necessarily confirm causation.
- The causative exposure/antigen is identified in <50% of cases.
- Corticosteroid therapy has been the classic mainstay of treatment for HP. However, careful attention should be paid toward identification of the offending antigen because antigenic avoidance, when identified, has been associated with significantly improved survival.[74]

Sarcoidosis

- Sarcoidosis is diagnosed by the presence of noncaseating granulomas on biopsy samples (lung or lymph nodes).
- Exclusion of infectious etiologies is of particular importance in patients with exposure to endemic fungi/mycobacteria.
- The incidence rate in the United States is 35.5/100,000 for blacks and 10.9/100,000 for whites.[75]
- The cause of sarcoidosis has not been identified, although there are likely both environmental and genetic factors.[76]
- Patients frequently present for evaluation of progressive dyspnea and cough.
- Löfgren syndrome is defined as an acute presentation of sarcoidosis characterized by arthritis, erythema nodosum, and bilateral hilar lymphadenopathy.[76]
- CXR imaging in sarcoidosis varies from hilar adenopathy to diffuse pulmonary fibrosis and is used to stage the disease (Table 10-7) (Figure 10-5).

TABLE 10-7 Staging of Sarcoidosis

CXR Findings
Stage 0: Normal
Stage 1: Hilar or mediastinal lymphadenopathy
Stage 2: Hilar or mediastinal lymphadenopathy with pulmonary infiltrates
Stage 3: Pulmonary infiltrates
Stage 4: End-stage fibrosis

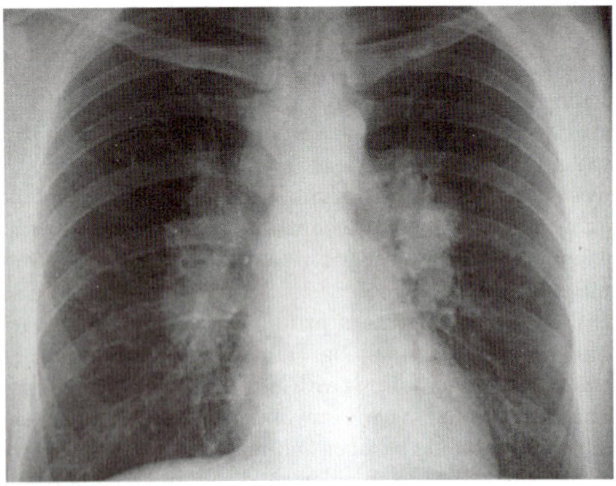

Figure 10-5 Chest X-ray showing bilateral hilar, subcarinal and right paratracheal adenopathy in sarcoidosis.

- On CT scan, parenchymal nodules appear in at least 80% of patients, typically following a bronchovascular distribution with intermittent coalescence into larger opacities.[77] Air trapping may be present.
- A granulomatous vasculitis may occur and predispose patients to the development of PH.
- Extrapulmonary manifestations are possible.
  - Most commonly include uveitis and skin disease such as erythema nodosum (raised, red, tender nodules on anterior legs) and lupus pernio (indurated plaques with associated discoloration of the nose, cheeks, lips, and ears).
  - Central nervous system involvement can manifest as central lesions (encephalopathy/vasculopathy, granulomatous meningitis), mononeuritis multiplex, or a host of other neurologic anomalies. Patients with these findings should be referred to specialists with experience in the treatment of this disorder.
  - Myocardial involvement may result in valvular dysfunction, cardiomyopathy, pericarditis, arrhythmia, and sudden cardiac death.[78]
  - Ocular involvement in the form of uveitis, keratoconjunctivitis sicca, and adnexal granuloma is common.
  - Endocrine involvement can manifest as hypercalcemia and hypercalciuria secondary to dysregulated production of calcitriol.[75] Also, infiltration of hypothalamus and thyroid is seen.
  - Interstitial nephritis and granulomatous nephritis have been associated with sarcoid.
- Annual ophthalmology evaluation should be considered a standard part of sarcoidosis care to monitor for ocular involvement. Referral to other specialists may be necessary as other visceral symptoms develop.

- For early stage disease, symptoms and radiographic changes may remit in the absence of treatment. In the setting of symptomatic disease or progression, corticosteroid therapy is typically first line. Many patients can be treated with intermittent steroid therapy alone, although those with advanced disease may be transitioned to nonsteroidal immunosuppression such as methotrexate or azathioprine. Infliximab is typically reserved for severe or progressive disease.[79]
- Prognosis is highly variable, ranging from indolent self-remitting disease to progressive fibrosis requiring transplantation. Indications for transplantation are reviewed in Table 10-6.

Organizing Pneumonia

- Organizing pneumonia is radiographically represented by decreased lung volumes and multifocal patchy consolidation and ground-glass opacities.
- Pathologically, organizing pneumonia represents a response to a proinflammatory stimulus. This is often infectious in nature, although a wide variety of pharmacologic agents and environmental exposures have been implicated as well. Idiopathic cases known as COP do occur.
- The typical clinical scenario is a patient with multiple episodes of "pneumonia" treated with antibiotics with absence of complete recovery.
- COP is a diagnosis of exclusion, and a comprehensive search for infectious or autoimmune etiology should be undertaken.
- Organizing pneumonia is typically responsive to steroid therapy.
- Recurrence, however, is common after steroid withdrawal, and long-term therapy (>6 months) is frequently necessary.

"Smoking-Related" ILD

- Smoking is associated with a number of ILDs.
- The risk of IPF is increased in smokers.
- RB-ILD presents in patients in the third to fifth decades of life with dyspnea, cough, and radiographic evidence of subtle upper lobe ground-glass nodules on HRCT. Prognosis is good with smoking cessation.
- DIP may represent a spectrum of disease along with RB-ILD. The predominant HRCT finding in DIP is ground-glass opacities, which may be peripheral, patchy, or diffuse in distribution. Small cystic spaces occasionally develop within the ground-glass opacities. Response to smoking cessation is generally favorable, although some patients require corticosteroid therapy. The disease occasionally persists despite therapy.[80] A more severe form of DIP may also be observed in occupational exposures, and a congenital form may be seen in children.
- PLCH is a parenchymal cystic lung disease characterized by irregular cysts associated with parenchymal nodules, often with sparing of the lung bases. Response to smoking cessation is generally considered good, although some patients have persistent, treatment-unresponsive disease. PLCH can be seen in the setting of systemic Langerhans cell histiocytosis as well, with treatment (usually chemotherapy) directed toward the systemic process.

Pneumoconiosis

- Pneumoconiosis are diseases of the lung parenchyma that result from exposure to inorganic dusts.
- Asbestos-induced lung disease arises from exposure to asbestos. Radiographic findings may range from pleural thickening and plaques to parenchymal changes resembling UIP. The presence of pleural plaques aids in differentiation from other ILDs, but asbestos-related fibrotic disease can exist in the absence of pleural manifestations. Treatment focuses on asbestos avoidance and supportive care. Prognosis is good in mild disease, although the risk of lung cancer (non-small cell and small cell carcinoma of the lung as well as malignant mesothelioma) is significantly increased in the setting of concomitant cigarette use.

- Silicosis results from exposure to silica crystals, which are found in stone and sand. Foundry workers, construction workers, sandblasters, and glassblowers are at increased risk. CXRs demonstrate small nodules in the upper and mid zones with hilar adenopathy in a manner similar to sarcoidosis. Patients who develop silicosis after a short time period are at increased risk for the later development of progressive massive fibrosis (PMF). Treatment is supportive, although close monitoring for development of tuberculosis (TB) is warranted given the increased risk of TB in these patients.[81]
- Berylliosis is caused by exposure to beryllium and beryllium compounds. Exposure occurs in the aerospace industry, atomic industry, beryllium mining, and fluorescent light bulb manufacturing. It is clinically indistinguishable from pulmonary sarcoidosis.

Cystic Lung Disease

- LAM is a progressive cystic disease of the lung seen exclusively in young women. LAM is seen frequently in patients with tuberous sclerosis where it can affect men too, although much less commonly. Imaging demonstrates diffuse, round, thin-walled cysts. Pneumothorax is a common initial presentation. Extrapulmonary manifestations may include renal tumors, specifically angiomyolipomas. Sirolimus has been shown to reduce disease progression, but disease recurs once therapy is stopped, and long-term effects are uncertain at this point.[82]
- Amyloidosis and light chain deposition disease can be associated with cystic lung disease in the setting of underlying systemic amyloidosis, long-standing CTD, or myeloma. Cysts are variable in size and distribution. Treatment focuses on the underlying condition.
- LIP is a rare disease, usually associated with CTDs (primarily Sjögren syndrome), lymphoproliferative diseases (such as lymphoma), and viral infections (such as HIV). Idiopathic cases also occur. Imaging demonstrates irregular cysts, multifocal ground-glass opacities, nodularity, and septal thickening. Treatment and prognosis are variable depending on the underlying condition.
- Birt–Hogg–Dubé syndrome is a rare cause of cystic disease associated with skin and renal neoplasms. Cysts are irregularly shaped and commonly localized to the lung bases. Treatment is supportive, and progression is generally slow.[83]
- PLCH is described under the "Smoking-Related" ILD section.

MANAGEMENT CONSIDERATIONS

- The medical management of selected ILDs is briefly reviewed in Table 10-8.
- All ILD patients should be monitored for the development of hypoxemia. Supplemental oxygenation should be provided to maintain oxyhemoglobin saturation by pulse oximetry (SpO_2) ≥89% both at rest and with exertion (measured by 6MW testing).
- Smoking cessation/avoidance should be strongly encouraged, and patients should avoid occupational/environmental triggers of their ILD, if identified.
- Pulmonary rehabilitation therapy should be prescribed for all patients if they meet eligibility criteria.
- Bone density assessment is recommended for patients receiving chronic systemic corticosteroid therapy, and periodic reassessment (e.g., every 1–2 years) should be performed.
- *Pneumocystis jirovecii* pneumonia prophylaxis should be considered in patients receiving chronic immunosuppressive therapy.[84]
- Patients should receive vaccinations against pneumococcus and influenza.
- Patients with ILDs should be considered for referral to centers with expertise in the diagnosis and treatment of these conditions, with particular consideration for participation in ongoing clinical trials.
- ILD increases the risk of PH.[85] Patients with dyspnea out of proportion to their parenchymal lung disease or those with symptoms of right heart failure should be screened

TABLE 10-8 Medical Treatment of Selected Interstitial Lung Diseases

ILD	Potential Therapeutic Interventions[a]
Medication-induced ILD	• Discontinue culprit medication • Corticosteroids
Connective tissue disease–associated ILD (UIP, NSIP, COP)	• Corticosteroids • Immunosuppressive therapy (e.g., cyclophosphamide, azathioprine, mycophenolate, rituximab)
IPF	• Pirfenidone • Nintedanib • Consideration for participation in a clinical trial
DIP, RB-ILD	• Smoking cessation • Corticosteroids (likely of limited benefit)
Sarcoidosis	• Corticosteroids • Immunosuppressive therapy (e.g., methotrexate, azathioprine, infliximab)
Chronic HP	• Avoid offending antigens • Corticosteroids (likely of limited benefit) • Immunosuppressive therapy

[a]Lung transplantation is a consideration for select patients with end-stage interstitial lung disease.

COP, cryptogenic organizing pneumonia; DIP, desquamative interstitial pneumonia; HP, hypersensitivity pneumonitis; ILD, interstitial lung disease; IPF, idiopathic pulmonary fibrosis; NSIP, nonspecific interstitial pneumonia; RB-ILD, respiratory bronchiolitis-interstitial lung disease; TNF, tumor necrosis factor; UIP, usual interstitial pneumonia.

with TTE. Although the use of pulmonary vasodilators in this population remains controversial, other therapies targeted at maintenance of euvolemia and optimization of RV function can be helpful in controlling symptoms.

- Several of the ILDs are associated with an increased incidence of malignancy. Rapid weight loss or radiographic changes (e.g., new solitary nodules or persistent consolidation) should raise suspicion and prompt further workup.
- Goals of care and expectations of therapy should be made clear to all patients.
- Palliative care is an ongoing part of disease management in many ILDs, and hospice care should be discussed with all patients with advanced disease who are not transplant candidates. Open discussions of goals of care are helpful in guiding management of acute exacerbations and progressive disease.[86]

Hemoptysis

GENERAL PRINCIPLES

Hemoptysis is the coughing up of blood or blood-stained mucus. It is a sign of an underlying pulmonary pathologic process. It can be life-threatening and as such requires rapid identification, workup, and treatment.

Definition

- **True hemoptysis** is expectoration of blood from the lower respiratory tract below the glottis.

- **Massive hemoptysis/life-threatening hemoptysis:**
  - Is usually defined by volume per unit time.
  - Definitions range from >100 mL in 16 hours to >1000 mL in 24 hours.
  - It is most commonly defined as **>600 mL of blood expectorated per 24 hours.**[87,88]
  - Volumes of >100 mL in 24 hours associated with gas exchange abnormality, airway obstruction, or hemodynamic instability are also considered life-threatening.

Classification

Clinically, hemoptysis is usually classified as being **massive/life-threatening or not (see above).** It may also be classified by the **anatomic location** of the bleeding.

- Airway
- Parenchyma
- Vascular
- Combination

There are various other classifications in the literature based on appearance, frequency, rate, volume, and potential for clinical consequences of the hemoptysis that may suggest an underlying etiology or predict outcome and thus help guide in diagnosis and management. However, considerable overlap exists in the clinical presentation both within and between etiologies.

Etiology

It is clinically useful to identify etiology according to anatomic location.

- Airway: **bronchitis (acute and chronic), bronchiectasis, malignancy**, foreign body, trauma, pulmonary endometriosis, broncholithiasis, and bronchovascular fistula.
- Parenchymal: **tuberculosis, pneumonia, lung abscess, vasculitides, and pulmonary hemorrhage syndromes** (antineutrophil cytoplasmic antibody [ANCA]–positive vasculitis, Goodpasture syndrome, systemic lupus erythematosus, diffuse alveolar hemorrhage, acute respiratory distress syndrome)
- Vascular: **elevated pulmonary venous pressure** (LV failure, mitral stenosis), pulmonary embolism, arteriovenous malformation (AVM), pulmonary arterial trauma (i.e., pulmonary arterial catheter balloon overinflation), varices/aneurysms, vasculitides, and pulmonary hemorrhage syndromes
- Etiologies involving multiple anatomic locations: **cavitary lung disease** (TB, aspergilloma, lung abscess), thrombocytopenia, disseminated intravascular coagulation, anticoagulants, antiplatelets, cocaine and other inhaled agents, lung biopsy, bronchovascular fistula, bronchopulmonary sequestration, and Dieulafoy disease
- **Idiopathic/undiagnosed lesions may occur in up to 50% of case series.** The prognosis in these cases is usually favorable, although up to 4% may eventually be diagnosed with malignancy.[89,90]

Epidemiology

The incidence of each cause of hemoptysis varies considerably. Listed are some of the most common causes of hemoptysis.[90,91]

- Bronchiectasis: 1%–37%
- Bronchitis: 2%–37%
- Malignancy: 2%–24%
- TB/cavitary lung disease: 2%–69%
- Pneumonia: 1%–16%
- Pulmonary embolus: 3%
- Pulmonary edema: 4%
- Idiopathic: 2%–50%

Pathophysiology

The source of hemoptysis depends on the etiology and location of the underlying pathologic process.

- **The pulmonary arterial circulation** supplies 99% of all blood flow to the lung parenchyma under low pressure. Disruption can result in minor hemoptysis or more life-threatening hemoptysis because of processes such as vasculitis, diffuse alveolar hemorrhage, pulmonary embolism, acute respiratory distress syndrome, AVM rupture, pulmonary artery catheter trauma, severe mitral stenosis, LV failure, or Rasmussen aneurysm (pulmonary artery aneurysm associated with TB).
- **The bronchial arterial circulation** arises from the aorta and intercostal arteries. It supplies high-pressure blood flow to the lungs but accounts for only 1% of pulmonary blood flow. Disruption by a foreign body, tumor invasion, fungal invasion, or denuded airway mucosa can result in massive, life-threatening hemoptysis. Bleeding from the bronchial circulation may account for up to 88% of all cases of massive hemoptysis.

DIAGNOSIS

Identifying and correcting the underlying pathologic process is the basis of diagnosis and management of hemoptysis (Figure 10-6).

Clinical Presentation

Hemoptysis may present in isolation or accompany other manifestations of an underlying disorder (Table 10-9). The appearance, timing, and volume of hemoptysis can provide important clues to narrowing the differential diagnosis.

- Appearance: gross blood, blood-tinged sputum, blood-streaking, foamy pink sputum

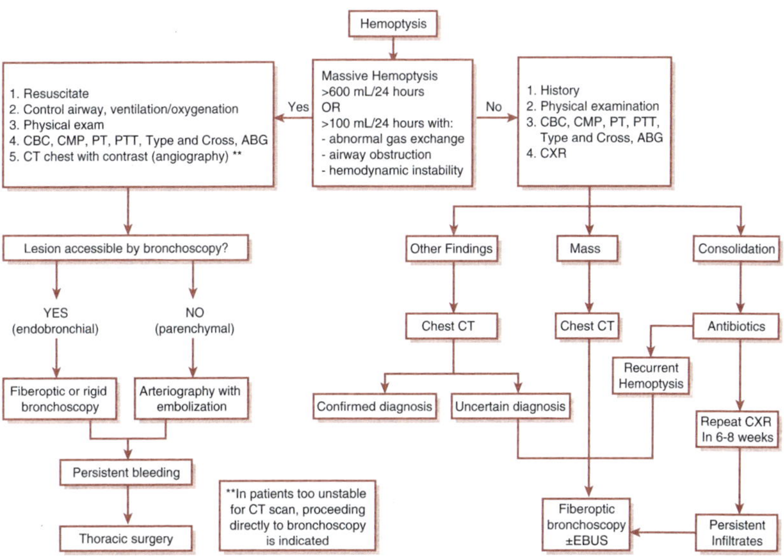

Figure 10-6 Algorithm for evaluation of hemoptysis. ABG, arterial blood gas; CBC, complete blood count; CMP, complete metabolic panel; CT, computed tomography; EBUS, endobronchial ultrasound; PT, prothrombin time; PTT, partial thromboplastin. (Adapted from Earwood JS, Thompson TD. Hemoptysis: evaluation and management. *Am Fam Physician*. 2015;91:243-249.)

TABLE 10-9 Clues to Diagnosing the Cause of Hemoptysis From the History and Physical Examination

Cause of Hemoptysis	Historical Clue	Physical Examination Finding
Bronchogenic carcinoma	Smoker, age >40 y; recurrent nonmassive hemoptysis, weight loss	Local chest wheezing
Chronic bronchitis/ bronchiectasis	Frequent, copious sputum production; frequent "pneumonias"	Scattered, bilateral, coarse crackles, wheezes; clubbing
TB, fungal lung disease, lung abscess	Subacute constitutional symptoms; travel and exposure history	Fever, focal coarse chest crackles, cachexia
Acute pneumonia	Acute fever, productive cough, pleurisy, rusty brown hemoptysis	Fever, focal coarse chest crackles, localized bronchial breath sounds
Vasculitis, hemorrhage syndrome	Subacute constitutional symptoms, hematuria, rash, arthralgias	Diffuse chest crackles, mucosal ulcers, rash
Heart failure	Orthopnea, lower extremity edema, history of valvular disease	Murmurs, S_3, loud P_2, lower extremity edema
AVM/hereditary hemorrhagic telangiectasia	Platypnea, epistaxis, family history of similar signs and symptoms	Mucosal telangiectasias, orthodeoxia
Pulmonary embolus	Acute dyspnea, pleurisy	Hypoxemia, pleural rub, unilateral lower extremity edema (DVT)

AVM, arteriovenous malformation; TB, tuberculosis; DVT, deep venous thrombosis.

- Timing: first episode, recurrent episodes, chronic small volumes, acute large volumes
- Volume: minor, submassive, massive

History

- The most important facts to gather include volume of hemoptysis, patient age, smoking history, prior lung disease, previous malignancy, risk factors for coagulopathy, and prior episodes of hemoptysis.
- Review of systems should focus on symptoms suggesting cardiopulmonary disease, active infection, underlying malignancy, and systemic inflammatory disorders.

Physical Examination

- Obtaining vital signs including oxygen saturation is the first step in patient examination.
- Thereafter one should pay attention to the patient's general state of health, lung examination noting focal or diffusely abnormal findings such as bronchial breath sounds, crackles, stridor, and/or expiratory wheezes. Cardiac examination for murmurs, loud P2, signs of deep vein thrombosis (DVT), and connective tissue disease should be performed.
- A thorough examination should always be performed, observing any manifestations suggesting underlying cardiopulmonary, infectious, immunologic, or malignant disease.

Differential Diagnosis

One must distinguish between **true hemoptysis** and **pseudohemoptysis**, which comes from the upper airway (above the glottis) or aspirated gastrointestinal tract bleeding that is later expectorated.

Diagnostic Testing

- A thorough **history and physical examination** is important to provide clues and guidance in additional testing.
- Additional testing is aimed at determining and localizing the bleeding source and identifying the underlying etiology.

Laboratories and Electrocardiography

- Basic labwork including CBC, comprehensive metabolic panel, and coagulation studies are indicated.
- Type and cross-matching of blood is indicated, especially in cases of massive hemoptysis.
- An ABG analysis may be indicated in cases of shortness of breath or respiratory compromise.
- Sputum studies may be helpful in cases of infection and can be analyzed with routine Gram stain and culture, fungal culture, and acid-fast bacilli (AFB) smear/culture as indicated.
- Serologic studies and urinalysis with microscopy may be clinically indicated based on the suspicion for rheumatologic disease or vasculitis. These may include ANA screen, ANCA screen, including reflex testing to myeloperoxidase (MPO) and proteinase 3 (PR3), anti–glomerular basement membrane antibodies, complement levels, cryoglobulins, double-stranded DNA antibodies, and others.
- BNP or pro-NT-BNP levels may be helpful when cardiac failure is suspected.
- ECG can help assess for underlying cardiac disease.

Imaging

- **Posteroanterior CXR** is performed in all cases of hemoptysis.
  - **Unfortunately, these may be normal or nonlocalizing in up to 50% of all cases.**[92,93]
  - **Furthermore, CXR may be normal in up to 10% of hemoptysis cases caused by bronchogenic carcinoma.**[92]
- **Chest CT:** CT should be performed if the diagnosis remains in doubt after initial clinical and CXR evaluation (see Figure 10-6). CT chest can be performed with or without contrast; however, CT angiography is increasingly useful in localizing the source of hemoptysis.
  - Advantages:
    - Can visualize parenchyma, vasculature, and airways to varying extent.
    - **Especially useful for hemoptysis resulting from bronchiectasis, cavitary lung disease, masses, and vascular malformations.**[94]
    - **Can detect up to 96% of CXR-occult malignancies.**[95]
    - CT visualizes tumors with efficacy comparable with bronchoscopy.[96]
    - CT angiography may be better than bronchoscopy in determining the etiology and source of hemoptysis.[97]
    - CT angiography is useful for planning embolization procedures.[98]
  - Disadvantages:
    - CT is less efficacious than bronchoscopy in recognizing subtle bronchial and mucosal lesions.[94]
    - It is nonspecific in cases of parenchymal/alveolar hemorrhage.
    - Delay in treatment places unstable patients at high risk.
- **Echocardiography** may be performed if structural or valvular cardiac disease is suspected.

Diagnostic Procedures

- **Fiber-optic (flexible) bronchoscopy:** Generally **localizes/lateralizes bleeding source** in over two-thirds of cases, depending on the setting.[99]
  - **Indications**
    - If the source is unclear after initial evaluation and imaging
    - Persistent or recurrent hemoptysis
    - To rule out infection
    - If the clinical presentation suggests an airway abnormality
    - To obtain biopsy specimens, if imaging suggests malignancy or is nonlocalizing in the **presence of at least two risk factors for bronchogenic carcinoma:**
      - Male sex
      - Age >40 years
      - >40 pack-year smoking
      - Duration of hemoptysis >1 week
      - Volume expectorated >30 mL[92,100,101]
    - To identify potential anatomic area for arterial embolization
    - To provide endobronchial treatments
    - To rule out alveolar hemorrhage
  - The timing of bronchoscopy is controversial, although yields increase when performed during or within 48 hours of bleeding.[102]
- **Bronchial and pulmonary arteriography is** performed in the setting of **persistent, recurrent, or massive hemoptysis**
  - Advantages:
    - Can be both diagnostic and therapeutic via simultaneous **embolization** of the visualized culprit vessel.
    - Useful in hemoptysis of varying degrees in the setting of different etiologies including bronchiectasis, malignancy, aspergilloma, and others.[103]
    - Can be preceded by CT angiography for procedure planning.[98]
  - Disadvantages:
    - **Variable and inexact localization** of the bleeding source depending on clinical setting.[99]
    - Anatomic variability.
    - Bleeding in cases where it is insufficient for contrast extravasation.

TREATMENT

The approach to hemoptysis is primarily aimed at **distinguishing massive/life-threatening hemoptysis from nonmassive hemoptysis.** The three main goals are

1. to stabilize the patient's airway and hemodynamics,
2. to diagnose the cause and localize the site of hemoptysis, and
3. to decide on need for and type of therapy in each case.

- **Nonmassive hemoptysis** is usually treated conservatively. Treatment may include the following:
  - Reversal of coagulopathy
  - Antitussives
  - Bronchoscopy if recurrent
  - Steroids and/or immunosuppression for rheumatologic conditions
  - Treatment for infection (fungal, TB, mycobacteria)
  - Diuretics and/or inotropes for heart disease (LV failure, mitral stenosis)

- **Massive hemoptysis:** management requires urgent action, intensive care monitoring, and an early multidisciplinary approach including an interventional pulmonologist, a thoracic surgeon, and an interventional radiologist (see Figure10-6).
  - **Initial stabilization:**
    - **Airway management** may require intubation, with a large (>8 mm) endotracheal tube.[104]
      - Single-lumen main stem intubation for selective ventilation of unaffected lung.
      - Double-lumen endotracheal intubation for selective ventilation of unaffected lung. Should be performed and managed only under appropriately skilled supervision.
    - **Lateral decubitus positioning** (affected lung down) to minimize aspiration into unaffected lung.
  - **Bronchoscopy** with directed airway therapy: **Rigid bronchoscopy** is favored if available because it provides optimal airway access and ventilatory control, easier suctioning, and allows for manipulation of instruments.
    - **Direct tamponade with the distal end of the bronchoscope.**
    - **Balloon tamponade:** left in place for 1–2 days. Monitor for ischemic mucosal injury or postobstructive pneumonitis.[105] Fogarty balloons, bronchial blockers, and pulmonary artery catheter balloons have all been described for tamponading bleeding.
    - **Endobronchial electrocautery**[106]
    - **Argon-plasma coagulation**[106,107]
    - **Endobronchial stent placement**[108]
    - **Topical hemostatic agents:** cold saline, epinephrine, vasopressin, thrombin, and oxidized regenerated cellulose have been used to control bleeding.[109-111]
- **Arteriography and embolization should be performed early** in massive or recurrent hemoptysis.
  - **Successful embolization** in more than **>85% of cases can be achieved** with careful localization.[103,112]
  - Embolization is particularly useful in cystic fibrosis (CF) patients.[113,114]
  - **Treatment failure is usually because of inadequate or incomplete source vessel identification.** Postembolization arteriography may identify additional systemic culprit vessels, most commonly from the intercostal and phrenic arteries.[115]
  - **Rebleeding is common** in embolized patients, occurring in up to 20% of cases over 1 year. Rebleeding appears to be more common in patients with sarcoidosis, malignancy, and aspergilloma.[112,116,117]
  - **Risks** include bronchial or partial pulmonary infarction and, rarely, ischemic myelopathy because of inadvertent embolization of a spinal artery.

Medications

Systemic procoagulants: These are used only in unstable massive hemoptysis as a temporizing measure. Alternatively, they may be required when conventional bronchoscopic, interventional, or surgical therapies are contraindicated and/or unavailable. Examples are administration of factor VII, vasopressin, and aminocaproic acid.

Surgical Management

Emergent surgery has high morbidity and mortality compared with elective surgery following patient stabilization.[87]

- **Lobectomy or pneumonectomy offers definitive cure.**
  - **Indications: persistent focal/unilateral massive hemoptysis despite other therapy.** It is particularly useful for stable patients with hemoptysis due to cavitary lung disease, localized bronchogenic carcinoma, AVM, or traumatic injuries.[118]
  - **Contraindications:** poor pulmonary reserve, advanced malignancy, active TB, diffuse lung disease, or diffuse alveolar hemorrhage.

REFERRAL/CONSULTATION

- Pulmonary (interventional for massive hemoptysis, if available)
- Thoracic surgery
- Interventional radiology

OUTCOME/PROGNOSIS

Mortality depends on etiology and volume of hemoptysis.[87,119,120]

- Mortality may be as high as 80% in cases of massive hemoptysis because of malignancy
- Mortality tends to be <10% with nonmassive hemoptysis
- Mortality in patients with bronchiectasis and lung infections is less than 1%

Cystic Fibrosis

GENERAL PRINCIPLES

Definition

CF is an **autosomal recessive disorder** caused by mutations of the cystic fibrosis transmembrane conductance regulator gene (*CFTR*), located on chromosome 7, which results in multisystem exocrine organ dysfunction.

Epidemiology

- In the United States, approximately 30,000 people are affected by CF, and about 1000 new cases are diagnosed every year.[121]
- CF is the most common life-shortening genetic disease in Caucasians; however, the diagnosis should be considered in patients of diverse ethnic backgrounds as well.
- Patients are typically diagnosed via newborn screening or during childhood, but there is increasing recognition of milder variants that may not present until later in life.
- In 2016, approximately 50% of patients with CF were ≥18 years old.
- There is a remarkable variation in the incidence rates of CF reported among native Asians. For example, CF incidence in Jordan is 1 in 2500 live births, followed by 1 in 5000 in Bahrain.[*,†,‡]
- In contrast, incidence rate of CF in Japan is as low as 1 in 350,000 live births. Furthermore, fewer than 30 CF cases have been reported over the past two decades from China.[§,¶]
- Mutation carrier frequency of CF in India is 1 in 238.[**]

Etiology

- CF is caused by **mutations in the *CFTR* gene**, a cyclic adenosine monophosphate (cAMP)–regulated chloride channel, which normally maintains hydration of exocrine organ secretions.

---

[*] Nazer HM. Early diagnosis of cystic fibrosis in Jordanian children. *J Trop Pediatr.* 1992;38:113–115.

[†] Kakish KS. Cystic fibrosis in Jordan: clinical and genetic aspects. *Bahrain Med Bull. 2001*;23:157–159.

[‡] Al-Mahroos F. Cystic fibrosis in Bahrain incidence, phenotype, and outcome. *J. Trop Pediatr.* 1998;44:35–39.

[§] Yamashiro Y, Shimizu T, Oguchi S, Shioya T, Nagata S, Ohtsuka Y. The estimated incidence of cystic fibrosis in Japan. *J Pediatr Gastroenterol Nutr.* 1997;24:544–547.

[¶] Liu Y, Wang L, Tian X, et al. Characterization of gene mutations and phenotypes of cystic fibrosis in Chinese patients. *Respirology.* 2015;20:312–318.

[**] Kapoor V, Shastri SS, Kabra M, et al. Carrier frequency of F508del mutation of cystic fibrosis in Indian population. *J Cyst Fibros.* 2006;5:43–46.

- Abnormal CFTR causes decreased chloride secretion and increased sodium absorption on the surface of epithelial cells with resulting thickened secretions in the airways, sinuses, pancreatic ducts, biliary tree, intestines, and reproductive tract.
- CFTR mutations are categorized into five classes: (1) **defective synthesis,** (2) **defective processing and maturation,** (3) **defective regulation,** (4) **defective conductance, and** (5) **reduced function/synthesis.**
- The most common mutation is **F508del**, a class II mutation resulting from the deletion of DNA coding for phenylalanine (F) amino acid at position 508. The majority of the resultant misfolded protein is destroyed intracellularly and does not reach the cell surface. Over 85% of patients in the United States have at least one copy of this mutation.[121]
- **G551D** and **R117H** mutations, present in 3%–5% of the patients, are class III mutations in which the defective regulation of the CFTR protein results in impaired opening of the channel.
- >2000 other potentially causative mutations in the CFTR gene have been identified.[121]

Pathophysiology

- CFTR normally regulates transport of chloride ions across the epithelium.
- The primary pulmonary manifestations of disease are related to the malfunction of chloride transport across the airway epithelium, resulting in diminished airway surface liquid and impaired mucociliary clearance.
- Poor mucociliary clearance results in an impaired ability to clear infection. Recurrent infection begets an inflammatory cascade that results in bronchiectasis, chronic infection, and, ultimately, respiratory failure and premature death.
- Similarly, thickened secretions in the pancreatic and biliary ducts lead to maldigestion, malabsorption, and, occasionally, liver disease and diabetes.[122]

DIAGNOSIS

Since 2010, newborn screening has become mandatory in all 50 states, and the proportion of patients diagnosed early has increased. Patients diagnosed early at the asymptomatic stage may have better nutritional outcomes and lung function later in their childhood.[123] In 2016, 62% of new diagnoses were the result of newborn screening.[121]

- A diagnosis of CF is made when there is[124]
  - Compatible clinical features of CF (see clinical features), or
  - A positive family history of CF, or
  - A positive newborn screening test

  and
  - Elevated (>60 mmol/L) sweat chloride or
  - Intermediate (30–59 mmol/L) sweat chloride, and
    - Presence of two disease-causing mutations in *CFTR* or
    - Abnormal CFTR functional assay
- A diagnosis of **cystic fibrosis–related metabolic syndrome** (CRMS) is made when there is a positive newborn screening test, and an intermediate sweat chloride level without two causative mutations, or a negative (<30 mmol/L) sweat chloride level with two *CFTR* mutations, at least one with unclear phenotypic consequences.
- Although genotyping may assist in the diagnosis, it alone cannot establish or rule out the diagnosis of CF, and the initial test of choice remains the sweat chloride test.

Clinical Presentation

- **Pulmonary manifestations**

  Cough with purulent sputum production, wheezing, hemoptysis, dyspnea, progressive airflow obstruction, bronchiectasis, and pneumothorax.

- **Extrapulmonary manifestations**
  Chronic rhinosinusitis, nasal polyposis, pancreatic insufficiency (vitamins A, D, E, and K deficiency), malnutrition, meconium ileus, distal intestinal obstruction syndrome, volvulus, intussusception, rectal prolapse, diabetes mellitus, liver, biliary) cirrhosis, portal hypertension, cholelithiasis, cholecystitis, nephrolithiasis, male infertility (bilateral absence of the vas deferens), epididymitis, growth retardation, recurrent venous thrombosis, aquagenic wrinkling, hypertrophic pulmonary osteoarthropathy, and osteopenia.

History

Presenting symptoms may include[125]

- Cough with purulent sputum production (40%)
- Failure to thrive (29%)
- Malnutrition
- Steatorrhea
- Meconium ileus

Physical Examination

- Underweight
- Inspiratory crackles on lung examination typically anterior and in the apices
- Digital clubbing

Differential Diagnosis

- **Primary ciliary dyskinesia:** bronchiectasis, sinusitis, and infertility, but limited gastrointestinal symptoms and normal sweat chloride levels, occasionally seen with dextrocardia or situs inversus totalis (Kartagener syndrome)
- **Immunodeficiency (e.g., severe combined immunodeficiency, common variable immunodeficiency):** recurrent sinus and pulmonary infections but typically no gastrointestinal symptoms and normal sweat chloride levels
- **Alpha-1 antitrypsin deficiency:** early-onset emphysema, airflow obstruction, chronic sputum production, panniculitis, chronic hepatitis, cirrhosis, hepatocellular carcinoma; bronchiectasis is a common radiographic feature[126] with normal sweat chloride levels
- **Shwachman–Diamond syndrome:** pancreatic insufficiency, cyclic neutropenia, and short stature, which may lead to lung disease, but normal sweat chloride levels[127]
- **Young syndrome:** bronchiectasis, sinusitis, and azoospermia, but mild respiratory symptoms, lack of gastrointestinal symptoms, and normal sweat chloride levels
- **Idiopathic bronchiectasis**

Diagnostic Testing

- **Skin sweat testing** with a standardized quantitative pilocarpine iontophoresis method remains the **gold standard for the diagnosis of CF.**[128]
  - A sweat chloride concentration of ≥60 mmol/L on two separate occasions is consistent with the diagnosis of CF.
  - Intermediate sweat test results (30–59 mmol/L sweat chloride) or nondiagnostic results should lead to repeat sweat testing, genetic testing, or nasal potential difference (NPD) testing. Sweat chloride ≤29 mmol/L is normal.
  - Sweat testing should be performed at a CF care center to ensure reliability of results.
  - Abnormal sweat chloride concentrations are rarely detected in non-CF patients.
- **Genetic tests** have detected >2000 putative CF mutations.
  - Two recessive mutations on separate alleles must be present to cause CF.
  - Commercially available CF screens identify >90% of the abnormal genes in a Caucasian Northern European population, although they test for only a minority of the known CF genes. Full gene sequencing is commercially available, but interpretation may be

complex. Information about specific mutations and reported clinical phenotype may be found at http://www.cftr2.org/.

- **CFTR Functional Assays**
  - Should be performed at specialized centers.
  - **Transepithelial NPD**
    - A test in which the voltage across the epithelial lining of the nose is measured at baseline, after inhibiting sodium channels with amiloride and after stimulating CFTR with a cAMP agonist.
    - Results may be affected by nasal polyposis or mucosal inflammation.
  - **Intestinal Current Measurements (ICM)**
    - More sensitive than NPD in milder forms of CF
    - Transepithelial current of intestinal tissue (obtained via biopsy) is measured after stimulation with chloride secretory agents.

Laboratories

- Sputum cultures typically identify multiple organisms, including *Staphylococcus aureus*, nontypeable *Haemophilus influenzae*, *Pseudomonas aeruginosa*, *Stenotrophomonas maltophilia*, and *Burkholderia cepacia* complex. Isolation of mucoid variants of *P. aeruginosa* from the respiratory tract occurs frequently. Use of special culture media for fastidious organisms is recommended.
- Nontuberculous mycobacteria are frequently isolated from the airways of persons with CF and may be pathogenic in some.
- **Testing for malabsorption** because of pancreatic exocrine insufficiency is often not formally performed because clinical evidence (the presence of foul-smelling, bulky, and loose stools; low fat-soluble vitamin levels [vitamins A, D, and E]; and a prolonged prothrombin time [vitamin K dependent]) and a clear response to pancreatic enzyme treatment are usually considered sufficient for the diagnosis. In some cases, low fecal elastase level or coefficient of fat absorption <85% on a formal 72-hour fecal fat collection may confirm pancreatic insufficiency.
- Tests that identify chronic sinusitis or infertility, especially obstructive azoospermia in men, also support the diagnosis of CF.

Testing

- CXR shows hyperinflation with cystic lung disease, bronchiectasis, and mucous plugging, especially in the upper lobes.
- High-resolution CT scan may be helpful in evaluating patients with early or mild disease by detecting early changes in the airways.
- Pulmonary function tests demonstrate expiratory airflow obstruction with increased residual volume and TLC.
- Impairment of alveolar gas exchange may be present later in the course of disease, progressing to hypoxemia and hypercapnia.

TREATMENT

- CF therapy aims to improve quality of life and functioning, decrease the number of exacerbations and hospitalizations, avoid complications associated with therapy, reduce the rate of decline in lung function, and decrease mortality.
- A comprehensive program addressing multiple organ system derangements, as provided at CF care centers, is recommended.
- **Pulmonary therapy**[129] primarily focused on clearing pulmonary secretions and controlling infection.

- **Inhaled bronchodilators:** β-Adrenergic agonists (albuterol metered-dose inhaler, two to four puffs bid–qid; salmeterol or formoterol, one dry powder inhalation bid). Used to treat the reversible components of airflow obstruction and facilitate mucus clearance.
- **Recombinant human deoxyribonuclease:** DNase, dornase-α, Pulmozyme (2.5 mg or one ampule per day inhaled using a jet nebulizer)
  - It digests extracellular DNA, decreasing the viscoelasticity of the sputum.
  - It improves pulmonary function and decreases the incidence of respiratory tract infections that require parenteral antibiotics.[130]
  - Adverse effects may include pharyngitis, laryngitis, rash, chest pain, and conjunctivitis.
- **Hypertonic saline:** (4 mL of inhaled 7% saline twice daily)
  - Because of high osmolality, water is drawn from the airway epithelium and can rehydrate the periciliary airway surface liquid.
  - Treatment results in fewer exacerbations and improvement in lung function.[131]
  - Inhaled bronchodilators should be administered prior to treatments to avoid treatment-induced bronchospasm.
- Antibiotics
  - A combination of an antipseudomonal β-lactam and an aminoglycoside is typically recommended during acute exacerbations.[132] Other antibiotics are indicated based on organism (e.g., for patients with MRSA).
  - Sputum culture and sensitivities should guide therapy. *P. aeruginosa* is the most frequent pulmonary pathogen.
  - The duration of antibiotic therapy is dictated by the clinical response. At least 14 days of antibiotics are typically needed to treat an exacerbation.
  - Home IV antibiotic therapy is common, but hospitalization may allow better access to comprehensive therapy and diagnostic testing. Oral antibiotics are recommended only for mild exacerbations.
  - The use of chronic or intermittent prophylactic antibiotics can be considered, especially in patients with frequent recurrent exacerbations, but antimicrobial resistance may develop.
  - In patients chronically infected with *P. aeruginosa*, the inhaled aerosolized antibiotics tobramycin (300 mg nebulized twice daily) and aztreonam lysinate (75 mg nebulized 3× daily) can be used via alternating 28 days on with 28 days off to improve pulmonary function, decrease the density of *P. aeruginosa*, and decrease the risk of hospitalization. Voice alteration (13%) and tinnitus (3%) are potential adverse events associated with long-term inhaled tobramycin, and pyrexia and airway irritation have been reported with inhaled aztreonam. More recently, continuous alternating inhaled antibiotic therapy has become the standard of care for many patients with chronic *Pseudomonas* infection and pulmonary impairment.
  - Patients with CF have atypical pharmacokinetics and often require higher drug doses at more frequent intervals during an acute exacerbation. In adult patients with CF, for example, cefepime is often dosed at 2 g IV q8h, and tobramycin is often dosed at 8 mg/kg IV daily (aiming for peak levels of >20 μg/mL and trough levels of <2 μg/mL).
  - Once-daily aminoglycoside dosing is preferred and should be guided by pharmacokinetic testing. Monitoring levels (peaks and troughs) of drugs such as aminoglycosides helps to ensure therapeutic levels and to decrease the risk of toxicity.
- **Anti-inflammatory therapy**
  - **Azithromycin** (500 mg oral 3×/week) used chronically shows mild improvement in lung function and reduces days in the hospital for treatment of respiratory exacerbations. Patients should be screened for nontuberculous mycobacteria (NTM) before initiation of macrolide antibiotics because chronic monotherapy can lead to macrolide resistant NTM.

    - **Glucocorticoids** used in short courses may be helpful to some patients with asthma-like symptoms, but long-term therapy should be avoided to minimize the side effects, which include glucose intolerance, osteopenia, and growth retardation.
    - **Ibuprofen** used in high doses has been used as a chronic anti-inflammatory agent in children age 6–17 with mild impairment of lung function.
  - **Restoration of CFTR function**
    - **Ivacaftor**: Ivacaftor is a CFTR potentiator that has initially been shown to improve lung function and decreases the risk of pulmonary exacerbations in patients with the G551D mutation.[133] Since its initial release, the FDA has expanded the use of ivacaftor in patients with more than 35 mutations with partially functioning CFTR protein ("residual function mutations").
    - **Lumacaftor–Ivacaftor**: Lumacaftor increases surface protein expression by partially correcting the CFTR folding defect in patients with the F508del mutation, the most common mutation in CF patients. Combined with ivacaftor, it has been shown to improve lung function and decrease the risk of pulmonary exacerbations in patients who are homozygous for the F508del mutation.[134]
    - **Tezacaftor–Ivacaftor**: Tezacaftor is a second-generation CFTR corrector. In combination with Ivacaftor, it has been shown to result in improvement in FEV_1 with fewer adverse events compared with lumacaftor–ivacaftor.[134,135] Tezacaftor–ivacaftor has recently been approved by the FDA for patients with F508del homozygous mutation and in patients with at least one residual function mutation.
    - Other CFTR corrector molecules, potentiators, and molecules that suppress *CFTR* nonsense mutations (premature stop codons) are in various phases of clinical development and testing.
  - **Mechanical airway clearance devices:** flutter valve, acapella device, high-frequency chest oscillation vests, low- and high-pressure positive expiratory pressure devices.
    - Can be used in combination with medical therapy to promote airway clearance.
    - Other alternatives include postural drainage with chest percussion and vibration, and breathing and coughing exercises.
  - **Pulmonary rehabilitation**
    Pulmonary rehabilitation may improve functional status and promote clearance of airway secretions.
  - **Oxygen therapy**
    - May be indicated based on standard recommendations used for the treatment of chronic obstructive pulmonary disease.
    - Rest and exercise oxygen assessments should be performed as clinically indicated.
  - **Noninvasive ventilation**
    - Used for chronic respiratory failure due to CF-related bronchiectasis.
    - Has not been clearly demonstrated to provide a survival benefit, although it may provide symptomatic relief or may be used as a bridge to transplantation.
- **Extrapulmonary therapy**
  - **Pancreatic insufficiency**
    - Primary management involves **pancreatic enzyme supplementation.**
    - Enzyme dose should be titrated to achieve one to two semisolid stools per day and to maintain adequate growth and nutrition.
    - Enzymes are taken immediately before meals and snacks.
    - Dosing of pancreatic enzymes should be initiated at 500 units lipase/kg/meal and should not exceed 2500 units lipase/kg/meal.
    - **High doses** (6000 units lipase/kg/meal or >24,000 units lipase/kg/day) have been associated with **chronic intestinal strictures.**
    - Gastric acid suppression may enhance enzyme activity.

- **Vitamin deficiency**
  - **Vitamins A, D, E, and K** can all be taken orally with meals and enzymes.
  - Iron deficiency anemia requires iron supplementation.
- **CF-related diabetes mellitus (CFRD)**
  - Related to pancreatic insufficiency and managed with **insulin**; oral hypoglycemics are not recommended.
  - CF patients should also be regularly screened for CFRD with an oral glucose tolerance test (OGTT). Hemoglobin A1c is not recommended as a screening test in CFRD.
  - Typical diabetic dietary restrictions are liberalized (high-calorie diet with unrestricted fat) to meet the increased energy requirements of patients with CF and to encourage appropriate growth and weight maintenance.
- **Bowel impaction/distal intestinal obstruction syndrome (DIOS)**
  - **Laxatives** such as senna, magnesium citrate, or polyethylene glycol can be tried initially.
  - Refractory cases may require a Hypaque enema with visualization of clearance of the obstruction.
  - Can be mistaken for appendicitis or gallbladder disease because the appendix can be enlarged in CF because of mucus inspissation and white blood cell counts and/or alkaline phosphatase elevations, which are common in CF.
  - Narcotic use and/or significant dehydration and/or nonadherence with pancreatic enzyme supplementation can precipitate severe bowel obstruction, so prophylactic laxatives such as daily polyethylene glycol (e.g., MiraLAX 17 g in 8 oz water) in post-surgical patients are often indicated.
- **CF-related liver disease (CFLD)**
  - Hepatobiliary manifestation ranges from mild abnormalities in liver function tests (LFT) over hepatic steatosis to cirrhosis.
  - Most cases of cirrhosis are diagnosed during childhood (<18 years).
  - Annual screening with physical examination and LFT and gamma-glutamyltransferase is recommended.
  - Sequelae of portal hypertension such as esophageal varies should be managed accordingly; however, studies evaluating the efficacy of band ligation or β-blockade in the CF population are lacking.
- **Osteopenia**

  Screening should be routinely performed on patients with CF, and if present, osteopenia may be managed with calcium, vitamin D supplementation, and bisphosphonate therapy as clinically indicated.
- **Chronic sinusitis**
  - Many patients will benefit from chronic **nasal steroid** administration.
  - Nasal saline washes may also be helpful.
  - Patients whose symptoms cannot be controlled with medical management may benefit from functional endoscopic sinus surgery and nasal polypectomy.
- **Mental Health**
  - Depression and anxiety are common among patients and caregivers of CF patients.
  - Depression was found in 13%–33% of adult CF patients and 20%–35% of caregivers. The prevalence of anxiety was ~30%.[136]
  - Psychological symptoms are associated with worse adherence, heath-related quality of life, decreased lung function, and lower body mass index.
  - Both patients and caregivers should be screened for depression and anxiety on a regular basis and referred for treatment.
  - Selective serotonin reuptake inhibitors (SSRIs) should be considered when there is no response to nonpharmacologic therapies; drug–drug interaction should be considered

with the use of SSRIs (e.g., lumacaftor is a strong CYP3A4 inducer and higher doses of citalopram or escitalopram may be needed).

Surgical Management

- **Massive hemoptysis**
  Treatment includes IV antibiotics and, in refractory cases, may require bronchial artery embolization. Surgical lung resection is rarely indicated.
- **Pneumothorax**
  Unless small, pneumothoraces are treated with chest tube placement. Surgical pleurodesis should be considered in cases of recurrent pneumothorax.
- **Lung transplantation**
  - The majority of patients with CF die from pulmonary disease.
  - FEV_1 <30% predicted, development of hypercarbia and/or PH, decreased exercise tolerance, increasing frequency, and severity of exacerbations are some of the indications for referral for transplantation.[137]
  - All patients undergoing transplant evaluation should be tested for the presence of NTM and *B. cepacia* complex in the sputum. The presence of *B. cenocepacia* is considered to be a contraindication to lung transplantation in most transplant centers.

Lifestyle/Risk Modification

- **Avoidance of irritating inhaled fumes, dusts, or chemicals**, including second-hand smoke, is recommended.
- **Yearly influenza vaccination** decreases the incidence of infection and subsequent deterioration.
- **Pneumovax** and **Prevnar 13** are recommended for all patients with CF.
- People with CF should avoid contact with others with the disease, unless they are members of the same household, to reduce the risk of transmission of infection from one person to another.
- Palivizumab is a humanized monoclonal antibody against respiratory syncytial virus (RSV), which is used to help prevent serious RSV infection in young children.

Diet

A high-calorie diet with vitamin supplementation is typically recommended.

Activity

- CF patients should maintain as much activity as possible.
- Exercise is an excellent form of airway clearance.

SPECIAL CONSIDERATIONS

- When in a healthcare setting, all personnel should implement contact precautions, whether in the clinic or in the hospital.
- **Patients with previous isolation of *B. cepacia* complex should be cared for in a separate area than those without this species.**
- Although fertility may be decreased in women with CF secondary to thickened cervical mucus, many women with CF have tolerated pregnancy well.
- Maternal and fetal outcomes are good for women with adequate pulmonary reserve (FEV_1 >50% predicted) and good nutritional status, and pregnancy does not appear to affect their survival.
- Screening for gestational diabetes with OGTT is recommended at both 12–16 weeks and at 24–48 weeks gestation in women without a prior diagnosis of CFRD.

- Pregnancies should be planned to optimize patient status and coordinate care with obstetrics. CF genetic screening should be offered to partners of patients with CF.

COMPLICATIONS

Other pulmonary complications of CF may include allergic bronchopulmonary aspergillosis, massive hemoptysis, acquisition of atypical mycobacterium, and pneumothorax.

REFERRAL

- CF patients or suspected CF patients should be referred to a national Cystic Fibrosis Foundation (CFF)–accredited care center.
- Tests such as sweat chloride testing, NPD, and ICM are best done at specialized CF care centers.
- A team of CF specialists, including physicians, nutritionists, respiratory therapists, and social workers, aid in the routine care of these patients.

PATIENT EDUCATION

Information can be found at the CFF website (www.cff.org).

MONITORING/FOLLOW-UP

All persons with CF should be followed in an accredited CF care center. Patients should follow-up as an outpatient every 3 months with pulmonary function tests and yearly laboratories including vitamin levels and screening for CF-related diabetes.

OUTCOME/PROGNOSIS

- Predictors of increased mortality include age, female gender, low weight, low FEV_1, pancreatic insufficiency, diabetes mellitus, infection with *B. cepacia*, and the number of acute exacerbations.
- With improved therapy, the median survival has been extended to over 47 years.[121]

Solitary Pulmonary Nodule

GENERAL PRINCIPLES

- The goal of a careful evaluation of the solitary pulmonary nodule (SPN) is to determine if the lesion is more likely **malignant or benign.**
- **A lesion >3 cm has a high likelihood of malignancy and should be treated as such, whereas lesions <3 cm need more careful assessment.**
- Nodules with benign characteristics should be closely followed so that invasive procedures with associated risks can be avoided.
- Identifying early lung cancer is of the utmost importance because there is a >60% survival rate of patients who have a malignant SPN removed.[138]

Definition

An SPN is defined as a rounded lesion <3 cm in diameter. It is completely surrounded by lung parenchyma, unaccompanied by atelectasis, intrathoracic adenopathy, or pleural effusion. Pulmonary nodules <8 mm remain within this definition; however, there is evidence to suggest that these nodules have a lower overall malignancy risk.[138] Lesions that measure >3 cm are considered masses.

Epidemiology

Historically the incidence of SPN has been cited to be 150,000 in the United States. A 2015, California based, integrated healthcare system's review extrapolated this value to be over 1.5 million. This value is susceptible to errors associated with this form of methodology. However, it does highlight that the incidence of SPN has increased with changes in clinical practice post National Lung Screening Trial.[139]

Etiology

- Although underlying etiologies for pulmonary nodules are varied, the most important designation clinically is deciphering between a malignant and a nonmalignant process.
- **Malignancy accounts for approximately 40% of SPNs, although this may vary geographically depending on the prevalence of nonmalignant processes such as histoplasmosis.**
- **Granulomas** (both infectious and noninfectious) may account for 50% of undiagnosed SPNs, depending on the prevalence of cancer in the particular population.
- The remaining 10% are composed of **benign neoplasms**, such as **hamartomas** (5%) and a multitude of other causes.

Risk Factors

- **Smoking** is the most important associated risk factor for almost all malignant SPNs. Other risk factors include family history, female sex, emphysema, prior malignancy, and asbestos exposure.
- For infectious etiologies, an immunocompromised state promotes an increased risk.
- The probability of malignancy rises with increasing age.

Lung Cancer Screening

Screening high-risk patients using low-dose chest CT resulted in a 20% relative reduction in mortality from lung cancer compared with screening with CXR.[140]

DIAGNOSIS

- Diagnosis of the SPN is made radiographically, usually via CXR or CT scan.
- Most frequently, the nodule is noted incidentally on a study performed for other reasons (e.g., chronic cough, chest pain).

Clinical Presentation

- As stated previously, the majority of SPNs are diagnosed incidentally by radiographic tests done for other reasons, so there may not be overt symptoms.
- There are instances when a nodule may precipitate cough, chest pain, hemoptysis, or sputum production depending on the etiology and location of the SPN.

History

- Ask typical screening questions for malignancy including **weight loss and night sweats.**
- **Hemoptysis** may indicate malignancy but may also prompt investigations for antineutrophil cytoplasmic antibody (ANCA)–associated vasculitis, tuberculosis (TB), and hereditary hemorrhagic telangiectasia (HHT).
- Ask about arthritis and arthralgias for possible undiagnosed rheumatoid arthritis or sarcoidosis.

- Take an exposure history including recent travel history related to endemic mycoses (histoplasmosis, coccidioidomycosis, etc.) as well as possible TB exposures.
- A history of previous malignancies increases the risk of metastatic disease of the lung.
- Patients who are immunosuppressed from HIV, organ transplant, or chronic steroids have increased risk of infectious causes.
- Smoking is linked to 85% of lung cancers. A patient's risk of lung cancer decreases significantly 5 years after smoking cessation, but it never truly returns to normal.
- An occupational history is important including possible exposure to asbestosis (associated with not only mesothelioma but also non–small-cell lung cancer), silica, beryllium, radon, and ionizing radiation, among others.

Physical Examination

- Although there are no specific physical examination findings related to SPNs, evidence for underlying etiologies might be discovered with a thorough examination.
- Note signs of weight loss or cachexia are suggestive of malignancy.
- Do a thorough lymph node examination. **A cervical lymph node might provide an easy diagnostic target to determine the etiology of an SPN.**
- Perform a breast examination in women and testicular examination in young men.
- A careful skin examination may reveal telangiectasias, erythema nodosum, rheumatoid nodules, or other findings that might suggest a cause.

Diagnostic Criteria

- As mentioned previously, an SPN is identified as a rounded lesion <3 cm in circumference. It is completely surrounded by lung parenchyma, unaccompanied by atelectasis, intrathoracic adenopathy, or pleural effusion.
- The first step in managing an SPN is to stratify the patient in terms of malignancy risk: low-, intermediate-, or high-risk categories (Table 10-10). Risk stratification can be accomplished either qualitatively via clinical judgment or quantitatively using validated risk assessment tools. These approaches appear to be complementary.[141]
- Once the risk of malignancy has been established, further management can proceed, as outlined in Figure 10-7.

TABLE 10-10 Assessment of the Probability of Malignancy

Assessment Criteria	Low (<5%)	Intermediate (5%–65%)	High (>65%)
Clinical factors alone (determined by clinical judgment and/or use of validated model)	Young, less smoking, no prior cancer, smaller nodule size, regular margins, and/or non–upper-lobe location	Mixture of low and high probability features	Older, heavy smoking, prior cancer, larger size, irregular spiculated margins, and/or upper-lobe location
FDG-PET scan results	Low-moderate clinical probability and low FGD-PET activity	Weak or moderate FDG-PET scan activity	Intensely hypermetabolic nodule
Nonsurgical biopsy results (bronchoscopy or TTNA)	Specific benign diagnosis	Nondiagnostic	Suspicious for malignancy

(Continued)

TABLE 10-10 Assessment of the Probability of Malignancy (Continued)

Assessment Criteria	Low (<5%)	Intermediate (5%–65%)	High (>65%)
Computed tomography scan surveillance	Resolution or near-complete resolution, progressive or persistent decrease in size, or no growth over ≥2 y (solid nodule) or ≥3–5 y (subsolid nodule)	Nonapplicable	Clear evidence of growth

FDG, 18-fluorodeoxyglucose; TTNA, transthoracic needle aspiration.
Reprinted from Gould MK, Donington J, Lynch WR, et al. Evaluation of individuals with pulmonary nodules: when is it lung cancer? Diagnosis and management of lung cancer, 3rd ed: American College of Chest Physicians evidence-based clinical practice guidelines. *Chest.* 2013;143: e93S–e120S; with permission from Elsevier.

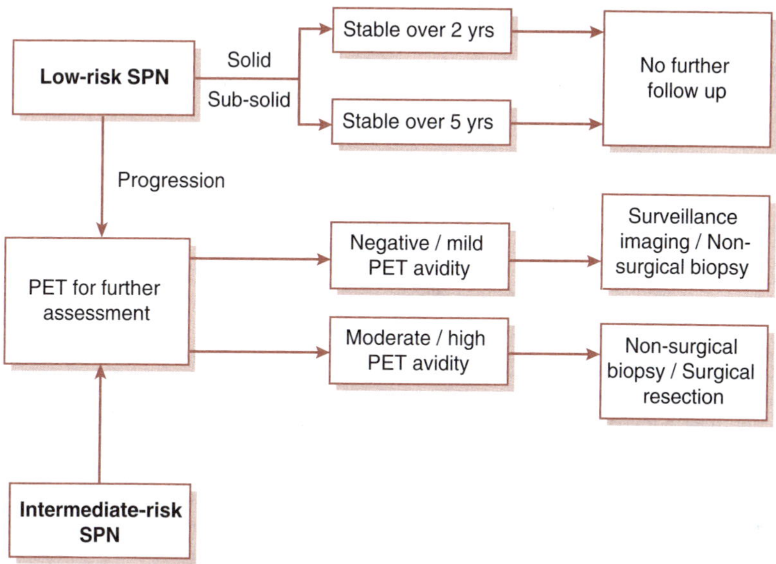

Figure 10-7 Diagnostic and therapeutic management of low- and intermediate-risk pulmonary nodules. PET, positron emission tomography; SPN, solitary pulmonary nodule; yrs, years.

Differential Diagnosis

Pulmonary nodules are divided primarily into malignant or benign etiologies, with benign processes further divided into infectious or noninfectious causes (Table 10-11).

TABLE 10-11	Differential Diagnosis of the Solitary Pulmonary Nodule (SPN)
Malignant	• Primary Pulmonary carcinoma (80% of all malignant SPNs) • Primary Pulmonary lymphoma • Primary Pulmonary carcinoid • Solitary Pulmonary metastasis • Melanoma, osteosarcoma, testicular, breast, prostate, colon, and renal cell carcinoma
Benign neoplasms	• Hamartoma (accounts for most benign neoplastic SPNs) • Arteriovenous malformations (consider HHT) • Others, including neural tumors (schwannoma, neurofibroma), fibroma, and sclerosing hemangioma
Granulomas	Infectious • Mycobacterial disease (most commonly tuberculosis) and fungal infections (histoplasmosis, coccidioidomycosis, blastomycosis, cryptococcosis, aspergillosis) Noninfectious granulomas associated with vasculitis • Granulomatosis with polyangiitis, eosinophilic granulomatosis with polyangiitis • Noninfectious granulomas not associated with vasculitis • Sarcoid granulomatosis, hypersensitivity pneumonitis, and berylliosis
Other etiologies	Infectious • Bacterial (nocardiosis, actinomycosis, round pneumonia), measles, abscess, septic embolus Noninfectious • Lipoid pneumonia, amyloidosis, subpleural lymph node, rheumatoid nodule, pulmonary scar or infarct, congenital malformations (bronchogenic cyst, sequestration), skin nodule, rib fracture, pleural thickening from mass or fluid

HHT, hereditary hemorrhagic telangiectasia.

Diagnostic Testing

Laboratories

- Routine laboratory testing is seldom helpful unless the history and physical examination strongly suggest an etiology.
- If CTDs or vasculitides are suspected, perform appropriate testing.
- Hyponatremia may suggest syndrome of inappropriate antidiuretic hormone (SIADH) associated with primary lung cancer, as well as other pulmonary processes.
- Hypercalcemia might suggest lung cancer as well as sarcoidosis.
- Anemia may indicate chronic pulmonary hemorrhage (e.g., HHT) or a chronic inflammatory disease.
- Microbiologic studies, particularly sputum culture, may aid in the diagnosis of an infectious SPN.
- Sputum cytology has limited use because yield is low for peripherally located, small lesions.

Imaging

The mainstay of diagnostic evaluation of an SPN is via radiographic studies, primarily **CXR, chest CT, and positron emission tomography (PET) scan.**

- CXR
    - A previous CXR is an important tool in the initial evaluation of an SPN.

- If an SPN has been present and unchanged on CXR for >2 years, then further evaluation may not be warranted. Subsolid lesions should be followed for longer periods because the volume-doubling time (VDT) is extended in certain types of non–small-cell lung cancers.
- If an SPN appears on a new radiograph in <30 days, it is likely not malignant and most likely infectious or inflammatory.
- There are radiographic findings that make it more likely that a lesion is **benign (calcifications, a laminated appearance)** or more likely **malignant (spiculated, irregular border)** (see Table 10-10).
- The CXR is easy to obtain and delivers a low dose of radiation; however, it has limitations in the initial characterization, and careful comparisons over time are required for SPN evaluation.
- The risk of malignancy rises with increasing size as follows: nodules <5 mm, <1%; nodules 5–9 mm, 2%–6%; nodules 8–20 mm, 18%; and nodules >20 mm, >50% (Figure 10-8).

- **Chest CT**
  - Chest CT is now considered the most important radiologic examination for SPN evaluation. With few exceptions, an SPN requires assessment by CT.
  - Accurate volumetric measurement of lesion size allows precise comparison to determine stability or growth.
  - Imaging allows a careful examination of mediastinal lymph nodes.
  - Thin cuts through the lesion are more sensitive than CXR for characterizing calcifications and lamination as well as the margins of the lesion.
  - **VDT**: most malignant nodules have a VDT between 20 and 400 days. So a nodule that has increased in size over a short period of time (<20 days) or is stable for a prolonged period of time on CT (>400 days) is likely to be benign.
- **PET scan**
  - 18-Fluorodeoxyglucose (FDG)-PET can help distinguish malignant and benign lesions because cancers are metabolically active and take up FDG avidly.

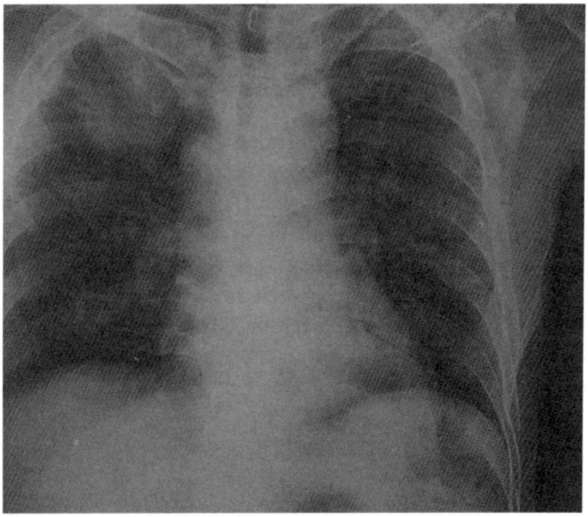

Figure 10-8 Chest X-ray showing a solitary pulmonary nodule in the right upper zone with erosion of ribs suggestive of malignancy.

- PET has a sensitivity of 80%–100% and specificity of 79%–100% for detecting malignancy.
- **False negatives** can occur in bronchoalveolar carcinoma, carcinoid, and mucinous neoplasms, whereas **false positives** are common in nonmalignant "inflammatory" conditions (infectious and autoimmune processes).
- Higher incidence of both false-positive and false-negative results occurs in nodules <10 mm, thus discouraging the use of PET scan in this situation.[142]
- PET scan is most commonly used in the evaluation of low- to moderate-risk indeterminate nodules for further risk stratification (see Figure 10-7).

- **Contrast-enhanced CT**
  - Technique using contrast enhancement and measurement of Hounsfield units to risk stratify an SPN for malignancy.
  - A multicenter analysis demonstrated high sensitivity but relatively low specificity for identifying malignant nodules.[143]
  - This method may be an important tool for risk assessment of an indeterminate SPN in centers that have experience with the technique.

Diagnostic Procedures

- **If a nodule is considered high risk and the patient is an appropriate surgical candidate, then the best approach is to forego biopsy and pursue resection.**
- Any change of an SPN on serial imaging warrants resection or invasive biopsy.
- If a lesion has low-risk characteristics, there is no indication to pursue biopsy and subjecting a patient to unneeded risk.
- **Biopsy** is most often pursued when there is discordance between clinical risk stratification and imaging tests. For example, when pretest suspicion for malignancy is significant but PET imaging is negative, biopsy may be indicated.
- In addition, for patients in whom surgery represents significant risk secondary to comorbidities, using a less-invasive biopsy strategy to determine the presence of malignancy is appropriate.
- There are primarily two options for biopsy of an SPN: transthoracic needle aspiration (TTNA) and flexible bronchoscopy. Choosing either modality is based on nodule and patient factors, as well as institutional experience. These factors include nodule size, location, and finding of emphysema on CT chest.
  - TTNA
    - This technique is usually performed under the guidance of fluoroscopy, ultrasound, or CT (more common).
    - This approach is most commonly used for nodules with a peripheral location and without anatomic impediment to a biopsy needle.
    - Sensitivity of TTNA for the diagnosis of lung cancer is 80%–90% in selected patients.
    - Specificity for identifying malignancy is high with TTNA; however, there is a significant rate of nondiagnostic biopsies, and sensitivity depends on many factors, including nodule size and distance from the pleura.
    - A nondiagnostic biopsy does not rule out malignancy.
    - The complications of TTNA are bleeding (1%), pneumothorax (15%), and 6%–7% incidence of pneumothorax requiring chest tube drainage.[144]
  - **Bronchoscopy**
    - Conventional flexible bronchoscopy is best suited for central airway lesions and has a sensitivity of 88% in malignancy. Advanced bronchoscopic techniques are recommended in the diagnosis of peripheral lesions where their diagnostic yield is superior to that of conventional bronchoscopy.

- Advanced bronchoscopic modalities include radial probe endobronchial ultrasound and electromagnetic navigation, with sensitivities of 73% and 71%, respectively, for the detection of malignancy in peripheral nodules.
- Complete mediastinal and hilar lymph node examination for pathological staging may also be performed during bronchoscopy for peripheral lesion diagnosis, obviating the need for additional procedures.
- The complications of bronchoscopy are bleeding (2%–5%) and pneumothorax (2%–4%).[144]

TREATMENT

- Management of low- and intermediate-risk SPNs is outlined in Figure 10-7.
- Overall treatment strategy is to identify lesions with significant malignancy risk and pursue surgical resection when possible.
- If a nodule has low-risk characteristics and has demonstrated stability over a period of 2 years, then no further treatment is warranted. Further follow-up of subsolid lesions is necessary because their VDTs may be prolonged.
- If a specific etiology for the SPN is diagnosed (e.g., a CTD or infection), then treatment is targeted toward the underlying process.

Other Nonpharmacologic Therapies

- Although **surgical resection is preferable in patients with either a high-risk lesion or biopsy-proven malignancy**, if surgical resection is not an option, there are other less effective therapies.
- **Stereotactic radiation** is currently the most widely used therapy in this clinical situation. This mode of external-beam therapy aims to decrease collateral radiation–induced damage to adjacent lung tissue.
- There are more experimental approaches, including brachytherapy and radiofrequency ablation, which are currently under development.

Surgical Management

- Surgical resection of an indeterminate SPN is indicated in the following situations:
  - The clinical probability of malignancy is moderate to high (>60%).
  - The nodule is hypermetabolic by PET imaging.
  - The nodule has been proven malignant by biopsy.
- A combination of surgical techniques, including VATS, mediastinoscopy, and thoracotomy, can lead to diagnosis (via intraoperative frozen section), staging, and potential cure during a single induction of anesthesia.

MONITORING/FOLLOW-UP

- For a low- or intermediate-risk pulmonary nodule for which resection is not warranted (see Figure 10-7), desired, or possible, routine follow-up with chest CT is standard practice.
- Follow-up of SPN depends on whether it is a solid or subsolid nodule. Solid nodules require 2 years of surveillance, and subsolid nodules require 5 years of surveillance to document stability.
- The updated 2017 Fleischner Society recommendations aim toward decreasing the number of chest CT scans for SPN follow-up and to provide greater flexibility to clinicians and patients for shared decision-making.[145]

Bronchiectasis

GENERAL PRINCIPLES

Definition

Bronchiectasis is defined as an irreversible (permanent), abnormal dilation of the cartilage-containing airway bronchi or bronchioles.

Classification

- According to the shape of the bronchial dilation: tubular (cylindrical), varicose (bulbous), and cystic (saccular/balloon appearance).
- According to the extent of involvement: diffuse (generalized) bronchiectasis or focal (localized) bronchiectasis.

Etiology

- Congenital
  - CF, ciliary dysfunction syndromes (Young syndrome, Kartagener syndrome), hypogammaglobulinemia, alpha-1 antitrypsin deficiency, pulmonary sequestration, Mounier-Kuhn syndrome or tracheobronchomegaly, and Williams–Campbell syndrome (bronchomalacia).
- Acquired
  - Infections: pulmonary tuberculosis, *M. avium* complex (MAC), suppurative pneumonia, ABPA, and pertussis.
  - Postobstructive bronchiectasis: endobronchial tumors or foreign bodies, enlarged hilar lymph nodes.
  - Autoimmune diseases: rheumatoid arthritis, Sjogren syndrome, systemic lupus erythematosus, and inflammatory bowel disease.
  - Others: repeated aspiration of gastric juice, inhalation of toxic gas (ammonia), interstitial lung fibrosis (traction bronchiectasis), radiation fibrosis, sarcoidosis, and chronic hypersensitivity pneumonitis.

Clinical Presentation

History

- Chronic productive cough with foul-smelling, thick, copious, tenacious sputum with streaks of blood. Rarely, massive hemoptysis occurs. Infective exacerbation is common.
- In severe/widespread bronchiectasis, the patient presents with anorexia, exertional breathlessness/dyspnea, and wheezing.
- Bronchiectasis sicca/dry bronchiectasis: occasionally, the patient is asymptomatic or has nonproductive cough and the only manifestation will be hemoptysis.

Physical Findings

Digital clubbing (2%), nasal polyps, signs of chronic sinusitis, coarse, leathery crackles (75%), and wheezing (20%) are seen on examination.

Diagnostic Investigations

- Blood: anemia, raised ESR, and leukocytosis.
- Sputum culture usually grows organisms, especially *Pseudomonas*.

Imaging

- Chest X-ray: parallel linear densities, tram-track opacities, or ring shadows reflecting thickened and abnormally dilated bronchial walls.

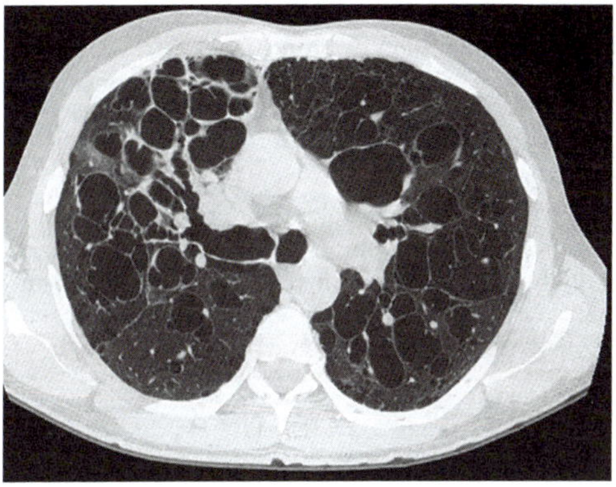

Figure 10-9 HRCT of cystic bronchiectasis.

- Chest CT: more specific, sensitive, and is the imaging modality of choice for the confirmation of bronchiectasis. HRCT findings include bronchoarterial ratio >1–1.5 (internal airway lumen/adjacent pulmonary artery, lack of tapering of bronchi [tram-track appearance]) and airway visibility within 1 cm of a costal pleural surface or touching the mediastinal pleura (Figure 10-9).
- Bronchoscopy: to identify the site of bleeding in patients with hemoptysis, therapeutically to remove secretions, and localized bronchiectasis.
- Pulmonary function test: it may detect mild-to-moderate airflow obstruction, but a restrictive pattern evolves with advanced disease.
- Sweat electrolytes: measurement of sodium and chloride concentrations in sweat is useful in CF.
- Serum immunoglobulins: up to 10% of adults with bronchiectasis have antibody class or subclass deficiency (mainly IgA). Its estimation is also useful when primary hypogammaglobulinemia is suspected.

Patients suspected of ciliary dysfunction syndrome: assessment of ciliary function may be done by the following ways:

- Mucociliary clearance (nasal clearance of saccharin): measure the time taken for a small pellet of saccharin placed in the anterior chamber of the nose to reach the pharynx, where the patient can taste it. Normally, it should be <30 minutes.

  A prolongation of this time (>60 minutes) is found in patients with ciliary dysfunction.
- Measurement of ciliary beat frequency: assessed by using biopsies taken from the nose.
- Electron microscopy: it can detect structural abnormalities of cilia.
- Study of the sperms.

Treatment

- Treatment of underlying diseases.
- Bronchial hygiene by chest physiotherapy (e.g., postural drainage), hydration and mucolytic administration, and aerosolization of bronchodilators.
- Antibiotic therapy.
  - Oral ciprofloxacin (500–750 mg twice daily) or ceftazidime by intravenous injection or infusion (1–2 g three times daily) for 7–10 days.
  - Suppressive antibiotics: inhaled antibiotics are safe and effective, for example, tobramycin and gentamicin.
- Specific therapy for organisms (MAC, etc.)
- Bronchodilators (β-adrenoreceptor agonists, anticholinergics), treatment of GERD.

- Surgical treatment only in refractory cases.
  - The procedure involved is excision of bronchiectatic areas. It is usually done in cases where the bronchiectasis is restricted to a single lobe or segment on CT.
- Other measures
  - Vaccination.
  - Promptly treat episodes of sinusitis.
  - Treat complicated ABPA with prednisolone and itraconazole.
  - Mucolytic dornase (DNase) is recommended in CF-related bronchiectasis. It reduces viscosity of sputum by breaking down the DNA released from neutrophils.

Pleural Diseases

GENERAL PRINCIPLES

- The pleural lining is a serous membrane covering the lung parenchyma, chest wall, diaphragm, and mediastinum.
- The presence of excess fluid or any amount of gas in the pleural space is abnormal.
- The pleural membrane covering the surface of the lung is known as the visceral pleura; the parietal pleura covers the remaining structures.
  - In between the visceral and parietal pleura of each lung is the pleural space, a potential space that contains a thin layer of fluid of approximately 10 mL in volume.
  - The parietal pleura secretes approximately 2400 mL of fluid daily, which is reabsorbed by the visceral pleura.[146]

Definition

- A pleural effusion is an accumulation of >10 mL of fluid in the pleural space.
  - A hemothorax refers to a pleural effusion that mainly comprises blood.[147]
  - Chylothorax is a collection of chyle within the pleural space. Chyle is a milky fluid consisting of lymph and fat droplets.[148]
  - A parapneumonic effusion is fluid collection in the pleural space as a result of a pneumonia/consolidation or bronchiectasis. The three types of parapneumonic effusions include uncomplicated effusion, complicated effusion, and empyema.[149,150]
  - An empyema refers to infected fluid within the pleural space.
- A pneumothorax is a collection of gas in the pleural space.
  - Primary spontaneous pneumothorax occurs when the lung parenchyma is normal without any obvious underlying lung disease.[151]
  - Secondary spontaneous pneumothorax is a complication of underlying parenchymal lung disease.[151]
  - Sometimes if air is trapped in the pleural space under high pressure, a tension pneumothorax develops which can be fatal if not recognized and treated.[152,153]

Epidemiology

- More than one million cases of pleural effusion occur annually in the United States.
- It is estimated that malignant pleural effusion affects about 150,000 people a year in the United States. Congestive heart failure and parapneumonic effusion are the predominant etiologies of pleural effusion in the United States.[150]
- Incidence of pneumothorax varies widely by gender, country, and race.

Etiology

- Pleural effusions have a variety of causes and are listed below (Table 10-12).
  - Empyema is generally caused by extension of an infection of the lung or surrounding tissue.

TABLE 10-12 Causes of Pleural Effusion

- Exudates
  - Infections
    - Bacteria
    - Tuberculosis
    - Fungi
    - Parasites
    - Viruses
    - Mycoplasma
  - Neoplasms
    - Metastatic carcinoma
    - Lymphoma
    - Leukemia
    - Mesothelioma
    - Bronchogenic carcinoma
    - Chest wall tumors
  - Intra-abdominal disease/gastrointestinal
    - Abdominal surgery
    - Pancreatitis
    - Meigs syndrome
    - Intrahepatic abscess
    - Incarcerated diaphragmatic hernia
    - Subdiaphragmatic abscess
    - Esophageal rupture
    - Endoscopic variceal sclerotherapy
    - Hepatitis
  - Collagen vascular diseases
    - Systemic lupus erythematosus
    - Rheumatoid arthritis
    - Drug-induced lupus
    - Sjogren syndrome
    - Granulomatosis with polyangiitis
    - Eosinophilic granulomatosis with polyangiitis
    - Immunoblastic lymphadenopathy
  - Drug-induced pleural disease
    - Nitrofurantoin
    - Dantrolene
    - Methysergide
    - Bromocriptine
    - Procarbazine
    - Amiodarone
  - Pulmonary infarction secondary to thromboembolic disease
  - Miscellaneous
    - Dressler syndrome (post-cardiac injury)
    - Sarcoidosis
    - Yellow nail syndrome
    - Trapped lung
    - Radiation therapy
    - Electrical burns
    - Iatrogenic injury
    - Ovarian hyperstimulation syndrome

(Continued)

TABLE 10-12 Causes of Pleural Effusion (Continued)

- Chronic atelectasis
- Asbestos exposure
- Familial Mediterranean fever
- Urinoma

- Idiopathic
- Lipid laden
  - Chylous
  - Pseudochylous
- Trauma

- Transudates
  - Increased hydrostatic pressure
    - Congestive heart failure
    - Constrictive pericarditis
    - Superior vena caval obstruction
  - Decreased oncotic pressure
    - Cirrhosis
    - Nephrotic syndrome
    - Hypoalbuminemia
    - Peritoneal dialysis
  - Miscellaneous
    - Acute atelectasis
    - Subclavian catheter misplacement
    - Myxedema
    - Idiopathic

- Common microbial pathogens are *Staphylococcus aureus, Streptococcus* species, and *Haemophilus influenza* and *oral anaerobes.*
- Empyemas are frequently polymicrobial in cases where aspiration is suspected, commonly because of oral flora.

- The three major grouped causes of chylothorax are malignancy (50% of cases),[148,154] trauma (25%), and idiopathic (15%).[155] Other rare causes such as LAM[156] and trauma to thoracic duct account for 10%.
  - 75% of chylous effusions associated with malignancy are due to lymphoma-related obstruction of pleural lymphatics preventing reabsorption of pleural fluid.[148]
- Trauma as a causative factor of chylothorax includes any cardiothoracic surgical procedure.
  - It may take 1–2 weeks post surgery for the chylothorax to become apparent.
- In a number of cases, chylothorax results from transdiaphragmatic leakage of chylous ascites.[148]
  - Causes of chylous ascites include nephrotic syndrome, hypothyroidism, and cirrhosis of the liver.[148]
- Hemothorax may result from trauma or an iatrogenic etiology and are rarely spontaneous.[147]
- Other causes of pleural effusion include heart failure, anasarca, and pulmonary embolism.

- Secondary pneumothorax is often seen in chronic obstructive pulmonary disease, AIDS, CF, tuberculosis, Pneumocystis jirovecii pneumonia, sarcoidosis, pulmonary fibrosis, asthma, Marfan disease, LAM, PLCH, trauma, or any cavitary or cystic lung disease.

Pathophysiology

- Pleural effusions can be categorized as transudates or exudates.
  - Transudates result primarily from passive fluid shifts that occur as a result of changes in the hydrostatic and/or oncotic pressures of the circulation.[157]
  - Exudates are indicative of an active pleural process such as inflammation of the pleura or underlying lung tissue.[157]
  - There are numerous causes of both transudates and exudates (Table 10-12).[157]
- Primary spontaneous pneumothorax is thought to result from rupture of subpleural apical blebs, with no obvious preceding cause.[158]
- Secondary pneumothorax results from rupture of pathologic lung architecture such as emphysematous bullae, cysts or cavity formation.[158]

Risk Factors

- Risk factors for pleural effusion reflect those of the underlying causative disease.
- Primary spontaneous pneumothoraces are more common in tall, thin males, and recur 50% of the time.
- Marfan disease is associated with a primary spontaneous pneumothorax.[158]

DIAGNOSIS

- Diagnosis of a pleural disease is based on history, physical examination, and radiographic imaging, which includes chest radiography, CT scan, and chest ultrasound.[159]
- Differentiation into a specific pathologic entity is based on history, imaging, and laboratory analysis (chemistry, microbiology, and cytology) of the pleural fluid if present.

Clinical Presentation

- Symptom onset may be chronic, subacute, or acute depending on the rapidity with which the pleural pathology developed (amount of gas or excess pleural fluid).
- If the effusion is very large in nature, it may cause a mass effect potentially progressing to a tension physiology and hemodynamic instability from cardiac tamponade resulting in a life-threatening hypotension.

History

- Dyspnea is the primary symptom of pleural disease, and pain may also be present.
  - Pain is generally pleuritic in nature.
  - Referred pain to the abdomen and ipsilateral shoulder are possible.
- Other symptoms depend on the specific etiology of the pleural disease:
  - Empyema may be associated with fevers, chills, and malaise.
  - Hemothorax may present with signs and symptoms of anemia such as acute or subacute dyspnea.[147]
  - Chylothorax contains large amounts of fat, protein, and lymphocytes, which accounts for nutritional and immunologic deficiencies observed when they are chronic in nature.

Physical Examination

- Decreased expansion on inspiration, dullness to percussion, and decreased or absent breath sounds on auscultation are all consistent with a pleural effusion.
- However, the examination finding that correlates best with presence of pleural effusion is asymmetric chest wall expansion.
- Asymmetric chest wall appearance, decreased breath sounds, decreased tactile fremitus, and hyperresonance to percussion are all consistent with a large pneumothorax.
- Hypotension may be the presenting sign if there is a mass effect from a large pleural effusion or tension pneumothorax.

Diagnostic Criteria

- There are no clinical criteria to definitively diagnose a pleural effusion or pneumothorax and radiographic imaging is generally needed.

Differential Diagnosis

- The differential diagnosis for pleural effusion or pneumothorax include other causes of dyspnea such as pulmonary edema, pneumonia, compressive or resorptive atelectasis, thromboembolic disease, or interstitial lung disease or central airway obstruction because of benign or malignant disease.

Diagnostic Testing

- Radiographic imaging and laboratory testing of pleural fluid are the two most useful diagnostic modalities for diagnosing pleural disease.

Laboratory Testing

- Categorization of pleural fluid as transudative or exudative assists with diagnosis and therapeutic management.[160]
  - Light's criteria compare levels of protein and lactate dehydrogenase in the effusion with those in the patient's serum to determine whether inflammation or fluid shift is responsible for the effusion.[161]
    - If one of the three criteria is met, the effusion is defined as an exudate (Table 10-13).[160,161]
- Heffner's criteria have similar sensitivity for identifying exudative pleural effusions when compared with Light's criteria and do not require concomitant serum values for comparison (Table 10-13).[162]
- On clinical examination if a patient is suspected to have a transudative effusion, but meets Light's criteria for an exudative effusion, measure serum–pleural fluid albumin gradient, or measure the serum–pleural protein gradient (Roth's criteria).
  - Serum-effusion albumin gradient of >1.2 g/dL: transudative.
  - Serum-effusion protein gradient >3.1 g/dL: transudative.
- Other useful studies to differentiate the type of pleural effusion include pH, glucose, cell count, Gram stain, culture, and triglycerides. Hematocrit should be sent if hemothorax is suspected.[160]
    - Empyema can be diagnosed by a positive Gram stain or culture.
  - Empyema is also characterized by a low pH and low glucose.
  - Hemothorax is defined by a pleural hematocrit/serum hematocrit of > 0.5.

TABLE 10-13 Criteria for Defining an Effusion

- Light's criteria
  - Pleural fluid protein to serum protein ratio of >0.5
  - Pleural fluid lactate dehydrogenase (LDH) to serum LDH ratio of >0.6
  - Pleural fluid LDH >2/3 serum upper limit of normal
- Heffner criteria
  - Pleural fluid protein >2.9 g/dL
  - Pleural fluid cholesterol >45 mg/dL
  - Pleural fluid LDH >45% of upper limits of normal serum value

Adapted from Light RW. Clinical manifestations and useful tests. In: Light RW, ed. *Pleural Diseases.* 4th ed. Baltimore: Lippincott Williams and Wilkins; 2001:42–86; Heffner JE, Brown LK, Barbieri CA. Diagnostic value of tests that discriminate between exudative and transudative pleural effusions. *Chest.* 1997;111:970–980.

- Chylothorax is diagnosed by pleural triglycerides >110 mg/dL or by the presence of chylomicrons in the pleural fluid.[148]
  - If chylothorax is suspected and triglycerides are 50–110 mg/dL, a lipoprotein electrophoresis can confirm the presence of chylomicrons.[148]
- Malignant pleural effusion is diagnosed by a positive fluid cytology, and though highly specific it is not sensitive. The sensitivity of diagnosis of a malignant pleural effusion increases with subsequent thoracentesis up to three times and with increasing amount of pleural fluid.[163]

- See Table 10-14 for other pleural fluid laboratory values associated with specific pleural effusions.
- **Tuberculous pleural effusion** is lymphocytic exudate. Smear for AFB is rarely +ve (10%). Culture for *M. tuberculosis* is positive in approximately 25%–50% of patients. Pleural concentration of adenosine deaminase (ADA) is a useful screening test, and TB can be excluded if the value is very low. Marked elevation in the levels of soluble interleukin-2 (IL-2) receptors and PCR for DNA of *M. tuberculosis* can aid in diagnosis.
- **Urinothorax** forms as a result of retroperitoneal leakage and accumulation of urine in the pleural cavity. The pleural fluid is a transudate with pH <7 and pleural fluid-to-serum creatinine ratio >1.

Imaging

- Chest radiograph is generally the first imaging study obtained when a patient presents with a suspected pleural effusion or pneumothorax.[164]
  - On a posteroanterior chest film, blunting of the costophrenic angle or blurring of the diaphragmatic margin suggests the presence of a pleural effusion.
    - Generally, 200–500 mL of fluid is needed to generate this finding (Figure 10-10).[165]
  - A lateral decubitus film of the affected side can reveal an effusion of approximately 100 mL and allows for assessment of a free-flowing versus loculated effusion.[164,165]

TABLE 10-14 Helpful Features of Exudative Pleural Effusions

- Malignancy
  - Fluid cytology positive for malignant cells
- Tuberculosis
  - Pleural fluid is lymphocytic
  - Positive acid-fast bacilli stain is very rare
  - Pleural fluid is sanguineous
- Connective tissue disease
  - Pleural fluid usually lymphocytic and will often have antinuclear antibody positivity
- Pancreatitis
  - Increased amylase
- Infection
  - Gram stain and culture often reveal specific infection
  - Empyema is accompanied by very low glucose and pH and a markedly elevated lactate dehydrogenase
- Drug related
  - Eosinophilic fluid
- Chylothorax
  - Milky fluid, triglyceride level >110 mg/dL
- Hemothorax
  - Sanguineous fluid
  - Hematocrit of pleural fluid is >50% of peripheral blood

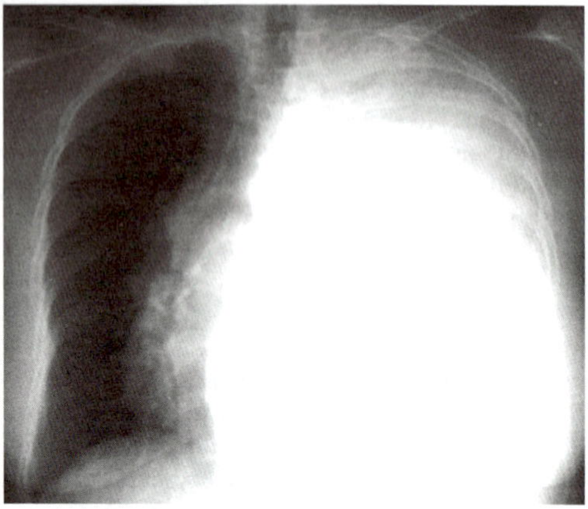

Figure 10-10 Chest X-ray showing homogenous opacity in the left hemithorax with obliteration of costophrenic and cardiophrenic angles with trachea and mediastinal shift to opposite side, suggestive of massive left sided pleural effusion.

- CT is more sensitive than radiography and can detect the presence of even a very small amount of fluid or air in the pleural space as well as the presence of loculations in the pleural fluid.[164]
- Ultrasound is a modality that is increasingly being used to image the pleural space.
  - Ultrasound can detect fluid or air and provides qualitative information regarding pleural fluid and detects small amounts of fluid as well as the presence of septations in the pleural space.
    - Ultrasound findings such as fluid echogenicity and the presence of septations indicate a complex loculated effusion potentially changing management and predicting clinical outcome.
    - Ultrasound guidance is often used to direct treatments such as drainage of fluid or chest tube insertion.

Diagnostic Procedures

- Thoracentesis should be performed for diagnosis in cases of pleural effusion of unknown etiology. Subsequent thoracentesis increase the diagnostic yield depending on etiology.[163]
- Therapeutic thoracentesis can lead to symptom relief and is indicated for dyspnea.
  - Thoracentesis should generally be performed after ultrasound localization of pleural fluid to decrease risk of complications such as pneumothorax.
  - CXR should be performed after the procedure to rule out a complicating pneumothorax.
  - Hemothorax is a rare complication.

TREATMENT

- Generally, treatment of a pleural effusion depends on the etiology.
  - Transudative pleural effusions are most appropriately managed by treating the underlying cause.
    - Symptomatic treatment may involve drainage of the effusion if the presenting symptom is dyspnea or acute respiratory failure.
  - Exudative pleural effusions should be evaluated for an underlying cause.
    - Treatment may involve drainage of the effusion or even pleurodesis to prevent re-accumulation of fluid.
    - Placement of an indwelling pleural catheter for malignant recurrent pleural effusions or hepatic hydrothorax that is persistent after diuresis is an option.[166]

- Treatment of pneumothorax generally involves draining the air from the pleural space by insertion of a chest tube.
- Pleurodesis should be considered after the first episode of secondary spontaneous pneumothorax because of high rate of recurrence.[151]

Medications

- Pleural effusions can sometimes be treated with medications depending on the cause.
- Parapneumonic effusions and empyema are treated with antibiotics in conjunction with fluid drainage.[150]
- Transudative pleural effusions can sometimes be treated effectively with diuretics in disease states such as congestive heart failure, anasarca, renal failure, and liver failure.
- There is no medical treatment for pneumothorax.

Other Nonpharmacologic Therapies

- Pleurodesis involves instillation of a sclerosing agent into the pleural space to cause scarring and restriction of the space itself.
    - This is generally performed for recurrent malignant effusion, recurrent pneumothorax once the lung has re-expanded, and occasionally chylothorax and after the first episode of secondary spontaneous pneumothorax.[151]
- When other modalities fail, total parenteral nutrition with complete bowel rest can cause chylothoraces to resolve as oral intake results in chyle formation.[148]
    - Medium-chain triglyceride diets have been tried, as chyle is derived from long-chain triglycerides in the diet, though this has yielded mixed results.[148]
- If a pneumothorax is <15% of the hemithorax volume, it is safe to observe and follow-up with radiographic studies.
    - High oxygen content (e.g., 100% nonrebreather mask) administration increases the rate of pleural air reabsorption by increasing the nitrogen gradient between the air in the pneumothorax and the pleural capillaries.
- In cases of persistent pneumothorax secondary to a bronchopleural fistula, fiberoptic bronchoscopy with placement of endobronchial valves causing atelectasis of the distal lung can be placed in a segmental or subsegmental bronchus if the bronchopleural fistula has been localized to one location via balloon catheter occlusion.[167]

Surgical Management

- Pleural effusion:
    - Chest tube insertion is often indicated for drainage of large pleural effusions.
    - Other indications for chest tube insertion include empyema, chylothorax, and hemothorax.[147]
    - As discussed, thoracentesis can be used as a therapeutic modality.
    - Malignant pleural effusion:
        - Tunneled pleural catheter is used for recurrent malignant pleural effusion and occasionally hepatic hydrothorax not amenable to diuresis.[166]
        - This catheter can be drained at home every other day with attachment to a vacuum-sealed device.
        - In our experience, approximately 50% of effusions are permanently drained by way of autopleurodesis allowing for removal of the tunneled pleural catheter.[168]
    - Empyema:
        - In cases where chest tube drainage does not effectively drain an empyema and there is continued evidence of infection, VATS with decortication is often indicated.
        - There is a role for intrapleural use of tissue plasminogen activator and recombinant deoxyribonuclease (DNAse) in pleural infections resulting in improved fluid drainage and decreased need for VATS.[169]

- Hemothorax:
  - Requires surgical stabilization in 30% of penetrating injuries and 15% of blunt injuries.[170]
  - Initial output of >1500 mL of blood or continued chest tube output or >200 mL of blood over 2 hours requires surgical intervention.
  - Clotted blood in the pleural space may require VATS to prevent development of empyema or fibrothorax.[171]
- Chylothorax:
  - For persistent chylothorax, surgical interventions include thoracic duct ligation via VATS in conjunction with pleurectomy or pleurodesis.[171]
  - Pleuroperitoneal shunting is also occasionally performed, though obviously not in cases in which the pleural disease is secondary to chylous ascites.[170]
  - Early surgical intervention for chylothorax should be considered when chest tube output is >1500 mL/day or in a patient with malnourishment or an immunocompromised state.[148]
- Pneumothorax:
  - Treated with chest tube insertion if they are large, symptomatic, under tension, recurrent, or bilateral.
    - In extreme circumstances where a large pneumothorax is causing cardiovascular collapse, immediate needle decompression is indicated by inserting a needle in the anterior chest above the nipple line in a parasternal location.
  - For recurrent pneumothorax, VATS may be indicated with endoscopic stapling and removal of the bulla or fistula, particularly if there is a bronchopleural fistula.[167]
  - Therapeutic success of bronchoscopic management of bronchopleural fistula with endobronchial valves, coils, glue or sealant has been variable and treatment must be individualized.[167]

SPECIAL CONSIDERATIONS

- The etiology of pleural effusions can often be discerned by their appearance.
  - A serous effusion is more likely to be transudative, while an exudative effusion is more likely to have other appearances, frequently with a cloudy or serosanguinous appearance.
  - If the fluid appears frankly bloody, a hemothorax should be suspected.
  - Pus indicates an empyema.
  - Milky white and opalescent pleural fluid is indicative of a chylothorax.
- In cases of massive hemothorax requiring surgical intervention, clamping the chest tube may result in tension hemothorax and cardiovascular collapse.[171]
- Chylothorax is nonirritating and bacteriostatic, thus secondary infection is extremely rare.[170]

COMPLICATIONS

- Disease recurrence.
- Cardiovascular compromise in extreme cases.
- Other complications are disease-specific.

REFERRAL

- Interventional pulmonology may be consulted for the placement of chest tubes, tunneled pleural catheters, or endobronchial valve placement.
- Surgical consultation may be needed as per the above section on surgical management.

Summary

- Pulmonary hypertension includes patients with mean pulmonary artery pressure >20 mm Hg measured by right heart catheterization.
- For patients with PAH without evidence of vasoreactivity, up-front therapy with the prostacyclin analogue treprostinil plus the phosphodiesterase type-5 inhibitor tadalafil and endothelin receptor antagonist ambrisentan is indicated.
- Common risk factors for the development of OSA are obesity (body mass index [BMI] ≥30 kg/m^2), the menopause, male gender, and increasing age.
- Snoring and daytime sleepiness are among the most common symptoms, but many patients with OSA are asymptomatic. Overnight polysomnography (PSG) is the gold standard for a proper diagnosis of OSA.
- Transbronchial cryobiopsy is an acceptable alternative to surgical lung biopsy in patients with ILD of undetermined type, in medical centers with appropriate expertise.
- The diagnosis of sarcoidosis relies on the presence of noncaseating granuloma on histopathologic examination, compatible clinical presentation, and exclusion of other causes of granulomatous inflammation.
- Due to the high etiological diversity and the potential for malignancy, pulmonary nodules represent a clinical challenge.

Scan the QR code to access chapter references.

11 Allergy and Immunology

Niharika Thota, Zhen Ren, Jennifer M. Monroy, and Shishir M. Upadya

Adverse Drug Reactions

GENERAL PRINCIPLES

Definition

- An **adverse drug reaction** (ADR) is an undesired pharmacological response that occurs when a drug is given for the appropriate purpose.
- The etiology of a drug reaction can be immunologic, toxic, or idiosyncratic in nature.
- Drug allergy is due to an immune response that is mediated by drug-specific antibody or T cells.

Classification

- *Type A* (Augmented) reactions are predictable, often dose dependent, and related to the pharmacokinetics of the drug. They comprise up to 80% of all ADRs (e.g., hepatic failure due to overdose of acetaminophen, sedative side effects of antihistamines, drug–drug interactions, and GI bacterial alteration after antibiotics).
- *Type B* (Bizarre) reactions are unpredictable and are not related to the dose or the drug's pharmacokinetics. They account for 10%–15% of all ADRs.
- *Type C* (Chronic) reactions are chronic, dose related and time related, uncommon, and related to cumulative dose (e.g., hypothalamic–pituitary–adrenal axis suppression by corticosteroids and osteonecrosis of the jaw with bisphosphonates).
- *Type D* (Delayed) reactions are time related and uncommon, and become apparent sometime after use of the drug (e.g., carcinogenesis, tardive dyskinesia, and teratogenesis).
- *Type E* (End of use) reactions are uncommon and occur soon after withdrawal of the drug (e.g., withdrawal syndrome with opiates or benzodiazepines).
- *Type F* (Failure) reactions are unexpected failure of therapy, common, dose related, and often caused by drug interactions (e.g., inadequate dosage of an oral contraceptive when used with an enzyme inducer and resistance to antimicrobial agents).
  - Immune-mediated adverse reactions can be from a variety of mechanisms. They usually occur on re-exposure to the offending drug.
  - **Pseudoallergic reactions,** formerly called anaphylactoid reactions, are caused by IgE-independent degranulation of mast cells.

Epidemiology

- ADRs are reported to account for 10%–15% of hospitalized patients.[1]
- Mortality from ADRs is significant and ranges from 0.14%–0.32%.[2]
- Lifetime prevalence of drug-induced anaphylaxis is 0.05%–2.0%.[1] The most common drugs causing IgE-mediated anaphylaxis are penicillins and anesthetic agents given during the perioperative period. Drug-induced anaphylaxis is seen predominantly in older age group.

Etiology

- **β-Lactam** antibiotics are the most common drug class allergy in United States, which includes penicillins, penicillin derivatives (ampicillin and amoxicillin), cephalosporins,

monobactams and carbapenems. Penicillin allergy is the most prevalent antibiotic allergy of this class. About 8% of patients in health-care report have a penicillin allergy.[3]
- About 90% patients with history of penicillin allergy will be able to tolerate penicillins, as most patients outgrow their allergy overtime.[4]
- Rate of penicillin-induced anaphylaxis after parenteral administration is approximately 1–2 per 10,000 treated patients.[5]

- Hospitalized patients with a history of penicillin allergy have been shown to have a longer hospital stay with increased incidence of vancomycin-resistant *Enterococcus*, methicillin-resistant *Staphylococcus aureus*, and *Clostridium difficile* infections compared to patients without a reported penicillin allergy.[6]
- The chemical structure of penicillins results in their high immunogenicity. Being immunologically inert, it spontaneously breaks down to reactive intermediates.
  - The core structure is composed of a reactive β-lactam ring that covalently binds with carrier proteins to form a hapten, which stimulates an immune response. The major determinant of immunogenicity of penicillin is the benzylpenicilloyl form seen in 93% of tissue-bound penicillin.
  - The minor antigenic determinants are all remaining penicillin conjugates. They comprise benzylpenicillin, benzylpenicilloate, and benzylpenilloate.
  - Most immediate reactions to penicillins are related to the major determinant. In other penicillins such as ampicillin, the R side chain is the antigenic determinant.
  - Penicillin can cause any of the four types of Gell–Coombs classification of adverse immune reactions. Most common clinical features being urticaria, pruritus, fever, and bronchospasm.
- The cross-reactivity between β-lactam antibiotics is variable and largely determined by their side-chain structure attached to the β-lactam ring.
- Before the 1980s, early first-generation cephalosporins had a higher cross-reactivity to penicillin because they were contaminated with a small amount of penicillin.[6] Based on recent studies, the treatment of cephalosporins without preceding penicillin skin testing in patients with a history of penicillin allergy showed a reaction rate of 0.1%.[7] Risk of a cross-reaction is 5.0%–16.5% with first-generation cephalosporins, 4% with second-generation, and 1%–3% with third- or fourth-generation.[6]
  - Although many of the reactions to second- and third-generation cephalosporins are directed at the side chains, skin testing to penicillin in these patients can be helpful because most severe anaphylactic reactions are directed against the reactive bicyclic core.
  - Patients with a history of a severe reaction to penicillin should be considered sensitive to cephalosporin unless they are skin test negative. Although patients with a history of a nonanaphylactic reaction to penicillin can often be given a second- or third-generation cephalosporin safely, it is advisable to precede the dose with an oral provocation challenge.
  - Selective reactions to piperacillin tazobactam may be identified by skin tests beforehand, and these patients may not have reactivity to other penicillins.[32]
- Skin test cross-reactivity has been documented between carbapenems and penicillins. Patients undergoing a graded carbapenem challenge with a positive penicillin skin test and a negative carbapenem skin test did not have any hypersensitivity reactions.[4]
- The monobactam aztreonam rarely cross-reacts with penicillins. Ceftazidime does share an identical R-group side chain to aztreonam and is highly cross-reactive.[8]
- **Sulfonamide allergy**
  - There is an increase in allergy to sulfonamides in patients with HIV compared to the general population. Trimethoprim–sulfamethoxazole hypersensitivity occurs in 60% of HIV-positive patients compared to 5% of HIV-negative patients.[9]
  - Type I IgE-mediated reactions to sulfonamides are not common. The most frequently seen reaction is a maculopapular rash (T cell-mediated) that develops 7–12 days after initiating the drug. Other reactions include urticaria and, less commonly, anaphylaxis,

Stevens–Johnson syndrome (SJS), and toxic epidermal necrolysis (TEN). Cross-reactivity between antibiotic and nonantibiotic sulfa-containing medications is low. Patients with sulfonamide antibiotic allergy were more likely to react to penicillin than a sulfonamide nonantibiotic.[10]

- **NSAIDs** and aspirin can cause IgE-mediated urticaria, angioedema, and anaphylaxis. It can also exacerbate urticaria in patients who have chronic urticaria. Exacerbation of respiratory symptoms in patients with underlying asthma is referred to as aspirin-exacerbated respiratory disease (AERD). Samter's triad is the combination of asthma, NSAID sensitivity, and nasal polyposis. COX2 inhibitors are generally safe to administer in these patients. Aspirin desensitization followed by daily aspirin therapy in AERD patients improves asthma exacerbations, oral steroid use, reduced nasal polyps, and sinus infections. In non-AERD aspirin allergy with acute cardiovascular need for aspirin administration, a 2-step aspirin challenge is suggested over desensitization.[32]

Pathophysiology

The immunologic mechanisms for drug hypersensitivity are demonstrated in the Gell and Coombs classification of hypersensitivity (Table 11-1).

Risk Factors

Factors that increase a patient's risk of an ADR include size and structure of drug, route of exposure (cutaneous most immunogenic), dose, duration, frequency, gender (women > men), genetic factors (HLA type, history of atopy), prior drug reaction, coexisting medical illnesses, and concurrent medical therapy.

DIAGNOSIS

Clinical Presentation

- A history is essential for making the diagnosis of an allergic drug reaction. Questions should be directed at establishing the following information: sign and symptoms, timing of the reaction, purpose of the drug, other medications the patient is receiving, prior exposure to drug or related drug, and history of other allergic drug reactions.
- Urticaria, angioedema, wheezing, and anaphylaxis are all characteristics of IgE-mediated (type 1) reactions.

TABLE 11-1 Immunologically Mediated Drug Reactions

Type of Reaction	Representative Examples	Mechanism
Anaphylactic (type 1)	Anaphylaxis Urticaria Angioedema	IgE-mediated degranulation of mast cells with resultant mediator release
Cytotoxic (type 2)	Autoimmune hemolytic anemia Interstitial nephritis	IgG or IgM antibodies against cell antigens and complement activation
Immune complex (type 3)	Serum sickness Vasculitis	Immune complex deposition and subsequent complement activation
Cell mediated (type 4)	Contact dermatitis Photosensitivity dermatitis	Activated T cells against cell surface–bound antigens

- Symptoms do not typically occur on the first exposure to the medication unless the patient has been exposed to a structurally related medication. On re-exposure, however, symptoms tend to manifest acutely (often <1 hour).
- IgE-mediated reactions tend to worsen with repeated exposure to the offending medication.
- Pseudoallergic reactions (non–IgE-mediated) can be clinically indistinguishable from IgE-mediated reactions because the final common pathway for their reaction is mast cell degranulation.

- **Maculopapular exanthemas** are the most common cutaneous manifestation of drug allergy.
  - These reactions are mediated by T cells and typically delayed in onset, first occurring between 2 and 14 days of exposure to culprit medications. It can occur sooner with subsequent exposures. Lesions typically begin on the trunk, especially in dependent areas, and spread to the extremities.
  - Rarely, these rashes can progress to a more serious drug reaction involving blistering of the skin and/or end-organ involvement.
- **DRESS** (**D**rug **R**eaction with **E**osinophilia and **S**ystemic **S**ymptoms) are a serious life-threatening ADR, often presenting as rash and fever with systemic involvement, can manifest as hepatitis, eosinophilia, pneumonitis, lymphadenopathy, and nephritis.
  - Symptoms tend to present 2–6 weeks after introduction of medication and resolve few weeks to months after stopping the offending agent. Certain viral infections such as EBV, HHV-6, HHV-7, and CMV are associated with increased risk of complications.
  - First described with antiepileptic (carbamazepine) agents but has also been reported to occur with abacavir, allopurinol, NSAIDs, dapsone, sulfonamides, minocycline, and β-blockers.
  - Atypical lymphocytosis (>5%) and eosinophilia (>1.5 × 10^9/L) are noted.
- **Erythema multiforme** (EM), **SJS, and TEN** are all serious drug reactions primarily involving the skin.
  - EM is characterized most typically by target lesions. SJS and TEN manifest with varying degrees of sloughing of the skin and mucous membranes (<10% in SJS and >30% in TEN). Risk factors being HIV, hematological malignancy, systemic lupus erythematosus, and bone marrow transplant.
  - **Readministration or future skin testing with the offending drug is absolutely contraindicated.**

PREVENTION AND TREATMENT

- Acute drug reactions such as anaphylaxis should be treated promptly and **discontinuation** of the suspected drug is the most important initial approach in managing an allergic drug reaction.
- HLA testing may be indicated in susceptible populations for prevention of a severe ADR for some drugs such as abacavir and carbamazepine.
- Future use of the drug in question should **always be avoided** unless there is no therapeutic alternative available.
- If use of the drug must be considered, a careful history of the reaction is helpful in defining the potential risk. Patients may lose their sensitivity to a drug over time, and determining the date of reaction is useful. Symptoms that occur with the start of a drug course are more likely to be IgE-mediated than symptoms that develop several days after the completion of a course.
- The types of symptoms are also important. Toxic reactions (e.g., nausea secondary to macrolide antibiotics or codeine) are not immunologic reactions and do not necessarily predict problems with other members in their respective class.

- If the patient is taking the drug for a life-threatening illness (e.g., meningitis with penicillin allergy) and the reaction is a mild skin reaction, it may be reasonable to continue the medication and treat the reaction symptomatically. **If the rash is progressive, however, the drug must be discontinued to avoid a desquamative process such as SJS.**

REFERRAL

- If no alternative drug is available and the patient has a history of an IgE-mediated reaction, the patient should be referred to an allergist for further evaluation.
- The allergist may perform one of several procedures if indicated depending on the medication, type of reaction, and availability of testing reagents.
  - **Skin testing** may be performed to assess for the presence of IgE to the medication.
    - Although skin testing may be performed to nearly any medication, sensitivity and specificity of the skin test results have been best established with penicillin.
    - Results of testing to drugs other than penicillin must be interpreted within the clinical context of the case.
  - **Graded dose challenge** assesses how the patient tolerates progressively larger doses of medication (e.g., 1/1000, 1/10, and full dose given 20 minutes apart).
  - **Drug desensitization** is defined as induction of temporary state of clinical unresponsiveness or tolerance to a suspected drug. It is performed when the patient has an identified IgE-mediated reaction but still requires the medication.
    - The exact mechanism by which desensitization prevents anaphylaxis is unclear.
    - The drug must be taken daily at a specified dose to maintain the "desensitized state."
    - If a dose of drug is missed for a period >48 hours following a desensitization procedure, the patient will often need to undergo a repeat desensitization.
  - Successful desensitization or graded challenge does not preclude the development of a non–IgE-mediated, delayed reaction (e.g., rash).

Anaphylaxis

GENERAL PRINCIPLES

Definition

Anaphylaxis is a rapidly developing, life-threatening systemic reaction mediated by the release of mast cell and basophil-derived mediators into the circulation. The peak severity is seen usually within 5–30 minutes.

Classification

Immunologic anaphylaxis

- Allergic IgE-mediated anaphylaxis (type 1 hypersensitivity)
- IgG-mediated anaphylaxis (rare)

Nonimmunologic anaphylaxis. Previously known as *anaphylactoid reactions.*

Epidemiology

Incidence of anaphylaxis is approximately 50–2000 episodes per 100,000 person-years. Fatality is estimated at 0.7%–2% per case of anaphylaxis. In the United States, the lifetime prevalence of anaphylaxis is reported to be 1.6%.[11]

Etiology

Immunologic causes

- Foods, especially peanuts, tree nuts, shellfish, finned fish, milk, and eggs

- Insect stings (bees, wasps, and fire ants)
- Medications
- Latex rubber
- Blood products

Nonimmunologic causes
- Radiocontrast media
- Medications (i.e., NSAIDs, opiates, vancomycin, muscle relaxants, rarely ACE inhibitors, and sulfating agents)
- Hemodialysis
- Physical factors (cold temperature or exercise)
- Idiopathic

Pathophysiology (Figure 11-1)

Immunologic
- Anaphylaxis is due to sensitization to an antigen and formation of specific IgE to that antigen. On re-exposure, the IgE on mast cells and basophils binds the antigen and cross-links the IgE receptor, which causes activation of the cells with subsequent systemic release of preformed mediators, such as histamine, tryptase, carboxypeptidase A, and proteoglycans. Slow-reacting substance of anaphylaxis, cysteinyl leukotrienes (LTC4 and LTD4) also play an important role.

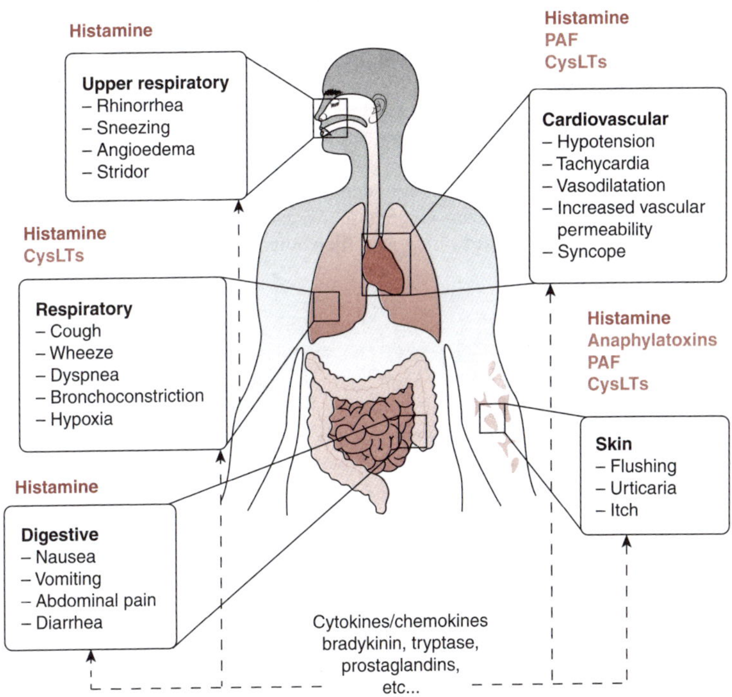

Figure 11-1 Pathophysiology of anaphylaxis. *PAF*, platelet activating factor; *CysLTs*, cysteinyl leukotrienes.

- The release of mediators ultimately causes capillary leakage, cellular edema, and smooth muscle contractions resulting in the constellation of physical symptoms.

Nonimmunologic. Non–IgE-mediated anaphylaxis is also mediated by direct degranulation of mast cells and basophils in the absence of immunoglobulins.

Risk Factors

- Persistent asthma: increased risk of fatal anaphylaxis if asthma is uncontrolled.
- Cardiovascular disease: increased risk for death in older age.
- Elevated baseline tryptase indicates possible mast cell disorder. Individuals with **mastocytosis**, a disease characterized by a proliferation of mast cells, are at higher risk for severe anaphylaxis from both IgE- and non–IgE-mediated causes.
- Previous sensitization and formation of antigen-specific IgE with history of anaphylaxis.
- Concomitant use drugs: beta-adrenergic blockers, ACE inhibitors, NSAIDs, alcohol, etc.
- Cofactors such as exercise, fever, acute infection, premenstrual status, and emotional.
- Sensitivity to seafood or iodine does not predispose to radiocontrast media reactions.

Prevention

- **For all types of anaphylaxis, recognition of potential triggers and avoidance are the best prevention.**
- **Self-injectable epinephrine and patient education for all patients with a history of anaphylaxis.**
- Radiocontrast sensitivity reactions
  - Use of low-ionic contrast media is strongly suggested.
  - Premedication before procedure.
    - Prednisone 50 mg PO given 13, 7, and 1 hour before procedure.
    - Diphenhydramine 50 mg PO given 1 hour before procedure.
    - H_2 blocker may also be given 1 hour before procedure.
- **Premedication is not 100% effective, and appropriate precautions for handling a reaction should be taken.**
- Anaphylaxis can be a presenting sign of underlying mastocytosis.
- Red man syndrome from vancomycin. Symptoms can usually be prevented by slowing the rate of infusion and premedicating with diphenhydramine (50 mg PO) 30 minutes before start of the infusion.

DIAGNOSIS

Diagnosis is based primarily on history and physical examination and the documentation of the presence of a specific IgE to the suspected allergen (if the trigger is IgE mediated). Confirmation of anaphylaxis can, in some cases, be provided by the laboratory finding of an elevated serum tryptase level. However, the absence of an elevated tryptase level does not exclude anaphylaxis.

Clinical Presentation

- The clinical manifestations of allergic and nonallergic anaphylaxis are the same.
- Most serious reactions occur within minutes after exposure to the antigen, but in some circumstances, the reaction may be delayed for hours.
- Some patients experience a biphasic reaction characterized by a recurrence of symptoms after resolution of initial anaphylactic episode. Time range is varied and typically occurs 1–8 hours.
- A few patients have a protracted course that requires several hours to days of continuous supportive treatment.

- Manifestations include pruritus, flushing, urticaria, angioedema, respiratory distress (due to laryngeal edema, laryngospasm, or bronchospasm), hypotension, uterine cramping, abdominal cramping, emesis, and diarrhea.

History

A thorough history is taken to help identify the potential trigger, such as new foods, medications, or other commonly known allergens. Also documenting the time of onset of symptoms—that is, minutes to hours or days after a suspected exposure—can help to classify the type of anaphylaxis.

Physical Examination

- Pay special attention to vital signs: Blood pressure, respiratory rate, and oxygen saturation.
- Airway and pulmonary: Assess for any evidence of laryngeal edema or angioedema. Auscultate lung fields to listen for evidence of wheezing. Continue to assess for need to protect the airway.
- Perform a focused cardiovascular examination.
- Skin: Urticaria or erythema.

Diagnostic Criteria

See Table 11-2 for diagnostic criteria for anaphylaxis.

Differential Diagnosis

- Anaphylaxis due to **preformed IgE and re-exposure:** Medications, insect sting, and foods are the most common causes of anaphylaxis. Galactose-α-1,3-galactose allergy is thought to be triggered by tick bites and is a cause of delayed anaphylaxis to red meats including beef, pork, and lamb.
- **Exercise-induced anaphylaxis:** anaphylaxis occurs exclusively in association with physical exertion and other cofactors. Triggers include food (wheat, celery, nuts, seafood) and NSAIDs.

TABLE 11-2 Anaphylaxis

Anaphylaxis is likely when one of the following three criteria occurs:

1. Acute skin and/or mucosal symptoms (e.g., hives, pruritus, flushing, lip/tongue/uvula swelling) and one of the following:
   a. Respiratory symptoms (e.g., wheezing, stridor, shortness of breath, hypoxia)
   b. Hypotension or associated end-organ dysfunction (e.g., hypotonia, syncope, incontinence)
2. Exposure to probable allergen for the patient and two or more of the following:
   a. Skin/mucosal tissue involvement
   b. Respiratory symptoms
   c. Hypotension or end-organ dysfunction
   d. Persistent gastrointestinal symptoms (e.g., emesis, abdominal pain)
3. Decreased blood pressure after exposure to known allergen for the patient:
   a. Adults: Systolic blood pressure <90 mm Hg or >30% decrease in systolic blood pressure
   b. Infants and children: Hypotension for age or >30% decrease in systolic blood pressure

Reprinted from Sampson HA, Munoz-Furlong A, Campbell RL, et al. Second symposium on the definition and management of anaphylaxis: Summary report—Second National Institute of Allergy and Infectious Disease/Food Allergy and Anaphylaxis Network symposium. *J Allergy Clin Immunol.* 2006;117:391–397 with permission from Elsevier.

- Treatment would be to avoid exercise immediately after eating. Advise all patients to carry 2 epinephrine autoinjectors and exercise with partner.
- Causes of **nonallergic anaphylaxis:**
  - **Radiocontrast sensitivity reactions** are thought to be from direct degranulation of mast cells in susceptible patients because of osmotic shifts. Reactions can occur in 5%–10% of patients, with fatal reactions occurring in 1 in 75,000 procedures. It is rare to have an IgE-mediated reaction to radiocontrast.
  - **Red man's syndrome** from vancomycin consists of pruritus and flushing of the face and neck.
  - **Mastocytosis** should be considered in patients with recurrent unexplained anaphylaxis or flushing, especially with previous reactions to nonspecific mast cell degranulators such as opiates and radiocontrast media.
  - **Ingestant-related reactions** can mimic anaphylaxis. This is usually due to sulfites or the presence of a histamine-like substance in spoiled fish (scombroidosis).
  - **Flushing syndromes** include flushing due to red man syndrome, carcinoid, vasointestinal peptide (and other vasoactive intestinal peptide–secreting tumors), postmenopausal symptoms, rosacea, use of niacin, and alcohol use.
- Other forms of shock such as hypoglycemic, cardiogenic, septic, and hemorrhagic.
- Vasovagal syncope can be distinguished from anaphylaxis by a presence of bradycardia; however, bradycardia can occur in anaphylaxis because of the Bezold–Jarisch reflex.
- Respiratory diseases such as acute laryngotracheitis and foreign body obstruction in trachea.
- Miscellaneous syndromes such as hereditary angioedema (C1 esterase inhibitor [C1 INH] deficiency syndrome), pheochromocytoma, neurologic (seizure, stroke), and capillary leak syndrome.
- Neuropsychiatric causes such as panic attacks or vocal cord dysfunction.
- Idiopathic.

Diagnostic Testing

- Epicutaneous skin testing and serum specific IgE testing when available to identify trigger allergens.
- Serum tryptase peaks at 1 hour after symptoms begin and may be present for up to 4 hours.

TREATMENT

- Early recognition of signs and symptoms of anaphylaxis is a critical first step in treatment.
- **Epinephrine is the medication of choice for treatment of anaphylaxis.**
- **Maintain recumbent position while assessing and starting therapy.**
- **Airway management is a priority.** Supplemental 100% oxygen therapy should be administered. Endotracheal intubation may be necessary. If laryngeal edema is not rapidly responsive to epinephrine, cricothyroidotomy or tracheotomy may be required.
- **Volume expansion with IV fluids may be necessary.**

Medications

Epinephrine should be administered immediately. There are no absolute contraindications for treatment with epinephrine in anaphylaxis.

- Adult: 0.3–0.5 mg (0.3–0.5 mL of a 1:1000 solution) IM in the lateral thigh, repeated at 10- to 15-minute intervals if necessary.
- Child: 1:1000 dilution at 0.01 mg/kg or 0.1–0.3 mL administered IM in the lateral thigh, repeated at 10- to 15-minute intervals if necessary.

- 0.5 mL of 1:1000 solution sublingually in cases of major airway compromise or hypotension.
- 3–5 mL of 1:10,000 solution via central line.
- 3–5 mL of 1:10,000 solution diluted with 10 mL of normal saline via endotracheal tube.
- For protracted symptoms that require multiple doses of epinephrine, an IV epinephrine drip may be useful; the infusion is titrated to maintain adequate BP.

Glucagon could reverse refractory bronchospasm and hypotension in patients who are taking β-adrenergic antagonists. Recommended dosage is 1–5 mg intravenously bolus slowly over 5 minutes followed by an infusion at 5–15 μg/min titrated to clinical response.

Inhaled β-adrenergic agonists should be used to treat resistant bronchospasm.

Glucocorticoids have no significant immediate effect but may prevent biphasic reactions. Methylprednisolone 1–2 mg/kg daily for 1–2 days.

Antihistamines relieve skin symptoms but have no immediate effect on the reaction. They may shorten the duration of the reaction.

- Adult: Diphenhydramine 25–50 mg IM or IV
- Child: Diphenhydramine 12.5–25.0 mg IM or IV

REFERRAL

Referrals to an allergist for further evaluation should be offered to all patients with a history of anaphylaxis. More importantly, patients with *Hymenoptera* sensitivity should be evaluated to determine eligibility for venom immunotherapy.

Eosinophilia

GENERAL PRINCIPLES

- Eosinophils are granulocytes that developed from bone marrow pluripotent progenitor cells.
- Eosinophil maturation is promoted by interleukin (IL)-5, IL-3, and granulocyte-macrophage colony-stimulating hormone (GM-CSF).
- Eosinophils are normally seen in peripheral tissue such as mucosal tissues in the gastrointestinal and respiratory tracts. They are recruited to sites of inflammation.
- Eosinophils can be involved in a variety of infectious, allergic, neoplastic, and idiopathic diseases.

Definition

- A value >500 eosinophils/μL is defined as having eosinophilia.
- The extent of eosinophilia can be categorized as mild (500–1500 cells/μL), moderate (1500–5000 cells/μL), or severe (>5000 cells/μL).
- The degree of eosinophilia is *not* a reliable predictor of eosinophil-mediated organ damage.
  - Hypereosinophilia: >1500 eosinophils/μL (with or without end-organ damage).

Classification

- Peripheral eosinophilia can be divided into primary, secondary, or idiopathic.
- Primary eosinophilia is seen with hematologic disorders where there may be a clonal expansion of eosinophils (chronic eosinophilic leukemia) or a clonal expansion of cells that stimulate eosinophil production (chronic myeloid or lymphocytic disorders).
- Secondary eosinophilia is also called reactive eosinophilia. It is a polyclonal expansion of eosinophils due to overproduction of IL-5. There are numerous causes such as parasites,

allergic diseases, autoimmune disorders, toxins, medications, and endocrine disorders such as Addison disease.
- Idiopathic eosinophilia is considered when primary and secondary causes are excluded.

Eosinophilia Associated With Atopic Disease

- Mild eosinophilia is more commonly seen in allergic rhinitis and asthma.
- In allergic rhinitis, increased nasal eosinophilia is more common than peripheral blood eosinophilia.
- Nonallergic rhinitis with eosinophilia syndrome is a form of chronic inflammatory rhinitis with persistent nasal eosinophilia (≥25%) in nonatopic patients. It has a propensity to develop nasal polyps, asthma, and aspirin intolerance (AERD).
- Sputum eosinophilia is a common feature of asthma and suggests responsiveness to corticosteroid treatment.

Eosinophilia Associated With Pulmonary Infiltrates

This classification is inclusive of the pulmonary infiltrates with eosinophilia syndromes and the eosinophilic pneumonias.

- **Allergic bronchopulmonary aspergillosis** (ABPA) is a hypersensitivity response to colonized *Aspergillus fumigatus* in the airways that occurs almost exclusively in asthmatics or cystic fibrosis patients. It is characterized by pulmonary infiltrates, central bronchiectasis, elevated serum IgE with peripheral eosinophilia, positive skin testing to *A. fumigatus*, and the presence of IgE or IgG antibody to *Aspergillus*.
- Disseminated coccidioidomycosis can lead to marked eosinophilia.
- **Eosinophilic pneumonias** consist of pulmonary infiltrates with lung eosinophilia and are only occasionally associated with blood eosinophilia.
  - Acute eosinophilic pneumonia is an idiopathic disease that presents with fever, cough, dyspnea, and hypoxemia occurring for days to weeks, typically in males and in individuals who have recently started to smoke tobacco.
  - Chronic eosinophilic pneumonia is an idiopathic disease that presents with fever, cough, dyspnea, and significant weight loss occurring for weeks to months, typically in females and nonsmokers. It is associated with peripheral blood eosinophilia. "The photographic negative of pulmonary edema" is a classic radiographic finding (radiographic pattern of predominately peripheral consolidation).
  - Löffler syndrome is a combination of blood eosinophilia and transient pulmonary infiltrates due to passage of helminthic larvae, usually *Ascaris lumbricoides*, through the lungs.
  - Tropical pulmonary eosinophilia is a hypersensitivity response in the lung to lymphatic filariae. Peripheral blood microfilariae are usually not detected.

HIV

Eosinophilia is seen in about 20% of patients with HIV infection. The causes can be due to reactions to highly active antiretroviral therapy medications, adrenal insufficiency associated with cytomegalovirus infection, eosinophilic folliculitis, or underlying parasitic infection.

Eosinophilia Associated With Parasitic Infection

Various multicellular parasites or helminths such as *Ascaris*, hookworm, or *Strongyloides* can induce blood eosinophilia, whereas single-celled protozoan parasites such as *Giardia lamblia* do not. The level of eosinophilia reflects the degree of tissue invasion by the parasite. Eosinophilia is usually of the highest grade during the early phase of infection.

- In cases of blood eosinophilia, ***Strongyloides stercoralis* infection must be excluded** because this helminth can set up a cycle of autoinfection leading to chronic infection with intermittent, sometimes marked, eosinophilia.

- Tissue eosinophilia may not be accompanied by blood eosinophilia when the organism is sequestered within tissues (e.g., intact echinococcal cysts) or is limited to the intestinal lumen (e.g., *Ascaris* and tapeworms).
- Among the helminths, the principal parasites that need to be evaluated are *S. stercoralis*, hookworm, and *Toxocara canis*. The diagnostic consideration can also vary according to geographic region.
- There are some important caveats that need to be considered when evaluating patients for parasitic diseases and eosinophilia: *Strongyloides* can persist for decades without causing major symptoms and can elicit varying degrees of eosinophilia ranging from minimal to marked eosinophilia.
- *T. canis* (visceral larva migrans) should be considered in children with a propensity to eat dirt contaminated by dog *Ascaris* eggs.

Eosinophilia Associated With Cutaneous Disease

- **Atopic dermatitis** is classically associated with blood and skin eosinophilia.
- **Eosinophilic fasciitis (Shulman syndrome)** is characterized by acute erythema, swelling, and induration of the extremities progressing to symmetric induration of the skin that spares the fingers, feet, and face. It can be precipitated by exercise.
- **Eosinophilic cellulitis (Wells syndrome)** presents with recurrent swelling of an extremity without tactile warmth and failure with antibiotic therapy.
- **Eosinophilic pustular folliculitis** is a pruritic skin eruption that can be seen in patients with HIV.
- **Episodic angioedema with eosinophilia (Gleich syndrome)** is a rare disease that leads to recurrent attacks of fever, angioedema, urticaria, weight gain, and blood eosinophilia without other organ damage.
- **Angiolymphoid hyperplasia with eosinophilia:** Presents with eosinophilia and papules, plaques, and nodules on the head and neck.
- **Kimura disease** presents with eosinophilia and large subcutaneous masses on the head or neck. Typically seen in Asian men.

Eosinophilia Associated With Multiorgan Involvement

- **Drug-induced eosinophilia.** Numerous drugs, herbal supplements, and cytokine therapies (e.g., GM-CSF and IL-2) can cause blood and/or tissue eosinophilia. Drug-induced eosinophilia typically responds to cessation of the culprit medication. Asymptomatic drug-induced eosinophilia does not necessitate cessation of therapy. However, end-organ involvement should always be investigated promptly.
- **Eosinophilic granulomatosis with polyangiitis (EGPA), also known as Churg–Strauss syndrome,** is a small- and medium-vessel vasculitis with chronic rhinosinusitis, asthma, and peripheral blood eosinophilia (typically >1500 cells/μL). The onset of asthma and eosinophilia may precede the development of EGPA by several years.
  - It is noted to have intravascular and extravascular eosinophilic granuloma formation and lung involvement with transient infiltrates on chest radiograph. Other manifestations include mononeuropathy or polyneuropathy, subcutaneous nodules, rash, gastroenteritis, renal insufficiency, cardiac arrhythmias, and heart failure.
  - Half of patients have antineutrophil cytoplasmic antibodies directed against myeloperoxidase (p-ANCA). Biopsy of affected tissue reveals a necrotizing vasculitis with extravascular granulomas and tissue eosinophilia.
  - Initial treatment involves high-dose glucocorticoids with the addition of cyclophosphamide if necessary. Maintenance therapy with azathioprine is recommended after remission is achieved. Mepolizumab has recently been approved by the Food and Drug Administration (FDA) for treatment of EGPA as it has prolonged time in remission.[12] Leukotriene modifiers, like all systemic steroid-sparing agents (including inhaled steroids and omalizumab), have been associated with unmasking of EGPA due to a

decrease in systemic steroid therapy; however, no evidence exists that these drugs *cause* EGPA.[13]

Mastocytosis

Systemic mastocytosis is characterized by infiltration of mast cells into various organs including the skin, liver, lymph nodes, bone marrow, and spleen. Peripheral eosinophilia can be seen in up to 20% of cases of systemic mastocytosis, and bone marrow biopsies often show an excess number of eosinophils.

Endocrine Disorders

Adrenal insufficiency (e.g., Addison disease) in critically ill patients is associated with low-grade eosinophilia.

Hypereosinophilic Syndrome

A proliferative disorder of eosinophils characterized by sustained eosinophilia >1500 cells/μL for ≥1 month documented on two occasions with eosinophil-mediated damage to organs such as the heart, gastrointestinal tract, kidneys, brain, and lung. All other causes of eosinophilia should be excluded to make the diagnosis.[14]

- Hypereosinophilic syndrome (HES) occurs predominantly in men between the ages of 20–50 years and presents with insidious onset of fatigue, cough, and dyspnea.
- Approximately 10%–15% HES patients have myeloproliferative disorders. Myeloproliferative variants of HES are characterized by constitutive expression of *FIP1L1/PDGFRA* fusion protein and elevated serum vitamin B_{12} levels. HES patients with FIP1L1/PDGFRA respond well to imatinib.
- Lymphocytic-variant HES (L-HES) accounts for 17%–26% HES patients. Unusual IL-5–producing T cells are found in L-HES.
- Cardiac disease is a major cause of morbidity and mortality in patients with HES. At presentation, patients typically are in the late thrombotic and fibrotic stages of eosinophil-mediated cardiac damage with signs of a restrictive cardiomyopathy and mitral regurgitation. An echocardiogram may detect intracardiac thrombi, endomyocardial fibrosis, or thickening of the posterior mitral valve leaflet. Neurologic manifestations range from peripheral neuropathy to stroke or encephalopathy. Bone marrow examination reveals increased eosinophil precursors.
- **Acute eosinophilic leukemia** is a rare myeloproliferative disorder that is distinguished from HES by several factors: an increased number of immature eosinophils in the blood (>50,000 AEC)[33] and/or marrow, >10% blast forms in the marrow, other cytopenias, and symptoms and signs compatible with an acute leukemia. Treatment is similar to other leukemias.
- **Lymphoma.** Eosinophilia can present in any T- or B-cell lymphoma. As many as 5% of patients with non-Hodgkin lymphoma and up to 15% of patients with Hodgkin lymphoma have modest peripheral blood eosinophilia. Eosinophilia in Hodgkin lymphoma has been correlated with IL-5 messenger RNA expression by Reed–Sternberg cells.
- **Atheroembolic disease.** Cholesterol embolization can lead to eosinophilia, eosinophiluria, renal dysfunction, livedo reticularis, purple toes, and increased erythrocyte sedimentation rate (ESR).
- **Immunodeficiency.** Hyper-IgE syndrome, autoimmune lymphoproliferative syndrome, and Omenn syndrome can present with recurrent infections, dermatitis, and eosinophilia.

Epidemiology

In industrialized nations, peripheral blood eosinophilia is most often due to atopic disease, whereas helminthic infections are the most common cause of eosinophilia in the rest of the world.

Pathophysiology

Eosinophilic granules contain basic proteins, which bind to acidic dye. Once activated, eosinophils produce major basic protein, eosinophil cationic protein, eosinophil-derived neurotoxin, and eosinophil peroxidase, which are toxic to bacteria, helminths, and normal tissue.

DIAGNOSIS

There are two approaches that are useful for evaluating eosinophilia, either by associated clinical context (Table 11-3) or by degree of eosinophilia (Table 11-4).

TABLE 11-3 Causes of Eosinophilia
Eosinophilia Associated With Atopic Disease
Allergic rhinitis
Asthma
Atopic dermatitis
Eosinophilia Associated With Pulmonary Infiltrates
Passage of larvae through the lung (Löffler syndrome)
Chronic eosinophilic pneumonia
Acute eosinophilic pneumonia
Tropical pulmonary eosinophilia
Allergic bronchopulmonary aspergillosis
Coccidioidomycosis
Eosinophilia Associated With Parasitic Infection
Helminths (*Ascaris lumbricoides, Strongyloides stercoralis, hookworm, Toxocara canis* or *Toxocara cati, Trichinella*)
Protozoa (*Dientamoeba fragilis, Sarcocystis,* and *Isospora belli*)
Eosinophilia Associated With Primary Cutaneous Disease
Atopic dermatitis
Eosinophilic fasciitis
Eosinophilic cellulitis
Eosinophilic folliculitis
Episodic angioedema with anaphylaxis
Eosinophilia Associated With Multiorgan Involvement
Drug-induced eosinophilia
Eosinophilic granulomatosis with polyangiitis or Churg–Strauss syndrome
Hypereosinophilic syndrome
Eosinophilic leukemia
Systemic mastocytosis
Lymphomas
Miscellaneous Causes
Eosinophilic gastroenteritis
Interstitial nephritis
Retroviral infections (HIV, human T-lymphotropic virus type 1)
Eosinophilia myalgia syndrome
Transplant rejection
Atheroembolic disease
Adrenal insufficiency

TABLE 11-4 Classification of Eosinophilia Based on the Peripheral Blood Eosinophil Count

Peripheral Blood Eosinophil Count (cells/μL)		
500–2000	2000–5000	>5000
Allergic rhinitis	Intrinsic asthma	Eosinophilia myalgia syndrome
Allergic asthma	Allergic bronchopulmonary aspergillosis	Hypereosinophilic syndrome
Food allergy	Helminthiasis	Episodic angioedema with eosinophilia
Urticaria	Eosinophilic granulomatosis with polyangiitis (EGPA) or Churg–Strauss syndrome	EGPA or Churg–Strauss syndrome
Addison disease	Drug reactions	Leukemia
Pulmonary infiltrates with eosinophilia syndromes	Vascular neoplasms	
Solid neoplasms	Eosinophilic fasciitis	
Nasal polyposis	HIV	

Clinical Presentation

History

- A history is important in narrowing the differential diagnosis of eosinophilia. It is important to determine if the patient has symptoms of atopic disease (rhinitis, wheezing, rash) or cancer (weight loss, fatigue, fever, night sweats) and to evaluate for other specific organ involvement such as lung, heart, or nerves. Prior eosinophil count can help determine the duration and magnitude of eosinophilia.
- A complete medication list, including over-the-counter supplements, and a full travel, occupational, and dietary history should be obtained.
- Any pet contact should be ascertained for possible exposure to toxocariasis.

Physical Examination

Physical examination should be guided by the history, with a special focus on the skin, upper and lower respiratory tracts, and cardiovascular and neurologic systems. Relevant physical examination findings include rash, nasal/sinus findings, signs of cardiac and/or respiratory abnormalities, lymphadenopathy, hepatomegaly/splenomegaly, or neurologic findings.[33]

Differential Diagnosis

- Various conditions can result in **eosinophilia associated with pulmonary infiltrates** (see Table 11-3). The presence of asthma should lead to consideration of ABPA or EGPA.
- The etiology of **eosinophilia associated with cutaneous lesions** (see Table 11-3) is guided by the appearance of the lesions and results of the skin biopsy. The diagnosis of EGPA cannot be made without a tissue biopsy showing infiltrating eosinophils and granulomas.
- When eosinophilia is marked and all other causes have been ruled out, the diagnosis of **HES** should be considered. Diagnosis requires a blood eosinophilia of >1500/μL on two occasions with associated organ involvement.

Diagnostic Testing

Laboratories

- Initial laboratory evaluations generally include complete blood count (CBC) with differential and eosinophil count, liver function tests, serum chemistries and creatinine, serum B12 level, troponin, markers of inflammation (e.g., ESR and/or C-reactive protein [CRP]), and urinalysis. Further diagnostic studies are based on clinical presentations and initial findings. Mild **eosinophilia associated with symptoms of rhinitis or asthma** is indicative of underlying atopic disease, which can be confirmed by skin testing.
- Depending on the travel history, **stool examination** for ova and parasites should be done on three separate occasions. Because only small numbers of helminths may pass in the stool and because tissue- or blood-dwelling helminths will not be found in the stool, **serologic tests** for antiparasite antibodies should also be sent. Such tests are available for strongyloidiasis, toxocariasis, and trichinellosis.
- Diagnosis at the time of presentation with Löffler syndrome can be made by detection of *Ascaris* larvae in respiratory secretions or gastric aspirates but not stool.
- Sinus CT, nerve conduction studies, and testing for p-ANCA may be helpful in the diagnosis of EGPA.
- Peripheral blood smear and flow cytometry of lymphocyte subpopulations can aid in the diagnosis of hematologic malignancy. Bone marrow biopsy for pathologic, cytogenetic, and molecular testing on bone marrow and/or peripheral blood (e.g., for *FIP1L1/PDGFRA* mutation by FISH) may be required. Serum vitamin B_{12} level may be elevated in myeloproliferative neoplasms and autoimmune lymphoproliferative syndrome.
- Evaluation for idiopathic HES should also consist of troponin measurement, echocardiogram, and ECG.
- Immunoglobulin levels are helpful if concerned for an immunodeficiency. Elevated immunoglobulin levels can be found in L-HES.
- A tryptase level is necessary if mastocytosis is considered as a cause of eosinophilia; however, it may also be elevated in cases of M-HES.[34]

Imaging

CXR findings may also help to narrow the differential diagnosis.

- Peripheral infiltrates with central clearing are indicative of chronic eosinophilic pneumonia.
- Diffuse infiltrates in an interstitial, alveolar, or mixed pattern may be seen in acute eosinophilic pneumonia as well as drug-induced eosinophilia with pulmonary involvement.
- Transient infiltrates may be seen in Löffler syndrome, EGPA, or ABPA.
- Central bronchiectasis is a major criterion in the diagnosis of ABPA.
- A diffuse miliary or nodular pattern, consolidation, or cavitation may be found in cases of tropical pulmonary eosinophilia.

Diagnostic Procedures

- If no other cause of pulmonary infiltrates has been identified, a **bronchoscopy** may be necessary for analysis of bronchoalveolar lavage (BAL) fluid and lung tissue. The presence of eosinophils in BAL fluid or sputum with eosinophilic infiltration of the parenchyma is most typical of acute or chronic eosinophilic pneumonia.
- Skin biopsy will aid in diagnosing the cutaneous eosinophilic diseases and EGPA.

TREATMENT

- Mild eosinophilia with no evidence of end-organ damage may not need treatment.
- Oral steroids are indicated when there is evidence of organ involvement. However, strongyloidiasis must be excluded before administration of steroids to prevent hyperinfection syndrome.

- When a drug reaction is suspected, discontinuation of the drug is both diagnostic and therapeutic. Other treatment options depend on the exact cause of eosinophilia because, with the exception of HES, eosinophilia is a manifestation of an underlying disease.
- **HES:** Patients with marked eosinophilia with no organ involvement may have a benign course. In contrast, those with organ involvement and *FIP1L1/PDGFRA*-associated disease may have an extremely aggressive course without treatment.
    - Monitoring and early initiation of high-dose intravenous glucocorticoids should be pursued in all patients except those who have the *FIP1L1/PDGFRA* fusion gene. Empirical treatment with ivermectin (200 μg/d for 2 days) may be considered in patients with high risk of strongyloides infestation.[34]
    - Patients with the *FIP1L1/PDGFRA* fusion mutation should be started on imatinib mesylate (Gleevec), a tyrosine kinase inhibitor. Treatment should be initiated promptly in these patients to prevent progression of cardiac disease and other end-organ damage. Imatinib has been shown to induce disease remission and halt progression.[15]
    - Hydroxyurea has been the most frequently used effective second-line agent and/or steroid-sparing agent for HES. Interferon-α2b in combination with glucocorticoids has been used to treat L-HES. Hematopoietic cell transplantation (HCT) may be considered in refractory HES.
    - In steroid refractory cases with HES, imatinib mesylate and vincristine (administered concomitantly with steroids) have also been tried and shown efficacy in a small group of patients.[34]
    - Mepolizumab, a humanized anti–IL-5 antibody, has shown corticosteroid-sparing effects in FIP1L1/PDGFRA-negative, corticosteroid-responsive subjects with HES.[16]
    - Alemtuzumab, an anti-CD52 antibody (CD52 is expressed on the surface of eosinophils), has been shown to be effective in treatment for patients with refractory idiopathic hypereosinophilic syndrome.[17] Other investigational agents include benralizumab (an anti-IL-5 antibody), Dupilumab (an IL-4 and IL-13 blocking antibody), and dexpramipexole.
- Primary eosinophilia disorders should be followed by a specialist; any cases of unresolved or unexplained eosinophilia warrant evaluation by an allergist/immunologist.

Urticaria and Angioedema

GENERAL PRINCIPLES

Definition

- **Urticaria** (hives) are raised, erythematous, well-demarcated pruritic skin lesions. Central clearing can cause an annular lesion and is often seen after antihistamine use. An individual lesion usually lasts minutes to hours.
- **Angioedema** is swelling of the deep dermis and subcutaneous tissue. It is often painful rather than pruritic and generally lasts less than 48 hours. It can be found anywhere on the body but most often involves the tongue, lips, eyelids, throat, bowels, and/or genitals. When angioedema occurs without urticaria, specific diagnoses must be entertained (see Differential Diagnosis section).

Classification

- **Acute urticaria (with or without angioedema)** is defined as the occurrence of hives and/or angioedema lasting <6 weeks. It can be caused by an allergic reaction to a medication, food, insect sting, or exposure (contact or inhalation) to an allergen. Patients can develop a hypersensitivity to a food, medication, or self-care product that previously had been used without difficulty. In many cases of acute urticaria, no identifiable trigger can be found.

- **Chronic urticaria (with or without angioedema)** is defined as the occurrence of hives and/or angioedema for >6 weeks. There are many possible causes of chronic urticaria and angioedema, including medications, autoimmunity, self-care products, and physical triggers. However, the etiology remains unidentified in >80% of cases.

Epidemiology

- Urticaria is a common condition that affects 15%–24% of the US population at some time in their life. Chronic idiopathic urticaria occurs in approximately 1% of the US population, and there does not appear to be an increased risk in persons with atopy.[18]
- Angioedema occurs in 40%–50% of patients with urticaria.

Etiology

- IgE-mediated: drugs, foods, stinging and biting insects, latex, inhalant, or contact allergen
- Non–IgE-mediated: narcotics, muscle relaxants, radiocontrast, vancomycin, NSAIDs, ACE inhibitors
- Transfusion reactions
- Infections (i.e., viral, bacterial, parasitic)
- Systemic disorders: autoimmune diseases, malignancy, mastocytosis, hypereosinophilic syndrome, cryoglobulinemia, and hereditary diseases
- Physical urticaria: dermographism, cold, cholinergic, pressure, vibratory, solar, and aquagenic
- Idiopathic

Pathophysiology

Most forms of urticaria and angioedema are caused by the degranulation of mast cells or basophils and the release of inflammatory mediators. Histamine is the primary mediator and elicits edema (wheal) and erythema (flare). Hereditary angioedema and related syndromes are mediated by the overproduction of bradykinin and are not responsive to antihistamines.

DIAGNOSIS

Diagnosis is based on complete history and physical examination with characteristic skin lesions.

Clinical Presentation

- Patients with an acute urticaria episode present with history of pruritic, raised, erythematous lesions. Individual lesions resolve over a period of 1–24 hours.
- Angioedema usually presents with painful swelling without pruritus. The swelling can take up to 72 hours to resolve.
- Physical urticaria is induced by environmental or physical stimuli. The common triggers are cold, heat, sweating, exercise, pressure, vibration, and sunlight. Dermographism, literally "skin writing," is the most common form of physical urticaria. It affects approximately 4% of the population and can be elicited by briskly stroking or scratching skin.

History

- A detailed history should elicit identifiable triggers and rule out any systemic causes. When the individual skin lesion lasts longer than 48 hours, the diagnosis of urticarial vasculitis must be investigated by a skin biopsy.
- Any changes in environmental exposures, foods, medications, personal care products, etc., should be determined.

- It is important to differentiate from anaphylaxis, which affects organs other than the skin, as this will be treated differently (see Anaphylaxis section).

Physical Examination

- Complete examination of the affected and nonaffected skin.
- Urticaria appears as erythematous, raised lesions that blanch with pressure.
- Angioedema appears as swelling; can often involve the face, tongue, extremities, or genitalia; and may be asymmetric.

Differential Diagnosis

- IgE-mediated allergic reaction to drugs, foods, insects, inhalant, or contact allergen.
- Non–IgE-mediated drug and food reactions (i.e., medications including NSAIDs, vancomycin, radioactive iodine, opiates, muscle relaxants, foods including tomatoes and strawberries).
- Pruritic urticarial papules and plaques of pregnancy.
- Mast cell release syndromes (i.e., systemic mastocytosis, cutaneous mastocytosis including urticaria pigmentosa).
- Cutaneous small-vessel vasculitis (i.e., urticarial vasculitis, systemic lupus erythematosus).
- Hypereosinophilic syndrome.
- Toxic drug eruptions.
- Allergic contact dermatitis (i.e., poison ivy, poison oak).
- Cryopyrin-associated periodic syndromes including familial cold autoinflammatory syndrome and Muckle–Wells syndrome.
- **Angioedema without urticaria** should lead to consideration of specific entities.
  - Use of ACE inhibitors or angiotensin II receptor blockers (ARBs) can be associated with angioedema at any point in the course of therapy.
  - **Hereditary angioedema** (HAE), **or C1 INH deficiency,** is inherited in an autosomal dominant pattern; 25% of cases arise from de novo mutations.
  - **Acquired C1 INH deficiency** presents similarly to HAE but is typically associated with an underlying lymphoproliferative disorder, connective tissue disease, or other neoplasias.

Diagnostic Testing

Epicutaneous skin testing and patch testing are only indicated when symptoms are associated with specific triggers.

Laboratories

- Routine laboratory testing in the absence of a clinical history is rarely helpful in determining an etiology in chronic urticaria.
- One can consider the following limited routine laboratory testing to evaluate for systemic disease that can lead to chronic urticaria: CBC with differential, CRP or ESR, thyroid-stimulating hormone, renal and liver profiles.
- Autologous serum skin testing, assays for basophil histamine release, and autoantibodies to IgE and the high-affinity IgE receptor are available, but the utility of these tests has not been established.
- All patients with **angioedema without urticaria should be screened with a C4 level, which is reduced during and between attacks of HAE.** If the C4 level is reduced, a quantitative and functional C1 INH assay should be performed. Measuring C1 INH levels alone is not sufficient because 15% of patients have normal levels of a dysfunctional C1 INH protein; therefore, it is important to also obtain the functional assay.
- Acquired C1 INH deficiency patients have reduced C1q, C1 INH level and function, and C4 levels due to an autoantibody to C1 INH.

Diagnostic Procedures

- A skin biopsy should be performed if individual lesions persist for >24 hours to rule out urticarial vasculitis.
  - Biopsy of acute urticarial lesions reveals dilation of small venules and capillaries located in the superficial dermis with widening of the dermal papillae, flattening of the rete pegs, and swelling of collagen fibers.
  - Chronic urticaria is characterized by a dense, non-necrotizing, perivascular infiltrate consisting of T lymphocytes, mast cells, eosinophils, basophils, and neutrophils.
  - Angioedema shows similar pathologic alterations in the deep, rather than superficial, dermis, and subcutaneous tissue.

TREATMENT

- The ideal treatment of acute urticaria with or without angioedema is identification and avoidance of specific causes. **All potential causes should be eliminated.** Most cases of acute urticaria are self-limited and resolve spontaneously. In some instances, it is possible to reintroduce an agent cautiously if it is believed not to be the etiologic agent. This trial should be done in the presence of a physician with epinephrine readily available.
- Careful consideration should be given to the **elimination or substitution of each prescription or over-the-counter medication** or supplement. If a patient reacts to one medication in a class, the reaction likely will be triggered by all medications in that class. Exacerbating agents (e.g., NSAIDs, opiates, vancomycin, and alcohol) should be avoided because they may induce nonspecific mast cell degranulation and exacerbate urticaria caused by other agents.
- In patients presenting with hereditary and acquired angioedema, a prompt assessment of airway is critical, especially in those presenting with a laryngeal attack.

Medications

If acute urticaria is associated with additional systemic symptoms such as hypotension, laryngeal edema, or bronchospasm, treatment with epinephrine (0.3–0.5 mL of a 1:1000 solution IM) should be administered immediately. See Anaphylaxis section for additional information.

Acute urticaria and/or angioedema

- **Second-generation antihistamines** such as cetirizine, fexofenadine, or loratadine should be administered to patients until the hives have cleared. Higher than conventional, US FDA–approved doses may provide more efficacy. A first-generation antihistamine such as hydroxyzine may be added as an evening dose if needed to obtain control in refractory cases. H_2 antihistamines, such as ranitidine, may also be added to the above treatment.
- **Oral corticosteroids** should be reserved for patients with moderate to severe symptoms. Corticosteroids will not have an immediate effect but may prevent relapse.
- If a patient presents with systemic symptoms, self-administered epinephrine (like a pen device) should be prescribed for use in the case of anaphylaxis.

Chronic urticaria

- A stepwise approach has been suggested for the treatment of chronic urticaria.[18]
- Step 1: Monotherapy with a second-generation H_1 antihistamine.
- Step 2: One or more of the following:
  - Dose advancement of the second-generation H_1 antihistamine, up to four times the conventional dose
  - Addition of another second-generation H_1 antihistamine
  - Addition of H_2 antihistamine
  - Addition of leukotriene receptor antagonist
  - Addition of first-generation H_1 antihistamine to be taken at bedtime

- Step 3: Dose advancement of a potent antihistamine (i.e., doxepin, hydroxyzine) as tolerated. This is limited by sedation; use with caution in the elderly.
- Step 4: Add an alternative agent.
  - Omalizumab: FDA approved for patients with chronic urticaria who have failed H1 antihistamine therapy.
  - Cyclosporine
  - Other anti-inflammatory agents, immunosuppressants, or biologics
- **Optimal duration of therapy has not been established; tapering medications after 3–6 months of symptom control has been suggested.**

Hereditary and acquired angioedema (disorder of C1 inhibitor)

- Laryngeal attacks or severe abdominal attacks: C1 inhibitor concentrate, icatibant (synthetic bradykinin B2-receptor antagonist), and ecallantide (recombinant plasma kallikrein inhibitor, not available outside the US) are first-line agents.
- If none of the first-line medications are available, other options are solvent/detergent (S/D)-treated plasma or fresh frozen plasma (FFP, 2 units every 2–4 hours until satisfactory response is obtained).[35] Symptomatic therapy and rehydration are also to be pursued.
- Preventative medications include C1 inhibitor replacement via IV or SC route, lanadelumab, attenuated androgens, and antifibrinolytics.

REFERRAL

All patients with chronic urticaria or a history of anaphylaxis should be referred to an allergy specialist for evaluation to identify potential allergic and autoimmune triggers.

Immunodeficiency

GENERAL PRINCIPLES

Definition

- Primary immunodeficiencies (PIDs) are disorders of the immune system that result in an increased susceptibility to infection.
- Secondary immunodeficiencies are also disorders of increased susceptibility to infection but are attributable to an external source.

Classification

PIDs can be organized by the defective immune components with considerable heterogeneity in each disorder.

- **Predominantly antibody deficiencies:** The defect is primarily in the ability to make antibodies.
  - Common variable immune deficiency (CVID)
  - X-linked (Bruton) agammaglobulinemia
  - IgG subclass deficiency
  - Specific antibody deficiency
  - Hyper IgM syndrome
  - Selective IgA deficiency
- **Combined immunodeficiencies and syndromes:** The defect results in deficiencies in both cellular and humoral immune responses.
  - Severe combined immunodeficiencies
  - DiGeorge syndrome
  - Hyper-IgE (Job) syndrome

- **Defects of innate immunity:** Defects in germline-encoded receptors and downstream signaling pathways
  - Deficiency of Toll-like receptor signaling
  - Mendelian susceptibility to mycobacterial diseases (MSMD)
  - Natural killer (NK) cell deficiency
  - Phagocytic cell deficiencies
  - Chronic granulomatous disease (CGD)
- **Complement deficiencies.**
- **Diseases of immune dysregulation:** Autoimmunity and lymphoproliferation are characteristic manifestations in these disorders.

Epidemiology

- Secondary immunodeficiency syndromes, particularly HIV/AIDS, are the most common immunodeficiency disorders.
- The estimated prevalence of PIDs is approximately 1 in 1200 live births.
- Most PIDs presenting in adulthood are humoral immune defects affecting antibody production.

Etiology

- Predominantly antibody immune deficiencies are thought to be caused by defects in B-cell maturation. Combined immunodeficiencies are caused by defective T-cell–mediated immunity and associated antibody deficiency.
- A variety of genetic mutations have been associated with specific PID syndromes.
- Secondary immunodeficiencies can be caused by medications (chemotherapy, immunomodulatory agents, corticosteroids), infectious agents (e.g., HIV), malignancy, antibody loss (e.g., nephrotic syndrome, protein losing enteropathy, or consumption during a severe underlying infection), autoimmune disease (e.g., systemic lupus erythematosus, rheumatoid arthritis), malnutrition (vitamin D), and other underlying diseases (e.g., diabetes mellitus, cirrhosis, uremia).

DIAGNOSIS

Clinical Presentation

- The hallmark of PID is recurrent infections. Clinical suspicion should be increased by recurrent sinopulmonary infection, deep-seated infections, opportunistic infections, or disseminated infections in an otherwise healthy patient.
- Specific PIDs are often associated with particular types of pathogens (e.g., catalase-positive infections in CGD or MSMD).
- Recurrent urinary tract infections are only rarely associated with PID.
- Patients with PIDs may also present with autoimmunity, immune dysregulation, allergic diseases, and malignancies.
- **Selective IgA deficiency** is the most common immune deficiency, with a prevalence of 1 in 300–500 people.
  - Most patients are asymptomatic. Some may present with recurrent sinus and pulmonary infections. Therapy is directed at early treatment with antibiotics because IgA replacement is not available.
  - Associated autoimmune diseases are observed in 20%–30% of cases. Absolute IgA-deficient patients (i.e., <7 mg/dL) are at risk for developing a severe transfusion reaction to blood products including IV immunoglobulin (IVIG), because of the presence of IgE anti-IgA antibodies in some individuals; therefore, these patients should be transfused with washed red blood cells or receive blood products only from IgA-deficient donors.

- **CVID** is the most common symptomatic PID, occurring with a frequency of 1/25,000. It includes a heterogeneous group of disorders in which most patients present in the second to fourth decade of life with recurrent sinus and pulmonary infections and are discovered to have low and dysfunctional IgG, IgA, and/or IgM antibodies with poor response to immunizations.
  - B-cell numbers are often normal, but there is decreased ability to produce immunoglobulin because of the lack of isotype-switched memory B cells. Some patients may also exhibit T-cell dysfunction.
  - CVID is largely idiopathic, although there are molecular defects in the B-cell signaling and development pathways (e.g., TACI, ICOS, BAFF-R, and CD19) with some forms of the disorder.
  - Patients with CVID are particularly susceptible to infection with encapsulated organisms.
  - Patients may have associated gastrointestinal disease or autoimmune abnormalities (most commonly autoimmune hemolytic anemia, idiopathic thrombocytopenic purpura, pernicious anemia, and rheumatoid arthritis).
  - There is an increased incidence of malignancy, especially lymphoid and gastrointestinal malignancy.
  - Therapy consists of IVIG or subcutaneous immunoglobulin (SCIG) replacement therapy as well as prompt treatment of infections with antibiotics.
- **Specific antibody deficiency** is defined as poor or absent antibody responses to polysaccharide antigens (i.e., 23-valent pneumococcal vaccine) in the setting of normal levels of immunoglobulins and IgG subclasses.
  - B-cell numbers and response to protein antigens (i.e., tetanus toxoid and diphtheria toxoid) are usually normal.
  - Patients have increased susceptibility to sinopulmonary infections. Allergic diseases are also common.
  - Therapeutic approaches include adequate antibiotic treatment for infections, pneumococcal conjugate vaccine, and sometimes immunoglobulin replacement.
- **X-linked (Bruton) agammaglobulinemia** clinically manifests very similarly to severe CVID and is typically diagnosed in childhood but can present in adulthood.
  - Patients usually have low levels of all immunoglobulin types and very low levels of B cells.
  - Specific genetic defect is in Bruton tyrosine kinase, which is involved in B-cell maturation.
- **Subclass deficiency.** Deficiencies of each of the IgG subclasses (IgG1, IgG2, IgG3, and IgG4) have been described.
  - These patients present with similar complaints as the CVID patients.
  - Total IgG levels may be normal. A strong association with IgA deficiency exists. There is disagreement as to whether this is a separate entity from CVID. In most cases, there is no need to evaluate IgG subclass levels.
  - Isolated subclass deficiency without recurrent infections is of unknown clinical significance.
- **Hyper IgM syndrome** is characterized by low IgA and IgG levels with normal or increased IgM and poor antibody function. There are several gene mutations reported, which cause defective class switching in immunoglobulins. Depending on the mutation, some patients may have poor T-cell function as well leading to increased opportunistic infections.
- **Hyper-IgE syndrome (Job syndrome)** is characterized by recurrent pyogenic infections of the skin and lower respiratory tract. This syndrome can result in severe abscess and empyema formation. Some forms of the disease are associated with autosomal dominant mutation of *STAT3*.

 - The most common organism involved is *S. aureus*, but other bacteria and fungi have been reported.
 - Patients present with recurrent infections and have associated pruritic dermatitis, coarse (lion-like) facies, growth retardation, scoliosis, retention of primary teeth, and hyperkeratotic nails.
 - Laboratory data reveal the presence of normal levels of IgG, IgA, and IgM but markedly elevated levels of IgE. A marked increase in tissue and blood eosinophils may also be observed.
- **Complement deficiencies** are a broad category of PID characterized by recurrent infections to a range of pathogens.
 - Recurrent disseminated neisserial infections are associated with a deficiency in the terminal complement system (C5–C9).
 - Systemic lupus-like disorders and recurrent infection with encapsulated organisms have been associated with deficiencies in other components of complement.
 - Factor H deficiency can lead to membranoproliferative glomerulonephritis and hemolytic uremic syndrome.
 - CH50 and AH50 are useful to screen for deficiencies of the classical pathway and alternative pathway, respectively.
 - Complement receptor 3 and 4 deficiency results from a deficiency of CD18 and causes leukocyte adhesion deficiency type 1, and CD59 deficiency causes **paroxysmal nocturnal hemoglobinuria**.
- **CGD** is characterized by defective killing of intracellular pathogens by neutrophils.
 - Patients usually present with frequent infection, often with abscesses, from *S. aureus* and other catalase-positive organisms. *Aspergillus* is a particularly troublesome pathogen for patients with CGD.
 - Diagnosis is made by demonstration of defective respiratory burst with flow cytometry assay using dihydrorhodamine.
- **MSMD** is caused by defects in Th1 immunity and is associated with mutations in genes involved in interferon-γ and IL-12 signaling. Characteristic infections include mycobacterial infections (including typical and atypical *Mycobacterium*) and *Salmonella* infections.

Diagnostic Testing

- Frequent sinopulmonary infections, recurrent and invasive infections requiring IV antimicrobial agents, infections with unusual pathogens, and family history of PID are warning signs for PIDs.
- Initial evaluation should focus on identifying possible secondary causes of recurrent infection such as allergy, medications, and anatomic abnormalities. Workup begins with a CBC with differential, HIV test, quantitative immunoglobulin levels, and complement levels. Often the evaluation will need to include enumeration of lymphocytes by flow cytometry if B-, T-, or NK-cell defects are suspected. Other specialized tests including genetic testing may be needed to make a definitive diagnosis.
- If clinical suspicion is high for an underlying antibody-predominant PID, B-cell function can be assessed by measuring immunoglobulin response to vaccinations. Preimmunization and postimmunization titers for both a protein antigen (i.e., tetanus) and a polysaccharide antigen (i.e., Pneumovax, the unconjugated 23-valent vaccine) are measured because proteins and polysaccharide antigens are handled differently by the immune system.
- Titers of specific antibodies are measured before and at 4–8 weeks after immunization.
- Genetic testing can also be performed.

TREATMENT

- Killed or subcomponent vaccines are safe for most patients with PID, although some patients may not produce full response. Live attenuated vaccines may be contraindicated in some individuals with PID and their families.
- Prophylactic antibiotics may be considered in some PID syndromes to prevent recurrent infections.
- IgA deficiency: No specific treatment is available. However, these patients should be promptly treated at the first sign of infection with an antibiotic that covers *Streptococcus pneumoniae* or *Haemophilus influenzae*.
- CVID should be treated with immunoglobulin replacement in forms of IVIG or SCIG. Numerous preparations of immunoglobulin are available, all of which undergo viral inactivation steps. Possible side effects include myalgias, vomiting, chills, and lingering headache (due to immune complex–mediated aseptic meningitis).

REFERRAL

Patients in whom a PID is being seriously considered should undergo evaluation by an allergist/clinical immunologist with expertise in diagnosing and treating PID.

Immunoglobulin G4-Related Disease (IgG4-RD)

DEFINITION

IgG4-RD is an immune-mediated fibroinflammatory condition affecting multiple organs. The hallmark of IgG4-RD is dense lymphoplasmacytic infiltrations with predominance of IgG4-positive plasma cells in the affected tissue; IgG4-RD is accompanied by some degree of fibrosis and obliterative phlebitis and increased number of eosinophils. Patients usually present with a subacute mass of the affected organ or with diffuse enlargement of an affected organ.[36]

Serum IgG4 levels are elevated in approximately two-thirds of the patients,[19] while rest of the patients have normal serum IgG4 levels.[20]

Pathogenesis

The pathogenesis of IgG4-RD remains incompletely understood, but there is growing evidence that the disease is autoimmune in character, with an important role for T cells, especially CD4+ and T-follicular helper cells, and that the IgG4 antibodies are not themselves pathogenic.

Epidemiology

The recognition of the disease continues to grow. The majority of the patients are men (62%–83%) and older than 50 years of age.[21] In Japan, the prevalence of the disease has been reported to be approximately 0.28–1.08 per 100,000 of population.[22]

DIAGNOSIS

Clinical Manifestations

Patients often present with subacute development of a mass in the affected organ (e.g., pancreas, nodular lesions in the lung). Multiple organs are affected in 60%–90% of patients. The affected tissues share particular pathologic features.

Following four main clinical phenotypes have been identified:

- **Group 1**: pancreatohepatobiliary disease.
- **Group 2**: retroperitoneal fibrosis/aortitis.
- **Group 3**: head and neck limited disease.
- **Group 4**: classic Mikulicz syndrome with systemic involvement.

Common manifestations of IgG4-RD include the following: type 1 autoimmune pancreatitis and IgG4-related sclerosing cholangitis, Mikulicz disease, Riedel's thyroiditis, interstitial pneumonitis, and tubulointerstitial nephritis.

Diagnostic Evaluation

IgG4-related disease should be suspected as a potential diagnosis in patients who have any of the following: Pancreatitis of unknown origin, sclerosing cholangitis, bilateral salivary and/or lacrimal gland enlargement, retroperitoneal fibrosis (RPF), orbital pseudotumor or proptosis, and the development of an otherwise unexplained mass lesion in organs such as pancreas, biliary tree, orbits, lungs, kidneys, major salivary gland, or lacrimal gland.[37]

Tissue biopsy is the gold standard for the diagnosis in most settings. The diagnosis is based on the combination of characteristic histopathologic, clinical, serologic, and radiologic findings. The commonly shared features include tumor-like swelling of involved organs, a lymphoplasmacytic infiltrate enriched in IgG4-positive plasma cells, and variable degree of fibrosis that has a characteristic "storiform" pattern. In addition, elevated serum concentrations of IgG4 are found in 60%–70% of the patients.

TREATMENT

The extent of disease should be evaluated before initiating treatment (computed tomography/PET of the chest, abdomen, and pelvis).

Prednisone, a glucocorticoid, at a dose of 0.6 mg/kg/d is the drug of choice, which is then tapered to discontinuation over a 2-month period. Responses are characterized by symptomatic improvement, reductions in the size of masses, improvement of organ function, and often a decrease in serum levels of IgG4. In patients who do not respond to prednisone or have contraindications to steroids, rituximab is the option rather than conventional antimetabolite immunosuppressive drugs such as azathioprine and methotrexate. The B-cell depletion leads to quick reduction in IgG4 levels and improvement in organ function.

Spontaneous improvement can be seen, but the disease often recurs without treatment. Most patients respond initially to steroids, but relapses are common following discontinuation of the therapy.

There may be a possibility of increased risk of malignancy in these patients; however, this is disputed by some studies and as such the issue remains controversial.[38]

Cytokine Release Syndrome

General Principles

Cytokine release syndrome (CRS) is an acute systemic inflammatory syndrome characterized by fever and multiple organ dysfunction that can be triggered by a variety of factors such as infections and certain drugs. It is associated with chimeric antigen receptor (CAR) T-cell therapy, therapeutic antibodies, and haploidentical allogeneic transplantation.

CRS was reported in the setting of haploidentical donor stem cell transplantation and graft-versus-host disease. Cytokine storm due to massive T-cell stimulation is also a proposed pathomechanism of severe viral infections such as influenza, SARS-CoV-2, and COVID-19.

Epidemiology

Significant CRS occurs in one-quarter to one-half of the patients treated with CAR T-cell therapy for relapsed or refractory acute lymphoblastic leukemia/lymphoma.[23] CRS is less common following immunotherapy with bispecific antibodies and in treatment of solid tumors.

A CRS-like syndrome that develops after a severe viral infection (e.g., influenza/COVID-19) or treatment with nonprotein-based drugs, such as oxaliplatin and lenalidomide, should be referred to as cytokine storm rather than CRS per se.[24]

Pathophysiology

CRS is a supraphysiologic response to immune therapy that activates or engages T cells or other immune effector cells. The systemic reaction is associated with increased levels of inflammatory cytokines and activation of T lymphocytes, macrophages, and endothelial cells.

Figure 11-2 depicts the pathophysiology and clinical manifestation of CRS.

DIAGNOSIS

Clinical Manifestations

These include fever, possibly accompanied by fatigue, headache, diarrhea, and arthralgia—resembling a mild flu-like syndrome.

Mild CRS can progress to a more severe syndrome which may include hypotension, hypoxia, and uncontrolled systemic inflammatory response with circulatory collapse, vascular leakage, cardiac dysfunction, and multiorgan system failure—a severe systemic inflammatory response syndrome (SIRS). Neuropsychiatric manifestations such as aphasia, altered level of consciousness, impaired cognitive skills, motor weakness, seizures, and cerebral edema may also develop in the patient. Usually, the neurologic toxicity occurs two to four days after the onset of severe CRS, may be progressive, and may even occur after the resolution of CRS symptoms.[39]

Diagnostic Testing

CRS should be suspected in a patient with fever, with or without tachypnea, tachycardia, hypotension, hypoxia, or other clinical findings, after receiving immune therapy such as CAR T-cell therapy, bispecific T-cell-engaging therapy, or haploidentical HCT.

CRS is a clinical diagnosis requiring fever, with or without hypotension, hypoxia, and other end-organ dysfunction, in the hours to days after treatment with immune therapy.

As such, leukocytosis may be present with activated or abnormal lymphocytes in peripheral blood due to CAR-T therapy, or pancytopenia due to chemotherapy/malignancy may also be seen.

Deranged renal/liver functions, as well as dyselectrolytemias are commonly seen. Hypophosphatemia, hypokalemia, and hyponatremia are the most frequently encountered.[40]

Nonspecific inflammatory markers, such as C-reactive protein and serum ferritin, are universally elevated; however, they are unreliable as they may lag behind clinical changes by >12 hours and also fall rapidly upon administering treatment like tocilizumab.[41] Specific inflammatory cytokines, including IL-6,10, soluble IL-2R alpha, and interferon gamma are also elevated, but are constrained by the limited availability of testing methods.

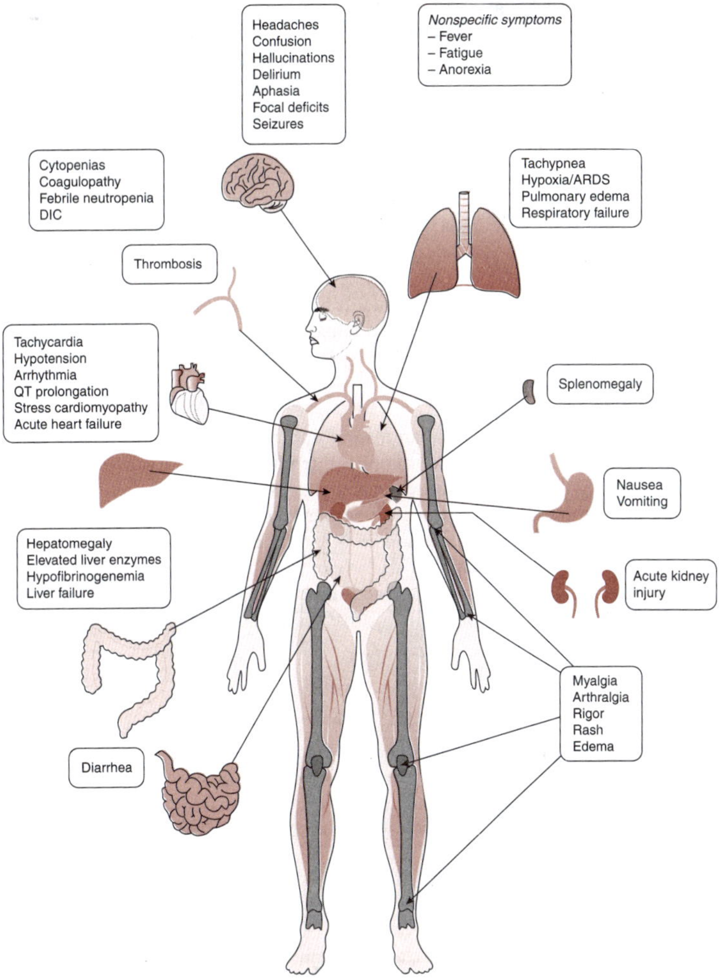

Figure 11-2 Clinical presentation of CRS.

TREATMENT

For mild CRS of any cause, symptomatic treatment with antihistamines, antipyretics, and fluids rather than with steroids or tocilizumab appears beneficial, but is based on risk–benefit ratio.

For severe CRS caused by CAR T-cell therapy, initial treatment with tocilizumab plus a corticosteroid rather than with a single agent alone appears beneficial. Tocilizumab should be given intravenously over 1 hour as follows: patients weighing <30 kg, 12 mg/kg; and patients weighing >30 kg, 8 mg/kg; total tocilizumab dose should not exceed 800 mg.

Steroid therapy includes hydrocortisone 100 mg every 8 hours, dexamethasone 10 mg four times daily, or methylprednisolone 1 mg/kg/d until there is improvement in CRS.

For severe CRS caused by blinatumomab, interrupting the infusion plus treating with a corticosteroid is favorable.

Hemophagocytic Lymphohistiocytosis

General Principles

Hemophagocytic lymphohistiocytosis (HLH) is an aggressive and life-threatening syndrome of excessive immune activation. It is most common in infants and young children but can affect patients of any age, with or without a predisposing familial condition. The term macrophage activation syndrome (MAS) refers to a form of HLH that occurs primarily in patients with juvenile idiopathic arthritis or other rheumatologic diseases. It has also been referred to as "reactive hemophagocytic syndrome."

Epidemiology

HLH is primarily a pediatric syndrome. Infants are most commonly affected, with highest incidence in those >3 months. The male-to-female ratio is close to 1:1.[25] In adults, there may be a slight male predisposition.[26]

Pathophysiology

HLH is a syndrome of excessive inflammation and tissue destruction due to abnormal immune activation. The dysregulated immune state is thought to be caused by the absence of normal downregulation by activated macrophages and lymphocytes. The cell types involved in the pathogenesis of HLH include the following: macrophages, natural killer (NK) cells, and cytotoxic lymphocytes. The NK cells and/or cytotoxic lymphocytes fail to eliminate activated macrophages. This lack of normal feedback regulation results in excessive CD8+ T cell and macrophage activation with highly elevated levels of interferon gamma and other cytokines, which drive the pathology of HLH leading to tissue destruction.

Genetics

Genetic defect plays a major role in childhood HLH and is increasingly found in adult cases. Most of the implicated genes encode components of the machinery for perforin-dependent cytotoxicity. These genes act in an autosomal recessive fashion and many cases are related to consanguinity. Mutations at familial hemophagocytic lymphohistiocytosis (FHL) loci include PRF1/perforin, UNC13D/Munc13-4, and STX11/syntaxin 11.

DIAGNOSIS

Clinical Features

HLH presents as a febrile illness associated with multiple organ involvement.

- The HLH-2004 study reported the following clinical findings[27]:
  - Fever: 95%
  - Splenomegaly: 89%
  - Bicytopenia: 92%
  - Hypertriglyceridemia or hypofibrinogenemia: 90%
  - Hemophagocytosis: 82%
  - Ferritin >500 µg/L: 94%
  - Low/absent NK-cell activity: 71%
  - Soluble CD25 elevation: 97%

Diagnostic Evaluation

The initial evaluation includes a CBC, coagulation studies, ferritin, liver function test, triglycerides, and blood cultures. The bone marrow should be examined for the cause of cytopenias, infectious organisms, and hemophagocytosis. CT/PET scan should be done to evaluate for possible malignancy. For those with a high clinical suspicion, specialized testing

TABLE 11-5 Diagnostic Criteria of HLH-2004

The diagnosis of HLH can be established if one of either 1 or 2 below is fulfilled:
1. A molecular diagnosis consistent with HLH is made.
2. Diagnostic criteria for HLH are fulfilled (five of the eight criteria below):
   (a) Fever
   (b) Splenomegaly
   (c) Cytopenias (affecting >2–3 lineages in the peripheral blood)
      i. Hemoglobin <9 g/dL (in infants >4 weeks of age, hemoglobin <10 g/dL)
      ii. Platelets $<100 \times 10^9$/L
      iii. Neutrophils $<1.0 \times 10^9$/L
   (d) Hypertriglyceridemia (fasting triglycerides >265 mg/dL) and/or hypofibrinogenemia (fibrinogen <150 mg/dL)
   (e) Hemophagocytosis in bone marrow, spleen, or lymph nodes
   (f) Low or absent NK-cell activity
   (g) Ferritin > 500 ng/mL
   (h) Elevated soluble CD25 (i.e., sIL2R) two standard deviations above age-adjusted laboratory specific norms

Adapted from Henter et al.[28]

The diagnosis of HLH syndrome is based on a compatible clinical presentation in the setting of elevated inflammatory markers. Ideally, the diagnosis of HLH is based on fulfilling the published diagnostic criteria used in HLH-2004 trial.[28] A scoring system has been developed to generate a diagnostic score referred to as an "**HScore**" that estimates the probability of HLH.[29]

of immunologic parameters and genetic testing are also indicated. Table 11-5 summarizes the diagnostic criteria of HLH.

TREATMENT

Untreated patients with HLH have a survival of months, due to progressive multiorgan failure. Often the greatest barrier is delayed diagnosis. Survival can be dramatically increased with HLH-specific therapy.

Among patients who are acutely ill or deteriorating, HLH-94-based therapy includes etoposide and dexamethasone given at tapering doses over 8 weeks, with intrathecal methotrexate and hydrocortisone for those with central nervous system (CNS) involvement.

Etoposide is given at a dose of 150 mg/m^2 for adults, and 5 mg/kg for children weighing <10 kg.

The dose is given twice weekly for the first 2 weeks and, once weekly till 8 weeks.

The HLH-2004 protocol incorporated cyclosporine as part of the initial therapy.

Patients should receive supportive care such as transfusions of red blood cells, platelets, and fresh frozen plasma. They may also require antibiotics for managing/preventing infections. For those with HLH gene mutation, refractory disease, CNS involvement, and hematologic malignancies that cannot be cured, HCT following induction therapy is recommended.

For patients with refractory or recurrent/relapsed HLH, treatment with emapalumab (interferon-gamma-blocking antibody), ruxolitinib (JAK inhibitor), or liposomal doxorubicin with etoposide and methylprednisolone and alemtuzumab (anti-CD52 antibody) can be tried.

Prognosis

Without therapy, mortality of patients with HLH is high. Patients treated on HLH-94 protocol had a median survival of 54% at 6.2 years. Those with neurological involvement had lesser survival rates than those without. No patient with familial HLH survived without HCT. Long-term sequelae included neurological ones, including intellectual disabilities, nerve palsies and other organ damage, such as renal impairment, obstructive bronchiolitis, and growth retardation.[30,31]

In adults, prognosis is worse in those with an underlying malignancy and older age. In a review study of adults with HLH, features associated with early death included underlying lymphoma, low platelet count, elevated aspartate aminotransferase (AST) and elevated lactate dehydrogenase (LDH), and age over 50 years.[42]

Summary

- Anaphylaxis is an acute, life-threatening hypersensitivity disorder, defined as a generalized, rapidly evolving, multisystemic allergic reaction. Treatment includes airway maintenance, decontamination, epinephrine 1:1000 0.3–0.5 mg IM, and a fluid bolus.
- Hemophagocytic lymphohistiocytosis (HLH) is a hyperinflammatory syndrome characterized by persistently activated cytotoxic lymphocytes and macrophages, which is characterized by three Fs—fever, falling blood counts, and raised ferritin, and if untreated, leads to multiorgan dysfunction and death.
- Immunoglobulin G4-related disease is a multiorgan, fibroinflammatory condition with tumefactive lesions and "storiform" fibrosis, affecting mostly pancreas, kidneys, orbital adnexal structures, salivary glands, and retroperitoneum.
- Primary immunodeficiency diseases are inherited defects in one or more component of the immune system making patients prone for infections, autoinflammation, autoimmunity, allergy, and malignancy.
- Hypereosinophilic syndrome is defined as an absolute eosinophil count greater than 1500/mm^3 on two occasions at least one month apart or marked tissue eosinophilia.

Scan the QR code to access chapter references.

12 Fluid and Electrolyte Management

Miraie Wardi, Steven Cheng, Madhav H. Hande, and Vivek K. Koushik

FLUID MANAGEMENT AND PERTURBATIONS IN VOLUME STATUS

- **Total body water (TBW):** Water comprises approximately 60% of total body weight in men and 50% in women and is distributed in two major compartments: two-thirds is **intracellular fluid** (ICF) and one-third is **extracellular fluid** (ECF). ECF is further subdivided into intravascular and interstitial spaces in a ratio of 1:4.
  - **Example:** For a healthy 70-kg man,

$$\text{TBW} = 0.6 \times 70 = 42\ \text{L}$$

    - ICF = 2/3 TBW = 0.66 × 42 = 28 L
    - ECF = 1/3 TBW = 0.33 × 42 =14 L
    - Intravascular compartment = 0.25 × 14 = 3.5 L
    - Interstitial compartment = 0.75 × 14 = 10.5 L
  - The distribution of water between intravascular and interstitial spaces can be affected by changes to the Starling balance of forces. Low oncotic pressure (i.e., low albumin states) and high hydrostatic pressure (i.e., Na^+-retentive states) increase the movement of fluid from vascular to interstitial compartments, which is an important step in the development of edema.
  - Because the majority of water is contained in the intracellular space, the loss of free water does not typically result in the hemodynamic changes associated with volume depletion. Instead, disturbances in TBW changes serum **osmolality** and electrolyte concentrations.
  - The intact kidney adapts to changes in TBW by increasing water excretion or reabsorption. This is mediated by the **antidiuretic hormone (ADH; vasopressin)**, which permits water movement across the distal nephron. Although vasopressin release is predominately responsive to osmotic cues, volume contraction can cause a nonosmotic release of ADH resulting in a reduction of renal water excretion.
- **Total body Na^+:** 85%–90% of **total body Na^+** is extracellular and constitutes the predominant solute in the ECF. Changes to the body's total Na^+ content typically results from a loss or gain of this Na^+-rich fluid, leading to contraction or expansion of the ECF space. Clinically, this manifests as volume depletion (hypotension, tachycardia) and volume expansion (peripheral or pulmonary edema).
  - Na^+ *concentration* is distinct from Na^+ *content.* Na^+ concentration reflects the amount of Na^+ distributed in a fixed quantity of water. An increase in TBW can decrease the Na^+ concentration even if the body's total Na^+ content remains unchanged (dilutional).
  - The intact kidney can respond to altered Na^+ content in the ECF space by increasing or decreasing Na^+ reabsorption. This response is mediated by cardiovascular, renal, hepatic, and central nervous system sensors of the effective circulating volume.
- **Plasma osmolality (pOsm):** The pOsm is determined by the ratio of plasma solute particles and plasma water. Most of the plasma solutes are dissociated sodium salts with lesser

contributions from other ions (e.g., potassium, calcium, glucose, and urea). The normal pOsm is 275–290 mOsmol/kg.

$$\text{Serum osmolality} = \{([Na^+] \times 2) + ([\text{glucose}] \div 18) + ([\text{BUN}] \div 2.8)\}$$

- **Plasma tonicity:** Plasma tonicity is the effective pOsm, which is sensed by osmoreceptors and determines the transcellular distribution of water. It reflects the concentration of solutes that do not easily cross cell membranes (mostly sodium salts) and thus affects the distribution of water between the cells and the ECF.

The Euvolemic Patient

- In a euvolemic patient, the goal of fluid and electrolyte administration is to maintain homeostasis. The best way to accomplish this is to allow free access to food and oral fluids. Patients who are unable to tolerate oral intake require maintenance fluids to replace renal, gastrointestinal (GI), and insensible fluid losses.
- The decision to provide maintenance IV fluid (IVF) should be thoughtfully considered and not administered by rote. Fluid administration should be reassessed *at least* daily. Patient weight, which may indicate net fluid balance, should be monitored carefully.
  - Clinical assessment of fluid status is challenging, especially in a critically ill patient; therefore, it is essential to complement clinical evaluation with objective measures of assessing fluid status such as Point-of-care ultrasound (POCUS), echocardiogram, and body composition monitoring (bio-impedance).
- When prescribing IV fluid therapy, it's crucial to consider the patient's water and electrolyte needs separately. Additionally, a thorough patient history, including comorbidities, medication history, and assessment of cardiac and renal status, will facilitate more precise guidance for fluid therapy.
  - Minimum **water** requirements for daily fluid balance can be approximated from the sum of the required urine output, stool water loss, and insensible losses.
    - The minimum urine output necessary to excrete the daily solute load is the amount of solute consumed each day (roughly 600–800 mOsm/d in an average individual) divided by the maximum amount of solute that can be excreted per liter of urine (maximum urine concentrating capacity is 1200 mOsm/L in healthy kidneys). The result is an obligate urine output of *at least* 0.5 L/d.
    - The water lost in stools is typically 200 mL/d.
    - **Insensible water losses** from the skin and respiratory tract amount to roughly 400–500 mL/d. The volume of water produced from endogenous metabolism (<250–350 mL/d) should be considered as well. The degree of insensible loss may vary tremendously depending on respiratory rate, metabolic state, and temperature (water losses increase by 100–150 mL/d for each degree of body temperature over 37°C).
    - Fluid from drain losses must be factored in as well.
    - After adding each of these components, the minimum amount of water needed to maintain homeostasis is roughly 1400 mL/d or 60 mL/h.
  - **Electrolytes** that are usually administered during maintenance fluid therapy are Na^+ and K^+ salts. Requirements depend on minimum obligatory and ongoing losses.
    - It is customary to provide **75–175 mEq Na^+/d** as NaCl. (A typical 2-g Na^+ (or 5 g of NaCl) diet provides 86 mEq Na^+/d.)
    - Generally, **20–60 mEq K^+/d** is included if renal function is normal (approximately 1 mEq/kg/d).
    - Carbohydrate in the form of **dextrose, 100–150 g/d**, is given to minimize protein catabolism and prevent starvation ketoacidosis.
  - Table 12-1 provides a list of common IV solutions and their contents. By combining the necessary components, one can derive an appropriate maintenance fluid regimen tailored for each patient.

TABLE 12-1 Commonly Used Parenteral Solutions

IV Solution	Osmolality (mOsm/L)	[Glucose] (g/L)	$[Na^+]$ (mEq/L)	$[Cl^-]$ (mEq/L)	HCO_3^- Equivalents (mEq/L)
D5W	278	50	0	0	0
0.45% NaCl[a]	154	–[b]	77	77	0
0.9% NaCl[a]	308	–[b]	154	154	0
3% NaCl	1026	–	513	513	0
Lactated Ringer's[c]	274	–[b]	130	109	28 (as lactate)

[a]NaCl 0.45% and 0.9% are half-normal and normal saline, respectively.
[b]Also available with 5% dextrose.
[c]Also contains 4 mEq/L K^+, 1.5 mEq/L Ca^{2+}, and 28 mEq/L lactate.
D5W, 5% dextrose in water.

- **Example:** A patient is admitted for a procedure and is given nothing by mouth. To maintain homeostasis, you must replace 2 L of water, 154 mEq Na^+, 40 mEq K^+, and 100 g dextrose over the next 24 hours (values are within **water** and **electrolyte** requirements described earlier).
  - 2 L of water: Dose fluid at 85 mL/h (2000 mL ÷ 24 hours)
  - 154 mEq of Na^+: Use 0.45% normal saline (NS) (77 mEq Na^+/L)
  - 40 mEq of K^+: Add 20 mEq/L KCl to each liter of IVF
  - 100 g dextrose: Use D5 (50 g of dextrose/L)
  - Order: **D5 0.45% NaCl with 20 mEq/L KCl at 85 mL/h**
  - Despite being called "normal saline," the fluid is neither completely "normal" nor physiological. Although the osmolality is 308 mOsm/L (approximates plasma), it contains approximately 10% more sodium than plasma (154 mEq/L in NS vs 140 mEq/L in plasma) and 50% more chloride than plasma (154 mEq/L in NS vs 100 mEq/L in plasma) and also the pH being acidic. Hence, care must be taken while administering any intravenous fluid.

The Hypovolemic Patient

GENERAL PRINCIPLES

- Volume depletion (hypovolemia) generally results from a deficit in **total body Na^+** content. This may result from **renal** or **extrarenal losses** of Na^+ from the ECF. **Free water loss** can also cause volume depletion, but the quantity required to do so is large as water is lost mainly from the ICF and not the ECF where volume contraction can be assessed.
- **Renal losses** may be secondary to enhanced diuresis, salt-wasting nephropathies, mineralocorticoid deficiency, or resolution of obstructive renal disease.
- **Extrarenal losses** include fluid loss from the GI tract (vomiting, nasogastric suction, fistula drainage, diarrhea), respiratory losses, skin losses (especially with burns), hemorrhage, and severe third spacing of fluid in critically ill patients.

DIAGNOSIS

Clinical Presentation

- **Symptoms** include complaints of thirst, fatigue, weakness, muscle cramps, and postural dizziness. Sometimes, syncope and coma can result with severe volume depletion.

- **Signs** of hypovolemia include low jugular venous pressure, postural hypotension, postural tachycardia, and the absence of axillary sweat. Diminished skin turgor and dry mucous membranes are poor markers of decreased interstitial fluid. Mild degrees of volume depletion are often not clinically detectable, whereas larger fluid losses can lead to mental status changes, oliguria, and hypovolemic shock (Table 12-2).

Diagnostic Testing

Laboratory studies are often helpful but must be used in conjunction with the clinical picture.

- **Urine sodium** is a marker for Na^+ avidity in the kidney.
  - Urine Na^+ <15 mEq is consistent with volume depletion as is a fractional excretion of sodium (FeNa) <1%. The latter can be calculated as

$$([\text{Urine Na}^+ \times \text{Serum Cr}] \div [\text{Urine Cr} \times \text{Serum Na}^+]) \times 100.$$

    This indicates that due to low circulating volume, the renin-angiotensin-aldosterone system is activated leading to renal reabsorption of sodium, resulting in low urinary sodium and low FeNa levels. In cases of acute kidney injury (AKI), FeNa proves useful in distinguishing between prerenal (volume contraction) and renal causes.
  - Concomitant metabolic alkalosis may increase urine Na^+ excretion despite volume depletion because of obligate excretion of Na^+ to accompany the bicarbonate anion. In such cases, a urine chloride of <20 mEq is often helpful to confirm volume contraction.
  - **Urine osmolality** and **serum bicarbonate** levels may also be elevated.
  - **Hematocrit** and **serum albumin** may be increased from hemoconcentration.

TREATMENT

- It is often difficult to estimate the **volume deficit** present. Owing to this, therapy is largely empiric, requiring frequent reassessments of volume status while resuscitation is under way.

TABLE 12-2 Assessment of Degrees of Hypovolemia

Finding	Mild (3%–5%)	Moderate (6%–9%)	Severe (≥10%)
Pulse	Normal	Rapid	Rapid and low volume or absent
Systolic pressure	Normal	Normal to low	Low
Respiration	Normal	Deep, rate may be increased	Deep, tachypnea or decreased to absent
Buccal mucosa	Tacky or slightly dry	Dry	Parched
Eyes	Normal	Sunken	Markedly sunken
Skin turgor	Normal	Reduced	Tenting
Skin	Normal	Cool	Cool, mottled, acrocyanosis
Urine output	Normal or mildly reduced	Markedly reduced	Anuria
In children, anterior fontanelle	Normal	Sunken	Markedly sunken

- Mild volume contraction can usually be corrected via the oral route. However, the presence of hemodynamic instability, symptomatic fluid loss, or intolerance to oral administration requires IV therapy.
- The primary therapeutic goal is to protect hemodynamic stability and replenish **intravascular volume** with fluid that will expand the ECF compartment. This can be accomplished with Na^+-based solutions because Na^+ will be retained in the ECF.
  - **Isotonic fluid,** such as NS (0.9% NaCl), contains a Na^+ content similar to that of plasma fluid in the ECF and thus remains entirely in the ECF space. It is the initial fluid of choice for replenishing **intravascular volume.**
    - The administration of solute-free water is largely ineffective, because the majority of water will distribute to the ICF space.
    - Half-NS (0.45% NS) has 77 mEq of Na^+ per liter, roughly half the Na^+ content of an equal volume in the ECF. Thus, half of this solution will stay in the ECF and half will follow the predicted distribution of water.
  - Fluids can be administered as a bolus or at a steady maintenance rate. In patients with symptomatic volume depletion, a 1–2 L bolus is often indicated to acutely expand the intravascular space. The bolus can be repeated if necessary, although close attention should be directed toward possible signs of volume overload. Smaller boluses should be used for patients with poor cardiac reserve or significant edema. Once the patient is stable, fluids can be administered at a maintenance rate to replace ongoing losses. In patients with hemorrhage or GI bleeding, **blood transfusion** can accomplish both volume expansion and concomitant correction of anemia.

The Hypervolemic Patient

The clinical manifestations of hypervolemia result from a surplus of **total body Na^+**. It can be caused by a primary disorder of renal Na^+ retention. Alternatively, it may be secondary to decreased **effective circulating volume**, as in heart failure, cirrhosis, or profound hypoalbuminemia.

DIAGNOSIS

Clinical Presentation

- Expansion of the **interstitial compartment** may result in peripheral edema, ascites, and pleural effusions. Expansion of the **intravascular compartment** may result in pulmonary rales, elevated jugular venous pressure, hepatojugular reflux, an S_3 gallop, and elevated blood pressure.
- Because overt signs of hypervolemia may not manifest until 3–4 L of fluid retention, a gradual rise in water weight is often the earliest indication of Na^+ retention.
- **Symptoms** may include dyspnea, abdominal distention, or swelling of extremities.

Diagnostic Testing

- Laboratory studies are generally not needed as hypervolemia is primarily a bedside diagnosis.
- **The urine** [Na^+] may be low (<15 mEq/L) with decreased **effective circulating volume** reflecting renal sodium retention.
- A CXR may show pulmonary edema or pleural effusions, but clear lung fields do not exclude volume overload.

TREATMENT

Treatment must address not only the ECF volume excess but also the underlying pathologic process. Alleviating the Na^+ excess can be accomplished by the judicious use of diuretics and by limiting Na^+ intake.

Medications

- Diuretics enhance the renal excretion of Na^+ by blocking the various sites of Na^+ reabsorption along the nephron.
  - **Thiazide diuretics (TDs)** block NaCl transporters in the distal convoluted tubule. They are often used for mild states of chronic Na^+ retention. Because of their specific site of action, TD impair urinary dilutional capacity (the ability to excrete water) and often stimulate a responsive increase in proximal tubule reabsorption.
  - **Loop diuretics (LDs)** block Na^+-K^+-$2Cl^-$ transporter in the thick ascending loop of Henle. They are often used in circumstances requiring a brisk and immediate diuresis, such as acute volume overload. LD impair urinary concentration (increase renal free water excretion) and enhance the excretion of divalent cations (Ca^{2+} and Mg^{2+}).
  - **Potassium-sparing diuretics** act by decreasing Na^+ reabsorption in the collecting duct. Although the overall diuretic effect of these agents is comparatively small, they serve as useful adjunctive agents. Furthermore, because aldosterone antagonists do not require tubular secretion, they can be particularly useful in those with decreased renal perfusion or impaired tubular function.
  - **Sequential nephron blockade** with either metolazone or chlorothiazide in ADHF, renal dysfunction, and diuretic resistance appears to be effective and safe, and is recommended for fluid overload refractory to loop diuretic monotherapy.
- Treatment of the underlying disease process is critical in preventing the continued Na^+ reabsorption in the kidney. Nephrotic syndrome is discussed in Chapter 13, Renal Diseases; treatment of heart failure is discussed in Chapter 5, Heart Failure and Cardiomyopathy; and cirrhosis is addressed in Chapter 19, Liver Diseases.

DISORDERS OF SODIUM CONCENTRATION

Hypernatremia and **hyponatremia** are primarily disorders of *water balance* or *water distribution*. The body is designed to withstand both drought and deluge with adaptations to renal water handling and thirst mechanism. A persistent abnormality in [Na^+] thus requires both an initial challenge to water balance as well as a disturbance of the adaptive response.

Hyponatremia

Hyponatremia is defined as a plasma [Na^+] **<135 mEq/L**. It is the most common electrolyte disorder in hospitalized patients and occurs in 15%–22% of the patients at admission.

GENERAL PRINCIPLES

- To maintain a normal [Na^+], the ingestion of water must be matched with an equal volume of water excretion. Any process that limits the elimination of water or expands the volume around a fixed Na^+ content may lead to a decrease in Na^+ concentration.
- Expansion of the space surrounding the Na^+ content can occur in a variety of ways:
  - **Pseudohyponatremia** refers to a laboratory anomaly in which high levels of plasma proteins and/or lipids expand the nonaqueous portion of the plasma sample and result in an errant report of a low ECF [Na^+]. This can be averted with Na^+-sensitive electrodes, and the normal ECF [Na^+] can be confirmed with a normal serum osmolality.

- ○ **Hyperosmolar hyponatremia** refers to circumstances in which an osmotically active solute other than Na^+ accumulates in the ECF, drawing water into the ECF and diluting the Na^+ content. This is most commonly caused by **hyperglycemia**, resulting in a fall in plasma [Na^+] of 1.6–2.4 mEq/L for every 100 mg/dL rise in plasma glucose.[1] Other solutes, such as glycine, mannitol, or sorbitol, can be absorbed into the ECF during bladder irrigation, leading to the transient hyponatremia seen in **post–transurethral resection of the prostate syndrome**. Prompt renal excretion and metabolism of the absorbed fluid usually corrects the hyponatremia rapidly, although symptomatic hyponatremia can occasionally be seen in the setting of renal insufficiency.
- ○ Rarely does the ECF water content rises simply because the ingested quantity of water exceeds the physiologic capacity of water excretion in the kidney. This is seen in psychogenic polydipsia, water intoxication, beer potomania, and the so-called "tea and toast" diet. Underlying each of these circumstances is the fact that there is a limit to renal water clearance. Urine cannot be diluted to an osmolality less than approximately 50 mOsm/L, meaning that a small amount of solute is required in even the most dilute urine. Ingestion of a high volume of water can therefore exceed the capacity for excretion, particularly in those with a solute-poor diet, because the solute load required to generate urinary water loss is quickly depleted. The excess water is retained, Na^+ concentrations falls, and hyponatremia results.

- Decreased clearance of water from the kidney can also occur through a variety of processes. As mentioned previously, renal water handling is largely controlled by ADH (or vasopressin).
- **"Appropriate"** ADH secretion occurs with a fall in effective circulating volume. In these conditions, thirst and water retention are stimulated, protecting volume status at the cost of the osmolar status. This category is classically subdivided based on the associated assessment of ECF status:
  - ○ **Hypovolemic hyponatremia** may result from **any** cause of net Na^+ loss, such as in thiazide use and cerebral salt wasting (CSW).
  - ○ **Hypervolemic hyponatremia** occurs in edematous states such as congestive heart failure (CHF), hepatic cirrhosis, and severe nephrotic syndrome. Despite the expanded interstitial space, the circulating volume is reduced. Alterations in Starling forces contribute to this apparent paradox, shifting fluid from the intravascular to interstitial space.
- **"Inappropriate"** secretion of ADH is characterized by the activation of water-conserving mechanisms, despite the absence of osmotic- or volume-related stimuli. Because the renal response to volume expansion remains intact, these patients are typically **euvolemic**. However, because of the rise in TBW, serum concentrations of Na^+ are decreased.
  - ○ The most common form of this is the **syndrome of inappropriate ADH (SIADH)**. This disorder is caused by the nonphysiologic release of vasopressin from the posterior pituitary or an ectopic source. Common causes of SIADH include neuropsychiatric disorders (e.g., meningitis, encephalitis, acute psychosis, cerebrovascular accident, head trauma), pulmonary diseases (e.g., pneumonia, tuberculosis, positive-pressure ventilation, acute respiratory failure), and malignant tumors (most commonly small-cell lung cancer).
    - ▪ **SIADH** is diagnosed by the criteria given in Table 12-3.
    - ▪ **Pharmacologic agents** may also stimulate inappropriate ADH secretion. Common culprits include antidepressants (particularly selective serotonin reuptake inhibitors), narcotics, antipsychotic agents, chlorpropamide, and NSAIDs.
    - ▪ A recent understanding is that it may be prudent to use the term SIAD (syndrome of inappropriate anti-diuresis) as opposed to SIADH because the underlying mechanisms may be any of the following: Increased ADH may or may not be related to malignancy due to loss of ADH regulation (Type A), neurohypophysis injury or osmoregulatory disorders (Type B), reset osmostat (Type C), V2 receptor or AQP2 gene mutations in the kidney (Type D), altered osmoregulation may be due to renal salt wasting (Type E).

TABLE 12-3	Diagnostic Criteria for SIADH
Essential criteria	• Hypo-osmotic hyponatremia—effective serum osmolality: <275 mOsm/kg • Urine osmolality >100 mOsm/L • Euvolemia • Urine sodium concentration >30 mmol/L with normal dietary salt and water intake • No recent use of diuretics • The absence of conditions that stimulate ADH secretion, including volume contraction, nausea, adrenal dysfunction, and hypothyroidism
Supplementary criteria	• Serum uric acid <4 mg/dL • Serum urea <21.6 mg/dL • Failure to correct hyponatremia after 0.9% saline infusion • Fractional sodium excretion >0.5% • Fractional urea excretion >55% • Fractional uric acid excretion >12% • Correction of hyponatremia through fluid restriction

 - **Reset osmostat** is a phenomenon in which the set point for pOsm is reduced. Thus, ADH and thirst responses, although functional, maintain pOsm at this new, lower level. This phenomenon occurs in almost all pregnant women (perhaps in response to changes in the hormonal milieu) and occasionally in those with a chronic decreased effective circulating volume.

- **Cerebral Salt Wasting** is often a differential diagnosis of SIADH in patients with hyponatremia, particularly in patients with CNS disease, such as subarachnoid hemorrhage. It is characterized by hypovolemic hyponatremia due to inappropriate urinary sodium wasting. Clinical differences between SIADH and CSW are listed in Table 12-4.

DIAGNOSIS

Clinical Presentation

The clinical features of hyponatremia are related to the osmotic intracellular water shift leading to cerebral edema. Therefore, the symptoms (Table 12-5) are primarily neurologic, with severity that is dependent on both the magnitude and rapidity of decrease in plasma [Na^+]. In **acute hyponatremia** (i.e., developing in <48 hours), patients may complain of nausea and malaise with [Na^+] of approximately 125 mEq/L. As the plasma [Na^+] falls further,

TABLE 12-4 Clinical Differences Between SIADH, Cerebral Salt Wasting (CSW), and Diabetes Insipidus (DI)

	SIADH	CSW	DI
Urine output	Decreased	Polyuric	Polyuric
Serum Na	Low	Low	High
Urine Na	High	High	Low
Serum osmolality	Low	Can be low or normal	High
Urine osmolality	High	Can be low or normal	Low
CVP	High	Low	Can be normal or low

CVP, central venous pressure.

TABLE 12-5 Classification of Hyponatremia According to Severity of Presenting Symptoms

Severity	Serum Sodium Level	Neurologic Symptoms	Typical Duration of Hyponatremia
Mild	<135 mmol/L	Headache, irritability, difficulty concentrating, altered mood, and depression	Chronic (several days to many weeks or months)
Moderate	<130 mmol/L	Nausea, confusion, disorientation, altered mental status, unstable gait, and falls	Intermediate or chronic (>24–48 h)
Severe	<125 mmol/L	Vomiting, seizures, obtundation, respiratory distress, and coma	Acute (<24–48 h)

symptoms may progress to include headache, lethargy, confusion, and obtundation. Stupor, seizures, and coma do not usually occur unless the plasma [Na^+] falls acutely below 115 mEq/L. In **chronic hyponatremia** (>48 h in duration), adaptive mechanisms designed to defend cell volume occur and tend to minimize the increase in ICF volume and its symptoms.

Diagnostic Testing

The underlying cause of hyponatremia can often be ascertained from an accurate history and physical examination, including an assessment of **ECF volume status** and the **effective circulating volume.**

Three laboratory analyses, when used with a clinical assessment of volume status, can narrow the differential diagnosis of hyponatremia: (1) the **pOsm**, (2) the **urine osmolality**, and (3) the **urine** [Na^+] (Figure 12-1; Table 12-6).

- **pOsm:** Most patients with hyponatremia have a low pOsm (<275 mOsm/L). If the pOsm is not low, **pseudohyponatremia** and **hyperosmolar hyponatremia** must be ruled out.
- **Urine osmolality:** The appropriate renal response to hypo-osmolality is to excrete a maximally dilute urine (urine osmolality <100 mOsm/L and specific gravity <1.003). A urine sample that is not dilute suggests impaired free water excretion due to appropriate or inappropriate secretion of the ADH.
- **Urine** [Na^+] adds laboratory corroboration to the bedside assessment of effective circulating volume and can discriminate between **extrarenal** and **renal losses** of Na^+. The appropriate response to decreased effective circulating volume is to enhance tubular Na^+ reabsorption such that urine [Na^+] is <10 mEq/L. A urine [Na^+] of >20 mEq/L suggests a normal effective circulating volume or a Na^+-wasting defect. Occasionally, the excretion of a nonreabsorbed anion obligates loss of the Na^+ cation despite volume depletion (ketonuria, bicarbonaturia).

TREATMENT

- **Rate of correction**
  - In *chronic* hyponatremia, the target rate of correction should not exceed 10 mEq/L over 24 hours.
    - The risk of iatrogenic injury is increased in patients with chronic hyponatremia because cells gradually adapt to the hypo-osmolar state. An abrupt normalization presents a dramatic change from the accommodated osmotic milieu.

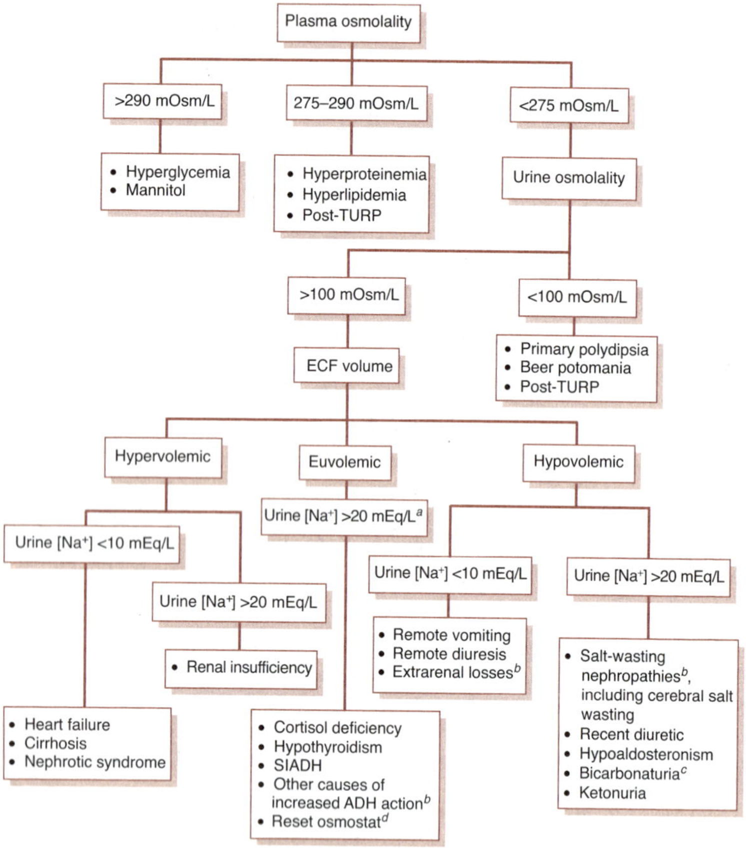

Figure 12-1 Algorithm depicting the diagnostic approach to hyponatremia. ADH, antidiuretic hormone; ECF, extracellular fluid; post-TURP, post–transurethral resection of the prostate syndrome; SIADH, syndrome of inappropriate antidiuretic hormone. [a]Urine [Na$^+$] may be <20 mEq/L with low Na$^+$ intake. [b]See text for details. [c]From vomiting-induced contraction alkalosis or proximal renal tubular acidosis. [d]Urine osmolality may be <100 mOsm/L after a water load.

- The primary risk of overcorrection is the development of **osmotic demyelination syndrome (ODS)**, formerly called central pontine myelinolysis (CPM). ODS results from damage to neurons due to rapid osmotic shifts. In its most overt form, it is characterized by flaccid paralysis, dysarthria, dysphagia, seizures, lethargy, confusion, disorientation, obtundation, and coma. It can be confirmed by CT scan or MRI of the brain. The risk of precipitating ODS is increased with correction of the [Na$^+$] by 10–12 mEq/L in a 24-hour period.[2] Other risk factors for developing ODS include pre-existing hypokalemia, malnutrition, liver disease, and alcoholism.

- In *symptomatic* hyponatremia, the serum [Na$^+$] should again be corrected cautiously. A targeted rise in serum [Na$^+$] by 4–6 mEq/L within the first 4–6 hours is generally sufficient to reverse the neurologic sequelae and avoid overcorrection. The total daily correction should not exceed 10 mEq/d. Table 12-7 gives the treatment recommendations.

TABLE 12-6 Differential Diagnosis and Features of Hyponatremia According to Volume Status, Urine Osmolality, and Urine [Na^+]

	Orthostatic Hypotension	Edema	$U_{[Na^+]}$ (mEq/L)	U_{Osm} (mOsm/L)	Common Causes
Normovolemic hyponatremia	Absent	No	>20	>100	Psychogenic polydipsia Glucocorticoid deficit Hypokalemia Drugs SIADH
Hypovolemic hyponatremia - renal losses	Normally present	No	>20	>100	Diuretics Mineralocorticoid deficit Salt-losing nephropathy
Hypovolemic hyponatremia - extrarenal losses	Normally present	No	<10	>100	Vomiting Diarrhea
Hypervolemic hypernatremia	Absent	Yes	Compensated: >20 Decompensated: <10	Compensated: <100 Decompensated: >100	CHF Cirrhosis Nephrotic syndrome Acute and chronic kidney disease

<table>
<tr><th colspan="2">TABLE 12-7 Recommendations for the Treatment of Hyponatremia</th></tr>
<tr><td colspan="2">Hyponatremia with Severe Symptoms</td></tr>
<tr><td colspan="2">First-hour management, regardless of whether acute or chronic</td></tr>
<tr><td colspan="2">Prompt IV infusion of 150 mL 3% hypertonic over 20 min
Recheck the serum sodium concentration after 20 min while repeating an infusion
Repeat the above steps twice or until a target of 5 mmol/L increase in serum sodium concentration is achieved</td></tr>
<tr><td>Follow-up management in case of improvement of symptoms after a 5 mmol/L increase</td><td>• Stop the infusion of hypertonic saline
• Limit the increase in serum sodium concentration to a total of 10 mmol/L during the first 24 h and an additional 8 mmol/L every 24 h thereafter until the serum sodium concentration reaches 130 mmol/L
• Check the serum sodium concentration after 6 and 12 h and daily afterwards</td></tr>
<tr><td>Follow-up management in case of no improvement of symptoms after a 5 mmol/L increase</td><td>• Continue an IV infusion of 3% hypertonic saline aiming for an additional 1 mmol/L/h increase in serum sodium concentration
• Stop the infusion of 3% hypertonic saline when the symptoms improve, the serum sodium concentration increases 10 mmol/L in total, or the serum sodium concentration reaches 130 mmol/L, whichever occurs first
• Monitor the serum sodium concentration every 4 h if an IV infusion of 3% hypertonic saline or equivalent is continued</td></tr>
<tr><td colspan="2">Hyponatremia with Moderately Severe Symptoms</td></tr>
<tr><td colspan="2">• Immediate treatment with a single IV infusion of 150 mL 3% hypertonic saline or equivalent over 20 min
• Aim for an increase of 5 mmol/L per 24 h in serum sodium concentration
• Limit the increase in serum sodium concentration to 10 mmol/L in the first 24 h and 8 mmol/L every 24 h thereafter, until a serum sodium concentration of 130 mmol/L is reached
• Monitor the serum sodium concentration after 1, 6, and 12 h</td></tr>
<tr><td colspan="2">Hyponatremia without Severe or Moderately Severe Symptoms</td></tr>
<tr><td>Acute
• If the acute decrease in serum sodium concentration exceeds 10 mmol/L, a single IV infusion of 150 mL 3% hypertonic saline or equivalent over 20 min is recommended
• Monitor the serum sodium concentration after 4 h</td><td>Chronic
• Treatment should be targeted to the cause of the disorder
• Avoid an increase in serum sodium concentration of >10 mmol/L during the first 24 h and >8 mmol/L every 24 h thereafter
• Monitor the serum sodium concentration every 6 h until the serum sodium concentration has stabilized under stable treatment</td></tr>
</table>

(Continued)

TABLE 12-7 Recommendations for the Treatment of Hyponatremia (Continued)

Indications to reverse therapy to prevent osmotic demyelination	
Acute	**Chronic**
Not usually necessary	If exceeding maximal rate of correction, options include: • Administer 2–4 μg of desmopressin every 8 h with 3 mL/kg/h IV D5W over 1 h • Repeat D5W until serum sodium within limit range • Stop vaptan • Follow serum sodium hourly

Type of intervention

- Hypertonic saline can also be infused at a rate calculated to achieve the desired amount of correction. This can be accomplished by:
- Step 1. Calculating the approximate change in [Na⁺] in mEq/L from the infusion of 1 L of fluid:

$$\Delta\,[Na^+] = \frac{[Na^+_i] + [K^+_i] - [Na^+_s]}{[TBW + 1]}$$

  - $[Na^+_i]$ and $[K^+_i]$ are the sodium and potassium concentrations in the infused fluid and $[Na^+_s]$ is the starting serum sodium.[3]
  - TBW is estimated by multiplying the lean weight (in kilograms) by 0.6 in men and 0.5 in women.
- Step 2. Determining the rate of administration (liters per hour) by dividing the desired rate of correction (mEq/L/h) by the Δ [Na⁺] calculated in the previous step (mEq/L/L of fluid).
- Step 3. Adjusting the starting rate based on concerns for overcorrection.
- Unfortunately, no equation can account for the daily dynamic fluctuations of water and solutes, and in patients with an unexpected water diuresis, this equation underestimates the degree of correction that is actually achieved. In one study, the ratio of actual to predicted change in [Na⁺] was, on average, 1.66.[4]
- If a continuous infusion of hypertonic saline is preferred, we suggest *initiating* the infusion at 60% of the calculated rate, then titrating the hourly rate based on frequent laboratory result checks.
- If the desired rate of correction is exceeded, hypertonic fluids should be discontinued and either hypotonic fluids or desmopressin can be given to re-lower the serum Na⁺ to achieve a 24-hour correction of less than 10 mEq.
- Example: A 100 kg man is brought to the hospital with mental status changes and a serum Na of 110. You would like to raise his Na by 1 mEq/L over the next 4–6 hours using hypertonic saline (3% saline: 513 mEq of Na, 0 mEq of K).
  - Δ [Na⁺] = (513 mEq/L – 110 mEq/L) / (60 + 1) = 6.61 mEq/L/L of 3% saline
  - Rate of infusion = 1 mEq/L/h ÷ 6.61 mEq/L/L of 3% saline = 151 mL/h
  - Adjusted starting rate (60% of calculated): 91 mL/h
- No algorithm or equation can replace the importance of **rechecking laboratory data** to ensure correction at an appropriate rate and adjust fluid administration.

- In asymptomatic hyponatremia, treatment should be targeted to the cause of the disorder.
  - **Hypovolemic hyponatremia.** In patients with asymptomatic hypovolemic hyponatremia, **isotonic** saline can be used to restore the intravascular volume. Restoration of a euvolemic state will reduce the impetus toward renal water retention, leading to normalization of [Na^+]. If the duration of hyponatremia is unknown, the process described earlier can be used to calculate the expected change from 1 L of 0.9% NS, the rate of administration, and the suggested adjustment to avoid overcorrection.
  - **Hypervolemic hyponatremia.** Hyponatremia in CHF and cirrhosis often reflects the severity of the underlying disease. The hyponatremia itself is typically asymptomatic. Because the *effective* circulating volume is decreased, the administration of fluid may worsen the volume overload state. Definitive treatment requires management of the underlying condition, although restriction of water intake and increasing water diuresis may help to attenuate the degree of hyponatremia and hypervolemia.
  - **SIADH.** This disorder should be distinguished from the previously listed conditions that stimulate vasopressin secretion. The standard first-line therapy is water restriction and correction of any contributing factors (nausea, pneumonia, drugs, etc.). If this fails or if the patient is symptomatic, the following can be attempted to promote water excretion:
  - **Water restriction.** The amount of fluid restriction necessary depends on the extent of water elimination. A useful guide to the necessary degree of fluid restriction is as follows:
    - If (Urine Na^+ + Urine K^+)/Serum Na^+ <0.5, restrict to 1 L/d.
    - If (Urine Na^+ + Urine K^+)/Serum Na^+ is 0.5–1.0, restrict to 500 mL/d.
    - If (Urine Na^+ + Urine K^+)/Serum Na^+ is >1, then the patient has a negative renal free water clearance and any amount of ingested water may be retained. In such situations, the following options may be required:
  - **A high dietary solute load** (using salt or urea tablets) increases the capacity for water excretion. The obligate water loss that accompanies the excretion of the high dietary solute load helps to alleviate water retention in SIADH.
  - **LDs** impair the urinary concentrating mechanism and can enhance free water excretion. Contrary to the popular opinion that all diuretics cause hyponatremia, LDs can actually lead to a rise in serum sodium. This phenomenon occurs because Na/K/2Cl channels in the loop of Henle are blocked and sodium is not reabsorbed here. However, when the excess sodium reaches the distal segment, paradoxical increase in Na reabsorption occurs.
  - **Vasopressin antagonists** promote a water diuresis and may be useful in the therapy of SIADH. Both IV (conivaptan) and oral (tolvaptan) preparations are approved for the treatment of euvolemic hyponatremia. However, given the risks of overcorrection, these agents should be initiated in a closely monitored inpatient setting.
  - Lithium and demeclocycline interfere with the collecting tubule's ability to respond to ADH, but are rarely used because of significant side effects. They should only be considered in severe hyponatremia that is unresponsive to more conservative measures.

Hypernatremia

GENERAL PRINCIPLES

- Hypernatremia is defined as a plasma [Na^+] **>145 mEq/L** and represents a state of **hyperosmolality** (see Disorders of Sodium Concentration section).
- Hypernatremia may be caused by a primary **Na^+ gain** or a **water deficit**, the latter being much more common. Normally, this hyperosmolar state stimulates thirst and the excretion of a maximally concentrated urine. For hypernatremia to persist, one or both of these compensatory mechanisms must be impaired.

- **Impaired thirst response** may occur in situations where access to water is limited, often due to physical restrictions (institutionalized, handicapped, postoperative, patients on nasogastric tube feeding or intubated patients) or mental impairment (delirium, dementia).
- **Hypernatremia due to water loss.** The loss of water must occur in excess of electrolyte losses to raise [Na^+].
    - **Nonrenal water loss** may be due to evaporation from the skin and respiratory tract (insensible losses) or loss from the GI tract. Diarrhea is the most common GI cause of hypernatremia. Osmotic diarrhea (induced by lactulose, sorbitol, or malabsorption of carbohydrate) and viral gastroenteritis, in particular, result in disproportional water loss.
    - **Renal water loss** results from either **osmotic diuresis** or **diabetes insipidus (DI)**.
        - **Osmotic diuresis** is frequently associated with glycosuria and high osmolar feeds. In addition, increased urea generation from accelerated catabolism, high-protein feeds, and stress-dose steroids can also result in an osmotic diuresis.
        - Hypernatremia secondary to nonosmotic urinary water loss is usually caused by impaired vasopressin secretion (**central diabetes insipidus** [**CDI**]) or resistance to the actions of vasopressin (**nephrogenic diabetes insipidus** [**NDI**]). Partial defects occur more commonly than complete defects in both types.
        - The most common cause of CDI is destruction of the neurohypophysis from trauma, neurosurgery, granulomatous disease, neoplasms, vascular accidents, or infection. In many cases, CDI is idiopathic.
        - NDI may either be inherited or acquired. Acquired NDI often results from a disruption to the renal concentrating mechanism due to drugs (lithium, demeclocycline, amphotericin), electrolyte disorders (hypercalcemia, hypokalemia), medullary washout (LDs), and intrinsic renal diseases.
- **Adipsic diabetes insipidus** is a rare hypothalamic disorder characterized by a loss of thirst in response to hypernatremia accompanied by diabetes insipidus.
- **Hypernatremia due to primary Na^+ gain** occurs infrequently because of the kidney's capacity to excrete the retained Na^+. However, it can rarely occur after repetitive **hypertonic saline** administration or chronic **mineralocorticoid excess** of some drugs, including antibiotics with high sodium content that can also cause primary sodium gain (e.g., fosfomycin).
- **Transcellular water shift** from ECF to ICF can occur in circumstances of transient intracellular hyperosmolality, as in seizures or rhabdomyolysis.

DIAGNOSIS

Clinical Presentation

- Hypernatremia results in contraction of brain cells as water shifts to attenuate the rising ECF osmolality. Thus, the most severe symptoms of hypernatremia are neurologic, including altered mental status, weakness, neuromuscular irritability, focal neurologic deficits, and occasionally, coma or seizures. Acute hypernatremia can result in focal intracerebral hemorrhage, subarachnoid hemorrhage, and osmotic demyelination. As with hyponatremia, the severity of the clinical manifestations is related to the *acuity* and *magnitude* of the rise in plasma [Na^+]. **Chronic hypernatremia** is generally less symptomatic as a result of adaptive mechanisms designed to defend cell volume.
- **CDI and NDI** generally present with complaints of polyuria and thirst. Signs of volume depletion or neurologic dysfunction are generally absent unless the patient has an associated thirst abnormality.

Diagnostic Testing

Urine osmolality and the **response to desmopressin acetate (DDAVP)** can help narrow the differential diagnosis for hypernatremia (Figure 12-2).

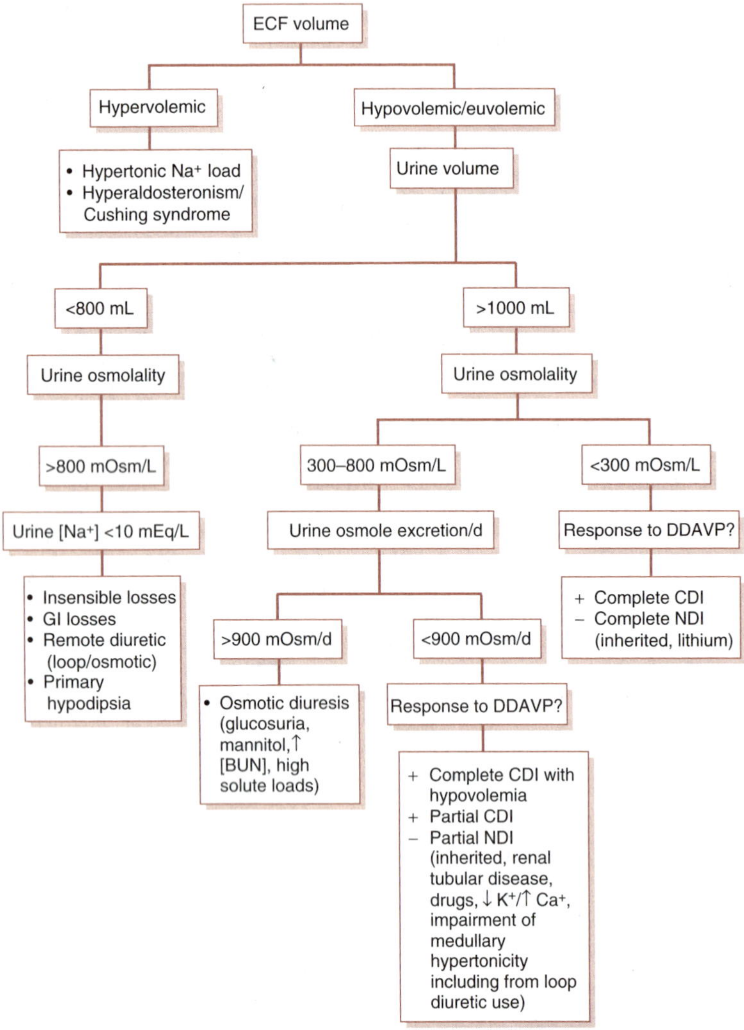

Figure 12-2 Algorithm depicting the diagnostic approach to hypernatremia. BUN, blood urea nitrogen; ↑Ca^+, hypercalcemia; CDI, central diabetes insipidus; DDAVP, desmopressin acetate; ECF, extracellular fluid; GI, gastrointestinal; NDI, nephrogenic diabetes insipidus; ↓K^+, hypokalemia; (+), conditions with increase in urine osmolality in response to desmopressin acetate; (–), conditions with little increase in urine osmolality in response to desmopressin acetate.

- The appropriate renal response to hypernatremia is a small volume of concentrated urine (urine osmolality >800 mOsm/L). **Urine osmolality** <800 mOsm/L suggests a defect in renal water conservation.
  - A urine osmolality <300 mOsm/L in the setting of hypernatremia suggests complete forms of CDI and NDI.

 - Urine osmolality between 300 and 800 mOsm/L can occur from partial forms of DI as well as osmotic diuresis. The two can be differentiated by quantifying the daily solute excretion (estimated by the urine osmolality multiplied by urine volume in 24 hours). A daily solute excretion >900 mOsm/L defines an osmotic diuresis.
- **Response to DDAVP.** Complete forms of CDI and NDI can be distinguished by administering the vasopressin analog DDAVP (10 μg intranasally) after careful water restriction. The urine osmolality should increase by at least 50% in complete CDI and does not change in NDI. The diagnosis is sometimes difficult when partial defects are present.

TREATMENT

- **Rate of Correction**
  - As in hyponatremia, aggressive correction of ***symptomatic*** **hypernatremia** is potentially dangerous. The rapid shift of water into brain cells increases the risk of seizures or permanent neurologic damage. Therefore, the water deficit should be reduced gradually and plasma [Na^+] levels should be reduced by no more than **10–12 mEq/L per day**.
  - In ***chronic*** **hypernatremia**, the risk of treatment-related complications is increased because of the cerebral adaptation to the chronic hyperosmolar state. The plasma [Na^+] should be lowered at a more moderate rate (between 5 and 8 mEq/L per day).
- **Intervention**
  - The mainstay of management is the administration of water, preferably by mouth or nasogastric tube. Alternatively, 5% dextrose in water (D5W) or quarter NS can be given via IV.
    - The extent of the **free water deficit** can be calculated by the equation:

$$\text{Free water deficit} = \{([Na^+] - 140)/140\} \times (\text{TBW})$$

    - This free water deficit provides a target amount of water that should be replaced to correct the hypernatremia.
    - The rate of water administration can be estimated by dividing this amount by the time frame over which hypernatremia should be normalized to achieve the target rate of correction outlined above.
      - Example: For a 3 L free water deficit that you wish to correct over 24 hours, the D5W can be run at 3 L/24 h = 125 mL/h.
  - It should be noted that this equation does NOT account for ongoing free water losses. Using this equation alone without considering ongoing losses through GI or renal excretion may result in an underestimation of the amount of water required to correct a patient's hypernatremia.
- **Acute hypernatremia:** 5% dextrose in water, intravenously, at a rate of 3–6 mL/kg/h till serum sodium reaches 145 mEq/L. Then the rate of infusion is reduced to 1 mL/kg/h and continued until a normal serum sodium (140 mEq/L) is reached.
  - No single equation adequately captures the dynamic input and output of free water in a patient. Because of this, it is critically important to **recheck laboratory data** to ensure that an appropriate rate of correction is being achieved.
  - If hypernatremia does not respond to standard corrective measures or the free water deficit is very large, renal replacement in the form of CRRT (continuous renal replacement therapy) can be considered especially in a critically ill patient to gradually bring down sodium levels.
- **Specific therapies for the underlying cause**
  - **Hypovolemic hypernatremia.** In patients with mild volume depletion, Na^+-containing solutions such as 0.45% NS can be used to replenish the ECF as well as the water deficit. If patients have severe or symptomatic volume depletion, correction of volume status with **isotonic fluid** should take precedence over correction of the hyperosmolar state. Once the patient is hemodynamically stable, hypotonic fluid can be given to replace the free water deficit.

- **Hypernatremia from primary Na^+ gain** is unusual. Cessation of iatrogenic Na^+ is typically sufficient.
- **DI without hypernatremia.** DI is best treated by removing the underlying cause. Despite the renal water loss, DI should not result in hypernatremia if the thirst mechanism remains intact. However, treatment is sometimes required to alleviate symptomatic polyuria.
  - **CDI.** Because the polyuria is the result of impaired secretion of vasopressin, treatment is best accomplished with the administration of DDAVP, a vasopressin analog.
  - **NDI.** A low Na^+ diet combined with TD will decrease polyuria by inducing mild volume depletion. This enhances proximal reabsorption of salt and water, thus decreasing urinary free water loss. Decreasing protein intake will further decrease urine output by minimizing the solute load that must be excreted.

POTASSIUM

- Potassium is the major **intracellular** cation. Of the 3000–4000 mEq of K^+ found in the average human, 98% is sequestered within cells. Thus, although ECF [K^+] is normally 3.5–5.0 mEq/L, the intracellular concentration is roughly 150 mEq/L. This difference in ICF and ECF K^+ content is maintained by the **Na^+/K^+ adenosine triphosphatase pump.**
- The K^+ intake of individuals on an average is approximately 40–120 mEq per day, 90% of which is absorbed by the GI tract. Maintenance of the steady state necessitates matching K^+ excretion with ingestion.
- The elimination of potassium occurs predominately through **renal excretion** at the distal nephron. K^+ secretion is enhanced by distal Na^+ reabsorption, which generates a **lumen-negative gradient** and **distal urine flow rate.**
- Renal potassium handling is responsive to **aldosterone,** which stimulates the expression of distal luminal Na^+ channels, and the **serum potassium concentration.** Aldosterone secretion is, in turn, responsive to angiotensin II and hyperkalemia.

Hypokalemia

GENERAL PRINCIPLES

- Hypokalemia is defined as a plasma [K^+] <3.5 mEq/L.
- **Spurious hypokalemia** may be seen in situations in which high numbers of metabolically active cells present in the blood sample absorb the ECF potassium.
- True hypokalemia may result from one or more of the following: (1) **decreased net intake,** (2) **shift into cells,** or (3) **increased net loss.**
  - **Diminished intake** is seldom the sole cause of K^+ depletion because urinary excretion can be effectively decreased to <15 mEq/d. However, dietary K^+ restriction may exacerbate the hypokalemia from GI or renal loss.
  - **Transcellular shift.** Movement of K^+ into cells may transiently decrease the plasma [K^+] without altering total body K^+ content. These shifts can result from alkalemia, insulin, catecholamine release, increased erythropoiesis (administration of methylcobalamin), hypothermia, and chloroquine toxicity. **Hypokalemic periodic paralysis** is a rare disorder that predisposes patients to transcellular K^+ shifts that result in episodic muscle weakness. The hypokalemic form can be triggered after a carbohydrate-rich meal.
  - **Nonrenal K^+ loss.** Hypokalemia may result from the loss of potassium-rich fluids from the lower GI tract (villous adenoma, VIPoma). Hypokalemia from the loss of upper GI contents is typically more attributable to renal K^+ secretion from secondary hyperaldosteronism. Rarely does, in excessive sweating, loss of K^+ through the integument can provoke hypokalemia.

- **Renal K^+ loss** accounts for most cases of *chronic* hypokalemia. This may be caused by any of the following factors:
  - **Augmented distal urine flow** occurs commonly with diuretic use and osmotic diuresis (e.g., glycosuria). Bartter and Gitelman syndromes mimic loop and thiazide diuretic use, respectively, and promote renal K^+ loss by the same mechanism.
  - **Hyperaldosteronism** can result in increased renal K^+ loss because aldosterone plays a central role in coupling the reabsorption of sodium with the excretion of potassium.
    - **Primary mineralocorticoid excess** can be the result of an adrenal adenoma or adrenocortical hyperplasia.
    - Cortisol also has an affinity for mineralocorticoid receptors but is typically converted quickly to cortisone, which has markedly less mineralocorticoid activity. Still, if cortisol is present in abundance (Cushing syndrome) or fails to be converted to cortisone (syndrome of mineralocorticoid excess), it may mimic hyperaldosteronism.
    - **Secondary hyperaldosteronism** can be seen in any situation with a decreased effective circulating volume.
    - Constitutive activation of the distal renal epithelial Na^+ channel can mimic hyperaldosteronism. This occurs in a number of monogenic disorders, including **Liddle syndrome**, and leads to hypertension and hypokalemia. Unlike primary or secondary hyperaldosteronism, aldosterone levels are often suppressed in disorders of the epithelial Na^+ channel.
- Increased distal delivery of a nonreabsorbable anion such as bicarbonate (metabolic alkalosis or type 2 renal tubular acidosis), ketones, and hippurate (from toluene intoxication or glue sniffing) can also potentiate the lumen-negative gradient that drives K^+ secretion.
- Amphotericin B can increase membrane permeability and cause luminal potassium secretion.

DIAGNOSIS

Clinical Presentation

- The clinical features of K^+ depletion vary greatly and their severity depends in part on the degree of hypokalemia. Symptoms seldom occur unless the plasma $[K^+]$ is <3.0 mEq/L.
- Fatigue, myalgias, and muscular weakness or cramps of the lower extremities are common. Smooth muscle function may also be affected and may manifest with complaints of constipation or frank paralytic ileus. Severe hypokalemia may lead to complete paralysis, hypoventilation, or rhabdomyolysis.

Diagnostic Testing

When the etiology is not immediately apparent, **renal K^+ excretion** and the **acid–base status** can help identify the cause.

- **Urine K^+.** The appropriate response to hypokalemia is to excrete <25 mEq/d of K^+ in the urine. Urinary K^+ excretion can be measured with a 24-hour urine collection or estimated by multiplying spot urine $[K^+]$ by the total daily urine output. A spot urine $[K^+]$ may be helpful (urine $[K^+]$ <15 mEq/L suggests appropriate K^+ conservation), but the results can be confounded by a variety of factors.
- Alternatively, the **transtubular potassium gradient** (TTKG), which estimates the potassium gradient between the urine and the blood in the distal nephron, can be calculated as follows:
  - **TTKG** = (Urine K × Plasma osm)/(Plasma K × Urine osm)
  - A TTKG <2 suggests a nonrenal source, whereas a TTKG >4 suggests inappropriate renal K excretion.
- **Urine potassium-to-creatinine ratio** less than 13 mEq/g creatinine (1.5 mEq/mmol creatinine) indicates transcellular potassium shifts, gastrointestinal losses, diuretic use,

or poor dietary intake. Urine potassium-to-creatinine ratio of more than 13 mEq/g indicates renal potassium wasting.

- **Acid–base status.** Intracellular shifting and renal excretion of K^+ are often closely linked with the acid–base status. Hypokalemia is generally associated with metabolic alkalosis and can play a critical role in the maintenance of metabolic alkalosis. The finding of metabolic acidosis in a patient with hypokalemia thus narrows the differential significantly, implying lower GI loss, distal RTA, or the excretion of a nonreabsorbable anion from an organic acid (diabetic ketoacidosis [DKA], hippurate from toluene intoxication).
- **ECG** changes associated with hypokalemia include flattening or inversion of the T wave, a prominent U wave, ST-segment depression, premature atrial complexes, premature ventricular beats, and a prolonged QU interval (Figure 12-3). Severe K^+ depletion may result in a prolonged PR interval, decreased voltage, and widening of the QRS complex. The risk of arrhythmia is more in older patients, patients with organic heart disease, and patients on digoxin or other antiarrhythmic drugs.

TREATMENT

The **therapeutic goals** are to safely correct the K^+ deficit and to minimize ongoing losses through treatment of the underlying cause. *Hypomagnesemia* should also be sought in all hypokalemic patients and corrected to allow effective K^+ repletion.

Total body potassium deficit of **200–400 mEq** is required to lower the serum potassium concentration by 1 mEq/L. Correction needs to be targeted to total body deficit.

- Correction of the K^+ deficit can be accomplished with either oral or IV therapy.

Oral therapy:

- Oral replacement with potassium chloride is the mainstay of therapy in hypokalemia.
- Potassium phosphate, oral or IV, may be appropriate in patients with combined hypokalemia and hypophosphatemia.
- Potassium bicarbonate or potassium citrate should be considered in patients with concomitant metabolic acidosis.
- It is generally safer to correct the K^+ deficit via the oral route when hypokalemia is mild and the patient can tolerate oral administration. Oral doses of 40 mEq are generally well tolerated and can be given as often as every 4 hours. Traditionally, 10 mEq of potassium

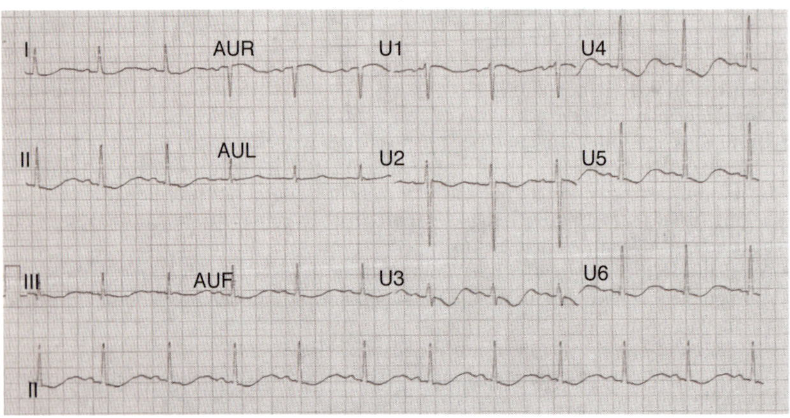

Figure 12-3 ECG showing prominent U waves and prolonged QU interval.

salts are given for each 0.10 mEq/L decrement in serum [K^+]. However, with increasing severity of hypokalemia, this grossly underestimates the K^+ necessary to normalize *total* K^+ content. Furthermore, as the K^+ shifts back to the intracellular space, it may appear as though K^+ supplementation is doing very little to correct ECF [K^+]. In such cases, potassium supplementation should be increased and continued until serum levels rise.

IV Therapy:

- Patients with imminently life-threatening hypokalemia and those who are unable to take anything by mouth require IV replacement therapy with KCl. The maximum concentration of administered K^+ should be no more than **40 mEq/L via a peripheral vein or 100 mEq/L via a central vein.** The rate of infusion should not exceed 20 mEq/h, unless paralysis or malignant ventricular arrhythmias are present. Ideally, KCl should be mixed in NS because dextrose solutions may initially exacerbate hypokalemia (as a result of insulin-mediated movement of K^+). Maximal daily dose is 240–400 mEq/day. The rate of infusion should not exceed 20 mEq/h unless paralysis or malignant ventricular arrhythmias are present. Continuous cardiac monitoring is recommended for infusion rates >10 mEq/h. If administering potassium through a central line, femoral veins are preferable because infusion through internal jugular or subclavian central lines can acutely increase the local concentration of K^+ and affect cardiac conduction.
- Potassium-sparing diuretics (spironolactone, amiloride, triamterene, and eplerenone) can be used.

Hyperkalemia

GENERAL PRINCIPLES

- Hyperkalemia is defined as a plasma [K^+] **>5.5 mEq/L.**
- **Pseudohyperkalemia** represents an artificially elevated plasma [K^+] due to K^+ movement out of cells immediately before or following venipuncture. Contributing factors include repeated fist clenching, hemolysis, and marked leukocytosis or thrombocytosis.
- True hyperkalemia occurs as a result of (1) **transcellular shift**, (2) **increased exposure to K^+**, and most commonly, (3) **decreased renal K^+ excretion**. Combinations of these mechanisms often underlie cases of hyperkalemia in clinical practice, and decreased renal excretion is nearly always some component of the pathophysiology.
    - **Transcellular shift.** Insulin deficiency, hyperosmolality, nonselective β-blockers, digitalis, metabolic acidosis (excluding those from organic acids, i.e., due to lactic acidosis or ketoacidosis), and depolarizing muscle relaxants, such as succinylcholine, release K^+ from predominate ICF stores into the ECF compartment. The release of intracellular K^+ can also be seen after severe exercise, rhabdomyolysis, hyperthermia, and tumor lysis syndrome. In the younger population, familial hyperkalemic periodic paralysis is a rare but important cause to consider as well.
    - **Increased exposure to K^+** is rarely the sole cause of hyperkalemia unless there is an impairment in renal excretion. Foods with a high content of K^+ include salt substitutes, red meat, dried fruits, nuts, tomatoes, potatoes, spinach, kiwis, mangoes, oranges, bananas, seaweed, avocados, and lima beans. Juices derived from these foods may be especially rich sources.
    - **Decreased renal K^+** excretion. In the setting of hyperkalemia, the kidney is capable of generating a significant urinary excretion of K^+. This process can be impaired by a number of processes, including intrinsic renal disease, decreased delivery of filtrate to the distal nephron, adrenal insufficiency, and hyporeninemic hypoaldosteronism (type 4 RTA). Rarer causes include pseudohypoaldosteronism types 1 and 2. Hyporeninemic hypoaldosteronism is usually seen in patients with diabetes.
- **Drugs** may also be implicated in the genesis of hyperkalemia through a variety of mechanisms. Common culprits include angiotensin-converting enzyme inhibitors, angiotensin receptor blockers, nicorandil, potassium-sparing diuretics, NSAIDs, digitalis (overdose),

tacrolimus, and cyclosporine. Heparin and ketoconazole can also contribute to hyperkalemia through the decreased production of aldosterone, although these agents alone are typically insufficient to sustain a clinically significant hyperkalemia.

DIAGNOSIS

Clinical Presentation

- The most serious effect of hyperkalemia is cardiac arrhythmogenesis, secondary to potassium's pivotal role in membrane potentials. Patients may present with palpitations, syncope, or even sudden cardiac death.
- Severe hyperkalemia causes partial depolarization of the skeletal muscle cell membrane and may manifest as weakness, potentially progressing to flaccid paralysis and hypoventilation if the respiratory muscles are involved.

Diagnostic Testing

- If the etiology is not readily apparent and the patient is asymptomatic, **pseudohyperkalemia** should be excluded by rechecking laboratory data.
- An assessment of **renal [K^+] excretion** and the **renin-angiotensin-aldosterone axis** can help narrow the differential diagnosis when the etiology is not immediately apparent.
  - Low aldosterone levels suggest either adrenal disease (renin levels elevated) or hyporeninemic hypoaldosteronism (renin levels low; occurs with type 4 RTA as well as chloride shunting or Gordon syndrome).
  - High aldosterone levels, typically accompanied by high renin levels, suggest aldosterone resistance (pseudohypoaldosteronism) but can also be seen in K^+-sparing diuretics.
- ECG changes are summarized in Table 12-8 and Figure 12-4.

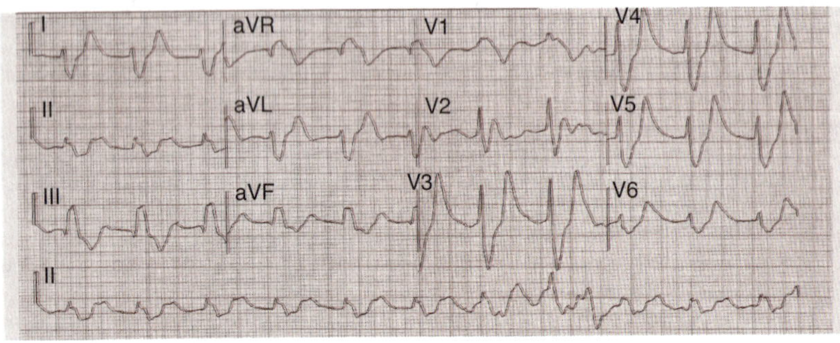

Figure 12-4 ECG showing absent P waves, wide QRS, and tall tented T waves.

TABLE 12-8 Sequential ECG Changes with Hyperkalemia

Serum Potassium (mEq/L)	ECG
5.5–6.5	Tall, peaked T waves
6.5–7.5	Loss of P waves
7–8	Widening of the QRS complex
8–10	Cardiac arrhythmias, sine wave pattern, and ventricular fibrillation/asystole

TREATMENT

Severe hyperkalemia with ECG changes is a medical emergency and requires immediate treatment directed at minimizing membrane depolarization and acutely reducing the ECF [K^+]. **Acute therapy** may consist of some or all of the following (the hypokalemic effect is additive):

- **Calcium gluconate** decreases membrane excitability but does not lower [K^+]. The usual dose is 1000 mg (10 mL) of a 10% solution infused for over 2–3 minutes. The effect begins within minutes but is short-lived (30–60 minutes), and the dose can be repeated if no improvement in the ECG is seen after 5–10 minutes.
- **Insulin** causes K^+ to shift into cells and temporarily lowers the plasma [K^+]. A commonly used combination is 10–20 units of regular insulin and 25–50 g of glucose-administered IV. Hyperglycemic patients should be given the insulin alone.
- **$NaHCO_3$** is effective for severe hyperkalemia associated with metabolic acidosis. In the acute setting, it can be given as an IV isotonic solution (three ampules of $NaHCO_3$ in 1 L of 5% dextrose).
- **β_2-Adrenergic agonists** promote cellular uptake of K^+. The onset of action is 30 minutes, lowering the plasma [K^+] by 0.5–1.5 mEq/L, and the effect lasts for 2–4 hours. Albuterol can be administered in a dose of 10–20 mg as a continuous nebulized treatment for over 30–60 minutes.
- **Longer term** means for [K^+] removal.
  - Increasing distal Na^+ delivery in the kidney enhances renal K^+ clearance. This can be achieved with the administration of saline in patients who appear volume depleted. Otherwise, LDs (furosemide) can be used if renal function is adequate.
  - **Cation exchange resins,** such as sodium polystyrene sulfonate (SPS), zirconium cyclosilicate, and patiromer, promote the excretion of K^+ in the GI tract and can be used in the management of chronic or resistant hyperkalemia. SPS is usually given as a 25–50 g dose. Because this particular cation exchange resin releases Na^+ in exchange for K^+, it should be used cautiously in patients with volume overload. Additional side effects of SPS include colonic necrosis, particularly when it is given as an enema. Newer agents such as patiromer appear to be effective, well tolerated, and safe. The usual dose is 8.4 g mixed with 100 mL of water, given daily.
- **Dialysis** should be reserved for patients with renal failure and those with severe life-threatening hyperkalemia who are unresponsive to more conservative measures. In patients with renal failure and refractory hyperkalemia, conventional hemodialysis lowers potassium faster than CRRT; hence, the former is preferred.
- **Chronic therapy** may involve dietary modifications to avoid high K^+ foods (see Potassium, Hyperkalemia, Etiology section), correction of metabolic acidosis with oral alkali, the promotion of kaliuresis with diuretics, and/or administration of exogenous mineralocorticoid in states of hypoaldosteronism.
- In type 4 RTA, oral fludrocortisone may be useful to treat hyperkalemia.

CALCIUM

- Calcium is essential for bone formation and neuromuscular function.
- Approximately 99% of body calcium is in the bone; most of the remaining 1% is in the ECF. Nearly 50% of serum calcium is ionized (free), whereas the remainder is complexed to albumin (40%) and anions such as phosphate (10%).
- **Calcium balance** is regulated by **parathyroid hormone** (PTH) and **calcitriol** (Figure 12-5).
  - **PTH** increases serum calcium by stimulating bone resorption, increasing calcium reclamation in the kidney, and promoting renal conversion of vitamin D to calcitriol. Serum calcium regulates PTH secretion by a negative feedback mechanism: Hypocalcemia stimulates and hypercalcemia suppresses PTH release.

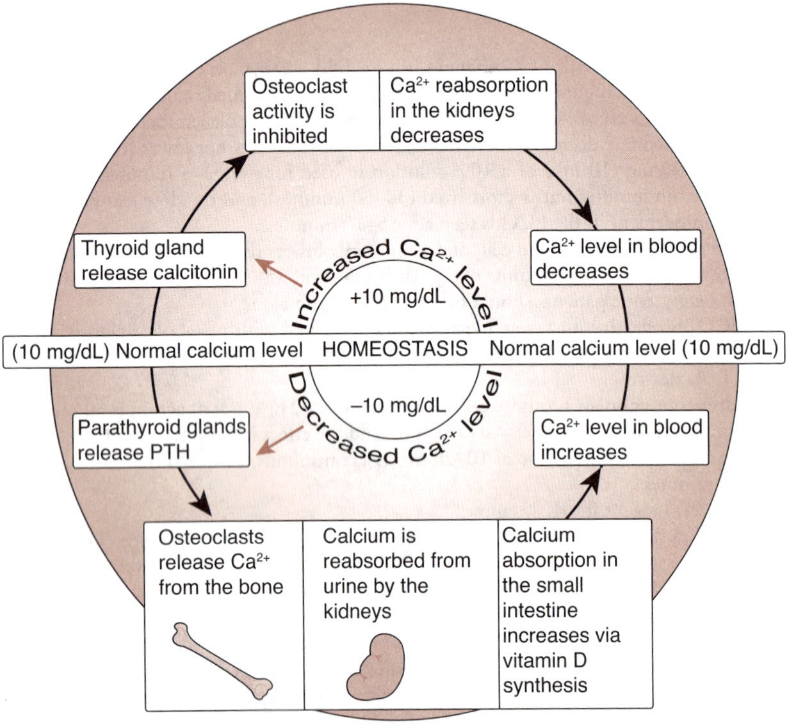

Figure 12-5 Calcium homeostasis.

- **Calcitriol** [1,25-dihydroxycholecalciferol, 1,25-dihydroxyvitamin D_3, or $1,25(OH)_2D_3$] is the active form of vitamin D. It stimulates intestinal absorption of calcium and is one of the many factors that provide feedback to the parathyroid gland.
- **Calcitonin** inhibits the osteoclast activity and the renal reabsorption of calcium, thus lowering serum calcium.
- Before interpreting calcium values, serum calcium must be corrected with respect to serum albumin, as hypoalbuminemia may falsely show low serum calcium levels.

$$\text{Corrected calcium (mg/dL)} = [0.8 \times (4.0 - \text{serum albumin})] + \text{serum calcium}$$

Hypercalcemia

GENERAL PRINCIPLES

- A serum calcium >**10.3 mg/dL** with a normal serum albumin or an ionized calcium >**5.2 mg/dL** defines hypercalcemia.
- Clinically significant hypercalcemia typically requires both an increase in ECF calcium and a decrease in renal calcium clearance. Underlying disturbances to calcium metabolism are thus often masked by compensatory mechanisms until the patient develops a concomitant disorder, such as decreased renal clearance from volume depletion. More than 90% of cases are due to **primary hyperparathyroidism** or **malignancy**.

- **Primary hyperparathyroidism** causes most cases of hypercalcemia in *ambulatory* patients. It is a common disorder, especially in elderly women, in whom the annual incidence is approximately 2 in 1000. Nearly 85% of cases are due to an **adenoma** of a single gland, 15% to **hyperplasia** of all four glands, and 1% to **parathyroid carcinoma**.
- **Malignancy** is responsible for most cases of hypercalcemia among *hospitalized* patients. Patients usually have advanced, clinically obvious disease. In these patients, hypercalcemia may develop from stimulation of osteoclast bone resorption from tumor cell products, tumor-derived **PTH-related peptides** (PTHrPs), and tumor calcitriol production.
- Less common causes account for about 10% of cases of hypercalcemia:
  - **Increased vitamin D activity** occurs with exogenous exposure to vitamin D or increased generation of calcitriol in chronic granulomatous diseases (e.g., sarcoidosis, tuberculosis).
  - The **milk-alkali syndrome** describes the acute or chronic development of hypercalcemia, alkalosis, and renal failure that may result from the ingestion of large quantities of calcium-containing antacids.
  - **Other.** Hyperthyroidism, adrenal insufficiency, prolonged immobilization, Paget disease, and acromegaly may be associated with hypercalcemia. **Familial hypocalciuric hypercalcemia** is a rare, autosomal dominant disorder of the calcium-sensing receptor, which is characterized by asymptomatic hypercalcemia from childhood and a family history of hypercalcemia. Drugs such as lithium, TD, teriparatide, and theophylline (toxicity) can cause hypercalcemia.
  - **Pseudohypercalcemia is** seen in conditions with hyperalbuminemia such as severe dehydration and paraproteinemias.

DIAGNOSIS

Clinical Presentation

Clinical manifestations generally are present only if serum calcium exceeds 12 mg/dL and tend to be more severe if hypercalcemia develops rapidly. Most patients with **primary hyperparathyroidism** have asymptomatic hypercalcemia that is found incidentally.

- Renal manifestations include polyuria and nephrolithiasis. If serum calcium rises above 13 mg/dL, renal failure with nephrocalcinosis and ectopic soft tissue calcifications are possible.
- GI symptoms include anorexia, vomiting, **constipation,** and rarely, signs of pancreatitis.
- Neurologic findings include weakness, fatigue, confusion, stupor, and coma.
- Osteopenia and frequent fractures may occur from the disproportional resorption of bone in hyperparathyroidism. Rarely, **osteitis fibrosa cystica** can develop when hyperparathyroidism is profound and prolonged, resulting in "brown tumors" and marrow replacement.

Diagnostic Testing

- The history and physical examination should focus on (1) the duration of symptoms of hypercalcemia, (2) clinical evidence of any of the unusual causes of hypercalcemia, and (3) symptoms and signs of malignancy (which almost always precede **malignant hypercalcemia**). If hypercalcemia has been present for more than 6 months without an obvious etiology, primary hyperparathyroidism is almost certainly the cause. Diagnostic algorithm is shown in Figure 12-6.
- **Serum calcium** should be interpreted with knowledge of the serum albumin, or an ionized calcium should be measured. **Corrected** $[Ca^{2+}] = [Ca^{2+}] + \{0.8 \times (4.0 - [albumin])\}$. Many patients with primary hyperparathyroidism will have a calcium level that is chronically within the high normal range.
- Intact **serum PTH** may be the most important first step in the evaluation of hypercalcemia.

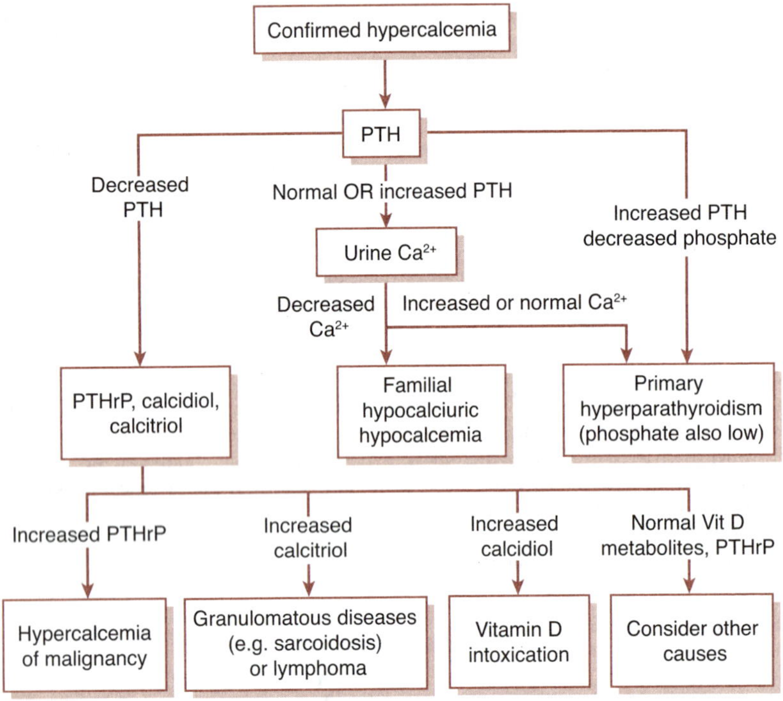

Figure 12-6 Diagnostic algorithm for hypercalcemia.

- Elevations in ECF calcium typically result in suppression of PTH. Thus, the finding of a normal or elevated intact PTH in the setting of hypercalcemia is suggestive of primary hyperparathyroidism.
- When the intact PTH is appropriately suppressed, **PTHrP** can be measured to investigate the possible humoral hypercalcemia of malignancy.

- $1,25(OH)_2D_3$ levels are elevated in granulomatous disorders, primary hyperparathyroidism, calcitriol overdose, and acromegaly; $25(OH)D_3$ levels are elevated with noncalcitriol vitamin D intoxication.
- **Serum phosphorus** is often decreased in hyperparathyroidism because of stimulation of phosphaturia, whereas Paget disease and vitamin D intoxication both tend to have increased phosphorus levels.
- **Urine calcium** may be elevated in primary hyperparathyroidism because of a filtered load of calcium that exceeds the capacity for renal reabsorption. If the family history and clinical picture are suggestive, patients with **familial hypocalciuric hypercalcemia** can be distinguished from patients with primary hyperparathyroidism by documenting a low calcium clearance by a 24-hour urine collection (<200 mg calcium per day) or fractional excretion of calcium (<1%).
- **ECG** may reveal a shortened QT interval and with very severe hypercalcemia, variable degrees of atrioventricular block.

TREATMENT

- **Acute management** of hypercalcemia is warranted if severe symptoms are present or with serum calcium >12 mg/dL. The following regimen is presented in the order that therapy should be given.
- **Correction of hypovolemia** with 0.9% saline fluid is mandatory in patients who demonstrate volume depletion, because hypovolemia prevents effective calciuresis. Maintenance fluids can be continued after achieving euvolemia to sustain a urine output of 100–150 mL/h. The patient should be monitored closely for signs of volume overload.
- Forced diuresis using LD may be considered once the volume status has been restored to normal, and is also useful in patients with underlying comorbidities such as heart failure or renal insufficiency to prevent volume overload.
- **IV bisphosphonates** can be used to decrease the liberation of calcium from bone in persistent hypercalcemia. Pamidronate 60 mg is infused over 2–4 hours; for severe hypercalcemia (>13.5 mg/dL), 90 mg can be given over the same duration. A hypocalcemic response is typically seen within 2 days and may persist for 2 weeks or longer. Treatment can be repeated after 7 days if hypercalcemia recurs. Zoledronate is a more potent bisphosphonate that is given as a 4 mg dose infused over at least 15 minutes. Hydration should precede bisphosphonate use. Renal insufficiency is a relative contraindication.
- Other options
  - **Calcitonin** inhibits bone resorption and increases renal calcium excretion. Salmon calcitonin, 4–8 IU/kg IM or SC q6–12h, lowers serum calcium 1–2 mg/dL within several hours in 60%–70% of patients. Although it is less potent than other inhibitors of bone resorption, it has no serious toxicity, is safe in renal failure, and may have an analgesic effect in patients with skeletal metastases. Also, calcitonin is better not administered for >3 days as tachyphylaxis can set in.
  - **Glucocorticoids** are effective in hypercalcemia because of hematologic malignancies and granulomatous production of calcitriol. The initial dose is 20–60 mg/d of prednisone or its equivalent. After serum calcium stabilizes, the dose should be gradually reduced to the minimum needed to control symptoms of hypercalcemia. Toxicity (see Chapter 25, Arthritis and Rheumatologic Diseases) limits the usefulness of glucocorticoids for long-term therapy.
  - **Denosumab** is a receptor activator of nuclear factor kappa-B ligand inhibitor that can be used in patients with hypercalcemia that is refractory to bisphosphonates or in patients with a contraindication to bisphosphonate therapy, such as patients with CKD. It is given at a dose of 120 mg SC weekly for 4 weeks and then monthly.
  - **Dialysis.** Hemodialysis and peritoneal dialysis using low calcium dialysate are effective for patients with very severe hypercalcemia (>16 mg/dL) and CHF or renal insufficiency.
- **Chronic management** of hypercalcemia
  - **Primary hyperparathyroidism.** In many patients, this disorder has a benign course, with minimal fluctuation in serum calcium concentration and no obvious clinical sequelae. Parathyroidectomy is indicated in patients with (1) corrected serum calcium >1.0 mg/dL above the upper limit of normal, (2) creatinine clearance <60 mL/min, (3) age <50 years, and (4) bone density at hip, lumbar spine, or distal radius >2.5 standard deviations below peak bone mass (T score <2.5) and/or previous fragility fracture.[5] Surgical intervention typically has a high success rate (95%) with low morbidity and mortality.
  - **Medical therapy** may be a reasonable option in asymptomatic patients who are not surgical candidates. Management consists of liberal oral hydration with a high-salt diet, daily physical activity to lessen bone resorption, and avoidance of TD. Oral bisphosphonates and estrogen replacement therapy or raloxifene in postmenopausal women can be considered in the appropriate clinical context. **Cinacalcet,** an activator of the

calcium-sensing receptor, has also been shown to reduce PTH secretion and serum calcium levels.

- **Malignant hypercalcemia.** Bisphosphonate and glucocorticoid therapy with a calcium-restricted diet (<400 mg/d) can be tried, although these maneuvers rarely yield long-term success unless the malignancy responds to treatment. **Denosumab** may be used in patients with persistent hypercalcemia of malignancy in whom bisphosphonates may be contraindicated because of renal failure.

Hypocalcemia

GENERAL PRINCIPLES

- A serum calcium **<8.4 mg/dL** with a normal serum albumin or an ionized calcium **<4.2 mg/dL** defines hypocalcemia.
- **Pseudohypocalcemia** describes the situation in which the total calcium is reduced because of hypoalbuminemia, but the **corrected** [Ca^{2+}] (see Calcium, Hypercalcemia, Diagnostic Testing section) and ionized calcium remain within the normal ranges.
- **Effective hypoparathyroidism.** Reduced PTH activity can result from decreased PTH release from autoimmune, infiltrative, HIV infection, or iatrogenic (e.g., post-thyroidectomy) destruction of parathyroid tissue. In rare patients, hypoparathyroidism is congenital, as in DiGeorge syndrome or **familial hypocalcemia.** Release of PTH is also impaired with both hypomagnesemia (<1 mg/dL) and severe hypermagnesemia (>6 mg/dL).
- **Vitamin D deficiency** lowers total body calcium, but does not usually affect serum calcium levels unless the deficiency is severe because the resultant secondary hyperparathyroidism often corrects serum calcium levels. Significant vitamin D deficiency can occur in the elderly or those with limited sun exposure, advanced liver disease (due to decreased synthesis of precursors), and nephrotic syndrome. Reduced activity in vitamin D activation via 1-α-hydroxylase activity can be seen with vitamin D-dependent rickets and chronic renal insufficiency.
- Serum calcium levels may also be reduced by profound elevations in serum phosphorus, which binds with the calcium and deposits in various tissues. Calcium can also be bound by citrate (during transfusion of citrate-containing blood products or with continual renal replacement using citrate anticoagulation) as well as by drugs such as foscarnet, bisphosphonates, cinacalcet, and fluoroquinolones. Increased binding to albumin can also be seen in the context of alkalemia, which increases the exposure of negatively charged binding sites on albumin.
- **Other.** A low serum-free calcium level is common in critically ill patients, perhaps due to a cytokine-mediated decrease in PTH and calcitriol release with target organ resistance to their effects.
- **Spurious hypocalcemia:** Gadolinium-based contrast agents gadodiamide and gadoversetamide interfere with the colorimetric assays for calcium, leading to false low values.

DIAGNOSIS

Clinical Presentation

- Clinical manifestations vary with the degree of hypocalcemia and rate of onset.
- Acute, severe hypocalcemia may cause laryngospasm, confusion, seizures, or vascular collapse with bradycardia and decompensated heart failure.
- Acute, moderate hypocalcemia may cause increased excitability of nerves and muscles, leading to circumoral or distal paresthesias and tetany.

- **Trousseau sign** is the development of carpal spasm when a blood pressure cuff is inflated above systolic pressure for 3 minutes. **Chvostek sign** refers to twitching of the facial muscles when the facial nerve is tapped anterior to the ear. The presence of these signs is known as **latent tetany.**
- Clues to the diagnosis may be provided by a bedside evaluation for (1) previous neck surgery (postoperative hypoparathyroidism), (2) systemic diseases (autoimmune, infiltrative disorders), (3) family history of hypocalcemia, (4) drug-induced hypocalcemia, and (5) conditions associated with vitamin D deficiency (e.g., uremia).

Diagnostic Testing

- Laboratory data should be used to evaluate the calcium-PTH axis as well as concurrent mineral abnormalities.
- **Albumin** should be measured when there is an abnormality in serum calcium levels to rule out pseudohypocalcemia, as mentioned earlier.
- **Serum PTH** that is low or inappropriately normal in the setting of hypocalcemia is indicative of hypoparathyroidism. A high PTH is often found with vitamin D deficiency, PTH resistance, and hyperphosphatemia.
- **Serum phosphorus** is often helpful in identifying vitamin D deficiency (low calcium, low phosphorus) or intravascular chelation of calcium (low calcium, high phosphorus).
- **Vitamin D** stores are usually assessed by measuring only $25(OH)D_3$ because calcitriol $[1,25(OH)_2D_3]$ levels can be normalized through the compensatory increase of 1-α-hydroxylase activity.
- **Magnesium** deficiency should always be ruled out during management of hypocalcemia.
- **ECG** may show a prolonged QT interval and bradycardia.

TREATMENT

Acute management of symptomatic hypocalcemia requires prompt and aggressive therapy.

- **Phosphorus** must first be checked. In severe hyperphosphatemia (>6.5 mg/dL), administration of calcium will increase the calcium–phosphorus product and may exacerbate the formation of ectopic calcifications. In acute, symptomatic hypocalcemia with severe hyperphosphatemia, dialysis may be needed to acutely manage the mineral abnormalities. If the hypocalcemia is asymptomatic, a reduction of phosphorus should precede aggressive calcium supplementation.
- **Hypomagnesemia,** if present, must be treated first to effectively correct the hypocalcemia. Two grams of magnesium sulfate can be given IV for over 15 minutes followed by an infusion (see Magnesium, Hypomagnesemia, Treatment section) and may even be given empirically if renal failure is not present.
- **Calcium supplementation.** IV calcium should be reserved for severe or symptomatic hypocalcemia and can be administered as calcium chloride or calcium gluconate. Calcium gluconate is typically favored because of reduced risk of tissue toxicity with extravasation. Calcium gluconate is often prepared as a 10% solution (100 mg of calcium gluconate per mL). One ampule (10 mL) of calcium gluconate thus contains 1000 mg of calcium gluconate and approximately 90 mg of elemental calcium.
  - When it is necessary to treat severe (<7.5 mg%) or symptomatic hypocalcemia (carpopedal spasm, QT prolongation), an initial dose of 90–180 mg of elemental calcium can be achieved with 1–2 g of **calcium gluconate** (equal to 10–20 mL or one to two ampules of 10% calcium gluconate) mixed in 50–100 mL of D5W administered over 10–20 minutes.
  - The effect of initial treatment is only *transient*, and maintenance of calcium levels typically requires a continuous infusion of 0.5–1.5 mg/kg/h of elemental calcium. A solution comprised 1 L D5W with 100 mL of 10% calcium gluconate contains approximately 900 mg of elemental calcium per liter, approximating 1 mg of elemental

calcium per milliliter of fluid. Infusion is typically begun at a rate of 50 mL/h (approximately 50 mg of elemental calcium per hour) and titrated up as needed.

- **Chronic management.** Treatment requires calcium supplements and vitamin D or its active metabolite to increase intestinal calcium absorption.
  - **Oral calcium supplements.** Calcium carbonate (40% elemental calcium) or calcium acetate (25% elemental calcium) can be given with the goal administration of 1–2 g of *elemental* calcium PO tid. Calcium supplementation should be given apart from meals to minimize binding with phosphorus and maximize enteric absorption. Serum levels should be checked once to twice per week to guide ongoing therapy.
  - **Vitamin D.** Simple dietary deficiency can be corrected by the use of ergocalciferol 400–1000 IU/d. However, in conjunction with other hypocalcemic disorders, larger doses may be required. A 6- to 8-week regimen of 50,000 IU should be dosed weekly in those with underlying impairments in vitamin D metabolism (i.e., renal insufficiency) and daily in patients with severe malnutrition or malabsorption.
  - In comparison, **calcitriol** has a much more rapid onset of action. The initial dosage is 0.25 μg daily, and most patients are maintained on 0.5–2.0 μg daily. The dose can be increased at 2- to 4-week intervals. Because calcitriol increases enteric absorption of phosphorus as well as calcium, phosphorus levels should be monitored and oral phosphate binders initiated if phosphorus exceeds the normal range.
- In the setting of chronic kidney disease (CKD) with hypocalcemia, hyperphosphatemia, and high PTH (secondary hyperparathyroidism), administration of calcium may cause pathological vascular calcification; hence, one must be careful in such a scenario.

COMPLICATIONS

Development of hypercalcemia. In the event that hypercalcemia develops, vitamin D and calcium supplements should be stopped. Once serum calcium falls to normal, both forms of supplementation should be restarted at lower doses. Hypercalcemia due to calcitriol usually resolves within 1 week.

PHOSPHORUS

- Phosphorus is critical for bone formation and cellular energy metabolism.
- Approximately 85% of **total body phosphorus** is in the bone and most of the remainder is within the cells. Thus, serum phosphorus levels may not reflect total body phosphorus stores.
- **Phosphorus balance** is determined primarily by four factors:
  - **PTH** regulates the incorporation and release of minerals from bone stores and decreases proximal tubular reabsorption of phosphate, causing urinary wasting.
  - The **phosphate concentration** itself regulates renal proximal reabsorption.
  - **Insulin** lowers serum levels by shifting phosphate into cells.
  - **Calcitriol** [$1,25(OH)_2D_3$] increases serum phosphate by enhancing intestinal phosphorus absorption.

Hyperphosphatemia

GENERAL PRINCIPLES

- A serum phosphate **>4.5 mg/dL** defines hyperphosphatemia.
- **Hyperphosphatemia** is caused by (1) **transcellular shift**, (2) **increased intake**, and most commonly, (3) **decreased renal excretion**. In clinical practice, renal insufficiency is usually present and serves as the major predisposing factor toward the development of hyperphosphatemia.

- **Transcellular shift** occurs in rhabdomyolysis, tumor lysis syndrome, and massive hemolysis as phosphorus is released from cells into the ECF. Metabolic acidosis (lactic/keto) and hypoinsulinemia reduce phosphorus flux into cells and contribute to the hyperphosphatemia sometimes seen in DKA.
- **Increased intake** leading to hyperphosphatemia usually occurs in the setting of renal insufficiency, either with dietary indiscretion in chronic kidney disease or as an iatrogenic complication. The latter can be seen when Phospho-Soda enemas (e.g., Fleet) or active vitamin D analogs are given to patients with renal insufficiency.
- **Decreased renal excretion** occurs most commonly in the setting of renal failure (acute and chronic). Occasionally, hypoparathyroidism and pseudohypoparathyroidism reduce renal phosphorus clearance as well.

DIAGNOSIS

Clinical Presentation

- Signs and symptoms are typically attributable to hypocalcemia and the metastatic calcification of soft tissues. Occasionally, skin deposition can result in severe pruritus. **Calciphylaxis** describes the tissue ischemia that may result from the calcification of smaller blood vessels and their subsequent thrombosis.
- Chronic hyperphosphatemia contributes to the development of renal osteodystrophy (see Chapter 13, Renal Diseases).

Diagnostic Testing

The elevated serum phosphorus can be accompanied by hypocalcemia as a result of **intravascular chelation** of calcium by phosphorus.

TREATMENT

- **Acute hyperphosphatemia** is treated by increasing renal excretion of phosphorus, and as such, treatment is limited when renal insufficiency is present.
  - **Recovery of renal function** will often correct the hyperphosphatemia in the patient within 12 hours. Saline and/or acetazolamide (15 mg/kg q4h) can be given to further encourage phosphaturia, if needed.
  - **Hemodialysis** may be required, especially if irreversible renal insufficiency or symptomatic hypocalcemia is present.
- **Chronic hyperphosphatemia** is almost always associated with chronic kidney disease. Its management consists of reducing phosphorus intake through dietary modification and the use of phosphate binders (discussed more in detail in Chapter 13, Renal Diseases).

Hypophosphatemia

GENERAL PRINCIPLES

- A serum phosphate **<2.8 mg/dL** defines hypophosphatemia.
- Hypophosphatemia may be caused by (1) **impaired intestinal absorption**, (2) **increased renal excretion**, or (3) **transcellular shift** into cells. Often, there are several mechanisms that work in concert to lower serum phosphate.
  - **Impaired intestinal absorption** occurs with the malabsorption syndromes, the use of oral phosphate binders, or vitamin D, deficiency from any cause (see Calcium, Hypocalcemia, Etiology section). Chronic alcoholism is often associated with poor intake of both phosphate and vitamin D, resulting in total body phosphorus depletion.

- **Increased renal excretion** occurs with high levels of PTH, as seen in hyperparathyroidism. This can be particularly pronounced in patients with secondary or tertiary hyperparathyroidism who undergo renal transplantation, because the high PTH causes a profound phosphaturic effect on the functional allograft. Hypophosphatemia may also occur from osmotic diuresis and disorders of proximal tubular transport such as familial X-linked hypophosphatemic rickets and Fanconi syndrome. In acutely ill patients on continuous renal replacement therapy, the removal of phosphorous by slow continuous dialysis can also result in hypophosphatemia.
- **Transcellular shift** is stimulated by respiratory alkalosis as well as insulin. The latter is responsible for the paradoxical reduction in phosphorus during treatment of malnutrition with hyperalimentation (the refeeding syndrome). The endogenous increase in insulin during treatment shifts phosphorus intracellularly, further reducing serum phosphorus in the malnourished individual. Phosphorus can also be rapidly absorbed into bone following parathyroidectomy for severe hyperparathyroidism (hungry bone syndrome).

DIAGNOSIS

Clinical Presentation

Signs and symptoms typically occur only if total body phosphate depletion is present and the serum phosphorus level is <1 mg/dL. These end-organ effects are due to the inability to form adenosine triphosphate and the impaired tissue oxygen delivery that occurs with a decrease in red blood cell 2,3-diphosphoglycerate. These include muscle injury (rhabdomyolysis, impaired diaphragmatic function, and heart failure), neurologic abnormalities (paresthesias, dysarthria, delirium, stupor, seizures, and coma), and rarely, hemolysis and platelet dysfunction (defective clot retraction).

Diagnostic Testing

- The cause is usually apparent from the clinical situation in which the hypophosphatemia occurs. If not, measurement of **urine phosphorus excretion** helps define the mechanism. Renal excretion of >100 mg by the 24-hour urine collection or a fractional excretion of phosphate >5% during hypophosphatemia indicates excessive renal loss.
- Low serum **25(OH)D_3** suggests dietary vitamin D deficiency or malabsorption. An elevated **intact PTH** may occur in primary or secondary hyperparathyroidism.

TREATMENT

- **Acute moderate hypophosphatemia** (1.0–2.5 mg/dL) is common in the hospitalized patient and is often due simply to **transcellular shifts**, requiring no treatment if asymptomatic, except correction of the underlying cause.
- **Acute severe hypophosphatemia** (<1.0 mg/dL) may require IV phosphate therapy when associated with serious clinical manifestations. IV preparations include potassium phosphate (1.5 mEq potassium/mmol phosphate) and sodium phosphate (1.3 mEq sodium/mmol phosphate).
  - An infusion of phosphate, 0.08–0.16 mmol/kg in 500 mL 0.45% saline, is given via IV for over 6 hours (1 mmol phosphate = 31 mg phosphorus). IV repletion should be stopped when the serum phosphorus level is >1.5 mg/dL and when the patient can tolerate oral therapy. Because of the need to replenish intracellular stores, 24–36 hours of phosphate administration may be required.
  - Extreme care must be taken to avoid hyperphosphatemia, which may lead to hypocalcemia. If hypotension occurs, acute hypocalcemia should be suspected, and the infusion

should be stopped or slowed. Further doses should be based on symptoms and on the serum calcium and phosphorus levels, which should be measured every 8 hours.

- **Chronic hypophosphatemia.** Vitamin D deficiency, if present, should be treated first (see Calcium, Hypocalcemia, Treatment section), followed by oral supplementation of 0.5–1.0 g elemental phosphorus PO bid to tid. Preparations include Neutra-Phos (250 mg elemental phosphorus and 7 mEq of Na+ and K+ per capsule) and Neutra-Phos K+ (250 mg elemental phosphorus and 14 mEq K+ per capsule). Contents of the capsules should be dissolved in water. Fleet Phospho-Soda (815 mg phosphorus and 33 mEq sodium per 5 mL) is an alternative oral agent. Limiting side effects include nausea and diarrhea.

MAGNESIUM

- **Magnesium** plays an important role in the neuromuscular function.
- Approximately 60% of body magnesium is stored in the bones, and most of the remainder is found in cells. Only 1% is in the ECF. As a result, the serum magnesium is a poor predictor of intracellular and total body stores and may grossly underestimate total magnesium deficits.
- The main determinant of magnesium balance is the **magnesium concentration** itself, which directly influences renal excretion. Hypomagnesemia stimulates tubular reabsorption of magnesium, whereas hypermagnesemia inhibits it.

Hypermagnesemia

GENERAL PRINCIPLES

- A serum magnesium **>2.2 mEq/L** defines hypermagnesemia.
- Most cases of clinically significant hypermagnesemia are iatrogenic, occurring with large doses of magnesium-containing antacids or laxatives and during treatment of preeclampsia with IV magnesium. Because renal excretion is the only means of lowering serum magnesium levels, the presence of significant renal insufficiency can lead to magnesium toxicity even with therapeutic doses of these antacids and laxatives.
- Mild, insignificant elevations in magnesium can occur in end-stage renal disease patients, theophylline intoxication, DKA, and tumor lysis syndrome.

DIAGNOSIS

Clinical Presentation

- Signs and symptoms are usually seen when the serum magnesium level is >4 mEq/L.
- Neuromuscular abnormalities usually include hyporeflexia (usually the first sign of magnesium toxicity), lethargy, and weakness that can progress to paralysis and diaphragmatic involvement, leading to respiratory failure (serum levels >15 mEq/L).
- Cardiac findings include hypotension, bradycardia, and cardiac arrest.

Diagnostic Testing

The **ECG** may reveal bradycardia and prolonged PR, QRS, and QT intervals with magnesium levels of 5–10 mEq/L. Complete heart block or asystole may eventually ensue with levels >15 mEq/L.

TREATMENT

- **Prevention.** In the setting of significant renal insufficiency, the inadvertent administration of magnesium-containing medications (e.g., Maalox, magnesium citrate) should be avoided.
- **Asymptomatic hypermagnesemia.** In the setting of normal renal function, normal magnesium levels will quickly be attained with the removal of the magnesium load.
- **Symptomatic hypermagnesemia**
  - Prompt supportive therapy is critical, including mechanical ventilation for respiratory failure and a temporary pacemaker for significant bradyarrhythmias.
  - The effects of hypermagnesemia can be antagonized quickly by the administration of 10% calcium gluconate 10–20 mL IV (1–2 g) for over 10 minutes.
  - Renal excretion can be encouraged with saline administration.
  - With significant renal insufficiency, hemodialysis is required for definitive therapy.

Hypomagnesemia

GENERAL PRINCIPLES

- A serum magnesium **<1.3 mEq/L** defines hypomagnesemia.
- Hypomagnesemia is most commonly caused by impaired intestinal absorption and increased renal excretion.
  - **Decreased intestinal absorption** occurs in malnutrition, as is common in chronic alcoholics or any malabsorption syndrome. Magnesium can also be lost through prolonged diarrhea and nasogastric aspiration. Hypomagnesemia has been described with chronic use of proton pump inhibitors, presumably due to impaired intestinal absorption.
  - **Increased renal excretion** of magnesium can occur from increased renal tubular flow (as occurs with osmotic diuresis) as well as impaired tubular function (as seen with resolving acute tubular necrosis, LD, Bartter, Gitelman, and EAST [epilepsy, ataxia, sensorineural deafness, mental retardation, and a renal salt-losing tubulopathy]) syndromes.
- **Drugs.** Several medications similarly induce defects in tubular magnesium transport, including aminoglycosides, amphotericin B, cisplatin, pentamidine, and cyclosporine.

DIAGNOSIS

Clinical Presentation

- Neurologic manifestations include lethargy, confusion, tremor, fasciculations, ataxia, nystagmus, tetany, and seizures.
- Atrial and ventricular arrhythmias may occur, especially in patients treated with digoxin.

Diagnostic Testing

- Low serum [Mg^{2+}] in conjunction with an appropriate clinical scenario is sufficient to establish the diagnosis of **magnesium deficiency**. However, because of the slow exchange of magnesium between the bone and intracellular pools (see Magnesium section), a normal serum level does not exclude total body **magnesium deficiency**.
- The etiology of hypomagnesemia usually is evident from the clinical context, but if there is uncertainty, measurement of **urine magnesium excretion** is helpful. A 24-hour urine magnesium of >2 mEq (or >24 mg) or a fractional excretion of magnesium of >2% during hypomagnesemia suggests **increased renal excretion**. The fractional excretion of magnesium is calculated by

$$(\text{Urine Mg}^{2+}/\text{Urine Cr}) \div [(\text{Serum Mg}^{2+} \times 0.7)/\text{Serum Cr}] \times 100$$

- Hypocalcemia (see Calcium, Hypocalcemia, Etiology section) and/or hypokalemia (see Potassium, Hypokalemia, Etiology section) can often be found as a result of hypomagnesemia-induced derangements in mineral homeostasis.
- ECG abnormalities may include a prolonged PR and QT interval with a widened QRS. **Torsades de pointes** is the classically associated arrhythmia.

TREATMENT

- In patients with normal renal function, excess magnesium is readily excreted, and there is little risk of causing hypermagnesemia with recommended doses. However, *magnesium must be given with extreme care in the presence of renal insufficiency.*
- The route of magnesium administration depends on whether clinical manifestations from magnesium deficiency are present.
  - **Asymptomatic hypomagnesemia** can be treated orally. Numerous preparations exist, including Mag-Ox 400 (240 mg elemental magnesium per 400 mg tablet), UroMag (84 mg per 140 mg tablet), and sustained-release Slow-Mag (64 mg per tablet). Typically, approximately 240 mg of elemental magnesium is administered daily for mild deficiency, whereas more severe hypomagnesemia may require up to 720 mg/d of elemental magnesium. The major side effect is diarrhea. Normalization of serum magnesium levels can be deceiving, because the administered magnesium slowly shifts to replete intracellular and bone stores. Furthermore, abrupt increases in serum levels stimulate renal excretion. Thus, serum levels should be followed closely and replacement should be maintained until patients demonstrate stable normalization of serum magnesium concentrations.
  - **Severe symptomatic hypomagnesemia** should be treated with 1–2 g magnesium sulfate (1 g magnesium sulfate = 96 mg elemental magnesium) IV for over 15 minutes. To account for gradual redistribution to severely depleted intracellular stores, replacement therapy may need to be maintained, often for 3–7 days. Serum magnesium should be measured daily and the infusion rate adjusted to maintain a serum magnesium level of <2.5 mEq/L. Tendon reflexes should be tested frequently because hyporeflexia suggests hypermagnesemia. Reduced doses and more frequent monitoring must be used even in mild renal insufficiency.

ACID–BASE DISTURBANCES

GENERAL PRINCIPLES

- The normal ECF **pH is 7.40 ± 0.03.** Perturbations in pH can occur with changes in the ratio of $[HCO_3^-]$ to partial pressure of carbon dioxide (pCO_2) (as described by the **Henderson–Hasselbalch equation**):

$$pH = 6.1 + \log([HCO_3^-] \div [pCO_2 \times 0.3])$$

- Maintenance of pH is essential for normal cellular function. Three general mechanisms exist to keep it within a narrow window:
  - **Chemical buffering** is mediated by $[HCO_3^-]$ in the ECF and by protein and phosphate buffers in the ICF. The normal $[HCO_3^-]$ is 24 ± 2 mEq/L.
  - **Alveolar ventilation** minimizes variations in the pH by altering the pCO_2. The normal pCO_2 is 40 ± 5 mm Hg.
  - **Renal H^+ handling** allows the kidney to adapt to changes in acid–base status via $[HCO_3^-]$ reabsorption and excretion of titratable acid (e.g., $H_2PO_4^-$) and NH_4^+.

- **Acidemia and alkalemia** refer to processes that lower and raise pH, regardless of mechanism. They can be caused by metabolic or respiratory disturbances:
  - **Metabolic acidosis** is characterized by a decrease in the plasma $[HCO_3^-]$ due to either HCO_3^- loss or the accumulation of acid.
  - **Metabolic alkalosis** is characterized by an elevation in the plasma $[HCO_3^-]$ due to either H^+ loss or HCO_3^- gain.
  - **Respiratory acidosis** is characterized by an elevation in pCO_2 resulting from alveolar hypoventilation.
  - **Respiratory alkalosis** is characterized by a decrease in pCO_2 resulting from hyperventilation.

DIAGNOSIS

Analysis should be systematic so that accurate conclusions are drawn and appropriate therapy initiated. Once the acid–base process is correctly identified, further diagnostic studies may be undertaken to determine the precise etiologies at play.

- **Step 1.** Check arterial blood gas. Acidemia is present when pH is <7.37 and alkalemia when pH >7.43.
- **Step 2.** Establish the primary disturbance by determining whether the change in $[HCO_3^-]$ or pCO_2 can account for the observed deflection in pH.
  - In acidemia, a decreased $[HCO_3^-]$ suggests metabolic acidosis and an elevated pCO_2 suggests respiratory acidosis. In alkalemia, an elevated $[HCO_3^-]$ suggests metabolic alkalosis, whereas a decreased pCO_2 suggests respiratory alkalosis.
  - A **combined disorder** is present when pH is normal, but the pCO_2 and $[HCO_3^-]$ are both abnormal. Changes in both pCO_2 and $[HCO_3^-]$ can cause the change in pH.
- **Step 3.** Determine whether compensation is appropriate.
  - The **compensatory mechanism** is an adaptation to the primary acid–base disturbance intended to stabilize the changing pH. A respiratory process that shifts the pH in one direction will be compensated by a metabolic process that shifts the pH in the other and vice versa.
  - The effect of compensation is to attenuate *but not completely correct* the primary change in pH.
  - The expected compensations for the various primary acid–base derangements are given in Table 12-9.
  - An inappropriate compensatory response suggests the presence of a combined disorder.
  - Example: In a patient with metabolic acidosis, respiratory compensation attenuates the metabolic disturbance to pH by lowering pCO_2. However, if the pCO_2 is higher than expected, respiratory compensation is insufficient, revealing a respiratory acidosis with the primary metabolic acidosis. If pCO_2 is lower than expected, compensation is excessive, revealing a concomitant respiratory alkalosis.
- **Step 4.** Determine the **anion gap (AG)**.
  - In normal individuals, the total serum cations are balanced with the total serum anions. Total cations comprise measured cations (MCs) and unmeasured cations, whereas total anions comprise measured anions (MAs) and unmeasured anions (UAs). Certain forms of acidosis are characterized by an increase in the pool of UAs. The **AG** is merely a way of demonstrating the accumulation of this UA.
  - $AG = [NH^+] - [Cl^-] + [HCO_3^-]$. The normal AG is 10 ± 2 mEq/L.

$$\begin{aligned} AG &= \text{the excess of unmeasured anions (vs. unmeasured cations)} \\ &= UA - UC \end{aligned}$$

Because total cations = total anions:

$$MC + UC = MA + UA$$

TABLE 12-9 Expected Compensatory Responses to Primary Acid–Base Disorders

Disorder	Primary Change	Compensatory Response	Limits of Compensation
Metabolic acidosis	↓ $[HCO_3^-]$	↓ pCO_2 1.2 mm Hg for every 1 mEq/L ↓ $[HCO_3^-]$ OR pCO_2 = last two digits of pH	$[PCO_2]$ = 15 mm Hg
Metabolic alkalosis	↑ $[HCO_3^-]$	↑ pCO_2 0.7 mm Hg for every 1 mEq/L ↑ $[HCO_3^-]$	$[PCO_2]$ = 55 mm Hg
Respiratory acidosis	↑ pCO_2		
Acute		↑ $[HCO_3^-]$ 1.0 mEq/L for every 10 mm Hg pCO_2	$[HCO_3^-]$ = 38 mEq/L
Chronic		↑ $[HCO_3^-]$ 3.5 mEq/L for every 10 mm Hg ↑ pCO_2	$[HCO_3^-]$ = 45 mEq/L
Respiratory alkalosis	↓ pCO_2		
Acute		↓ $[HCO_3^-]$ 2.0 mEq/L for every 10 mm Hg ↓ pCO_2	$[HCO_3^-]$ = 18 mEq/L
Chronic		↓ $[HCO_3^-]$ 5.0 mEq/L for every 10 mm Hg ↓ pCO_2	$[HCO_3^-]$ = 15 mEq/L

Rearranging the equation:

$$MC + UC = MA + UA$$

MCs are Na^+; MAs are Cl^- and HCO_3^-.

- Because albumin is the principal UA, the AG should be corrected if there are gross changes in serum albumin levels.

$$\mathbf{AG_{correct} = AG + \{(4\text{-}[albumin]) \times 2.5\}}$$

- An elevated AG suggests the presence of metabolic acidosis with a circulating anion (Table 12-10).

- **Step 5.** Assess the delta gap.
  - To maintain a stable total anion content, every increase in an UA should be met with a decrease in HCO_3^-. Comparing the change in the AG (ΔAG) with the change in the $[HCO_3^-]$ ($\Delta[HCO_3^-]$) is a simple way of making sure that each change in the AG is accounted for.
  - If the $\Delta AG = \Delta[HCO_3^-]$, this is a simple AG metabolic acidosis.
  - If the $\Delta AG > \Delta[HCO_3^-]$, $\Delta[HCO_3^-]$ did not decrease as much as expected. This is a metabolic alkalosis **and** AG metabolic acidosis.
    Example: A patient with DKA has been vomiting before admission. He has an AG of 20 and an $\Delta[HCO_3^-]$ of 20. His ΔAG = 10 and $\Delta[HCO_3^-]$ = 4, revealing an AG metabolic acidosis (DKA) with a metabolic alkalosis (vomiting).
- If the $\Delta AG < \Delta[HCO_3^-]$, $[HCO_3^-]$ decreased more than expected. This is a nongap metabolic acidosis **and** AG metabolic acidosis.

TABLE 12-10 The Four Primary Acid–Base Disorders and Their Common Etiologies

	Acidosis	Alkalosis
Metabolic	Gap • Ketoacids (starvation, alcoholic, diabetic) • Exposures (methanol, ethylene glycol, salicylates) • Lactic acid (shock, drug related) • Profound uremia	Generation • Loss of H^+-rich fluids (GI loss) • Contraction alkalosis • Alkali administration
	Nongap • Nonrenal HCO_3^- loss (diarrhea) • Renal $HCO_3$2 loss (type 2 RTA) • ↓ H secretion (type 1 RTA) • Hypoaldosteronism (type 4 RTA)	Maintenance • Volume contraction • Chloride depletion • Hypokalemia
Respiratory	Depression of respiratory center Neuromuscular failure Lung disease	CNS stimulation Hypoxemia Anxiety

	Type 1 RTA	Type 2 RTA	Type 4 RTA
Serum [K]	↓ or nl	↓ or nl	↑
Serum $[HCO_3]$	<10	15–20	>15
Urine pH	>5.3	Varies	<5.3

CNS, central nervous system; GI, gastrointestinal; nl, normal; RTA, renal tubular acidosis.

Example: A patient is admitted with fevers and hypotension after a prolonged course of diarrhea. She has an AG of 15 and an $[HCO_3^-]$ of 12. Her ΔAG is 5 and her $\Delta[HCO_3^-]$ is 12, revealing a nongap metabolic acidosis (diarrhea) and an AG metabolic acidosis (lactic acidosis).

- **Step 6**. Urine anion gap (discussed later).
- **NOTE**
  - Even in the presence of normal pH:
    - *Abnormal PCO_2 and HCO_3 is a telltale evidence of acid–base disorder.*
    - *Abnormal serum AG suggests the presence of an acid–base disorder.*
    - *Suspect an acid–base disorder if K is abnormal.*

Metabolic Acidosis

GENERAL PRINCIPLES

- The causes of a metabolic acidosis can be divided into those that cause an **elevated AG** and those with a **normal AG**. Many of the causes seen in clinical practices can be found in Table 12-10.
- AG acidosis results from exposure to acids, which contribute an UA to the ECF. Common causes are DKA, lactic acidosis, and toxic alcohol ingestions.

- Non–AG acidosis can result from the loss of [HCO_3^-] from the GI tract. Renal causes due to renal excretion of [HCO_3^-] or disorders of renal acid handling are referred to collectively as **RTAs.**
- Enteric [HCO_3^-] loss occurs most commonly in the setting of severe diarrhea.
- The three forms of RTA (Table 12-11) correlate with the three mechanisms that facilitate renal acid handling: proximal bicarbonate reabsorption, distal H^+ secretion, and generation of NH_3, the principle urinary buffer. Urinary buffers reduce the concentration of free H^+ in the filtrate, thus attenuating the back leak of H^+, which occurs at low urinary pH.
  - **Proximal (type 2) RTA** is caused by impaired proximal tubular HCO_3^- reabsorption. Causes include inherited mutations (cystinosis), heavy metals, drugs (tenofovir, ifosfamide, carbonic anhydrase inhibitors), and multiple myeloma and other monoclonal gammopathies.
  - **Distal (type 1) RTA** results from impaired distal H^+ secretion. This may occur because of impairment in H^+ secretion, as seen with a variety of autoimmune (Sjögren syndrome, lupus, rheumatoid arthritis) or renal disorders. Hypercalciuria is another main cause of distal RTA in adults. It can also be caused by a back leak of H^+ due to increased membrane permeability, as seen with amphotericin B.
  - **Distal hyperkalemic (type 4) RTA** may result from either low aldosterone levels or from aldosterone resistance. The resulting hyperkalemia reduces the availability of NH_3 to buffer urinary H^+. Hyporeninemic hypoaldosteronism is seen with some frequency in patients with diabetes. Certain drugs, including NSAIDs, β-blockers, and cyclosporine, have also been implicated.

TABLE 12-11 Overview of Renal Tubular Acidosis

	Type 1 RTA (Distal RTA)	Type 2 RTA (Proximal RTA)	Type 4 RTA (Hyperkalemic RTA)
Incidence	Rare	Very rare	Common
Pathophysiology	Inability of the intercalated cells of the distal tubule to secrete H^+	Inability of the proximal convoluted tubule cells to reabsorb HCO_3^-	Aldosterone deficiency and/or resistance
Serum potassium levels	Decreased or normal	Decreased or normal	Increased
Urine pH	>5.3	<5.3	<5.3
Urine anion gap	Positive	Negative	Positive
Calcium excretion	↑	Normal	Normal or ↓
Bone involvement	Bone demineralization without overt rickets or osteomalacia	Vitamin D-resistant rickets/ osteomalacia	Bone demineralization without overt rickets or osteomalacia
Nephrolithiasis	Usually present	Absent	Absent
Treatment	Alkali therapy with sodium bicarbonate or sodium citrate	Alkali therapy with orally administered potassium citrate	Furosemide Fludrocortisone Low potassium diet

- Occasionally, the kidney is unable to secrete sufficient H^+ because of an impaired luminal gradient. In these situations, poor filtrate delivery or impaired Na^+ reabsorption in the distal nephron is responsible for decreasing the voltage gradient, which augments H^+ secretion. This can be seen with marked volume depletion, urinary tract obstruction, sickle cell nephropathy, and amiloride or triamterene use.

DIAGNOSIS

The first step in narrowing the differential diagnosis for a metabolic acidosis is to calculate the **AG**.

- The specific cause of an **elevated AG** can usually be determined by clinical history. However, specific laboratory studies are available to identify certain anions such as lactate, acetoacetate, acetone, and β-hydroxybutyrate. (It should be noted that the use of nitroprusside to detect ketones may fail to identify ketoacidosis due to β-hydroxybutyrate.) The presence of alcohol (methanol, ethanol, ethylene glycol) can also be determined with laboratory assays. Clinical suspicion for toxic alcohol ingestion is corroborated by an increased **osmolal gap**. This gap is the difference between measured and calculated serum osmolality:

$$[\text{Osm}]_{\text{meas}} - \{([\text{Na}^+] \times 2) + ([\text{glucose}] \div 18) + ([\text{BUN}] \div 2.8)\}$$

- If a **normal AG** is present, the GI HCO_3^- losses can be differentiated from RTAs via the **urine anion gap** (UAG). The **UAG** is the difference between the major measured anions and cations in urine: $[Na^+]_u + [K^+]_u - [Cl^-]_u$. Because Na^+_4 is the major unmeasured urinary cation, a negative UAG reflects high Na^+_4 excretion, an appropriate response to a metabolic acidosis. Conversely, a positive UAG signifies low Na^+_4 excretion, which in the face of a metabolic acidosis suggests a defect in distal renal acidification.
- Serum $[K^+]$ and urine pH can be helpful in distinguishing between the RTAs.
  - Types 1 and 2 are typically associated with hypokalemia, whereas type 4 is characterized by hyperkalemia.
  - Urine pH is low (usually <5.3) in type 4 RTA, because the defect is in the generation of the NH_3 buffer and the mechanism for H^+ secretion is intact. In contrast, urine pH is inappropriately high in type 1 RTA (urine pH >5.3). In type 2 RTA, urine pH is variable. It is elevated during the initial bicarbonaturia, when filtered bicarbonate exceeds the threshold for reabsorption and low when the filtered load is below this threshold.

TREATMENT

- **Ketoacidosis** attributable to ethanol abuse and starvation can be corrected with the resumption of caloric intake through oral intake or dextrose-containing fluids and by correction of any volume depletion that may be present. The treatment of DKA is described in Chapter 23, Diabetes Mellitus and Related Disorders.
- **Lactic acidosis** will resolve once the underlying cause is treated and tissue perfusion is restored. Often, this involves aggressive therapeutic maneuvers for the treatment of shock as described in Chapter 8, Critical Care. The administration of alkali does not appear to have clear benefit in lactic acidosis and may lead to rebound metabolic alkalosis once the underlying cause is managed. Its use in dire circumstances or severe acidosis remains controversial.
- Management of toxic ingestions is described in Chapter 28, Toxicology.
- **Normal AG metabolic acidosis.** Treatment with $NaHCO_3$ is appropriate for patients with a normal AG metabolic acidosis. The HCO_3^- deficit can be calculated in mEq:

$$HCO_3^- \text{ deficit} = \{0.5 \times \text{lean weight} \times [24 - (HCO_3^-)]\}$$

However, this assumes a volume of distribution equal to 50% of total body weight. In reality, the distribution of HCO_3^- increases with the severity of the acidosis and may exceed 100% of total body weight in very severe acidosis. It should be noted that the standard 650 mg tablet of oral $NaHCO_3$ provides only 7 mEq of HCO_3^-, whereas one ampule of IV $NaHCO_3$ contains 50 mEq. Still, parenteral $NaHCO_3$ should always be prescribed with caution because of the potential adverse effects, including pulmonary edema, hypokalemia, and hypocalcemia.

- **Treatment of the RTAs.** Correction of the chronic acidemia with alkali administration is warranted to prevent its catabolic effect on bone and muscle.
  - In *distal (type 1) RTA*, correction of the metabolic acidosis requires oral HCO_3^- replacement to the order of 1–2 mEq/kg/d with $NaHCO_3$ or sodium citrate. Potassium citrate replacement may be necessary for patients with hypokalemia, nephrolithiasis, or nephrocalcinosis. Underlying conditions should be sought and treated.
  - In *proximal (type 2) RTA*, much larger amounts of alkali (10–15 mEq/kg/d) are required to reverse the acidosis. Administration of potassium salts minimizes the degree of hypokalemia associated with alkali therapy.
  - Management of *type 4 RTA* requires correction of the underlying hyperkalemia. This consists of dietary K^+ restriction (40–60 mEq/d) and possibly LDs with or without oral $NaHCO_3$ (0.5–1 mEq/kg/d). Mineralocorticoid administration (fludrocortisone, 50–200 μg PO daily) should be used in patients with primary adrenal insufficiency and may be considered in other causes of hypoaldosteronism.

Metabolic Alkalosis

GENERAL PRINCIPLES

- Development of a persistent metabolic alkalosis requires both generation (an inciting cause) and maintenance (a persistent impairment of the corrective renal response).
- Generation often occurs with a primary increase in the plasma HCO_3^- and may be due to either **HCO_3^- gain** from alkali administration or more commonly, **excessive H^+ loss.** The latter may result from the loss of H^+-rich fluids, including upper GI secretions. **Contraction alkalosis** refers to the contraction of volume around a fixed content of bicarbonate.
- Maintenance requires a concomitant impairment in renal HCO_3^- excretion because the kidney normally has a large capacity to excrete HCO_3^-. This occurs as a result of a **decreased glomerular filtration rate** or enhanced tubular HCO_3^- reabsorption from **chloride depletion, volume contraction**, and **hypokalemia.** A decrease in filtered chloride is sensed by the macula densa and as a result of tubuloglomerular feedback, reduces filtered HCO_3^- and stimulates aldosterone release. It also limits adaptive distal HCO_3^- secretion. Metabolic alkalosis is often described as being **chloride responsive** or **chloride unresponsive**.

DIAGNOSIS

Clinical Presentation

- Because key causes of metabolic alkalosis are related to volume contraction, patients may present with signs of volume depletion. Occasionally, patients demonstrate hypertension or mild ECF expansion as a result of mineralocorticoid excess.

Diagnostic Testing

- The etiology of metabolic alkalosis is often obvious from the history. Common causes include loss of upper GI secretions through vomiting or excessive urinary H^+ loss from diuretics.

- Urine electrolytes are generally useful in identifying the etiology of a metabolic alkalosis when the history and physical examination are unrevealing.
  - A **urine** $[Cl^-]$ <20 mEq/L is consistent with **chloride-responsive** metabolic alkalosis and usually indicates volume depletion. A urine $[Cl^-]$ >20 mEq/L indicates a chloride-unresponsive cause (see Table 12-10).
  - Urine $[Na^+]$ is not reliable in predicting the effective circulating volume in these conditions because *bicarbonaturia obligates renal* Na^+ *loss* even in volume depletion.
- **Serum potassium** levels are often low in metabolic alkalosis because of transcellular shifts. Furthermore, hypokalemia contributes to alkalosis by increasing tubular H^+ secretion and Cl^- wasting.

TREATMENT

- **Chloride-responsive** metabolic alkaloses are most effectively treated with saline resuscitation until euvolemia is achieved. The increase in filtered chloride leads to improved renal handling of the bicarbonate load.
- **Chloride-unresponsive** metabolic alkaloses do not respond to saline administration and are often associated with a normal or expanded ECF volume.
  - Mineralocorticoid excess can be managed with a K^+-sparing diuretic (amiloride or spironolactone) and repletion of the K^+ deficit.
  - Alkalosis from excessive alkali administration will quickly resolve once the HCO_3^- load is withdrawn, assuming normal renal function.
  - Given that the presence of hypokalemia will continue to perpetuate some degree of alkalosis regardless of other interventions, potassium must be repleted in all cases of metabolic alkalosis.
  - Acetazolamide can be used if alkalosis persists despite the above interventions or if saline administration is limited by a patient's volume overload. This therapy promotes bicarbonaturia, although renal K^+ loss is enhanced as well. Acetazolamide can be dosed at 250 mg q6h × 4 or as a single dose of 500 mg.
  - Severe alkalemia (pH >7.70) with ECF volume excess and/or renal failure can be treated with isotonic (150 mEq/L) HCl administered via a central vein. The amount of HCl required can be calculated as follows: (0.5 × lean weight in kg) × ($[HCO_3^-]$ − 24). Correction should occur over 8–24 hours.

Respiratory Acidosis

GENERAL PRINCIPLES

The causes of respiratory acidosis can be divided into hypoventilation from (1) **respiratory center depression**, (2) **neuromuscular failure**, (3) **decreased respiratory system compliance**, (4) **increased airway resistance**, and (5) **increased dead space** (see Table 12-10).

Diagnosis

- Symptoms of respiratory acidosis result from changes in the cerebrospinal fluid (CSF) pH. A very severe hypercapnia may be well tolerated if it is accompanied by renal compensation and a relatively normal pH. Conversely, a modest rise in pCO_2 can be very symptomatic if acute.
- Initial symptoms and signs may include headache and restlessness, which may progress to generalized hyperreflexia/asterixis and coma.

TREATMENT

- Treatment is directed at correcting the underlying disorder and improving ventilation (see Chapter 10, Pulmonary Diseases).
- Administration of $NaHCO_3$ to improve the acidemia may *paradoxically worsen the pH* in situations of limited ventilation. The administered HCO_3^- will combine with H^+ in the tissues and form pCO_2 and water. If ventilation is fixed, this extra CO_2 generated cannot be blown off and worsening of hypercapnia will result. Therefore, HCO_3^- should, in general, be avoided in *pure* respiratory acidosis.

Respiratory Alkalosis

GENERAL PRINCIPLES

The common causes of hyperventilation resulting in respiratory alkalosis are given in Table 12-10.

DIAGNOSIS

Clinical Presentation

- The rise in CSF pH that occurs with **acute respiratory alkalosis** is associated with a significant reduction in cerebral blood flow that may lead to light headedness and impaired consciousness. Generalized membrane excitability can result in seizures and arrhythmias. Symptoms and signs of acute hypocalcemia (see Calcium, Hypocalcemia, Clinical Presentation section) may be evident from the abrupt fall in ionized calcium that can occur.
- **Chronic respiratory alkalosis** is usually asymptomatic because a normal pH is well defended by compensation.

Diagnostic Testing

The rise in pH from **acute respiratory alkalosis** can cause a reduced ionized calcium, a profound hypophosphatemia, and hypokalemia.

TREATMENT

- Treatment of respiratory alkalosis should focus on identifying and treating the underlying disease.
- In intensive care unit patients, this may involve changing the ventilator settings to decrease ventilation (see Chapter 8, Critical Care).

Summary

- Crystalloid solutions are typically preferred as the first-line treatment, whereas colloid solutions are not the recommended initial option for hypovolemia, unless it is not due to bleeding.
- Isotonic IV maintenance fluids reduce the risk of hyponatremia and are a more appropriate choice.
- Degree and duration of hyponatremia, along with the severity of symptoms, determine the management algorithm and the rapidity to correct sodium.

- Patients with neuromuscular weakness, paralysis, or ECG changes and elevated potassium of >5.5 mEq/L in patients at risk for ongoing hyperkalemia or confirmed hyperkalemia of 6.5 mEq/L should have aggressive treatment.
- Answering four questions will help determine the acid base disorder present in the clinical scenario: What is the pH? What is the bicarbonate? What is the $PaCO_2$? What is the anion gap?

Scan the QR code to access chapter references.

13 Renal Diseases

Seth Goldberg, Daniel W. Coyne, and Madhav H. Hande

Evaluation of the Patient with Renal Disease

DIAGNOSIS

Clinical Presentation

- Most patients with renal disease are asymptomatic. Renal disease is often detected through abnormal laboratory data, such as elevated serum creatinine. Abnormal urinalysis with proteinuria, hematuria, or pyuria may also indicate renal disease. Anatomic kidney abnormalities may be incidentally discovered through imaging studies.
- The presentation of acute kidney injury (AKI) can vary widely, ranging from constitutional symptoms of generalized malaise to more concerning symptoms such as decreasing urine output, worsening hypertension, dependent or generalized edema, foamy urine, weight changes, or decreased appetite.
- With advanced chronic kidney disease (CKD), patients may begin to experience nausea, vomiting, a metallic taste in the mouth, generalized itching, intractable hiccups, alterations in sensorium, edema, breathlessness, and lethargy. A wide range of electrolyte abnormalities, including hyperkalemia, hypocalcemia, hyperphosphatemia, and metabolic acidosis, may also develop.

Diagnostic Testing

The focus of the initial evaluation of the patient with renal disease is to determine the need for emergent dialysis. Then, investigations to identify the etiology are undertaken while differentiating components of acute and chronic disease.

- **Basic diagnostic testing**
  - A basic evaluation includes electrolytes (with calcium and phosphorus), Cr, blood urea nitrogen (BUN), and albumin. When Cr is stable over days to weeks, it can be used to calculate an estimated glomerular filtration rate (eGFR), which can be calculated using the Chronic Kidney Disease Epidemiology Collaboration (CKD-EPI) equation using the age, gender, race (African American or non-African American), and serum creatinine of the patient. The Modification of Diet in Renal Disease (MDRD) formula is similar to the CKD-EPI formula, but tends to overdiagnose CKD.
  - With both equations, CKD is not considered present when the eGFR is >60 mL/min/1.73 m^2 unless other evidence of renal damage (e.g., proteinuria) is present for at least 3 months.
  - Use of cystatin C to estimate the GFR may be better able to accurately classify patients in the 45–60 mL/min/1.73 m^2 range, although this has not been shown to improve outcomes or to provide better predictions of risk.[1]
  - Unlike the complex formulae above, the Cockcroft-Gault equation can be calculated manually and yields an estimated creatinine clearance, which is equal to ((140 – Age)/(serum creatinine in mg/dL)) × (weight in kg/72). The equation should be multiplied by 0.85 for females.

- **Urine studies**
  - Routine urine studies include a urine dipstick (for protein, blood, glucose, leukocyte esterase, nitrites, pH, and specific gravity) as well as a freshly voided specimen for microscopic examination (for cells, casts, and crystals). The urine sample is centrifuged at 2100 rpm for 5 minutes, and then most of the supernatant is poured off. The pellet is resuspended by gently tapping the side of the tube.
    - **Proteinuria** can be estimated from a spot urine protein-to-creatinine ratio in patients whose serum creatinine level is in the steady state. A normal ratio is <250 mg of protein per gram of Cr. A 24-hour urine collection for protein can be obtained when the serum Cr is not at a stable baseline and is a more precise assessment of proteinuria.
    - **Hematuria** (more than three red blood cells [RBCs] per high-power field on an unspun specimen) can represent an infectious, inflammatory, or malignant process anywhere along the urinary tract. Dysmorphic RBCs (with rounded protuberances) suggest a glomerular source of bleeding and can be accompanied by RBC casts formed within the tubules. The absence of RBCs in a patient with a positive dipstick for blood suggests hemolysis or rhabdomyolysis (forms of pigment nephropathy).
    - **White blood cells** (WBCs) in the urine represent an infectious or inflammatory process. This may be seen with a urinary tract infection (UTI), parenchymal infections such as pyelonephritis or abscess, or acute interstitial nephritis (AIN). WBC casts are consistent with AIN and pyelonephritis, but can also be seen as part of an active sediment in inflammatory glomerular diseases.
    - **Additional biochemistry tests can be ordered to evaluate for specific etiologies and discussed in the individual sections below.**
- **Imaging**
  - **Renal ultrasonography** can document the presence of two kidneys, assess size, and identify hydronephrosis or renal cysts. Small kidneys (<9 cm) generally reflect chronic disease, although kidneys may be large (generally >13 cm) in diabetes, HIV, deposition disorders, and polycystic kidney disease. A discrepancy in kidney size of >2 cm suggests chronic disease in a unilateral kidney, such as that seen in renal artery stenosis with atrophy of the affected kidney. The presence of hydronephrosis suggests obstructive nephropathy. Retroperitoneal fibrosis can encase the ureters and prevent dilation despite the presence of an obstruction.
  - **CT** has less utility in the evaluation of kidney disease because the iodinated contrast dye can be nephrotoxic and may cause worsening renal function. However, noncontrast helical CT scanning has become the test of choice in evaluating nephrolithiasis.
  - **MRI** and magnetic resonance angiography (MRA) can be helpful in evaluating renal masses, detecting renal artery stenosis, and diagnosing renal vein thrombosis. Unlike standard arteriography, MRA does not require the administration of nephrotoxic contrast agents but does employ gadolinium-based contrast agents, which are associated with the development of nephrogenic systemic fibrosis (NSF) in patients with advanced renal failure or dialysis dependence.[2] Guidelines that limit the use of gadolinium in at-risk patients have decreased the incidence of NSF. The available contrast agents should be used with caution when necessary.
  - **Radionuclide scanning** uses technetium isotopes to assess the contribution of each kidney to the overall renal function, providing important information if unilateral nephrectomy is being considered for malignancy or for living donation. Renal scanning is also useful in transplantation, where renal uptake and excretion of the tracer can be followed.
- **Diagnostic procedures**
  - **Kidney biopsy** can determine diagnosis, classify disease, guide therapy, and provide prognostic information in many settings, particularly in the evaluation of glomerular

or deposition diseases. Biopsy of a native kidney may be indicated in adults with unexplained proteinuria, hematuria, or renal dysfunction. Biopsy of a renal transplant allograft may be necessary to distinguish acute rejection from medication toxicity and other causes of renal dysfunction.

- Small echogenic kidneys with loss of renal corticomedullary differentiation generally imply an advanced stage of renal parenchymal disease and are unlikely to yield useful diagnostic information; they also have an increased risk of postprocedural bleeding, and biopsy should generally be avoided in these cases.
- Preparative measures for native kidney biopsy include avoiding aspirin and antiplatelet agents for 5–7 days and reversing anticoagulation before procedure, ultrasonography (to document the presence of two kidneys and assess size and location), urinalysis or urine culture to exclude infection, and blood pressure control. If uremic platelet dysfunction is suspected by an elevated bleeding time (>10 minutes) or abnormal platelet function assays, IV desmopressin acetate (DDAVP at 0.3 µg/kg) can be infused 30 minutes before biopsy. Patients on dialysis should not receive heparin immediately after the biopsy. If body habitus precludes a percutaneous approach, a transjugular renal biopsy can be performed.
- A hemoglobin drop of approximately 10% is common after the procedure. Difficulty voiding after the procedure may represent urethral clot obstructing the flow of urine.

Acute Kidney Injury

GENERAL PRINCIPLES

Definition and Classification

- According to KDIGO 2012 guidelines 4, AKI is defined as any of the following:
  - Increase in SCr by ≥0.3 mg/dL within 48 hours; or
  - Increase in SCr to ≥1.5 times baseline, which is known or presumed to have occurred within the prior 7 days; or
  - Urine output <0.5 mL/kg/h for 6 hours
- Stage 1 AKI is defined as a Cr 1.5–1.9 times baseline, an increase in Cr ≥0.3 mg/dL within 48 hours, or a urine output <0.5 mL/kg/h for 6–12 hours.
- Stage 2 AKI is defined as a Cr 2–2.9 times baseline or a urine output <0.5 mL/kg/h for at least 12 hours.
- Stage 3 AKI is defined as a Cr ≥3 times baseline, a Cr increase to ≥4 mg/dL, initiation of renal replacement therapy, urine output <0.3 mL/kg/h for at least 24 hours, or anuria for at least 12 hours.
- Renal failure can be classified as oliguric or nonoliguric, based on the amount of urine output. Cutoffs of approximately 500 mL/d or 25 mL/h for 4 hours are frequently used in clinical practice (Table 13-1).
- The Acute Disease Quality Initiative suggested an expanded diagnostic AKI criterion to enhance the accuracy of diagnosing AKI. The proposed classification involves using damage and functional biomarkers, along with clinical information, to recognize different pathophysiological processes, identify AKI causes, and determine AKI severity.[3] The AKI stages were delineated in the subsequent manner:
  - Stage 1S: Subclinical AKI—Biomarker positive, change in serum creatinine level <0.3 mg/dL, and no urine output criteria met.
  - Stage 1A: Biomarker negative and increase of serum creatinine level by ≥0.3 mg/dL for 48 hours or ≥150% for 7 days and/or urine output <0.5 mL/kg/h for >6 hours.
  - Stage 1B: Biomarker positive and increase in serum creatinine level by ≥0.3 mg/dL for 48 hours or ≥150% for 7 days and/or urine output <0.5 mL/kg/h for >6 hours.

TABLE 13-1 Classification Systems for Acute Kidney Injury

Acute Kidney Injury Network (AKIN) Staging		Urine Output (Common to Both)	RIFLE Classification	
Serum Creatinine			**Class**	**Serum Creatinine or GFR**
Stage 1	1.5–1.9 times baseline **or** ≥0.3 mg/dL (≥26.5 μmol/L) increase	<0.5 mL/kg/h for 6–12 hours	**R**isk	Increase in serum creatinine ×1.5 times **or** GFR decrease >25%
Stage 2	Increase of 2.0–2.9 times baseline	<0.5 mL/kg/h for ≥12 hours	**I**njury	Serum creatinine ×2 **or** GFR decrease >50%
Stage 3	3.0 times baseline **or** Increase in serum creatinine to ≥4.0 mg/dL (≥353.6 μmol/L) **or** Initiation of renal replacement therapy **or** In patients <18 years, decrease in eGFR to <35 mL/min per 1.73 m^2	<0.3 mL/kg/h for ≥24 hours **or** Anuria for ≥12 hours	**F**ailure	Serum creatinine ×3 **or** Serum creatinine >4 mg/dL (>354 μmol/L) with an acute rise >0.5 mg/dL (>44 μmol/L) **or** GFR decreased >75%
			Loss	Persistent acute renal failure = complete loss of kidney function for longer than 4 weeks
			End-stage kidney disease	ESRD >3 months

Modified from The Kidney Disease Improving Global Outcomes (KDIGO) Working Group. Definition and classification of acute kidney injury. Kidney Int. 2012;(Suppl 2):19–36.

- Stage 2A: Biomarker negative and increase of serum creatinine level by >200% and/or urine output <0.5 mL/kg/h for >12 hours.
- Stage 2B: Biomarker positive and increase of serum creatinine level by >200% and/or urine output <0.5 mL/kg/h for >12 hours.
- Stage 3A: Biomarker negative and increase of serum creatinine level by >300% (≥4 mg/dL with an acute increase of ≥0.5 mg/dL) and/or urine output <0.3 mL/kg/h for >24 hours or anuria for >12 hours and/or acute renal replacement therapy.
- Stage 3B: Biomarker positive and increase of serum creatinine level by >300% (≥4 mg/dL with an acute increase of ≥0.5 mg/dL) and/or urine output <0.3 mL/kg/h for >24 hours or anuria for >12 hours and/or acute renal replacement therapy.

Etiology

Etiologies of AKI are classically divided according to the anatomic location of the physiologic defect. **Prerenal** disease involves a disturbance of renal perfusion, whereas **postrenal** disease involves obstruction of the urinary collecting system. **Intrinsic** renal disease involves the glomeruli, microvasculature, tubules, or interstitium of the kidneys. Table 13-2 lists some of the common causes of AKI.

Prerenal

- The term **prerenal azotemia** implies preserved intrinsic renal function in the setting of renal hypoperfusion and reduced GFR. The effective circulating volume is decreased, resulting from intravascular volume depletion, low cardiac output, or disordered vasodilation (hepatic cirrhosis).
- When the cause is true volume depletion, presentation involves a history of excessive fluid loss, reduced intake, or orthostatic symptoms. Physical examination may reveal dry mucous membranes, poor skin turgor, and orthostatic vital signs (drop in blood pressure by at least 20/10 mm Hg or an increase in heart rate by 10 bpm after standing from a seated or lying position). The central venous pressure is typically <8 cm H_2O.
- Low cardiac output causes prerenal azotemia via a drop in the effective circulating volume, despite total body volume overload. Sympathetic and neurohormonal systems are activated, stimulating the renin–angiotensin–aldosterone system for sodium reclamation as well as antidiuretic hormone (ADH) promoting further water retention. This can lead to increased reabsorption of urea nitrogen in relation to creatinine and patients present with a prerenal pattern on laboratory investigations. In heart failure, diuresis may paradoxically improve the prerenal azotemia by unloading the ventricles and improving cardiac function and renal perfusion (see Chapter 5, Heart Failure and Cardiomyopathy). The use of ultrafiltration (UF) was evaluated and found to be inferior to pharmacologic therapies, resulting in more adverse events in the treatment of acute decompensated heart failure.[4]

TABLE 13-2 Causes of Acute Kidney Injury

Prerenal	Intrinsic	Postrenal
Hypovolemia Hypotension (including sepsis) Loss of autoregulation (NSAIDs, RAAS blockers) Abdominal compartment syndrome Renal artery stenosis Heart failure Hepatic cirrhosis	**Tubular:** Ischemic ATN, toxic ATN (contrast, pigment, uric acid) **Vascular:** Glomerulonephritis, dysproteinemia, thrombotic microangiopathy (HUS, TTP), atheroembolic disease **Interstitial:** Acute interstitial nephritis, pyelonephritis **Infections** such as malaria, leptospirosis, scrub typhus, dengue, yellow fever; snake bite (viperidae species); arthropod bites (bees, wasps, and spiders); herbal medicines and alternate medicine preparations such as yellow oleander, rhubarb, djenkol beans, and Chinese yew	Urethral obstruction Ureteral obstruction (bilateral, or unilateral if solitary kidney)

ATN, acute tubular necrosis; HUS, hemolytic-uremic syndrome; RAAS, renin–angiotensin–aldosterone system; TTP, thrombotic thrombocytopenic purpura.

- Hepatic failure leads to splanchnic vasodilation and venous pooling, which diminishes the effective circulating volume and activates the renin–angiotensin–aldosterone system along with ADH secretion despite total body volume overload. This can progress to the **hepatorenal syndrome** (HRS), which is characterized by a rise in serum creatinine of >0.3 mg/dL within 48 hours or ≥1.5 times from baseline that is not reduced with administration of albumin (1 g/kg of body weight) and after a minimum of 2 days off diuretics. The diagnosis of HRS should be in the absence of shock, nephrotoxic agents, or findings of renal parenchymal disease.[5] Spontaneous bacterial peritonitis, aggressive diuresis, gastrointestinal bleeding, or large-volume paracentesis can precipitate HRS in a cirrhotic patient. Management of the renal disease is supportive, and if definitive treatment of the liver disorder (either through recovery or via transplantation) can occur, renal recovery is common. Temporizing measures include treatment of the underlying precipitating factor (e.g., proteinuria >500 mg/d, peritonitis, gastrointestinal bleeding) and withholding diuretics. Dialytic support can be used as a bridge to transplantation in appropriate candidates, with anticipation of renal recovery if the period of dialysis dependence is shorter than 6 weeks. Additional treatment options are discussed further in Chapter 19, Liver Diseases.
- In the volume-depleted patient, certain medications can block the ability of the kidney to autoregulate blood flow and GFR. NSAIDs inhibit the counterbalancing vasodilatory effects of prostaglandins at the afferent arteriole and can induce AKI in volume-depleted patients. Angiotensin-converting enzyme (ACE) inhibitors and angiotensin receptor blockers (ARBs) can cause efferent arteriolar vasodilation and a drop in the GFR.
- Abdominal compartment syndrome, from intestinal ischemia, obstruction, or massive ascites, can compromise flow through the renal vasculature via increased intra-abdominal pressure (IAP). An IAP >20 mm Hg, measured via a pressure transducer attached to the bladder catheter, suggests the diagnosis.

Postrenal

- Postrenal failure occurs when the flow of urine is obstructed within the collecting system. Common causes include **prostatic enlargement, bilateral kidney stones, or malignancy.** The increased intratubular hydrostatic pressure leads to diminished GFR. Bilateral involvement (or unilateral obstruction to a solitary functioning kidney) is generally required to produce a significant change in the Cr level. When the diagnosis is suspected, a renal ultrasound should be performed early to evaluate for hydronephrosis. However, hydronephrosis may be less pronounced when there is concomitant volume depletion or if retroperitoneal fibrosis has encased the ureters, preventing their expansion.
- Treatment depends on the level of obstruction. When urethral flow is impeded (usually by prostatic enlargement in men), placement of a bladder catheter can be both diagnostic and therapeutic; **a postvoid residual urine volume >300 mL** suggests the diagnosis. When the upper urinary tract is involved, urologic or radiologic decompression is necessary, with stenting or placement of percutaneous nephrostomy tubes.
- Relief of bilateral obstruction is frequently followed by a **postobstructive diuresis**. Serum electrolytes need to be closely monitored if polyuria ensues, and replacement of approximately half of the urinary volume with 0.45% saline is recommended.
- Crystals may cause micro-obstructive uropathy within the tubules. IV acyclovir and the protease inhibitor indinavir can induce AKI by this mechanism. The urine may show evidence of crystals, although sometimes not until urine flow is reestablished. Treatment is typically supportive after the offending agent is discontinued. As with relief of other forms of obstructive uropathy, a polyuric phase may occur.

Intrinsic Renal Failure

Causes of intrinsic renal failure can be divided anatomically into tubular, glomerular/vascular, and interstitial categories. Disease can be primarily renal in nature or part of a systemic process.

- **Tubular**
  - **Ischemic acute tubular necrosis** (ATN) is the most common cause of renal failure in the intensive care setting and is the end result of any process that leads to significant hypoperfusion of the kidneys, including sepsis, hemorrhage, or any prolonged prerenal insult.
    - The injury results in the sloughing of renal tubular cells, which can congeal with cellular debris in a matrix of Tamm–Horsfall protein to form granular casts. These have a "muddy brown" appearance and are strongly suggestive of ATN in the proper context. The fractional excretion of sodium (FE_{Na}) (>1%) and fractional excretion of urea (FE_{Urea}) (>35%) are typically elevated as the tubules lose their ability to concentrate the urine.
    - Management of ATN is supportive, with avoidance of further nephrotoxic insults. Fluid management is aimed at maintaining euvolemia. Volume deficits, if present, should be corrected. If volume overload and oliguria become evident, a diuretic challenge is reasonable, typically with IV furosemide (40–120 mg boluses or a continuous drip at 10–20 mg/h). This has not been shown to hasten recovery but can simplify overall management.
    - Recovery from ATN may take days to weeks to occur but can be expected in >85% of patients with a previously normal Cr. Dialysis may be necessary to bridge the time to recovery.
  - Toxic ATN can result from endogenous chemicals (e.g., hemoglobin, myoglobin) or exogenous medications (e.g., iodinated contrast, aminoglycosides). These forms share many of the diagnostic features of ischemic ATN.
    - **Iodinated contrast** is a potent renal vasoconstrictor and is toxic to renal tubules. When renal injury occurs, the Cr typically rises 24 hours after exposure and peaks in 3–5 days. Risk factors for contrast nephropathy include underlying CKD, age >75 years, diabetes, albuminuria, volume depletion, heart failure, anemia, higher contrast volumes, intra-arterial contrast, use of hyperosmolar contrast, and multiple contrast exposures in <72 hours. Preventative measures include periprocedure IV volume expansion and discontinuation of diuretics within 24 hours of the procedure. Normal saline at 150 mEq/L can be given at 3 mL/kg/h for 1 hour before exposure, then at 1 mL/kg/h for 6 hours after the procedure. In a recent large, randomized, controlled trial, sodium bicarbonate was not found to be superior to normal saline, whereas acetylcysteine was not shown to be better than placebo.[3]
    - **Aminoglycoside nephrotoxicity** is typically nonoliguric, occurs from direct toxicity to the proximal tubules, and results in the renal wasting of potassium and magnesium. Replacement of these electrolytes may become necessary. A similar pattern of potassium and magnesium loss is seen in cisplatin toxicity. A prolonged exposure to the aminoglycoside of at least 5 days is required. Peak and trough levels correlate poorly with the risk of developing renal injury. Risk may be minimized by avoiding volume depletion and by using the extended-interval dosing method (see Chapter 15, Antimicrobials).
    - **Pigment nephropathy** results from direct tubular toxicity by hemoglobin and myoglobin. Vasoconstriction may also play a role. The diagnosis may be suspected by a positive urine dipstick test for blood but with an absence of RBCs on microscopic examination. Myoglobinuria can be distinguished from hemoglobinuria by utilizing the rapid ammonium sulfate precipitation test in which hemoglobin precipitates resulting in a clear supernatant, while the supernatant remains reddish in the presence of myoglobin. In **rhabdomyolysis**, the creatine kinase (CK) level is elevated to at least

10 times the upper limit of normal with a disproportionate rise in Cr, potassium, and phosphorus. Aggressive IV fluid administration with normal saline should be initiated immediately, and large volumes are required to replace the fluid lost into necrotic muscle tissue. Urinary alkalinization with sodium bicarbonate (150 mEq/L, three ampules) is not generally recommended as it may worsen the hypocalcemia.

- In **tumor lysis syndrome**, acute uric acid nephropathy can result. In addition to the elevated Cr, there is typically hyperuricemia, hyperphosphatemia, and hypocalcemia. A ratio of urine uric acid to urine Cr that is >1 is consistent with this diagnosis, as is the finding of uric acid crystals in the urine sediment. Prophylaxis with allopurinol 600 mg can decrease uric acid production. Rasburicase (15 mg/kg IV) is highly effective at depleting uric acid levels and can be given as prophylaxis or as treatment. Alkalinization of the urine should be avoided if hyperphosphatemia is present, because this could increase the risk of calcium phosphate precipitation in the urine.

- **Glomerular/vascular**
  - The finding of **dysmorphic urinary RBCs, RBC casts, or proteinuria in the nephrotic range (>3.5 g/d)** strongly suggests the presence of a glomerular disease. Glomerular diseases are described individually in further detail later on in this chapter.
  - A small subgroup of glomerular diseases can present with rapidly deteriorating renal function, over days to weeks, termed **rapidly progressive glomerulonephritis.** A nephritic picture is common, with RBC casts, edema, and hypertension. A renal biopsy may reveal the specific underlying disease, but crescent formation in >50% of glomeruli is usually present. For those deemed to have salvageable renal function, management is with high-dose pulse glucocorticoid therapy (IV methylprednisolone 7–15 mg/kg/d for 3 days), followed by a course of oral prednisone (1 mg/kg/d for 1 month, then tapered over the next 6–12 months). Cyclophosphamide is typically added to this regimen, with monthly IV doses (1 g/m^2) having less cumulative toxicity than the daily oral dosing strategy (2 mg/kg/d).
- **Thrombotic microangiopathy** encompasses a broad spectrum of diseases that can result in hemolytic anemia, platelet consumption, and intracapillary thrombi, typically with associated endothelial cell injury. Differentiating among the various causes of this entity can allow for better targeted therapy.
- **Thrombotic thrombocytopenic** purpura (TTP) can result from a reduced activity of ADAMTS 13 (due to deficiency or inhibitory antibodies) leading to von Willebrand factor-rich microthrombi secondarily affecting arterioles and capillaries of a variety of organs. **Infection-associated TMA** results from diarrheal bacterial toxins (e.g., Shiga and Shiga-like toxin), neuraminidase from *Streptococcus pneumoniae,* or complement dysregulation from SARS-CoV-2, all of which cause direct injury to the endothelial cells. **Complement mediated TMA** (Atypical HUS) has been described in patients with mutations or inhibitors in proteins that regulate the complement cascade, such as factor H and factor I, responsive to treatment with eculizumab, a C5 inhibitor.[6] Malignant hypertension, autoimmune diseases (e.g., antiphospholipid syndrome, scleroderma renal crisis, and systemic lupus erythematosus), pregnancy, malignancies, and a variety of medications (mitomycin C, clopidogrel, cyclosporine, tacrolimus) have also been associated with TMA. Classification, diagnosis, and therapy are discussed in Chapter 20, Disorders of Hemostasis and Thrombosis.
  - **Atheroembolic disease** can be seen in patients with diffuse atherosclerosis after undergoing an invasive aortic or other large artery manipulation, including cardiac catheterization, coronary bypass surgery, aortic aneurysm repair, and placement of an intra-aortic balloon pump. Physical findings may include retinal arteriolar plaques, lower extremity livedo reticularis, and areas of digital necrosis. Eosinophilia, eosinophiluria, and hypocomplementemia may be present, and WBC casts may be found in the urine sediment. However, in many cases, the only laboratory abnormality is a

rising Cr that follows a stepwise progression. Renal biopsy shows cholesterol clefts in the small arteries. Anticoagulation may worsen embolic disease and should be avoided if possible. No specific treatment is available. Many patients progress to CKD and even to end-stage renal disease (ESRD).

- **Interstitial**
  - **AIN** involves inflammation of the renal parenchyma, typically caused by medications or infections. The classic triad of **fever, rash, and eosinophilia** is seen in less than one-third of patients, and its absence does not exclude the diagnosis. Pyuria and WBC casts are also suggestive of AIN. β-Lactam antibiotics are the most frequently cited causative agents, but nearly all antibiotics can be implicated. The time course typically requires exposure for at least 5–10 days before renal impairment occurs. Other medications, such as proton pump inhibitors, 5-aminosalicyaltes, and allopurinol, have been associated with AIN. NSAIDs can produce a chronic interstitial nephritis with nephrotic range proteinuria. Streptococcal infections, leptospirosis, and sarcoidosis have all been implicated in AIN.
  - Treatment is principally the withdrawal of the offending agent. Renal recovery typically ensues, although the time course is variable, and temporary dialytic support may be necessary in severe cases. A short course of prednisone at 1 mg/kg/d may hasten recovery.
  - Parenchymal infections with **pyelonephritis or renal abscesses** are uncommon causes of AKI. Bilateral involvement is usually necessary to induce a rise in Cr. Urine findings include pyuria and WBC casts, and antibiotic therapy is guided by culture results.

AKI IN TROPICS

- AKI in tropics is predominantly community acquired and affects young individuals who were previously in good health.
- AKI is often due to a single cause, that is, infections, toxins, environmental factors, or obstetric complications, and are often preventable.[7]
- Important infectious causes include vector-borne infections such as malaria, dengue fever, and scrub typhus; direct infections such as leptospirosis; diarrhoeal diseases and other infections like melioidosis, typhoid, chlamydia, and HIV.
- Toxins include animal poisons such as snake bite, scorpion sting, carp gallbladder, or bile; plant and fungal toxins such as herbal medicines, star fruit, Djenkol beans, and mushrooms; and chemical nephrotoxins such as ethylene glycol, copper sulphate, and paraquat.
- Environmental factors such as heat stroke and natural disasters and obstetric complications, including postabortal/puerperal sepsis, pre-eclampsia, and ante- and postpartum hemorrhage also contribute to AKI in tropical regions.
- Low levels of income, poor access to healthcare, and social or cultural practices (such as the use of traditional herbal medicines and treatments) contribute to poor outcomes in these cases.

DIAGNOSIS

- Uncovering the cause of AKI requires careful attention to the events preceding the rise in Cr. In the hospitalized patient, blood pressure patterns, hydration status, medications, and iodinated contrast use must be investigated. Antibiotic dose and duration as well as PRN medications should not be overlooked.
- Evidence of ongoing hypovolemia or hypoperfusion is suggestive of prerenal disease. Most causes of postrenal disease are identified on ultrasound by dilation of the collecting system or by massive urine output on placement of a bladder catheter. When promptly corrected, prerenal and postrenal disorders can show a rapid decrease in the serum Cr, and failure of this to occur can suggest an alternative diagnosis.

- **Urinary casts** point toward an intrinsic cause of AKI. Granular casts ("muddy brown") suggest ATN, WBC casts suggest an inflammatory or infectious interstitial process, and RBC casts strongly suggest glomerular disease. Identification of crystals in the urine sediment may be supportive of kidney disease related to intoxication of ethylene glycol, uric acid excretion, tumor lysis syndrome, or medications such as acyclovir and indinavir. This underscores the importance of examining fresh urinary sediment in the evaluation of AKI.
  - Scoring systems which include urine microscopy for identification of renal tubular epithelial cells and granular casts are useful in differentiating between acute tubular necrosis (ATN) and prerenal acute kidney injury as well as in predicting the severity and prognosis of AKI.

Various laboratory parameters can be used to differentiate prerenal states from ATN in oliguric patients and are summarized in Table 13-3. The basis for these tests is to evaluate tubular integrity, which is preserved in prerenal disease and lost in ATN. In states of hypoperfusion, the kidneys should avidly reabsorb sodium, resulting in a low FE_{Na}: $FE_{Na} = [(U_{Na} \times P_{Cr})/(P_{Na} \times U_{Cr})] \times 100$, where U is urine and P is plasma.

- **A value <1% suggests renal hypoperfusion with intact tubular function.** Loop diuretics and metabolic alkalosis can induce natriuresis, increase FE_{Na}, and mask the presence of renal hypoperfusion. The FE_{Urea} can instead be calculated in these settings, where a value of <35% suggests a prerenal process.
- Contrast and pigment nephropathy can result in a low FE_{Na} because of early vasoconstriction ("prerenal" drop in glomerular perfusion), as can glomerular diseases because of intact tubular function. The FE_{Na} also has limited utility when AKI is superimposed on CKD because the underlying tubular dysfunction makes the test difficult to interpret.
- With hypoperfusion, the urine is typically concentrated, containing an osmolality >500 mOsm/kg and a high specific gravity (>1.020). In ATN, concentrating ability is lost and the urine is usually osmolar to the serum (isosthenuria). In the blood, the ratio of BUN to Cr is normally <20:1, and an elevation is consistent with hypovolemia.
- The Food and Drug Administration has approved a kit that detects two biomarkers of acute kidney injury, TIMP-2 and IGFBP-7 in urine. A positive test identifies patients at increased risk of AKI in the next 12 hours, while a negative test makes AKI unlikely.[8] The clinical utility of this test in critically ill patients at risk for AKI is unclear.
- Serum and urine biomarkers have the potential for detecting AKI early; identifying subclinical AKI; identifying the cause, site, and degree of injury; and monitoring therapeutic benefits of interventions. Serum NGAL and serum cystatin care markers of glomerular filtration and proximal tubular function. Urine interleukin-18 (IL-18), kidney injury molecule-1 (KIM-1), L-type fatty acid binding protein (L-FABP) are early detection biomarkers indicating proximal tubular injury. Tissue inhibitor metalloproteinase-2/insulin-like growth factor-binding protein 7 (TIMP-2/IGFBP-7) are markers

TABLE 13-3 Laboratory Findings in Oliguric Acute Kidney Injury

Diagnosis	BUN:Cr	FENa (%)	Urine Osmolality (mOsm/kg)	Urine Na	Urine SG	Sediment
Prerenal azotemia	>20:1	<1%	>500	<20	>1.020	Bland
Oliguric ATN	<20:1	>1%	<350	>40	Variable	Granular casts

ATN, acute tubular necrosis; BUN, blood urea nitrogen; Cr, creatinine; FENa, fractional excretion of sodium; SG, specific gravity.

of cell cycle arrest which are highly upregulated after kidney injury and are designed to predict the risk of developing stage 2–3 AKI within 12 hours of assessment.

TREATMENT

- Disease-specific therapies are covered in their respective sections. In general, treatment of AKI is primarily supportive in nature. Volume status must be evaluated to correct for hypovolemia or hypervolemia. Volume deficits, if present, should be corrected, after which the goal of fluid management should be to keep input equal to output. In the oliguric volume-overloaded setting, a trial of diuretics (usually high-dose loop diuretics in a bolus or as a continuous drip) may simplify management, although it has not been shown to hasten recovery.
- Electrolyte imbalances should be corrected in the setting of AKI. Hyperkalemia, when mild (<6 mEq/L), may be treated with dietary potassium restriction and potassium-binding resins (e.g., sodium polystyrene sulfonate). When further elevated or accompanied by ECG abnormalities, immediate medical therapy is indicated, with calcium gluconate, insulin and glucose, inhaled β-agonists, and possibly bicarbonate (see Chapter 12, Fluid and Electrolyte Management). Severe hyperkalemia that is refractory to medical management is an indication for urgent dialysis.
- Mild **metabolic acidosis** can be treated with oral sodium bicarbonate, 650–1300 mg thrice daily. Severe acidosis (pH <7.2) can be temporized with IV sodium bicarbonate but requires monitoring for volume overload, rebound alkalosis, and hypocalcemia. Acidosis that is refractory to medical management is an indication for urgent dialysis.

SPECIAL CONSIDERATIONS

- All patients with AKI require daily assessment to determine the need for renal replacement therapy. Severe acidosis, hyperkalemia, or volume overload refractory to medical management mandates the initiation of dialysis. Certain drug and alcohol intoxications (methanol, ethylene glycol, or salicylates) should be treated with hemodialysis. Uremic pericarditis (with a friction rub) or encephalopathy should also be treated promptly with renal replacement therapy. Patients suffering from acute oliguric renal failure who are not expected to recover promptly likely benefit from earlier initiation of dialysis.
- In the absence of one of these acute indications, the timing of initiating dialytic therapy is less certain. Five studies analyzed this subject in ICU patients in a randomized controlled fashion, but provided somewhat contradictory results. **The ELAIN study showed a** survival advantage for patients beginning dialysis with a two- to threefold increase in Cr compared to patients with more severe elevations.[9] However, subsequent studies, that is AKIKI, IDEAL-ICU, and STARRT-AKI, suggested that there was no benefit in an earlier versus a later strategy for initiating renal replacement therapy. The AKIKI 2 trial included patients with AKI KDIGO stage 3, with oliguria for more than 72 hours or a blood urea nitrogen concentration higher than 112 mg/dL. It compared the "delayed strategy" as employed in prior strategies to a "more delayed strategy." The study concluded that longer postponing of RRT initiation did not confer additional benefit and was associated with potential harm.[10]

Glomerulopathies

GENERAL PRINCIPLES

- Classically, the presentation of glomerular diseases have been described as existing on a continuum with the nephrotic syndrome on one end, characterized by proteinuria

>3.5 g/d and accompanied by hypoalbuminemia, hyperlipidemia, and edema, and the nephritic syndrome on the other end, characterized by hematuria, hypertension, edema, and renal insufficiency. However, disease entities typically present somewhere in between with overlapping features. Specific diseases do present with a tendency to feature one syndrome over the other, related to the predominant site of glomerular injury.

- Minimal change disease (MCD), focal segmental glomerulosclerosis (FSGS), membranous nephropathy (MN), diabetic nephropathy (DN), and deposition dysproteinemias typically present with nephrotic features. IgA nephropathy, postinfectious glomerulonephritis, anti-GBM antibody disease, and antineutrophil cytoplasmic antibody (ANCA)-associated vasculitis typically present with nephritic features. Lupus nephritis and membranoproliferative glomerulonephropathy (MPGN) can present with overlapping features of both nephrotic and nephritic disease.
- Nephrotic diseases typically show injury along the filtration barrier with thickening of the glomerular basement membrane (GBM) or fusion of the podocyte foot processes. By comparison, nephritic diseases generally show varying degrees of mesangial cell proliferation and mesangial deposition. With a more aggressive disease, crescents may be seen within Bowman capsule.
- When a nephrotic process is suspected, it may be useful to check antinuclear antibodies (ANA), complement levels (C3, C4), cryoglobulins, and viral serologies [HIV, hepatitis B and C, parvovirus, cytomegalovirus (CMV), Epstein-Barr virus (EBV)]. It is important to review the medication profile and rule out malignancy or other systemic infectious or inflammatory conditions. A serum protein electrophoresis (SPEP) and urine immunofixation can be performed in proteinuric patients to evaluate for a monoclonal gammopathy and may be suspected by a large protein-albumin gap. Biomarkers such as anti-phospholipase A2 receptor (anti-PLA2R) antibodies may help to noninvasively diagnose membranous nephropathy (see later).
- When a nephritic process is suspected, testing for anti-GBM antibodies, antineutrophil cytoplasmic antibodies (ANCA), and antistreptolysin-O (ASO) titers may be helpful in narrowing the differential diagnosis. As with nephrotic processes, testing for ANA, C3, C4, cryoglobulins, and viral serologies can also provide useful information.
- Complement levels may be decreased in certain nephritic disorders such as postinfectious glomerulonephritis, lupus nephritis, MPGN, C3 glomerulopathy, and subacute bacterial endocarditis. Others, such as IgA nephropathy, ANCA vasculitis, and anti-GBM antibody disease, typically have normal complement levels.

TREATMENT

- Many disorders share the same features, and general therapeutic maneuvers can be addressed as a group. Specific therapies for individual glomerular diseases are discussed in the following text.
- Glomerular disease presenting with proteinuria should rely on treatment with **ACE inhibitors or ARBs** to reduce the intraglomerular pressure. Efficacy can be monitored by serial urine protein to Cr ratios. Electrolytes and Cr should be checked within 1–2 weeks of initiation of therapy or an increase in dose to document stability of renal function and potassium. Modest dietary protein restriction to 0.8 g/kg/d may slow progression, but this remains controversial.
- Edema and volume overload can usually be effectively managed with **diuretics** combined with **sodium restriction**. Aggressive treatment of hypertension can also slow progression of renal disease.
- The hyperlipidemia associated with the nephrotic syndrome responds to dietary modification and **statins (3-hydroxy-3-methylglutaryl–coenzyme A [HMG-CoA] reductase inhibitors)**.

- The nephrotic syndrome produces a hypercoagulable state and can predispose to thromboembolic complications. Deep venous thrombi and renal vein thrombosis may occur and should be treated with heparin anticoagulation followed by long-term oral anticoagulation. Prophylactic anticoagulation is controversial and may be beneficial in severely nephrotic patients, particularly with MN. Exact mechanisms of thrombosis remain controversial but likely include urinary loss of anticlotting proteins, increased synthesis of clotting factors, or local activation of the glomerular hemostasis system.
- When immunosuppression is considered, the risk of therapy should always be weighed against the potential benefit. Renal salvageability should be addressed, and patients with advanced disease on presentation who are unlikely to benefit from such treatment may be better served by avoiding the risks of high-dose immunosuppression. Corticosteroids are used for induction and maintenance regimens for minimal change disease, FSGS, ANCA-associated vasculitis, lupus nephritis, C3 glomerulopathies, and crescentic/rapidly progressive forms of IgA nephropathy. Cytotoxic agents (e.g., cyclophosphamide) have shown efficacy in minimal change disease, membranous nephropathy, ANCA-associated vasculitis, anti-GBM disease, and lupus nephritis. They require close monitoring of WBC counts, checked at least weekly at the initiation of therapy. Dose adjustments may be needed to maintain the WBC count >3500 cells/μL. Rituximab, a monoclonal antibody directed against CD20, has shown promise in a variety of immune-mediated disorders, including membranous nephropathy, ANCA-associated vasculitis, minimal change disease, lupus nephritis, and cryoglobulinemia.[11] Other immunosuppressive agents include calcineurin inhibitors (e.g., cyclosporine, tacrolimus, voclosporin), antimetabolites (azathioprine and mycophenolate mofetil), belimumab, and complement inhibitors (e.g., eculizumab, ravulizumab, avacopan). Therapeutic plasma exchange has a role in only specific circumstances, as described in more detail below.

Minimal Change Disease

GENERAL PRINCIPLES

Epidemiology

MCD is the most common cause of the nephrotic syndrome in children but has a second peak in adults aged 50–60 years. Typically, there is sudden onset of proteinuria with hypertension and edema as well as the full nephrotic syndrome, although renal insufficiency is unusual.

Associated Conditions

Secondary forms of MCD may accompany certain malignancies (Hodgkin disease and solid tumors being the most common). A form of interstitial nephritis associated with NSAID use may also be associated with MCD.

DIAGNOSIS

The kidney biopsy reveals normal glomeruli on light microscopy and negative immunofluorescence. Electron microscopy shows effacement of the foot processes as the only histologic abnormality.

TREATMENT

- In adults, treatment with oral prednisone at 1 mg/kg/d may induce remission (decrease in proteinuria) in 8–16 weeks. Once in remission, the steroids can be tapered over 3 months and then discontinued. The urine protein excretion should be followed during this taper.

- Relapse may occur in up to 75% of adults. Reinstitution of prednisone is often effective. If the patient is steroid dependent or steroid resistant, cytotoxic agents may be needed, with cyclophosphamide 2 mg/kg/d or chlorambucil 0.2 mg/kg/d. Cyclosporine 5 mg/kg/d is an alternative therapy. Rituximab may be beneficial in frequently relapsing or glucocorticoid-dependent MCD.[12]

Membranous Nephropathy

GENERAL PRINCIPLES

MN usually presents with heavy proteinuria and nephrotic syndrome. Disease progression is variable, with one-third remitting spontaneously, one-third progressing to ESRD, and one-third with an intermediate course.

Secondary etiologies of MN include autoimmune or collagen vascular diseases (systemic lupus erythematosus [SLE] class V, Sjögren syndrome, rheumatoid arthritis), infections (viral hepatitis, HIV, syphilis), and medications (penicillamine, NSAIDs, mercury, gold). Additionally, malignancy may play a role; therefore, patients with MN should undergo age-appropriate cancer screening.

DIAGNOSIS

Kidney biopsy reveals thickening of the GBM without significant hypercellularity on light microscopy. Additionally, "spikes" along the GBM are observed on silver stain, representing areas of normal basement membrane interposed between subepithelial deposits.[13–16] Immunofluorescence represents granular staining along the GBM with IgG and C3. On electron microscopy, subepithelial deposits are seen.

Antibodies to the podocyte antigen phospholipase A2 receptor have been implicated in 70% of adult idiopathic MN. Antibodies against thrombospondin type-1 domain-containing 7A (THSD7A) are seen in 10% of patients with MN and have been linked to malignancy.[1] Lupus nephritis may be associated with staining for Exostosin 1/Exostosin 2 (EXT1/EXT2), neural cell adhesion molecule 1 (NCAM 1), or transforming growth factor beta receptor 3 (TGFBR3). Additional podocyte antigens include neural EGFL like 1 (NELL 1) (5%–7%), semaphorin 3B (SEMA 3B), protocadherin 7 (PCDH7), and serine protease HTRA1 (HTRA1).

TREATMENT

Up to 30% of patients with MN will go into spontaneous remission.[2] KDIGO guidelines recommend conservative therapy as an initial approach with ACE inhibitors or ARBs for proteinuria and blood pressure control, diuretics for volume management, with or without anticoagulation.

Because of the generally favorable prognosis, specific therapy should be reserved for patients at higher risk for progression (e.g., heavy proteinuria, reduced GFR, low serum albumin, increased PLA2R titres >50 RU/mL, urinary IgG >1 μg/min, urinary alpha 1 microglobulin >40 μg/min, urinary beta 2 microglobulin >250 mg/d, selectivity index >0.20).

When immunosuppression is considered, a variety of regimens have been studied. One option is to use alternating months of a corticosteroid and a cytotoxic agent for 6 months (prednisone 0.5 mg/kg/d for months 1, 3, and 5 and cyclophosphamide 2.5 mg/kg/d for months 2, 4, and 6).

Rituximab has been shown to provide a more durable remission when compared to cyclosporine at 24 months of treatment.

Focal Segmental Glomerulosclerosis

GENERAL PRINCIPLES

FSGS is not a single disease but rather a pattern of glomerular injury with various mechanisms. It typically presents with nephrotic syndrome, hypertension, and sometimes renal insufficiency.

FSGS can be classified into primary (idiopathic), secondary, and genetic forms.[1] Secondary forms of FSGS are associated with obesity, vesicoureteral reflux, sickle cell disease, medications (pamidronate, α-interferon, sirolimus, anabolic steroids, tyrosine kinase inhibitors), and infections (HIV, parvovirus, CMV, EBV).

DIAGNOSIS

The kidney biopsy reveals segmental sclerosis of some glomeruli under light microscopy. The degree of interstitial fibrosis and tubular atrophy (rather than glomerular scarring) correlates with prognosis. Immunofluorescence shows deposition of IgM and C3 in areas of sclerosis, representing areas of trapped immune deposits. Electron microscopy shows effacement of the podocyte foot processes similar to that seen in MCD. Lesions can be classified into distinct histomorphological variants (collapsing, cellular, perihilar, tip, and NOS), though their clinical significance is uncertain. The tip variant tends to have the most favorable prognosis while the collapsing variant is associated with the poorest outcomes.

TREATMENT

Management is similar to MCD. For patients with nephrotic range proteinuria, a trial of high-dose oral prednisone at 1 mg/kg daily (not exceeding 80 mg daily) or 2 mg/kg on alternate days (not exceeding 120 mg every other day) may induce remission and then be tapered off over a 6-month period. Patients who relapse after a period of apparent responsiveness may benefit from a repeat course of steroids. Nonresponders and relapsers may respond to treatment with calcineurin inhibitors (cyclosporine 3–5 mg/kg/d or tacrolimus 0.05–0.1 mg/kg/d). Mycophenolate mofetil, rituximab, high-dose dexamethasone, and ACTH have been considered in patients who are unable to tolerate or have contraindications for calcineurin inhibitors. Induction of a complete remission (<0.3 g/d of proteinuria) or a partial remission (50% reduction in proteinuria and <3.5 g/d) is associated with significantly slower loss of renal function.

Diabetic Nephropathy

GENERAL PRINCIPLES

DN is the most common cause of ESRD in the United States. Albuminuria correlates with the risk of progression and is classified as absent (<30 mg/g Cr), microalbuminuria (30–300 mg/g Cr), or macroalbuminuria (>300 mg/g Cr). Early disease has glomerular hyperfiltration with an elevated GFR, followed by a linear decline that may progress to ESRD.

DIAGNOSIS

Diagnostic Testing

Kidney biopsy is not usually performed unless the rate of renal decline is more rapid than would be anticipated or other diagnoses are suspected. Histology for DN shows glomerular sclerosis with nodular mesangial expansion (Kimmelstiel-Wilson nodules) on light microscopy. Immunofluorescence does not reveal immune deposition. Electron microscopy may show GBM thickening.

TREATMENT

Treatment is centered on aggressive control of glucose and blood pressure. Specific hyperglycemic therapy is discussed further in Chapter 23, Diabetes Mellitus and Related Disorders. An ACE inhibitor or ARB is considered the first-line agent in the treatment of hypertension in diabetic patients and can offer better control of proteinuria. Studies combining ACE inhibitors with an ARB or the direct renin inhibitor aliskiren have shown worse renal and cardiovascular outcomes.[7]

Deposition Disorders/Dysproteinemias

GENERAL PRINCIPLES

Dysproteinemias—including those observed in multiple myeloma—encompass **amyloidosis, light chain deposition disease** (LCDD), **and heavy chain deposition disease** (HCDD). These disorders can affect the kidney in a variety of ways, including glomerular or tubular deposition, formation of insoluble protein casts in the tubules (micro-obstructive cast nephropathy), or through hypercalcemia and volume depletion. Glomerular deposition is typically associated with heavy proteinuria due to overflow as well as disruption of filtration barrier integrity.

DIAGNOSIS

Diagnostic Testing

Diagnosis is suggested by an abnormal monoclonal protein found in the SPEP, urine protein electrophoresis, or serum free light chains. Routine urine dipstick tests for negatively charged albumin and therefore may miss the positively charged immunoglobulin (Ig) chains, unless glomerular involvement has led to a generalized protein leakage. In some cases, all of these tests are negative, and only tissue biopsy can make the diagnosis.

Diagnostic Procedures

- Biopsy of the kidney can show characteristic deposits. For amyloidosis, this appears as Congo Red-positive β-pleated fibrils of 10 nm in diameter under electron microscopy. Immunofluorescence can identify the specific Ig chains for amyloidosis (more likely to be lambda light chains), LCDD (more likely to be kappa light chains), and HCDD. **Fibrillary glomerulopathy** and **immunotactoid glomerulopathy** are distinct deposition diseases that possess Congo Red-negative deposits. The fibrils of fibrillary glomerulopathy (12–20 nm) are typically thicker than those for amyloid, whereas the microtubules of immunotactoid glomerulopathy are even wider (20–60 nm) with a visible lumen in cross section. Immunotactoid glomerulonephropathy has a strong association with myelodysplastic disorders.
- When cast nephropathy is implicated in a dysproteinemic disorder, the biopsy shows enlarged tubules filled with proteinaceous material. Immunofluorescence can identify the specific components of these casts.

TREATMENT

Chemotherapy aimed at the underlying disease can be effective in reversing renal disease and may be particularly important in myeloma when cast nephropathy is present on biopsy.

Small studies have previously suggested renal functional benefit with plasmapheresis to effect an aggressive reduction in light chain burden. However, with recent improvements in chemotherapeutic options to accomplish this same goal, the added benefit of plasmapheresis or high cutoff hemodialysis for short-term outcomes is lost as compared to conventional supportive measures.[9] There is no specific treatment for fibrillary or immunotactoid glomerulopathy, although addressing an underlying malignancy, if present, may slow progression in the latter.

Membranoproliferative Glomerulonephropathy

GENERAL PRINCIPLES

Primary idiopathic MPGN is uncommon. Hepatitis C accounts for most cases of secondary MPGN, frequently in association with cryoglobulinemia. Other secondary causes include HIV, SLE, chronic infections, and various malignancies.

DIAGNOSIS

Clinical Presentation

MPGN can present with the nephrotic syndrome, nephritic syndrome, or a combination of both. Tradition classification of this disease was divided into three subtypes (I, II, and III); however, as its molecular basis has been elucidated, an alternate classification is now used, distinguishing between immunoglobin and nonimmunoglobulin forms.[17]

- MPGN results from immune complex-mediated activation of the classical complement pathway, with the finding of both immunoglobulin and complement on immunofluorescence staining of the biopsy specimen. IgM and C3 are most commonly seen, particularly in hepatitis C-associated cases.
- A newer entity, termed **C3 glomerulonephritis** (C3GN), is defined by the dominant staining for C3 on immunofluorescence in the absence of immunoglobulin. This pattern is suggestive of alternate pathway complement activation. The antibody C3 nephritic factor may be present in C3GN, stabilizing the C3-convertase and promoting complement consumption. Deficiencies of or antibodies against the complement regulators (factor H, factor I, complement factor H-related proteins) or a gain of function mutation in factor B may also activate the complement cascade.
- A related disorder, named **dense deposit disease** (**DDD**), also shows complement deposition in the absence of immunoglobulin but is characterized by electron-dense deposits in the GBM.

Diagnostic Testing

Kidney biopsy shows mesangial proliferation and hypercellularity on light microscopy with "lobulization" of the glomerular tuft. Accumulation of debris along the filtration barrier may lead to a damage-repair cycle that results in duplication of the GBM, giving a double-contour or "tram track" appearance on silver stain. Immunofluorescence can show granular mesangial and capillary wall deposits of Ig in the immune complex-mediated forms, whereas only the C3 staining is positive in C3GN or DDD. Electron microscopy can show subendothelial or intramembranous deposits.

TREATMENT

- In adult idiopathic MPGN, treatment with immunosuppression has not shown a consistent benefit, although this may have been a result of the lumping together of pathophysiologically dissimilar diseases under the older classification scheme.

- Treatment of the secondary forms is targeted at the underlying disease. If renal function is rapidly deteriorating in the presence of cryoglobulins, plasmapheresis may help stabilize disease. Case reports have demonstrated possible efficacy of eculizumab, an anti-C5 monoclonal antibody, in the treatment of C3GN.[11]

IgA Nephropathy/Henoch–Schönlein Purpura

GENERAL PRINCIPLES

- IgA nephropathy is typically idiopathic, characterized by a nephritic picture with microscopic (and less commonly macroscopic) hematuria and mild non-nephrotic range proteinuria.
- Presentation is most commonly in the second or third decade of life, generally following a slowly progressive course. Some patients may exhibit a crescentic form with a rapid decline in renal function resulting in ESRD.
- Henoch–Schönlein purpura is a related disorder that may represent a systemic form of the same disease, with vasculitic involvement of the skin (palpable purpura of the lower trunk and extremities), gastrointestinal tract, and joints.

DIAGNOSIS

Diagnostic Testing

Kidney biopsy shows increased mesangial cellularity on light microscopy, with predominant IgA and C3 deposition on immunofluorescence. On electron microscopy, there are electron-dense deposits in the mesangium. The revised Oxford classification, which includes mesangial (M) and endocapillary (E) hypercellularity, segmental sclerosis (S), interstitial fibrosis/tubular atrophy (T), and crescents (C) reliably prognosticates the clinical outcomes.

The international IgAN prediction tool, which combines clinical and histological data at diagnosis, predicts the risk of worsening kidney function (defined by a 50% decline in eGFR or development of end-stage renal disease) within five years from kidney biopsy.

TREATMENT

Aggressiveness of therapy depends on the severity of disease. For patients with a benign course, conservative management with ACE inhibitors or ARBs is recommended. Recent studies have demonstrated that SGLT2 inhibitors are beneficial in reducing renal adverse outcomes. Sparsentan, a dual blocker of the angiotensin II and endothelin A receptor, has demonstrated that it effectively reduces proteinuria while maintaining safety. The benefit of omega-3 fatty acid fish oil remains controversial.

For patients with persistent proteinuria of >1 g/d, despite maximally tolerated RAAS blockade, corticosteroids have been shown to provide benefit with reduction of proteinuria and slowed decline in GFR.[1] Long-term sustained benefit with immunosuppression is less well established.[2] The incidence of adverse events was higher in subjects receiving immunosuppression rather than conservative therapy alone; thus treatment decisions need to be individualized.

Targeted release budesonide, which is designed to release the drug in the ileocecal region, where the majority of Peyer patches are found, has been shown to effectively reduce proteinuria and the rate of decline in eGFR when compared to placebo.[18,19] Mycophenolate mofetil can be considered as a glucocorticoid sparing agent in Chinese patients. Hydroxychloroquine can also be considered in Chinese patients at high risk of progression despite optimized ACEi/ARBS. Tonsillectomy (with or without glucocorticoids) has been performed in Japan for patients with IgA nephropathy.

Patients with rapidly progressive IgAN should be offered treatment with cyclophosphamide and glucocorticoids in accordance with treatment for ANCA-associated vasculitis.

Postinfectious Glomerulonephropathy

GENERAL PRINCIPLES

- Postinfectious glomerulonephropathy classically presents with the nephritic syndrome, hematuria, hypertension, edema, and renal insufficiency. Proteinuria may be present and is usually in the subnephrotic range.
- The risk of nephritis is more with pyoderma strains of *Streptococcus* (M types 47, 49, 55, and 57) than with the pharyngitis strains (M types 1, 2, 4, and 12). Early antibiotic therapy reduces the risk of developing nephritis.
- It is classically associated with streptococcal infection, which typically affects children under the age of 10, after a latent period of 2–4 weeks from onset of pharyngitis or skin infection. However, bacterial endocarditis, visceral abscesses, and ventriculoperitoneal shunt infections can also lead to this immune complex-mediated disease.
- Low complement levels are usually seen. ASO titers may be elevated serially, as may anti-DNase B antibodies in streptococcal-associated disease.

Pathogenesis

Postinfectious glomerulonephritis is caused by subendothelial and mesangial deposition of immune complexes which trigger off an inflammatory cascade, causing diffuse proliferative GN.

DIAGNOSIS

Kidney biopsy reveals subepithelial humps on light and electron microscopy corresponding to the deposits on immunofluorescence (IgG, C3). There is widespread mesangial proliferation as well as an infiltration of polymorphonuclear cells. Positive cultures for *Streptococcus* may be obtained during epidemics. ASO titers are increased after throat infections and anti-DNAse B titers are elevated in postpyoderma cases. Serum C3 levels are often decreased early in the course of the disease.

TREATMENT

Treatment is primarily supportive. Treatment is given for any residual streptococcal infection with benzathine penicillin single IM injection of 1.2 million units in adults and half-dose in children with oral penicillin, erythromycin, or cephalosporins 6 hourly for 7–10 days. This will help in sodium and fluid restriction and control of hypertension. Resolution of the underlying infection typically leads to renal recovery in 2–4 weeks, even in cases where dialytic support was needed. A brisk diuresis should be anticipated in the recovery period. Complications include cerebral vasogenic edema, cerebral vasculitis, and posterior reversible encephalitis.

Lupus Nephritis

GENERAL PRINCIPLES

LN can manifest as proteinuria of varying degrees with dysmorphic RBCs and RBC casts and renal insufficiency. Positive lupus serology (e.g., ANA, anti-double-stranded DNA antibodies) and hypocomplementemia are often present during acute flares.

DIAGNOSIS

Renal biopsy can provide diagnostic and prognostic information. The World Health Organization classification has five major categories based on histologic appearance. Class I has normal glomeruli, classes II to IV have increasing degrees of mesangial proliferation, and class V has an appearance similar to MN. Immunofluorescence is usually positive for IgG, IgA, IgM, C1q, and C3 for the "full-house" fluorescence pattern.

TREATMENT

Aggressiveness of therapy considers the renal and extrarenal manifestations of the disease.

- Classes I and II LN rarely require specific treatment, and therapy is directed at the extrarenal manifestations.
- Class III LN, when mild or moderate, can generally be treated with a short course of high-dose steroids (prednisone 1 mg/kg/d).
- Patients with severe class III LN, class IV and V LN, or severe nephritic syndrome should undergo pulse IV methylprednisolone (7–15 mg/kg/d for 3 days) followed by oral prednisone at 0.5–1.0 mg/kg/d. A second agent such as cyclophosphamide or oral mycophenolate mofetil is usually employed. Cyclophosphamide may be given as a larger monthly dose of 0.5–1.0 g/m^2 for 6 cycles or a lower 500 mg dose every 2 weeks for 6 cycles. Remission can be maintained for several years with mycophenolate mofetil 1000 mg twice daily, which was shown to be superior to azathioprine 2 mg/kg/d in preventing relapse.[20] Rituximab therapy has also been shown to have treatment efficacy.

Pulmonary-Renal Syndromes

GENERAL PRINCIPLES

Several distinct clinical entities make up the pulmonary-renal syndromes where there is vasculitic involvement of the alveolar and glomerular capillaries. Typically, this results in rapidly progressive renal failure often with concurrent pulmonary involvement in the form of alveolar hemorrhage. A nephritic picture predominates, with dysmorphic RBCs and RBC casts in the urine. Arthralgias, abdominal pain, and fever may represent other systemic manifestations.

DIAGNOSIS

- In **anti-GBM antibody disease**, circulating antibody to the α-3 chain of type IV collagen is deposited in the basement membrane of alveoli and glomeruli, resulting in linear staining on immunofluorescence. **Goodpasture syndrome** includes pulmonary involvement and can present with life-threatening alveolar hemorrhage. The presence of anti-GBM antibody in the serum supports the diagnosis, and 10%–30% of patients will have a positive ANCA serology as well.
- In **granulomatosis with polyangiitis** (GPA; formerly known as Wegener granulomatosis), vasculitic lesions involve the small vessels of the kidneys and may also involve the lungs, skin, and gastrointestinal tract. As in anti-GBM antibody disease, pulmonary hemorrhage may be life-threatening. Biopsy findings include a small-vessel vasculitis with noncaseating granuloma formation in the kidneys, lungs, or sinuses.
    - GPA is part of a group of diseases known as **ANCA-positive vasculitis**, or *pauci-immune glomerulonephritis* (referring to the absence of immunostaining deposits), which includes Churg–Strauss syndrome (asthma and eosinophilia) and microscopic polyangiitis.

- ◦ In GPA, there is a positive cytoplasmic ANCA (c-ANCA) directed against serine proteinase-3, whereas in microscopic polyangiitis and Churg–Strauss syndrome, there is a positive perinuclear ANCA (p-ANCA) directed against myeloperoxidase.

TREATMENT

- In anti-GBM antibody disease, the goal of therapy is to *clear the pathogenic antibody* while suppressing new production. Treatment is with daily total volume plasmapheresis for approximately 14 days in conjunction with cyclophosphamide 2 mg/kg/d and glucocorticoids (IV methylprednisolone 7–15 mg/kg/d for 3 days, followed by oral prednisone 1 mg/kg/d). Immunosuppression is tapered over 8 weeks. Serial measurement of the anti-GBM antibody level is useful to monitor therapy, with plasmapheresis and immunosuppression continuing until it is undetectable.
- Poor response to therapy is predicted by the presence of oliguria, Cr >5.7 mg/dL, or dialysis dependence on presentation. Even if the likelihood of renal recovery is low, evidence of pulmonary involvement warrants aggressive therapy.
- Treatment of ANCA-positive vasculitis is with combined prednisone 1 mg/kg/d (with taper) and cyclophosphamide (IV at 1 g/m^2 monthly or orally at 2 mg/kg/d) for at least 3 months to induce remission. Therapy should then continue with oral steroids for 1 year to prevent relapse. Rituximab given IV as four weekly doses of 375 mg/m^2, in combination with steroids, has also been approved for treatment of GPA.[6] Addition of plasmapheresis does not appear to improve outcomes compared to prednisone/cyclophosphamide or prednisone/rituximab therapy alone. Double-strength sulfamethoxazole–trimethoprim given twice daily has been shown to reduce extrarenal relapses and to prevent *Pneumocystis (carinii) jirovecii* infection in patients on high-dose immunosuppression.

Polycystic Kidney Disease

GENERAL PRINCIPLES

- Autosomal-dominant polycystic kidney disease (ADPKD) is a hereditary disorder resulting in cystic enlargement of the kidneys. The incidence is estimated to be 1 in 500–1000 live births. Approximately 20% of patients with ADPKD do not have a positive family history. ADPKD currently accounts for up to 10% of patients with ESRD.
- There are two well-described mutations in the polycystin genes, PKD1 and PKD2, which encode for polycystin (PC) 1 and 2, respectively. PKD1 is more common, accounting for approximately 85% of ADPKD. PKD2 is associated with later progression of disease.
- The mechanism by which cysts form is unclear; a proposed "two-hit" hypothesis implicates a second somatic mutation that inactivates the wild-type allele in individual cells. The polycystin gene products localize to the primary cilium of the apical membrane of tubular cells. Disordered cell division and aberrant planar cell polarity may lead to overgrowth of the tubular segment, eventually pinching off from the rest of the collecting system and forming discrete cysts. In abnormal cells, cyclic AMP imparts a proliferative phenotype as well as inducing chloride extrusion into the cyst lumen.

DIAGNOSIS

Clinical Presentation

- Hypertension is an early feature of ADPKD and occurs even prior to a reduction in the GFR in approximately 60% of patients. As the affected tubules enlarge, they impinge on the blood flow to neighboring glomeruli, rendering them ischemic. This, in turn, leads to

RAAS activation and systemic hypertension. Onset of kidney failure is highly variable, with half of patients reaching ESRD by the age of 60.

- Kidney stones develop in approximately 25% patients with ADPKD, with a higher proportion of uric acid composition as compared to the general population.
- Cerebral aneurysms, hepatic cysts, mitral valve prolapse, and colonic diverticula are associated with ADPKD. As cysts grow, they may lead to the development of a palpable flank mass. Symptoms such as gross hematuria and pain can indicate cyst hemorrhage into the collecting system. Flank pain may also be caused by cyst infection or stretching of the renal capsule.

Diagnostic Testing

- Differentiation from other renal cystic diseases (acquired cystic kidney diseases, medullary sponge kidney, medullary cystic kidney disease, glomerulocystic kidney disease) can be made by the presence of enlarged cystic kidneys rather than shrunken or normal-sized cystic kidneys.
- Ultrasonography reveals multiple cysts. In the setting of a positive family history, a diagnosis of ADPKD can be made from ultrasound findings, with criteria differing according to age. Three or more cysts (unilateral or bilateral) are required for diagnosis in patients between the ages of 15 and 39. From ages 40 to 59, two or more cysts in each kidney are required. From age 60 and older, more than four cysts in each kidney are required to make the diagnosis.
- Patients with a family history of cerebral aneurysms or with symptoms attributable to a cerebral aneurysm should undergo evaluation with brain MRI/MRA; imaging can be performed without the use of gadolinium contrast.
- Genetic testing may be considered if patients have equivocal imaging results or a definitive diagnosis is required.

TREATMENT

- Treatment of hypertension consists of reduction in sodium intake and pharmacologic therapy when indicated. A large randomized controlled trial of patients with ADPKD suggested improved preservation of renal function at blood pressure targets of 95–110/60–75, but tolerability was limited by symptomatic hypotension.[1] Thus, guidelines for blood pressure control in patients with ADPKD are similar to those in other patients with CKD, targeting a systolic pressure of <120 mm Hg using standardized office measurements.
- In 2018, tolvaptan was approved in the United States for the treatment of ADPKD. Blockade of the vasopressin-2 receptor inhibits cyclic AMP production. Large randomized controlled trials of tolvaptan have revealed a reduction of the cyst growth rate and a decreased rate of GFR decline as compared to placebo.[2,3] Treatment can be offered to patients with a GFR >25 mL/min/1.73 m^2 and evidence of disease progression (e.g., GFR decline, enlarged kidney volume, increased kidney length). Of note, subjects between the ages of 56 and 65 who were enrolled in the clinical trial did not show a benefit beyond that of placebo. Polyuria and polydipsia are frequently experienced by patients on this medication, and it may limit dose escalation to the goal of 90 mg in the morning and 30 mg in the afternoon. Close monitoring of hepatic enzymes is mandatory, with measurements at baseline, at 2 weeks, 4 weeks, monthly through the first 18 months, then every 3 months afterward.
- Gross hematuria from cyst hemorrhage can usually be managed with bed rest, hydration, and analgesia. Resolution may take 5–7 days.

- Cyst infections are generally treated with antibiotics that achieve good penetration into the cysts. Sulfamethoxazole–trimethoprim and ciprofloxacin are the antibiotics of choice. The absence of bacterial growth in urine does not dismiss the possibility of infection, as the cystic fluid does not necessarily communicate with the rest of the collecting system.
- Pain that persists without an obvious hemorrhagic or infectious cause may respond to targeted cyst drainage or cyst reduction surgery. Drained cysts often exhibit recurrence, thereby limiting the long-term effectiveness of this procedure.[21–23]

Nephrolithiasis

GENERAL PRINCIPLES

- **Calcium-based stones** are the most common and appear predominantly as calcium oxalate or calcium phosphate salts. These stones are radiopaque. Calcium phosphate stones can appear as elongated, blunt crystals and form in alkaline urine. Calcium oxalate stones can be found in acidic or alkaline urine and can be dumbbell shaped or appear as paired pyramids (giving them an envelope appearance when viewed on end).
- **Uric acid stones** can be idiopathic or develop as part of hyperuricosuric states such as gout and myeloproliferative disorders. These stones are radiolucent and are found in acidic urine. Uric acid crystals exhibit a variety of shapes, with needles and rhomboid forms being the most common.
- **Struvite stones** contain magnesium, ammonium, and phosphate, and develop in alkaline urine associated with urea-splitting organisms (e.g., *Proteus, Klebsiella*). They are radiopaque and can extend to fill the renal pelvis, taking on a staghorn configuration. On microscopy, struvite crystals have a characteristic coffin lid shape.
- **Cystine stones** are uncommon and can form as the result of an autosomal recessive disorder. These stones have an intermediate radiolucency and appear as hexagonal crystals in the urine.

DIAGNOSIS

Clinical Presentation

Patients often present with costovertebral angle or flank pain, which can radiate to the scrotum or labia. Hematuria with nondysmorphic RBCs may be noted. Oliguria and AKI are uncommon, but can result if there is bilateral obstruction or if a solitary functioning kidney is affected.

Diagnostic Testing

- Basic laboratory investigation should include urine culture, pH, microscopy, serum calcium, phosphate, parathyroid hormone, and uric acid levels. Urine should be strained and passed stones analyzed for composition.
- A plain abdominal film may reveal the radiopaque stones composed of calcium salts, struvite, or cystine; however, noncontrast CT scanning has replaced other imaging modalities as the study of choice for suspected nephrolithiasis.
- Recurrent stone formers should undergo a more extensive evaluation, with 24-hour urine collections for volume, calcium, sodium, phosphate, uric acid, citrate, oxalate, and cysteine, and pH measurement. This collection should not be done during an acute episode in a hospitalized patient, but rather reserved for when the patient is on his or her usual outpatient diet.

TREATMENT

- General treatment consists of **volume expansion** to increase urine output and analgesia. If the stone is obstructing outflow or is accompanied by infection, removal is indicated with urgent urologic or radiologic intervention.
- After passage of a stone, treatment is directed at **prevention of recurrent stone formation**. Regardless of stone type, the foundation of therapy is maintenance of high urine output (2–3 L/d) and a low-sodium diet (<3 g/d).
- For calcium oxalate stones, a low-calcium diet is no longer recommended, given the risks of osteoporosis. Instead, patients should be on a normal calcium diet with no added calcium supplements. Oxalate-rich foods (e.g., spinach, rhubarb) should be avoided. Thiazide diuretics may reduce calciuria and potassium citrate may be added in patients with hypocitraturia.
- Uric acid stones can be prevented or reduced in size by urinary alkalinization, preferentially with potassium citrate 10 mEq, 2–6 tablets divided twice or thrice daily, to target a urine pH of 6–6.5. A low-protein diet or allopurinol may also help in the management of these stones, although the predominant factor in uric acid precipitation remains a low pH.
- Struvite calculi frequently require surgical intervention for their removal. Extracorporeal shock wave lithotripsy can be used as adjunctive therapy. Monthly urine cultures should be obtained, and if positive, aggressive antibiotic treatment is indicated.
- Cystine stones require extensive urinary alkalinization to a pH of 7.0–7.5 to induce solubility, aggressive sodium restriction (<2 g/d). Tiopronin can further increase solubility through breakage and exchange of disulfide bonds. Side effects include fever, rash, arthritis, myelosuppression, and hepatotoxicity.

Management of Chronic Kidney Disease

GENERAL PRINCIPLES

- CKD is divided into five stages based on the estimated GFR (Figure 13-1). To be classified as stage 1 or stage 2, *there must be an accompanying structural or functional defect* (e.g., proteinuria, hematuria) because the GFR is normal or near normal in these stages.
- Patients are usually asymptomatic until significant renal function is lost (late stage 4 and stage 5). However, *complications, including hypertension, anemia, and mineral bone disorders* (renal osteodystrophy and secondary hyperparathyroidism), often develop during stage 3 and thus must be investigated and addressed before patients become symptomatic.
- The decline in GFR may be followed by plotting the reciprocal of Cr versus time, revealing a linear decrement. This can be useful in end-stage planning and in predicting when renal replacement therapy will be needed. A steeper than anticipated decline in GFR suggests a superimposed renal insult.
- In the setting of CKD, initiation of dialysis based solely on a target GFR has not shown a mortality benefit.[24] Dialysis should be started before the worsening of the patient's metabolic or nutritional status.

Risk Factors

- **Decreased renal perfusion** can lead to a decline in GFR. This can occur with true volume depletion or diminished effective circulating volume (e.g., congestive heart failure, hepatic cirrhosis). **NSAIDs** can be particularly deleterious in this setting because they block the renal autoregulatory mechanisms to preserve GFR. ACE inhibitors or ARBs also produce a reversible decrement in GFR through alterations in hemodynamics.
- Few of the common etiology are increasing age, low birth weight, **diabetes mellitus (most common)**, obesity, smoking, and ADPKD.

Prognosis of CKD by GFR and albuminuria category

Prognosis of CKD by GFR and Albuminuria Categories: KDIGO 2012				Persistent albuminuria categories Description and range		
				A1	**A2**	**A3**
				Normal to mildly increased	Moderately increased	Severely increased
				<30 mg/g <3 mg/mmol	30–300 mg/g 3–30 mg/mmol	>300 mg/g >30 mg/mmol
GFR categories (mL/min/1.73 m²) Description and range	G1	Normal or high	≥90	Low	Moderate	High
	G2	Mildly decreased	60–89	Low	Moderate	High
	G3a	Mildly to moderately decreased	45–59	Moderate	High	Very high
	G3b	Moderately to severely decreased	30–44	High	Very high	Very high
	G4	Severely decreased	15–29	Very high	Very high	Very high
	G5	Kidney failure	<15			

Figure 13-1 Stages of chronic kidney disease. CKD, chronic kidney disease; GFR, glomerular filtration rate. (Reprinted from Summary of recommendation statements. Kidney Int Suppl (2011). 2013;3(suppl):5-14 with permission from Elsevier.)

- **Uncontrolled hypertension** leads to hyperfiltration, which may lead to worsening proteinuria and further damage to the glomeruli.
- **Albuminuria has also been identified as a risk factor for progression of renal disease. A prognostic scale has been developed incorporating both the GFR and degree of albuminuria to predict the likelihood to renal failure** (see Figure 13-1).
- **Nephrotoxic agents,** such as iodinated contrast agents, NSAIDs, traditional herbal medicine, heavy metals (lead), and aminoglycosides, should be avoided when possible. Careful attention to drug dosing is mandatory, frequently guided by the estimated GFR or CKD stage. Drug levels should be monitored where appropriate.
- Patients undergoing coronary angiography are at particular risk for worsening CKD. **Contrast nephropathy and atheroembolic disease** are potential complications of coronary angiography, and the risks and benefits of the procedure must be weighed with the patient before proceeding.
- **UTI or obstruction** should be considered in all patients with an unexplained drop in renal function. Some of the obstructions and disorders are chronic glomerulonephritis, nephrolithiasis, and congenital renal diseases, for example, ADPKD.
- **Worsening renal artery stenosis** may also lead to a more rapid decline in GFR as well as sudden worsening in previously controlled hypertension.
- **Renal vein thrombosis** may occur as a complication of the nephrotic syndrome and can exacerbate CKD. Hematuria and flank pain may be present (Table 13-4).

TABLE 13-4 Clinical Features of CKD

System	Clinical Features
Renal	Polyuria or oliguria
Musculoskeletal	Muscle wasting, bone tenderness, and pathological fractures
Metabolic	Tetany (hypocalcemia), symptoms of electrolyte imbalance, and malnourishment
Immune system	Recurrent infections due to immunosuppression
Gastrointestinal	Diarrhea, loss of appetite, nausea, and vomiting
Reproductive system	Loss of libido, amenorrhea, menorrhagia, and erectile dysfunction
Cardiovascular	Atherosclerosis and hypertension
Serosa	Pericardial effusion, pleural effusion, and ascites
Nervous system	Peripheral neuropathy and encephalopathy
Dermatologic	Pruritus and calciphylaxis
Hematological	Anemia

TREATMENT

Treatment of CKD is focused on avoidance of risk factors (listed above), dietary modification, blood pressure control, adequate treatment of the associated conditions, and ultimately, preparation for renal replacement therapy.

- **Dietary restrictions**
  - **Sodium restriction** to <3 g/d is usually adequate for most CKD patients. Restriction to <2 g/d should be used if heart failure or refractory hypertension is present. A 24-hour urine sodium level of 100 mEq roughly correlates with a 2.4 g/d diet.
  - Fluid restriction is generally not required in CKD patients, and if excessive, may lead to volume depletion and hypernatremia. Restriction is appropriate in patients with dilutional hyponatremia.
  - **Potassium should be restricted** to 60 mEq/d in individuals with hyperkalemia. Tomato-based products, bananas, potatoes, and citrus drinks are high in potassium and should be avoided in these patients.
  - **Dietary phosphate restriction** should be 800–1000 mg/d. Dairy products, dark colas, and nuts should be avoided in hyperphosphatemia. Oral binders (calcium carbonate or acetate, lanthanum carbonate, sevelamer carbonate) can be taken with meals if dietary restrictions are unable to control phosphate levels.
- **Hypertension**
  - Uncontrolled hypertension accelerates the rate of decline of renal function. Blood pressure control <140/90 mm Hg is recommended for patients with CKD.[25]
  - **ACE inhibitors or ARBs** should be used preferentially in the CKD population. They lower intraglomerular pressure and possess renoprotective properties beyond their antihypertensive effect, particularly in proteinuric states. Because of their effects on intrarenal hemodynamics, a 30% rise in serum Cr should be anticipated and tolerated; a further rise should prompt a search for possible renal artery stenosis. The Cr and serum potassium should be checked approximately 1–2 weeks after a dose adjustment. Combined therapy with ACE inhibitors and ARBs is not recommended because of an increased risk of hyperkalemia and AKI without statistical benefit in mortality or long-term renal protection.[26]

- **Diuretics** are also beneficial in achieving euvolemia in hypertensive CKD patients. Thiazide diuretics become less effective as the GFR falls below 30 mL/min, whereas loop diuretics retain their efficacy, although higher doses may be required for the desired effect.

- **Anemia**
  - A normocytic anemia is common in CKD and should be evaluated once the GFR falls below 60 mL/min/1.73 m^2 (stage 3).
  - Alternate causes for an anemia should be entertained in the appropriate setting and iron stores assessed. If the transferrin saturation is <30% and there is no evidence of iron overload (ferritin <1000 ng/mL), consideration should be given to iron repletion with 1 g of an IV preparation of iron dextran (1000 mg once with test dose of 25 mg), ferric gluconate (125 mg, 8 doses), or iron sucrose (100 mg, 10 doses).
  - Erythropoiesis-stimulating agents (ESAs), such as epoetin and darbepoetin, can effectively reduce but do not prevent the need for RBC transfusions. ESA therapy increases the risk of stroke and thrombotic and cardiovascular events and worsens outcomes in patients with cancer. These agents should not be started in CKD unless the hemoglobin is <10 g/dL, other causes of anemia such as iron deficiency are addressed, and reduction in transfusions is a goal. The minimum dose that maintains the hemoglobin above the need for transfusion and *below 11 g/dL* should be used. Correction of iron deficiency frequently decreases the ESA dose requirement and may defer the need for ESA. Targeting the hemoglobin to higher levels has been associated with increased cardiovascular mortality, and this risk may be related to the higher doses of ESA.[27]

- **Bone mineral disorders**
  - CKD bone mineral disorders increase in prevalence as the GFR declines through stage 3 and more advanced disease. They include disorders of bone turnover and secondary hyperparathyroidism.
  - **Osteitis fibrosa cystica** is commonly associated with secondary hyperparathyroidism and increased bone turnover, resulting in bone pain and increased fracture risk. Adynamic bone disease is a low turnover state with suppressed parathyroid hormone (PTH) levels. Osteomalacia can involve deposition of aluminum into bone and is less commonly seen today with the decreased use of aluminum-based phosphate binders.
  - In CKD, starting in stage 3, vitamin D deficiency, low calcium, and elevated phosphate can all contribute to **secondary hyperparathyroidism**. The general goal of therapy is to suppress PTH toward normal while maintaining normal serum calcium and phosphate. This can be addressed in three steps: repletion of vitamin D stores (25-OH vitamin D), control of dietary phosphate with binders, and administration of active vitamin D (1,25-dihydroxyvitamin D or an analog).
    - Deficient stores (25-OH vitamin D <30 ng/mL) should be corrected with oral ergocalciferol 50,000-IU capsule weekly or every other week or cholecalciferol 2000–4000 IU daily. The duration of treatment depends on severity of the deficiency, with levels <5 ng/dL warranting at least 12 weeks of treatment. Once at goal, maintenance therapy can rely on either monthly ergocalciferol 50,000 IU or daily cholecalciferol 1000–2000 IU.
    - Phosphate control can be difficult as GFR declines, even with appropriate dietary restriction. Phosphate binders inhibit gastrointestinal absorption. Calcium-based binders are effective when given with meals as calcium carbonate (200 mg of elemental calcium per 500 mg tablet) or calcium acetate (169 mg of elemental calcium per 667 mg tablet). In general, the total daily elemental calcium administered should be <1500 mg. Lanthanum carbonate and sevelamer carbonate are non-calcium-based alternatives.
    - Active vitamin D (1,25-dihydroxyvitamin D) and its synthetic analogs are potent suppressors of PTH and can be administered if serum PTH remains elevated. Options include daily calcitriol (0.25–1 μg), paricalcitol (1–5 μg), or doxercalciferol (1–5 μg).

Calcium levels need to be monitored regularly and doses adjusted to avoid hypercalcemia.

- Cinacalcet is a calcimimetic that acts on the parathyroid gland to suppress PTH release. It should be used only in dialysis patients and usually in conjunction with active vitamin D because it may induce significant hypocalcemia and is relatively ineffective as monotherapy.

- **Metabolic acidosis.** As renal function deteriorates, the kidney is unable to appropriately excrete sufficient acid, resulting in metabolic acidosis (mixed high and normal anion gap). To compensate, alkaline buffer is released from the skeleton but can ultimately worsen bone mineral disease.
  - Treatment with **sodium bicarbonate** 650–1300 mg thrice daily can help maintain the serum bicarbonate level at 22 mEq/L. Such therapy, however, can increase the sodium load and contribute to edema or hypertension.
  - Citrate, another alkaline source, should not be used in the CKD or ESRD population because it can dramatically enhance gastrointestinal absorption of aluminum and lead to aluminum toxicity or osteomalacia.
- **Hyperlipidemia.** Therapy with statins combined with ezetimibe has shown improved cardiovascular outcomes with fewer major atherosclerotic events in patients with moderate to severe CKD and in the dialysis population, although the benefit in patients on dialysis was less.[28] Use of lipid-lowering therapy is appropriate in patients with atherosclerotic disease at all stages of CKD.
- **Preparation for renal replacement therapy**
  - Patients should be counseled at an early stage to determine preferences for renal replacement therapies, including hemodialysis, peritoneal dialysis (PD), and eligibility for renal transplantation.
  - In stage 4 CKD, preparation for the creation of a permanent vascular access for hemodialysis should be initiated by protecting the nondominant forearm from IV catheters and blood draws. Timely referral for vein mapping and to an access surgeon can facilitate the creation and maturation of an arteriovenous (AV) access.

RENAL REPLACEMENT THERAPIES

Approach to Dialysis

TREATMENT

- **Modalities**
  - Renal replacement therapy is indicated when conservative medical management is unable to control the metabolic derangements of kidney disease. This applies to the acute and chronic settings. Common acute indications include **hyperkalemia**, **metabolic acidosis**, and **volume overload** that are refractory to medical management. Uremic **encephalopathy** or **pericarditis** as well as certain **intoxications** (methanol, ethylene glycol, or salicylates) can all be indications to initiate dialytic therapy acutely. In the chronic setting, renal replacement therapy is typically begun before the worsening of the metabolic or nutritional status of the patient (Table 13-5).
  - Dialysis works by solute diffusion and water transport across a selectively permeable membrane. In hemodialysis, blood is pumped counter-currently to a dialysis solution within an extracorporeal membrane. This can be performed intermittently (3–4 hours during the day) or in a continuous 24-hour fashion, depending on hemodynamic stability or goals of therapy. PD uses the patient's peritoneal membrane as the selective filter, and dialysis fluid is instilled into the peritoneal cavity.

TABLE 13-5 Indications for Renal Replacement Therapy

AKI	CKD
Refractory hyperkalemia	When eGFR falls below 10–15 mL/min/1.72 m^2
Metabolic acidosis	Signs of uremia (pericarditis, encephalopathy, etc.)
Pulmonary edema	Worsening nutritional status (anorexia, loss of weight, nausea)
Uremic complications (pericarditis, bleeding, etc.)	Refractory volume overload
Volume control (in oliguric/anuric patients)	Fatigue, malaise, and cognitive impairment

  - Transplantation offers the best long-term survival and most completely replaces the filtrative and endocrine functions of the native kidney. However, it carries the risks that accompany long-term immunosuppression.
- **Diffusion**
  - The selectively permeable membrane contains pores that allow electrolytes and other small molecules to pass by diffusion while holding back larger molecules and cellular components of the blood. Movement relies on the molecular size and the concentration gradient. Potassium, urea, Cr, and other waste products of metabolism pass into the dialysis solution while alkaline buffers (bicarbonate or lactate) enter the blood from the dialysis solution.
- **Ultrafiltration/convection**
  - Removal of volume is termed ultrafiltration. It can be achieved in hemodialysis via a transmembrane hydrostatic pressure that removes excess fluid from the blood compartment. In PD, water follows its osmotic gradient into the relatively hyperosmolar dialysis solution (usually with dextrose providing the osmotic driving force).
  - As water is removed from the vascular compartment, it drags along solute in proportion to its concentration in the blood. This usually accounts for only a small fraction of the total clearance but can be significantly increased if a physiologic "replacement fluid" is infused into the patient concurrently to prevent hypovolemia, a process termed convective clearance. This strategy is frequently employed by continuous hemodialysis modalities.

Hemodialysis

GENERAL PRINCIPLES

- Hemodialysis is by far the most commonly used form of renal replacement therapy in the United States. Intermittent hemodialysis (IHD) typically runs for 3–4 hours per session and is performed three times weekly. Outpatient, in-center hemodialysis for ESRD generally uses this modality, although variations are available for patients undergoing home treatments.
- Continuous renal replacement therapy (CRRT) can be used in specialized circumstances, particularly when the patient's hemodynamic status would not tolerate the rapid fluid shifts of IHD. Although less efficient (with slower blood flows) and using slower UF rates, CRRT can achieve equivalent clearances of both solute and fluid compared to IHD due to its continuous, 24-hour nature. The slower blood flows usually necessitate anticoagulation (with systemic heparin or regional citrate) to prevent the filter from clotting. Continuous modalities require specialized nursing and an intensive care setting.

- The most frequently employed form of CRRT is continuous venovenous hemodiafiltration (CVVHDF).
- In CVVHDF, blood is slowly pumped counter-currently to a dialysis solution (diffusion), and a replacement fluid (a "cleansed" physiologic solution devoid of uremic toxins) is infused into the circuit to balance most of the ultrafiltrate (convection).

- Sustained low-efficiency dialysis is a hybrid form of IHD and CRRT used in an intensive care setting. Intermediate blood flows lower the clotting risk if anticoagulation is not used while intermediate treatment lengths (8–10 hours) still allow for adequate clearances. Patients also spend a significant portion of the day off the machine to allow for nonbedside testing, procedures, and physical therapy.
- **Prescription and adequacy**
  - IHD typically runs for 3–4 hours and can ultrafilter 3–4 L safely in hemodynamically stable patients. In the chronic setting, IHD is generally performed three times weekly, although the longer interdialytic interval on the weekend has been associated with a heightened mortality risk.[29] In the acute setting, the appropriate interval is not clearly known, although a thrice-weekly schedule is likely adequate.
  - Adequacy is assessed by calculating the clearance of BUN, which serves as a surrogate marker of the "uremic factors." The urea reduction ratio can be calculated by the following:

$$\text{URR} = \left[(\text{predialysis BUN} - \text{postdialysis BUN})/(\text{predialysis BUN})\right] \times 100$$

A reduction rate of >65% is considered adequate in the chronic setting.[30] An adequacy target is less well defined for AKI.

  - Intensive daily hemodialysis was not shown to be superior to standard thrice-weekly treatments.[31]
  - Clearance is measured differently in CRRT where dialytic therapy is taking place around the clock, effectively providing an extracorporeal "GFR." Drug dosing needs to be adjusted accordingly; an estimate of this clearance can be calculated by the sum of the dialysis fluid, replacement fluid, and net UF rates and then converted into milliliters per minute. For most circumstances, this approximates a clearance of 20–50 mL/min.
  - With CRRT, the net UF rate can be adjusted as needed, according to the patient's hemodynamic status. One must be vigilant in checking electrolyte levels (particularly calcium and phosphorus) to ensure they remain within the desired ranges. Ionized calcium levels are especially important to follow when regional citrate anticoagulation is being used.
  - Phosphate, which is predominantly intracellular, is generally poorly removed by IHD; however, in CRRT, there is continuous efflux of this anion, and significant hypophosphatemia can occur.

COMPLICATIONS

- Nontunneled catheters are typically placed in the internal jugular or femoral vein and carry the same risks as other central venous catheters (infection, bleeding, pneumothorax). They are almost exclusively used in the inpatient setting and are generally used for 1–2 weeks. Tunneled catheters have lower rates of infection and can be used for 6 months while a more definitive access is maturing (AV fistula or graft).
  - Fevers and rigors, particularly during dialysis, should prompt a search for an infectious cause, and empiric antibiotic coverage for staphylococci and gram-negative bacteria should be administered.
  - The catheter should then be replaced after a period of defervescence and sterilization of the blood (at least 48 hours). Documented bacteremia should be treated with antibiotics for at least several weeks.

- Thrombosis of an AV fistula or graft can frequently be recanalized by thrombolysis or thrombectomy. Stenotic regions can be evaluated by a fistulogram, and treatment may encompass angioplasty or stent deployment.
- Intradialytic hypotension is most commonly due to intravascular volume depletion from rapid UF. Antihypertensive medications may also contribute. Infectious causes should be sought in the appropriate setting. Acute treatment of the drop in blood pressure includes infusion of normal saline (as 200 mL boluses) and reduction of the UF rate.
- Dialysis disequilibrium is an uncommon syndrome that may occur in severely uremic patients undergoing their first few treatments. Rapid clearance of toxins is thought to induce cerebral edema by osmolar shifts and can present as nausea, emesis, headache, confusion, or seizures. Occurrence can be prevented or ameliorated by initiating patients on dialysis with slower blood flows and shorter treatments.

Peritoneal Dialysis

GENERAL PRINCIPLES

- There are two modalities in use: manual exchanges and automated cycler exchanges.
  - The manual modality, also called continuous ambulatory peritoneal dialysis (CAPD), has the patient instill dialysis fluid into the peritoneum for a specified length of time, after which the dialysate is drained and replaced by another dwell.
  - The automated modality, also called continuous cycling peritoneal dialysis (CCPD), typically operates overnight where a machine runs a preprogrammed set of exchanges while the patient sleeps. A final fill usually remains in the peritoneum and is carried during the daytime for continued solute exchange.
- Both PD modalities require strict adherence to sterile technique, and careful patient selection is necessary. Generally, PD should not be used if there is a history of recent abdominal surgery or if multiple peritoneal adhesions are present.
- **Prescription and adequacy**
  - The choice between CAPD and CCPD usually depends on patient preference and on the transport characteristics of the peritoneal membrane. Manual exchanges (i.e., CAPD) can be used as a backup modality, particularly in the hospital where nurse staffing or machine availability may be limited.
  - In writing PD orders, the following variables must be specified: dwell volume, dwell time, number of exchanges, and dextrose concentration of the dialysis solution. The dwell volume is typically between 2 and 3 L. The dextrose concentration can be 1.5%, 2.5%, or 4.25%, providing the osmotic gradient for fluid removal. Higher dextrose concentrations allow for greater UF but also lead to more inward glucose diffusion and worsening control of diabetes. Icodextrin is a glucose polymer preparation that can be used in longer dwell because it is minimally absorbed and thus maintains an effective osmotic gradient up to 18 hours. Commercially available PD solutions may have color-coded tabs, and patients may know these better than the actual concentrations (yellow for 1.5%, green for 2.5%, red for 4.25%). A sample order set for manual CAPD would be 2.5 L dwells, four exchanges per day, 6 hours per dwell, with 2.5% dextrose.
  - PD is less efficient than conventional hemodialysis. However, given its continuous nature, solute clearance and UF can approximate that of other modalities. Larger volumes and more frequent exchanges can assist with solute exchange. Increasing the concentration of dextrose can promote greater UF in volume-overloaded patients.
  - *Residual renal function is very important in the PD population, and avoidance of nephrotoxins should be practiced.*[32]

COMPLICATIONS

- **Peritonitis** typically presents with diffuse abdominal pain and cloudy peritoneal fluid. A sample should be sent for cell count, differential, Gram stain, and culture. A WBC count of >100 cells/μL, of which at least 50% are neutrophils, supports the diagnosis.
  - Empiric intraperitoneal antibiotics should cover for both gram-positive and gram-negative organisms, with a first-generation cephalosporin (cefazolin or cephalothin) and ceftazidime at 15–20 mg/kg of each in the longest dwell of the day.[33] If a methicillin-resistant organism is suspected, vancomycin (30 mg/kg every 5–7 days) should be used for gram-positive coverage, along with a third-generation cephalosporin for gram-negative coverage, including *Pseudomonas*.
  - The intraperitoneal route is the preferred method of administration, unless the patient is overtly septic, in which case IV antibiotics should be used. Antibiotics can be tailored once culture results are known and should be continued for 2–3 weeks. Multiple organisms, particularly if gram-negative, should prompt a search for intestinal perforation.
- Tunnel or exit site infections may present with local erythema, tenderness, or purulent drainage, although crusting at the exit site alone does not necessarily indicate infection. Treatment can be with oral cephalosporins (gram-positive) or fluoroquinolones (gram-negative). However, infections can be difficult to eradicate, and catheter removal may be required with a temporary transition to hemodialysis.
- Failure of PD fluid to drain is termed outflow failure. This may result from kinking of the catheter, constipation, or plugging of the catheter with fibrin strands. Conservative treatment should aim at resolving constipation if present and instilling heparin into the PD fluid at a dose of 500 units/L.
- Small hernias are at particularly high risk for incarceration and should be corrected surgically while the patient is temporarily treated with hemodialysis. Fluid leaks can lead to abdominal wall and genital edema and typically result from anatomic defects. Hydrothorax usually occurs on the right side and can be diagnosed by a markedly elevated glucose concentration in the pleural fluid. Pleurodesis can eliminate the potential space and permit continuation of PD.
- **Sclerosing encapsulating peritonitis** is a complication of long-term PD. The peritoneal membrane becomes thickened and entraps loops of bowel, leading to symptoms of bowel obstruction. A bloody drainage may be present. Treatment is supportive with the focus on bowel rest and surgical lysis of adhesions. A trial of immunosuppression with prednisone 10–40 mg/d may have limited benefit.
- Hyperglycemia results from the systemic absorption of glucose from the dialysis fluid. Because peritoneal uptake of insulin is unpredictable, treatment with subcutaneous insulin is preferred.
- Hyperlipidemia is common in the PD population, and treatment should be reserved for those with specific cardiac indications.
- Unlike hemodialysis, patients on PD tend to experience hypokalemia, likely due to a continuous potassium exodus in the dialysate as well as from an intracellular shift from the increased endogenous insulin production. Oral replacement is usually sufficient, either with relaxation of prior dietary restrictions or with low-dose supplementation (10–20 mEq/d of potassium chloride).
- Protein loss can be high, and the dietary protein intake should be 1.2–1.3 g/kg/d. Episodes of peritonitis can make the membrane even more susceptible to protein losses.

Transplantation

GENERAL PRINCIPLES

- Renal transplantation offers patients an improved quality of life and survival as compared to other renal replacement modalities.
- Pretransplant evaluation focuses on cardiopulmonary status, vascular sufficiency, and human lymphocyte antigen typing. Structural abnormalities of the urinary tract need to be addressed. Contraindications include most malignancies, active infection, or significant cardiopulmonary disease.
- In adult recipients, the renal allograft is placed in the extraperitoneal space, in the anterior lower abdomen. Vascular anastomosis is typically to the iliac vessels, whereas the ureter is attached to the bladder through a muscular tunnel to approximate sphincter function.
- Immunosuppression protocols vary among institutions. A typical regimen would include prednisone along with a combination of a calcineurin inhibitor (cyclosporine or tacrolimus) and an antimetabolite (mycophenolate derivative, azathioprine, or rapamycin).
- Evaluation of allograft dysfunction frequently requires kidney biopsy. Current laboratory and radiologic tests cannot reliably distinguish acute rejection from drug toxicity, the two most common causes of a rising Cr in the transplant population. Post-transplant lymphoproliferative disease, interstitial nephritis, and infections such as cytomegalovirus, *Polyomavirus* (BK virus), and pyelonephritis may present similarly to acute allograft dysfunction and should be excluded.
- Complications and long-term management of transplant recipients are discussed further in Chapter 17, Solid Organ Transplant Medicine and Stem Cell Transplantation.

Summary

- Creatinine clearance is more helpful in evaluating renal function than creatinine levels. This can be calculated using some equations, such as the modification of diet in renal disease (MDRD), CKD-EPI equation, and the Cockcroft-Gault formula.
- Urine albumin measurement is an important component in screening for chronic kidney disease. The presence of proteinuria is an independent risk factor for cardiovascular disease, end-stage renal disease, stroke, and death in the general population, and in patients with chronic kidney disease.
- AKI is a complex syndrome that include pre-renal AKI, acute tubular necrosis, acute interstitial nephritis, acute glomerular diseases, and acute obstructive nephropathy.
- Chronic kidney disease (CKD) is defined as the presence of kidney damage or an estimated glomerular filtration rate (eGFR) less than 60 mL/min/1.73 mt^2, persisting for 3 months or more, irrespective of the cause.
- Up to 60% of SLE patients develop lupus nephritis, which has a significant impact on their quality of life and prognosis.

Scan the QR code to access chapter references.

14 Treatment of Infectious Diseases

Carlos Mejia-Chew, Nigar Kirmani, Stephen Y. Liang, Jeco Jacob Kuttykandathil, and Gauri Malavalli Girish

Principles of Therapy

GENERAL PRINCIPLES

- Infections are caused by bacteria, viruses, fungi, or parasites and can involve any organ system.
- Antimicrobials should be used carefully and only when indicated. Antimicrobial stewardship is necessary to combat drug resistance, avoid adverse effects, and curb excess cost.
- The World Health Organization (WHO) estimates that infectious diseases account for more than 17 million deaths per year worldwide. It is estimated that at least 30 new infectious diseases have emerged within the past two decades. Southeast Asia bears the highest risk and burden of many of these diseases. In 2021, approximately 1.65 billion individuals required treatment for neglected tropical diseases.[1]
- Several emerging and re-emerging infections have been identified from Asia. There is an urgent need of good surveillance network and robust public health interventions to identify and control any potential outbreak at the earliest.
- Infectious disease consultation reduces mortality for many infections and can aid with the diagnosis and management of complicated infectious diseases and monitoring of antimicrobial therapy.[2] Infectious disease consultation and training need to be strengthened in many parts of Asia.
- The COVID-19 disease caused by coronavirus SARS-CoV2 infected over 760 million cases and 6.9 million deaths since 2019, though actual numbers are expected to be much higher. This global pandemic highlighted the importance of focused diagnostic approach and targeted therapy.

DIAGNOSIS

- **History and physical examination** are critical, particularly for diagnostic dilemmas such as fever of unknown origin (FUO). Eliciting exposures, occupation, travel history, and recreational activities informs and often helps broaden the differential diagnosis.
- **Gram stain** from potentially infected patient specimens can facilitate a rapid presumptive diagnosis and guide empiric antibiotic selection.
- **Aerobic, anaerobic, fungal, or acid-fast bacilli (AFB) microbiologic cultures** should be performed on patient specimens as indicated. Appropriate sample collection and its proper transport are crucial to reach a correct diagnosis. The microbiology laboratory should be consulted if organisms with special growth requirements are suspected to ensure appropriate transport and processing of cultures.
- **Antimicrobial susceptibility testing** of cultures facilitates the selection of antimicrobial agents and reduces the incidence of polypharmacy.
- **Rapid diagnostic testing** (e.g., polymerase chain reaction [PCR], antigen detection) has become increasingly widespread and helps provide early confirmation of an infectious etiologic agent.

TREATMENT

- **Choice of initial antimicrobial therapy**
  - Overuse of antimicrobials has led to an epidemic of antimicrobial-resistant organisms, some multidrug-resistant organisms (MDRO) with few remaining treatment options. Therefore, the first question one should ask is, "Does an infection exist that needs to be treated?"
  - Empiric antimicrobial therapy should be directed against the most likely infecting organism(s).
  - Antimicrobial susceptibility patterns should be considered in selecting empiric therapy. Antibiograms provide important insight into trends in local antimicrobial resistance.
  - Drug allergies, previous microbiologic cultures, prior antimicrobial exposure, and drug–drug interactions should also guide antimicrobial selection.
  - De-escalate to an antimicrobial regimen with the narrowest spectrum of activity once the infectious etiologic agent has been identified and susceptibility data are available.
- **Timing for the initiation of antimicrobial therapy**
  - In acute clinical scenarios, empiric therapy should begin immediately and ideally after appropriate microbiologic cultures have been obtained. Urgent therapy is indicated in febrile patients who are neutropenic or asplenic, and in patients with sepsis, meningitis, or rapidly progressive necrotizing infections.
  - In clinically stable patients, empiric antimicrobials can be withheld pending further evaluation, allowing for more targeted therapy.
- **Route of administration**
  - Patients with serious infections should receive IV antimicrobial agents.
  - Oral therapy is acceptable in less-urgent circumstances if adequate drug concentrations can be achieved at the site of infection.
  - **Type of therapy**
  - Renal and hepatic function should guide antimicrobial dosing regimens.
  - Always assess for drug–drug interactions before starting treatment to avoid adverse events and ensure effectiveness of therapy.
- **Assessment of outcomes on antimicrobial therapy**
  - If there is concern for potential treatment failure, ask the following questions:
    - Is the isolated organism the etiologic agent? Is there a superinfection?
    - Has an appropriate antimicrobial regimen been selected?
    - Are adequate concentrations of the antimicrobial achieved at the site of infection?
    - Has adequate source control been accomplished?
- **Duration of therapy**
  - Use the shortest duration of therapy for the infection identified.[3]
  - Treatment of acute uncomplicated infections should be continued until the patient is afebrile and clinically well, usually for a minimum of 72 hours.
  - Certain infections (e.g., endocarditis, septic arthritis, osteomyelitis) require prolonged therapy.

SPECIAL CONSIDERATIONS

- **Immunosuppressed hosts**
  - In patients with HIV/AIDS, transplant recipients (solid organ and hematopoietic stem cell), patients undergoing chemotherapy, and patients on glucocorticoids or other immune-modulating agents, consider opportunistic infections. Neutropenic patients require broader empiric antimicrobial therapy.

- **Pregnancy and the postpartum patient**
  - There are no Class A antimicrobials. Penicillins and cephalosporins (Class B) are frequently used. **Tetracyclines and fluoroquinolones are contraindicated.** Sulfonamides and aminoglycosides should not be used if alternative agents are available.
  - Many antimicrobials are excreted in breast milk and should be used with caution in breastfeeding women.

TOXIN-MEDIATED INFECTIONS

Clostridium Difficile Infection

GENERAL PRINCIPLES

Frequently seen after systemic antimicrobial therapy. Those patients who are elderly, immunocompromised, or receiving multiple and long-term antibiotics are at a higher risk.

DIAGNOSIS

Clinical Presentation

- Symptoms may range from mild or moderate watery diarrhea to severe and potentially fatal pseudomembranous colitis.
- Patients suspected to have *C. difficile* infection should be assessed for disease severity as follows:
  - Nonsevere disease: Watery diarrhea (≥3 episodes/24 hours) along with lower abdominal pain, nausea, low-grade fever, WBC ≤15,000 cells/mL, and creatinine <1.5 mg/dL.
  - Severe and fulminant colitis: Diarrhea, localized/diffuse abdominal pain and distension, fever, leukocytosis (>15,000 cells/mL), deranged renal parameters (creatinine >1.5 mg/dL) and electrolytes, increased lactic acid and hypotension. Fulminant disease can manifest as colonic ileus or toxic megacolon leading to bowel perforation.
  - Recurrent disease: Characterized by the resolution of symptoms while on appropriate therapy and the reemergence of symptoms a few weeks after stopping treatment (Figure 14-1).

Differential Diagnosis

Antibiotic-associated osmotic diarrhea without *Clostridium difficile* infection should be considered and will resolve after withdrawal of the antibiotic.

Diagnostic Testing

- Testing for *C. difficile* infection is recommended in patients with unexplained and new-onset ≥3 unformed stools in 24 hours. Diagnosis is made by detection of toxigenic *C. difficile* in diarrheal stool through nucleic acid amplification test (NAAT) or enzyme immunoassay.
- Visualization of pseudomembranes on colonoscopy or sigmoidoscopy with biopsy can also be diagnostic for *C. difficile* infection.

TREATMENT

- For an initial episode of *C. difficile* infection (severe or nonsevere), treatment should consist of vancomycin 125 mg PO q6h for 10 days and discontinuation of the offending antibiotic if possible.[4] Oral fidaxomicin (200 mg PO q12h for 10 days) is an alternate first-line drug. If the above-mentioned drugs are not available, metronidazole can be used.

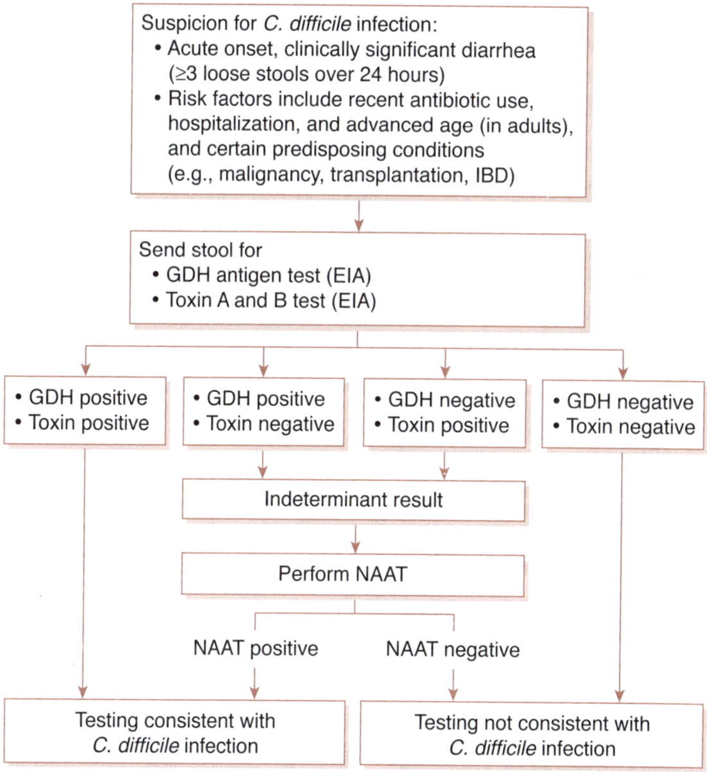

Figure 14-1 Approach to a patient suspected to have *C. difficile* infection. *Source*: Adapted from Graphic 100540 Version 10.0 UptoDate – Clostridioides difficile infection.

- For fulminant infections complicated by ileus, toxic megacolon, hypotension, or shock, surgery consultation should be obtained along with treatment consisting of vancomycin 500 mg PO or by nasogastric tube q6h in combination with metronidazole 500 mg IV q8h. If ileus is present, consider adding rectal instillation of vancomycin. In some cases, colectomy may be necessary.[4]
- Endpoint of therapy is cessation of diarrhea; **do not retest stool for toxin clearance.**
- Avoid antimotility agents in severe disease.
- Recurrence is common and is treated with vancomycin using tapered and pulsed regimens. Adjunctive therapy with oral rifaximin is sometimes used. Bezlotoxumab 10 mg/kg intravenously can be used as a single-dose adjunctive therapy.
- Fecal microbiota transplantation may be considered for patients with multiple recurrences (at least 3) despite appropriate antibiotic treatment.[4]

Tetanus

GENERAL PRINCIPLES

- Caused by *Clostridium tetani* toxin (tetanospasmin) from wound contamination with spores and affecting the nervous system.

- Tetanus is best prevented by immunization. For high-risk wounds, additional prophylaxis with human tetanus immunoglobulin 250 units IM is recommended.[5]

DIAGNOSIS

Classically presents with intensely painful muscle spasms and rigidity, followed by autonomic dysfunction. Symptoms often begin in the face (trismus, risus sardonicus) and neck muscles. Spasms of the glottis and respiratory muscles may cause acute asphyxia. Delirium and high fever are usually absent. Diagnosis is clinical.

Differential Diagnosis

- Drug-induced dystonias secondary to drugs like phenothiazines
- Strychnine poisoning
- Trismus from a dental infection
- Malignant neuroleptic syndrome

TREATMENT

- General supportive care includes nursing in a quiet, dark, well-ventilated room.
- Passive immunization with human tetanus immunoglobulin 3000–6000 units IM (in divided doses with part infiltrated around the wound) to neutralize unbound toxin is warranted. Active immunization with tetanus toxoid should be given at a separate site.
- Surgical debridement of the wound is critical.
- Antibiotic therapy, usually consisting of metronidazole 500 mg IV q6–8h or penicillin G 2–4 million units IV q4–6h, for 7–10 days is recommended. If a mixed infection is suspected, initiate the patient on a first- to third-generation cephalosporin, e.g., ceftriaxone 1–2 g q24h or cefazoline 1–2 g q8h.
- Benzodiazepines or neuromuscular blocking agents such as vecuronium, and magnesium sulphate may be used to control spasms.

TOXIC SHOCK SYNDROME

Toxic shock syndrome (TSS) is a life-threatening systemic disease caused by exotoxin superantigens produced by *Staphylococcus aureus* or group A β-hemolytic *Streptococcus* (GABHS) (Table 14-1).

Staphylococcal Toxic Shock Syndrome

GENERAL PRINCIPLES

Most often associated with colonization of surgical wounds, burns, vaginitis, or tampon use in young women. Cases are also seen after nasal packing for epistaxis. Mortality is low (<3%) in menstrual cases as compared to in nonmenstrual cases (6%).

DIAGNOSIS

Clinical Criteria

- **Fever:** Temperature ≥38.9°C (102.0°F)
- **Rash:** Diffuse macular erythroderma
- **Desquamation:** 1–2 weeks after onset of rash

TABLE 14-1 Treatment of Toxic Shock Syndromes

Etiology	Antibiotic Therapy	Adjunctive Therapy	Notes
Group A β-hemolytic *Streptococcus* (GABHS)	Penicillin G 4 million units IV q4h + clindamycin 900 mg IV q8h for 10–14 d	IVIG 1 g/kg on day 1, then 0.5 g/kg on days 2 and 3	Surgical debridement is almost always indicated for necrotizing infections. Clindamycin is added to decrease toxin production.
Staphylococcus aureus	Oxacillin 2 g IV q4h or vancomycin 1 g IV q12h + clindamycin 900 mg IV q8h for 10–14 d + one of the following: • Cefepime 2 g IV q8H • A carbapenem (meropenem/imipenem)	IVIG as per GABHS may be useful in severe cases, but higher doses may be needed	Surgical debridement may be necessary for wounds. Tampons and other foreign bodies should be removed and avoided in future, especially if TSST-1 antibody titres are negative.

IVIG, intravenous immunoglobulin; *TSST-1*, toxic shock syndrome toxin-1.

- **Hypotension**
    - **For adults:** Systolic blood pressure ≤90 mm Hg
    - For children <16 years of age: Systolic blood pressure <5th percentile by age
- **Multisystem involvement** (3 or more of the following organ systems)
    - **Gastrointestinal:** Vomiting or diarrhea at onset of illness
    - **Muscular:** Severe myalgia or creatine phosphokinase elevation >2 times the upper limit of normal
    - **Mucous membranes:** Vaginal, oropharyngeal, or conjunctival hyperemia
    - **Renal:** Blood urea nitrogen or serum creatinine >2 times the upper limit of normal or pyuria (>5 leukocytes/high-power field) in the absence of urinary tract infection
    - **Hepatic:** Bilirubin or transaminases >2 times the upper limit of normal
    - **Hematologic:** Platelets <100,000/μL
    - **Central nervous system:** Disorientation or alterations in consciousness without focal neurologic signs when fever and hypotension are absent

Laboratory Criteria

Cultures (blood or cerebrospinal fluid) negative for alternative pathogens (blood cultures may be positive for *S. aureus*)

Serologic tests negative (if obtained) for Rocky Mountain spotted fever, leptospirosis, or measles

Case Classification

- **Probable case:** A case which meets the laboratory criteria and 4 of the 5 clinical criteria

- **Confirmed case:** A case which meets the laboratory criteria and all 5 of the clinical criteria, including desquamation (unless the patient dies before desquamation occurs)

Diagnostic Testing

- Blood cultures are usually negative. Creatine kinase (CK) is often elevated.
- Staphylococcal isolates can be tested for toxin production, including toxic shock syndrome toxin-1 (TSST-1). Serum antibodies against TSST-1 may protect against future recurrences.[6]

TREATMENT

See Table 14-1.

Streptococcal Toxic Shock Syndrome

GENERAL PRINCIPLES

Associated with invasive GABHS infections, particularly necrotizing fasciitis or myositis (80% of cases). Mortality is much higher (30%–70%) compared to staphylococcal TSS.

DIAGNOSIS

Clinical Presentation

Initial presentation is typically abrupt onset of severe diffuse or localized pain. Systemic manifestations are otherwise similar to staphylococcal TSS, but the desquamating erythroderma is much less common.

Clinical Criteria

- **Hypotension:** systolic blood pressure ≤90 mm Hg in adults
- **Multiorgan involvement** characterized by two or more of the following:
  - **Renal impairment:** In adults, creatinine ≥2 mg/dL; in patients with pre-existing renal disease, ≥2 times elevation over baseline
  - **Coagulopathy:** Platelets ≤100,000/mm^3 (100 × 106/L) or disseminated intravascular coagulation, defined by prolonged clotting times, low fibrinogen level, and the presence of fibrin degradation products.
  - **Liver involvement:** Alanine aminotransferase, aspartate aminotransferase, or total bilirubin levels ≥2 times the upper limit of normal for the patient's age; in patients with pre-existing liver disease, ≥2 times elevation over baseline
  - **Acute respiratory distress syndrome**
  - **Erythematous macular rash** may desquamate
  - **Soft tissue necrosis,** such as, necrotizing fasciitis, myositis, or gangrene

Diagnostic Testing

Blood cultures are usually positive, and antistreptolysin O titres are elevated.

TREATMENT

See Table 14-1.

SKIN, SOFT TISSUE, AND BONE INFECTIONS

Purulent Skin and Soft Tissue Infections (Furuncles, Carbuncles, Abscesses)

GENERAL PRINCIPLES

S. aureus infections are common. Methicillin-resistant *S. aureus* (MRSA) is a growing concern.

TREATMENT

- Incision and drainage (I&D) alone is usually adequate, especially for abscesses measuring <5 cm.
- Parenteral antibiotic therapy is needed for extensive disease; systemic illness; rapid progression with associated cellulitis; comorbid diseases (diabetes mellitus); immunosuppression; inability to tolerate or absorb oral therapy; or lack of response to I&D.
- Empiric antibiotic therapy should cover community-acquired MRSA.
- Empiric IV antibiotics include vancomycin (20–35 mg/kg one-time loading dose followed by 15–20 mg/kg IV q8h), or daptomycin 4–6 mg/kg od PLUS
  - Cefepime 2 g q8h
  - Meropenem 1 g q8h (if ESBL positive organism suspected)
- Oral antibiotics include clindamycin 300–450 mg q8h, trimethoprim-sulfamethoxazole (TMP-SMX) 1–2 double-strength tablets q12h, doxycycline 100 mg q12h, and linezolid 600 mg q12h.
- Duration of antibiotic therapy is usually 5–7 days[7] and can be extended up to 14 days if the clinical response is slow.

Nonpurulent Skin and Soft Tissue Infections

Erysipelas

GENERAL PRINCIPLES

Erysipelas appears as a painful, superficial, erythematous, sharply demarcated lesion that is usually found on lower extremities. In normal hosts, GABHS is responsible for this infection.

TREATMENT

Penicillin V 250–1000 mg PO q6h or penicillin G 2.0–4.0 million units IV q6h, depending on the severity of illness. In patients who are penicillin allergic, macrolides and clindamycin are alternatives.

Cellulitis

GENERAL PRINCIPLES

- Common organisms include β-hemolytic streptococci and *S. aureus* (MSSA and MRSA).
- Severe cellulitis is sometimes seen after exposure to fresh (*Aeromonas hydrophila*) or salt (*Vibrio vulnificus*) water.

TREATMENT

- If streptococci or MSSA are suspected, a β-lactam antibiotic (cephalexin or dicloxacillin 500 mg PO q6h) or clindamycin can be used.
- If there is a strong concern for community-acquired MRSA, empiric antibiotic coverage may consist of clindamycin or linezolid. TMP-SMX can also be used in combination with a β-lactam antibiotic (e.g., cephalexin) to provide streptococcal coverage.
- Coverage for waterborne pathogens should initially consist of ceftazidime 2 g IV q8h, cefepime 2 g IV q8h, or ciprofloxacin 750 mg PO q12h in combination with doxycycline 100 mg IV/PO q12h. Duration of therapy is usually 5–7 days, with extension up to 14 days in case of severe infection.
- For patients with soft tissue infection following water exposure, the following antibiotics are used for initial empiric therapy:
  - First-generation cephalosporin, cephalexin (500 mg orally four times daily) or cefazolin (1 g intravenously every eight hours).
    PLUS
  - fluoroquinolone, e.g., levofloxacin (750 mg once daily).
    PLUS (if there is an epidemiologic risk present)
  - For individuals exposed to seawater: Doxycycline (100 mg twice daily) for Vibrio species.
- In cases of soil-contaminated wounds or exposure to sewage-contaminated water: Metronidazole (500 mg four times daily) for anaerobic coverage.[8]

Complicated Skin and Soft Tissue Infections

GENERAL PRINCIPLES

Deep soft tissue infections, surgical and traumatic wound infections, large abscesses, complicated cellulitis, and infected ulcers and burns fall under this classification.

DIAGNOSIS

Cultures of abscesses and surgical debridement specimens should be obtained to guide antibiotic therapy.

TREATMENT

- Patients should be hospitalized to receive IV antibiotics (including MRSA coverage) and undergo surgical intervention as necessary. Vancomycin 15–20 mg/kg IV q12h, teicoplanin 6 mg/kg IV loading followed by maintenance dosage, linezolid 600 mg PO/IV q12h, daptomycin 4 mg/kg IV qday, clindamycin 900 mg IV q8h, and ceftaroline 600 mg IV q12h are all acceptable antibiotic options.[7]

Infected Decubitus Ulcers and Limb-Threatening Diabetic Foot Ulcers

GENERAL PRINCIPLES

- Infections are usually polymicrobial. **Superficial swab cultures are unreliable.** Instead, deep tissue cultures obtained after wound debridement are preferred.
- Osteomyelitis is a frequent complication and should be excluded.

TREATMENT

- Wound care and debridement are important first-line therapies.
- **Mild diabetic foot infections** are usually due to *S. aureus* and streptococci and can be treated with cephalexin or amoxicillin-clavulanate (875 mg/125 mg PO q12h).[9] If MRSA is suspected, either TMP-SMX or doxycycline is recommended.
- **Moderate to severe infections** require systemic antibiotics covering *S. aureus* (including MRSA), anaerobes, and enteric gram-negative organisms. Options include
  1. Vancomycin plus a β-lactam/β-lactamase inhibitor combination (e.g., piperacillin tazobactam) or a carbapenem (e.g., meropenem)
  2. Vancomycin with metronidazole combined with either ciprofloxacin or a third-generation cephalosporin.

Necrotizing Fasciitis

GENERAL PRINCIPLES

- This is an infectious disease emergency with high mortality manifested by extensive soft tissue infection and thrombosis of the microcirculation with resulting necrosis. Infection spreads quickly along fascial planes and may be associated with sepsis or TSS. Fournier gangrene is necrotizing fasciitis of the perineum.
- Bacterial etiology is either mixed (aerobic and anaerobic organisms) or monomicrobial (GABHS or *S. aureus*, including community-acquired MRSA).
- It is associated with high mortality.

DIAGNOSIS

Clinical Presentation

May present initially like simple cellulitis rapidly progressing to necrosis with dusky, hypoesthetic skin and bulla formation in association with severe pain. Pain out of proportion to examination should raise concern for necrotizing fasciitis. It most commonly affects the extremities, with the lower extremities being more commonly affected than the upper.

Diagnostic Testing

- Diagnosis is clinical. High suspicion should prompt **immediate surgical exploration** where lack of resistance to probing is diagnostic.
- Cultures of operative specimens and blood should be obtained. Creatine kinase may be elevated.
- CT and plain films may demonstrate gas and fascial edema early in the disease process.

TREATMENT

- Aggressive surgical debridement is critical, along with IV antibiotics and volume support.
- Initial broad-spectrum empiric antibiotic therapy should consist of a β-lactam/β-lactamase inhibitor/high-dose penicillin/carbapenem/fluoroquinolone in combination with clindamycin. Vancomycin should also be added until MRSA can be excluded.
- Adjunctive hyperbaric oxygen may be useful.

Anaerobic Myonecrosis (Gas Gangrene)

GENERAL PRINCIPLES

It is a life-threatening muscle infection due to *Clostridium perfringens*, *Clostridium septicum*, *S. aureus*, GABHS, or other anaerobes. Distinguishing this condition from necrotizing fasciitis requires gross inspection of the involved muscle at the time of surgery.

Gas gangrene presents with sudden onset of severe muscle pain, followed by purple or red discoloration of skin, with bullae and tenderness.

TREATMENT

Treatment requires prompt surgical debridement and combination antimicrobial therapy with IV penicillin (3–4 million units IV q4h) plus clindamycin (900 mg IV q8h). A third-generation cephalosporin, ciprofloxacin, or an aminoglycoside should be added until a gram-negative infection can be excluded.

Osteomyelitis

GENERAL PRINCIPLES

- Osteomyelitis is an infection of bone. It should be considered when skin or soft tissue infections overlie bone and when localized bone pain accompanies fever or sepsis.
- See Table 14-2.

DIAGNOSIS

- Diagnosis is made by detection of exposed bone through a skin ulcer or by imaging with plain films, bone scintigraphy, or MRI.[10]
- Biopsy and cultures of the affected bone should be performed (before initiation of antimicrobials when possible) for pathogen-directed therapy.
- Erythrocyte sedimentation rate and C-reactive protein are usually markedly elevated and can be used to monitor the response to therapy.

TREATMENT

- See Table 14-2.
- Parenteral β-lactam antibiotics (oxacillin, cefazolin) are effective against MSSA. Vancomycin, daptomycin, and linezolid are used to treat MRSA osteomyelitis. Oral agents capable of achieving reasonable bone levels include TMP-SMX, clindamycin, and doxycycline.
- Gram-negative osteomyelitis can be treated with parenteral or oral fluoroquinolones, which have excellent bone penetration and bioavailability, or with a third-generation cephalosporin.
- Cure typically requires at least 4–6 weeks of high-dose antimicrobial therapy. Parenteral therapy should be given initially; oral regimens may be considered after 2–3 weeks if the pathogen is susceptible and adequate bactericidal levels can be achieved.[11]
- If peripheral vascular disease is present, revascularization may be helpful.

TABLE 14-2 Treatment of Osteomyelitis

Etiology of Osteomyelitis	Organism	Treatment Considerations
Acute hematogenous	• *Staphylococcus aureus*	• Antibiotic therapy alone may be sufficient if no foreign body is present.
Vertebral	• *S. aureus* • Gram-negative bacilli • *Mycobacterium tuberculosis*	• Biopsy off antibiotics (preferred) to guide therapy. • Antibiotic therapy alone may be sufficient.
Associated with a contiguous focus of infection	• *S. aureus* • Gram-negative bacilli • Coagulase-negative staphylococci (surgical site infections) • Anaerobes/polymicrobial (infected sacral decubitus ulcers, diabetics)	• Diabetics and patients with peripheral vascular disease seldom are cured with antibiotics alone. Revascularization, debridement, or amputation is often required. • Long-term, suppressive antimicrobial therapy can be used if surgery is not feasible. • Hyperbaric oxygen may be a useful adjunct.
Presence of an orthopedic device	• *S. aureus* • Coagulase-negative *Staphylococcus species*	• Rarely eradicated by antimicrobials alone, and typically requires removal of the device. • If removal is impossible, the addition of rifampcin 300 mg PO q8-12h is recommended and long-term, suppressive antimicrobial therapy may be needed.
Associated with hemoglobinopathies	• *S. aureus* • *Salmonella species*	
Chronic osteomyelitis	• Gram-negative pathogens (necrotic sequestrum) • *S. aureus*	• Surgical removal of sequestrum is recommended in addition to antibiotics.
Culture-negative osteomyelitis	• Review above pathogens	• Empiric therapy should cover *S. aureus* and all other likely pathogens.

CENTRAL NERVOUS SYSTEM INFECTIONS

Meningitis

GENERAL PRINCIPLES

- Meningitis (inflammation of the meninges) is caused by bacterial, fungal, or viral infections or by noninfectious causes such as medications.
- Bacterial meningitis is a medical emergency and requires immediate therapy without delay for diagnostic procedures. Rapid initiation of antimicrobial treatment decreases mortality.

- *Streptococcus pneumoniae* is the most common bacterial etiology in adults, followed by *Neisseria meningitidis*, group B *Streptococcus*, and *Haemophilus influenzae. Listeria monocytogenes* is more frequent in the elderly and in immunocompromised hosts.[12]
- Healthcare-associated meningitis (after neurosurgical procedures or head trauma) and intraventricular shunt infections are caused by staphylococci (*S. aureus* and coagulase-negative staphylococci) and gram-negative bacilli.

DIAGNOSIS

Clinical Presentation

- Meningitis should be considered in any patient with fever, headache, and stiff neck or neurologic symptoms, especially altered mental status.
- **Aseptic meningitis** (meningitis with negative bacterial cultures) is usually milder and may be preceded by upper respiratory symptoms or pharyngitis. Enteroviruses, and occasionally arboviruses, are the most common cause; drugs such as nonsteroidal anti-inflammatory agents and TMP-SMX are less common causes.
- Bacterial, viral, and noninfectious etiologies cannot be distinguished clinically.

Diagnostic Testing

- Diagnosis requires a **lumbar puncture** with measurement of opening pressure; cerebrospinal fluid (CSF) protein, glucose, and cell count with differential; and Gram stain with culture (Table 14-3). Blood cultures should always be obtained. Head CT scan before lumbar puncture is **not** necessary for immunocompetent patients unless there are focal neurologic abnormalities, seizures, or diminished level of consciousness.[13]
- In **bacterial meningitis**, CSF findings include a neutrophilic pleocytosis, markedly elevated CSF protein, and decreased glucose level.
- In **aseptic meningitis**, a lymphocytic CSF pleocytosis is common (although neutrophils may predominate early), along with a normal glucose. CSF PCR can detect enteroviruses,

TABLE 14-3 Typical Cerebrospinal Fluid Findings in Meningitis[13]

	Opening Pressure ($mm\ H_2O$)	White Cells (/μL)	Glucose (mg/dL)	Protein (mg/dL)	Laboratory Diagnosis
Normal	<180	0–5	50–75	15–40	None
Bacterial meningitis	↑	100–5000 neutrophils	<40	100–500	Gram stain, culture
Tuberculous meningitis	↑	50–300 lymphocytes	<45	50–300	Acid-fast bacilli smear, culture, polymerase chain reaction (PCR) for *Mycobacterium tuberculosis*
Cryptococcal meningitis	↑↑	20–500 lymphocytes	<40	>45	Cryptococcal antigen, India ink stain, fungal culture
Viral meningitis	↑	10–1000 lymphocytes	Normal	50–100	Virus-specific PCR

herpes simplex virus (HSV), varicella zoster, CMV, EBV, and HIV. CSF lymphocytosis with profoundly decreased glucose level should prompt a workup for tuberculous or fungal meningitis.

- Depending on the clinical scenario, other useful CSF studies include Venereal Disease Research Laboratory to diagnose neurosyphilis, acid-fast stain and culture, cryptococcal antigen (CrAg) and fungal culture, and arbovirus antibodies.

TREATMENT

Empirical Antimicrobial Therapy for Bacterial Meningitis

High-dose parenteral antimicrobial therapy should be started immediately after lumbar puncture (without delay for imaging). An empiric regimen should be based on patient risk factors and Gram stain of the CSF.

1. **Adults aged less than 50 years**
    - Cefotaxime 2 g IV 4 times daily or
    - Ceftriaxone 2 g IV twice daily or
    - Cefepime 2 g IV thrice daily
      PLUS
    - Vancomycin 15–20 mg/kg IV twice daily
2. **Patients in whom penicillin-resistant pneumococcal infection is suspected, or in areas with a significant incidence of penicillin resistance in the community**
   As for (1) but add:
    - Vancomycin 15–20 mg/kg IV twice daily or
    - Rifampicin 600 mg IV or orally twice daily
3. **Adults aged >50 years and those in whom *Listeria monocytogenes* infection is suspected (brainstem signs, immunosuppression, diabetic, alcohol misuser)**
   As for (1) but add:
    - Ampicillin 2 g IV 6 times daily or amoxicillin 2 g IV 6 times daily
4. **Adults aged >60 years, or with risk factors in (3) above, in areas with a significant incidence of penicillin resistance in the community**
   As for (2) but add:
    - Ampicillin 2 g IV 6 times daily or
    - Amoxicillin 2 g IV 6 times daily
5. **Patients with a clear history of anaphylaxis to β-lactams**
    - Chloramphenicol 25 mg/kg IV 4 times daily
      PLUS
    - Vancomycin 15–20 mg/kg IV twice daily

   If over the age of 60 years, add: cotrimoxazole 10–20 mg/kg (of the trimethoprim component) in four divided doses
6. **Hospital-acquired meningitis, posttraumatic or postneurosurgery meningitis, neutropenic patients, or patients with impaired cell-mediated immunity**
    - Ampicillin + ceftazidime or
    - Meropenem + vancomycin
7. **Immunocompromised patients**
    - Vancomycin plus ampicillin plus cefepime 2 g IV q8h or meropenem 2 g IV q8h
8. **Adjunctive treatment:** Started just before or with initial antibiotics and continued for 4 days reduces the risk of a poor neurologic outcome in patients with meningitis caused by *S. pneumoniae*. Glucocorticoids should not be used if a different pathogen is isolated.[14]
    - Dexamethasone 10 mg 4 times daily for 2–4 days
    - **Therapy for specific infections (Table 14-4)**

TABLE 14-4 Antimicrobial Therapy of Central Nervous System Bacterial Infections Based on Pathogens

Organism	Antibiotic
Streptococcus pneumoniae	
Vancomycin should be discontinued if the isolate is susceptible to ceftriaxone (minimum inhibitory concentration [MIC] <1.0 μg/mL). For penicillin-sensitive isolates (MIC <0.1 μg/mL), penicillin G 4 million units IV q4h can be used. Dexamethasone should be given early in treatment.	
Penicillin-sensitive	Penicillin G 4 million units IV q4H or ampicillin
Penicillin-intermediate	Ceftriaxone or cefotaxime or cefepime
Penicillin-resistant	Ceftriaxone (or cefotaxime or cefepime) + vancomycin
Neisseria meningitides	
Patients should be placed in droplet isolation for at least the first 24 hours of treatment. Close contacts (e.g., persons living in the same household and health-care personnel having close contact with secretions, such as performing endotracheal intubation) should receive prophylaxis with either ciprofloxacin 500 mg PO once; rifampicin 600 mg PO bid for 2 days; or ceftriaxone 250 mg IM. Terminal component complement deficiency (C5–C9) should be ruled out in patients with recurrent meningococcal infections.	
Penicillin-sensitive	Penicillin G or ampicillin
Penicillin-resistant	Ceftriaxone or cefotaxime. Alternatives are meropenem and chloramphenicol
Listeria monocytogenes	
Seen in immunosuppressed adults, pregnant women, and the elderly.	
Penicillin-sensitive	Ampicillin 2 g IV q4H + gentamicin
Penicillin-allergic	TMP-SMX (TMP 5 mg/kg IV q6h) or meropenem (2 g IV q8h)
Gram-negative bacilli	
Gram-negative bacillary meningitis is usually a complication of head trauma or neurosurgical procedures.	
(Susceptible organism except Pseudomonas spp.)	Ceftriaxone or cefotaxime
Pseudomonas aeruginosa	Ceftazidime or cefepime 2 g IV q8h or meropenem
Staphylococci spp.	
S. aureus meningitis is usually a result of high-grade bacteremia, direct extension from a parameningeal focus, or recent neurosurgical procedure.	
Methicillin-sensitive	Oxacillin and Nafcillin 2 g IV q4H. Ceftriaxone is alternative. Avoid first- and second-generation cephalosporin as they do not penetrate the CSF
Methicillin-resistant/penicillin allergic	Vancomycin 15–20 mg/kg/dose every 8–12 hours
Enteroviral meningitis	Supportive care
Moderate-to-severe HSV meningitis	Acyclovir 10 mg/kg IV q8h

Encephalitis

GENERAL PRINCIPLES

- Encephalitis is inflammation of the brain parenchyma, usually due to viral infections.
- **HSV-1** is the most common and most important cause of sporadic infectious encephalitis. Other causes include arboviruses such as West Nile virus (WNV), Japanese encephalitis (JE), enteroviruses, other herpesviruses, and rabies.
- Nonviral causes include *Mycobacterium tuberculosis*, syphilis, fungi, *Mycoplasma pneumoniae*, and *Bartonella henselae*. In the summer months, tick-borne illness (e.g., *Ehrlichia*, Rocky Mountain spotted fever [RMSF] and Lyme disease) should be considered.
- Noninfectious causes include vasculitis, collagen vascular disease, paraneoplastic syndromes, autoimmune encephalitis, and acute disseminated encephalomyelitis, which can occur after an infection or immunization.

DIAGNOSIS

Clinical Presentation

- Presenting complaints include fever, **altered mental status**, and neurologic abnormalities, particularly with personality change or seizures, usually without meningeal signs.
- The presence of features such as parotitis suggest mumps encephalitis.
- Acute-onset rapid progression of symptoms, such as altered sensorium, hydrophobia, aerophobia, pharyngeal spasms could indicate rabies encephalitis.
- The presence of vesicles grouped together in a dermatomal pattern may suggest varicella zoster encephalitis.

Diagnostic Testing

- CSF analysis is important and should include PCR testing for HSV and enteroviruses and measurement of CSF and serum arbovirus antibodies. A positive PCR for HSV-1 confirms the diagnosis, but a negative PCR does not rule it out. Other PCR tests (*Ehrlichia*, *Bartonella*, *Mycoplasma*, varicella-zoster virus, cytomegalovirus) are sent if there is clinical suspicion. The diagnosis of WNV and JE is made by detecting IgM antibodies in the CSF. Viral cultures are routinely done. Refer to Table 14-3.
- MRI is the most sensitive neuroimaging and may show temporal lobe enhancement in HSV encephalitis.
- EEG can show focal abnormalities in encephalitis.
- Brain biopsy is often done as a last resort.
- In case nonviral causes are ruled out, one must exclude tuberculous meningitis, syphilis, and brain abscess.

TREATMENT

- Acyclovir 10 mg/kg IV q8h should be started on **all** patients with suspected encephalitis and continued for 14–21 days, until HSV is definitively ruled out. Delayed therapy greatly increases the risk of poor neurologic outcomes.
- Treatment of other viral causes is mainly supportive.
- Antibiotic therapy for presumed bacterial meningitis (see above) should be initiated if clinically indicated and discontinued once CSF cultures are negative.
- Doxycycline 100 mg q12h should be added if there is suspicion for tick-borne illness or if the patient is from an endemic area.[15]

Japanese Encephalitis

GENERAL PRINCIPLES

- JE is the leading cause of viral encephalitis in Asia.
- The disease is primarily acquired by children younger than 15 years and is historically more common in rural and agricultural areas.
- The JE virus (JEV) is mainly transmitted by the mosquito *Culex tritaeniorhynchus*, which prefers to breed in irrigated rice paddies.
- Wading ardeid water birds (e.g., herons and egrets) serve as virus reservoirs, but the virus regularly spills over into pigs that act as amplifier host.

DIAGNOSIS

Clinical Presentation

- Most JE infections are asymptomatic.
- Common presenting features include high fever, chills, headache, myalgia, and confusion.
- In children, gastrointestinal complaints (pain and vomiting) can dominate initially and 75% will experience seizures.
- Neurologic manifestations: Mental status changes, focal neurologic deficits (e.g., hemiplegia, quadriplegia, paresis, or cranial nerve palsies), weakness, and even movement disorders (especially parkinsonian features) have been described. Some patients present with Guillain–Barré syndrome.[16]
- The case fatality rate is 20%–30%, and 30%–40% of survivors suffer from permanent neurologic sequelae.

Diagnostic Testing

- JE is most commonly diagnosed by testing for JEV IgM in the CSF, which is reliably positive if the CSF sample is taken at least 5–8 days into illness. Serum antibodies can be detected by ELISA in almost all samples after 9 days of symptom onset.[17]
- CSF pressures can be elevated with lymphocyte predominant increased counts, mild elevated protein, and deranged CSF: plasma glucose.
- Imaging: MRI is the preferred modality, often revealing involvement in the thalamus.
- EEG: Findings may include theta and delta coma, burst suppression, epileptiform activity, and alpha coma.

TREATMENT

- Supportive measures. No definite antiviral is known.

PREVENTION

- Vaccination and vector control measures are the cornerstone of JE control and prevention measure.
- The WHO recommends integration of JE vaccination into national immunization schedules in all areas where the disease is a public health priority. For adults aged 18–65 years, the primary immunization schedule for JE-VC involves two doses (0.5 mL each) administered intramuscularly 7–28 days between doses. The two-dose series should be completed at least one week prior to travel.

Nipah Virus Disease

- Nipah virus, an enveloped ribonucleic acid virus, has been a major cause of encephalitis outbreaks in various parts of Asia.
- The name "Nipah" comes from a Malaysian village where the first outbreak was reported in 1998–1999. A recent outbreak occurred in Kerala, India in September 2023.
- Nipah outbreaks have been associated with high secondary attack rates and high mortality. It is critical to emphasize on appropriate infection control measures to prevent the spread.
- Humans acquire Nipah virus disease as a result of spillover transmission from bats or human–human interaction.

DIAGNOSIS

Clinical Presentation

- Clinical presentation of Nipah typically includes fever, headache, myalgia, nausea, and vomiting. Meningismus can be observed. Cardiac involvement such as left ventricular hypokinesia, myocardial involvement can be seen. Rapid deterioration with encephalitis and/or respiratory involvement can occur.

Diagnostic Testing

- PCR testing for diagnosis of Nipah infection in infected fluid/sample is the mainstay of diagnosis.
- IgM ELISA is the first-line serological investigation.
- CSF analysis: Elevated WBC, protein
- Neuroimaging: Multiple, small focal lesions in subcortical and deep white matter without surrounding edema.
- EEG: Diffuse slow wave pattern with or without periodic bitemporal independent sharp wave discharges.

TREATMENT

- Treatment of Nipah virus disease is mostly limited to supportive care and syndromic management of acute encephalitis syndrome.
- Ribavirin has shown some encouraging evidence for treatment and postexposure prophylaxis (PEP).
- Monoclonal antibody m102.4 and favipiravir are being studied for their potential role in Nipah.

Brain Abscess

GENERAL PRINCIPLES

- Brain abscess in the immunocompetent host is usually bacterial in origin and a result of spread from a contiguous focus (mastoiditis, sinusitis, dental infection) or from septic emboli from endocarditis or bacteremia or related to trauma or surgery.
- Infection is often polymicrobial, with viridans streptococci, *S. aureus*, and anaerobes being the most common pathogens; staphylococci and gram-negative bacilli predominate after surgery. In immunocompromised hosts, etiologies include invasive fungal infection, *Nocardia*, and tuberculosis; in HIV-infected patients, toxoplasmosis is a leading consideration.[18]

TABLE 14-5 Neurological Deficits Based on Site of Lesion
Temporal Lobe
Wernicke's aphasia
Homonymous superior quadrantanopia
Mild contralateral facial muscle weakness
Frontal Lobe
Drowsy
Inattentive
Disturbed judgment
Mutism
Seizures
Presence of grasp, suck, and snout reflexes
Contralateral hemiparesis (when the abscess is large)
Parietal Lobe
Impaired position sense, two-point discrimination, and stereognosis
Focal sensory and motor seizures
Homonymous hemianopsia
Impaired opticokinetic nystagmus
Cerebellar
Ataxia
Nystagmus (coarser on gaze toward the lesion)
Ipsilateral incoordination of arm and leg movements with intention tremor
Brainstem
Facial weakness and dysphagia
Multiple other cranial nerve palsies
Contralateral hemiparesis

CLINICAL PRESENTATION

Neurologic deficits will vary with the location of the lesion (Table 14-5).

DIAGNOSIS

- Diagnosis is radiographic, with ring-enhancing lesions seen on MRI or contrast-enhanced CT scan. Differential diagnoses include the following:
  - Epidural and subdural empyema
  - Septic dural sinus thrombosis
  - Mycotic cerebral aneurysms
  - Septic cerebral emboli with associated infarction

  - Acute focal necrotizing encephalitis (most commonly due to herpes simplex virus)
  - Metastatic or primary brain tumors
  - Pyogenic meningitis
- A microbiologic etiology should be determined by aspiration, biopsy, or at the time of surgery.

TREATMENT

- Empiric therapy should cover the most likely pathogens based on the primary infection site. When the source is unknown, a third-generation cephalosporin (ceftriaxone) combined with metronidazole and vancomycin is started in immunocompetent hosts, and it is modified when culture data are available. Cefepime or ceftazidime should be substituted for ceftriaxone after neurosurgical procedures or penetrating head trauma.
- Neurosurgical consultation is imperative for drainage; cultures **must** be sent to enable pathogen-directed therapy, as a prolonged course of antibiotic therapy is often needed.
- Follow-up imaging to assess improvement determines length of therapy.

Neurocysticercosis

- Three human *Taenia* species, *Taenia solium*, *Taenia saginata*, and *Taenia asiatica*, have been identified to cause human infections.
- The pork tapeworm, *T. solium*, is the most pathogenic to humans, causing cysticercosis and neurocysticercosis (NCC). The parasitic cysticercosis/taeniasis has been prioritized as a neglected tropical disease (NTDs) by the WHO.
- The infection is common in people from Latin America, Southeast Asia, and sub-Saharan Africa. It has an important impact on public health in many Asian countries including Cambodia, Indonesia, Japan, Lao PDR, Malaysia, India, Nepal, Thailand, the Philippines, PR China, Bali, and Vietnam.
- NCC has been identified as a single leading cause for seizures or epilepsy in areas where it is endemic.
- Ingested eggs of *T. solium* differentiate into larvae, which disseminate to brain and other tissues and form cysts.
- Brain imaging reveals characteristic multiple unilocular cysts that eventually calcify.

DIAGNOSTIC CRITERIA FOR NEUROCYSTICERCOSIS[19]

Absolute Criteria

- Demonstration of the parasite from biopsy of lesion from brain or spinal cord histologically.
- Presence of subretinal cysticercus.
- Demonstration of a scolex within a cystic lesion on neuroimaging.

Neuroimaging Criteria

Major Criteria

- Cystic lesions with no discernible scolex
- Enhancing lesions
- Multilobulated cystic lesions in the subarachnoid space.
- Typical parenchymal brain calcifications

Confirmation Criteria

- Resolution of cystic lesions after treatment with cysticidal drugs
- Resolution of single small enhancing lesion spontaneously
- Sequential neuroimaging studies demonstrating migration of ventricular cysts

Minor Criteria

- Abnormal enhancement of basal leptomeninges or obstructive hydrocephalus

Clinical/Epidemiologic Exposure Criteria

Major Criteria

- Detection of specific anticysticercal antibodies or cysticercal antigens by standardized immunodiagnostic tests
- Cysticercosis outside the central nervous system
- Household contact with *Taenia solium* infection

Minor Criteria

- Clinical manifestations suggestive of neurocysticercosis
- Individuals with prior or current residence in an area endemic to cysticercosis

TREATMENT

- Prior to initiating treatment tailored for neurocysticersosis, one must rule out ocular cysticercosis. Otherwise, the inflammatory reaction to the degenerating cysticerci can result in worsening vision. Those who require long-term corticosteroid should have been examined for any evidence of tuberculosis.
- Treatment consists of anticonvulsants, albendazole (15 mg/kg/d in two divided doses for 10–14 days), or praziquantel (50 mg/kg/d for 10–14 days), with concomitant glucocorticoids to decrease the inflammatory response, and/or surgery.[20]

CARDIOVASCULAR INFECTIONS

Infective Endocarditis

GENERAL PRINCIPLES

Epidemiology

- Yearly incidence of infective endocarditis has increased from 9.91/100,000 people in 1990 to 13.8 in 2019 which constitutes a 39.3% increase.[21]
- Rheumatic heart disease remains the key risk factor for infective endocarditis in developing countries and underlies up to two-thirds of cases.
- Patients are usually young adults and infection is caused predominantly by community-acquired, penicillin-sensitive streptococci entering via the oral cavity.
- Rising incidence of acute bacterial endocarditis (ABE) and healthcare-associated endocarditis (related to IV catheters and invasive procedures) in recent times has been driven by increased rates of *S. aureus* bacteremia.
- **Prosthetic valve endocarditis** (PVE) occurs in 3%–6% of patients with prosthetic heart valves.

Etiology

- **Infective endocarditis** (IE) is usually caused by gram-positive cocci. *S. aureus* is the most common pathogen followed by viridans group streptococci, enterococci, and coagulase-negative staphylococci.
- *Enterococcus* species cause 5%–10% of cases of **subacute bacterial endocarditis** (SBE).

- Gram-negative and fungal IE occur infrequently and are usually associated with injection drug use or prosthetic heart valves.
- Bacteremia from distant foci of infection or dental procedures are frequent seeding events.
- Early PVE (within the first year of surgery) commonly occurs in the first 2 months and is typically caused by *S. aureus*, coagulase-negative staphylococci, gram-negative bacilli, and *Candida* spp.
- Late-onset PVE is caused by the same organisms seen in native valve endocarditis.

Risk Factors

Structural heart disease (e.g., degenerative valve disease), IV drug use, prosthetic heart valves, intravascular devices, chronic hemodialysis, HIV, and a prior history of endocarditis are predisposing factors for endocarditis.

DIAGNOSIS

The 2023 Duke-International Society for Cardiovascular Infectious Disease (ISCVID) (see Table 6-4) criteria for diagnosis of IE, incorporating microbiologic, pathologic, echocardiographic, and clinical findings, are widely used but should not replace clinical judgment.

Clinical Presentation

- Clinical presentation is protean, ranging from acute sepsis, commonly seen in ABE, to an indolent low-grade febrile illness, malaise, and anorexia in SBE. Heart failure or stroke is another form of presentation.
- Immune complex-mediated manifestations (nephritis, arthralgias, Osler nodes) and embolic phenomenon (renal, splenic, and cerebral infarcts; petechiae; Janeway lesions) are more commonly seen in SBE.
- **PVE** must be considered in any patient with persistent bacteremia after heart valve surgery or new valve dehiscence with secondary hemolysis.

Diagnostic Testing

- The most reliable diagnostic criterion for IE is persistent bacteremia in a compatible clinical setting. Three blood cultures should be taken from separate sites over at least a 1-hour period before empiric antimicrobial therapy. Blood cultures are negative in 10%–15% of patients, most commonly because of prior receipt of antibiotics.
- Echocardiography plays an important role in establishing the diagnosis of IE and determining the need for surgical intervention.
- Patients with IE and vegetations seen by transthoracic echocardiography (TTE) are at higher risk of embolism, heart failure, and valvular disruption. However, a negative TTE cannot rule out IE.
- Transesophageal echocardiography (TEE) has higher sensitivity and should be the first test in patients with prosthetic valves, rated at least possible IE by clinical criteria, or complicated IE (i.e., paravalvular abscess). In every other situation, TTE should be done first.[23]
- True **culture-negative IE** is rare and usually caused by fastidious pathogens, such as nutritionally deficient streptococci (*Abiotrophia* and *Granulicatella*), HACEK organisms, *Coxiella burnetii* (Q fever), *Bartonella*, *Brucella*, *Tropheryma whipplei* (Whipple disease), and fungi. Empiric therapy can be initiated despite negative cultures (Table 14-6).
- **HACEK** is an acronym for a group of fastidious, slow-growing, gram-negative bacteria (*Haemophilus*, *Aggregatibacter*, *Cardiobacterium*, *Eikenella*, and *Kingella* species) that account for 5%–10% of community-acquired cases of IE.
- Routine investigations for the evaluation of a case of IE reveals elevated ESR, CRP, normocytic normochromic anemia, positive rheumatoid factor, hypocomplementemia. Urinalysis shows microscopic hematuria, proteinuria, and/or pyuria.

TABLE 14-6 Treatment of Endocarditis Caused by Specific Organisms[23]

Organism	Antibiotic Regimen	Duration	Notes
Viridans Group Streptococci and *Streptococcus gallolyticus*			
MIC <0.12 μg/mL	• Penicillin G (12–18 million units IV qday) or ceftriaxone (2 g IV qday) ± gentamicin (3 mg/kg IV qday) for the first 2 wk • Vancomycin (15 mg/kg IV q12h)	4-wk If used, gentamicin is given only during the first 2-wk	• PVE, major embolic or extended symptoms require a 6-wk course of treatment + gentamicin • Gentamicin may be ototoxic and nephrotoxic
MIC 0.12–0.5 μg/mL	• Penicillin G (4 million units IV q4h) or ceftriaxone + gentamicin • Vancomycin if PCN allergic + gentamicin	4-wk total with 2-wk of gentamicin	• Vancomycin is reserved for patients with true β-lactam allergy and unable to be desensitized
MIC >0.5 μg/mL	• Treat as enterococcal endocarditis	6-wk	
Enterococcus Species			
Penicillin-susceptible	• Ampicillin (2 g IV q4h) + gentamicin (3 mg/kg ideal body weight in 2–3 equally divided doses) • Ampicillin + ceftriaxone (2 g IV q12h)	4–6-wk	• If high-level gentamicin resistance, substitute streptomycin (15 mg/kg IV qday IV in two divided doses based on ideal body weight) or ceftriaxone (4 g IV qday in two divided doses)
Penicillin-resistant	• Vancomycin (15 mg/kg IV q12h) + gentamicin (3 mg/kg in 3 equally divided doses)	6-wk	
Vancomycin (VRE) and ampicillin resistant	• Linezolid (600 mg IV/PO q12h) • Daptomycin (≥10–12 mg/kg qday)	≥6-wk	• This should be managed in conjunction with an infectious diseases consultant
Staphylococcus aureus			
NVE MSSA	• Oxacillin or nafcillin (2 g IV q4h) • Cefazolin (2 g IV q8h) if penicillin allergy without anaphylaxis	6-wk	• Initial 3–5 d gentamicin for synergy may not be beneficial. • Penicillins are superior to vancomycin, and desensitization is preferred when possible.

(Continued)

TABLE 14-6 Treatment of Endocarditis Caused by Specific Organisms[23] (Continued)

Right-sided only NVE MSSA (IV drug user)	• Oxacillin or nafcillin (2 g IV q4h) • Daptomycin (6 mg/kg IV qday)	2-wk	• 2-wk is only recommended in HIV negative patients without vascular prosthesis or embolic disease, other than septic pulmonary emboli. • CK must be monitored in patients on daptomycin.
NVE, MRSA	• Vancomycin (15 mg/kg IV q12h) or daptomycin (≥8 mg/kg IV qday)	6-wk	
***Staphylococcus Species* (Prosthetic Valve)**			
MSSA/MSSE	• Oxacillin + rifampicin (300 mg PO q8h) + gentamicin (3 mg/kg per 24 h IV in 2 or 3 equally divided doses)	≥6-wk total	Gentamicin given only during the first 2-wk
MRSA/MRSE	• Vancomycin + rifampicin + gentamicin or • Daptomycin 6 mg/kg every 24 hours + rifampicin/gentamicin	≥6-wk total 4 weeks	Gentamicin given only during the first 2-wk
HACEK organisms	• Ceftriaxone (2 g IV qday) Alternatives: • Ampicillin (2 g IV q4h) • Ciprofloxacin (400 mg IV q12h)	4-wk for NVE 6-wk for PVE	HACEK stands for *Haemophilus, Aggregatibacter, Cardiobacterium, Eikenella, Kingella.*
Culture-negative IE	Consultation with an infectious diseases specialist to define the most appropriate choice of therapy is recommended		

Baseline and weekly audiometry recommended for patients receiving aminoglycosides for >7 days. Monitor aminoglycoside and vancomycin levels. Goal vancomycin trough levels are 15–20 μg/mL.

CK, creatinine kinase; IE, infective endocarditis; MIC, minimum inhibitory concentration; MRSA, methicillin-resistant *Staphylococcus aureus*; MRSE, methicillin-resistant *Staphylococcus epidermidis*; MSSA, methicillin-sensitive *Staphylococcus aureus*; MSSE, methicillin-sensitive *Staphylococcus epidermidis*; NVE, native valve endocarditis; PCN, penicillin; PVE, prosthetic valve endocarditis; VRE, vancomycin-resistant *Enterococcus*.

- Patient should undergo a thorough dental evaluation to look for periodontal inflammation, caries, pulpal infection.

TREATMENT

- **Standard of care consists of targeted IV antimicrobials for 4–6 weeks, starting from the day that source control and blood culture clearance are achieved.**[23]
- Antimicrobial susceptibility testing of the causative organism is essential for optimal treatment.
- **IE** often requires empiric antimicrobial treatment before culture results become available. Initial treatment for *S. aureus* should consist of vancomycin 15 mg/kg IV q12h. Therapy should then be modified based on culture and susceptibility data. For methicillin-sensitive isolates, oxacillin 2 g IV q4h is superior to vancomycin.
- In selected cases of **SBE**, if the patient is clinically stable, therapy can usually be delayed until culture data and susceptibilities are available.
- **PVE** requires aggressive combination of antimicrobials for at 6 weeks or longer and surgery because of the increased risk for treatment failure and relapse. Initial empiric therapy pending culture data include the addition of rifampicin and gentamicin to improve biofilm penetration.
- Baseline audiometry is recommended for patients who will receive ≥7 days of aminoglycoside therapy, with weekly repeat testing while on treatment.
- **Antibiotic therapy for specific organisms** is described in Table 14-6.
  - *Streptococcus gallolyticus* bacteremia and endocarditis are associated with lower gastrointestinal tract disease, including neoplasms. Groups B and G streptococcal endocarditis may also be associated with lower intestinal pathology.
  - Coagulase-negative *Staphylococcus* (e.g., *Staphylococcus epidermidis*) IE primarily occurs in patients with prosthetic heart valves, although native valve endocarditis is increasing, particularly in health-care settings. *Staphylococcus lugdunensis* IE is associated with a high rate of perivalvular extension and metastatic spread.
- **Response to antimicrobial therapy**
  - Clinical improvement is frequently seen within 3–10 days of initiating therapy.
  - Blood cultures should be obtained daily until clearance of bacteremia has been documented.
  - Persistent or recurrent fever usually represents extensive cardiac infection but also may be due to septic emboli, drug hypersensitivity, or subsequent nosocomial infection.[24]

Surgical Management

- **Native valve endocarditis** indications for surgery include: persistent vegetation after systemic embolization, mobile vegetations ≥10 mm, ≥1 embolic event in the first 2 weeks of treatment, or increase in the size of the vegetation despite antimicrobial therapy; refractory heart failure and aortic or mitral regurgitation with ventricular failure; heart block, annular or aortic abscess, fistula, or perforation; and infection with fungi or other highly resistant organisms, and persistent bacteremia or fever lasting >5–7 days, provided that other sites of infection and fever have been excluded.
- For **PVE**, besides the indications listed above, valve dehiscence, intracardiac fistula, or severe prosthetic valve dysfunction resulting in heart failure and relapsing PVE also require surgery.[23]

SPECIAL CONSIDERATIONS

American Heart Association recommendations for prophylaxis for IE are outlined in Table 14-7.

TABLE 14-7 Endocarditis Prophylaxis[25]

I. Endocarditis prophylaxis is recommended for the following cardiac conditions: prosthetic valves; previous endocarditis; unrepaired cyanotic congenital heart disease or repaired congenital heart disease with prosthetic material during the first 6 mo after procedure, or with residual defects at or adjacent to the site of the prosthetic device; and cardiac valvulopathy in transplant recipients.	
II. Regimens for dental, oral, or respiratory tract procedures (including dental extractions, periodontal or endodontic procedures, professional teeth cleaning, bronchoscopy with biopsy, rigid bronchoscopy, surgery on respiratory mucosa, and tonsillectomy):	
Standard prophylaxis	Amoxicillin 2 g PO 1 h before procedure
Unable to take PO	Ampicillin 2 g IM or IV, or cefazolin or ceftriaxone 1 g IM or IV within 30 min before procedure
Penicillin-allergic patient	Cephalexin 2 g PO, or clarithromycin or azithromycin 500 mg PO 1 h before procedure
Penicillin allergic and unable to take PO	Cefazolin or ceftriaxone 1 g IV within 30 min before procedure
III. Gastrointestinal and genitourinary procedures do not require routine use of prophylaxis. High-risk patients infected or colonized with enterococci should receive amoxicillin, ampicillin, or vancomycin to eradicate the organism before urinary tract manipulation.	
IV. Prophylaxis is recommended for procedures on infected skin, skin structures, or musculoskeletal tissue ONLY for patients with cardiac conditions outlined above. An antistaphylococcal penicillin or cephalosporin should be used.	

Myocarditis

GENERAL PRINCIPLES

- Myocarditis is an inflammatory disease of the myocardium often but not always caused by an infectious agent.
- Causes of infectious myocarditis include viruses, bacteria, rickettsia, fungi, and parasites.
- Viruses are the most frequent etiologic organism and include enteroviruses (Coxsackie B and echovirus), adenovirus, human herpesvirus 6, parvovirus B-19, dengue, and many others. Many cases of myocarditis associated with dengue, scrub typhus, Lyme disease, and influenza have been reported from the Indian subcontinent. Diphtheritic myocarditis should be considered as a differential especially in unvaccinated children.
- Noninfectious causes of myocarditis include alcohol, arsenics, cyclophosphamide, carbon monoxide, and radiation.

CLINICAL PRESENTATION

Chest pain, fever, exercise intolerance, tachypnea, heart sounds such as S3, S4, or summation gallop, heart failure, and fever are the classical manifestations of infectious myocarditis.

DIAGNOSIS

- ECG shows atrial or ventricular arrhythmia, partial or complete heart block, new-onset bundle branch block, and diffuse ST-segment abnormalities in the EKG.

- Abnormal echocardiogram.
- The diagnostic "gold standard" is endomyocardial biopsy for histological, immunological, and immunohistochemical criteria, including specific viral PCR.
- Cardiac magnetic resonance imaging can be useful for the diagnosis and monitoring of disease progression.
- Viral culture and serologic testing are rarely helpful.
- Elevated cardiac enzymes (e.g., troponin).

TREATMENT

- Supportive care is the mainstay of treatment.
- NSAIDs should be avoided. Restriction of alcohol consumption as it can worsen the severity of myocarditis. AHA recommends 3–6 months abstinence from competitive sports after myocarditis.[26]
- Patients diagnosed to have myocarditis with heart failure should receive standard therapy of heart failure.
- Antiarrhythmics such as amiodarone and dofetilide can be used with caution as indicated. Pacing can be done for those patients with complete heart block and/or symptomatic bradycardia.
- Anticoagulation can be added for patients with atrial fibrillation, systemic embolism, or in the presence of a left ventricular thrombus.
- Mechanical circulatory support with a ventricular assist device (VAD) can be considered in hemodynamically unstable patients who have refractory symptoms despite medical line of treatment. VADs can serve as a bridge to transplantation.
- The role of IV immunoglobulin and antiviral agents such as ribavirin in viral-mediated myocarditis remains anecdotal.[27] The role of immunosuppressive therapy has been shown to be beneficial in studies.

UPPER RESPIRATORY TRACT INFECTIONS

Pharyngitis

GENERAL PRINCIPLES

Viruses are the most common cause of pharyngitis. GABHS pharyngitis is responsible for merely 5%–15% of cases in adults, with other bacteria responsible to a lesser extent. Unfortunately, 60% of adults with pharyngitis receive antibiotics.[29]

DIAGNOSIS

Clinical Presentation

Fever, nasal congestion, coryza, conjunctivitis, cervical lymphadenopathy, tonsillar exudates, and throat pain are the most common clinical manifestations. Distinguishing bacterial from viral pharyngitis on clinical grounds alone is difficult.

Differential Diagnosis

- **Acute HIV infection** should be considered in the setting of pharyngitis with atypical lymphocytosis and negative *Streptococcus* and Epstein–Barr virus testing.
- **Epiglottitis** should be considered in the febrile patient with severe throat pain, odynophagia, new-onset drooling, and dysphagia.

- Suppurative complications including **peritonsillar or retropharyngeal abscess** should be considered in the patient with severe unilateral pain, muffled voice, trismus, and dysphagia.

Diagnostic Testing

- Diagnostic testing is usually reserved for symptomatic patients with exposure to a case of streptococcal pharyngitis, those with signs of significant infection (fever, tonsillar exudates, and cervical adenopathy) or whose symptoms persist despite symptomatic therapy, and patients with a history of rheumatic fever.
- Rapid antigen detection testing (RADT) is useful for diagnosing **GABHS** (>90% sensitivity and specificity), which requires antimicrobial therapy to prevent suppurative complications and rheumatic fever. A negative test does not reliably exclude GAS, making throat culture necessary if clinical suspicion is high.
- Serology for **Epstein–Barr virus** (e.g., heterophile agglutinin or monospot) and examination of a peripheral blood smear for atypical lymphocytes should be performed when infectious mononucleosis is suspected.

TREATMENT

- Symptomatic therapy of reducing pain in acute pharyngitis by administering analgesics such as acetaminophen. NSAIDs and aspirin can also be used. Topical therapy for symptomatic relief in the form of lozenges can be used.
- Most cases of pharyngitis are self-limited and do not require antimicrobial therapy.

Treatment for **GABHS** is indicated with a positive culture or RADT, if the patient is at high risk for development of rheumatic fever, or if the diagnosis is strongly suspected, pending culture results. Treatment options include penicillin V 500 mg PO q12h for 10 days, clindamycin 300 mg PO q8h for 10 days, azithromycin 500 mg PO on day 1 followed by 250 mg qday on days 2–5, or benzathine penicillin G 1.2 million units IM as a one-time dose.[30] In some communities up to 15% of the **GABHS** isolates are resistant to macrolides.

- Gonococcal pharyngitis is treated with ceftriaxone 250 mg IM as a single dose, plus azithromycin or doxycycline.

Epiglottitis

GENERAL PRINCIPLES

- Epiglottitis is a respiratory emergency, as inflammation of the epiglottis can lead to airway obstruction.
- *H. influenzae* type B, *S. pneumoniae*, *S. aureus*, and GABHS are common bacterial causes of epiglottitis, although viral and fungal pathogens may also be implicated. Non-infectious etiologies include caustic injury, thermal injury, local trauma.

DIAGNOSIS

Clinical Presentation

Fever, sore throat, odynophagia, drooling, muffled voice, and dysphagia in a patient with a normal oropharyngeal examination should prompt a clinical diagnosis of epiglottitis. Inspiratory stridor is a sign of impending respiratory compromise. **"Tripod" positioning (trunk leaning forward, neck hyperextended, chin thrust forward) is caused by epiglottitis and represents the patient's attempt to maximize the patency of a significantly obstructed upper airway.**

Diagnostic Testing

- Throat and blood cultures are useful in determining the etiology.
- Soft tissue lateral radiographs of the neck may demonstrate the "thumb print" sign.
- Bedside ultrasound can aid in the diagnosis and show the "alphabet P sign."
- Definitive diagnosis is made by visualization of the epiglottis with direct laryngoscopy.

TREATMENT

- Airway stabilization is the priority. Assess for the patency of the airway. In case of complete airway obstruction, begin bag-valve-mask ventilation with 100% oxygen. If saturation continues to decline, initiate RSI and attempt endotracheal intubation. Avoid laryngeal mask airway. If unsuccessful, seek emergency otolaryngologist consult and proceed for surgical cricothyrotomy. In case of partial obstruction, administer supplemental oxygen.
- Obtain cultures prior to starting empirical antibiotics.
- Antimicrobial therapy should include an agent that is active against *H. influenzae*, such as ceftriaxone 2 g IV qday or cefotaxime 2 g IV q6-8h. Vancomycin or clindamycin should be added if there is concern for MRSA. Glucocorticoids are often also given.

Rhinosinusitis

GENERAL PRINCIPLES

- **Acute rhinosinusitis** is referred to the symptomatic inflammation of the nasal cavity and paranasal sinuses lasting <4 weeks. Based on etiology, it is classified as acute viral rhinosinusitis, uncomplicated bacterial rhinosinusitis caused by *S. pneumoniae*, *H. influenzae*, *Moraxella catarrhalis*, and anaerobes are involved in <2% of cases and should be considered only if symptoms persist for >10 days. In immunosuppressed patients, fungal causes (i.e., *Mucor*, *Rhizopus* and *Aspergillus* species) should be considered. Complicated bacterial rhinosinusitis is when there is clinical evidence of extension beyond the paranasal sinuses and nasal cavity.
- **Chronic rhinosinusitis** may be caused by any of the etiologic agents responsible for acute sinusitis, as well as *S. aureus*, *Corynebacterium diphtheriae*, and many anaerobes (e.g., *Prevotella* spp., *Veillonella* spp.). Possible contributing factors include asthma, nasal polyps, allergies, or immunodeficiency.

DIAGNOSIS

Clinical Presentation

- **Acute rhinosinusitis** presents with purulent nasal discharge, nasal obstruction, and sinus tenderness with or without fever, lasting <4 weeks. Patients may develop erythema or edema over bony area covering the sinuses, cheek tenderness, or tenderness on percussing the upper teeth.
- **Subacute rhinosinusitis:** Symptoms last for 4–12 weeks
- **Chronic rhinosinusitis** is defined by symptoms lasting >12 weeks including mucopurulent drainage, nasal obstruction, facial pain or pressure, and decreased sense of smell with documented signs of inflammation.
- **Recurrent rhinosinusitis** is when patient has had four or more episodes of acute rhinosinusitis.
- Patients can develop complications such as periorbital/orbital cellulitis, subperiosteal abscess, osteomyelitis of the sinus bones, meningitis, or a septic cavernous sinus thrombosis.

Diagnostic Testing

- Diagnosis requires objective evidence of mucosal disease, usually with rhinoscopy and nasal endoscopy. If radiological imaging is done, limited sinus CT should be used. Plain films are not recommended.
- Sinus cultures should be obtained from nasal endoscopy or sinus puncture. Nasal swabs are not helpful.

TREATMENT

- The goals of medical therapy for acute and chronic rhinosinusitis are to control infection, reduce tissue edema, facilitate drainage, maintain patency of the sinus ostia, and break the pathologic cycle that leads to chronic sinusitis.
- **Acute rhinosinusitis**
  - **Symptomatic treatment** is the mainstay of therapy, including oral decongestants and analgesics with or without a short course of topical decongestant or intranasal glucocorticoid.[31]
  - **Empiric antibiotic therapy** is indicated only for severe persistent symptoms (≥10 days) or failure of symptomatic therapy. First-line therapy should consist of a 5–7-day course of amoxicillin-clavulanate 875 mg/125 mg PO q12h. Doxycycline or a respiratory fluoroquinolone (e.g., moxifloxacin, levofloxacin) may be used as alternative therapy in case of β-lactam allergy or primary treatment failure. TMP-SMX and macrolides are not recommended for empiric therapy owing to high rates of resistance.
- **Chronic rhinosinusitis.** Treatment usually includes topical and/or systemic glucocorticoids; the role of antimicrobial agents is unclear. If they are used, amoxicillin-clavulanate is the first-line treatment, with clindamycin for penicillin-allergic patients. Some chronic cases may require endoscopic surgery.

Influenza Virus Infection

GENERAL PRINCIPLES

Influenza is an acute febrile respiratory illness, caused by influenza A or B virus, which is readily transmissible and associated with outbreaks of varying severity during the winter months.

DIAGNOSIS

Clinical Presentation

In immunocompetent patients, influenza virus infection causes an acute, self-limited febrile illness associated with headache, myalgias, cough, coryza, and malaise. These symptoms may last up to 2 weeks. Although GI symptoms are not common in adults, vomiting and diarrhea were common features in adults during the 2009–2010 H1N1 influenza pandemic.

Diagnostic Testing

Diagnosis is usually made clinically during influenza season, with confirmation by nasopharyngeal swab for rapid antigen testing, PCR (higher sensitivity), molecular assay (nucleic acid amplification test), or direct fluorescent antibody test and culture. Immunocompromised and those at an increased risk of influenza complications can be tested.

TREATMENT

- Treatment is usually symptomatic.
- Antiviral medications may shorten the duration of illness but must be initiated within 24–48 hours of the onset of symptoms to be effective in immunocompetent patients.[32] Antiviral therapy should not be withheld from patients presenting >48 hours after symptom onset requiring hospitalization or at high risk for complications (see Complications section).
  - The **neuraminidase inhibitors** (oseltamivir 75 mg PO q12h or zanamivir 10 mg inhaled q12h, each for 5 days, or peramivir, 600 mg single dose IV) are approved by the US Food and Drug Administration for the treatment of Influenza A and B.
  - **M2 inhibitors** (amantadine and rimantadine, each 100 mg PO q12h) are **not** recommended owing to high rates of resistance.
  - Circulating strains change annually with varying resistance patterns to both classes of antivirals. **Treatment decisions must be based on annual resistance data**, available from the Centers for Disease Control and Prevention (CDC) (http://www.cdc.gov).
- **Vaccination** is the most reliable prevention strategy. Annual vaccination is recommended for all individuals 6 months of age and older. Efficacy of vaccination varies annually from 50% to 90% depending on prevailing outbreak and circulating influenza strains.

COMPLICATIONS

- Adults >65 years old, residents of nursing homes and other long-term care facilities, pregnant women (and those up to 2 weeks postpartum), and patients with chronic medical conditions (e.g., pulmonary disease, cardiovascular disease, active malignancy, diabetes mellitus, chronic renal insufficiency, chronic liver disease, immunosuppression including HIV and transplantation, morbid obesity) are at greater risk of complications.
- Influenza pneumonia and secondary bacterial pneumonia, typically due to *S. aureus*, are the most common complications of influenza infection.
- Viral antigenic drift and shift can cause emergence of strains with enhanced virulence or the potential for pandemic spread, requiring modified therapy or heightened infection control measures.

LOWER RESPIRATORY TRACT INFECTIONS

Acute Bronchitis

GENERAL PRINCIPLES

Acute bronchitis involves inflammation of the bronchi without evidence of pneumonia, that occurs in the absence of chronic obstructive pulmonary disease. It is most often caused by viruses such as coronavirus, rhinovirus, influenza, or parainfluenza. Uncommon causes include *M. pneumoniae*, *Chlamydophila pneumoniae*, and *Bordetella pertussis*. Unfortunately, 60%–90% of patients with acute bronchitis are given antibiotics.[29]

DIAGNOSIS

Clinical Presentation

Symptoms include cough with or without sputum production lasting >5 days. It is sometimes associated with wheezing or rhonchi on physical examination. Up to half of the patients have purulent sputum production; however, fever is uncommon.

Diagnostic Testing

- Diagnosis is made clinically. Sputum cultures are not recommended.
- In febrile, systemically ill, or older patients with abnormal vital signs, pneumonia should be ruled out radiographically, and diagnostic tests for influenza should be performed depending on the season and local disease trends.
- Cough lasting >2 weeks in an adult should be evaluated for pertussis with a nasopharyngeal swab for culture or PCR.

TREATMENT

- Treatment is symptomatic and should be directed towards controlling cough (dextromethorphan 15 mg PO q6h).
- Multiple studies have shown no benefit in antimicrobial therapy for generally healthy patients with acute, non–pertussis-related bronchitis.
- Pertussis treatment consists of azithromycin 500 mg PO single dose followed by 250 mg PO qday for 4 more days, or clarithromycin 500 mg PO q12h for 14 days.
- Pertussis cases should be reported to the local health department for contact tracing and administration of PEP with azithromycin when indicated.

Community-Acquired Pneumonia (CAP)

GENERAL PRINCIPLES

- CAP refers to an acute infection of the pulmonary parenchyma that the patient has developed outside of a hospital setting or develops within 48 hours of hospitalization.
- The predominant organism involved is *S. pneumoniae*; other bacterial etiologies are *H. influenzae* and *M. catarrhalis*. Pneumonia caused by atypical agents, such as *Legionella pneumophila*, *C. pneumoniae*, or *M. pneumoniae*, cannot be reliably distinguished clinically. Influenza and other respiratory viruses may also cause pneumonia in adults. The COVID-19 pandemic is an important cause for CAP.
- Community-acquired MRSA is an important cause of severe, necrotizing pneumonia.
- Patients aged 65 or older, and those with certain medical conditions, should receive the pneumococcal vaccination with both the 23-valent and the 13-valent vaccine, as recommended per CDC guidelines.[26]

DIAGNOSIS

Clinical Presentation

- The presentation of community acquired pneumonia (CAP) is extremely variable. Fever and respiratory symptoms, including cough with sputum production, dyspnea, and pleuritic chest pain, are common in immunocompetent patients. Signs include tachypnea, rales, or evidence of consolidation on auscultation.
- CAP presents acutely, over a matter of hours to days. If a patient has symptoms for more than 2–3 weeks, particularly if accompanied by weight loss or night sweats, this should raise the question of an alternate diagnosis, such as mycobacterial or fungal infection.

Diagnostic Testing

- Blood
  - Full blood count: Neutrophilic leukocytosis, hemolytic anemia (occasional complication of *M. pneumonia*)
  - Urea and electrolytes: >20 mg/dL: marker of severity, hyponatremia

- LFT: Abnormal if basal pneumonia induces inflammation of liver, hypoalbuminemia: marker of severity
- Procalcitonin: Elevation suggests bacterial > viral etiology
- CRP/ESR: Nonspecific elevation

• Blood culture
  - ABG: Perform when saturation <93% or clinical features severe enough to assess ventilatory failure or acidosis

• Sputum
  - Sputum sample: Gram stain, culture & sensitivity
  - Pharyngeal swab: NAAT for respiratory viruses and bacteria

• Urine
  - Urine routine: Pneumococcal and legionella antigen

• Chest X-ray
  - Lobar pneumonia: Progresses from patchy opacification to homogenous consolidation of affected lobe, presence of air bronchogram
  - Bronchopneumonia: Patchy and segmental shadowing
  - Complications: Parapneumonic effusions, intrapulmonary abscess, empyema
  - *S. aureus* pneumonia: Presence of multilobular shadowing, cavitations, pneumatoceles, abscesses
  - Pleural fluid: Thoracocentesis aspirate sent for Gram stain and culture
  - Fiberoptic bronchoscopy: Used for detection of less common organisms, especially in immunocompromised patients, or if the patient is not responding to adequate therapy
  - Tuberculosis: Sputum for acid-fast stain and culture should be obtained, and the patient should be placed on airborne isolation

TREATMENT

• All patients should be assessed for hospitalization and evaluated for comorbid factors, oxygenation and severity of illness using validated severity scales such as the Pneumonia Severity Index or CURB-65 (Figure 14-2).

CURB-65 Severity Score	
Feature	Point
C: Confusion	1
U: Urea >7 mmol/L	1
R: Respiratory rate ≥30 breaths/min	1
B: Blood pressure (systolic <90 mm Hg, or diastolic ≤60 mm Hg)	1
65: Age ≥65 years	1

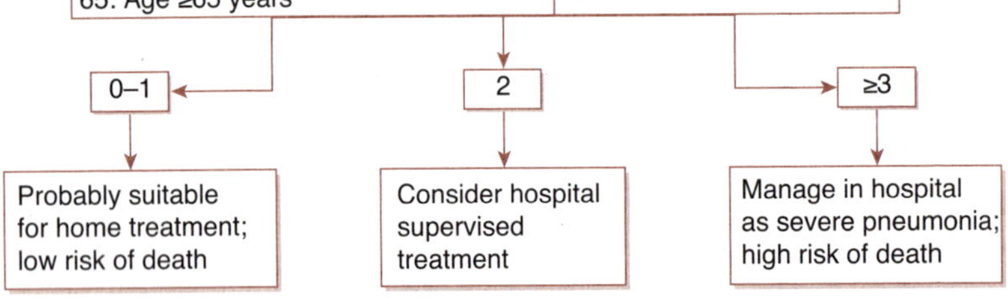

Figure 14-2 Assessment of Pneumonia severity.

- Antibiotics should be given as soon as CAP is diagnosed, ideally within 4 hours of arrival to the hospital, as delays lead to higher mortality. Antibiotic therapy should be narrowed once a specific microbiologic etiology has been identified.
- **Immunocompetent outpatients** with no recent antibiotic exposure and no comorbidities should receive a macrolide, such as azithromycin 500 mg PO single dose followed by 250 mg PO qday for 4 more days, or doxycycline 100 mg q12h for at least 5 days.
- **Outpatients with recent antibiotic exposure or comorbidities** should receive a macrolide (azithromycin or clarithromycin) with high-dose amoxicillin 1 g PO q8h for at least 5 days. Flouroquinone should be avoided in TB endemic areas in view of growing resistance to this reserve drug.
- **Hospitalized patients** should be treated with ceftriaxone 1 g IV qday or cefotaxime 1 g IV q8h PLUS a macrolide (azithromycin or clarithromycin). Duration of therapy should be at least 5 days for low severity pneumonia, provided that the patient has been afebrile for >48 hours and has demonstrated clinical improvement. For severe pneumonia, duration of therapy is 7 days, with longer courses indicated in select cases.
- In **critically ill patients**, the addition of azithromycin or a respiratory fluoroquinolone to a β-lactam (ceftriaxone, cefotaxime, ampicillin-sulbactam) is necessary to provide coverage for *L. pneumophila.* MRSA coverage with vancomycin, teicoplanin, or linezolid should also be considered. If *P. aeruginosa* is a concern, an antipseudomonal β-lactam (cefepime, piperacillin-tazobactam, meropenem, imipenem) in combination with an antipseudomonal fluoroquinolone (ciprofloxacin, levofloxacin) is recommended. Once *Pseudomonas* has been isolated and antibiotic susceptibilities are available, monotherapy is an option.
- **Thoracentesis** of pleural effusions should be performed, with analysis of pH, cell count, Gram stain and bacterial culture, protein, and lactate dehydrogenase (see Chapter 10, Pulmonary Diseases). Empyemas should be drained.

Lung Abscess

GENERAL PRINCIPLES

- Lung abscess is a circumscribed area of necrosis in the pulmonary parenchyma that typically results from aspiration of oral flora. It can occur due through hematogenous route via septic emboli seeding, direct extension of empyema, endobronchial obstruction, or superinfection of a pulmonary infarct.
- Polymicrobial infections are common and involve oral anaerobes (*Prevotella* spp., *Peptostreptococcus*, *Fusobacterium*, *Bacteroides* spp., and *Actinomyces* spp.). Microaerophilic streptococci (*Streptococcus milleri*), enteric gram-negative bacilli (*Klebsiella pneumoniae*), and *S. aureus*, including community-acquired MRSA, are less frequent causes.
- Risk factors include periodontal disease and conditions that predispose patients to aspiration of oropharyngeal contents (alcohol intoxication, sedative use, seizures, stroke, and neuromuscular disease).

DIAGNOSIS

Clinical Presentation

Infections are indolent and may be reminiscent of pulmonary tuberculosis, with fever, chills, night sweats, weight loss, dyspnea, and cough productive of putrid or blood-streaked sputum for several weeks.

Diagnostic Testing

- Chest radiography is sensitive and typically reveals infiltrates with cavitation and air–fluid levels in dependent areas of the lung, such as the lower lobes or the posterior segments of the upper lobes. Chest CT can provide additional anatomic detail.
- Respiratory isolation and sputum testing for tuberculosis should be performed on all patients with cavitary lung lesions.
- Routine lab tests, such as complete blood count, renal and liver function test, and electrolytes, are commonly conducted.

TREATMENT

- Antibiotic therapy should consist of clindamycin or a β-lactam/β-lactamase inhibitor (ampicillin-sulbactam, piperacillin-tazobactam, amoxicillin-clavulanate) or a carbapenem (ertapenem). For MRSA cavitary lung lesions, linezolid or vancomycin should be used. Metronidazole monotherapy is ineffective due to the presence of microaerophilic nonculturable organisms in the oral microbiota, and thus, it should be combined with penicillin. For patients at risk for drug-resistant gram-negative infections, it is advisable to start the patient on imipenem or meropenem.
- Percutaneous drainage or surgical resection is rarely necessary and should be reserved for antibiotic-refractory disease, usually involving large abscesses (>6 cm) or infections with resistant organisms.

Tuberculosis

GENERAL PRINCIPLES

- Globally, in 2022, an estimated 10.6 million people were diagnosed as having TB, with an estimated 1.13 million TB deaths among HIV-negative people. TB remains one of the leading infectious diseases causing of death worldwide.[34] The incidence rate for TB rose by 3.9% between 2020 and 2022.
- Geographically, 4.85 million TB cases in 2022 were in the WHO regions of Southeast Asia. Eight countries accounted for two-thirds of the global total with India, China, Indonesia, the Philippines, Pakistan, Bangladesh, Nigeria, and Democratic Republic of Congo being the most affected countries.[35]
- Drug-resistant TB is a serious public health threat. In 2022, there were about 4,10,000 million new cases of multidrug/rifampicin-resistant TB with a treatment success rate of 63% globally.[36]
- Latent tuberculosis infection (LTBI) is a misnomer referring to someone who has infection, but not disease (clinical and radiological evidence of active disease). The lifetime risk of progression to active disease is 10% (5% within 2 years of infection and an additional 5% thereafter). In poorly controlled HIV and other immunosuppressed patients, the annual progression rate from latent to active tuberculosis is 10%. Adequate treatment of LTBI can reduce the risk of disease up to 90%.[37]

DIAGNOSIS

Clinical Presentation (Figure 14-3)

- The most frequent clinical presentation is pulmonary disease. Symptoms are often indolent and may include cough for >14 days, hemoptysis, dyspnea, fever, night sweats, weight loss, or fatigue. Misdiagnosis and treatment with a fluoroquinolone for presumed CAP can lead to treatment delay and fluoroquinolone resistance.[38]

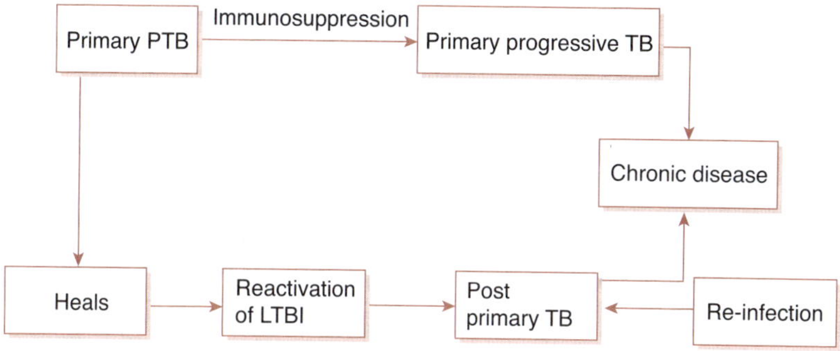

Figure 14-3 Natural history of tuberculosis.

- Extrapulmonary disease is increasingly being recognized as an important manifestation of tuberculosis. It can present as cervical lymphadenopathy, genitourinary disease, osteomyelitis, miliary dissemination, meningitis, peritonitis, or pericarditis.

Diagnostic Testing (Figure 14-4)

- Chest radiography may reveal focal infiltrates, nodules, cavitary lesions, miliary disease, pleural effusions, or hilar/mediastinal lymphadenopathy. Reactivation disease classically involves the upper lobes.
- Respiratory sample (sputum/induced sputum/BAL/gastric aspirate in children) should be sent for AFB smears, CBNAAT, and cultures. In suspected EPTB, an appropriate biopsy/fluid/pus/other sample should be tested for histopathology along with AFB smears, CBNAAT, and cultures. A diagnosis of active tuberculosis is made with a positive AFB smear, a positive NAAT for *M. tuberculosis* complex, or positive culture. Nontuberculous mycobacteria (NTM) may be positive on smear but negative on NAAT. On smear-negative samples, sensitivity of these assays can be up to 90%, if 3 sputum samples are tested.
- All patients with confirmed or suspected tuberculosis should undergo HIV testing.
- Antimicrobial susceptibility testing should be performed on all initial isolates and on isolates obtained from patients who do not respond to standard therapy. Rapid detection of rifampicin resistance, possible with molecular techniques (Cepheid Gene Xpert MTB/RIF), correlates with MDR-TB.
- LTBI may be diagnosed by a positive tuberculin skin test (TST) or interferon-γ release assay (IGRA).
- Diagnostic algorithm for tuberculosis and extrapulmonary tuberculosis summarized in Figures 14-4 and 14-5.

TREATMENT

Active Tuberculosis

- Hospitalized patients with active tuberculosis should be placed in airborne isolation in a **negative-pressure room.** Health-care personnel should use a N95 or powered air purifying respiratory during patient care.[39]
- The local health department should be notified of all tuberculosis cases so that contacts can be identified and directly observed therapy (DOT) administered when the patient is discharged. DOT is essential to ensure adherence and prevent emergence of drug resistance.

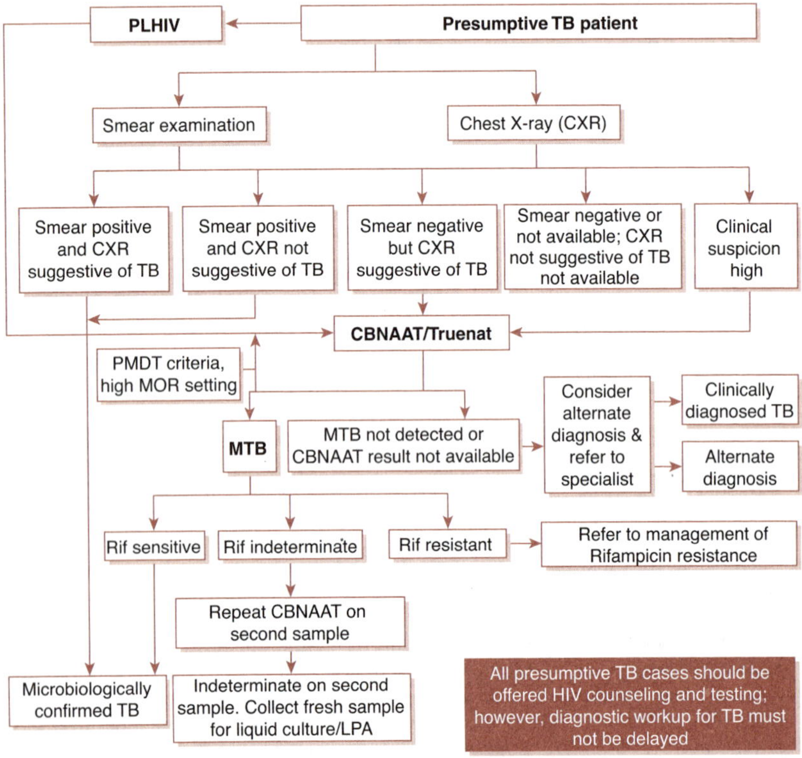

Figure 14-4 Algorithmic approach to a suspected case of tuberculosis. LPA, line probe assay; Rif, rifampicin. Adapted from NTEP Training module (1–4) for Medical Officers, July 2020.

- **Multidrug anti-TB treatment regimens** are required because drug resistance develops when a single drug is administered. Extended therapy is necessary because of the prolonged generation time of mycobacteria.

Intensive Phase (4-Drug Regimen) Duration – 8 Weeks	Dose
Rifampicin (RIF/R)	10 mg/kg; maximum, 600 mg PO qday
Isoniazid (INH/H)	5 mg/kg; maximum, 300 mg PO qday
Pyrazinamide (PZA/Z)	15–25 mg/kg; maximum, 2 g PO qday
Ethambutol (EMB/E)	15–25 mg/kg PO qday

- Pyridoxine (vitamin B_6) 25–50 mg PO qday should be used with INH to prevent sensory neuropathy.
- **Continuation phase** consists of 16 weeks of INH, RIF, and EMB to reach a standard total of 6 months of therapy for pulmonary tuberculosis. Patients at high risk for relapse (cavitary pulmonary disease or positive AFB cultures after 2 months of therapy) should be treated for an additional 28 weeks beyond the 8-week initial phase, for a total of 9 months.

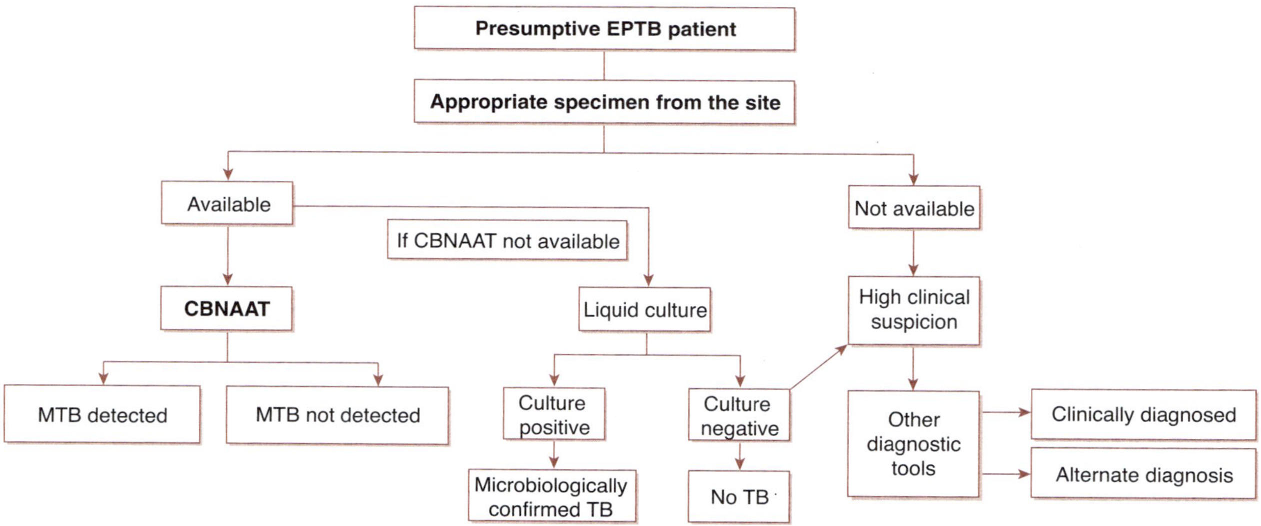

Figure 14-5 Diagnostic approach to a suspected case of extra-pulmonary tuberculosis. Adapted from NTEP Training module (1–4) for Medical Officers, July 2020.

- Daily therapy is the most efficacious regimen and it is strongly recommended in patients with HIV.
- Therapy for **MDR TB** often requires individualized drug regimens, and consultation with an expert in the treatment of tuberculosis is strongly recommended.
- **Shorter all oral MDR TB regimen:** 4–6 $Bdq_{(6\ m)}$-Lfx/Mfx-Cfz-Z-E-Hh-Eto/5 Lfx/Mfx-Cfz-Z-E
  Initial phase: 4–6 $Bdq_{(6\ m)}$-Lfx/Mfx-Cfz-Z-E-Hh-Eto
  Continuation phase: 5 Lfx/Mfx-Cfz-Z-E
- **BPaLM regimen** (regimen of choice for MDR/RR-TB with absence of unknown fluoroquinolone resistance): As per WHO 2022 regimen, new recommendation of a 6-month treatment regimen composed of bedaquiline, pretomanid, linezolid (600 mg), and moxifloxacin (BPaLM) rather than the 9-month or longer (18-month) regimens in MDR/RR-TB patients. This regimen is under study in a select group of patients in India.
- In countries like India, an **all oral longer MDR-TB regimen** (18–20 Lfx $Bdq_{[6\ months\ or\ longer]}$ Lzd Cfz Cs) is still preferred. Examples of a replacement regimen is 18Bdq-Lzd-Cfz-Cs-Dlm-[PZA]: the treatment lasts 18 months with 6 individual drugs; Z is used, but not considered as a likely effective drug.[40] The replacement sequence for Group C for a longer oral M/XDR TB regimen was recommended in the order or factors such as delamanid, amikacin, pyrazinamide, ethionamide, PAS, ethambutol, and penems. These drugs are replaced as per their efficacy, resistance patterns, prior use, and side effects.
- **Extrapulmonary disease** in adults can be treated in the same manner as pulmonary disease, with 6-month regimens, except for bone and joint infection (9–12 months) and central nervous system (CNS) tuberculosis (12 months).[41]
- **Pregnant women** should not receive PZA and should be treated with a 9-month regimen. INH, RIF, and EMB, with pyridoxine, should be administered during the initial 8-week phase, until susceptibilities are known, with continuation of INH and RIF for the remainder of therapy.
- **Glucocorticoids** in combination with antituberculous drugs are recommended in tuberculous meningitis. Prednisone 1 mg/kg (maximum, 60 mg) PO qday or dexamethasone 12 mg IV qday is tapered over several weeks.
- An integrated diagnostic and treatment algorithm for drug-resistant TB followed in India is given in Figure 14-6 and Table 14-8.

Latent Tuberculosis

- Chemoprophylaxis for LTBI should be administered only after active disease has been ruled out by clinical assessment, chest radiography, and sputum collection.
- Risk factors for progression include a positive conversion within 2 years of a previously negative TST or IGRA; a history of untreated tuberculosis or radiographic evidence of previous fibrotic disease (calcified granulomas in the absence of fibrosis do not confer increased risk); patients with HIV infection, diabetes mellitus, end-stage renal disease, hematologic or lymphoreticular malignancy, chronic malnutrition, or silicosis or who are receiving immunosuppressive therapy; and close contacts (household members) of patients with active disease who have been diagnosed with LTBI.
- Persons with advanced **HIV** infection or other severely immunocompromised states (e.g., transplant) who have had known contact with a patient with active tuberculosis should be treated for LTBI.
- INH 300 mg PO qday for 9 months is the most studied regimen for LTBI who have risk factors for progression to active disease, regardless of age. However, less than 60% of patients complete the 9-month treatment course.
- Shorter regimens may improve compliance. RIF 600 mg qday for 4 months, or INH 900 mg PO plus rifapentine 900 mg PO (with dose adjustment for patients <50 kg) once weekly for 12 weeks are as effective as daily INH, even when self-administered.[37]

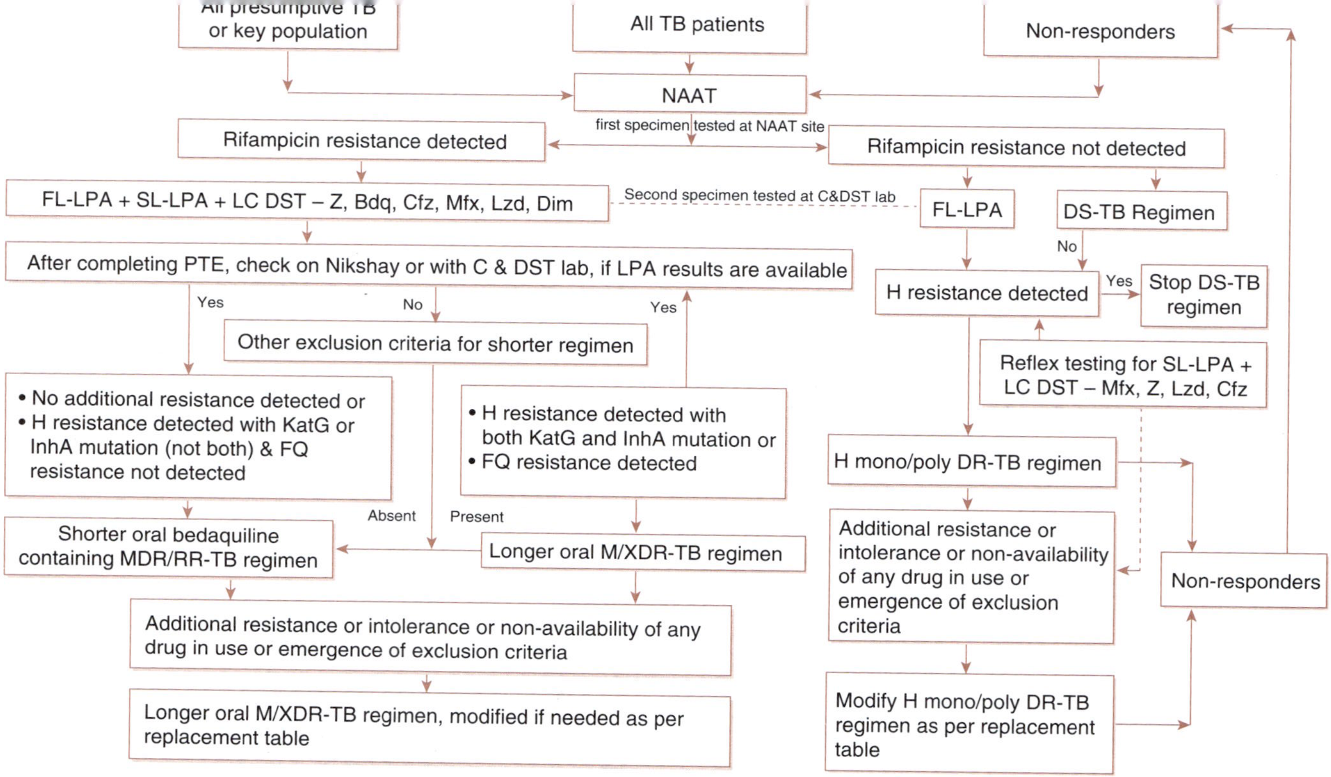

Figure 14-6 Integrated diagnostic and treatment algorithm for drug-resistant tuberculosis. Adapted from https://tbcindia.gov.in/WriteReadData/l892s/8368587497Guidelines%20for%20PMDT%20in%20India.pdf. C&DST, culture and drug susceptibility testing; DST, drug susceptibility testing; FL-LPA, first line, line probe assay; FQ, fluoroquinolones; LC, liquid culture; RR, rifampicin resistance; SL-LPA, second line, line probe assay.

TABLE 14-8 Treatment Options for Drug-Resistant TB (WHO 2016 Classification)

WHO 2016 TB Drugs Classification		
Group A Fluoroquinolones		• Levofloxacin • Moxifloxacin • Gatifloxacin
Group B Second-line injectable agents		• Amikacin • Capreomycin • Kanamycin (Streptomycin)
Group C Other core second-line agents		• Ethionamide/prothionamide • Cycloserine/terizidone • Linezolid • Clofazimine
Group D Add-on agents (not core MDR-TB regimen components)	D1	• Pyrazinamide • Ethambutol • High-dose isoniazid
	D2	• Bedaquiline • Delamanid
	D3	• *p*-Aminosalicylic acid • Imipenem-cilastatin • Meropenem • Amoxicillin-clavulanate • (Thioacetazone)

Groups and Steps	Medicine	Abbreviation
Group A **Include all three medicines**	Levofloxacin or	Lfx
	Moxifloxacin	Mfx
	Bedaquiline	Bdq
	Linezolid	Lzd
Group B **Add one or both medicines**	Clofazimine	Cfz
	Cycloserine or	Cs
	Terizidone	Trd
Group C **Add to complete the regimen and when medicines from Group A and B cannot be used**	Ethambutol	E
	Delamanid	Dlm
	Pyrazinamide	Z
	Imipenem-cilastatin or	Ipm-Cln
	Meropenem	Mpm
	Amikacin	Am
	(OR Streptomycin)	(S)
	Ethionamide or	Eto
	Prothionamide	Pto
	p-aminosalicylic acid	PAS

Adapted from WHO treatment guidelines for drugresistant tuberculosis. Available at https://iris.who.int/bitstream/handle/10665/250125/9789241549639-eng.pdf

TB PREVENTIVE THERAPY

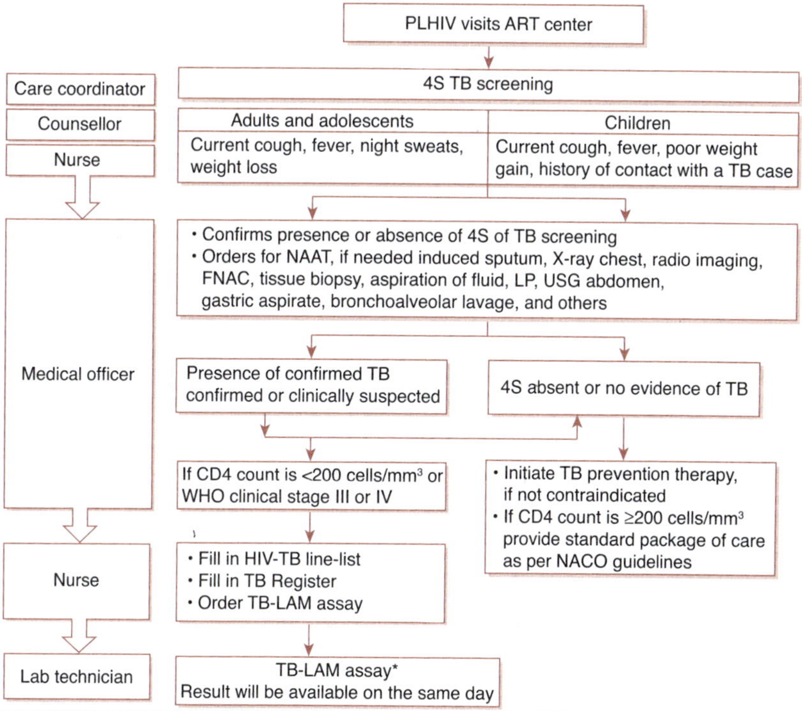

Medical officer: Management of TB

NAAT	TB-LAM**	Interpretation	Action
Positive	Positive	**Microbiologically confirmed TB case**	Start ATT, exclude DR-TB
Positive	Negative		
Negative/ Not available	Positive	Clinically diagnosed TB case	Start ATT
Negative/ Not available	Negative	Will depend on correlation with TB signs and symptoms	• Consider other diagnosis • If TB is unlikely, start TPT

#Negative TB-LAM test does not rule out active TB

ART should be initiated as soon as possible within two weeks for initiating TB treatment, regardless of CD4 cell count (except when signs and symptoms of meningitis are present)

*Currently TB-LAM assay is not available in the programme
Adapted from National Guidelines for HIV Care and Treatment, 2021. Available at https://naco.gov.in/sites/default/files/National_Guidelines_for_HIV_Care_and_Treatment_2021.pdf

Monitoring

- **Response to therapy.** Patients with initial positive sputum AFB smears should submit sputum for AFB smear and culture every 1–2 weeks until AFB smears become negative. Sputum should then be obtained monthly until two consecutive negative cultures are documented. Conversion of cultures from positive to negative is the most reliable indicator of response to treatment. Continued symptoms or persistently positive cultures after 3 months of treatment should raise the suspicion of drug resistance or lack of adherence and prompt referral to an expert in the treatment of TB.

- **Adverse reactions.** Most patients should have a baseline laboratory evaluation at the start of therapy that includes hepatic enzymes, bilirubin, complete blood count, and serum creatinine. Routine laboratory monitoring for patients with normal baseline values is probably unnecessary except in the setting of HIV (particularly if receiving concurrent antiretroviral therapy), alcohol abuse, chronic liver disease, or pregnancy. Monthly clinical evaluations with specific inquiries about symptoms of drug toxicity are essential. Patients taking EMB should be tested monthly for visual acuity and red–green color perception (Ishihara test).
- Referral to the public health department is recommended to ensure adherence by DOT and to monitor for medication-related complications.

GASTROINTESTINAL AND ABDOMINAL INFECTIONS

Infectious Gastroenteritis

- Acute infectious diarrhea can be caused by viruses, bacteria, and parasites. It is usually of <2 weeks duration.
- A careful history of food ingestion, water supply, travel, antibiotic use, and illness in family members should be elicited.
- Infectious diarrhea can be categorized as either dysentery (invasive or inflammatory diarrhea) or watery diarrhea (noninflammatory diarrhea) (Table 14-9).
  - Dysenteric diarrhea involves the colon and may be associated with fever and bloody stools. Etiologies include *C. difficile*, *Campylobacter*, nontyphoid *Salmonella*, *Shigella*, enterohemorrhagic *E. coli* 0157:H7 (which can lead to hemolytic-uremic syndrome, HUS), and *Yersinia*.[42]

TABLE 14-9 Inflammatory Diarrhea vs Noninflammatory Diarrhea

Inflammatory Diarrhea	Noninflammatory Diarrhea
Bloody diarrhea, may be associated with pus	Watery, nonbloody
Associated with fever, nausea, and vomiting	Usually mild, self-limited
Usually caused by an invasive or toxin-producing bacterium	Caused by a virus or noninvasive, toxin-producing bacterium
Stool examination for bacteria is required in all patients	Diagnostic evaluation is limited to patients with severe or persistent (>7 days) diarrhea
Causes: **Viral:** Cytomegalovirus Protozoal: *Entamoeba histolytica* **Bacteria:** Enterohemorrhagic (O157:H5) and enteroinvasive (O157:H7) *E. coli*, *Shigella, Campylobacter, Salmonella, Chlamydia, Neisseria gonorrhoeae*	Causes: **Viruses:** norovirus, rotavirus, adenovirus, Protozoal: Giardia lamblia, *Cryptosporidium, Cyclospora* **Bacteria:** Enterotoxigenic *E. coli* (ETEC), *Bacillus cereus, Vibrio cholerae*

DIAGNOSIS

Stool testing is indicated if there is fever, bloody stools, immunocompromise, severe disease, or symptoms for >7 days. Stools should be sent for fecal leukocytes, culture, *C. difficile* toxin testing, antigen testing, and parasite examination (as indicated) (Figure 14-7).

TREATMENT

- Fluid and electrolyte replacement is the mainstay of therapy.
- Antimotility agents should be avoided in dysenteric diarrhea.

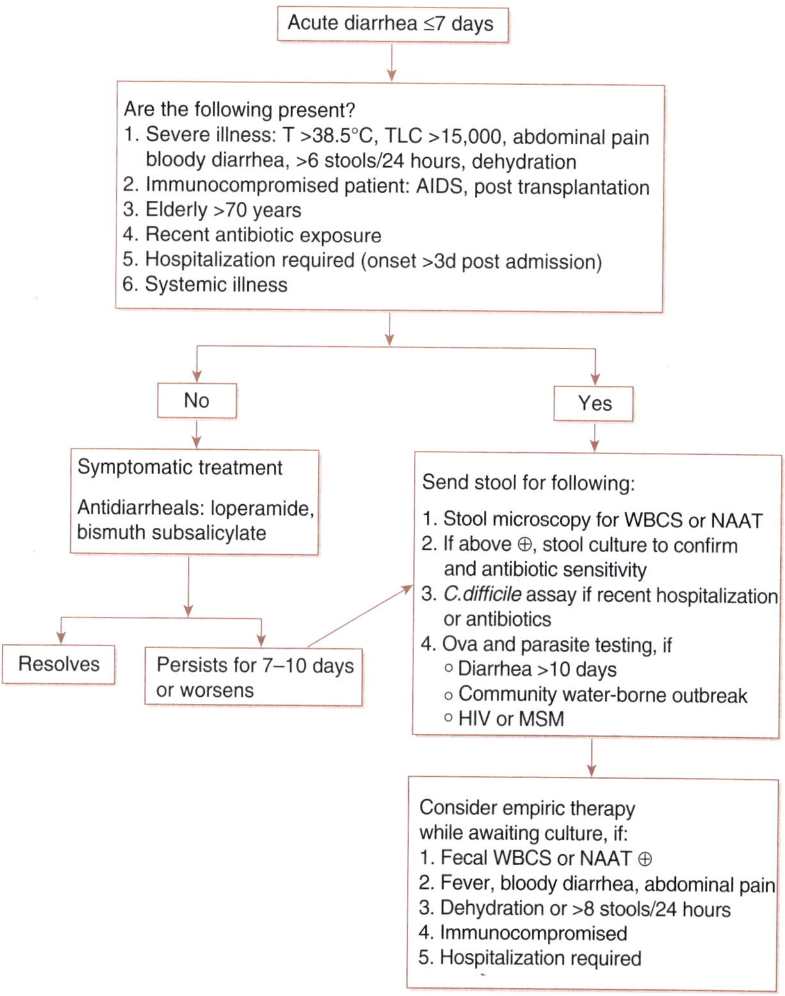

Figure 14-7 Approach to acute diarrhea.

- Antibiotics can be used in dysenteric diarrhea for severe disease, bloody stools, and in high-risk patients.
- Azithromycin 1 g single dose or 500 mg PO qday for 3 days or ciprofloxacin 750 mg PO single dose or 500 mg PO bid for 3 days is often used.
- If symptoms persist 24 hours after a single-dose regimen, complete a three-day course using multiple-dose regimen.
- Antibiotics are contraindicated in enterohemorrhagic *E coli*, as they increase the risk of HUS.
- Traveler's diarrhea can be treated with ciprofloxacin or TMP-SMX without stool testing.
- Treat empirically if there is suspicion of *C. difficile* infection.

Chronic Diarrhea

- Diarrhea lasting >30 days is defined as chronic.
- Infectious causes are usually parasitic, including *Cryptosporidium* (see Chapter 16 section on Opportunistic Infections in HIV), *Giardia*, and *Entamoeba.*
  - Giardiasis is diagnosed by stool antigen testing or microscopic examination. Treatment is metronidazole 500 mg PO q12h for 7 days and tinidazole 2 g PO single dose or nitazoxanide 500 mg PO q12h for 3 days.
  - Amebiasis is diagnosed by stool microscopy, antigen testing and serology. Treatment is metronidazole 500 mg q8h for 7–10 days, followed by iodoquin or paromomycin to eradicate cysts (Figure 14-8).

Intra-Abdominal Infection

- Intra-abdominal infections occur because of inflammation or disruption of the gastrointestinal tract that allows normal bowel flora to inoculate the abdominal cavity. They can be classified as low risk (uncomplicated) or high risk (complicated).
- Infections are typically polymicrobial with enteric gram-negative bacilli (e.g., *E. coli*, *Klebsiella* spp.), *Enterococcus* spp., and especially anaerobes such as *Bacteroides fragilis.*
- Low-risk community–acquired infections are of mild-to-moderate severity and include acute diverticulitis, colitis, or appendiceal abscess, provided there are no risk factors for antibiotic resistance or treatment failure. These can be treated with
  1. A single β-lactam/β-lactamase inhibitor combination like piperacillin-tazobactam, or
  2. A third-generation cephalosporin (e.g., ceftriaxone)/fluoroquinolone plus metronidazole.
- High-risk community infections are severe infections and occur in patients at risk for adverse outcomes or resistant pathogens (e.g., age >70 years, comorbidities, immunocompromise, sepsis, delay in source control). An agent with activity against *P. aeruginosa* and resistant *Enterobacteriaceae* such as meropenem, imipenem, or piperacillin-tazobactam, or a combination of cefepime/ceftazidime with metronidazole can be used.
- Local resistance patterns must be taken into consideration for antibiotic selection.
- Healthcare-associated infections (HAIs) may be caused by MDRO and require additional antibiotics if ESBL-producing organisms or MRSA are a consideration.
- Source control with abscess drainage or surgical resection is critical.
- Avoid clindamycin, cefoxitin, and moxifloxacin owing to high rates of resistance among *B. fragilis.*
- Empiric antifungal coverage is usually not indicated unless yeast is grown from a sterile site.[43] See Table 14-10.

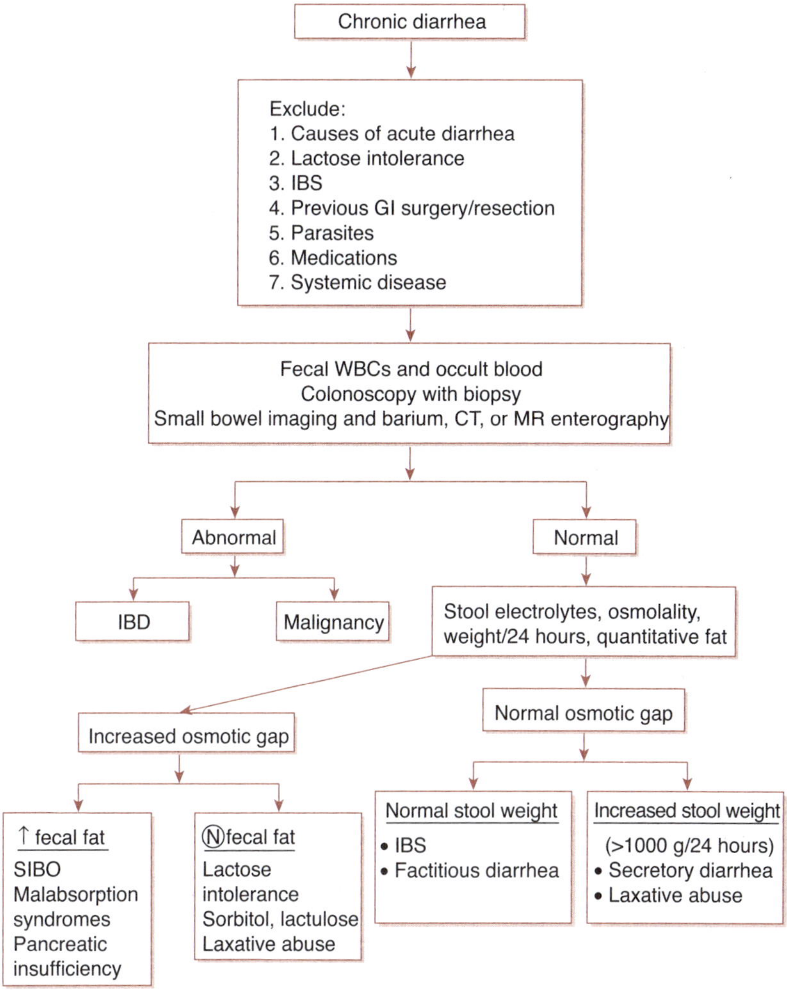

Figure 14-8 Approach to chronic diarrhea.

Peritonitis

GENERAL PRINCIPLES

- **Primary** or **spontaneous bacterial peritonitis (SBP)** is a common complication of cirrhosis and ascites. *M. tuberculosis* and *Neisseria gonorrhoeae* (Fitz-Hugh–Curtis syndrome) also can occasionally cause primary peritonitis (see Chapter 16, Sexually Transmitted Infections, HIV, and AIDS). *E. coli*, *Klebsiella pneumonia*, and *S. pneumoniae* are common pathogens.

TABLE 14-10 Empiric Therapy Examples for Intra-Abdominal Infections[43]

Oral Regimens
- Ciprofloxacin 500–750 mg PO q12h + metronidazole 500 mg PO q8h
- Moxifloxacin 400 mg PO qday

Parenteral Regimens
Low risk—no concern for *Pseudomonas aeruginosa*
- Ertapenem 1 g IV q24h
- Ceftriaxone 1–2 g IV qday + metronidazole 500 mg IV q8h
- Piperacillin/tazobactam 4.5 g IV q6h

High risk—concern for P. *aeruginosa*
- Piperacillin/tazobactam 4.5 g IV q6h
- Cefepime 1–2 g IV q8h + metronidazole 500 mg IV q8h
- Ciprofloxacin 400 mg IV q8–12h + metronidazole 500 mg IV q8h
- Meropenem 1 g IV q8h or imipenem-cilastatin 500 mg IV q6h

Concern for *Enterococcus* spp
- Add ampicillin 2 g IV every 4 hours or vancomycin 15–20 mg/kg IV every 8–12 hours

Concern for vancomycin-resistant *Enterococcus* spp.[a]
- Add linezolid 600 mg PO/IV q12h or daptomycin 6–8 mg/kg IV qday to above regimens

Concern for yeast[a]
- Add echinocandin (e.g., micafungin 100 mg IV qday) or fluconazole 400 mg PO/IV qday to above regimens

[a]If isolated from a sterile site.

- **Secondary peritonitis** may be caused by a perforated viscus in the gastrointestinal or genitourinary tract or contiguous spread from a visceral infection, usually resulting in an *acute* surgical abdomen.
- Peritonitis related to **peritoneal dialysis** is addressed in Chapter 13, Renal Diseases.

DIAGNOSIS

Clinical Presentation

SBP may present with subtle abdominal symptoms without typical signs of infection. SBP should be ruled out with a diagnostic paracentesis in patients admitted with cirrhosis and ascites presenting with gastrointestinal bleeding, encephalopathy, acute kidney injury (AKI), or other decompensation of liver disease. Patients with secondary peritonitis may appear acutely ill with abdominal tenderness and peritoneal signs. Suspect SBP in a patient with ascites with any of the following[44]:
- Temperature >37.8°C
- Abdominal pain and/or tenderness
- A change in mental status
- Ascitic fluid neutrophil count >250 mm^3

Diagnostic Testing

- Send blood cultures and ascites fluid for culture (directly inoculate culture bottles at bedside), cell count, and differential. **SBP** is diagnosed when ascites fluid has

>250 neutrophils/mm, culture results are positive and secondary causes of peritonitis are excluded.[44]

- Diagnosis of **secondary peritonitis** is made clinically and with imaging to evaluate for free air (perforation) and the source of infection. Blood cultures should be obtained.

TREATMENT

- First-line treatment typically includes either a third-generation cephalosporin (e.g., cefotaxime 2 g IV q8h) or a fluoroquinolone (e.g., ciprofloxacin 400 mg IV q12h). Administration of IV albumin on days 1 and 3 of treatment may improve survival.[37]
- Treatment should be continued for 5 days. Extended courses may be needed for *P. aeruginosa* or resistant organisms.
- **SBP prophylaxis** may be initiated after the first episode of SBP or after variceal bleeding in individuals afflicted with cirrhosis and ascites, provided their ascitic fluid protein level is <1.5 g/dL with renal impairment or liver failure. Double strength TMP-SMX, ciprofloxacin, or norfloxacin od can be given for the same.
- Nonselective β-blockers must be permanently discontinued once SBP develops because use of these drugs in the setting of SBP has been associated with decreased transplant-free survival, increased rates of hepatorenal syndrome and increased duration of hospitalization.[44]
- Secondary peritonitis may require surgical intervention if there is perforation or intraabdominal abscess formation. Antibiotics are continued until imaging demonstrates resolution of the abscess.
- Treatment of chronic tuberculous peritonitis is the same as that of pulmonary tuberculosis.

Hepatobiliary Infections

GENERAL PRINCIPLES

- **Acute cholecystitis** is associated with cholelithiasis and is caused by intestinal flora such as *E. coli*, *Klebsiella*, *Enterobacter*, etc. Acalculous cholecystitis occurs in 5%–10% of cases.
- **Ascending cholangitis** is an infectious complication of an obstructed common bile duct, often following pancreatitis or cholecystitis.

DIAGNOSIS

Clinical Presentation

Tenderness and guarding of the RUQ on deep inspiration (Murphy's sign) is a common sign of a hepatobiliary infection. Ascending cholangitis presents as the **Charcot triad** of fever, RUQ pain, and jaundice. **Reynolds pentad** adds symptoms of confusion and hypotension and warrants rapid intervention. Bacteremia and shock are common.

Diagnostic Testing

- Liver enzyme abnormalities are seen in acute cholangitis.
- Diagnosis of biliary tract infections is usually made by ultrasonography. Technetium-99m-hydroxy iminodiacetic acid scanning and CT scanning may also be useful.
- Endoscopic retrograde cholangiopancreatography allows for diagnosis as well as therapeutic intervention in the case of common bile duct obstruction and should be considered in patients with common bile duct dilation, jaundice, or liver enzyme abnormalities.

TREATMENT

- Management of **acute cholecystitis** includes parenteral fluids, restricted PO intake, analgesia, and surgery. Advanced age, severe disease, or complications such as gallbladder ischemia or perforation, peritonitis, or bacteremia mandate broad-spectrum antibiotics such as ampicillin/sulbactam 3 g IV q6h, piperacillin/tazobactam 3.375 g IV q6h, ertapenem 1 g IV qday or meropenem 500 mg IV q8h. Immediate surgery is usually necessary for severe disease, but surgery may be delayed up to 6 weeks if there is an initial response to medical therapy. After cholecystectomy, perioperative antibiotics may be discontinued.[45]
- The mainstay of therapy for **ascending cholangitis** is aggressive supportive care, including broad-spectrum antibiotics as above. Surgical or endoscopic decompression and drainage is necessary. Development of an abscess requires surgical drainage.

OTHER INFECTIONS

- **Viral hepatitis** (see Chapter 19, Liver Diseases)
- ***Helicobacter pylori*–associated** disease (see Chapter 18, Gastrointestinal Diseases)

Liver Fluke

GENERAL PRINCIPLES

- Liver fluke infection is a chronic parasitic inflammatory disease of the bile ducts.
- The most well-known species that cause human infection are *Clonorchis sinensis*, *Opisthorchis viverrini*, and *Opisthorchis felineus*.
- Infection occurs through the ingestion of fluke-infested freshwater raw fish.
- Throughout the world, particularly in Southeast Asia, more than 35 million people are infected.

DIAGNOSIS

Clinical Presentation

- Acute infection is usually asymptomatic. Symptoms are seen only in older patients from endemic areas due to increased worm burden.
- It may present as fever, nausea, vomiting, abdominal pain, or generalized fatigue.
- Chronic infection may lead to suppurative cholangitis, formation of bile duct stone, and development of cholangiocarcinoma.

Diagnostic Testing

- Stool routine and microscopy is done for flukes' egg detection.
- PCR-based method for the detection of liver fluke's genetic materials in the stool can be used.
- Detection of liver fluke's specific antibodies in the serum, saliva, and urine could be performed.
- A monoclonal antibody-based ELISA (Mab-ELISA) has been developed to detect *O. viverrini* metabolic antigen in the feces.

TREATMENT

- Praziquantel (75 mg/kg in three divided doses) is the drug of choice for the treatment of fluke infection including opisthorchiasis and clonorchiasis. Tribendimidine is one of the promising agents.

GENITOURINARY INFECTIONS

- The spectrum of genitourinary tract infections varies from uncomplicated to complicated, depending on host factors and underlying conditions. Diagnostic and therapeutic approaches to adult genitourinary infections are determined by gender-specific anatomic differences, prior antimicrobial exposures, and the presence of catheters, stents, etc. Infections are primarily caused by Enterobacteriaceae (*E. coli*, *Proteus mirabilis*, and *K. pneumoniae*) and *Staphylococcus saprophyticus*.
- Workup typically includes urinalysis and microscopic examination of a fresh, unspun, clean-voided, or catheterized urine specimen. Pyuria (positive leukocyte esterase or ≥8 leukocytes per high-power field) or bacteriuria (positive nitrites or ≥1 organism per oil-immersion field) suggests active infection. A high number of epithelial cells indicates an inadequate sample. A urine Gram stain can be helpful in guiding initial antimicrobial choices. Quantitative culture often yields $>10^5$ bacteria colony forming units (CFU)/mL, but colony counts as low as 10^2–10^4 bacteria/mL may indicate infection in women with acute dysuria.

Asymptomatic Bacteriuria

- Asymptomatic bacteriuria is defined as the isolation of $>10^5$ CFU/mL of a single bacterial species in a specimen (men, catheters) or 2 consecutive specimens (in women, within 2 weeks) in appropriately collected urine obtained from a person **without** symptoms of urinary infection.
- **Asymptomatic bacteriuria** is of limited clinical significance and **should not be treated except in pregnant women or patients undergoing urologic surgery.** Pregnant women should have screening urine culture near the end of the first trimester and be treated if positive. Treatment is **not** recommended for asymptomatic bacteriuria in the elderly, diabetics, institutionalized patients, spinal cord injury patients, or catheterized patients.

Cystitis

- Uncomplicated cystitis is defined as infection of the bladder or lower urinary tract in otherwise healthy, nonpregnant adult women.
- Complicated cystitis is defined based on several risk factors including anatomic abnormality, immunosuppression, pregnancy, indwelling catheters, or unusual pathogens.
- Recurrent cystitis may be seen in women and is usually due to reinfection rather than recurrence.[46]

DIAGNOSIS

Clinical Presentation

- Lower urinary tract infection (UTI) is diagnosed based on clinical history of dysuria, urgency, frequency, or suprapubic pain associated with pyuria and bacteriuria on urine analysis and positive urine culture. Fever is more likely if there is associated pyelonephritis.
- Dysuria without pyuria in sexually active patients warrants consideration of sexually transmitted infection (see Chapter 16, Sexually Transmitted Infections).

Diagnostic Testing

- **Acute uncomplicated cystitis in women:** Many women are treated empirically without a urine culture. A pretreatment urine culture is recommended for diabetics, patients who are symptomatic for >7 days, individuals with recurrent UTI, women who use a contraceptive diaphragm, and individuals older than 65 years.

- **Sterile pyuria:** Prior antimicrobials may result in negative cultures. Differential diagnosis includes chronic interstitial nephritis, interstitial cystitis, or infection with atypical organisms including *Chlamydia trachomatis*, *Ureaplasma urealyticum*, *N. gonorrhoeae*, or rarely, *M. tuberculosis*. Specific cultures of the endocervix for sexually transmitted infections should be performed.

TREATMENT

- See Tables 14-11 and 14-12.
- **Acute uncomplicated cystitis in women:** A 5-day course of nitrofurantoin, a 3-day course of TMP-SMX, or a single dose of fosfomycin are recommended for empiric treatment. Fluoroquinolones should **not** be used as first-line treatment. Therapy should be extended to 7 days in pregnant patients and diabetics. Post-treatment urine culture should only be obtained if symptoms do not improve within 48 hours. Foreign bodies including stents and catheters should be removed.[47]

TABLE 14-11 Empiric Therapy for Urinary Tract Infections[46]

Disease	Empiric Therapy	Notes
Simple Cystitis		
Women	*First line:* • TMP-SMX DS PO bid × 3 d • Nitrofurantoin PO 100 mg bid × 5 d • Fosfomycin 3 g PO × 1 dose *Alternative:* • FQ (not first line) × 3 d *Pregnancy:* • Nitrofurantoin PO 100 mg bid × 7 d • Cephalexin PO 500 mg bid × 7 d • Cefuroxime axetil × 7 d	• Choose antibiotics based on local susceptibility patterns. • Extend therapy to 7 d for diabetics and older patients. • Fosfomycin and β-lactams have lower efficacy; avoid if early pyelonephritis is suspected. • Treat asymptomatic bacteriuria in pregnancy.
Men	*First line:* • TMP-SMX DS PO bid × 7 d • FQ × 5 d	• Treat 7–14 d. • Avoid nitrofurantoin and β-lactam in men due to low tissue concentrations. • Consider urologic evaluation for recurrent disease or pyelonephritis.
Pyelonephritis, complicated UTI	*Outpatient, mild–moderate illness:* • FQ × 7 d *Inpatient, severe illness:* • FQ • Aminoglycoside • β-Lactam/β-lactamase inhibitor[a] • Third- or fourth-generation cephalosporin[b]	• Consider IV until afebrile followed by outpatient oral therapy in stable patients to complete 10–14 d. • Can consider shortening if complicating factor is resolved (i.e., removal of stone). • Do not use FQ in pregnancy.

(Continued)

TABLE 14-11 Empiric Therapy for Urinary Tract Infections[46] (Continued)

Disease	Empiric Therapy	Notes
Recurrent cystitis	*Postcoital prophylaxis:* TMP-SMX SS × 1 or nitrofurantoin 100 mg × 1 or cephalexin 250 mg × 1 *Continuous prophylaxis:* TMP-SMX 0.5 SS qday or every other day × 6 mo or nitrofurantoin 50–100 mg qhs × 6 mo *Intermittent self-treatment:* TMP-SMX DS PO q12h × 3 d or ciprofloxacin 250 mg PO q12h × 3 d	• Topical vaginal estrogen in postmenopausal women, and methenamine hippurate may have a role in preventing recurrent UTI. • Cranberry products and D-mannose have been recommended as prophylactic agents, but their efficacy is controversial.

[a]β-lactam/β-lactamase inhibitors: ampicillin/sulbactam 1.5–3 g IV q6h, piperacillin/tazobactam 3.75–4.5 g IV q6h.
[b]Third- or fourth-generation cephalosporins include ceftriaxone 1–2 g IV qday (third-generation) or cefepime 1 g IV q8h (fourth-generation).
DS, double strength; FQ, fluoroquinolone; GU, genitourinary; SS, single strength; TMP, trimethoprim; TMP-SMX, trimethoprim-sulfamethoxazole; UTI, urinary tract infection.

TABLE 14-12 Dosing Examples for Urinary Tract Infections

Class	Oral (Less Severe)	Parenteral (More Severe)
Folate inhibitors	• TMP-SMX DS 160 mg/800 mg PO q12h • Trimethoprim 100 mg PO q12h	N/A
Fluoroquinolone	• Ciprofloxacin 250–500 mg PO q12h • Levofloxacin 250–750 mg PO qday	• Ciprofloxacin 400 mg IV q12h • Levofloxacin 250–750 mg IV qday
β-lactam/β-lactamase inhibitor	• Amoxicillin-clavulanate 500 mg/125 mg PO q12h or q8h	• Ampicillin-sulbactam 1.5–3 g IV q6h • Piperacillin-tazobactam 3.375–4.5 g IV q6h
Cephalosporins	• Cephalexin 200–500 mg PO q6h • Cefpodoxime proxetil 100 mg PO q12h	• Cefazolin 1 g IV q8h • Ceftriaxone 1 g IV qday • Cefepime 1 g IV q8h
Carbapenems	N/A	• Ertapenem 1 g IV q8h • Imipenem 500 mg IV q6h • Meropenem 1 g IV q8h
Aminoglycoside	N/A	• Gentamicin 5 mg/kg qday
Fosfomycin[a]	• Fosfomycin 3 g PO once	N/A
Nitrofurantoin[a]	• Nitrofurantoin 100 mg PO bid	N/A

[a]Uncomplicated cystitis.
DS, double strength; N/A, not applicable; TMP-SMX, trimethoprim-sulfamethoxazole.

- **Recurrent cystitis in women** is usually due to reinfection (with a different organism) and may be challenging to manage. Risk factors include frequency of intercourse and spermicide use in young women and urologic abnormalities such as incontinence and cystocele in older women. Relapses (with the original infecting organism) that occur within 2 weeks of cessation of therapy should be treated for 2 weeks and may indicate a urologic abnormality.
- Prophylaxis may be considered for patients with frequent reinfection using continuous, postcoital, or self-initiated antibiotics. Estrogen therapy in postmenopausal women may also have a role in prevention; cranberry products have not been shown to help.[48]

Genitourinary Infections in Men

CYSTITIS

Cystitis is uncommon in young men; *E. coli* is the most frequent pathogen. Risk factors include urologic abnormality, anal intercourse, and lack of circumcision. Pyuria may also be an indication of sexually transmitted infections. A pretreatment urinalysis and culture should be sent. Other urologic studies are appropriate if there are no underlying risk factors, when treatment fails, in recurrent infections, or when pyelonephritis occurs.

PROSTATITIS

- **Acute prostatitis** usually presents with fever, chills, dysuria, pelvic pain, obstructive symptoms, and a boggy, tender prostate on examination. It is caused by *E. coli* and other gram-negative organisms. Diagnosis is made by physical examination and urine Gram stain and culture. Prostatic massage is contraindicated as it can lead to bacteremia.
- **Chronic prostatitis** is defined as presence of urinary symptoms for >3 months. It is frequently noninfectious. Chronic bacterial prostatitis is caused by enteric gram-negative organisms. Symptoms include frequency, dysuria, urgency, perineal discomfort, and recurrent UTIs. Urine cultures should be obtained when the patient is symptomatic. Referral to a urologist for quantitative cultures before and after prostatic massage may be necessary. Transrectal ultrasound can be used if prostatic abscess is suspected.

Treatment

- **Acute bacterial prostatitis** should be treated with a 6-week course of either ciprofloxacin 500 mg PO q12h or TMP-SMX 160 mg/800 mg (double strength) PO q12h.
- Chronic prostatitis is difficult to treat. Culture-positive **chronic bacterial prostatitis** should receive prolonged therapy (for at least 4–6 weeks with fluoroquinolones or TMP-SMX).

EPIDIDYMITIS

Epididymitis presents as a unilateral scrotal ache with swollen and tender epididymis on examination. Causative organisms are usually *N. gonorrhoeae* or *C. trachomatis* in sexually active young men and gram-negative enteric organisms in older men. Diagnosis and therapy should be directed according to this epidemiology, with NAAT testing and ceftriaxone and doxycycline in young men, and levofloxacin in men older than 35 years.[49]

PYELONEPHRITIS

Pyelonephritis is infection of the kidney, usually due to ascending infection from the lower urinary tract. The causative agents are typically Enterobacteriaceae such as *E. coli* or *Proteus* spp. The incidence of MDRO is rising, especially in patients with recent use of broad-spectrum antibiotics or exposure to health-care facilities. It is by definition considered as complicated UTI.

Diagnosis

Clinical Presentation

Patients present with fever, chills, flank pain, nausea/vomiting, and costovertebral angle tenderness, often along with cystitis symptoms. Patients may present with sepsis or multiorgan dysfunction, especially if they have urinary obstruction and recent instrumentation or are elderly or diabetic.

Diagnostic Testing

- Urinalysis reveals significant bacteriuria, pyuria, red blood cells, and occasional leukocyte casts. A urine culture should be sent. Blood cultures should be obtained in hospitalized patients as bacteremia is present in 15%–20% of cases.
- Imaging may be considered if symptoms persist despite 48–72 hours of appropriate antibiotics or for suspected urinary tract obstruction. Ultrasonography, CT scan, or IV pyelogram may demonstrate the presence of a renal abscess or renal calculi, which may require more invasive management.

Treatment

- Patients with **mild-to-moderate illness** who are able to take oral medications can typically be treated in the outpatient setting. Patients with more **severe illness** should be treated initially with IV therapy.
- Indications for hospitalization include sepsis, persistently high fever or pain, marked debility, urinary tract obstruction, and inability to tolerate orally. Start empiric antibiotics promptly.
- See Tables 14-11 and 14-12.

SYSTEMIC MYCOSES AND ATYPICAL ORGANISMS

- Clinical presentations are protean and not pathogen-specific. Consider systemic mycoses in normal hosts with unexplained chronic pulmonary pathology, chronic meningitis, lytic bone lesions, chronic skin lesions, FUO, or cytopenias. In immunocompromised patients, besides the above presentations, the development of new pulmonary, cutaneous, funduscopic, or head and neck signs and symptoms should prompt consideration of these pathogens.
- The mycoses can often be identified by taking into account epidemiologic clues (many are geographically restricted), site of infection, inflammatory response, and microscopic fungal appearance. These infections can be complex and difficult to treat, and infectious disease consultation is recommended in all cases.
- Antifungal agents have variable doses, depending on the severity of infection and the patient's renal and hepatic function. Lipid formulations of amphotericin B (Amb) are preferred over the deoxycholate formulation owing to its more favorable toxicity profile. Significant drug–drug interactions exist between azole antifungals and many other medications, including immunosuppressant drugs. Loading doses of azole antifungals may be recommended in certain circumstances. Because treatment may be prolonged (weeks to months), it is recommended to check therapeutic levels of several antifungals to minimize toxicity. Levels may be checked for flucytosine, itraconazole, posaconazole, and voriconazole but not for isavuconazole or fluconazole.
- For details on treatment of fungal pathogens, *Nocardia*, and *Actinomyces*, see Table 14-13.

TABLE 14-13 Treatment of Fungal Infections, *Nocardia*, and *Actinomyces*

Pathogen and Therapy	Additional Comments
***Candida* spp.** *Mucosal* • Thrush: Clotrimazole troche, nystatin suspension or Fluc 100 mg qday × 7–14 d • Esophageal: Fluc 200 mg qday × 14–21 d • Vaginal: Topical azole × 3–7 d or Fluc 150 mg PO once • Frequent recurrence: Fluc 150 mg/wk × 6 mo *Invasive Candiasis* • Empirical treatment: Echinocandin • Targeted: based on species and susceptibilities • Average duration: 14 d	• *Prophylaxis*: May be beneficial in select patients with solid organ transplant, chemotherapy-induced neutropenia, or stem cell transplants. • *Candidemia*: Treat from first negative blood culture. Perform ophthalmologic examination to rule out endophthalmitis. Central lines must be removed. • *Complicated infection*: Duration may be extended if metastatic foci present or continued neutropenia.
Cryptococcus neoformans *Nonmeningeal, local, or mild–moderate disease* • Fluc 400 mg PO/IV qday × 6–12 mo *Meningeal, disseminated, or moderately severe–severe disease* • Induction phase: Amb + 5-FC × 2 wk • Consolidation phase: Fluc 800 mg PO qday × 8 wk • Maintenance phase: Fluc 200 mg qday × 6–12 mo	• Perform LP to rule out meningitis. • HIV: Initiate ART 2–10 wk after starting Tx. Continue Fluc 200 mg PO qday for at least 12 mo and until CD4 count ≥100 for 6 mo. • Check baseline CSF opening pressure. If ≥25 cm of CSF, reduce by 50% (up to 30 mL). Perform daily serial LPs if pressure elevated (≥25 cm H_2O)

(Continued)

TABLE 14-13 Treatment of Fungal Infections, *Nocardia*, and *Actinomyces* (Continued)

Histoplasma capsulatum *Pulmonary* • Acute, mild–moderate: Observation. May Tx if symptoms >1 mo • Acute, moderately severe to severe: Amb for 1–2 wk or until clinically improved, then Itra for 12 wk • Chronic cavitary: Itra for 12–24 mo *Progressive disseminated histoplasmosis (PDH)* • Mild–moderate: Itra for 12 mo • Moderately severe to severe: Amb for 1–2 wk (4–6 wk if CNS involvement) or until clinically improved, then Itra for 12 mo *Mediastinal fibrosis* • Antifungal treatment is not recommended	• Steroids may be considered for respiratory distress, hypoxemia, or severe mediastinal lymphadenitis. • HIV: Itra 200 mg PO qday ppx in areas of high endemicity if CD4 count <150. • PDH: Check urine antigen levels during/after Tx to monitor for relapse. • TDM for itraconazole is recommended.
Blastomyces dermatitidis *Pulmonary or Disseminated Extrapulmonary* • Mild to moderate: Itra for 6–12 mo • Moderately severe to severe: Amb for 1–2 wk or until clinically improved, then Itra for 6–12 mo • Immunosuppressed: Treat as severe disease for 12 mo *CNS:* Amb for 4–6 wk then Fluc 800 mg PO qday for 12 mo *Suppression:* Itra lifelong if continued immunosuppression	• For CNS disease, Itra or Vori can be used instead of Fluc.

(Continued)

TABLE 14-13 Treatment of Fungal Infections, *Nocardia*, and *Actinomyces* (Continued)

Pathogen and Therapy	Additional Comments
Coccidioides immitis *Pulmonary* • Uncomplicated pneumonia, asymptomatic pulmonary nodule: May not need Tx. If Tx, Fluc 400 mg PO qday for 6–12 wk • Diffuse pneumonia: Amb for 1–2 wk or until clinically improved, then Fluc 400–800 mg PO qday for 12–24 wk, can extend up to 12 mo *Disseminated/Extrapulmonary* • Nonmeningeal: Fluc 800–1200 mg IV/PO qday • Meningeal: Fluc 800–1200 mg IV/PO qday—if not improving, consider intrathecal Amb; followed by Fluc lifelong	• Can follow serum CF titres during/after treatment. Rising titres suggest recurrence. • Consider surgery if pulmonary cavitary disease >2 yr or rupture. • HIV: Continue Tx until CD4 count ≥250. • After meningeal disease improves, lifelong Fluc. • Hydrocephalus may require shunt for decompression.
• ***Talaromycosis*** • Mild: Itra for 12 wk • Moderately severe to severe: Amb for 2 wk (induction) or until clinically improved, then Itra for 10 wk (consolidation)	• Maintenance with Itra or Vori in HIV until viral suppression and CD4 count >100
Sporothrix *Lymphocutaneous/Cutaneous: Itra × 3–6 mo* *Severe Systemic* • Pulmonary/disseminated/osteoarticular: Amb for 1–2 wk or until clinically improved, then Itra for 12 mo • Meningeal: Amb for 4–6 wk then Itra for 12 mo	• If no initial response, can use higher doses of Itra or add topical saturated solution of potassium iodide.

(Continued)

TABLE 14-13 Treatment of Fungal Infections, *Nocardia*, and *Actinomyces* (Continued)

Aspergillus *Pulmonary aspergilloma:* Surgical resection or arterial embolization in cases of severe hemoptysis *Invasive pulmonary aspergillosis:* Vori for at least 6–12 wk until lesions and immunosuppression resolve *Invasive sinonasal aspergillosis:* Amb or Vori. Surgical debridement is adjunctive and often required for cure *Allergic bronchopulmonary aspergillosis:* Itra or intermittent steroids may decrease exacerbations. *Prophylaxis:* Posa in high-risk patients may be considered	• Amb to cover mucormycosis as initial therapy for sinus disease pending confirmation of diagnosis. • If immunosuppression recurs, may need to restart ppx or Tx.
Mucormycosis *Cutaneous, Rhinocerebral:* Aggressive surgical resection and debridement with clean margins followed + Amb at upper dose range until improvement *Pulmonary:* Amb	• Mortality is very high in immunosuppressed patients with disseminated disease. • Posa and Isa are alternative Tx, after initial induction therapy with Amb.
Nocardia *Cutaneous:* TMP-SMX *Severe Infection (including CNS):* Induction regimen typically includes two or three drugs including TMP-SMX, imipenem or linezolid for 4–6 wk with stepdown to oral therapy for 6–12 mo *Suppression/prophylaxis:* TMP-SMX	• TMP-SMX is drug of choice but typically combined with other agents in disseminated disease. • Use susceptibility results to guide treatment.
Actinomyces Penicillin G 18–24 million units IV per day × 4–6 wk then penicillin V 1 g PO tid × 6–12 mo	• Surgery or drainage may be helpful in some cases. • Clindamycin or doxycycline can be used if penicillin allergy.

5-FC, flucytosine; Amb, amphotericin B; ART, antiretroviral therapy; CF, complement fixation; CNS, central nervous system; CSF, cerebrospinal fluid; Fluc, fluconazole; Isa, Isavuconazole; Itra, Itraconazole; LP, lumbar puncture; Posa, posaconazole; ppx, prophylaxis; TDM, therapeutic drug monitoring; TMP-SMX, trimethoprim-sulfamethoxazole; Tx, treatment; Vori, voriconazole.

Candidiasis

GENERAL PRINCIPLES

- *Candida* species are the most common cause of invasive fungal infections in humans.
- Infections ranging from uncomplicated mucosal disease to life-threatening invasive disease affecting any organ can occur. Infections are often associated with concurrent antibiotic use, contraceptive use, immunosuppressant and cytotoxic therapy, and indwelling foreign bodies. Mucocutaneous disease may resolve after elimination of the causative condition (e.g., antibiotic therapy) or may persist and progress in the setting of immunosuppressive conditions (AIDS).
- *Candida* species are the most commonly recovered yeast in the Asian countries, with non–*Candida albicans* species constituting 50%–80% of all isolates. The epidemiology of candidemia varies among countries in the region.
- Candidemia is the most common form of invasive candidiasis, the incidence of which varies from 1 to 12/1000 admissions in India.
- Serious complications of candidemia include skin lesions, ocular disease, endocarditis, and osteomyelitis.[51]

DIAGNOSIS

- Diagnosis of **mucocutaneous candidiasis** is usually based on clinical findings but can be confirmed by a potassium hydroxide preparation of exudates.
- Cultures can be obtained in refractory cases to exclude the presence of non–*C. albicans* species. **Invasive candidiasis** is diagnosed by positive cultures of blood or tissue.

TREATMENT

See Table 14-13.

Cryptococcosis

GENERAL PRINCIPLES

- *Cryptococcus neoformans* is a ubiquitous yeast associated with soil and pigeon excrement.
- Disease is principally meningeal (headache and mental status changes) and pulmonary (ranging from asymptomatic nodular disease to fulminant respiratory failure). Disseminated disease can involve any organ with predilection for the CNS, lungs, skin (umbilicated lesions mimicking molluscum), bone, and prostate.[52]
- Infection typically affects patients with impaired cellular immunity and carries high morbidity and mortality.

DIAGNOSIS

- Diagnosis via culture and histology tissue evaluation with the use of specific fungal stains are considered the gold standard.
- CrAg testing by latex agglutination or lateral flow assay is highly sensitive and specific in both serum and CSF.[53]
- Distinguishing between disseminated disease and localized pulmonary and asymptomatic disease is fundamental to guide therapy. Any patient with CNS disease, positive blood cultures, or elevated serum CrAg and those with severe pulmonary disease should be

considered to have disseminated disease. Disseminated disease warrants a lumbar puncture to exclude coexistent CNS involvement. HIV infection must be ruled out in cases of cryptococcosis. Always measure opening pressure, as elevated opening pressure (≥25 cm H_2O) has poor prognostic implications and must be managed with decompression, usually with serial lumbar punctures or a lumbar drain.[54]

TREATMENT

Treatment is dependent on the patient's immune function and site of infection (see Table 14-13). **Management of elevated intracranial pressure is critical.** An infectious disease consultation is recommended and has been associated with decreased 90-day mortality.[55]

Endemic Mycoses

Endemic mycoses identified in the Asian continent are histoplasmosis, talaromycosis (penicilliosis), and sporotrichosis. Blastomycosis has been infrequently reported from the Asia-Pacific region. Unlike Latin American countries, autochthonous (i.e., indigenous) coccidioidomycosis and paracoccidioidomycosis are not reported in the Asia-Pacific region, except as imported mycoses.[56]

GENERAL PRINCIPLES OF ENDEMIC MYCOSES

- Endemic mycoses are a group of diseases caused by diverse fungi that share common characteristics:
  - These fungi occupy a specific etiologic niche in the environment.
  - They are dimorphic in nature (yeast or spherule form in the tissue and mycelial form in the environment).
  - Endemic fungi can produce infection and disease in healthy hosts.
- The most common endemic mycoses in the Asia region are histoplasmosis, caused by *Histoplasma capsulatum*; talaromycosis (penicilliosis), caused by *Penicillium marneffei*; and sporotrichosis, caused by *Sporothrix schenckii*.

HISTOPLASMOSIS

- *H. capsulatum var. capsulatum* is a dimorphic fungus (yeast in tissues; mold in the environment) that grows in soil contaminated by bat or bird droppings.[57]
- *Histoplasmosis* has classically been associated with highest areas of endemicity along the Ohio and Mississippi River Valleys and Latin America. In Asia, it is increasingly being reported from India (Ganges belt in particular), China, Malaysia, and other Southeast Asian countries.

DIAGNOSIS

- Clinical manifestations are extremely varied, including acute flu-like symptoms, chronic granulomatous pulmonary disease, disseminated infection or fulminant multiorgan failure in immunocompromised patients (AIDS).
- Histoplasmosis may mimic tuberculosis and should be considered a close differential of the same in endemic areas.
- Despite adrenal enlargement which may be associated in individuals with histoplasmosis, these cases infrequently report clinical adrenal failure.

- Histoplasmosis may be associated with oral ulcers or mucocutaneous lesions, which may facilitate early diagnosis on biopsy.
- Diagnosis is based on culture or histopathology, antigen assay (urine, blood, or CSF), or antibody detection assays using a complement fixation (CF) test; with titres of 1:8 seen in most patients and titres ≥1:32 highly suggestive of active infection. The urine antigen assay is the most sensitive test for detecting acute and disseminated disease and is helpful in following response to therapy. Antibody assays are useful in subacute and chronic disease; antigen assays are less sensitive.

TREATMENT

See Table 14-13.

TALAROMYCOSIS (PENICILLIOSIS)

- Talaromycosis (penicilliosis) is an endemic disease found only in Southeast and Eastern Asia, including Thailand, Northeast India, China, Hong Kong, Laos, Cambodia, Malaysia, Myanmar, Vietnam, and Taiwan.
- Some studies have established bamboo rats as enzootic reservoirs for this fungus.
- HIV patients in endemic region may present with disseminated infection.

DIAGNOSIS

- Clinical manifestations are extremely varied, including mild to severe disease. Talaromycosis may present with fever, weight loss, cough, anemia, lymphadenopathy, and hepatosplenomegaly.
- Cutaneous lesions related to penicilliosis frequently occur on the face, upper trunk, and extremities, and may consist of necrotic or generalized papules or nodules and may have central umbilication.
- Talaromycosis may mimic tuberculosis and should be considered a close differential of the same in endemic areas.
- Diagnosis is based on culture or histopathology.

TREATMENT

See Table 14-13.

Sporotrichosis

GENERAL PRINCIPLES

S. schenckii is a globally endemic fungus that causes disease following traumatic inoculation with soil or plant material; most cases are occupational. Infection can also be associated with spread from infected cats or other digging animals.

DIAGNOSIS

Clinical Presentation

Lymphocutaneous disease is the usual manifestation with localization to skin and soft tissues. Pulmonary and disseminated forms of the infection are rarely seen from inhalation of the fungus.

Diagnostic Testing

Diagnosis requires culture or histopathological demonstration of yeast in tissue or body fluids.[56]

TREATMENT

See Table 14-13.

Blastomycosis

GENERAL PRINCIPLES

- *Blastomyces dermatitidis* is dimorphic fungus that is endemic to the Ohio and Mississippi River valleys, as well as the upper midwestern, south central, and southeastern United States.
- It is not clear whether blastomycosis is endemic in the Asia-Pacific region because very few autochthonous cases have been reported; these cases were isolated cases mostly from India where the fungus was isolated from pulmonary, cutaneous, and cerebral lesions.
- The organism commonly disseminates, affecting the lungs, skin, bone, brain, and genitourinary tract. Aggressive pulmonary and CNS disease can occur in both immunocompromised and immunocompetent patients.

DIAGNOSIS

Diagnosis is based on culture, histopathology, or antigen assay. Serologic studies cross-react with tests for *Histoplasma* and *Cryptococcus* species and are unreliable for diagnosis but can be used to assess early response to therapy when positive.

TREATMENT

See Table 14-13.

Aspergillosis

GENERAL PRINCIPLES

- *Aspergillus* species are ubiquitous environmental fungi that cause a broad spectrum of disease, usually affecting the respiratory system and sinuses.
- Invasive aspergillosis (IA) remains, overall, the most frequently reported mold infection in immunocompromised individuals within the Asia-Pacific region. It has also been reported in immunocompetent persons.
- IA is a serious condition associated with vascular invasion, thrombosis, and ischemic infarction of involved tissues and progressive disease after hematogenous dissemination. IA is usually seen in severely immunocompromised patients, especially allogeneic hematopoietic stem cell transplant recipients (HSCT).
- **Pulmonary aspergillomas** arise in the setting of preexisting bullous lung disease and are easily recognized by characteristic radiographic presentation and *Aspergillus* serology.
- **Allergic bronchopulmonary aspergillosis** is a chronic relapsing and remitting respiratory syndrome associated with *Aspergillus* colonization.

DIAGNOSIS

- Diagnosis can be very difficult given the varied manifestations of IA, and a high index of suspicion should be applied to patients with prolonged severe immunosuppression.
- Radiographic findings can be highly suggestive of pulmonary IA, particularly the halo-crescent sign on CT.
- Histopathology/cytology and culture examination of tissue and fluid specimens is recommended.
- Serum and bronchoalveolar lavage (BAL) galactomannan assay are accurate markers for the diagnosis of IA and can be followed prospectively in at-risk patients (e.g., hematologic malignancy, HSCT).[57]

TREATMENT

See Table 14-13.

Mucormycosis

GENERAL PRINCIPLES

- Zygomycetes are a class of ubiquitous environmental fungi found in decaying organic substrates. They have been reclassified into two orders, Mucorales and Entomophthorales.
- Mucorales contains the genera most commonly involved in human disease. These include *Mucor* spp., *Rhizopus* spp., and *Cunninghamella* spp. Disease manifestations vary depending on the affected organ, but the main clinical presentations include sinus (rhino-orbital or rhinocerebral), pulmonary, cutaneous, gastrointestinal, and disseminated infections. Angioinvasion and multiorgan infarction are rapidly progressive.
- In India, a rapid increase in the number of mucormycosis cases has recently been noted, especially associated with uncontrolled diabetes. Other risk factors include immunosuppression, iron overload, high-dose glucocorticoid therapy, and penetrating trauma.

DIAGNOSIS

- Clinical manifestations vary depending on which organ is affected. Invasive mucormycosis is devastating with rapid development of tissue necrosis from vascular invasion and thrombosis.
- Early identification and urgent measures are required.
- Sinus endoscopy should be performed if there is concern for invasive fungal sinusitis.
- Diagnosis requires tissue culture and silver stain with care to avoid disrupting fungal architecture.
- Head CT or MRI is helpful in head and neck disease to identify the involved structures.

TREATMENT

Urgent care and aggressive measures must be taken. Early debridement followed by medical management is the treatment approach of choice. Timely surgery can be lifesaving and should be sought as early as possible.

See Table 14-13.

Nocardiosis

GENERAL PRINCIPLES

- *Nocardia* is a ubiquitous group of aerobic gram-positive branching filamentous bacteria that causes severe local and disseminated disease in the setting of impaired cell-mediated immunity.[58]
- Typical infection tends to be pulmonary infiltrate, abscess, or empyema, but dissemination is common and tends to favor CNS infection, causing abscess.

DIAGNOSIS

- Clinical presentation can be acute, subacute, or chronic pneumonia.
- Chest imaging can reveal a variety of findings such as infiltrates, nodules, pleural effusions, or cavities.[59]
- Diagnosis requires sputum or tissue Gram stain and culture (including AFB), often needing multiple samples because yields are low.
- Brain MRI is recommended to evaluate for concurrent CNS infection in patients with pulmonary disease.

TREATMENT

See Table 14-13.

Actinomycosis

GENERAL PRINCIPLES

Actinomyces is a microaerophilic gram-positive bacillus that usually causes soft-tissue swelling of the oropharynx, face, or neck, typically over or underneath the mandible (orocervicofacial actinomycosis). Pulmonary and gastrointestinal disease can also be seen. Classic infections are chronic, indurated soft tissue lesions associated with draining fistulae that pass through tissue planes. Unlike *Nocardia*, infection is not limited to immunocompromised hosts.

DIAGNOSIS

Clinical presentation varies depending on what site is affected. Orocervicofacial infection is the most common form. Rare sites include the CNS and bones. Diagnosis is made by histopathology (Gram-positive branching bacilli) or observation of "sulfur granules" in drainage.[60]

TREATMENT

See Table 14-13.

Nontuberculous Mycobacteria

- NTM are ubiquitous environmental organisms that cause a spectrum of disease primarily involving the lungs (80%), skin and soft tissues, lymph nodes, and disseminated disease. Susceptibility testing and an infectious disease consultation are recommended to guide treatment. Different species are commonly associated with specific clinical presentations:

- **Pulmonary infection:** *Mycobacterium avium complex* (isolated in 85% of the cases), *M. kansasii*, and *M. abscessus* are the most common pathogens involved.
- **Skin, soft tissues, and bone infection:** *M. fortuitum*, *M. chelonae*, *M. scrofulaceum*, *M. marinum* ("fish tank granuloma"), and *M. ulcerans* (Buruli ulcer).
- **Lymphadenitis:** *M. avium complex* and *M. scrofulaceum*.
- **Disseminated:** *M. avium, M. kansasii, M. abscessus, M. chelonae,* and *M. haemophilum* (see Chapter 16, Sexually Transmitted Infections, Human Immunodeficiency Virus, and Acquired Immunodeficiency Syndrome).[61]

- ***Mycobacterium leprae*** has been covered under Leprosy.

TICK-BORNE INFECTIONS

- Tick-borne infections are common in many parts of Asia; prevalence of specific diseases depends on the local population of vector ticks and animal reservoirs.
- Risk should be assessed by outdoor activity in endemic regions and careful clinical examination which may reveal a clue such as an eschar in scrub typhus.

Lyme Disease

GENERAL PRINCIPLES

- Lyme borreliosis is a systemic illness of variable severity caused by the spirochete species *Borrelia burgdorferi*. It is one of the most common vector-borne diseases in the United States and Europe. It is increasingly being reported from Asia including China, India, and other Asian countries.

DIAGNOSIS

Clinical Presentation

Lyme disease has three distinct clinical stages, following an incubation period of 7–10 days:

- Stage 1 (early localized disease) is characterized by mild constitutional symptoms (fatigue, malaise, lethargy, mild headache, mild neck stiffness, myalgias, arthralgias, regional lymphadenopathy) and erythema *migrans*, a slowly expanding macular rash >5 cm in diameter, classically with central clearing (often not seen).
- Stage 2 (early disseminated disease) occurs within several weeks to months and includes multiple erythema *migrans* lesions, neurologic symptoms (e.g., seventh cranial nerve palsy, meningoencephalitis), cardiac symptoms (atrioventricular block, myopericarditis), lymphadenopathy, eye involvement, and asymmetric oligoarticular arthritis, most commonly affecting the knee.
- Stage 3 (late disease) occurs after months to years and includes chronic dermatitis, neurologic disease, and asymmetric monoarticular or oligoarticular arthritis. Chronic fatigue is not seen more frequently in patients with Lyme borreliosis than in control subjects.

Diagnostic Testing

Diagnosis rests on clinical suspicion in the appropriate setting but can be supported by two-tiered serologic testing (screening enzyme-linked immunosorbent assay followed by Western blot) with acute and convalescent serologies. In the acute phase of the illness, sensitivity of the serological testing is below 50%.[62]

TREATMENT

- Treatment depends on stage and severity of disease. Oral therapy (doxycycline 100 mg PO q12h, amoxicillin 500 mg PO q8h, or cefuroxime axetil 500 mg PO q12h for 10–21 days) is used for early localized or disseminated disease without neurologic or cardiac involvement. The same agents, given for 28 days, are recommended for late Lyme disease. Doxycycline has the added benefit of covering potential coinfection with ehrlichiosis. In the setting of true β-lactam allergy and if doxycycline cannot be given, macrolides are an alternative with a lower cure rate (~80%).
- Parenteral therapy (e.g., ceftriaxone 2 g IV qday, cefotaxime 2 g IV q8h, penicillin G 3–4 million units IV q4h) for 14–28 days is preferred for severe neurologic or cardiac disease, regardless of stage, although there are data to suggest that oral doxycycline is effective in this setting as well.[63]

Rocky Mountain Spotted Fever

GENERAL PRINCIPLES

RMSF is an acute febrile illness caused by *Rickettsia rickettsia* and transmitted by a variety of ticks, most commonly *Dermacentor variabilis* (dog tick). RMSF occurs throughout the United States, Canada, Mexico, Central America, and in parts of South America (Bolivia, Argentina, Brazil, and Colombia). It mostly occurs in spring and early summer when outdoor activity is frequent.[64]

CLINICAL PRESENTATION

The classic triad of fever, headache, and rash is often not present in the early phases of the disease. The typical petechial rash with centripetal distribution (starting on the distal extremities and extending to the trunk) will be present in <50% of patients in the first 3 days of illness, but it will develop in >90% between the third and fifth days of illness. A presumptive diagnosis based on the clinical syndrome and warrants immediate treatment.

DIAGNOSIS

Acute and convalescent serologies support the diagnosis, but early treatment may abolish the appearance of antibodies in the convalescent phase. PCR or immunostaining of tissue samples, such as skin biopsies, are highly specific.

TREATMENT

Antibiotic treatment of choice is doxycycline 100 mg IV/PO q12h for 7 days or continued for 3 days after the patient defervesce. Chloramphenicol is an alternative.

OUTCOME/PROGNOSIS

If treatment is delayed, RMSF is the most likely tick-borne illness to result in death or serious sequelae.[65]

Ehrlichiosis and Anaplasmosis

GENERAL PRINCIPLES

Ehrlichiosis and anaplasmosis are systemic tick-borne infections caused by obligate intracellular bacteria of the *Anaplasmataceae* family. Two similar syndromes are recognized:

- **Human monocytic ehrlichiosis** (HME) caused by *Ehrlichia chaffeensis* and transmitted by the lone star tick, is endemic to the southern and south-central United States.
- **Human granulocytic anaplasmosis** (HGA), caused by *Anaplasma phagocytophilum*, is found in the same regions as Lyme disease and shares the same tick vector (*Ixodes* spp.).

DIAGNOSIS

Clinical Presentation

Illness ranges from mild disease to septic shock. Clinical onset of illness usually occurs 1–2 weeks after tick bite with fever, headache, myalgias, and arthralgias. Rash is uncommon in adults. Leukopenia, thrombocytopenia, and elevated liver transaminases are important clues to the diagnosis. Severe disease can result in respiratory failure, renal insufficiency, and meningoencephalitis. CNS involvement is uncommon in HGA.

Diagnostic Testing

- Identification of morulae (intracytoplasmic inclusions) in circulating monocytes (HME) or granulocytes (HGA) on a blood smear are uncommonly seen but diagnostic.
- Acute and convalescent serologies obtained 3–6 weeks apart remain the diagnostic gold standard, but cross-reactivity among *Ehrlichial spp.* and reduced antibody response due to early treatment are common.
- PCR of the blood has high specificity (60%–85%) and sensitivity (60%–90%).

TREATMENT

Treatment should be started promptly based on clinical suspicion. Doxycycline 100 mg PO/IV q12h for 10–14 days (up to 3–5 days after defervescence, whichever is longer) is the drug of choice.[66] Rifampicin 300 mg PO q12h for 7–10 days is an option for patients with contraindications to doxycycline therapy.[67] Lack of defervescence after 72 hours of treatment suggests an alternative diagnosis.

Tularemia

GENERAL PRINCIPLES

- Tularemia is a zoonosis caused by the gram-negative bacteria *Francisella tularensis* and is endemic to south central United States. It is associated with exposure to infected animals (particularly rabbits) and transmitted via tick bite or aerosolized droplets.
- *F. tularensis* is one of the most infectious pathogens known, with as few as 10 organisms necessary to cause disease. Owing to its extreme infectivity, ease of dissemination, and capacity to cause illness with subsequent death, tularemia is considered a potential bioterrorism agent.

DIAGNOSIS

Clinical Presentation

Fever and malaise occur 2–5 days after exposure. Six clinical presentations are recognized, depending on the route of transmission: ulceroglandular (painful regional lymphadenitis with a skin ulcer), glandular (focal or regional lymphadenopathy alone), oculoglandular, and pharyngeal (conjunctival and oral mucosae involved), typhoidal (systemic disease with high fever and hepatosplenomegaly), and pneumonia. Systemic and pneumonic diseases have high mortality if not treated promptly.[68]

Diagnostic Testing

- Clinical suspicion in appropriate setting is required to make the diagnosis.
- Culture isolation in blood, sputum, or pleural fluid lacks sensitivity. Before sending specimens, the microbiology laboratory must be notified given the high infectivity of *F. tularensis* (biosafety level 3 facilities are required).
- Acute and convalescent serologic studies provide a retrospective diagnosis.

TREATMENT

Aminoglycosides are the treatment of choice. Streptomycin 1 g IM q12h or Gentamicin 5 mg/kg IV divided q8h for 10 days are preferred. Doxycycline 100 mg IV/PO q12h for 14–21 days is an alternative but is more likely to result in relapse. Ciprofloxacin 500–750 mg PO q12h for 14–21 days is also an alternative.[69]

Babesiosis

GENERAL PRINCIPLES

- Babesiosis is a malaria-like illness that is caused by the intraerythrocytic parasite *Babesia microti*, a tick-borne protozoan.
- Coinfection with Lyme disease can occur because both are transmitted by the same tick vector (*Ixodes* spp.).
- Although endemic to northwestern United States, cases have been reported in Europe and Asia as well.[70]

DIAGNOSIS

- Clinical disease ranges from subclinical to severe, with fever, chills, myalgias, and headache. Severity depends on infecting species and host immunity. Complications of severe disease include renal failure, respiratory distress, and multiorgan dysfunction.
- Hemolytic anemia, elevated lactate dehydrogenase (LDH), transaminitis, and thrombocytopenia are typical laboratory findings.
- Diagnosis is made by visualization of the parasite in erythrocytes on thin blood smears.
- Blood PCR is the most sensitive test.

TREATMENT

- For mild disease, atovaquone 750 mg PO q12h for 7–10 days plus azithromycin 500 mg PO on day 1, then 250 mg qday for 7–10 days, is the treatment of choice.

- Severe disease (organ dysfunction, parasitemia >5% or immunosuppressed) should be treated with atovaquone and IV azithromycin (500 mg daily) until symptoms abate; then transfer to all oral regimen as for mild disease. Alternative regimen includes clindamycin 600 mg IV q8h plus quinine 650 mg PO q8h for 7–10 days. Exchange transfusion may also be needed.
- Longer durations of therapy may be necessary in patients with persistent symptoms or until parasitemia has cleared.[71]

Heartland and Bourbon Virus

GENERAL PRINCIPLES

Bourbon and Heartland virus are rare systemic emerging tick-borne infections recently identified in the Midwest and southern United States.

CLINICAL PRESENTATION

- *Heartland virus disease:* Fever, malaise, headache, **confusion, leukopenia, and thrombocytopenia.**[72]
- *Bourbon fever:* Fever, malaise, headache, **nausea, vomiting, diarrhea, and maculopapular rash.** Bone marrow suppression and acute respiratory distress syndrome reflect severe disease.[73]

DIAGNOSIS

Protocols exist facilitating testing through state health departments and the CDC in the USA.

TREATMENT

No specific treatments for Bourbon or Heartland virus infection exist. Treatment is supportive.

MOSQUITO-BORNE INFECTIONS

Arboviruses

GENERAL PRINCIPLES

- Arboviruses are arthropod-borne viruses; their major vectors are mosquitoes and ticks. Vector control is important for disease control.
- Worldwide, the most prevalent arboviral diseases per year are dengue fever (DENV; 96 million cases), chikungunya virus (CHIKV; 693,000 cases), Zika virus (ZIKV; 500,000 cases), yellow fever (130,000 cases), Japanese encephalitis (42,500 cases), and West Nile virus (2,588 cases).[74]
- Other emergent or reemergent arboviral diseases are Eastern equine encephalitis, St. Louis encephalitis, La Crosse encephalitis, Rift Valley fever, Spondweni, Mayaro, Usutu, O'nyong-nyong, and Sindbis.[75]
- Infections usually occur in the summer months, and most are subclinical. Encephalitis is the most common clinical syndrome.

West Nile Virus

West Nile virus (WNV) is an arbovirus with a potential of neuroinvasion. It is transmitted by *Culex* mosquitoes. Infections peak in late summer and early fall. It is distributed throughout Africa, the Middle East, parts of Europe, South Asia, and Australia.

CLINICAL PRESENTATION

- Most infections are asymptomatic. Symptomatic cases of WNV infection range from a mild febrile illness with or without a maculopapular rash to aseptic meningitis, fulminant encephalitis, or a poliomyelitis-like presentation with flaccid paralysis. Extrapyramidal symptoms are common. Long-term neurologic sequelae are common with severe disease (fatigue, memory impairment, weakness, headache, gait abnormalities).
- Risk factors for neuroinvasive disease include age >60 years, malignancy, organ transplantation, and genetic factors.

DIAGNOSTIC TESTING

Diagnosis is usually clinical or by acute and convalescent serologic studies. Specific IgM antibody detection in CSF is diagnostic for acute WN virus infection.

TREATMENT

- Treatment is supportive care as for other arboviral encephalitides.[76]
- Patients who develop neuroinvasive disease may have serious adverse outcomes.
- Personal protective measures include the use of mosquito repellents. Mosquito control programs involve eliminating breeding sites.

Chikungunya

GENERAL PRINCIPLES

Chikungunya virus is an arthropod-borne alphavirus that is transmitted to humans by the bite of an infected *Aedes* mosquito. The virus has disseminated from its origins in West Africa and has now surfaced in regions across Asia, Europe, the Americas, as well as islands scattered throughout the Indian and Pacific Oceans.

Clinical Presentation

Illness begins after an incubation period of 3–7 days. Fever and malaise are the earliest symptoms progressing to polyarthralgia 2–5 days after the onset of fever. Multiple distal joints are involved (symmetric), with pain that can be disabling. Maculopapular rash may appear. Acute illness lasts 7–10 days. Severe complications like meningoencephalitis, cardiopulmonary decompensation, acute renal failure, and death are more frequent in those with comorbidities and in patients older than 65 years.[77] Following acute illness, some patients may experience chronic or relapsing joint pain for several months.

Diagnostic Testing

Serology is the primary tool for diagnosis. PCR has high sensitivity and specificity within the first 5 days of symptoms.

TREATMENT

- Supportive care with rest and anti-inflammatory agents.[78]
- Patients with chronic arthritis may require corticosteroids or DMARDs if symptoms are severe and refractory to NSAIDs.
- Preventing exposure to mosquitoes is the mainstay of prevention.

Dengue

- Dengue viruses (DENVs) are members of the family Flaviviridae and consist of 4 antigenically related but distinct viruses. They are transmitted by *Aedes* mosquitoes. Infection with these viruses causes Dengue fever, which is endemic in Asia, the Pacific, Africa, South and Central America, and the Caribbean.[79]

DIAGNOSIS

Clinical Presentation

Fever, headache, myalgia, bone pain, rash, leukopenia, and thrombocytopenia are the predominant symptoms. Increased vascular permeability and plasma leakage lead to dengue hemorrhagic fever characterized by bleeding manifestations. Hypotension and circulatory collapse occur in dengue shock syndrome.

Signs of impending critical illness called "warning signs" include persistent vomiting, severe abdominal pain, tender hepatomegaly, pleural effusion, ascites, mucosal bleeding, and lethargy or restlessness. Physical examination may reveal narrowed pulse pressure followed by hypotension and shock. Laboratory findings may include a high or increasing hematocrit (≥20% from baseline), a rapid decrease in platelets, increased activated partial-thromboplastin time, and decreased fibrinogen levels.

The three clinical phases of dengue are febrile phase, critical phase, and recovery phase. The critical phase is not seen in all infections.

1. **Febrile phase:** Usually lasts 3–7 days. Symptoms include fever (>38.5°C), headache, retro-orbital pain, and marked myalgia and arthralgia. A transient macular rash may develop 2–5 days after onset of fever. A tourniquet test reveals petechiae. Leukopenia, thrombocytopenia, and elevated transaminases are noted.
2. **Critical phase:** At defervescence, a small proportion of patients (usually children and young adults) develop plasma leakage, bleeding, shock, and organ impairment or failure, which usually lasts 24–48 hours (about 2 days). The extent of plasma leakage varies, and mild plasma leakage is not always associated with shock or organ failure.
3. **Recovery phase:** During the recovery phase, plasma leakage and hemorrhage resolve, vital signs stabilize, and accumulated fluids are resorbed. A pruritic confluent, erythematous eruption with small islands of unaffected skin may appear. The recovery phase typically lasts two to four days, but adults may have profound fatigue for days to weeks after recovery.[80]

Diagnostic Testing

A provisional diagnosis is based on clinical manifestations. Virus can be detected by PCR during the first 5 days, and by acute and convalescent serology later in the course of illness. Testing for NS1 antigen in the initial days of illness and IgM antibodies after days 5–7 is suggested.

Expanded dengue syndrome was coined by WHO in the year 2012 to describe cases which do not fall into either dengue shock syndrome (DSS) or dengue hemorrhagic fever (DHF).

The atypical manifestations noted in expanded dengue are multisystemic and multifaceted with organ involvement, such as liver, brain, heart, kidney, and CNS. Patients with involvement of gastrointestinal and hepatic system may present with features of asymptomatic elevation of liver enzymes, fulminant hepatic failure, acute pancreatitis, acalculous cholecystitis, peritonitis, subacute intestinal obstruction, or rupture of spleen.

WHO Grading for Severity of DHF	
DHF Grade I	Fever and hemorrhagic manifestation (positive tourniquet test) and evidence of plasma leakage
DHF Grade II	Grade I plus spontaneous bleeding
DHF Grade III	DHF Grade III refers to Grade I or Grade II plus circulatory failure
DHF Grade IV	Grade III plus profound shock with undetectable blood pressure and pulse

DSS consists of DHF Grade III and DHF Grade IV. Shock refers to normal systolic pressure but rising diastolic pressure with narrowing pulse pressure.

TREATMENT

Maintenance of adequate intravascular volume is critical. There is no antiviral treatment; avoid aspirin and NSAIDs (Figure 14-9).[81]

Zika Virus

- Zika virus is an arthropod-borne flavivirus transmitted to humans by the bite of an infected Aedes mosquito. It is related to other flaviviruses, including dengue virus, yellow fever virus, and West Nile virus.
- Since 2007, large outbreaks of Zika infection have occurred in the Pacific Islands, Central/South America, Mexico, Africa, and Asia.
- In addition to the *Aedes* mosquito, Zika is also transmitted vertically from a pregnant woman to her fetus, sexually and by blood transfusion.

DIAGNOSIS

Clinical Presentation

Incubation period is 2–14 days. Most infections are asymptomatic. Fever, maculopapular rash, conjunctivitis, arthralgias (small joints and feet), and headache are common. Complications include neurologic disease (including Guillain–Barre syndrome) and microcephaly and fetal loss in pregnant women (congenital Zika infection).

Diagnostic Testing

PCR testing for acute infection, and Zika virus serology.

TREATMENT

Treatment is symptomatic. Preventive measures include personal protective measures to prevent mosquito bites and institution of measures to eliminate and control mosquito breeding sites. Pregnant women should avoid travel to Zika-infected areas.

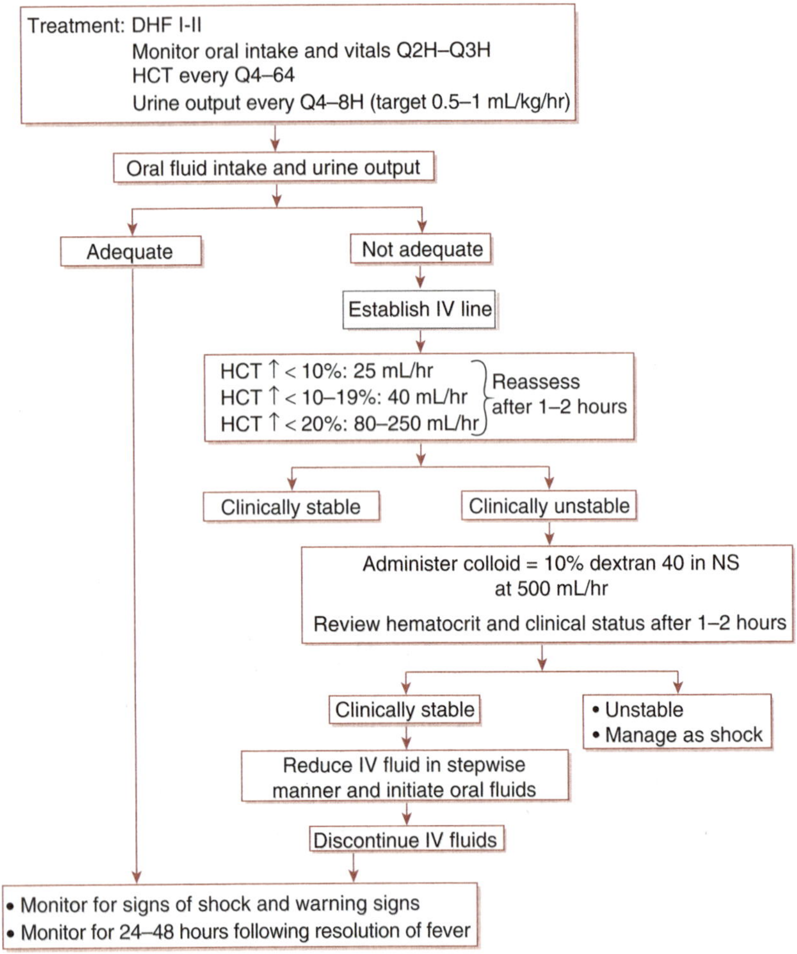

Figure 14-9 (*Continued*)

Malaria

GENERAL PRINCIPLES

- Malaria is a systemic parasitic disease that is endemic to most of the tropical and subtropical world. In 2023, the World Health Organization (WHO) reported 249 million cases (up from 245 million in 2020) and 608,000 deaths (down from 631,000 in 2020) due to malaria.[82] It is transmitted by the female *Anopheles* mosquito. Five species are known to cause human disease: *Plasmodium falciparum, Plasmodium vivax, Plasmodium ovale, Plasmodium malariae,* and *Plasmodium knowlesi.*

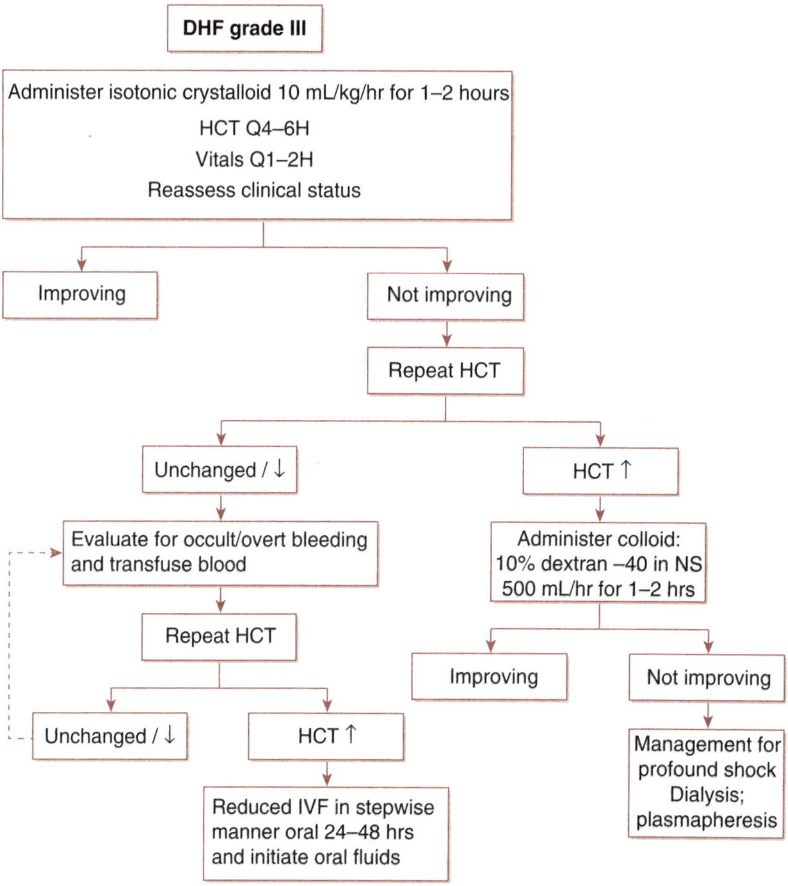

Figure 14-9 (*Continued*) Treatment algorithm for a patient with dengue.

DIAGNOSIS

Clinical Presentation

- Patients present with nonspecific symptoms, including fever, headache, myalgias, and fatigue.
- *P. falciparum* malaria, the most severe form, is a potential medical emergency. Complicated, or severe, falciparum malaria is diagnosed in the setting of hyperparasitemia (>5%), cerebral malaria, hypoglycemia, lactic acidosis, renal failure, acute respiratory distress syndrome, or coagulopathy. Many cases of severe and complicated *P. vivax* infection are being reported.
- Paroxysmal fever every other day can be seen in *P. vivax* and *P. ovale,* and every 3 days with *P. malariae.*
- Diagnosis of severe falciparum malaria is provided in Table 14-14.

TABLE 14-14 Diagnosis of Severe Falciparum Malaria

Severe Malaria Signs	Manifestations
i. Unarousable/coma, cerebral malaria	Failure to respond to appropriate stimuli, coma > 30 mins following seizure
ii. Acidosis/Acidemia	pH < 7.25 HCO_3 < 15 mmol/L BE >8, venous lactate >5 mmol/L deep labored breathing - respiratory distress
iii. Severe normocytic normochromic anemia	Hb < 5 g/dL, HCT <15%, with parasite level >10,000/μL
iv. Renal failure	Creatinine >3 g/dL, urine output <400 mL, failure to improve with hydration
v. Pulmonary edema/ ARDS	Noncardiogenic pulmonary edema, aggravated by fluid overload
vi. Hypoglycemia	Plasma glucose level <40 mg/dL
vii. Hypotension shock	systolic BP<80 mm Hg, skin/core temp >10°C capillary refill > 2 sec
viii. Bleeding/DIC	Bleeding/hemorrhage from gums, nose, GI tract, e/o DIC
ix. Convulsions	≥ 2 generalized seizures within 24 hours
x. Hemoglobinuria	Microscopic brown/black/red urine not a/w effect of oxidant drugs and red cell membrane defects (G6PD def)
xi. Extreme weakness	Prostration, inability to sit unaided
xii. Jaundice	Bilirubin >3 mg/dL combined with parasite density of >100,000/μL
xiii. Hyperparasitemia	Parasitemia levels <5% in nonimmune patients

Diagnostic Testing

- Malaria should be excluded in all persons with fever who live in or have traveled to an endemic area.
- Diagnosis is made by visualization of parasites on Giemsa-stained thick and thin blood smears, preferably obtained during febrile episodes.
- Rapid diagnostic tests such as *Plasmodium falciparum* HRP2 dipstick/card test and Plasmodium LDH dipstick/card test targeting antigens common to all *Plasmodium* species as well those specific to *P. falciparum* are available but should be confirmed with microscopy. Microtube concentration method with acridine orange stain can process large number of samples.

Complete blood counts	Normocytic normochromic anemia, total counts are usually normal but can be elevated in severe infections. Slight monocytosis, lymphopenia, eosinpenia followed by reactive lymphocytosis, and eosinophilia in the following weeks. Severe infection can cause thrombocytopenia
Inflammatory markers	Increased CRP, ESR
PT, aPTT	Prolonged
Antithrombin III	Decreased
Severe infections	Metabolic acidosis, hypoglycemia, reduced bicarbonate, phosphate, albumin, hypogammaglobulinemia, raised BUN, lactate, creatinine, muscle, and liver enzymes

TREATMENT

- Treatment is dependent on the type of malaria, severity, and risk of chloroquine resistance where the infection was acquired (Figure 14-10).
- **Uncomplicated malaria (*P. falciparum, P. ovale, P. vivax, P. malariae,* and *P. knowlesi*) from chloroquine-sensitive areas:** Chloroquine 600 mg base PO single dose followed by 300 mg base PO at 6, 24, and 48 hours.
- **Uncomplicated *P. falciparum* from chloroquine-resistant areas and *P. vivax* from Indonesia, or Papua New Guinea:**
  - Artemether-lumefantrine (20 mg artemether, 120 mg lumefantrine) 4 tablets PO at 0 and 8 hours, followed by 4 tablets q12h × 2 days.
  - Quinine sulfate 542 mg base PO q8h plus doxycycline 100 mg PO q12h or clindamycin 20 mg base/kg/d divided into 3 daily doses for 7 days.
  - Atovaquone-proguanil (250 mg atovaquone/100 mg proguanil) four tablets PO qday for 3 days.
- ***P. ovale* or *P. vivax*:** Add primaquine phosphate 30 mg base PO qday for 14 days to prevent relapse, after ruling out glucose-6-phosphate dehydrogenase deficiency.
- **Complicated severe malaria (most commonly *P. falciparum*):** Quinidine gluconate 6.25 mg base/kg loading dose IV over 1–2 hours followed by 0.0125 base/kg/min as a continuous infusion plus doxycycline or clindamycin for at least 24 hours; switch to oral as above when tolerated.
- IV artesunate is indicated in complicated falciparum malaria.[83] It is given as 2.4 mg/kg at admission followed by at 12, 24 hours and then once a day.
- Malaria in pregnancy (Figure 14-11)
- WHO recently approved the use of R21/Matrix-M vaccine for malaria prevention.[84]

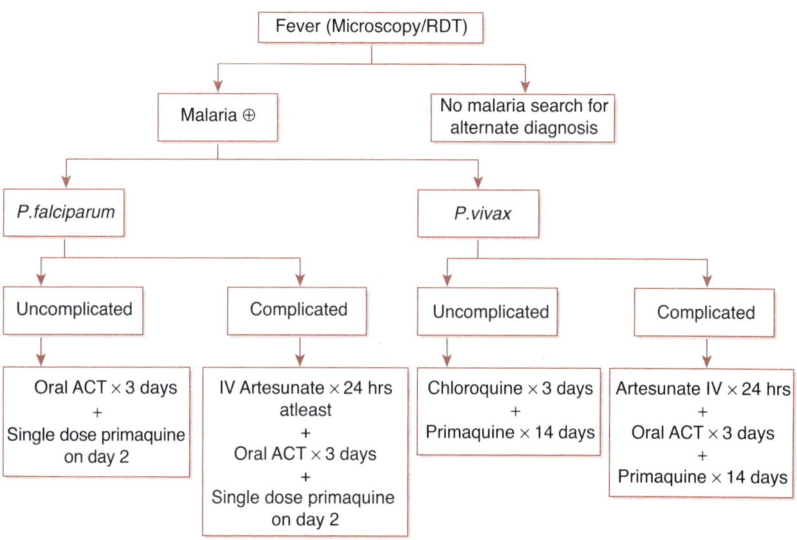

Figure 14-10 Treatment of malaria.

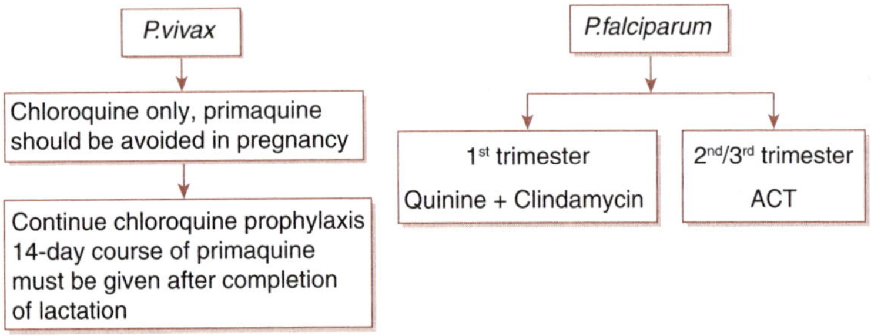

Figure 14-11 Treatment of malaria in pregnancy.

MALARIA VACCINE

- Mosquirix (RTS, S/AS01) is a recombinant vaccine against pre-erythrocytic stage of the parasite in which regions of *P. falciparum* circumsporozoite protein are fused to hep B surface antigen.
- It is administered IM for those >5 months of age. Three doses are given with an interval of 4 weeks while the 4th dose is given 15–18 months later.
- It has an efficacy of 30–45%. Protection wanes 18 months after use and must be readministered after 3 year

Zoonoses

Avian and Swine Influenza (see the Bioterrorism and Emerging Infections section)

Anthrax (see the Bioterrorism and Emerging Infections section)

Plague (see the Bioterrorism and Emerging Infections section)

Echinococcus

GENERAL PRINCIPLES

Echinococcosis is a zoonosis caused by cestodes of the genus *Echinococcus* (family Taeniidae). Four species cause infection in humans (Figure 14-12).

E. granulosus and *E. multilocularis* cause cystic echinococcosis (CE) and alveolar echinococcosis (AE), respectively.

E. vogeli and *E. oligarthus,* cause polycystic echinococcosis but are less frequently associated with human infection.

The pattern of distribution for CE is based on factors such as contact with dogs and raising livestock. Western China, Central Asia, South America, Middle East and eastern, Mediterranean countries, and Eastern Africa have been identified as endemic areas. However, several other cases from nonendemic areas of Asia are reported too.[85]

DIAGNOSIS

Clinical Presentation

Patients with CE are usually asymptomatic. Symptomatic CE is associated with damage or dysfunction of the target organs, particularly the liver (70%) and lungs (20%), with the

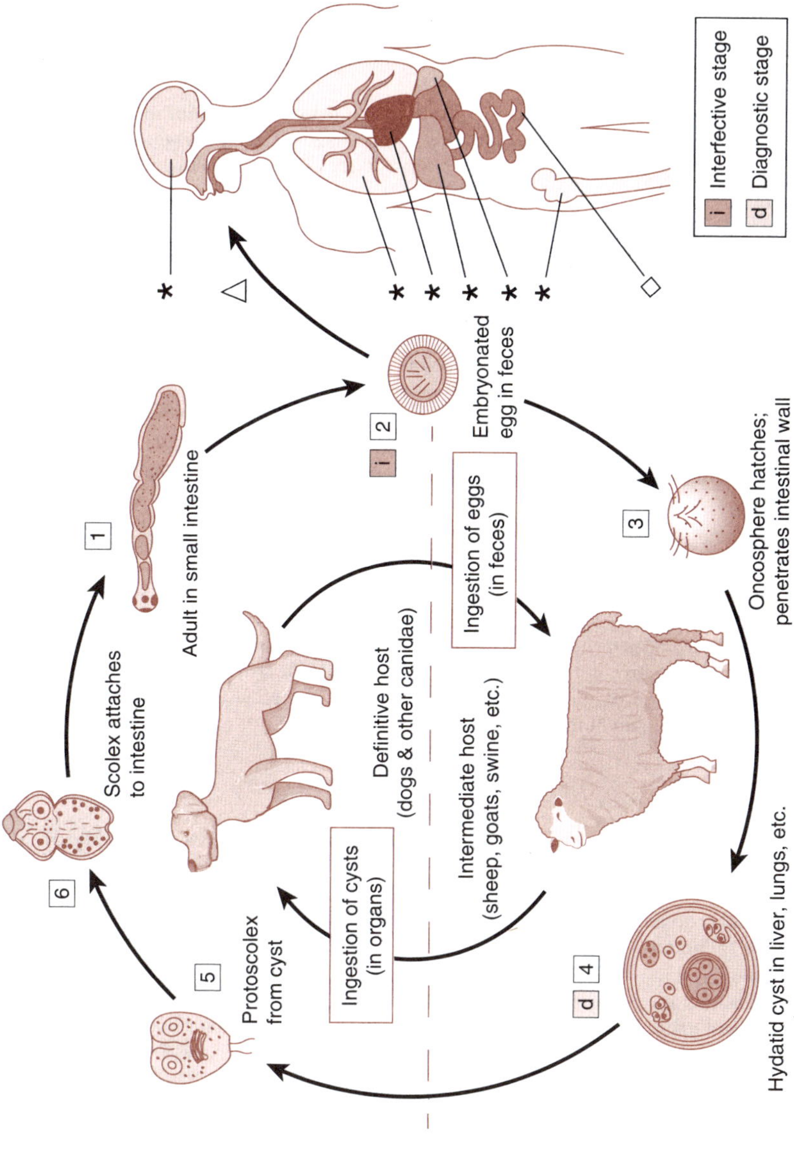

Figure 14-12 Life cycle of Echinococcus.

remainder including the brain, spleen, kidney, and heart. Symptomatic CE patients with liver cysts most often present with upper abdominal discomfort, poor appetite, and weight loss; compression of bile ducts may lead to jaundice. Clinical picture may mimic hepatocellular carcinoma.

Diagnostic Testing

The uses of imaging, serology, and molecular identification of the metacestode can help in diagnosis.

Ultrasound (USG) is primarily used to diagnose liver lesions and remains the mainstay to diagnose and classify the disease (snowflake sign or water lily sign). X-ray may be used for identifying lung cysts. Serologic assays are less likely to be positive in the setting of calcified or nonviable cysts.

TREATMENT

Mortality in untreated or inadequately treated AE patients is >90% within 10–15 years of diagnosis.

In CE, treatment is based on cyst type according to the size, location, and presence/absence of complications, as well as available medical expertise and equipment.

Various options are possible, alone or combined, for the treatment of both CE and AE, including surgery; puncture, aspiration, injection, and reaspiration (PAIR) technique; nonsurgical interventions; or use of anti-infective benzimidazole drug treatment.

Cat-Scratch Disease (CSD, Bartonellosis)

GENERAL PRINCIPLES

In the immunocompetent host, cat-scratch disease is usually a self-limiting disease. It is caused by the facultative intracellular coccobacillus *Bartonella henselae*. It can spread via cat scratch or bite, as well as a flea bite. Transmission can also occur if cat saliva comes in contact with broken skin or mucosal surfaces.[86]

CLINICAL PRESENTATION

- Usually presents with few papulovesicular lesions appearing 3–10 days after a cat bite or scratch, followed by regional lymphadenitis (usually cervical or axillary) and mild constitutional symptoms. Atypical presentations include oculoglandular disease (Parinaud's syndrome), encephalopathy, retinitis (stellate exudates), arthritis, FUO, and culture-negative endocarditis.
- In immunocompromised hosts, especially HIV-infected patients with a CD4 count <200 cells/mL, it can cause bacillary angiomatosis (angioproliferative nodules involving the skin and multiple organs) and bacillary peliosis (hepatosplenic cystic lesions).

DIAGNOSIS

Diagnosis is made by exclusion of other causes of lymphadenitis, detection of high antibody titres to *B. henselae*, PCR of infected tissue, or histopathological visualization of the bacilli using Warthin–Starry stain.

TREATMENT

- Localized disease spontaneously resolves in 2–4 months without treatment.
- If antimicrobial therapy is prescribed, azithromycin 500 mg PO single dose followed by 250 mg PO for 4 more days is recommended for lymphadenitis. Alternatives include clarithromycin 500 mg PO bid or TMP-SMX DS PO bid.
- In case of hepatosplenic disease, rifampicin 300 mg bid (IV or PO) is administered along with azithromycin or gentamycin.
- For neuroretinitis, rifampicin is prescribed, with either doxycycline (100 mg bid), azithromycin, or TMP-SMX.
- Needle aspiration of suppurative lymph nodes may provide symptomatic relief.[87]
- Culture-negative endocarditis due to *B. henselae* has been discussed in the Cardiovascular Infections section.

Leptospirosis

GENERAL PRINCIPLES

- Leptospirosis is an acute febrile illness with varying presentations caused by *Leptospira interrogans*, a ubiquitous pathogen of wild and domestic mammals, reptiles, and amphibians.
- Rodents are the main reservoir and symptoms appear 5–14 days after contact with the infected animal or water contaminated with their urine (Figure 14-13).

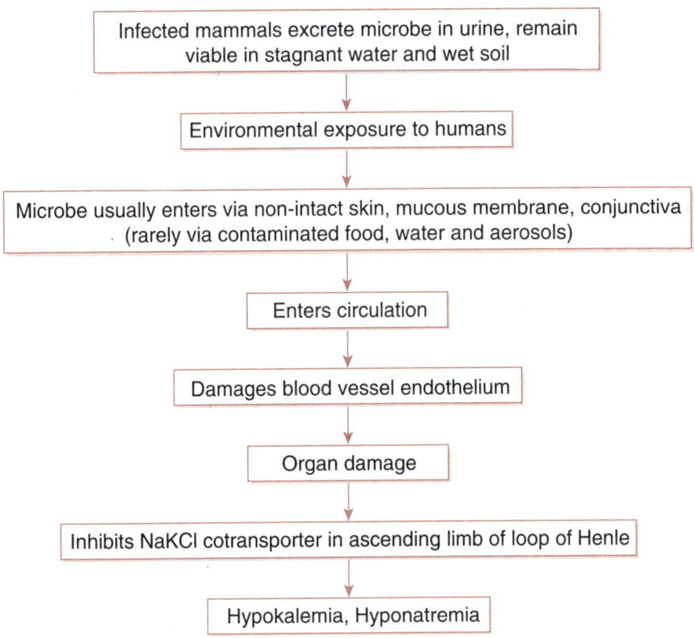

Figure 14-13 Pathogenesis of Leptospirosis.

CLINICAL PRESENTATION

- Anicteric leptospirosis is most commonly self-limited. Some patients develop a **biphasic illness** that starts with influenza-like symptoms and conjunctival suffusion (**septicemic phase**) progressing to aseptic meningitis or Weil's disease (**immune phase**) after a brief period of defervescence.
- A minority of cases progress directly to **Weil disease (icteric leptospirosis)**, with multiorgan failure manifested by severe jaundice, uremia, and hemorrhagic pneumonitis.

DIAGNOSIS (TABLE 14-15)

TABLE 14-15	Investigation in a Case of Leptospirosis
Complete blood counts	Leukocytosis with left shift
Blood cultures	Before day 10 of illness
Electrolytes	Hypokalemia, hyponatremia (nonoliguric hypokalemia, renal insufficiency: early manifestations)
Liver function test	Elevated bilirubin and transaminases
Inflammatory markers	Elevated CRP, ESR, procalcitonin
Urinalysis	Proteinuria, pyuria, granular cast, hematuria, raised creatinine, urine PCR, and culture
CSF analysis	Neutrophilic leukocytosis, raised protein
ELISA IgM	Fourfold increase in titres
Microscopic agglutination test (MAT)	Fourfold increase in titres
Chest x-ray	Nodular densities/consolidation, ground glass opacities

TREATMENT

For anicteric disease with mild symptoms, doxycycline 100 mg PO q12h or amoxicillin 500 mg PO q6h for 7 days is recommended. Penicillin G 1.5 million units IV q6h or a third-generation cephalosporin such as ceftriaxone 2 g/d IV or cefotaxime 1g IV q6h are used for patients with severe disease, during which a Jarisch–Herxheimer reaction is possible.[88] Doxycycline has been used for prophylaxis in several outbreaks during floods in endemic areas. Azithromycin 250 mg PO once-twice/week is alternate chemoprophylaxis.

Hantavirus

GENERAL PRINCIPLES

- Hantaviruses are a family of viruses spread mainly by wild rodents and can cause varied disease syndromes in people worldwide.
- Hantaviruses in the Americas are known as "New World" hantaviruses and may cause hantavirus cardiopulmonary syndrome (HCPS). Other hantaviruses, known as

"Old World" hantaviruses, are found mostly in Europe and Asia and may cause hemorrhagic fever with renal syndrome (HFRS). HFRS frequently occurs in China, South Korea, and Eurasia, such as East Asia, Europe, and Russia.

- Humans can become infected with hantaviruses through the inhalation of aerosols contaminated with the virus concealed in the excreta, saliva, and urine of infected animals.

DIAGNOSIS

Clinical Presentation

Hantavirus may cause asymptomatic or a nonspecific mild infection with fever and malaise.

HFRS: Five clinical phases are manifested in typical HFRS patients, including fever, hypotensive shock, and oliguric, polyuric, and convalescent phases.

Nephropathia endemica (NE) is a mild form of HFRS that is characterized by AKI and thrombocytopenia.

HCPS usually presents with cough and progressive dyspnea. The primary organ affected is lungs.

Diagnostic Testing

Serology is commonly used for diagnosis. Detection of hantavirus antigen in tissues by immunohistochemical staining and microscopic examination, or evidence of hantavirus RNA sequences in blood or tissue can aid the diagnosis.

TREATMENT

Supportive care is the mainstay of treatment.

- In HFRS, dialysis may be required to correct severe fluid overload.
- Intravenous ribavirin, an antiviral drug, has been shown to decrease illness and death associated with HFRS if used very early in the disease.

Brucellosis

GENERAL PRINCIPLES

Brucellosis is a zoonotic infection caused by members of the *Brucella* genus of gram-negative coccobacilli (*B. melitensis, B. abortus,* and *B. suis*). It is transmitted by direct contact with body fluids of livestock animals, by eating unpasteurized dairy foods, or by inhalation of infected aerosolized particles. Endemic areas for brucellosis include countries of the Mediterranean basin, Middle East, Central Asia, China, the Indian subcontinent, sub-Saharan Africa, and parts of Mexico and Central and South America. Annually 500,000 cases are reported worldwide.[89]

DIAGNOSIS

Clinical Presentation

- Incubation period is usually 2–4 weeks; it may be as long as several months.
- Symptoms are initially nonspecific but usually include constitutional symptoms such as fever and perspiration. **Malodorous, moldy perspiration** is almost pathognomonic.
- **Malta fever** is an undulant form of infection characterized by relapsing fever, night sweats, arthritis, back pain, and fatigue.
- Physical examination may be nonspecific, although **sacroiliitis** in young patients and spondylodiskitis or peripheral arthritis in older patients are the most common localized

forms of presentation. Lymphadenopathy, hepatomegaly, or splenomegaly may be present, and complications involving every organ system can occur (e.g., diarrhea, meningitis, endocarditis, pneumonia, hepatitis).

Diagnostic Testing

- A definitive diagnosis may be made by culture of the organism (from blood, body fluids, or tissue), or ≥4-fold rise in Brucella antibody titre between acute and convalescent phase serum specimens obtained ≥2 weeks apart. A presumptive diagnosis may be made by antibody titre ≥1:160 via standard tube agglutination test or by polymerase chain reaction detection of Brucella DNA in a clinical specimen.
- Isolation of the organism from blood or tissue culture remains the gold standard.

TREATMENT

- Doxycycline 100 mg PO q12h for 6 weeks for uncomplicated, nonfocal disease, or for 12 weeks in osteoarticular disease; along with streptomycin 15 mg/kg IM for the first 2–3 weeks (1 g max.) remains the treatment of choice. Rifampicin, fluoroquinolones, and co-trimoxazole are alternative options if doxycycline or streptomycin/gentamicin cannot be used.[90]
- In neurobrucellosis, ceftriaxone 2 g IV bd is given for the first 4-6 weeks, along with rifampicin and doxycycline which are given for at least 12 weeks. In brucella endocarditis, streptomycin or gentamicin can be given for 4 weeks along with 12 weeks of doxycycline and rifampicin.
- In brucella endocarditis, streptomycin or gentamicin can be given for 4 weeks along with 12 weeks of doxycycline and rifampicin.

Q Fever

GENERAL PRINCIPLES

- Q fever is a systemic infection caused by the gram-negative coccobacillus, *Coxiella burnetti*, which is shed in the urine, feces, milk, and especially the placenta of infected livestock (e.g., cattle, sheep, and goats).
- Close contact to the infected animal (most common exposure) is not required for development of human infection, given that an inoculum of a single bacteria can cause disease.

CLINICAL PRESENTATION

- Q fever can be acute or chronic. Incubation period averages from 18 to 21 days.
- Commonly it presents acutely as a mild, self-limiting, fever which usually affects the respiratory system. It is a well-known cause of FUO. Fever may rise to 40°C and persist for 1–3 weeks.
- **Atypical pneumonia** with fever and headache are the predominant presenting symptoms. Chest radiography demonstrating a coin-shaped pulmonary infiltrate (round pneumoniae) is a classic finding. Rarely it manifests as meningoencephalitis. Acute hepatic involvement resembles viral hepatitis. Post-Q fever fatigue syndrome has been reported to occur in up to 20% of patients with acute Q fever. Patients report severe fatigue, muscle pains, headache, photophobia, and/or mood and sleep changes.
- **Endocarditis** is the most well-characterized chronic form of Q fever, presenting with subacute constitutional symptoms. In the right epidemiological setting, the presence of

a heart valve vegetation with negative blood cultures should always prompt diagnostic testing for Q fever.

DIAGNOSTIC TESTING

Diagnosis is based on detection of phase I and II, IgM and IgG antibodies, as *C. burnetti* does not grow in standard routine cultures. Acute infection is characterized by a fourfold rise of phase II antibodies between serum samples taken 3–6 weeks apart. Phase I antibodies become dominant as the infection becomes chronic and a single **phase I IgG titre >1:800 is diagnostic in chronic Q fever.**[91] Histopathologic examination of tissues may reveal ring-shaped "donut granuloma."

TREATMENT

- **Acute Q fever** pneumonia and hepatitis are treated with doxycycline 100 mg PO q12h for 14 days (or until patient improves and is afebrile for at least 5 days). Macrolides, fluoroquinolones, and TMP-SMX are alternative drugs.
- **Chronic Q fever**, including endocarditis, is treated with doxycycline 100 mg PO q12h and hydroxychloroquine 200 mg PO q8h for 18–24 months. Repeat serological testing every 3 months to document response is recommended. Cure is established when phase I IgG titres fall below 1:800.

BITE WOUNDS

Animal Bites

GENERAL PRINCIPLES

- Management includes copious irrigation of the wound with tap water or sterile saline, debridement of necrotic material, culturing visibly infected wounds, and obtaining imaging to exclude fracture, foreign body, or joint space involvement.
- Most wounds should not be sutured unless they occur on the face and have been thoroughly irrigated.

TREATMENT

- Antimicrobial therapy is given to treat infection and as prophylaxis for high-risk bite wounds based on severity (Figure 14-14) (e.g., moderate to severe), location (e.g., hands, genitalia, near joints), type of animal, immune status (e.g., diabetes mellitus, asplenia, immunosuppression), and mechanism of injury (e.g., puncture, crush injury). Tetanus toxoid should be administered if the patient has been previously vaccinated but has not received a booster in the last 5 years.
- Prophylactic antibiotic therapy with amoxicillin-clavulanate 875 mg/125 mg PO q12h for 3–5 days should usually be administered.

SPECIAL CONSIDERATIONS

- **Dog bites:** Normal oral flora includes *Pasteurella multocida*, streptococci, staphylococci, and *Capnocytophaga canimorsus*. Dog bites comprise 80% of animal bites, but only 5% of such bites become infected. For infected dog bite wounds, amoxicillin-clavulanate, or clindamycin plus ciprofloxacin, is effective.

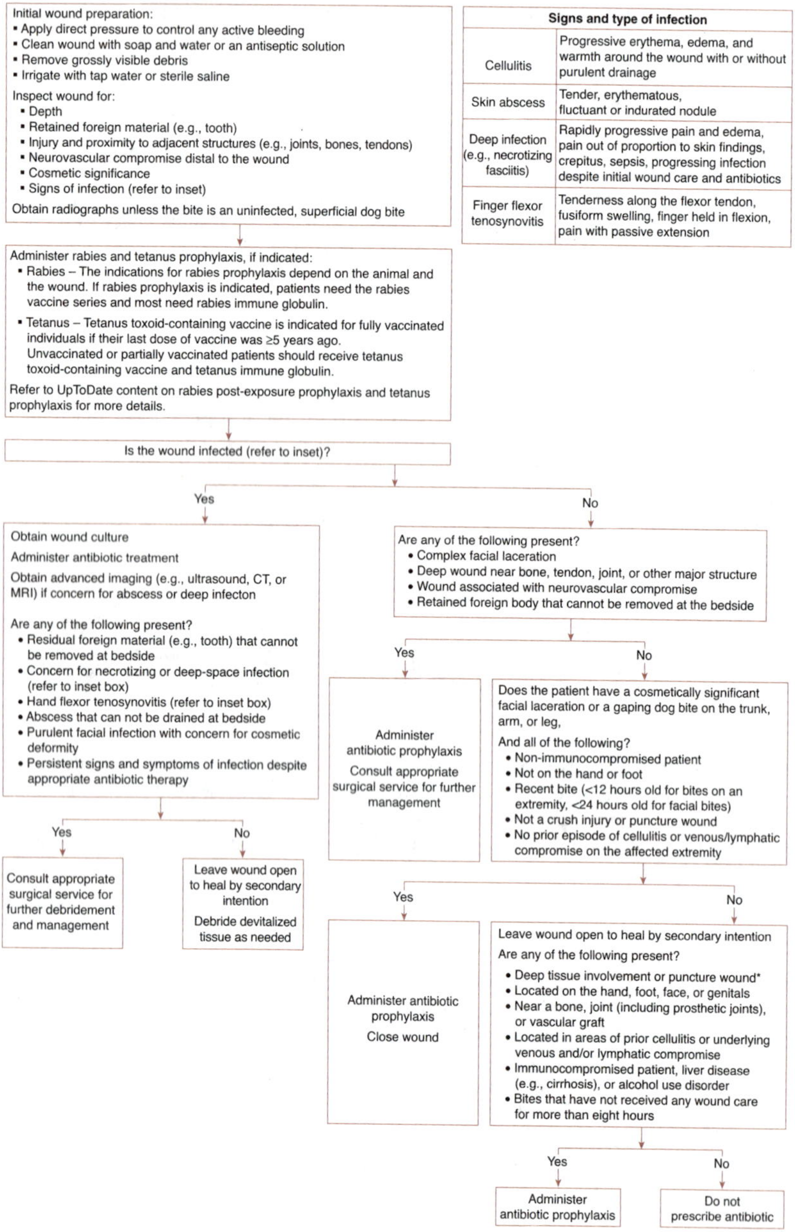

Signs and type of infection	
Cellulitis	Progressive erythema, edema, and warmth around the wound with or without purulent drainage
Skin abscess	Tender, erythematous, fluctuant or indurated nodule
Deep infection (e.g., necrotizing fasciitis)	Rapidly progressive pain and edema, pain out of proportion to skin findings, crepitus, sepsis, progressing infection despite initial wound care and antibiotics
Finger flexor tenosynovitis	Tenderness along the flexor tendon, fusiform swelling, finger held in flexion, pain with passive extension

Figure 14-14 Management of animal bite.

- **Cat bites:** Normal oral flora includes *P. multocida* and *S. aureus*. Because more than 80% of cat bites become infected, prophylaxis with amoxicillin-clavulanate should be routinely provided. Cephalosporins should not be used. Bartonellosis can also develop after a cat bite.
- **Wild animal bites:** Amoxicillin-clavulanate is a good choice for prophylaxis and empiric treatment for most animal bites. Monkey bites should be treated with acyclovir because of the risk of *Herpesvirus simiae* (B virus).

Rabies

- Rabies is a fatal disease caused by the neurotropic Rabies virus of the Rhabdoviridae family. Almost all cases of rabies are transmitted from rabid animals through a bite. In rare cases, rabies may result from a nonbite exposure (e.g., saliva contact with open skin or mucous membranes) or via transplantation of tissue or organs from a donor with unrecognized rabies.
- The virus is first amplified near the site of inoculation and subsequently enters local motor and sensory nerves. It then migrates centrally in a retrograde direction within the axoplasm of peripheral nerves until it reaches the spinal cord and brain.
- Risk of rabies depends on the animal species and geographic location. Infection is usually caused by dog bites in Asia and Africa and by bat bites in North America.
- The average incubation period is 1–3 months.
- The disease can present as two clinical forms: encephalitic (more common) and paralytic forms. The encephalitic form is typically divided into three stages—the prodrome, the acute neurologic phase, and coma/death.
- The prodrome consists of nonspecific flu-like symptoms, including malaise, anorexia, irritability, low-grade fever, sore throat, headache, nausea, and vomiting. There may also be specific neurologic signs and symptoms at the site of virus entry that are suggestive of rabies, including paresthesia, pain, and pruritus.
- An acute neurologic syndrome of either encephalitic or paralytic rabies follows the prodrome and typically lasts for 2–7 days without supportive care. Manifestations may include hyperactivity, persistent fever, fluctuating consciousness, painful pharyngeal or inspiratory spasms, autonomic stimulation (hypersalivation), hydrophobia, and seizures. Paralytic rabies is characterized by quadriparesis and sphincter involvement.
- Atypical rabies has been most often described in patients with bat-associated rabies. Atypical features include neuropathic pain, choreiform movements of the bitten limb during the prodromal phase, focal brainstem signs, cranial nerve palsies, myoclonus, and seizures.
- Diagnosis widely relies on history taking and clinical presentation in most developing countries. It may require more than a single test as sensitivity of a single test is low.
- Rabies antibodies in CSF are diagnostic. Serum antibodies in paired titre or unimmunized individual can aid diagnosis. Testing of viral DNA by reverse transcription PCR can detect virus in the saliva, CSF, or tissue (skin biopsy from the nape of the neck). Direct fluorescent antibody testing can be used for diagnosis.
- There is no known effective treatment for symptomatic rabies. However, the disease can be very effectively prevented after recognized exposures using recommended courses of postexposure rabies prophylaxis (Table 14-16).
- Any wound by an animal bite should be washed thoroughly with soap and water. Treatment relies mostly on PEP with rabies immunoglobulin (if skin breach) and rabies vaccine before the development of symptoms.
- The need for rabies vaccination and immunoglobulin prophylaxis (see Appendix A, Immunizations and Post-exposure Therapies) should be determined after any animal bite.
- Regardless of species, if the animal is rabid or suspected to be rabid, the human diploid vaccine and rabies immunoglobulin should be administered immediately.

TABLE 14-16 WHO Post-Exposure Rabies Management

Category	PEP Vaccine Regimen	RIG	Comments
Category I - Touching or feeding animals, animal licks on intact skin	Not required	Not required	Exposed skin surfaces should be washed
Category II - Nibbling of uncovered skin, minor scratches or abrasions without bleeding	**Patients who have NOT been previously immunized:** Immediate vaccination with one of the following regimens: • 2-sites ID on days 0, 3, and 7 • 1-site IM on days 0, 3, 7, and between days 14 and 28 • 2-sites IM on day 0 and 1-site IM on days 7 and 21	Not required	Exposed skin surfaces should be washed
	Patients who have been previously immunized:* • 1-site ID on days 0 and 3 • 4-sites ID on day 0 • 1-site IM on days 0 and 3	Not required	Exposed skin surfaces should be washed
Category III - Single or multiple transdermal bites or scratches, contamination of mucous membrane or broken skin with saliva from animal licks, exposures due to direct contact with bats	**Patients who have NOT been previously immunized:** Immediate vaccination with one of the following regimens: • 2-sites ID on days 0, 3, and 7 • 1-site IM on days 0, 3, 7, and between days 14 and 28 • 2-sites IM on day 0 and 1-site IM on days 7 and 21	RIG should be administered[†]	Exposed skin surfaces should be washed
	Patients who have been previously immunized:* • 1-site ID on days 0 and 3 • 4-sites ID on day 0 • 1-site IM on days 0 and 3	Not required	Exposed skin surfaces should be washed

(Continued)

TABLE 14-16 WHO Post-Exposure Rabies Management (Continued)

This table describes regimens recommended by the World Health Organization (WHO) for post-exposure prophylaxis after a potential rabies exposure and are intended for areas that may have limited resources. Refer to the topic that discusses rabies vaccine and immunoglobulin for information on regimens recommended by the Centers for Disease Control and Prevention's Advisory Committee on Immunization Practices (ACIP) for use in the United States, as well as information on vaccine and immunoglobulin formulations and administration.

Advisory Committee on Immunization Practices: ACIP; ID: intradermal; IM: intramuscular; PEP: post-exposure prophylaxis; RIG: rabies immune globulin.

*Previously immunized patients include those who have received pre-exposure prophylaxis and those who have completed a post-exposure vaccine regimen >3 months ago. Post-exposure prophylaxis (except for wound care) is not recommended for individuals who have a rabies exposure <3 months after completing a post-exposure vaccine series.

†RIG should be infiltrated into and around the wound. For small wounds, the maximal quantity that is anatomically feasible should be administered. Similarly, for bat bites or scratches, which are not readily visible, RIG should be injected around the site of the exposure to the degree that is anatomically feasible. The WHO no longer recommends injecting the remainder of the RIG IM at a site distant from the wound, which differs from ACIP recommendations in the United States. Refer to the topic that discusses rabies immunoglobulin for ACIP recommendations.

Human Bites

- Human bites, particularly clenched-fist injuries, are prone to infection and other complications. The normal oral flora of humans includes viridans streptococci, staphylococci, *Bacteroides* spp., *Fusobacterium* spp., peptostreptococci, and *Eikenella corrodens.*
- **Prophylaxis** with amoxicillin-clavulanate 875 mg/125 mg PO q12h for 5 days is recommended for uninfected wounds.
- Infected wounds may require **parenteral therapy**, such as ampicillin-sulbactam 1.5 g IV q6h, piperacillin tazobactam 3.375 g q8h or ceftriaxone 1 g q12h plus metronidazole 500 mg q8h or clindamycin 600 mg 8 h. Therapy should be extended to 4–6 weeks if osteomyelitis is present.

HEALTH CARE-ASSOCIATED INFECTIONS

HAIs substantially contribute to morbidity, mortality, and excess health-care costs. The global incidence has been variable across and this attributable to lack of official guidelines in the management of an indwelling catheter. Efforts to control and prevent the spread of HAIs require an institutional assessment of resources, priorities, and commitment to infection control practices (see Appendix B, Infection Control and Isolation Recommendations).

Central Line-Associated Bloodstream Infections

GENERAL PRINCIPLES

- *S. aureus, S. epidermidis* (coagulase-negative staphylococci), aerobic gram-negative species, and *Candida* spp. are the most common organisms associated with central line-associated bloodstream infections (CLABSI), also known as catheter-related bloodstream infections (CRBSIs).
- Subclavian central venous catheters (CVCs) are associated with lower CLABSI rates than internal jugular CVCs, whereas femoral CVCs have the highest rates and should be removed within 72 hours of placement.
- Strategies for decreasing the incidence of CLABSI include proper hand hygiene, skin antisepsis using an alcohol-based chlorhexidine solution, maximal sterile barrier precautions during insertion, strict adherence to aseptic technique, and removal of nonessential CVCs as soon as possible.[92] Subcutaneous tunneling and use of antiseptic-impregnated CVCs may further reduce the incidence of CLABSIs. Routine exchange of CVCs over a guide wire is not recommended.

DIAGNOSIS

Clinical Presentation

CLABSI should be suspected in any febrile patient with a CVC. Clinical findings that increase the suspicion of CLABSI include local inflammation or phlebitis at the CVC insertion site, sepsis, endophthalmitis, lack of another source of bacteremia, and resolution of fever after catheter removal.

Diagnostic Testing

- Diagnosis is established by obtaining two or more blood cultures from both the CVC and a peripheral vein before initiation of antibiotics.

- Repeat blood cultures should be obtained after starting antibiotic therapy to demonstrate clearance of bacteremia.
- TEE is recommended to rule out endocarditis if the patient has an implantable cardiac pacemaker or defibrillator, a prosthetic heart valve, persistent bacteremia or fungemia, or persistent fever >3 days after initiation of appropriate antibiotic therapy and catheter removal, or if *S. aureus* is involved and <4 weeks of therapy is being considered.

TREATMENT

- Host factors, including comorbidities, severity of illness, MDR colonization, prior infections, and current antimicrobial agents, are important considerations when selecting an antimicrobial regimen.[93]
- **Empiric therapy**
  - Vancomycin 15–20 mg/kg IV q12h is appropriate for empiric therapy because a majority of CLABSIs are caused by staphylococci. The dose should be adjusted to achieve a vancomycin trough between 15 and 20 μg/mL.
  - Gram-negative bacilli, including *Pseudomonas*, should be covered broadly until species identification and antibiotic susceptibilities are known. Fourth-generation cephalosporins (e.g., cefepime), carbapenems, or a β-lactam/β-lactamase inhibitor combined with or without an aminoglycoside are potential options.
  - Recommended duration of therapy depends on whether the infection is complicated or uncomplicated, beginning from the date of the first negative blood culture or removal of the infected CVC, whichever came later.
- **Pathogen-specific therapy:** Once the pathogen has been identified, antimicrobial therapy should be narrowed to the most effective regimen.
  - ***S. aureus*:** **MSSA** CLABSI should be treated with oxacillin 2 g IV q4h or cefazolin 1–2 g IV q8h. First-line therapy for **MRSA** is vancomycin 15–20 mg/kg IV q12h with a target vancomycin trough between 15 and 20 μg/mL. Linezolid 600 mg PO/IV q12h or daptomycin 6 mg/kg IV qday are alternatives. Several reports have also shown successful usage of teicoplanin. Routine use of gentamicin for synergy in *S. aureus* bacteremia is not recommended.[94] TEE should be considered to evaluate for endocarditis. The recommended duration of therapy is generally 4–6 weeks. A 2-week course is acceptable for uncomplicated MRSA bacteremia, as defined by a negative TEE, negative blood cultures, and defervescence within 72 hours of starting effective therapy, absence of prosthetic material (e.g., pacemaker, valve), and no evidence of metastatic infection.[95]
  - ***S. epidermidis* (coagulase-negative staphylococci)** CLABSI is treated similarly to MRSA, with vancomycin being the drug of choice in most cases. Duration of therapy is 7 days after CVC removal or 14 days if the CVC is retained.
  - Sensitive ***Enterococcus*** CLABSI should be treated with ampicillin. Vancomycin should be used in the setting of ampicillin resistance. Vancomycin-resistant enterococci may require therapy with daptomycin or linezolid. Duration of treatment should be 7–14 days.
  - Therapy against **gram-negative bacilli** should be guided by antibiotic susceptibility testing. Duration may range from 7 to 14 days.
  - **Candidemia** should be treated with an echinocandin (e.g., micafungin 100 mg IV qday) in cases of moderate to severe illness pending species identification, after which therapy can be tailored. Fluconazole 400 mg IV/PO qday may be appropriate for stable patients who have not had any recent azole exposure. Duration of antifungal treatment should be for 14 days after the last positive blood culture. A dilated ophthalmologic examination is advised to look for *Candida* endophthalmitis.[51]

- **CVC removal** is always preferable. At a minimum, it is recommended that CVCs be removed in the following situations:
  - Any CLABSI involving *S. aureus*, most gram-negative bacilli, or *Candida* spp.
  - Insertion site or tunnel site infection (pus or significant inflammation at the site).
  - Immunocompromised patients with fever, neutropenia, and hemodynamic instability (e.g., sepsis).
- Antibiotic lock therapy in combination with an extended course of antibiotics may be an option in certain situations where CVC salvage is absolutely necessary.

Hospital- and Ventilator-Associated Pneumonia

GENERAL PRINCIPLES

The most frequently implicated pathogens are gram-negative bacilli and *S. aureus*.

DIAGNOSIS

Clinical Presentation

- Hospital-acquired pneumonia (HAP) is defined as pneumonia occurring ≥48 hours after admission that was not incubating at the time of admission.
- Ventilator-associated pneumonia (VAP) is defined as HAP developing >48–72 hours after endotracheal intubation and mechanical ventilation.
- To suspect HAP when a hospitalized patient develops purulent sputum (or endotracheal secretions), new radiological infiltrates, an otherwise unexplained increase in oxygen, temperature >38.3°C, with labs showing leukocytosis/leucopenia.

Diagnostic Testing

- Diagnosis is made by clinical criteria as well as microbiologic testing.
- Noninvasive respiratory sampling (e.g., spontaneous expectoration, sputum induction, nasotracheal suctioning) is preferred to establish a microbiologic diagnosis of HAP. Likewise, noninvasive sampling comprised of endotracheal aspiration with semiquantitative culture is favored over bronchoscopy aspirates (e.g., BAL, blind bronchial sampling) with quantitative culture to aid in diagnosis of VAP.[96]

TREATMENT

- Initial empiric antimicrobial therapy should cover *S. aureus* (including MRSA) and *P. aeruginosa*. Targeted therapy should be based on culture results and in vitro sensitivity testing.[96]
- Empyemas require drainage.

Treatment

Oral

- Co-amoxiclav – 500/125 mg q8h × 5 days

Alternative

- Doxycycline – 200 mg loading followed by 100 mg/d × 5 days
- Cefalexin – 500 mg Q12H × 5 days
- Cotrimoxazole – 800/160 mg Q12H × 5 days
- Levofloxacin – 500 mg Q12H × 5 days

IV

- Piperacillin tazobactam – 4.5 g Q8H (Q6H if severe infection)
- Ceftazidime – 2 g Q8H
- Ceftriaxone – 2 g qday
- Meropenem – 0.5–1 g Q8H
- Ceftazidime + avibactam – 2.5 g Q8H
- Levofloxacin – 500 g Q12H
- Cefuroxime – 750 mg TID-QID

Alternative if MRSA

- Vancomycin – 15–20 mg/kg/Q12H-Q8H, mol 2 g/dose
- Teicoplanin – 6 mg/kg BD × 3 doses then 6 mg/kg daily
- Linezolid – 600 mg Q12H

Prevention

- Regular hand washing
- Limit use of stress ulcer prophylaxis with PPI
- Antiseptic wash (chlorhexidine 2%) maybe used to decontamination the upper airway
- Selective decontamination of digestive tract when the anticipated requirement for ventilation exceeds 48 hours

Catheter-Associated Urinary Tract Infection

GENERAL PRINCIPLES

- Catheter-associated urinary tract infection (CAUTI) is the most common HAI.
- *E. coli,* other gram-negative enterics, *P. aeruginosa*, gram-positives (staphylococci, enterococci), and yeast are commonly isolated from catheterized urine.
- Aseptic technique during insertion of a catheter is of utmost importance for prevention of CAUTI as well as **prompt removal of the catheter** when no longer needed.

DIAGNOSIS

Clinical Presentation

Fever is the most common symptom. Suprapubic and/or flank pain are helpful localizing symptoms, although nonspecific presentations (e.g., altered mental status) are also possible.

Diagnostic Testing

- Urinalysis and urine culture should be performed before starting antibiotics.
- The Infectious Diseases Society of America (IDSA) guidelines define catheter-associated bacteriuria as follows:
  - Symptomatic bacteriuria (urinary tract infection [UTI]) – Culture growth of $\geq 10^3$ colony forming units (cfu)/mL of uropathogenic bacteria in the presence of symptoms or signs compatible with UTI without other identifiable source in a patient with indwelling urethral, indwelling suprapubic, or intermittent catheterization. Compatible symptoms include fever, suprapubic, or costovertebral angle tenderness, and otherwise unexplained systemic symptoms such as altered mental status, hypotension, or evidence of a systemic inflammatory response syndrome.
  - Asymptomatic bacteriuria – Culture growth of $\geq 10^5$ cfu/mL of uropathogenic bacteria in the absence of symptoms compatible with UTI in a patient with indwelling urethral, indwelling suprapubic, or intermittent catheterization.

- Pyuria and bacteriuria occur in **all** in patients with chronic indwelling catheters and **should not be treated** in absence of symptoms (unless there are complicating factors, as mentioned previously).

TREATMENT

- Symptomatic CAUTI should be managed with removal or exchange of the catheter and treatment with 7–10 days of antibiotic therapy. Refer to Table 14-11 for empiric therapy.
- Candiduria should be treated with catheter removal and should **not** be treated unless the patient is immunocompromised and at high risk for candidemia.[78]
- Emphasis should be given on optimum catheter care comprising meatal care, managing leakage, managing obstruction, or preventing back flow. Patients who require long-term catheter care can be planned for clean intermittent catheterization.

Methicillin-Resistant *Staphylococcus Aureus* (MRSA) Infections

GENERAL PRINCIPLES

MRSA infection should be distinguished from MRSA colonization, especially when isolated from nonsterile sites such as sputum. Contact precautions are indicated as transmission occurs via contact with colonized individual or contaminated fomite. Risk factors for infection due to hospital-acquired MRSA (HA-MRSA) include antibiotic use, prolonged hospitalization, intensive care, invasive devices, hemodialysis, MRSA colonization, and proximity to others with MRSA colonization or infection.

By definition, all MRSA isolates carry the mecA gene or a related variant known as mecC. Strains lacking a mec gene are not methicillin resistant. They can be detected by conventional culture techniques, cefoxitin disk diffusion (most accurate phenotypic assay), and rapid culture with chromogenic agar.

TREATMENT

- First-line therapy for most MRSA bacteremia is monotherapy with vancomycin (dosed to therapeutic trough levels). Teicoplanin 6–12 mg/kg q12h for 2 days followed by qday may be used as an alternative agent. Other alternative agents include linezolid 600 mg IV/PO q12h, daptomycin 8–10 mg/kg IV qday, ceftaroline, and telavancin. Daptomycin should not be used to treat pneumonia owing to inactivation by pulmonary surfactant.
- Patients with unfavorable clinical response to initial treatment (persistent bacteremia beyond 48–72 hours, persistent fever and lack of clinical improvement) warrant further evaluation for occult focus of infection that may require drainage, guided by clinical history and physical examination. In addition, antibiotic susceptibility results (on the original isolate as well as the breakthrough isolate) should be reviewed carefully for susceptibility to vancomycin as well as alternative agents.
- The duration of treatment of uncomplicated MRSA bacteremia is for 14 days. If deep focus of infection is suspected, IV therapy is extended based on the nature of the underlying infection.
- Eradication of MRSA nasal carriage can sometimes be achieved with a 5-day course of twice-daily intranasal mupirocin. Other regimens include chlorhexidine soap products, bleach baths, and oral antibiotic treatment with TMP-SMX with or without rifampicin. However, mupirocin resistance can develop, and carriage often recurs. Eradication efforts should target patients with recurrent MRSA infections.[95]

- Principles of prevention include attention to careful hand hygiene, environmental cleaning, appropriate use of antibiotics, and contact precautions during care of patients with MRSA infection.

Vancomycin-Resistant *Enterococcus* Infections

GENERAL PRINCIPLES

Vancomycin-resistant enterococci (VRE) are differentiated from other strains of *Enterococcus* by an increased minimum inhibitory concentration for vancomycin and the presence of vancomycin-resistance gene clusters such as vanA. Most VRE-related lower UTIs can be treated with nitrofurantoin, ampicillin, ciprofloxacin, or other agents that achieve high urinary concentrations. Contact precautions are indicated. Eradication of enteric VRE colonization has been attempted without success.

TREATMENT

- The majority of patients with VRE BSI are treated with daptomycin, linezolid, or quinupristin/dalfopristin.
- Healthcare-associated VRE is transmitted by hands of healthcare workers and good hand hygiene is considered essential to limit spread of disease.
- Refer to Table 14-17 for treatment regimens

TABLE 14-17 Monotherapy Regimens for Treatment of Bacteremia Due to Resistant Enterococci in Adults

Regimen	Dose and Route
Isolate is ampicillin susceptible and vancomycin resistant	
Preferred agents	
Ampicillin	1 to 2 g IV every 4 to 6 hours
Penicillin G	18 to 30 million units IV per 24 hours either continuously or in 6 equally divided doses
Alternate agents	
Daptomycin	8 to 12 mg/kg IV every 24 hours
Linezolid (alternative agent to daptomycin)	600 mg IV every 12 hours
Isolate is ampicillin resistant and vancomycin susceptible	
Preferred agents	
Vancomycin	Initially 15 mg/kg/dose IV every 12 hours, not to exceed 2 g per dose; subsequent dosing guided by serum trough concentration or AUC monitoring
Daptomycin (alternative agent to vancomycin)	8 to 12 mg/kg IV every 24 hours
Linezolid (alternative agent to daptomycin)	600 mg IV every 12 hours

(Continued)

TABLE 14-17 Monotherapy Regimens for Treatment of Bacteremia Due to Resistant Enterococci in Adults (Continued)

Regimen	Dose and Route
Alternate agents	
High-dose ampicillin (if ampicillin MIC is ≤32 mcg/mL)	3 to 4 g IV every 4 hours
Ampicillin-sulbactam (if ampicillin resistance is due to beta-lactamase production)	3 g IV every 6 hours
Isolate is ampicillin resistant and vancomycin resistant	
Preferred agents	
Daptomycin	8 to 12 mg/kg every 24 hours
Linezolid (alternative agent to daptomycin)	600 mg IV every 12 hours
Alternate agents	
High-dose ampicillin (if ampicillin MIC is ≤32 mcg/mL)	18 to 30 g per day
Ampicillin-sulbactam (if ampicillin resistance is due to beta- lactamase production)	3 g IV every 6 hours

Adapted from Monotherapy regimens for treatment of bacteremia due to resistant enterococci in adults. Available at https://www.uptodate.com/contents/image?csi=8de211ee-945e-4634-b6ef-db58d382e659&source=contentShare&imageKey=ID%2F59332

Multidrug-Resistant Gram-Negative Infections

GENERAL PRINCIPLES

- Highly resistant gram-negative organisms (e.g., *Klebsiella, Acinetobacter, Pseudomonas* species) have become increasingly common causes of HAI. Contact precautions are indicated.
- Gram-negative bacillary sepsis with septic shock is associated with a high risk of mortality. There has been a notable rise in the prevalence of extended spectrum β-lactamases (ESBL) and carbapenemases. ESBL confer resistance to β-lactam antibiotics and are susceptible to β-lactamase inhibitors.
- Risk factors for ESBL and carbapenem resistance occur due to hospitalization, residence in long-term care facility, hemodialysis, prior antibiotic therapy, use of steroids, percutaneous feeding tube.

DIAGNOSTIC TESTING

Disk diffusion, broth dilution, automated systems, double disk test, Elast strip, pyrosequencing, and microassay.

TREATMENT

- Antimicrobial choices are often limited. Options include broad-spectrum agents such as β-lactam/β-lactamase inhibitor combinations, carbapenems, tigecycline, and polymyxins. Infectious disease consultation is recommended.
- ESBL-preferred antibiotics:
  - Carbapenems (meropenem, imipenem, ertapenem)
  - Ceftolozane-tazobactam (clinical data required for further evaluation)
  - Ceftazidime-avibactum (clinical data required for further evaluation)
  - Tetracycline-eravacycline
  - Tigecycline, if β-lactam allergy
  - Plazomycin is an advanced aminoglycoside recommended for complicated UTIs
  - Fosfomycin for UTIs
- Carbapenem resistance: Individualized combination regimen with two or more agents is recommended.

BIOTERRORISM AND EMERGING INFECTIONS

- Changing patterns in human behavior and demographics, natural phenomena, and microbial evolution lead to new infections within a population or increased incidence or geographic range of known pathogens (emerging infections) (Table 14-18). Included in this category are several highly fatal and easily produced microorganisms, which have the potential to be used as agents of bioterrorism and produce substantial illness in large populations via an aerosol route of exposure. Most of these diseases are rare, so a high index of suspicion is necessary to identify the first few cases.
- A bioterrorism-related outbreak should be considered if an unusually large number of patients present simultaneously with a respiratory, gastrointestinal, or febrile rash syndrome; if several otherwise healthy patients present with unusually severe disease; or if an unusual pathogen for the region is isolated.

Anthrax

GENERAL PRINCIPLES

Spores from the gram-positive *Bacillus anthracis* germinate at the site of entry into the body.

DIAGNOSIS

Clinical Presentation

- **Cutaneous anthrax** (<2% case-fatality rate), also known as "woolsorter's disease," usually results from skin contact with spores from infected animals or animal products (e.g., wool, hides). Infection is characterized by a painless black eschar with surrounding tissue edema.
- **Systemic anthrax can assume the following forms:**
  - **Inhalational anthrax** (45% case-fatality rate) stems from inadvertent aerosolization of spores from contaminated animal products or an intentional release such as a bioterrorism event. Infection presents initially with an influenza-like illness causing hemorrhagic necrosis of the thoracic lymph nodes draining the lung and resulting in hemorrhagic mediastinitis or rarely necrotizing pneumonia, gastrointestinal symptoms, or both, followed by fulminant respiratory distress and multiorgan failure.[97]

TABLE 14-18 Emerging Infectious Diseases

Pathogen	Epidemiology	Clinical Presentation and Diagnosis	Management
ESKAPE Pathogens ***E****nterococcus faecium* ***S****taphylococcus aureus* ***K****lebsiella pneumoniae* ***A****cinetobacter baumannii* ***P****seudomonas aeruginosa* ***E****nterobacter species*	Group of antibiotic-resistant bacteria that are the leading cause of nosocomial infections worldwide. They are selected by inappropriate antimicrobial use. Most are MDROs via acquired plasmid-mediated resistance (e.g., colistin-resistance by the *mcr-1* gene).	Multiple clinical presentations, but most commonly cause nosocomial BSI, VAP, IAI, and hardware-associated infections. Diagnosis is based on cultures with susceptibility testing and/or detection of β-lactamase, carbapenamase, PBP2A, or other mechanism or resistance via molecular or biochemical tests.	Treatment is organism-specific and should be based on antimicrobial susceptibility testing results. An ID consultation should always be obtained as this has shown to decrease mortality in these infections.[2]
Candida auris	Multidrug-resistant *Candida i.e.*, hard to identify in the laboratory. Commonly misidentified as *Candida haemulonii*.	Healthcare-associated BSI, wound, and ear infections. Fungal cultures with susceptibilities allow the diagnosis.	Pending susceptibilities and echinocandin should be used. Consultation with an ID specialist is highly recommended
Zoonotic influenza viruses	Emergence of influenza A strains previously confined to avian/swine host via antigenic shifts, with the potential to cause a pandemic. Acquired via exposure to infected live or dead poultry/pigs (e.g., live animal markets).	Ranges from a mild upper respiratory infection (fever and cough) to a rapid progression to severe pneumonia, ARDS, shock, and even death. Nasopharyngeal swabs for PCR is the most sensitive diagnostic test. If PCR is not available, a rapid antigen detection immunoassay should be done.	A neuraminidase inhibitor (oseltamivir, or zanamivir) for a minimum of 5 d is the treatment of choice. Infection control measures and close communication with public health authorities are critical.

(Continued)

TABLE 14-18 Emerging Infectious Diseases (Continued)

Vaccine-preventable diseases	The antivaxxer movement has contributed to the rise of preventable infections in countries with established vaccination programs. 19.5 million people did not received routine life-saving vaccinations in 2016. Around 90,000 people died from measles in 2016.	See Lower Respiratory Tract Infections section in this chapter for details about pertussis. Measles presents with high fever, coryza, cough, conjunctivitis, and small white spots inside the cheeks (Koplik's spots). After several days, a descending rash affecting palms and soles appears. Specific serological and/or PCR testing establish the diagnosis.	Prevention through vaccination per recommended ACIP guidelines is key. Patients with measles should be placed on respiratory isolation Close contacts of patients with *B. pertussis* should receive antimicrobial prophylaxis with a macrolide.
Viral hemorrhagic fever **Filoviruses** (Ebola and Marburg) **Flaviviruses** (dengue, yellow fever) **Bunyaviruses** (hantaviruses, Congo–Crimean hemorrhagic fever, Rift Valley fever) **Arenaviruses** (South American hemorrhagic fever, Lassa fever)	Caused by many different RNA viruses in endemic areas. Most are transmitted by aerosol or contact with infected body fluids. Ebola has been shown to also have sexual transmission via semen.	Fever, headache, joint and muscle aches, diarrhea/vomiting, and unexplained bleeding or bruising are common to all of these infections Specific serological and/or molecular testing establish the diagnosis.	There is currently no antiviral drug licensed by the FDA for any of these infections. A tetravalent live, attenuated dengue vaccine gives persistent protective benefit in those who had previously been infected with the virus, but it's under safety review by FDA and WHO. WHO endorses the use of the recombinant vesicular stomatitis virus (rVSV) vaccine for the Zaire Ebola virus, if an Ebola outbreak occurs.

ARDS, acute respiratory distress syndrome; BSI, bloodstream infection; FDA, US Food and Drug Administration; IAI, intra-abdominal infections; ID, Infectious Diseases; MDRO, multidrug-resistant organism; PBP2A, penicillin-binding protein 2A; PCR, polymerase chain reaction; VAP, ventilator-associated pneumonia; WHO, World Health Organization.

- ◦ **Gastrointestinal anthrax** (≥40% case-fatality rate) commonly results from consumption of undercooked infected animal meat. Symptoms include nausea, vomiting, abdominal pain, ascites, and gastrointestinal hemorrhage related to necrotic mucosal ulcers.
- ◦ **Anthrax meningitis** (nearly always fatal) can arise from cutaneous, inhalational, or gastrointestinal anthrax, manifesting with parenchymal brain hemorrhage, seizures, delirium, or coma.

Diagnostic Testing

Diagnosis of inhalational disease is suggested by a widened mediastinum without infiltrates on chest radiograph and confirmed by blood culture and PCR. Acute and convalescent serum samples are utilized for serologic testing. Plasma can be tested for anthrax lethal factor toxin. Pleural fluid or bronchial biopsies can be tested for Gram stain, culture, and PCR analysis. In systemic anthrax, evaluation of CSF can be done. In cases of cutaneous anthrax, lesion specimens can be tested. Notify local infection control and public health department immediately for confirmed cases.

TREATMENT

- Empiric therapy for systemic anthrax with possible or confirmed meningitis is ciprofloxacin 400 mg IV q8h and meropenem 2 g IV q8h and linezolid 600 mg IV q12h for 2–3 weeks until clinically stable. Transition to oral therapy with ciprofloxacin 500 mg PO q12h *or* doxycycline 100 mg PO q12h *and* one other active agent can occur thereafter and continued to complete a total 60-day course antimicrobial therapy to reduce the risk of delayed spore germination.
- Systemic anthrax with meningitis excluded should be treated with ciprofloxacin 400 mg IV q8h *and* clindamycin 900 mg IV q8h or linezolid 600 mg IV q12h for 2 weeks until clinically stable, followed by transition to oral therapy to complete a total 60-day course of antimicrobial therapy as above. Antitoxin, including monoclonal antibodies (raxibacumab, obiltoxaximab) and anthrax immunoglobulin, may be requested from the CDC in select circumstances to treat inhalational anthrax in combination with antimicrobial therapy.[98,99]
- Uncomplicated cutaneous anthrax can be treated with oral ciprofloxacin 500 mg q12h *or* doxycycline 100 mg q12h for 7–10 days for naturally acquired cases and 60 days for bioterrorism-related cases.
- PEP for individuals at risk for inhalational anthrax consists of oral ciprofloxacin 500 mg q12h or doxycycline 100 mg q12h for 60 days after exposure.

Plague

GENERAL PRINCIPLES

- Plague is a murine zoonosis caused by the gram-negative bacillus *Yersinia pestis.*
- Infection may occur after exposure to infected animals (e.g., through scratches, bites, direct handling, inhalation of aerosolized respiratory secretions) and via rodent flea bites.

DIAGNOSIS

Clinical Presentation

There are three forms of plague.

- **Bubonic:** Local painful lymphadenitis (bubo) and fever (14% case-fatality rate), chills, weakness and headache.

TABLE 14-19 Antibiotics for Treatment of Plague (*Yersinia Pestis* Infection)

Drug	Adult Dosing
Aminoglycosides	
Gentamicin	IV/IM: 5 mg/kg every 24 hours
Streptomycin	IV/IM: 1 g every 12 hours
Fluoroquinolones	
Ciprofloxacin	IV: 400 mg every 8 hours Oral: 750 mg every 12 hours
Levofloxacin	IV/oral: 750 mg every 24 hours
Moxifloxacin	IV/oral: 400 mg every 24 hours
Tetracyclines	
Doxycycline	IV/oral: 200 mg loading dose then 100 mg every 12 hours

Source: Adapted from Nelson CA, Meaney-Delman D, Fleck-Derderian S, et al. Antimicrobial Treatment and Prophylaxis of Plague: Recommendations for Naturally Acquired Infections and Bioterrorism Response. MMWR Recomm Rep 2021; 70:1.

- **Septicemic:** Can cause peripheral necrosis and disseminated intravascular coagulation (DIC) ("black death"). Usually from progression of bubonic disease (30%–50% case-fatality rate).
- **Pneumonic:** Severe pneumonia with hemoptysis preceded by initial influenza-like illness (57% case-fatality rate, nearing 100% when treatment is delayed). Pneumonic disease can be transmitted from person to person and would be expected after inhalation of aerosolized *Y. pestis.*

Diagnostic Testing

Diagnosis is confirmed by isolation of *Y. pestis* from blood, sputum, or CSF. Treat all diagnostic samples as highly infectious. Notify local infection control and public health departments immediately.

TREATMENT

- Treatment should start at first suspicion of plague because rapid initiation of antibiotics improves survival (Table 14-19).
- PEP is indicated after unprotected face-to-face contact with patients with known or suspected pneumonic plague and consists of doxycycline 100 mg PO q12h or ciprofloxacin 500 mg PO q12h for 7 days.

Botulism

GENERAL PRINCIPLES

- The anaerobic gram-positive bacillus *Clostridium botulinum*, produces the toxin botulinum which causes botulism.
- Modes of acquisition include ingestion of the neurotoxin from improperly canned food and contamination of wounds with *C. botulinum* from the soil. Inhalational botulism could result from an intentional release of aerosolized toxin.

- Mortality is low when botulism is recognized early but may be very high in the setting of mass exposure and limited access to mechanical ventilation equipment.

CLINICAL FEATURES

- The classic triad consists of
  - An absence of fever,
  - Clear sensorium,
  - And symmetric descending flaccid paralysis with cranial nerve involvement, beginning with ptosis, diplopia, and dysarthria, and progressing to loss of gag reflex and diaphragmatic function with respiratory failure, followed by diffuse skeletal muscle paralysis. Sensation remains intact. Paralysis can last from weeks to months.
- Heart rate can be slow or normal with normal blood pressure.
- Diagnosis is confirmed by detection of toxin in serum. Notify local infection control and public health departments.

DIAGNOSIS

- Constellation of findings that should prompt consideration of botulism is provided in Table 14-20.

TABLE 14-20 Clinical Criteria of Botulism

At least one of the following symptoms of cranial neuropathy:
Blurred vision
Double vision
Difficulty speaking, including slurred speech
Any change in sound of voice, including hoarseness
Dysphagia/pooling of secretions/drooling
Thick tongue sensation
PLUS at least one of the following signs of neuropathy:
Ptosis
Signs suggestive of extraocular neuropathy
Extraocular palsy
Decreased tracking of objects
Fatigability manifested by avoiding light shining in the eye
Signs suggestive of facial neuropathy
Facial paresis
Loss of facial expression
Poor feeding or poor suck using pacifier
Fatigability while eating
Fixed pupils (not including abnormally or sluggishly reactive pupils)
Descending paralysis, beginning with cranial nerves
PLUS lack of fever (temperature ≤37.8°C or ≤100.4°F)

- These clinical criteria have been proposed as a tool to improve identification of patients with botulism. When all three are present, the sensitivity for botulism is approximately 78%–89%. The specificity is unknown.[100]
- Complete blood counts are usually within normal limits.
- CSF analysis is usually within normal limits, sometimes associated with elevated proteins.
- Electromyographic studies (EMG): Reduced compound muscle action potential (CMAP) and M-wave amplitudes, excessive action potentials, and frequency varying response to repetitive nerve stimulation (RMS).

Differential Diagnosis

Myasthenia gravis	Brainstem stroke	Guillain–Barré syndrome
Lambert-Eaton myasthenic syndrome	Poliomyelitis	Heavy metal poisoning

TREATMENT

- Treatment is primarily supportive and may require mechanical ventilation in the setting of respiratory failure. Wound botulism requires extensive surgical debridement.
- Further progression of paralysis can be halted by early administration of botulinum antitoxin, available through the state public health department or the CDC. Antitoxin is reserved only for cases where there is a high suspicion for botulism based on clinical presentation and exposure history. Routine PEP with antitoxin is not recommended because of the high incidence (10%) of hypersensitivity reactions and limited supply.

Viral Hemorrhagic Fevers: Ebola Virus Disease

GENERAL PRINCIPLES

- Viral hemorrhagic fever is caused by many different RNA viruses, including filoviruses (Ebola and Marburg), flaviviruses (dengue, yellow fever), bunyaviruses (Hantaviruses, Congo–Crimean hemorrhagic fever [CCHF], Rift Valley fever [RVF]), and arenaviruses (South American hemorrhagic fevers, Lassa fever).
- The 2014–16 West African Ebola Virus Disease (EVD) epidemic and subsequent outbreaks in Guinea in early 2021 demonstrate that sustained human-to-human transmission of EVD is possible in vulnerable populations.[101]
- Case-fatality rates are variable but can be as high as 90% for EVD in resource-limited settings. In the recent outbreak in Sudan that ended in 2023, the case fatality rate averaged around 50%.[102]

DIAGNOSIS

Clinical Presentation

- Early symptoms include abrupt onset of fevers and chills, myalgias, and malaise, with varying severity and symptomatology depending on the virus, but all can severely disrupt vascular permeability and cause DIC.
- A diffuse erythematous, nonpruritic maculopapular rash may form within 5–7 days of disease onset.
- Thrombocytopenia, leukopenia, leading to petechiae and ecchymosis or mucosal bleeding, and hepatitis are common.

- Vomiting and severe diarrhea (up to 10 L per day) leading to significant dehydration and mortality, as evidenced by the West African EVD epidemic, can also be a prominent feature.[101,103]
- Patients can occasionally develop neurological symptoms like meningoencephalitis.
- During the acute phase of illness cardiac manifestations such as relative bradycardia and pulse temperature dissociation have been observed.
- Conjunctival injection or uveitis can occur.

Diagnostic Testing

- Diagnosis requires consideration of epidemiology and patient risk factors, especially travel to endemic areas.
- Complete blood counts: Leukopenia, thrombocytopenia, and variable hematocrit
- Liver function test: Transaminitis
- Renal function test: Renal insufficiency causing elevated blood urea nitrogen and creatinine
- Serum electrolytes: Severe diarrhea can lead to significant electrolyte abnormalities (hyponatremia, hypokalemia, hyperkalemia, hypomagnesemia, and hypocalcemia)
- Serology performed by reference laboratories can confirm diagnosis. Nucleic acid testing (RTPCR) is considered the standard tests. Rapid immunoassay tests are now available. Notify local infection control and public health departments immediately.

Differential Diagnosis

• Malaria	• Meningococcal disease	• Measles
• Typhoid	• Influenza	• Traveler's diarrhea

TREATMENT

- Treatment is primarily supportive with attention to infection control.
- A recombinant vesicular stomatitis virus–Zaire Ebola virus (rVSV-ZEBOV) vaccine offered protection against EVD after exposure during the West African EVD epidemic. Investigation of multiple EVD vaccines remains ongoing.[104]
- Ribavirin (2 g IV × 1, then 1 g q6h × 4 days, then 500 mg q8h × 6 days) has been used for CCHF, Lassa, and RVF.[105,107]
- Exposed contacts should monitor temperature twice daily for 3 weeks. PEP with oral ribavirin can be administered to febrile CCHF, Lassa, and RVF contacts.
- Ebola specific therapies such as atoltivimab, maftivimab, and odesivimab (triple monoclonal antibody product) have been approved by the FDA in October 2020.
- Ansuvimab has been approved for use in December 2020.
- The above monoclonal antibodies are administered as a single dose.
- Empiric antibiotic coverage for gram-negative coverage should be initiated in those who have a clinical evidence of bacterial sepsis, which may be a late complication.

Leishmaniasis

GENERAL PRINCIPLES

Leishmaniasis is a disease with a worldwide distribution and is endemic to Asia, Africa, the Americas, and the Mediterranean region.

As per the WHO 2022 fact sheet, majority of visceral leishmaniasis (90%) occurs in India, Brazil, and east Africa. The annual incidence is estimated at 50,000 to 90,000 out of which only 25%–45% are reported to the WHO.

Most cases of cutaneous leishmaniasis (95%) occur in the Americas, the Mediterranean basin, the Middle East, and central Asia. Annual incidence is estimated to be around 600,000 to 1 million but only a small fraction ~ 200,000 are reported to the WHO.

TRANSMISSION

Leishmania parasites are transmitted through the bite of an infected phlebotomine sandfly.

DIAGNOSIS

Clinical Presentation

According to the clinical manifestations, leishmaniasis can be divided into the following: (1) cutaneous (localized and disseminated), (2) mucocutaneous, and (3) visceral leishmaniasis or kala-azar.

Visceral leishmaniasis may typically present with fever, fatigue, and splenomegaly in a patient from an endemic area. Mild hepatomegaly may occur in later stages. Laboratory investigations may reveal anemia or pancytopenia. In the early stages, leishmaniasis induces specific immunosuppression. In the early stages, leishmaniasis induces specific immunosuppression.

Diagnostic Testing

Diagnosis often relies on observing the parasites in the smear or in the imprint stained with Giemsa or Wright stain. Scraping from the border of a cutaneous or mucosal ulcer or biopsy from an active lesion may reveal the parasites in free form or inside macrophages or less frequently in polymorphonuclear leukocytes, ranging in number from 2 to 20 in a single cell.

In visceral leishmaniasis, the diagnosis is performed by observing protozoans through the microscope in a tissue sample obtained by aspiration from the spleen, bone marrow, or lymph node with a sensitivity of 95%, 55%–97%, or 60%, respectively.

Determination of serum anti-*Leishmania* IgG and the determination of anti-K39 antibodies are also widely used for diagnosis.

Treatment

Liposomal amphotericin B (AmBisome) is FDA-approved for the treatment of visceral leishmaniasis and generally is the treatment of choice. The Kala-azar Elimination Programme (KAEP), initiated jointly by India, Nepal, and Bangladesh, advises administration of a single dose of liposomal amphotericin (10 mg/kg).

Amphotericin B deoxycholate has powerful anti-leishmanial activity and can also be administered (0.75–1.00 mg/kg) for 15–20 doses.

Miltefosine is an orally approved drug for VL caused by *Leishmania donovani*. As per the weight bracket, patients weighing ≥25 kg should be administered with 50 mg twice daily and <25 kg with 50 mg once daily for a duration of 28 days. It is contraindicated in pregnant and breast-feeding females.

Pentavalent antimonial (SbV) therapy is widely used for visceral leishmaniasis (except in parts of South Asia, especially in the Indian state of Bihar, a majority of cases are refractory to Sb treatment). Administered as 20 mg/kg body weight, intravenously or intramuscularly, for 28–30 days.

Alternative agents which have been used successfully include paromomycin sulfate (administered as 11 mg/kg for 3 weeks) and pentamidine isethionate. Azoles have been used in CL with variable results.

Due to various limitations of monotherapy, such as limited number of antileishmanial drugs, long half-life of drugs like miltefosine, poor maintenance of cold chain, and general noncompliance, there is an increased risk of development of drug resistance.

Multidrug therapy includes a short-course combination:

- Single dose of AmBisome 5 mg/kg + 7 days of miltefosine/10 days of paromomycin OR
- 10 days of miltefosine + paromomycin

Patients require 6–12 months of regular follow-up as some may experience a relapse of the disease despite compliant treatment.

Leprosy

GENERAL PRINCIPLES

Leprosy is a chronic granulomatous disease affecting skin and nerves and is caused by *M leprae*. Even now, it remains a public health problem in many countries.

Early diagnosis is very important. The timely and proper implementation of treatment will prevent sequelae and physical disabilities

Transmission occurs via droplet infection and skin to skin contact.

CLASSIFICATION (TABLE 14-21)

TABLE 14-21 Classification of Leprosy

Ridley and Jopling Classification	WHO Classification
It is based on clinical, immunological, and histopathological criteria	It is for operational and therapeutic purposes. It is based on the bacterial index (BI).
Tuberculoid leprosy (TT)	Paucibacillary leprosy (2–5 skin lesions) (PB)
Borderline tuberculoid leprosy (BT)	Multibacillary leprosy (≥6 skin lesions; all of which are smear positive)
Mid borderline leprosy (BB)	
Borderline lepromatous leprosy (BL)	
Lepromatous leprosy (LL)	

DIAGNOSIS

Clinical Presentation

Clinical manifestations depend more on the cellular immune response of the host to *M. leprae* than on the bacillary penetration and proliferation.

Clinical manifestations are usually preceded by a long incubation period. The diagnosis of leprosy is established based on careful skin and neurologic examination of the patient.

General physical examination should include careful search for anesthetic patches, thickened nerves, and signs of peripheral neuropathy.

Tuberculoid Leprosy

The disease is limited due to the good cellular immune response of the host to *M. leprae,* with the patients showing single skin lesion or a small number of asymmetric lesions.

Sensitive change in the nerve path such as loss of sweating with impaired or absent sensations, with or without nerve thickening, may be the only manifestation, characterizing the primary neural form of the disease.

Lepromatous Leprosy

Skin lesions tend to be multiple and symmetrical (located more in the colder areas). Multiple peripheral nerves may be involved. Clinical appearance of leonine facies, eyelash loss (madarosis), ear lobule, and skin thickening may be the telltale signs for identifying leprosy.

Lepra Reaction

- Type 1 lepra reaction or reversal reaction (RR): It is a delayed hypersensitivity reaction. It occurs often in borderline patients and can cause improvement (reversal reaction) or worsening of the disease.
- Type 2 reaction or erythema nodosum leprosum (ENL): It is related to humoral immunity. It is manifested by sudden worsening, especially during treatment in the LL individuals (rarely, in BL patients).
- It may present as fever, malaise, myalgia, edema, arthralgia, and lymphadenomegaly. Neuritis and internal involvement, such as liver or kidney damage, may also occur.

Diagnostic Testing

Skin smear microscopy is used to detect alcohol-acid-resistant bacilli (AARB) in skin smears collected from standard sites (skin lesions, ear lobes, elbows).

It is performed using the Ziehl–Neelsen staining and used to assess the morphology index (MI) and the BI.

Histopathological examination of fragments of skin lesions or nerves may clinch the diagnosis.

Histopathological examination of biopsied skin lesion is mainly indicated for multibacillary cases with negative slit-skin smears and in cases of indeterminate leprosy. Nerve biopsy is needed to diagnose pure neuritic leprosy.

Serological tests for leprosy include fluorescent antibody adsorption test, glycolipid-1 antibody, monoclonal antibody-based test, genomic probes, and PCR techniques.

Differential Diagnosis (Table 14-22)

TABLE 14-22 Differential Diagnosis of Leprosy

Hypopigmented Macules	Plaque and Annular Lesions	Nodular Lesions	Nerve Thickening	Peripheral Neuropathy
• Vitiligo • Tinea versicolor • Pityriasis alba	• Lupus vulgaris • Tinea corporis • Sarcoidosis	• Syphilis • Leukemia cutis • Mycosis fungoides	• Hereditary sensory motor neuropathy type III • Amyloidosis	• Diabetes • Alcoholism • Nutritional deficiencies

TREATMENT

The WHO recommends a year of multidrug therapy treatment in MB leprosy.

Cases of neuritis are treated with prednisone (1–1.5 mg/kg/d); additionally, it is important to keep the affected limb at rest and monitor neural function. Corticosteroid therapy is

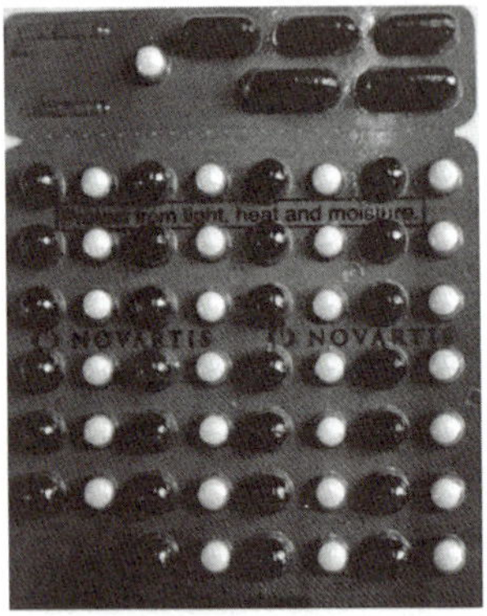

Multibacillary adult treatment

Once a month: Day 1
- 2 Capsules of rifampicin (300 mg × 2)
- 3 Capsules of clofazimine (100 mg × 3)
- 1 Tablet of dapsone (100 mg)

Once a day: Days 2–28
- 1 Capsule of clofazimine (50 mg)
- 1 Tablet of dapsone (100 mg)

Full course: 12 blister packs

MDT includes a combination of 600 mg of rifampicin once per month, 300 mg of clofazimine once per month, and daily doses of clofazimine (50 mg) and dapsone (100 mg) for a total of 12 months.

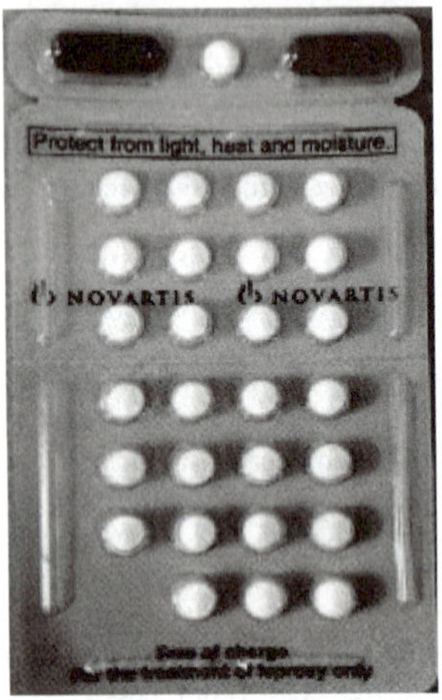

Paucibacillary adult treatment

Once a month: Day 1
- 2 Capsules of rifampicin (300 mg × 2)
- 1 Tablet of dapsone (100 mg)

Once a day: Days 2–28
- 1 Tablet of dapsone (100 mg)

Full course: 6 blister packs

The recommendation for PB patients is a 600-mg dose of rifampicin once per month and daily 100-mg doses of dapsone for 6 months.

Figure 14-15 Treatment of leprosy.

also recommended in cases of ENL, erythema polymorphous-like reaction, dermatoses like Sweet syndrome, ocular lesions, reactive hands and feet, glomerulonephritis, epididymo-orchitis, arthritis, and vasculitis (Figure 14-15).

Melioidosis

GENERAL PRINCIPLES

- *B. pseudomallei*, a gram-negative bacillus found in the environment of some tropical and subtropical regions, is the etiologic agent of melioidosis.
- South Asia is predicted to be the area with the greatest burden of disease, but the exact incidence is unknown due to limited awareness and laboratory constraints. Most cases are reported from northeastern Thailand, Southeast Asia and northern Australia.

- Patients with diabetes mellitus, in particular, have a high incidence of melioidosis. Other identified risk factors include soil/water exposure, thalassemia, renal disease, chronic lung disease, and excessive alcohol consumption.
- The predominant route of transmission is percutaneous inoculation during exposure to wet soil or contaminated water. Transmission via inhalation occurs in severe weather conditions.

DIAGNOSIS

Clinical Presentation

Clinical diagnosis is exceptionally challenging due to the varied clinical presentations, especially as the disease can mimic other infections such as tuberculosis. Pneumonia is the most common presentation of melioidosis. Other manifestations include prostatic infection or abscess, renal abscess, urinary tract infection, and bone and joint involvement. Melioidosis can rarely cause encephalitis.

Diagnostic Testing

Isolation of *B. pseudomallei* from bodily fluids of patients remains the "gold standard" in diagnosis.

IHA, latex agglutination, and immunofluorescence are used to diagnose melioidosis.

TREATMENT

Ceftazidime (50 mg/kg up to 2 g IV every 6–8 hours) or carbapenem antibiotics (imipenem and meropenem) are the drug of choice for acute phase.

Treatment regimen includes an induction phase (2–6 weeks), followed by a 2- to 6-month eradication phase using oral TMP/SMX or doxycycline.

Lung Fluke

GENERAL PRINCIPLES

Paragonimiasis is a food-borne parasitic zoonosis caused by the genus *Paragonimus*.

It is endemic in many parts of Asia. *P. westermani* has been reported from many countries such as Japan, Korea, Taiwan, China, Vietnam, Thailand, Myanmar, Laos, Cambodia, Indonesia, Nepal, Pakistan, Papua New Guinea, Malaysia, Philippines, Sri Lanka, and Northeast India.

Fresh water snails and crabs or crayfish are the first and second intermediate hosts, respectively. Humans acquire this infection by ingesting uncooked/undercooked crustaceans.

DIAGNOSIS

Clinical Presentation

The patients may present with signs and symptoms of mild pleural effusion, pneumonitis, bronchiectasis, or bronchopneumonia. The common presenting symptoms are pain or tightness in the chest, difficulty in breathing, rusty brown or blood-stained sputum, or recurrent hemoptysis. Chronic infection presents with fever, anemia, weakness, and weight loss.

Extrapulmonary paragonimiasis is caused by immature flukes migrating to various distant sites like brain, abdomen, and lymph nodes.

Diagnostic Testing

Laboratory diagnosis of paragonimiasis is done by demonstration of ova in the sputum/feces/pleural fluid or by serology. Radiological imaging may reveal one or more lesions at the sites of encysted flukes. Lesions are located more peripherally and in the mid and lower lung zones.

Differential Diagnosis

Pulmonary paragonimiasis presenting with hemoptysis is commonly misdiagnosed as pulmonary tuberculosis. Other differentials include Loeffler's syndrome, coccidioidomycosis, aspergillosis, histoplasmosis, nocardiosis, bronchiectasis, and malignancies.

TREATMENT

Praziquantel is the drug of choice and is given at a dose of 25 mg/kg/day in three divided doses for three days.

Enteric Fever

GENERAL PRINCIPLES

- Enteric fever (typhoid) is the commonest bacterial bloodstream infection and important public health concern in South Asia.
- It is caused by *Salmonella enterica* serovars Typhi and Paratyphi A.
- According to estimates, around 10.3 million people are affected each year in South Asia with India accounting for 8.3 million cases annually, and these figures may be grossly underestimated because of limitations in population-based surveillance systems and reliable diagnostic methods.

DIAGNOSIS

Clinical Presentation

- Typhoid presents with undifferentiated fever in the initial stages and is often confused with other common causes of acute fever in tropical regions.
- In the first week, patients develop rising (stepwise) fever associated with chills. Relative bradycardia may be observed. In the second week, patients develop abdominal pain and "rose spots" over the trunk and abdomen. In the following week, they progressively develop hepatosplenomegaly, intestinal bleeding, and perforation. Patients may worsen and develop encephalopathy and septic shock.
- There is also a risk of relapse and chronic fecal carriage. The mortality from untreated typhoid has been estimated at 10% or more.

Diagnostic Testing

- Isolation of *Salmonella* Typhi on blood culture is required for a definitive diagnosis and antibiotic susceptibility pattern. Bone marrow culture is the most sensitive diagnostic modality but is rarely indicated.
- Widal test (serological test) is widely used by clinicians in South Asia to diagnose typhoid. It relies on fourfold or greater rise in antibody titre against the H and O antigens of *Salmonella* Typhi between the acute and convalescent stages of disease to reach the diagnosis. However, it is not reliable to interpret results, particularly when it is used as a stand-alone test.

- Rapid antibody-based tests: Tubex, which measures immunoglobulin IgM antibodies to *S. Typhi* lipopolysaccharide and Typhidot, which measures IgM or IgG responses to an outer membrane protein have moderate diagnostic accuracy.
- Newer tests like detecting serum IgA against hemolysin E are under development.
- ELISA for antibodies to capsular polysaccharide Vi antigen are useful for detecting carriers in high-risk populations.

TREATMENT

- With appropriate antimicrobial treatment, symptoms typically resolve within a week and risk of mortality is less than 1%.
- Fluoroquinolones such as ciprofloxacin and ofloxacin are the drugs of choice for empiric therapy in fluoroquinolone susceptible individuals
- Azithromycin remains an effective oral option.
- Third-generation cephalosporins such as ceftriaxone and cefixime are commonly used in many parts of the world. In case of suspected ceftriaxone resistance, empiric carbapenems can be started while awaiting sensitivity testing.

Drug Resistance

- Since 2016, outbreaks of extensively drug-resistant *Salmonella* Typhi strains that are resistant to ceftriaxone and cefixime have been reported in parts of Pakistan.
- Rapid global spread of variants resistant to ampicillin, trimethoprim-sulfamethoxazole, and chloramphenicol have been observed.
- Near-universal resistance to ciprofloxacin has been observed in recent isolates from India.

Prevention

Several typhoid vaccines are available:

- Live attenuated vaccine: An oral vaccine (Ty21a vaccine) supplied in enteric-coated capsules taken once daily for 3 days
- Typhoid conjugate vaccine: Injectable Vi polysaccharide vaccine (ViCPS vaccine) given intramuscularly in a single dose
- Typhibev, containing Vi conjugated to CRM_{197} was approved by WHO in 2020.

Fever of Unknown Origin

GENERAL FEATURES

Definitions

- FUO is currently defined as:
  - fever (>38.3°C or >101°F) on at least two occasions
  - with an illness lasting for ≥ 3 weeks
  - in a patient who is not immunosuppressed,
  - the diagnosis remains uncertain after thorough history taking, examination, and reasonable investigation.
- The earlier classification of FUO as classical, nosocomial, HIV related, and immune deficient is no longer of interest as the current approach is to work up each patient as an individual entity.

ETIOLOGY (TABLE 14-23)

TABLE 14-23 Etiology of FUO

Infections	
Bacterial	Abscesses in the abdomen, epidural space, pharyngeal space, intracranial, liver, kidney, spleen, lungs, and muscles Appendicitis, peritonitis, cholecystitis, endocarditis, and septic arthritis Urinary tract infections Mastoiditis and osteomyelitis Melioidosis Atypical pneumonias Infected catheters, devices, and prosthesis Rickettsial fevers Sexually transmitted infections—chlamydia, LGV, and syphilis
Viral	Dengue virus, EBV, hepatitis viruses, HIV, CMV, and herpes simplex
Fungal	Aspergillosis, coccidioidomycosis, paracoccidioidomycosis, histoplasmosis, and candidiasis
Parasites	Malaria, filariasis, babesiosis, hydatid cysts, toxoplasmosis, trypanosomiasis, and leishmaniasis
Mycobacterial	Tuberculosis and leprosy
Noninfections	
Inflammation	*Autoimmune diseases:* SLE, Sjögren, rheumatoid arthritis, APLA syndrome, vasculitis, rheumatic fever, seronegative spondyloarthropathies, inflammatory bowel disease, autoimmune hepatitis, and autoimmune hemolytic anemias Granulomatous: Sarcoidosis *Inflammatory syndromes:* Still disease, hemophagocytic syndrome, familial Mediterranean fever, and periodic fever syndromes
Neoplasms	Hematologic cancers, solid tumors, and myelomas
Endocrine	Hyperthyroidism, Cushing syndrome, Addison disease, and thyroiditis
Miscellaneous	Acute disseminated encephalomyelitis, amyloidosis, Kikuchi disease, Castleman disease, Rosai–Dorfman disease, pulmonary embolism, deep vein thrombosis, fume fever, factitious fevers, complex status epilepticus, cerebrovascular accident, hypothalamic dysfunction, heat hyperpyrexia, malignant neuroleptic syndrome, malignant hyperthermia, and serum sickness
Drugs	Any drug can cause drug fever. Exceptions are drugs such as digoxin.
Substance abuse	Alcohol, cannabis, cocaine, heroin, and methanol
Poisoning	Organophosphate poisoning, fish poisoning, snake bite, yellow phosphorus, and copper sulfate

BASIC WORKUP (FIGURE 14-16)

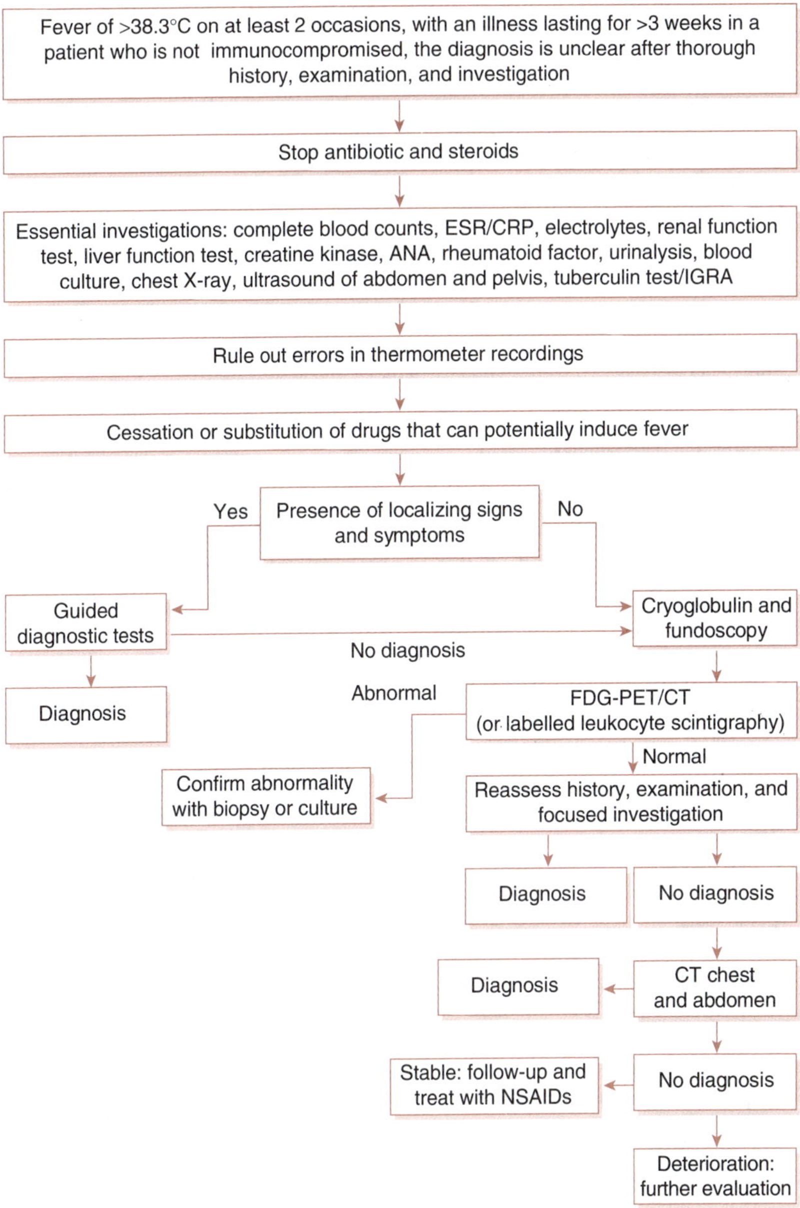

Figure 14-16 Algorithmic approach to FUO.

STRUCTURED APPROACH TO A PATIENT WITH FUO (TABLE 14-24)

TABLE 14-24 Structured Approach to a Patient with FUO
Initial diagnostic testing should include: Complete blood count with differential • Complete metabolic panel (LFT with PT INR, RFT, CPK, LDH) • Urine analysis with microscopy and urine culture • Erythrocyte sedimentation rate (ESR) • C-reactive protein (CRP) • HIV immunoassay • Glycosylated hemoglobin • Thyroid profile • Stool analysis
Chest X-ray
Ultrasound abdomen (venous Doppler of limbs if indicated)
Cardiac echocardiography - culture-negative endocarditis or atrial myxoma.
Cultures and Microbiology • Blood, sputum, urine, stool, ascitic fluid, CSF, pleural fluid, pericardial fluid, pus from abscess, joint space, swabs from soft tissue, endotracheal tube suction tip, central line catheter tip, bronchoalveolar lavage, removed prosthetic device, and crushed lymph node biopsy samples can be sent. Aerobic, anaerobic, and fungal cultures are usually done. • Three sets of blood cultures (from different sites, several hours apart, and prior to initiation of antibiotic therapy) • KOH mount and SDA medium are used to identify fungal elements. • Special preparations such as India ink are used for Cryptococcus. • AFB stain can be used to identify mycobacteria, Nocardia, and Cryptosporidium oocyst. • Serological testing: For HIV and hepatitis B and C. IgM ELISA is available for most viral and bacteriological infections. • Galactomannan tests are available for fungal identification, and they are species specific. • DNA and nucleic acid detection is available for tuberculosis, herpes, CMV, and hepatitis B and C. • Skin tests: Mantoux test is available for tuberculosis, lepromin test for leprosy, Casoni test for hydatid cyst, and Montenegro test for leishmaniasis.
Other Blood Investigations ANA, RA factor, anti-CCP antibody, ANCA, anticardiolipin antibody, HLA-B27, and serum ferritin are all used as markers for rheumatologic diseases.
Advanced Imaging CT chest and abdomen – effusions, collections, lymph node enlargement, granulomas, organomegaly, cysts, minor lung infiltrates, small cavities in the lung, and retroperitoneal masses and nodes. CT/MRI brain with contrast and angiography/venogram - space-occupying lesions such as tuberculoma, NCC, toxoplasmosis, cryptococcomas, encephalitis, brain abscess, mycotic aneurysms, CNS lymphomas, CNS tumors, ADEM, cerebral venous thrombosis, paranasal sinus infections, middle ear infections, skull bone, and skull base osteomyelitis.

(Continued)

TABLE 14-24 Structured Approach to a Patient with FUO (Continued)
Fluorodeoxyglucose positron emission tomography (FDG-PET)/CT - occult malignancies and metastasis; granulomatous diseases such as tuberculosis.
Biopsies Lymph node biopsies, solid organ biopsies such as liver biopsy, pleural biopsy, kidney biopsy and brain biopsy Bone marrow biopsy with flow cytometry -hematologic malignancies. Endoscopic examination of the upper and lower gastrointestinal tract – Crohn's disease, biliary tract disease, and gastrointestinal tumors Temporal artery biopsy – giant cell arteritis

Acute Undifferentiated Fever (AUF)

GENERAL PRINCIPLES

- AUF is a common cause of patients seeking healthcare in developing countries. It is defined as fever of <14 days duration with nonlocalizing signs and symptoms.[106]
- Acute undifferentiated febrile illness (AUFI) has a wide spectrum of causes ranging from infectious to noninfectious. A number of viruses, bacteria, protozoa, and rickettsia can cause AUFI.
- The most notable infectious etiologies include scrub typhus, dengue fever, malaria, enteric fever, and leptospirosis, all leading to significant morbidity and mortality. Nonspecific symptoms and signs along with the lack of accurate diagnostics often leads to irrational use of antibiotics and antimalarials.
- Concurrent infection with more than one etiologic agent results in illness with overlapping symptoms. It further makes the diagnosis and management of such patients challenging.

DIAGNOSIS

- Algorithmic approach to a patient with AUFI

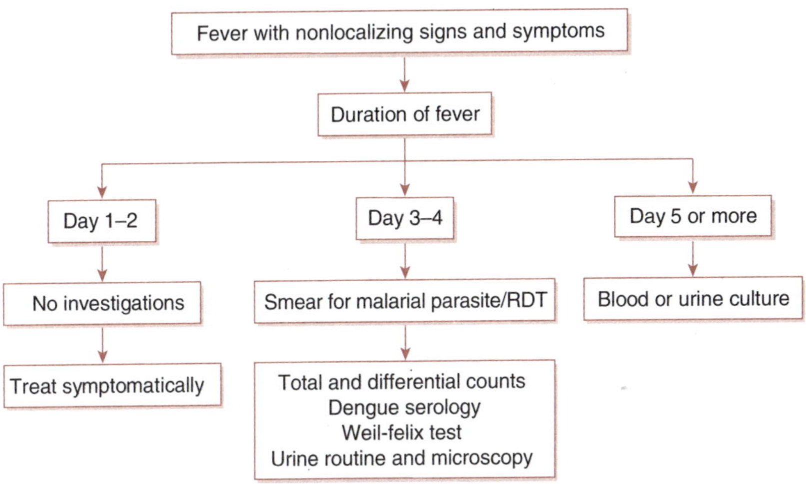

TABLE 14-25 Common Differential Diagnosis for AUFI

	Malaria	Dengue	Leptospirosis	Typhoid	Typhus
Hemoglobin	Decreased	Increased	Normal/ decreased	Normal	Normal/ decreased
Total counts	Normal	Decreased	Increased	Decreased	Increased
Platelets	Decreased	Decreased	Decreased	Normal	Mildly decreased
Hyperbilirubinemia	Present (mild)	Nil	Present (severe)	Nil	Present (mild)
Transaminitis	Mild	Mild to moderate	Severe	Mild	Mild to moderate
Renal failure	Present	Rare	Common	Rare	Present
Rash	Rare	Common (petechiae)	Common (petechiae/ ecchymosis)	Rare (rose spots)	Eschar
ARDS	Common	Common	Common	Rare	Common
Amylase	Normal	Normal	Increased	Normal	Normal

- The clinical features across the spectrum of different coinfection categories (Table 14-25) are nonspecific. Fever with chills and myalgia are common symptoms.

SARS-CoV-2

The coronavirus pandemic caused by the SARS-CoV-2 (Severe Acute Respiratory Syndrome CoronaVirus-2) began in March 2020 in India and has currently claimed more than 3 million lives globally. The virus was first identified in Wuhan, China. The origin of the virus is unknown; however, the earliest cases isolated in China could be traced back to the Huanan Seafood Market in Wuhan. It was later speculated that the virus is of zoonotic origin, most closely related to the coronavirus species seen in bats and pangolins.

As we move into the fourth year with the virus taking over the global ecosystem, it is both important and interesting to learn more about the virus that pushed our healthcare to its limits.

GENERAL PRINCIPLES

- COVID-19 is caused by infection with an enveloped betacoronavirus, SARS-CoV-2.

STRUCTURE OF SARS-COV-2

SARS-CoV-2 is a positive stranded RNA virus.

The viral genome is surrounded by:

- Nucleocapsid (N) protein
- Spike (S) protein
- Envelope (E) protein
- Membrane (M) proteins
- Hemagglutinin esterase (HE) glycoprotein

Over time, SARS-CoV-2 has developed several mutations in its genome, and each of these variants are denoted as variants of concern (VOC). Some of them are associated with increased risk of transmissibility. The B.1.1.7 (Alpha), B.1.351 (Beta), P.1 (Gamma), B.1.427 (Epsilon), B.1.429 (Epsilon), B.1.617.2 (Delta), and B.1.1.529 (Omicron) variants are classified as variants of concern.

TRANSMISSION

- Person to person transmission through respiratory particles.
- Aerosols that are generated during certain procedures (use of nebulizers).
- Fomites/air borne transmission may not play a major role.

Higher risks of transmission are observed with increased closeness of contact and prolonged duration of contact.

PATHOGENESIS (FIGURE 14-17)

(1) The S1 subunit of the spike protein of the virus contains the receptor binding domain (RBD) that binds to angiotensin-converting enzyme 2 (ACE 2) on the host cell. Other than respiratory epithelium, the ACE 2 receptors are found on intestinal epithelium and endothelium of blood vessels, which explains the gastrointestinal symptoms and cardiovascular complications.
(2) Viral binding to the host target cell receptor is followed by membrane fusion and releases the viral genome into the host cytoplasm.
(3) Translation.

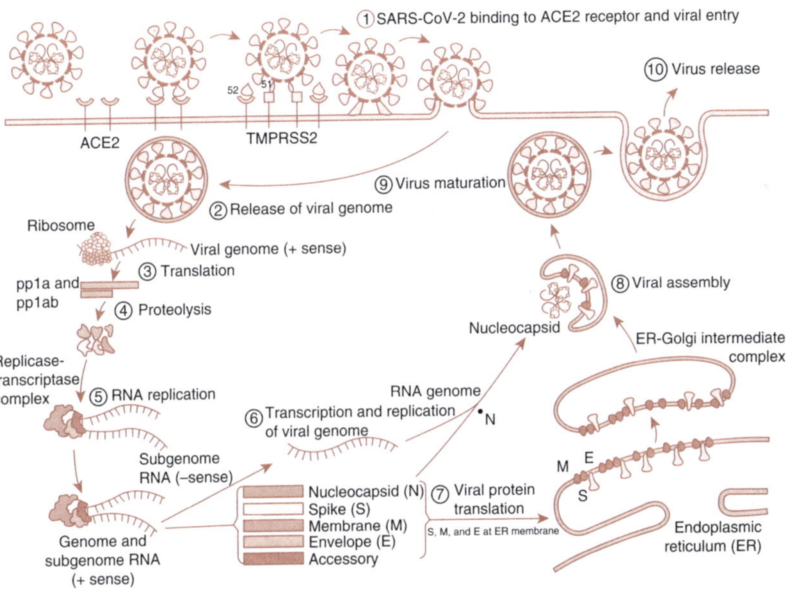

Figure 14-17 Pathogenesis of SARS-CoV-2.

(4) Proteolysis.
(5) RNA replication.
(6) Transcription and replication of viral genome.
(7) Viral protein translation.
(8) Viral assembly.
(9) Maturation.
(10) Release of infectious viral particles.

DIAGNOSIS

Clinical Presentation

The incubation period is up to 14 days following exposure. The median time duration from exposure to symptom onset is 4 to 5 days.

The clinical spectrum ranges from asymptomatic cases to severe and fatal COVID-19 infection. Common clinical presentations include the following:

- Fever
- Sore throat
- Nasal congestion or rhinorrhea
- Cough
- Shortness of breath
- Fatigue
- Myalgia
- Headache
- New loss of taste (ageusia) or smell (anosmia)
- Nausea or vomiting
- Diarrhea

Some patients develop severe disease with multiorgan dysfunction syndrome. Risk factors for severe COVID-19 illness include the following:

- Older age
- Cancer
- Cerebrovascular disease
- Chronic kidney disease
- Chronic obstructive pulmonary disease
- Diabetes mellitus
- Heart conditions (such as heart failure, coronary artery disease, or cardiomyopathies)
- Obesity
- Pregnancy
- Smoking (current and former)
- Immunocompromised state

Postacute Sequelae of SARS-CoV-2 Infection (PASC)/Post-COVID Conditions

Symptoms that are present for more than 4 weeks after acute infection has resolved. These include the following:

- Undue fatigue
- Difficulty concentrating ("brain fog")
- Sleep disturbances
- Dyspnea and post-COVID pulmonary fibrosis have also been reported.

"Long-COVID," also referred to as postacute COVID-19, chronic COVID-19 refers to symptoms that develop during or after acute COVID-19 illness, continue for ≥12 weeks, and are not explained by an alternative diagnosis.

Complications

- Acute respiratory distress syndrome: Acute inflammatory exudation involves lung parenchyma. Type 1 respiratory failure is a common finding. However, the development of acute type 2 respiratory failure is a sign of impending respiratory arrest.
- Venous thromboembolism: COVID-19 is associated with a hypercoagulable state. The risk for venous thromboembolism, notably DVT and pulmonary embolism, is markedly increased in patients admitted to the intensive care unit.
- Cardiovascular complications include arrythmias, myocarditis, heart failure, and cardiac arrest. The major risk factors for arrythmias include hypoxia, shock, and electrolyte disturbances.
- Disseminated intravascular coagulation and its sequelae.
- Acute kidney injury: The incidence of AKI is higher in acutely ill hospitalized patients with COVID-19. Many patients may require renal replacement therapy. Major pathogenic mechanisms include hemodynamic instability, thrombotic complications, and direct tubular injury.
- Neurological complications:
  - Delirium, meningoencephalitis, stroke, ADEM, and Guillain–Barre syndrome.
  - The postulated mechanisms are direct neuroinvasion, hypoxemia, molecular mimicry between SARS-CoV2 epitope, and myelin basic protein.
- Cytokine release syndrome:
  - Immune dysregulation is characterized by elevated cytokine levels, systemic inflammation, capillary leak syndrome, and multiorgan dysfunction. Immune hyperactivation coupled with inadequate negative regulation is thought to be the underlying mechanism involved in cytokine storm.
- Multisystem inflammatory syndrome in adults (MIS-A):
  - Children with recent COVID-19 infection present with Kawasaki-like illness, which was termed MIS-C. A similar condition has been described in adults, wherein, they present with fever, gastrointestinal symptoms, LV dysfunction, and elevated inflammatory markers. This is termed as multisystem inflammatory syndrome in adults (MIS-A).
- Infections related to immunosuppression: Mucormycosis and Aspergillosis
  - Opportunistic infections developing in COVID-19 patients on immunosuppression with steroids. It is more common in the presence of risk factors like diabetes mellitus/post-transplant, etc.

Diagnostic Testing

- Complete blood count—lymphopenia is commonly seen.
- Liver function test (LFT)—elevated transaminase levels
- Baseline renal function test
- Lactate dehydrogenase
- D-dimer
- Inflammatory markers (ferritin, C-reactive protein, and erythrocyte sedimentation rate)
- Chest X-ray (CXR) may not reveal any abnormality in mild cases. CXR in moderate to severe cases may reveal consolidation and ground-glass opacities in bilateral, peripheral, and lower lung zones. These findings are not unique to COVID-19 and are frequently seen with other viral pneumonias as well.
- Chest CT is reserved for hospitalized patients with COVID-19, whenever it is expected to make a difference in the management.

CT severity score: Each of the five lung lobes is scored on a scale of 0 to 5. Total score is the sum of lobar scores. Maximum score is 25.

Score of <8 is considered mild, 9–15 moderate, and >15 severe.

MANAGEMENT

For patients with mild disease, only supportive care is recommended, with close monitoring for clinical worsening. Treatment algorithm is discussed in Figure 14-18.

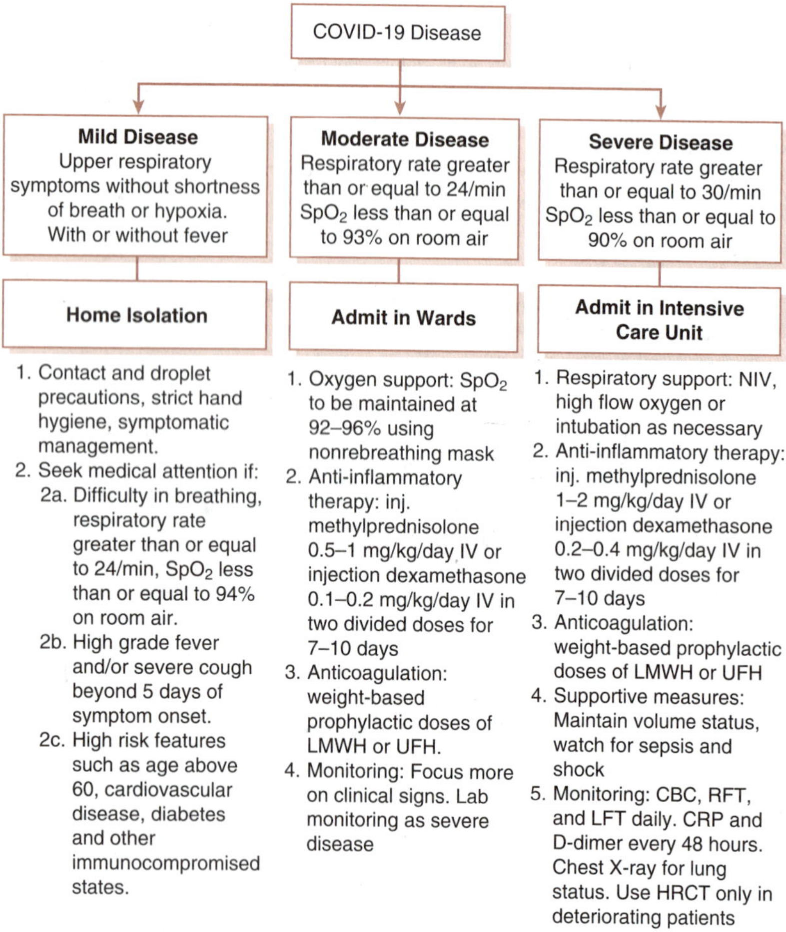

Figure 14-18 Treatment of COVID-19.

COVID-19 Specific Therapies

STEROIDS

The use of dexamethasone is reserved for severely ill patients with COVID-19 who are on supplemental oxygen or ventilatory support. Dexamethasone is given at a dose of 6 mg daily for 10 days or until discharge, whichever is shorter.

In the Randomized Evaluation of COVID-19 Therapy (RECOVERY) trial, dexamethasone group had a 17% relative reduction in the 28-day mortality among hospitalized patients compared with usual care alone.[108]

However, dexamethasone is not recommended in patients with nonsevere disease.

REMDESIVIR

In the SOLIDARITY trial, among patients hospitalized with COVID-19, there was no difference in overall 28-day mortality between remdesivir group compared to standard care.[109]

However, in the ACTT-1 trial, among patients who were on oxygen supplementation (but did not require high-flow oxygen or ventilatory support), there was a statistically significant mortality benefit with remdesivir.[110] The study also found a nonstatistically significant trend towards higher mortality among patients who did not require oxygen or ventilatory support.

Hence remdesivir is recommended for those requiring low-flow supplemental oxygen. The recommended dose is 200 mg intravenously on day 1, followed by 100 mg daily for 5 days (with extension to 10 days if there is no clinical improvement and in patients on mechanical ventilation or ECMO).

Remdesivir is not recommended in patients with an estimated glomerular filtration rate (eGFR) <30 mL/min per 1.73 m^2 unless the benefit outweighs the risk.

It is recommended to monitor LFT while on remdesivir. It should be discontinued if alanine aminotransferase (ALT) elevation is >10 times the upper limit of normal.

TOCILIZUMAB

Tocilizumab is an IL-6 receptor antagonist, given at a dose of 8 mg/kg as a single dose infusion over 60 minutes. Recommendations on its use are summarized below:

Guidelines	Recommendations to Add Tocilizumab to Dexamethasone
The National Institutes of Health[111]	In hospitalized patients who are on high-flow oxygen or greater support and have been admitted to the ICU within the past 24 h Or Have significantly increased inflammatory markers
The Infectious Diseases Society of America[112]	For hospitalized adults who have progressive severe COVID-19 and have elevated inflammatory markers

BARICITINIB

An oral Janus kinase inhibitor, baricitinib, which was used for treatment of rheumatoid arthritis, is thought to interfere with the SARS-CoV-2 viral entry. The US-FDA has issued emergency use authorization (EUA) for baricitinib 4 mg orally once daily for up to

14 days to be given in combination with remdesivir, in patients with COVID-19 who require oxygen or ventilatory support, as an alternative to tocilizumab.[113] Another similar molecule is tofacitinib.

Other molecules used in the past which now have questionable efficacy:

1. Convalescent plasma
2. Monoclonal antibodies (was useful in the past variants of SARS-CoV-2)
3. **Hydroxychloroquine:** In the RECOVERY trial, hydroxychloroquine did not decrease mortality among hospitalized patients, as compared with standard care.[114]
4. **Azithromycin**
5. **Lopinavir-ritonavir**
6. **Favipiravir** (RNA polymerase inhibitor)
7. Ivermectin
8. Inhaled interferon beta
9. Anakinra

GENERAL MEASURES

- Isolation of the patient
- Antipyretics
- Fluid and electrolytes management
- Thromboprophylaxis:
  - Hospitalized patients with COVID-19 (including those admitted to ICU) should receive prophylactic dose of anticoagulation.
  - The American Society of Hematology has recommended prophylactic dose of anticoagulation rather than high dose in individuals with COVID-19 acute and critical illness.[115]
  - Drugs used: Enoxaparin 40 mg once daily (for patients with creatinine clearance > 30 mL/min). In those with CrCl <30 mL/min, unfractionated heparin can be used.
  - There are no recommendations for routine postdischarge thromboprophylaxis.
  - However, extended thromboprophylaxis may be considered based on modified IMPROVE (International Medical Prevention Registry on Venous Thromboembolism) VTE risk score and D-dimer levels. Tablet Apixaban 2.5 mg BD for 2 to 3 weeks may be considered if the following criteria are met:

• Modified IMPROVE VTE risk score ≥4 OR
• Modified IMPROVE VTE risk score ≥2 and D-dimer levels ≥2 times upper limit of normal
• With low-bleeding risk

MANAGEMENT OF HYPOXIA

- Awake self-proning
- Modes of oxygenation:
  - Nasal cannula for low-flow oxygen delivery
  - Nonrebreather mask (NRBM)
  - Venturi masks
  - High-flow nasal cannula (HFNC)
  - Noninvasive ventilation (NIV)
  - Intubation and mechanical ventilation: Rapid sequence intubation (RSI)

- WHO suggests titrating oxygen to a target SpO_2 of ≥94% during initial resuscitation and ≥90% for maintenance oxygenation. Individualization of this goal is important, as some patients may require a lower target (for example, those with COPD)
- ARDS management as per protocol: Low tidal volume ventilation
- For refractory hypoxemia: Prone ventilation/recruitment maneuvers
- Use of in-line metered dose inhalers for delivering bronchodilators

COVID-19 Vaccine

Ever since the WHO declared COVID-19 as a global pandemic in 2019, several attempts have been made to develop a preventive vaccine against the disease. The aim of the COVID-19 vaccine is to induce protective immunity to prevent symptomatic infection and further to prevent severe illness, hospitalization, and death.

VACCINE TYPES

- mRNA-based vaccines: Moderna (mRna-1273) and Pfizer-BioNTech (Bnt162b2).
- Viral vector-based vaccines: chimpanzee adenovirus ChAdox1 based Oxford/AstraZeneca (Vaxzevria, Covishield), human adenoviruses type 26 and type 5 based Sputnik V and human adenovirus type 26 based Johnson & Johnson (Janssen).
- Inactivated/killed virus vaccines: Bharat Biotech Covaxin and Sinovac Biotech.
- Subunit (spike-protein) vaccine: Novavax.

DOSING

- Moderna vaccine: 0.5 mL per dose for two doses administered 28 days apart.
- Pfizer–BioNTech vaccine: 0.3 mL per dose for two doses administered 21 days apart.
- AstraZeneca vaccine/Covishield*: 0.5 mL per dose for 2 doses 4–12 weeks apart. The WHO recommends a dosing interval of 8–12 weeks due to increased immunogenicity observed with longer dosing intervals.
- Janssen vaccine: 0.5 mL as a single dose.
- Bharat Biotech Covaxin*: 0.5 mL per dose for two doses 4 to 12 weeks apart.
- Sputnik V vaccine: 0.5 mL per dose for two doses 3 weeks apart.
- Sinovac Biotech vaccine: 0.5 mL per dose for two doses 2 to 4 weeks apart.

Eligible age groups: All persons aged 18 and above.

As limited data is available in children less than 18 years of age, the WHO does not recommend vaccination in this age group, even if they belong to the high-risk group. The Pfizer–BioNTech, Moderna, Covishield, and Covaxin vaccine were previously authorized for use in age groups 16 years and above. This has been amended by the FDA on May 10, 2021 to include adolescents between 12 and 15 years of age.

CONTRAINDICATIONS

- History of severe allergic reaction to the previous dose or to a component of the vaccine.
- History of immediate allergic reaction within 4 hours of vaccine administration regardless of the severity of the reaction.
- Known allergy to any component of the vaccine (e.g., polysorbate 80).

*Recently, longer dosing intervals of 12 to 16 weeks have been recommended by national authorities (NTAGI and NEGVAC) in India.

- Pregnancy and lactation: The WHO does not recommend routinely vaccinating pregnant and lactating women. However, vaccination is recommended in all pregnant and lactating women belonging to the high-risk group for example, healthcare workers.
- Avoid vaccinating persons with moderate to severe acute febrile illness.
- Vaccination should be deferred in patients with active current COVID-19 infection till the person has recovered from the acute illness and no longer requires isolation. Prior history of COVID-19 infection is not a contraindication for vaccination irrespective of the severity of illness.

WARNINGS AND PRECAUTIONS

- Use with caution in patients with bleeding disorders as there is risk of hematoma following intramuscular injection. Vaccination should be scheduled shortly after antihemophilic therapy in those receiving the same.
- Patients on standard intensity anticoagulation with warfarin (target INR 2.0 – 3.0) can receive intramuscular injections as long as the most recent INR is <3.0.
- Patients on maintenance therapy with direct oral anticoagulants (Apixaban, Dabigatran, Edoxaban, and Rivaroxaban) can delay the dose on the day of vaccination until after the intramuscular injection but do not need to miss any doses.
- Patients on single agent antiplatelet therapy (e.g., aspirin or clopidogrel) can continue these medications without any adjustment.
- Patients with higher intensity antithrombotic treatment, for example warfarin with a target INR > 3.0 or dual antithrombotic medications, should be managed on an individual basis.
- Allow a minimum period of 14 days before or after administration of other vaccines.
- HIV and immunocompromised persons: Data regarding efficacy and safety is lacking in this population group. However, the CDC recommends vaccination in all persons with immunocompromised state included those with HIV or receiving immunosuppressive therapy if there is no contraindication. Ideally, complete vaccination ≥2 weeks prior to the immunosuppressive therapy if possible.

EFFICACY

All approved vaccines have an efficacy of almost 100% in preventing hospitalization and death. Data regarding vaccine efficacy is limited and studies are still underway.

The mRNA-1273 vaccine showed an overall efficacy of 94.1% at preventing COVID-19 illness, including severe disease after 2 standard doses.

The Bnt162b2 (Pfizer–BioNTech) vaccine was 100% effective against severe COVID-19 disease as defined by the CDC, USA and 95.3% effective against severe COVID-19 as defined by the FDA.

The overall vaccine efficacy after 2 standard doses of the ChAdox1 vaccine was 66.7% according to one study and 70.4% according to another. Those with longer dosing intervals between the two doses had higher efficacy at preventing symptomatic disease (81.3% at ≥12 weeks vs. 55.1% at <6 weeks).

Only the mRNA vaccines have studies conducted with proven efficacy against variant viruses.

ADVERSE EFFECTS

Common adverse effects include injection site pain, chills, fatigue, headache, and body aches.

They can be treated with acetaminophen when required. Avoid routinely using this medication prophylactically before or during vaccination, as it may diminish the therapeutic effect of the vaccine.

Very few cases of severe allergic reactions, anaphylaxis, and angioedema have been reported. Routine use of antihistamines prophylactically for allergic reactions should be avoided as it may mask the symptoms of anaphylaxis and delay diagnosis and treatment.

The Strategic Advisory Group of Experts on Immunization (SAGE) recommends that all vaccines be observed for 15 minutes after vaccination and that no further doses be given to those who develop an immediate severe allergic reaction to the first dose.

A very rare new type of adverse event called thrombosis with thrombocytopenia syndrome (TTS, also called vaccine induced immune thrombotic thrombocytopenia [VITT] or vaccine induced prothrombotic immune thrombocytopenia [VIPIT]), has been reported after vaccination with COVID-19 vaccines Vaxzevria and Covishield. It is characterized by unusual and severe blood clotting events associated with decreased platelet counts, in the absence of heparin exposure. Incidence of this rare syndrome is around 1/100,000 to 250,000 as per data from EU and UK reports. Most patients present within 5 to 30 days of vaccination with thrombosis, particularly cerebral venous thrombosis, splanchnic vein thrombosis, adrenal vein thrombosis and less commonly, pulmonary embolism and ischemic stroke. The TTS syndrome has not been linked to mRNA-based vaccines (such as Comirnaty or the Moderna mRNA-1273 vaccine). The exact pathophysiological mechanism by which these vaccines trigger TTS is not known, but it is likened to spontaneous heparin-induced thrombocytopenia (HIT) and is believed to be due to antibodies directed against platelet factor 4.

Management includes administration of therapeutic doses of anticoagulants, preferably a nonheparin-based anticoagulant without delay in all patients, if the suspicion for TTS is high. Additionally, treatment with intravenous immune globulin (IVIG) should be considered in all patients with TTS. Platelet transfusions are generally avoided to minimize the risk of further thrombosis and reserved for those patients with critical bleeding. FFPs and cryoprecipitates may be transfused in TTS patients with critical bleeding and hypofibrinogenemia.

Summary

- Overuse of antimicrobials has led to an epidemic caused by antimicrobial-resistant organisms, including some multidrug-resistant organisms (MDRO) with few remaining treatment options.
- Empiric antimicrobial therapy should be directed against the most likely infecting organism(s). Antibiograms provide important insight into trends in local antimicrobial resistance.
- De-escalate to an antimicrobial regimen with the narrowest spectrum of activity once the infectious etiologic agent has been identified and susceptibility data are available.
- Use the shortest duration of therapy for the infection identified.
- Toxin-mediated infections include *C. difficile* infection, tetanus, and toxic shock syndrome.
- Hospital-acquired infections (HAI) infections include central line-associated bloodstream infections (CLABSI), catheter-associated urinary tract infections (CAUTI), surgical site infections (SSI), hospital-acquired pneumonia (HAP), ventilator-associated pneumonia (VAP), and *C. difficile* infections (CDI).
- Molecular drug sensitivity tests should be obtained for all TB cases for rapid detection of mutations associated with resistance. When rifampin resistance is detected,

additional drug susceptibility testing (DST) should be performed immediately for first-line drugs, fluoroquinolones, and aminoglycosides. Resistance to fluoroquinolones should be excluded whenever isoniazid resistance is found.

- Pyrexia of unknown origin continues to be a diagnostic and management challenge for clinicians around the globe.
- Acute undifferentiated febrile illness (AUFI) is a term used to define a fever of less than two weeks (fourteen days) of duration without any evident focus of infection on initial physical examination or in basic laboratory tests.

Scan the QR code to access chapter references.

15 Antimicrobials

David J. Ritchie, Nigar Kirmani, Pranavjith A, and Kunal Seth

Introduction

As microbial resistance is increasing among many pathogens, a review of institutional as well as local, regional, national, and global susceptibility trends can assist in the development of empiric therapy regimens. Antimicrobial therapy should be modified based on results of culture and sensitivity testing to definitive therapy agent(s) that have the narrowest spectrum possible. In many cases, shorter durations of therapy have been shown to be as effective as traditionally longer courses. As many oral agents have excellent bioavailability, switching from parenteral to oral therapy whenever possible is recommended. Several antibiotics have major drug interactions or require alternate dosing in renal or hepatic insufficiency, or both. For antiretroviral, antiparasitic, and anti-hepatitis agents, see Chapter 16, Sexually Transmitted Infections, Human Immunodeficiency Virus, and Acquired Immunodeficiency Syndrome; Chapter 14, Treatment of Infectious Diseases; and Chapter 19, Liver Diseases, respectively.

ANTIBACTERIAL AGENTS

Penicillins

GENERAL PRINCIPLES

- Penicillins (PCNs) irreversibly bind PCN-binding proteins in the bacterial cell wall, causing osmotic rupture and death. Acquired resistance in many bacterial species through alterations in PCN-binding proteins or expression of hydrolytic enzymes has limited their use.
- PCNs remain among the drugs of choice for syphilis and infections caused by PCN-sensitive streptococci, methicillin-sensitive *Staphylococcus aureus* (MSSA), *Listeria monocytogenes, Pasteurella multocida*, and *Actinomyces*. These are effective against spirochetes (*Leptospira* spp., *Treponema pallidum*) and anaerobes (*Bacteroides*, *Actinomyces*, *Clostridia* spp. [except *C. difficile*]).

USES

- **Aqueous PCN G** (2–5 million units IV q4h or 12–30 million units daily by continuous infusion) is an IV preparation of PCN G and the drug of choice for most PCN-susceptible streptococcal infections and neurosyphilis.
- **Procaine PCN G** is an IM repository form of PCN G that can be used as an alternative treatment for neurosyphilis at a dose of 2.4 million units IM daily in combination with probenecid 500 mg PO qid for 10–14 days
- **Benzathine PCN** is a long-acting IM repository form of PCN G that is used for treating early latent syphilis (<1 year duration [one dose, 2.4 million units IM]) and late latent syphilis (unknown duration or >1 year [2.4 million units IM weekly for three doses]). It is occasionally given for group A streptococcal pharyngitis and prophylaxis after acute rheumatic fever.

- **PCN V** (250–500 mg PO q6h) is an oral formulation of PCN that is typically used to treat group A streptococcal pharyngitis.[1]
- **Ampicillin** (1–3 g IV q4–6h) is the drug of choice for treatment of infections caused by susceptible *Enterococcus* species or *L. monocytogenes*. Oral ampicillin (250–500 mg PO q6h) may be used for uncomplicated sinusitis, pharyngitis, otitis media, and urinary tract infections (UTIs), but amoxicillin is generally preferred.
- **Ampicillin/sulbactam** (1.5–3.0 g IV q6h) combines ampicillin with the β-lactamase inhibitor sulbactam, thereby extending the spectrum to include MSSA, anaerobes, and many Enterobacteriaceae. The sulbactam component also has unique activity against some strains of *Acinetobacter*. The agent is appropriate for treatment of head and neck infections; upper and lower respiratory tract infections; genitourinary tract infections; and abdominal, pelvic, and polymicrobial soft tissue infections, including those due to human or animal bites.[2]
- **Amoxicillin** (250–1000 mg PO q8h, 875 mg PO q12h, or 775 mg extended-release q24h) is an oral antibiotic similar to ampicillin that is used for uncomplicated sinusitis, pharyngitis, otitis media, community-acquired pneumonia (CAP), and UTIs.
- **Amoxicillin/clavulanic acid** (875 mg PO q12h, 500 mg PO q8h, 90 mg/kg/d divided q12h [Augmentin ES-600 suspension], or 2000 mg PO q12h [Augmentin XR]) is an oral antibiotic similar to ampicillin/sulbactam that combines amoxicillin with the β-lactamase inhibitor clavulanate. It is useful for treating complicated sinusitis and otitis media and for prophylaxis of human or animal bites after appropriate local treatment.
- **Nafcillin and oxacillin** (1–2 g IV q4–6h) are penicillinase-resistant synthetic PCNs that are drugs of choice for treating MSSA infections. Dose reduction should be considered in decompensated liver disease.
- **Dicloxacillin** (250–500 mg PO q6h) is an oral antibiotic with a spectrum of activity similar to that of nafcillin and oxacillin, which is typically used to treat localized skin infections.
- **Piperacillin/tazobactam** (3.375 g IV q6h or the higher dose of 4.5 g IV q6h for *Pseudomonas*) combines piperacillin with the β-lactamase inhibitor tazobactam. This combination is active against most Enterobacteriaceae, *Pseudomonas*, MSSA, ampicillin-sensitive enterococci, and anaerobes, making it useful for intra-abdominal and complicated polymicrobial soft tissue infections.
- **Carbenicillin** (382 mg PO q4–6h) and ticarcillin (18 g/d) penetrate the porin channel of gram-negative bacteria and are used for the treatment of UTI.
- Sulbactam, a β-lactam antibacterial and a β-lactamase inhibitor, along with durlobactam, a β-lactamase inhibitor, is indicated for the treatment of hospital-acquired bacterial pneumonia and ventilator-associated bacterial pneumonia (HABP/VABP) in patients 18 years of age and older. This combination is effective against infections caused by susceptible isolates of *Acinetobacter baumannii-calcoaceticus* complex.

SPECIAL CONSIDERATIONS

Adverse events: All PCN derivatives have been associated with anaphylaxis, urticaria, angioedema, interstitial nephritis, elevated liver function tests (LFTs), anemia, leukopenia, and phlebitis. Prolonged high-dose therapy (>2 weeks) is typically monitored with weekly serum creatinine and complete blood count (CBC). Monitoring LFTs is especially important with oxacillin/nafcillin, as these agents can cause hepatitis. All patients should be asked about PCN, cephalosporin, or carbapenem allergies. These agents should not be used in patients with a reported serious PCN allergy without prior skin testing or desensitization, or both.

Cephalosporins

GENERAL PRINCIPLES

- Cephalosporins exert their bactericidal effect by interfering with cell wall synthesis by the same mechanism as PCNs.
- These agents are clinically useful because of their broad spectrum of activity and low toxicity profile. All cephalosporins are devoid of clinically significant activity against enterococci when used alone. Within this class, only ceftaroline is active against methicillin-resistant *S. aureus* (MRSA).

USES

- **First-generation cephalosporins** have activity against staphylococci, streptococci, *Escherichia coli*, and many *Klebsiella* and *Proteus* species. These agents have limited activity against other enteric gram-negative bacilli and anaerobes. **Cefazolin** (1–2 g IV/IM q8h) is the most commonly used parenteral preparation, and **cephalexin** (250–500 mg PO q6h) and **cefadroxil** (500 mg–1 g PO q12h) are oral preparations. These agents are commonly used for treating skin/soft tissue infections, UTIs, MSSA infections, and for surgical prophylaxis (cefazolin).
- **Second-generation cephalosporins** have expanded coverage against enteric gram-negative rods and can be divided into above-the-diaphragm and below-the-diaphragm agents.
  - **Cefuroxime** (1.5 g IV/IM q8h) is useful for treatment of infections above the diaphragm. This agent has reasonable antistaphylococcal and antistreptococcal activity in addition to an extended spectrum against gram-negative aerobes and can be used for skin/soft tissue infections, complicated UTIs, and some community-acquired respiratory tract infections. It does not cover *Bacteroides fragilis*.
  - **Cefuroxime axetil** (250–500 mg PO q12h), **cefprozil** (250–500 mg PO q12h), and **cefaclor** (250–500 mg PO q12h) are oral second-generation cephalosporins typically used for bronchitis, sinusitis, otitis media, UTIs, local soft tissue infections, and oral step-down therapy for pneumonia or cellulitis responsive to parenteral cephalosporins.
  - **Cefoxitin** (1–2 g IV q4–8h) and **cefotetan** (1–2 g IV q12h) are useful for treatment of infections below the diaphragm. These agents have activity against gram negatives and anaerobes, including *B. fragilis*, and are commonly used for intra-abdominal or gynecologic surgical prophylaxis and infections, including diverticulitis and pelvic inflammatory disease.
- **Third-generation cephalosporins** have broad coverage against aerobic gram-negative bacilli and retain significant activity against streptococci and MSSA (except ceftazidime and MSSA). They have moderate anaerobic activity, but generally not against *B. fragilis*. Ceftazidime is the only third-generation cephalosporin that is useful for treating serious *P. aeruginosa* infections. Third-generation cephalosporins are also effective against *Borrelia burgdorferi*. Some of these agents (ceftriaxone, cefotaxime, ceftazidime) have substantial central nervous system (CNS) penetration and are useful in treating meningitis (see Chapter 14, Treatment of Infectious Diseases). Third-generation cephalosporins are not reliable for the treatment of serious infections caused by organisms producing AmpC β-lactamases regardless of the results of susceptibility testing. These resistant pathogens should be treated empirically with carbapenems, cefepime, or fluoroquinolones.
  - **Ceftriaxone** (1–2 g IV/IM q12–24h) and **cefotaxime** (1–2 g IV/IM q4–12h) are very similar in spectrum and efficacy. They can be used as empiric therapy for pyelonephritis, urosepsis, pneumonia, intra-abdominal infections (combined with metronidazole), gonorrhea, and meningitis. They can also be used for osteomyelitis, septic arthritis, endocarditis, and soft tissue infections caused by susceptible organisms. **Ceftriaxone** 2 g

IV q12h in combination with ampicillin IV is appropriate for treatment of ampicillin-sensitive *Enterococcus faecalis* endocarditis, especially when aminoglycosides need to be avoided.

- **Cefpodoxime proxetil** (100–400 mg PO q12h), **cefdinir** (300 mg PO q12h), **ceftibuten** (400 mg PO q24h), and **cefditoren pivoxil** (200–400 mg PO q12h) are oral third-generation cephalosporins useful for the treatment of bronchitis and complicated sinusitis, otitis media, and UTIs. These agents can also be used as step-down therapy for CAP. **Cefixime** (400 mg PO once) is no longer recommended as a first-line therapy for gonorrhea but may be used as alternative therapy for gonorrhea with a close 7-day test-of-cure follow-up.
- **Ceftazidime** (1–2 g IV/IM q8h) may be used for treatment of infections caused by susceptible strains of *P. aeruginosa*, but it is only weakly active against MSSA.

- **The fourth-generation cephalosporin cefepime** (500 mg–2 g IV/IM q8–12h) has excellent aerobic gram-negative coverage, including *P. aeruginosa* and other bacteria producing AmpC β-lactamases. Its gram-positive activity is similar to that of ceftriaxone and cefotaxime. **Cefepime** is routinely used for empiric therapy in febrile neutropenic patients. It also has a prominent role in treating infections caused by antibiotic-resistant gram-negative bacteria and some infections involving both gram-negative and gram-positive aerobes in most sites. Antianaerobic coverage should be added where anaerobes are suspected. Cefepime can be used in combination with enmetazobactam for the treatment of complicated UTIs. Cefiderocol (Fetroja) is a siderophore cephalosporin antibacterial drug that has been developed to combat a wide range of bacterial pathogens, including β-lactam-resistant and carbapenem-resistant organisms. It is administered as an IV infusion, 2 g every 8 hours, for 7–14 days.
- **The fifth-generation cephalosporin ceftaroline** (600 mg IV q12h) is a cephalosporin with anti-MRSA activity that is US Food and Drug Administration (FDA) approved for acute bacterial skin and skin structure infections and community-acquired bacterial pneumonia. **Ceftaroline's** unique MRSA activity is because of its affinity for PCN-binding protein 2a (PBP2a), the same cell wall component that renders MRSA resistant to all other β-lactams. **Ceftaroline** has similar activity to ceftriaxone against gram-negative pathogens, with virtually no activity against *Pseudomonas* spp., *Acinetobacter*, and other organisms producing AmpC β-lactamase, extended-spectrum β-lactamase (ESBL), or *Klebsiella pneumoniae* carbapenemase (KPC). Like all other cephalosporins, it is relatively inactive against *Enterococcus* spp.[3]
- **Ceftolozane-tazobactam** (1 g ceftolozane/0.5 g tazobactam IV q8h) is a combination product consisting of a cephalosporin and a β-lactamase inhibitor tazobactam. This agent is FDA approved for treatment of complicated intra-abdominal infections and complicated UTIs (cUTIs), including pyelonephritis. Ceftolozane-tazobactam has activity against many gram-negative bacteria, including many *P. aeruginosa* that are resistant to antipseudomonal carbapenems, antipseudomonal cephalosporins, and piperacillin-tazobactam. Ceftolozane-tazobactam is also active against some ESBL-producing organisms, especially ESBL-producing *E. coli*, but is not reliably active against MSSA, enterococci, and anaerobes.
- **Ceftazidime-avibactam** (2 g ceftazidime/0.5 g avibactam IV q8h) is a combination product consisting of ceftazidime plus the novel β-lactamase inhibitor avibactam. This agent is FDA approved for treatment of complicated UTIs, complicated intra-abdominal infections, and hospital-acquired/ventilator-associated pneumonia (HABP/VABP). Ceftazidime-avibactam is active against gram-negative bacteria, including some *P. aeruginosa* that are resistant to other antipseudomonal β-lactams. This agent is also active against ESBL- and AmpC-producing strains and possesses unique activity against KPC-producing Enterobacteriaceae (but not against metallo-β-lactamases). Ceftazidime-avibactam is not reliably active against MSSA, enterococci, and anaerobes.

SPECIAL CONSIDERATIONS

Adverse events: All cephalosporins have been rarely associated with anaphylaxis, interstitial nephritis, elevated liver function tests, anemia, thrombocytosis, hemolysis, and leukopenia. **PCN-allergic patients have up to a 5%–10% incidence of a cross-hypersensitivity reaction to cephalosporins.** These agents should not be used in a patient with a reported severe PCN allergy (i.e., anaphylaxis, hives) without prior skin testing or desensitization, or both. Prolonged therapy (>2 weeks) is typically monitored with a weekly serum creatinine and CBC. Because of its biliary elimination, ceftriaxone may cause biliary sludging. Cefepime has been associated with CNS side effects, including delirium and seizures. Cefotetan causes hypoprothrombinemia and disulfiram-like reaction.

Monobactams

GENERAL PRINCIPLES

- **Aztreonam** (1–2 g IV/IM q6–12h) is a monobactam that is active **only** against aerobic gram-negative bacteria, including *P. aeruginosa.*
- It is useful in patients with known serious β-lactam allergy because there is no apparent cross-reactivity.
- Aztreonam is also available in an inhalational dosage form (75 mg inhaled q8h for 28 days) to improve respiratory symptoms in cystic fibrosis patients infected with *P. aeruginosa.*

Carbapenems

GENERAL PRINCIPLES

- **Imipenem** (500 mg–1 g IV/IM q6–8h), **meropenem** (1–2 g IV q8h or 500 mg IV q6h), **doripenem** (500 mg IV q8h), and **ertapenem** (1 g IV q24h) are the currently available carbapenems.
- **Meropenem-vaborbactam** (2 g meropenem/2 g vaborbactam q8h) is a combination product consisting of meropenem plus the β-lactamase inhibitor vaborbactam. This agent is FDA approved for treatment of complicated urinary tract infections, including acute pyelonephritis. Meropenem-vaborbactam possesses unique activity against KPC-producing Enterobacteriaceae (but not against metallo-β-lactamases). However, vaborbactam does not appreciably enhance the activity of meropenem against *Pseudomonas* or *Acinetobacter*. Because of the meropenem component, this agent is reliably active against MSSA and anaerobes.
- Imipenem, cilastatin, and relebactam (Recarbrio): Recarbrio is a regimen comprising imipenem, a penem antibacterial; cilastatin, an inhibitor of the renal dehydropeptidase; and relebactam, a β-lactamase inhibitor. Approved by the FDA in July 2019 for the treatment of cUTIs, including pyelonephritis, and cIAI in patients 18 years of age. It is administered as a 30-minute IV infusion: 500 mg/500 mg/250 mg per vial (1.25 g/vial): 1.25 g IV every 6 hours for 4–14 days (for cUTI) and 1.25 g IV every 6 hours for 4–14 days (for cIAI).
- Carbapenems exert their bactericidal effect by interfering with cell wall synthesis, similar to PCNs and cephalosporins, and are active against most gram-positive and gram-negative bacteria, including anaerobes. They are among the antibiotics of choice for infections caused by organisms producing AmpC or ESBLs.[4]

USES

- Carbapenems are important agents for treatment of many antibiotic-resistant bacterial infections at most body sites. These agents are commonly used for severe polymicrobial infections, including Fournier's gangrene, intra-abdominal catastrophes, and sepsis in immunocompromised hosts.
- Notable bacteria that are **resistant** to carbapenems include ampicillin-resistant enterococci, MRSA, *Stenotrophomonas*, and KPC- and metallo-β-lactamase-producing gram-negative organisms. In addition, ertapenem does not provide reliable coverage against *P. aeruginosa, Acinetobacter*, or enterococci; therefore, imipenem, doripenem, or meropenem would be preferred for empiric treatment of nosocomial infections when these pathogens are suspected. **Meropenem** is the preferred carbapenem for treatment of CNS infections.
- **Faropenem medoxomil** (200 mg PO q12h) is a new orally administered penem antibiotic which has been tried for acute bacterial sinusitis (ABS), acute exacerbations of chronic bronchitis (AECB), CAP, and uncomplicated skin and skin structure infections (uSSSIs). FDA approval is awaited.

SPECIAL CONSIDERATIONS

- **Adverse events:** Carbapenems can precipitate seizure activity, especially in older patients, individuals with renal insufficiency, and patients with preexisting seizure disorders or other CNS pathology, and should be avoided in these patients unless there is no alternative therapy. Like cephalosporins, carbapenems have been rarely associated with anaphylaxis, interstitial nephritis, elevated liver function tests, anemia, and leukopenia.
- **Patients who are allergic to PCNs/cephalosporins may have a cross-hypersensitivity reaction to carbapenems,** and these agents should be avoided in patients with severe PCN allergy without prior skin testing, desensitization, or both. Prolonged therapy (>2 weeks) is typically monitored with a weekly serum creatinine, liver function tests, and complete blood count.

Aminoglycosides

GENERAL PRINCIPLES

- Aminoglycosides exert their bactericidal effect by binding to the bacterial ribosome, causing misreading during translation of bacterial messenger RNA into proteins. These drugs are often used in combination with cell wall–active agents (i.e., β-lactams and vancomycin) for treatment of some severe infections caused by gram-positive and gram-negative aerobes. Some are also active against *Mycobacterium tuberculosis* (MTB) and *MAC* (tobramycin, streptomycin, and amikacin), protozoa (paromomycin), and *Neisseria gonorrhoeae* (spectinomycin).
- Aminoglycosides tend to be synergistic with cell wall–active antibiotics such as PCNs, cephalosporins, and vancomycin. However, they do not have activity against anaerobes, and their activity is impaired in the low pH/low oxygen environment of abscesses. Cross-resistance among aminoglycosides is common, but not absolute, and susceptibility testing with each aminoglycoside is recommended. Use of these antibiotics is limited by **significant nephrotoxicity** and ototoxicity.
- Aminoglyoside antibiotics demonstrate concentration-dependent killing, synergistic effect with other antibiotics, and post-antibiotic effect.

USES

- Traditional dosing of aminoglycosides involves daily divided dosing with the upper end of the dosing range reserved for life-threatening infections. Peak and trough concentrations should be obtained with the third or fourth dose and then every 3–4 days, along with regular serum creatinine monitoring. **Increasing serum creatinine or peak/troughs out of the acceptable range requires immediate attention.**
- **Extended-interval dosing of aminoglycosides** is an alternative method of administration and is more convenient for most indications. Extended-interval doses are provided in the following specific drug sections. A drug concentration is obtained 6–14 hours after the first dose, and a nomogram (Figure 15-1) is consulted to determine the subsequent dosing interval. Monitoring includes obtaining a drug concentration 6–14 hours after the dosage at least every week and a serum creatinine at least three times a week. In patients who are not responding to therapy, a 12-hour concentration should be checked, and

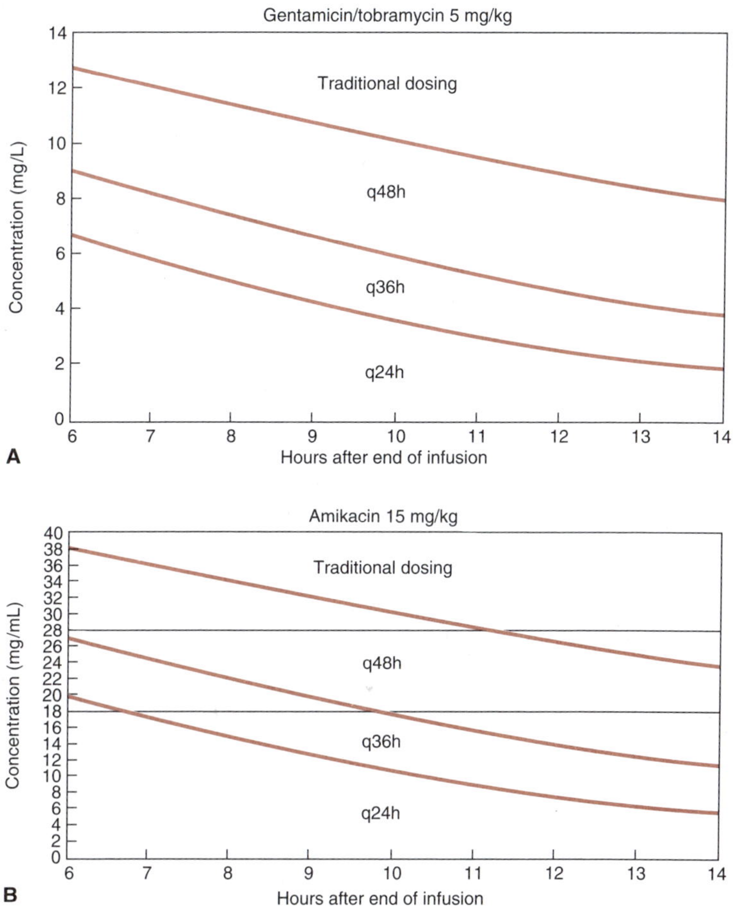

Figure 15-1 Nomograms for extended-interval aminoglycoside dosing. A, Gentamicin/tobramycin. B, amikacin.

if that concentration is undetectable, extended-interval dosing should be abandoned in favor of traditional dosing.

- For **obese patients** (actual weight >20% above ideal body weight [IBW]), an obese dosing weight (IBW + 0.4 × [actual body weight − IBW]) should be used for determining doses for both traditional and extended-interval methods. Traditional dosing, rather than extended-interval dosing, should be used for patients with endocarditis, burns that cover more than 20% of the body, anasarca, and creatinine clearance (CrCl) of <30 mL/min.
- **Gentamicin and tobramycin** traditional dosing is administered with an initial loading dose of 2 mg/kg IV (2–3 mg/kg in the critically ill), followed by 1.0–1.7 mg/kg IV q8h (peak, 4–10 μg/mL; trough, <1–2 μg/mL). Extended-interval dosing is administered with an initial loading dose of 5 mg/kg, with the subsequent dosing interval determined by a nomogram (see Figure 15-1). Tobramycin is also available as an inhaled agent for adjunctive therapy for patients with cystic fibrosis or bronchiectasis complicated by *P. aeruginosa* infection (300 mg inhalation q12h).
- **Amikacin** has an additional unique role for mycobacterial and *Nocardia* infections. Traditional dosing is an initial loading dose of 5.0–7.5 mg/kg IV (7.5–9.0 mg/kg in the critically ill), followed by 5 mg/kg IV q8h or 7.5 mg/kg IV q12h (peak, 20–35 μg/mL; trough, <10 μg/mL). Extended-interval dosing is 15 mg/kg, with the subsequent dosing interval determined by a nomogram (see Figure 15-1).
- Plazomicin sulfate (Zemdri) is a semisynthetic aminoglycoside bactericidal antibiotic drug, acting similarly to other aminoglycosides, by suppressing the 30S bacterial ribosomal subunit. Notably, while other aminoglycosides can be inactivated by aminoglycoside-modifying enzymes, plazomicin is resistant to the action of these enzymes. It targets infections with gram-negative aerobic bacteria in complicated urinary tract infections. Plazomicin is administered intravenously (IV) every 24 hours for 4–7 days; it is primarily active against gram-negative aerobic bacteria (e.g., *Enterobacteriaceae* family), to be used in patients over 18 years of age with cUTIs, including pyelonephritis, caused by susceptible *Escherichia coli, Klebsiella pneumoniae, Proteus mirabilis,* or *Enterobacter cloacae.*[5]

SPECIAL CONSIDERATIONS

- **Nephrotoxicity** is the major adverse effect of aminoglycosides. Nephrotoxicity is reversible when detected early but can be permanent. Aminoglycosides should be used cautiously or avoided, if possible, in patients with decompensated kidney disease. Concomitant administration of aminoglycosides with other known nephrotoxic agents (i.e., amphotericin B formulations, foscarnet, NSAIDs, pentamidine, polymyxins, cidofovir, and cisplatin) should be avoided if possible.
- **Ototoxicity** (vestibular or cochlear) is another possible adverse event that necessitates baseline and weekly hearing tests with extended therapy (>14 days).
- **Neuromuscular blockade** is a rare but a very serious toxicity of aminoglycoside treatment.

Vancomycin

GENERAL PRINCIPLES

- **Vancomycin** (usual starting dose is 15 mg/kg IV q12h) is a glycopeptide antibiotic that interferes with cell wall synthesis by binding to D-alanyl-D-alanine precursors that are critical for peptidoglycan cross-linking in most gram-positive bacterial cell walls. Vancomycin is bactericidal for staphylococci but bacteriostatic for enterococci.

  Vancomycin-resistant *Enterococcus faecium* (VRE) and vancomycin intermediate-resistant *S. aureus* (VISA) present increasing treatment challenges. Vancomycin-resistant *S. aureus* has been reported but remains rare.[6]

TABLE 15-1 Indications for Vancomycin Use
Treatment of serious infections caused by documented or suspected methicillin-resistant *Staphylococcus aureus* (MRSA)
Treatment of serious infections caused by ampicillin-resistant, vancomycin-sensitive enterococci
Treatment of serious infections caused by gram-positive bacteria in patients who are allergic to other appropriate therapies
Surgical prophylaxis for placement of prosthetic devices at institutions with known high rates of MRSA or in patients who are known to be colonized with MRSA
Empiric use in suspected gram-positive meningitis until an organism has been identified and sensitivities confirmed
Oral treatment of *Clostridium difficile* colitis

USES

- Indications for use are listed in Table 15-1.
- The **goal trough** concentration is 15–20 μg/mL for treatment of serious infections.

SPECIAL CONSIDERATIONS

- Vancomycin is typically administered by slow IV infusion over at least 1 hour per gram dose. More rapid infusion rates can cause the **red man syndrome**, which is a histamine-mediated reaction that is typically manifested by flushing and redness of the upper body.
- **Adverse events:** Nephrotoxicity, neutropenia, thrombocytopenia, and rash may also occur.

Fluoroquinolones

GENERAL PRINCIPLES

- Fluoroquinolones exert their bactericidal effect by inhibiting bacterial enzymes DNA gyrase and topoisomerase IV, which are critical for DNA replication. In general, these antibiotics are well absorbed orally, with serum concentrations that approach those of parenteral administration.
- Concomitant administration with aluminum- or magnesium-containing antacids, sucralfate, bismuth, oral iron, oral calcium, oral zinc, and metallic cation-containing enteral nutrition preparations can markedly impair absorption of oral fluoroquinolones.

USES

- **Ciprofloxacin** (250–750 mg PO q12h. 500 mg PO q24h [Cipro XR], or 200–400 mg IV q8–12h) and **ofloxacin** (200–400 mg IV or PO q12h) are active against gram-negative aerobes including many AmpC β-lactamase–producing pathogens. These agents are commonly used for UTIs, pyelonephritis, infectious diarrhea, prostatitis, and intra-abdominal infections (with metronidazole). Ciprofloxacin is the most active quinolone against *P. aeruginosa* and is the quinolone of choice for serious infections with that pathogen. However, ciprofloxacin has relatively poor activity against gram-positive pathogens and anaerobes and should not be used as empiric monotherapy for CAP, skin and soft tissue infections, or intra-abdominal infections. Oral and IV ciprofloxacin give similar maximum serum levels at their respective doses, thus oral therapy is appropriate unless contraindicated.[7]

- **Levofloxacin** (250–750 mg PO or IV q24h), **moxifloxacin** (400 mg PO/IV q24h daily), and **gemifloxacin** (320 mg PO q24h daily) have improved coverage of streptococci but generally less gram-negative activity than ciprofloxacin (except levofloxacin, which does cover *P. aeruginosa*). Moxifloxacin may be used as monotherapy of intra-abdominal or skin and soft tissue infections because of its antianaerobic activity, although resistance among *B. fragilis* is increasing. Each of these agents is useful for treatment of sinusitis, bronchitis, CAP, and UTIs (except moxifloxacin, which is only minimally eliminated in the urine). Some of these agents have activity against mycobacteria and have a potential role in treating drug-resistant TB and atypical mycobacterial infections. Levofloxacin may be used as an alternative for treatment of chlamydial urethritis.
- **Delafloxacin** (300 mg IV q12h or 450 mg PO q12h) is FDA approved for acute bacterial skin and skin structure infections. This agent is reliably active against MRSA, streptococci, some enterococci, gram-negative bacteria including *Pseudomonas*, and anaerobes. Unlike other fluoroquinolones, delafloxacin does not appear to prolong the QTc interval on the electrocardiogram and may be less prone to causing phototoxicity and central nervous system adverse effects.

SPECIAL CONSIDERATIONS

- **Adverse events** include nausea, CNS disturbances (headache, restlessness, and dizziness, especially in the elderly), rash, and phototoxicity. These agents can cause prolongation of the QT_c interval (excluding delafloxacin) and should not be used in patients who are receiving class I or class III antiarrhythmics, in patients with known electrolyte or conduction abnormalities, or with other medications that prolong the QT_c interval or induce bradycardia. These agents should also be used with caution in the elderly, in whom asymptomatic conduction disturbances are more common. Fluoroquinolones should not be routinely used in patients younger than 18 years or in pregnant or lactating women because of the risk of arthropathy in pediatric patients. They may also cause tendinitis or tendon rupture, especially of the Achilles tendon, particularly in elderly. Peripheral neuropathy and myasthenia gravis exacerbations may also occur. An increase in the international normalized ratio (INR) may occur when used concurrently with warfarin.
- **This class of antimicrobials has major drug interactions.** Before initiating use of these agents, it is necessary to review concomitant medications.

Macrolide and Lincosamide Antibiotics

GENERAL PRINCIPLES

- Macrolide and lincosamide antibiotics are bacteriostatic agents that block protein synthesis in bacteria by binding to the 50S subunit of the bacterial ribosome.
- This class of antibiotics has activity against gram-positive cocci, including streptococci and staphylococci, and some upper respiratory gram-negative bacteria, but minimal activity against enteric gram-negative rods.

USES

- Macrolides are commonly used to treat pharyngitis, otitis media, sinusitis, and bronchitis, especially in PCN-allergic patients, and are among the drugs of choice for treating

Legionella, *Chlamydia*, and *Mycoplasma* infections. Azithromycin and clarithromycin can be used as monotherapy for outpatient CAP and have a unique role in the treatment and prophylaxis against *Mycobacterium avium* complex (MAC) infections. Many PCN-resistant strains of pneumococci are also resistant to macrolides.

- **Clarithromycin** (250–500 mg PO q12h or 1000 mg XL PO q24h)[8] has enhanced activity against some respiratory pathogens (especially *Haemophilus*). It is commonly used to treat bronchitis, sinusitis, otitis media, pharyngitis, soft tissue infections, and CAP. It has a prominent role in treating MAC infection and is an important component of regimens used to eradicate *Helicobacter pylori* (see Chapter 18, Gastrointestinal Diseases).
- **Azithromycin** (500 mg PO for 1 day, then 250 mg PO q24h for 4 days; 500 mg PO q24h for 3 days; 2000-mg microspheres PO for one dose; 500 mg IV q24h) has a similar spectrum of activity as clarithromycin and is commonly used to treat bronchitis, sinusitis, otitis media, pharyngitis, soft tissue infections, and CAP. It has a prominent role in MAC prophylaxis (1200 mg PO every week) and treatment (500–600 mg PO q24h) in HIV patients. It is also commonly used to treat *Chlamydia trachomatis* infections (1 g PO single dose). A major advantage of azithromycin is that it has much fewer drug interactions than erythromycin and clarithromycin.[9]
- **Telithromycin** is the first ketolide available for the treatment of adults with sinusitis, AECB, and CAP due to *Streptococcus* spp.
- **Clindamycin** (150–450 mg PO q6–8h or 600–900 mg IV q8h) is a lincosamide (related to macrolides), with activity against staphylococci and streptococci, as well as anaerobes, including *B. fragilis*. It has excellent oral bioavailability (90%) and penetrates well into the bone and abscess cavities. It is also used for treatment of aspiration pneumonia and lung abscesses. Clindamycin has activity against most community-associated strains of MRSA and is used for skin and soft tissue infections caused by this organism. Clindamycin may be used as a second agent in combination therapy for invasive streptococcal and clostridial infections to decrease toxin production. It may also be used for treatment of suspected anaerobic infections of the head and neck (peritonsillar or retropharyngeal abscesses, necrotizing fasciitis), although metronidazole is used more commonly for intra-abdominal infections (clindamycin has less reliable activity against *B. fragilis*). Clindamycin has additional uses, including treatment of babesiosis (in combination with quinine), toxoplasmosis (in combination with pyrimethamine), and *Pneumocystis jirovecii* pneumonia (in combination with primaquine).
- Lefamulin (Xenleta) is a semisynthetic pleuromutilin antibiotic that binds to the peptidyl transferase center of the 50S bacterial ribosomal subunit, inhibiting protein synthesis within bacteria. It can be administered either as an IV infusion or PO. The recommended dosage is 600 mg orally every 12 hours for 5 days or 150 mg-infused IV for over 60 minutes every 12 hours for 5–7 days for the treatment of the community-acquired bacterial pneumonia.

SPECIAL CONSIDERATIONS

Adverse events: Macrolides and clindamycin are associated with nausea, abdominal cramping, and LFT abnormalities. Liver function profiles should be checked intermittently during extended therapy. Hypersensitivity reactions with prominent skin rash are more common with clindamycin, as is pseudomembranous colitis secondary to *Clostridium difficile*. Clarithromycin and azithromycin may cause QT_c interval prolongation and myasthenia gravis exacerbations. **Clarithromycin has major drug interactions** caused by inhibition of the cytochrome P450 system.

Sulfonamides and Trimethoprim

GENERAL PRINCIPLES

Sulfadiazine, sulfamethoxazole, and trimethoprim slowly kill bacteria by inhibiting folic acid metabolism. This class of antibiotics is most commonly used for uncomplicated UTIs, sinusitis, and otitis media. Some sulfonamide-containing agents also have unique roles in the treatment of *P. jirovecii, Nocardia, Toxoplasma*, and *Stenotrophomonas* infections.

USES

- **Trimethoprim** (100 mg PO q12h) is occasionally used as monotherapy for treatment of UTIs. Trimethoprim is more often used in the combination preparations outlined below. Trimethoprim in combination with dapsone is an alternate therapy for mild *P. jirovecii* pneumonia.
- **Trimethoprim/sulfamethoxazole** is a combination antibiotic (IV or PO) with a 1:5 ratio of trimethoprim to sulfamethoxazole. The IV preparation is dosed at 5 mg/kg IV q8h (based on the trimethoprim component) for serious infections. The oral preparations (160 mg trimethoprim/800 mg sulfamethoxazole per double-strength [DS] tablet) are extensively bioavailable, with similar drug concentrations obtained with IV and PO formulations. The combination has a broad spectrum of activity but does not inhibit *P. aeruginosa*, anaerobes, or group A streptococci. It is the therapy of choice for *P. jirovecii* pneumonia, *Stenotrophomonas maltophilia, Tropheryma whipplei*, and *Nocardia* infections. It is commonly used for treating sinusitis, otitis media, bronchitis, prostatitis, and UTIs (one DS tab PO q12h). Trimethoprim/sulfamethoxazole is active against MRSA and is widely used for uncomplicated cases of skin and soft tissue infections caused by this organism (often two DS tabs PO q12h). It is used as *P. jirovecii* pneumonia prophylaxis (one DS tab PO twice a week, three times a week, or single-strength or DS daily) in HIV-infected patients, solid organ transplant patients, bone marrow transplant patients, and in patients receiving fludarabine. IV therapy is routinely converted to the PO equivalent for patients who require prolonged therapy.
  - For serious infections, such as *Nocardia* brain abscesses, drug levels should be monitored with sulfamethoxazole peaks (100–150 μg/mL) and troughs (50–100 μg/mL) and dose adjusted accordingly. In patients with renal insufficiency, doses can be adjusted by following trimethoprim peaks (5–10 μg/mL). Prolonged therapy can cause bone marrow suppression, possibly requiring treatment with leucovorin (5–10 mg PO q24h) until cell counts normalize.
- **Sulfadiazine** (1.0–1.5 g PO q6h) in combination with pyrimethamine (200 mg PO followed by 50–75 mg PO q24h) and leucovorin (10–20 mg PO q24h) is the regimen of choice for toxoplasmosis. Sulfadiazine is also occasionally used to treat *Nocardia* infections.
- **Dapsone** is a sulfa drug used presently for the treatment of *Mycobacterium leprae*.

SPECIAL CONSIDERATIONS

Adverse events: These drugs are associated with cholestatic jaundice, bone marrow suppression, hyperkalemia (with trimethoprim/sulfamethoxazole), interstitial nephritis, "false" elevations in serum creatinine, and severe hypersensitivity reactions (Stevens-Johnson syndrome/erythema multiforme). Nausea is common with higher doses. **All patients should be asked whether they are allergic to "sulfa drugs,"** and specific commercial names should be mentioned (e.g., Bactrim or Septra). Hemolysis and methemoglobinemia in the setting of glucose-6-phosphate dehydrogenase (G6PD) deficiency may also occur.

Tetracyclines

GENERAL PRINCIPLES

- Tetracyclines are bacteriostatic antibiotics that bind to the 30S ribosomal subunit and block protein synthesis.
- These agents have unique roles in the treatment of *Rickettsia*, *Ehrlichia*, *Chlamydia*, and *Mycoplasma* infections. They are used as therapy for most tick-borne infections and Lyme disease–related arthritis, alternate therapy for syphilis, and therapy for *P. multocida* infections in PCN-allergic patients. Minocycline and doxycycline also have activity against some multidrug-resistant gram-negative pathogens and may be used in this setting based on results of susceptibility testing.

USES

- **Tetracycline** (250–500 mg PO q6h) is commonly used for severe acne and in some *H. pylori* eradication regimens. It has largely been replaced by doxycycline for other infections (see below). Aluminum- and magnesium-containing antacids and preparations that contain oral calcium, oral iron, or other cations can significantly impair oral absorption of tetracycline and should be avoided within 2 hours of each dose.
- **Doxycycline** (100 mg PO/IV q12h) is the most commonly used tetracycline and is standard therapy for *C. trachomatis*, Rocky Mountain spotted fever, ehrlichiosis, and psittacosis. This agent also has a role for malaria prophylaxis and for treatment of CAP. It is also used for uSSSIs caused by community-associated MRSA.
- **Minocycline** (200 mg IV/PO, then 100 mg IV/PO q12h) is similar to doxycycline in its spectrum of activity and clinical indications. Among the tetracyclines, minocycline is most likely to provide coverage against *Acinetobacter*. Minocycline can also be used for treating pulmonary nocardiosis, cervicofacial actinomycosis, and *Stenotrophomonas maltophilia* infections.[10]
- Eravacycline dihydrochloride (Xerava) is a fully synthetic bacteriostatic fluorocycline and a tetracycline-class antibacterial agent that binds bacterial 30S ribosomal subunit. Compared to other tetracyclines, it has two structural substitutions, enabling it to work on certain strains of gram-positive and gram-negative bacteria that typically possess tetracycline-specific resistance mechanisms. Notably, eravacycline can be used (at least in cell culture) against *Enterobacteriaceae* in the presence of certain β-lactamases. Eravacycline is administered IV in 60-minute infusions, given once every 12 hours for a total of 4–14 days. The dose is dependent on patient's weight (1 mg/kg), and it is intended for use in individuals over 18 years of age with complicated intra-abdominal infections.
- Sarecycline hydrochloride (Seysara) is a new, narrow-spectrum tetracycline derivative. It demonstrates antibacterial activity against skin and soft tissue pathogens, including *Cutibacterium acnes* (anaerobic gram-positive bacterium related to acne development). The drug is administrated as 1.5 mg/kg/day orally with food, in patients aged 9 and older, as a once-daily antibiotic, with statistically significant improvement seen as early as the third week.
- Omadacycline (Nuzyra) is an aminomethylcycline antibiotic belonging to the tetracycline class. It inhibits the 30S bacterial ribosomal subunit. Compared to other tetracycline antibiotics, omadacycline has structural modifications at the C9 and C7 positions of the core tetracycline rings, enabling ribosomal protection mechanisms and stability

in the efflux pump related to resistance to the tetracycline antibiotics. It is used for the treatment of community-acquired bacterial pneumonia (CABP) and acute bacterial skin and skin structure infections (ABSSI).

SPECIAL CONSIDERATIONS

Adverse events: Nausea and photosensitivity are common side effects, so patients should be warned about direct sun exposure. Rarely, these medications are associated with pseudotumor cerebri. **They should not routinely be given to children or to pregnant or lactating women** because they can cause tooth enamel discoloration in the developing fetus and young children. Minocycline is associated with vestibular disturbances and blue-black hyperpigmentation of skin and mucous membranes. Oral formulations of tetracyclines may cause esophageal ulceration if not properly swallowed.

MISCELLANEOUS ANTIMICROBIAL AGENTS

Colistin and Polymyxin B

GENERAL PRINCIPLES

- **Colistimethate sodium** (colistin; 2.5–5 mg/kg/d IV divided q12h) and **polymyxin B** (15,000–25,000 units/kg/d IV divided q12h) are bactericidal polypeptide antibiotics that kill gram-negative bacteria by disrupting the cell membrane. These drugs have reemerged in the treatment of multidrug-resistant gram-negative bacilli but are inactive against *Proteus*, *Providencia*, and *Serratia*.[11]
- **These medications should only be given under the guidance of an experienced clinician** because parenteral therapy has significant CNS and nephrotoxicity. Inhaled colistin (75–150 mg q12h given by nebulizer) is better tolerated than the IV formulation, generally causing only mild upper airway irritation, and has some effectiveness as adjunctive therapy for multidrug-resistant *P. aeruginosa* or *Acinetobacter* pulmonary infections.

SPECIAL CONSIDERATIONS

Adverse events with parenteral therapy include paresthesias, slurred speech, peripheral numbness, tingling, and significant dose-dependent nephrotoxicity. The dosage should be carefully reduced in patients with renal insufficiency because overdosage can result in neuromuscular blockade and apnea. Serum creatinine should be monitored daily early in therapy and then at a regular interval for the duration of therapy. **Concomitant use with aminoglycosides, other known nephrotoxins, or neuromuscular blockers should be avoided.**

Dalbavancin

GENERAL PRINCIPLES

Dalbavancin (1500 mg single dose or 1000 mg IV on day 1 followed by 500 mg IV on day 8 to complete the course of therapy) is a long-acting lipoglycopeptide (terminal half-life of 346 hours) that inhibits cell wall biosynthesis and demonstrates concentration-dependent bactericidal activity. It has a half-life of **170–210 hours**, making once-weekly dosing feasible. Dalbavancin has activity against many gram-positive aerobic bacteria, including staphylococci (including MRSA) and streptococci, and is FDA approved for acute bacterial skin and skin structure infections.

SPECIAL CONSIDERATIONS

Adverse events include nausea, diarrhea, vomiting, headache, insomnia, dizziness, and pruritus. In clinical trials, more dalbavancin-treated patients had alanine aminotransferase elevation greater than three times the upper limit of normal than patients treated with a comparative agent.

Daptomycin

GENERAL PRINCIPLES

Daptomycin (4 mg/kg IV q24h for skin and skin structure infections; 6–10 mg/kg IV q24h for bloodstream infections) is a cyclic lipopeptide. The drug exhibits rapid bactericidal activity against a wide variety of gram-positive bacteria, including enterococci, staphylococci, and streptococci. Daptomycin is FDA approved for treatment of complicated skin and skin structure infections as well as *S. aureus* bacteremia and right-sided endocarditis. The drug should **not** be used to treat lung infections as activity is decreased in the presence of pulmonary surfactant. Nonsusceptibility to daptomycin can develop, making it imperative that susceptibility of isolates be verified.

SPECIAL CONSIDERATIONS

Adverse events include gastrointestinal (GI) disturbances, injection site reactions, elevated LFTs, eosinophilic pneumonitis, and elevated creatine phosphokinase. Serum creatine phosphokinase (CK) should be monitored at baseline and weekly because daptomycin has been associated with skeletal muscle effects, including rhabdomyolysis. Patients should also be monitored for signs of muscle weakness and pain, and the drug should be discontinued if these symptoms develop in conjunction with marked CK elevations (5–10 times the upper limit of normal with symptoms or 10 times the upper limit of normal without symptoms). Concomitant use of 5-hydroxy-3-methylglutaryl–coenzyme A (HMG-CoA) reductase inhibitors should be avoided, if possible, because of the potential increased risk of myopathy.

Fosfomycin

GENERAL PRINCIPLES

Fosfomycin (3-g sachet dissolved in cold water PO once) is a bactericidal oral antibiotic that kills bacteria by inhibiting an early step in cell wall synthesis. It has a spectrum of activity that includes most urinary tract pathogens, including *P. aeruginosa*, *Enterobacter* spp., and enterococci (including VRE), and some multidrug-resistant gram-negative bacteria.

- It is most useful for treating **uncomplicated** UTIs in women with susceptible strains of *E. coli* or *E. faecalis*. It should not be used to treat pyelonephritis or systemic infections.[12]

SPECIAL CONSIDERATIONS

Adverse events include diarrhea. It should not be taken with metoclopramide, which interferes with fosfomycin absorption.

Oxazolidinones

GENERAL PRINCIPLES

- Oxazolidinones block assembly of bacterial ribosomes and inhibit protein synthesis.
- **Linezolid** (600 mg IV/PO q12h) IV and oral formulations produce equivalent serum concentrations. It has potent activity against gram-positive bacteria, including drug-resistant enterococci, staphylococci, and streptococci, but not against Enterobacteriaceae.
- Linezolid is useful for serious infections with VRE, as an alternative to vancomycin for treatment of MRSA infections, in patients with intolerance to vancomycin therapy, and as oral therapy of MRSA infections when IV access is unavailable. Linezolid should generally be avoided for catheter-related bloodstream or catheter site infections. Resistance can develop to this antibiotic, and it is imperative that organism susceptibility is verified.[13]

Tedizolid (mg PO/IV q24h) is an oxazolidinone antibiotic which inhibits bacterial protein synthesis. It is FDA approved for treating acute bacterial skin and skin structure infections. Tedizolid has activity against staphylococci (including MRSA), streptococci, and enterococci (including some strains resistant to linezolid).

SPECIAL CONSIDERATIONS

- **Adverse events** associated with linezolid include diarrhea, nausea, and headache. Thrombocytopenia occurs frequently in patients who receive more than 2 weeks of therapy, and serial platelet count monitoring is indicated. A CBC should be checked every week. Prolonged therapy has also been associated with peripheral and optic neuropathy. Lactic acidosis may also rarely occur.
- Linezolid has **several important drug interactions**. It is a mild monoamine oxidase inhibitor, and patients should be advised not to take selective serotonin reuptake inhibitors or other antidepressants, fentanyl, or meperidine while on linezolid to avoid the serotonin syndrome. Ideally, patients should be off antidepressants for at least a week before initiating linezolid. Coadministration of pseudoephedrine or phenylpropanolamine with linezolid can elevate blood pressure and should be avoided. Linezolid does not require dose adjustments for renal or hepatic dysfunction.
- **Adverse events** associated with tedizolid include nausea, diarrhea, vomiting, headache, and dizziness. Whether it is less prone to adverse effects characteristic of linezolid, such as hematologic disturbances and peripheral and optic neuropathy, if used beyond 6 days, is uncertain. Tedizolid phosphate appears less likely to inhibit monoamine oxidase as compared with linezolid; however, patients on serotonergic agents were excluded from tedizolid phase III clinical trials.

Metronidazole

GENERAL PRINCIPLES

- Metronidazole (250–750 mg PO/IV q6–12h) is only active against anaerobic bacteria and some protozoa. The drug exerts its bactericidal effect through accumulation of toxic metabolites that interfere with multiple biologic processes. It has excellent tissue penetration, including abscess cavities, bone, and the CNS.
- It has greater activity against gram-negative than gram-positive anaerobes but is active against *Clostridium perfringens* and *C. difficile*. It is a treatment of choice for bacterial vaginosis and can be used in combination with other antibiotics to treat intra-abdominal

infections and brain abscesses. However, it is no longer a preferred treatment for *C. difficile* colitis. Protozoal infections that are routinely treated with metronidazole include *Giardia*, *Entamoeba histolytica*, and *Trichomonas vaginalis*. Dose reduction may be warranted for patients with decompensated liver disease.[14]

SPECIAL CONSIDERATIONS

Adverse events include nausea, dysgeusia, disulfiram-like reactions to alcohol, and mild CNS disturbances (headache, restlessness). Rarely, metronidazole causes peripheral neuropathy, encephalopathy, and seizures.

Nitrofurantoin

GENERAL PRINCIPLES

- **Nitrofurantoin** (50–100 mg PO macrocrystals q6h or 100 mg PO dual-release formulation q12h for 5–7 days) is a bactericidal oral antibiotic used for uncomplicated UTIs except those caused by *Proteus*, *P. aeruginosa*, or *Serratia*. The drug is metabolized by bacteria into toxic intermediates that inhibit multiple bacterial processes. It has had a modest resurgence in use, as it is frequently effective for uncomplicated VRE UTIs.
- Prolonged therapy is associated with chronic pulmonary syndromes that can be fatal and should be avoided. Nitrofurantoin should not be used for pyelonephritis or any other systemic infections and should be avoided in patients with renal dysfunction.[15]

SPECIAL CONSIDERATIONS

Adverse events: Nausea is the most common adverse effect, and the drug should be taken with food to minimize this problem. Patients should be warned that their urine may become brown secondary to the medication. Neurotoxicity, hepatotoxicity, hemolytic anemia, hepatitis, and pulmonary fibrosis may also rarely occur with nitrofurantoin. It should not be used in patients with CrCl <60 mL/min because of increased risk for development of treatment-associated adverse effects. Probenecid decreases the concentration of nitrofurantoin in the urine and should be avoided.

Oritavancin

GENERAL PRINCIPLES

Oritavancin (1200 mg IV administered once to complete therapy) is a long-acting lipoglycopeptide (terminal half-life, 245 hours) that inhibits cell wall biosynthesis through multiple mechanisms. Oritavancin has activity against many gram-positive aerobic bacteria, including staphylococci (including MRSA) and streptococci, as well as some enterococci (including some strains resistant to vancomycin).

SPECIAL CONSIDERATIONS

Adverse events include nausea, diarrhea, vomiting, headache, insomnia, dizziness, and pruritus.

Quinupristin/Dalfopristin

GENERAL PRINCIPLES

- **Quinupristin/dalfopristin** (7.5 mg/kg IV q8h) is the first FDA-approved drug in the streptogramin class.
- This agent has activity against antibiotic-resistant gram-positive organisms, especially VRE, MRSA, and antibiotic-resistant strains of *Streptococcus pneumoniae*. It has some activity against gram-negative upper respiratory pathogens (*Haemophilus* and *Moraxella*) and anaerobes, but more appropriate antibiotics are available to treat these infections. Quinupristin/dalfopristin is bacteriostatic for enterococci and can be used for treatment of serious infections with VRE (only *E. faecium* because it is inactive against *E. faecalis*).

SPECIAL CONSIDERATIONS

Adverse events include arthralgias and myalgias, which occur frequently and can necessitate discontinuation of therapy. IV site pain and thrombophlebitis are common. It has also been associated with elevated LFTs and dose should be adjusted in patients with hepatic impairment. Quinupristin/dalfopristin is similar to clarithromycin with regard to drug interactions.

Telavancin

GENERAL PRINCIPLES

Telavancin (7.5–10 mg/kg q24–48h, based on CrCl) is a lipoglycopeptide antibiotic that is FDA approved for treatment of hospital-acquired and ventilator-associated bacterial pneumonia caused by *S. aureus* and for complicated skin and skin structure infections. Telavancin is broadly active against gram-positive bacteria, including MRSA, VISA, heteroresistant VISA (hVISA), daptomycin- and linezolid-resistant *S. aureus*, streptococci, vancomycin-sensitive enterococci, and some gram-positive anaerobes. The agent is not active against gram-negative bacteria, vancomycin-resistant *S. aureus*, and VRE.

SPECIAL CONSIDERATIONS

Adverse events include nausea, vomiting, metallic or soapy taste, foamy urine, and nephrotoxicity (which necessitates serial monitoring of serum creatinine). Prehydration with normal saline may mitigate the nephrotoxicity observed with the use of this drug. Telavancin can also cause a minor prolongation of the QT_c interval. Women of childbearing potential require a negative serum pregnancy test prior to receiving telavancin because of teratogenic effects noted in animals.

Tigecycline

GENERAL PRINCIPLES

Tigecycline (100 mg IV loading dose, then 50 mg IV q12h) is the only FDA-approved antibiotic in the class of glycylcyclines. Its mechanism of action is similar to that of tetracyclines; the addition of the glycyl side chain expands its activity against bacterial pathogens that are normally resistant to tetracyclines. It has a broad spectrum of bactericidal activity against gram-positive, gram-negative, and anaerobic bacteria except *P. aeruginosa* and some

Proteus isolates. It is FDA approved for treatment of complicated skin and skin structure infections, complicated intra-abdominal infections, and CAP, but it should be reserved for use when alternative treatments are not suitable. It may be used for treatment of infections due to susceptible strains of VRE and some multidrug-resistant gram-negative bacteria. Because of low achievable blood concentrations, tigecycline should not be used to treat primary bacteremia.

SPECIAL CONSIDERATIONS

Adverse events: Nausea and vomiting are the most common adverse events. Tigecycline has not been studied in patients younger than 18 years and is contraindicated in pregnant and lactating women. Because it has a similar structure to tetracyclines, photosensitivity, tooth discoloration, and, rarely, pseudotumor cerebri may occur. Pancreatitis may also occur.

ANTIMYCOBACTERIAL AGENTS

Effective therapy of MTB infections requires combination chemotherapy to prevent the emergence of resistant organisms and maximize efficacy. Increased resistance to antituberculous agents has led to the use of more complex regimens and has made susceptibility testing an integral part of TB management (see Chapter 14, Treatment of Infectious Diseases).

Isoniazid

GENERAL PRINCIPLES

Isoniazid (INH; 300 mg PO q24h) exerts bactericidal effects by interfering with the synthesis of lipid components of the mycobacterial cell wall. INH is a component of most TB treatment regimens and can be given twice a week in directly observed therapy (15 mg/kg/dose; 900 mg maximum). INH remains the drug of choice for treatment of latent TB infection (300 mg PO q24h for 9 months, or combined with rifapentine in a 12-week regimen).

SPECIAL CONSIDERATIONS

Adverse events include elevations in liver transaminases (20%). This effect can be idiosyncratic but is usually seen with advanced age, underlying liver disease, or concomitant consumption of alcohol and may be potentiated by rifampin. Transaminase elevations to greater than threefold the upper limit of the normal range necessitate holding therapy. Patients with known liver dysfunction should have weekly LFTs during the initial stage of therapy. INH also antagonizes vitamin B_6 metabolism and potentially can cause a peripheral neuropathy. This can be minimized by coadministration of pyridoxine, 25–50 mg PO daily, especially in the elderly, in pregnant women, and in patients with diabetes, renal failure, alcoholism, and seizure disorders.

Rifamycins

GENERAL PRINCIPLES

Rifamycins exert bactericidal activity on susceptible mycobacteria by inhibiting DNA-dependent RNA polymerase, thereby halting transcription.

- **Rifampin** (600 mg PO q24h or twice a week) is an integral component of most TB treatment regimens. It is also active against many gram-positive and gram-negative bacteria.

Rifampin is used as adjunctive therapy in staphylococcal prosthetic valve endocarditis and prosthetic bone and joint infections (300 mg PO q8h) and for prophylaxis of close contacts of patients with *Neisseria meningitidis* infection (600 mg PO q12h). The drug is well absorbed orally and is widely distributed throughout the body including the cerebrospinal fluid (CSF).

- **Rifabutin** (300 mg PO q24h) is primarily used to treat TB and MAC infections in HIV-positive patients who are receiving highly active antiretroviral therapy because it has fewer drug–drug interactions and less deleterious effects on protease inhibitor metabolism than does rifampin (see Chapter 16, Sexually Transmitted Infections, Human Immunodeficiency Virus, and Acquired Immunodeficiency Syndrome).
- **Rifapentine** (usual dose between 600 and 900 mg PO weekly based on body weight) is primarily used in combination with isoniazid for 12-week once-weekly treatment of latent tuberculosis infection.

SPECIAL CONSIDERATIONS

Adverse events: Patients should be warned about reddish-orange discoloration of body fluids, including contact lenses. Rash, GI disturbances, hematologic disturbances, hepatitis, and interstitial nephritis can occur. Uveitis has also been associated with rifabutin. **This class of antibiotics has major drug interactions.**

Pyrazinamide

GENERAL PRINCIPLES

- **Pyrazinamide** (15–30 mg/kg PO q24h [maximum, 2 g] or 50–75 mg/kg PO twice a week [maximum, 4 g/dose]) kills mycobacteria by an unknown disruption of membrane transport.
- It is well absorbed orally and widely distributed throughout the body, including the CSF. Pyrazinamide is typically used for the first 2 months of therapy.

SPECIAL CONSIDERATIONS

Adverse events include hyperuricemia and hepatitis.

Ethambutol

GENERAL PRINCIPLES

- **Ethambutol** (15–25 mg/kg PO q24h or 50–75 mg/kg PO twice a week; maximum, 2.4 g/dose) is bacteriostatic and inhibits arabinosyltransferase (involved in cell wall synthesis).
- Doses should be reduced in the presence of renal dysfunction.

SPECIAL CONSIDERATIONS

Adverse events may include **optic neuritis**, which manifests as decreased red-green color perception, decreased visual acuity, or visual field deficits. Baseline and monthly visual examinations should be performed during therapy. Renal function should also be carefully monitored because drug accumulation in the setting of renal insufficiency can increase risk of ocular effects.

Streptomycin

Streptomycin is an aminoglycoside that can be used as a substitute for ethambutol and for drug-resistant MTB. It does not adequately penetrate the CNS and should not be used for TB meningitis.

Antitubercular agents have been listed in Table 15-2.

Antibiotic Resistance

Antimicrobial resistance is on a tsunamic rise. A safe and effective strategy for antibiotic use involves prescribing an antibiotic only when it is needed and selecting an appropriate and effective medicine at the recommended dose, with the narrowest spectrum of antimicrobial activity and fewest adverse effects. Common resistant infections and their management have been enlisted in Table 15-3.

TABLE 15-2 Antitubercular Agents

First-line agents: isoniazid, rifampicin, ethambutol, pyrazinamide, streptomycin
Second-line agents: **Oral agents:** thioacetazone, ethionamide/prothionamide, *para*-aminosalicylic acid, fluoroquinolones (levofloxacin or moxifloxacin), cycloserine **Injectable agents:** fluoroquinolones, aminoglycosides (amikacin, kanamycin), and capreomycin
Other agents: carbapenems plus clavulanate, linezolid, clofazimine, amoxicillin–clavulanate, clarithromycin
Newer agents: bedaquiline, delamanid, pretomanid, delpazolid, sutezolid

TABLE 15-3 Common Resistant Infections and Their Management

Infections	Etiology	Treatment
Community-acquired pneumonia	*Streptococcus pneumoniae*, *Haemophilus influenzae*, *Moraxella catarrhalis*, aerobic gram-negative bacteria	• Inpatient (CURB-65 ≥2): – Inj. ceftriaxone 1–2 g IV BD or – Inj. ampicillin–sulbactam 3 g IV QID PLUS – Azithromycin 500 mg (IV/PO) OD for 5 d • Outpatient (CURB-65 ≤1): – Tab amoxicillin–clavulanic acid 625 mg TDS PLUS – Tab azithromycin 500 mg OD for 5 d • When risk of *Pseudomonas*/resistant gram-negative bacteria is present (COPD, bronchiectasis): – Replace ceftriaxone with any of the following: ▪ Piperacillin–tazobactam 4.5 g IV QID or

(*Continued*)

TABLE 15-3 Common Resistant Infections and Their Management (Continued)

Infections	Etiology	Treatment
		▪ Cefepime 2 g IV TDS or ▪ Imipenem 500 mg QID or ▪ Meropenem 1g TD PLUS ▪ Ciprofloxacin or levofloxacin
Culture-proven VAP/HAP	*Acinetobacter baumannii, Klebsiella pneumoniae, Pseudomonas aeruginosa*	Choose any one according to culture sensitivity: • Piperacillin–tazobactam 4.5 g IV QID • Cefoperazone–sulbactam (3 g IV BD) • Imipenem–cilastatin 500 mg IV QID • Meropenem 1 g IV TDS Carbapenemase-producing gram-negative bacilli: • Colistin 9 MU IV stat followed by 4.5 MU IV BD • Polymyxin B (20,000–25,000 units/kg loading f/b 25,000 units/kg/d IV in two divided doses) MSRA: • Preferred: – Inj. vancomycin 1 g IV DB or – Inj. linezolid 600 mg IV BD • Alternative: – Inj. teicoplanin (400 mg IV BD for three doses followed by 400 mg IV OD)
Spontaneous bacterial peritonitis	Gram-negative bacilli (*E. coli* > *Klebsiella*) more common than gram-positive organisms	Inj. cefotaxime 2 g IV TDS for at least 5 d
Acute uncomplicated cystitis	Enterobacteriaceae, enterococci	Ciprofloxacin 500 mg BD or levofloxacin 750 mg OD for 7 d Alternatives: • Nitrofurantoin 100 mg PO BD for 7 d • OR fosfomycin (3 g) sachet every other day for up to three doses
Enteric fever	*Salmonella* Typhi and Paratyphi	Inj. ceftriaxone 100 mg/kg/d and shift to oral Oral cefixime 20 mg/kg/d for 14 d Azithromycin 10–20 mg/kg/d for 7–10 d

(*Continued*)

TABLE 15-3 Common Resistant Infections and Their Management (Continued)

Infections	Etiology	Treatment
		Second line: • Ofloxacin 15 mg/kg/d in two divided doses for 10–14 d • Chloramphenicol 50–75 mg/kg/d orally for 14 d • TMP-SMX 8 mg/kg/day orally for 14 d
Bacillary dysentery	*Shigella* sp., *Campylobacter*, nontyphoidal salmonellosis, *E. coli*	Ceftriaxone 2 g IV OD for 5 d or oral cefixime 10–15 mg/kg/day × 5 d Azithromycin 1 g OD × 3 d
Bacterial meningitis	*S. pneumoniae*, *H. influenzae*, *Neisseria meningitidis*	Ceftriaxone 2 g IV 12 hourly/cefotaxime 2 g IV 4–6 hourly for 10–14 d
Skin and soft tissue infections	*Streptococcus pyogenes* (common), *S. aureus*	Amoxicillin–clavulanate 1.2 g IV TDS/625 mg oral TDS or ceftriaxone 2 g IV OD for 5–7 d Clindamycin 600–900 mg IV TDS for 5–7 d

ANTIVIRAL AGENTS

Current antiviral agents only suppress viral replication. Viral containment or elimination requires an intact host immune response. Anti-HIV agents will be discussed in Chapter 16, Sexually Transmitted Infections, Human Immunodeficiency Virus, and Acquired Immunodeficiency Syndrome.

Antiinfluenza Agents (Neuraminidase Inhibitors)

Zanamivir, oseltamivir, and peramivir block influenza A and B neuraminidases. Neuraminidase activity is necessary for successful viral egress and release from infected cells. These drugs have shown modest activity in clinical trials, with a 1- to 2-day improvement in symptoms in patients who are treated within 48 hours of the onset of influenza symptoms. At the onset of each influenza season, a consultation with local health department officials is recommended to determine the most effective antiviral agent. Although oseltamivir and zanamivir are effective for prophylaxis of influenza, annual influenza vaccination remains the most effective method for prophylaxis in all high-risk patients and healthcare workers (see Appendix A, Immunizations and Post-exposure Therapies).

- **Zanamivir** (10 mg [two inhalations] q12h for 5 days, started within 48 hours of the onset of symptoms) is an inhaled neuraminidase inhibitor that is active against influenza A and B. It is indicated for treatment of uncomplicated acute influenza infection in adults and children 7 years of age or older who have been symptomatic for <48 hours. The drug is also indicated for influenza prophylaxis in patient's age 5 years and older.
  Adverse events such as headache, GI disturbances, dizziness, and upper respiratory symptoms are sometimes reported. Bronchospasms or declines in lung function, or both, may

occur in patients with underlying respiratory disorders and may require a rapid-acting bronchodilator for control.

- **Oseltamivir** (75 mg PO q12h for 5 days) is an orally administered neuraminidase inhibitor that is active against influenza A and B. It is indicated for treatment of uncomplicated acute influenza in adults and children 1 year of age or older who have been symptomatic for up to 2 days. This agent is also indicated for prophylaxis of influenza A and B in adults and children 1 year of age or older.

  Adverse events include nausea, vomiting, and diarrhea. Dizziness and headache may also occur.
- **Peramivir** (600 mg IV single-dose therapy) is an IV neuraminidase inhibitor that is active against influenza A and B. It is FDA approved for single-dose treatment of acute, uncomplicated influenza in adults who have been symptomatic for up to 2 days. The agent has not been proven to be effective for serious influenza requiring hospitalization.

  Adverse events include diarrhea and rare cases of skin reactions, behavioral disturbances, neutrophils <1000/μL, hyperglycemia, creatine phosphokinase elevation, and elevation of hepatic transaminases.
- **Baloxavir** is a new oral selective inhibitor of influenza cap-dependent endonuclease that blocks influenza proliferation by inhibiting the initiation of mRNA synthesis and is effective against influenza A and B viruses.
- **Amantadine and rimantadine** target the M2 protein of influenza A only, which forms a proton channel in the viral membrane that is essential for efficient viral replication, and are not used for routine prophylaxis.

Antiherpetic Agents

GENERAL PRINCIPLES

Antiherpetic agents are nucleotide analogs that inhibit viral DNA synthesis.

- **Acyclovir** is active against herpes simplex virus (HSV) and varicella-zoster virus (VZV) (400 mg PO q8h for HSV, 800 mg PO five times a day for localized VZV infections, 5–10 mg/kg IV q8h for severe HSV infections, and 10 mg/kg IV q8h for severe VZV infections and HSV encephalitis).[16]
  - It is indicated for treatment of primary and recurrent genital herpes, severe herpetic stomatitis, and herpes simplex encephalitis. It can be used as prophylaxis in patients who have frequent HSV recurrences (400 mg PO q12h). It is also used for herpes zoster ophthalmicus, disseminated primary VZV in adults (significant morbidity compared to the childhood illness), and severe disseminated primary VZV in children.
  - **Adverse events.** Reversible crystalline nephropathy may occur; pre existing renal failure, dehydration, and IV bolus dosing increase the risk of this effect. Rare cases of CNS disturbances, including delirium, tremors, and seizures, may also occur, particularly with high doses, in patients with renal failure and in the elderly.
- **Valacyclovir** (1000 mg PO q8h for herpes zoster, 1000 mg PO q12h for initial episode of genital HSV infection, and 500 mg PO q12h or 1000 mg PO q24h for recurrent episodes of HSV) is an orally administered prodrug of acyclovir used for the treatment of acute herpes zoster infections and for treatment or suppression of genital HSV infection. It is converted to acyclovir in the body. An advantage over oral acyclovir is less frequent dosing. The most common **adverse effect** is nausea. Valacyclovir can rarely cause CNS disturbances, and high doses (8 g/d) have been associated with development of hemolytic-uremic syndrome/thrombotic thrombocytopenic purpura in immunocompromised patients.
- **Famciclovir** (500 mg PO q8h for herpes zoster, 250 mg PO q8h for the initial episode of genital HSV infection, and 125 mg PO q12h for recurrent episodes of genital HSV

infection) is an orally administered antiviral agent used for the treatment of acute herpes zoster reactivation and for treatment or suppression of genital HSV infections.

Adverse events include headache, nausea, and diarrhea.

Anticytomegalovirus Agents

- **Ganciclovir** (5 mg/kg IV q12h for 14–21 days for induction therapy of cytomegalovirus [CMV] retinitis, followed by 6 mg/kg IV for 5 days every week or 5 mg/kg IV q24h) is used to treat CMV infections.
  - It has activity against HSV and VZV, but safer drugs are available to treat those infections. The drug is widely distributed in the body, including the CSF.
  - It is indicated for treatment of CMV retinitis and other serious CMV infections in immunocompromised patients (e.g., transplant and AIDS patients). Chronic maintenance therapy is required to suppress CMV disease in patients with AIDS until CD4 count is >200 cell/μL.
  - **Adverse events:** Neutropenia is the main therapy-limiting adverse effect and may require treatment with granulocyte colony-stimulating factor for management (300 μg SC daily to weekly). Thrombocytopenia, rash, confusion, headache, nephrotoxicity, and GI disturbances may also occur. Blood counts and electrolytes should be monitored weekly while the patient is receiving therapy. Concomitant use of other agents with nephrotoxic or bone marrow suppressive effects should be avoided, if possible.
- **Valganciclovir** (900 mg PO q12–24h) is the oral prodrug of ganciclovir. This agent has substantial bioavailability and can be used for treatment of CMV retinitis. Adverse events are the same as those for ganciclovir.
- **Foscarnet** (60 mg/kg IV q8h or 90 mg/kg IV q12h for 14–21 days as induction therapy, followed by 90–120 mg/kg IV q24h as maintenance therapy for CMV; 40 mg/kg IV q8h for acyclovir-resistant HSV and VZV) is used to treat acyclovir-resistant HSV/VZV infections and ganciclovir-resistant CMV infections. It can be used in patients who are not tolerating or not responding to ganciclovir.

  Adverse events: Nephrotoxicity is a major concern. CrCl should be determined at baseline, and electrolytes (PO_4, Ca^{2+}, Mg^{2+}, and K^+) and serum creatinine should be checked at least twice a week. Normal saline (500–1000 mL) should be given before and during infusions to minimize nephrotoxicity. Foscarnet should be avoided in patients with a serum creatinine of >2.8 mg/dL or baseline CrCl of <50 mL/min. Concomitant use of other nephrotoxins should be avoided. Foscarnet chelates divalent cations can cause tetany even with normal serum calcium levels. Use of foscarnet with pentamidine can cause severe hypocalcemia. Other side effects include seizures, phlebitis, rash, and genital ulcers. **Prolonged therapy with foscarnet should be monitored by physicians who are experienced with administration of home IV therapy and can systematically monitor patients' laboratory results.**
- **Cidofovir** (5 mg/kg IV q wk for 2 weeks as induction therapy, followed by 5 mg/kg IV q14d chronically as maintenance therapy) is used primarily to treat CMV retinitis in patients with AIDS who are not responding to ganciclovir or foscarnet. It can be administered through a peripheral IV line.
  - **Adverse events:** The most common adverse event is nephrotoxicity. It should be avoided in patients with a CrCl of <55 mL/min, a serum creatinine >1.5 mg/dL, significant proteinuria, or a recent history of receipt of other nephrotoxic medications.
  - **Each cidofovir dose should be administered with probenecid** (2 g PO 3 hours before the infusion and then 1 g at 2 and 8 hours after the infusion) along with 1 L normal saline IV 1–2 hours before the infusion to minimize nephrotoxicity. Patients should have a serum creatinine and urine protein check before each dose of cidofovir is given.

This drug requires systematic monitoring of laboratory studies and close physician follow-up.

- **Letermovir** (480 mg IV or PO q24h) is a CMV DNA terminase inhibitor that is FDA approved for CMV prophylaxis in allogeneic hematopoietic stem cell transplant through 100 days posttransplant. It has been anecdotally utilized for treatment of CMV infection, although this is not an established indication. Letermovir is contraindicated with pimozide and ergot alkaloids. Concomitant use of cyclosporine mandates dose reduction of letermovir to 240 mg q24h. The drug appears to be well-tolerated.

Others

Remdesivir is an investigational antiviral agent under evaluation for COVID-19. The novel nucleotide analogue prodrug was first used to treat Ebola virus disease. The recommended adult dose is 200 mg intravenously on day 1 followed by 100 mg daily for 10 days total in patients on mechanical ventilation or ECMO and 5 days total in other patients.

ANTIFUNGAL AGENTS

Amphotericin B

GENERAL PRINCIPLES

Amphotericin B is fungicidal by interacting with ergosterol and disrupting the fungal cell membrane. Reformulation of this agent in various lipid vehicles has decreased some of its adverse side effects. Amphotericin B formulations are not effective for *Pseudallescheria boydii, Candida lusitaniae,* or *Aspergillus terreus* infections.

- **Amphotericin B deoxycholate** (0.3–1.5 mg/kg q24h as a single infusion over 2–6 hours) was once widely used but has now been supplanted by lipid-based formulations of the drug as a result of their improved tolerability.
- **Lipid complexed preparations** of amphotericin B, including liposomal amphotericin B (3–6 mg/kg IV q24h) and amphotericin B lipid complex (5 mg/kg IV q24h), have decreased nephrotoxicity and are generally associated with fewer infusion-related reactions than amphotericin B deoxycholate. Liposomal amphotericin B has the most FDA-approved uses and also appears to be the best tolerated lipid amphotericin B formulation overall.

SPECIAL CONSIDERATIONS

- The major **adverse event** of all amphotericin B formulations, including the lipid formulations, is **nephrotoxicity.** Patients should receive 500 mL of normal saline before and after each infusion to minimize nephrotoxicity. Irreversible renal failure appears to be related to cumulative doses. Therefore, concomitant administration of other nephrotoxins should be avoided if possible.
- Common **infusion-related effects** include fever/chills, nausea, headache, and myalgias. Premedication with 500–1000 mg of acetaminophen and 50 mg of diphenhydramine may control many of these symptoms. More severe reactions may be prevented by premedication with hydrocortisone 25–50 mg IV. Intolerable infusion-related chills can be managed with meperidine 25–50 mg IV.
- Amphotericin B therapy is associated with **potassium and magnesium wasting** that generally requires supplementation. Serum creatinine and electrolytes (including Mg^{2+} and K^{+}) should be monitored at least two to three times a week.

Azoles

GENERAL PRINCIPLES

Azoles are fungistatic agents that inhibit ergosterol synthesis.

- **Fluconazole** (100–800 mg PO/IV q24h) is the drug of choice for many *Candida* infections, such as UTIs, thrush, vaginal candidiasis (150-mg single dose), esophagitis, peritonitis, hepatosplenic infection, and can also be used for severe disseminated candidal infections (e.g., candidemia). It is the treatment of choice for consolidation therapy of cryptococcal meningitis following an initial 14-day course of an amphotericin B product or as a second-line agent for primary treatment of cryptococcal meningitis (400–800 mg PO q24h for 8 weeks, followed by 200 mg PO q24h thereafter for chronic maintenance treatment).

Fluconazole does not have activity against *Aspergillus* spp. or *Candida krusei*. *Candida glabrata* also has intrinsically low susceptibility to fluconazole.

- **Itraconazole** (200–400 mg PO q24h) is a triazole with broad-spectrum antifungal activity.
  - It is used to treat endemic mycoses such as coccidioidomycosis, histoplasmosis, blastomycosis, and sporotrichosis.
  - It is an alternative therapy for *Aspergillus* and can also be used to treat infections caused by dermatophytes, including onychomycosis of the toenails (200 mg PO q24h for 12 weeks) and fingernails (200 mg PO q12h for 1 week, with a 3-week interruption, and then a second course of 200 mg PO q12h for 1 week).
  - The capsules require adequate gastric acidity for absorption and, therefore, should be taken with food or carbonated beverage. The liquid formulation is preferred as it is not significantly affected by gastric acidity and is better absorbed on an empty stomach.
- **Posaconazole** (delayed-release tablet and IV doses are 300 mg PO/IV q12h on day 1, followed by 300 mg PO/IV q24h; oral suspension dose is 200 mg PO q8h for prophylaxis and 100–400 mg PO q12–24h for oropharyngeal candidiasis treatment) is an oral azole agent that is used for prophylaxis of invasive aspergillosis and candidiasis in hematopoietic stem cell transplant patients with graft-versus-host disease or in patients with hematologic malignancies experiencing prolonged neutropenia from chemotherapy as well as treatment of oropharyngeal candidiasis. It has also been used for treatment of mucormycosis, although it is not FDA approved for this use.
  - Each suspension dose should be administered with a full meal, liquid supplement, or acidic carbonated beverage (e.g., ginger ale). Acid-suppressive therapy may reduce absorption of the oral suspension, but not the delayed-release tablets.
  - Rifabutin, phenytoin, and cimetidine reduce posaconazole concentrations and should not be used concomitantly.
  - Posaconazole increases bioavailability of cyclosporine, tacrolimus, and midazolam, necessitating dosage reductions of these agents. Dosage reduction of vinca alkaloids, statins, and calcium channel blockers should also be considered.
  - Terfenadine, astemizole, pimozide, cisapride, quinidine, and ergot alkaloids are contraindicated with posaconazole.
- **Voriconazole** (loading dose of 6 mg/kg IV [two doses 12 hours apart], followed by a maintenance dose of 4 mg/kg IV q12h or 200 mg PO q12h [100 mg PO q12h if <40 kg]) is a triazole antifungal with a wide range of activity against pathogenic fungi. It is active against all clinically important species of *Aspergillus*, as well as *Candida* (including most non-*albicans*), *Scedosporium apiospermum*, and *Fusarium* spp.
  - It is the treatment of choice for most forms of invasive aspergillosis, for which it demonstrates response rates of 40%–50% and superiority over conventional amphotericin B.

It is also effective in treating candidemia, esophageal candidiasis, and *Scedosporium* and *Fusarium* infections.

  - An advantage of voriconazole is the easy transition from IV to PO therapy because of excellent bioavailability. For refractory fungal infections, a dose increase of 50% may be useful. The maintenance dose is reduced by 50% for patients with moderate hepatic failure.
  - Because of its metabolism through the **cytochrome P450 system** (enzymes 2C19, 2C9, and 3A4), there are several **clinically significant drug interactions** that must be considered. Rifampin, rifabutin, carbamazepine (markedly reduced voriconazole levels), sirolimus (increased drug concentrations), and astemizole (prolonged QT_c) are contraindicated with voriconazole. Concomitantly administered cyclosporine, tacrolimus, and warfarin require more careful monitoring.

- **Isavuconazonium sulfate, the prodrug of isavuconazole** (372 mg isavuconazonium sulfate [equivalent to 200 mg isavuconazole] PO/IV q8h for 48 hours, then 372 mg isavuconazonium sulfate [equivalent to 200 mg isavuconazole] PO/IV q24h), is an azole with broad-spectrum antifungal activity that is FDA approved for treatment of invasive aspergillosis and invasive mucormycosis.
  - The oral formulation has a 98% oral bioavailability that is unaffected by food.
  - The IV formulation does not contain a cyclodextrin-based solubilizing vehicle and can be safely used in patients with CrCl ≤50 mL/min.
  - It is not associated with QT_c prolongation, but rather a minor QT_c shortening.
  - Rifampin, carbamazepine, long-acting barbiturates, and St. John's wort significantly reduce isavuconazole concentrations and are contraindicated.
  - High-dose ritonavir and ketoconazole can significantly increase isavuconazole concentrations and are contraindicated.

SPECIAL CONSIDERATIONS

Nausea, diarrhea, and rash are mild side effects of the azoles. Hepatitis is a rare but serious complication. LFTs should be monitored regularly with chronic use and especially with compromised liver function. These agents may prolong the QT_c interval (excluding isavuconazole). Serum level monitoring is also advisable with use of itraconazole, posaconazole, and voriconazole. The IV formulations of voriconazole and posaconazole should not be used in patients with a CrCl of <50 mL/min because of accumulation and potential toxicity from the cyclodextrin vehicle. Transient visual disturbance is a common adverse effect (30%) of voriconazole. **This class of antibiotics has major drug interactions.**

Echinocandins

This class of antifungals inhibits the enzyme (1,3)-β-D-glucan synthase that is essential in fungal cell wall synthesis.

- **Caspofungin acetate** (70 mg IV loading dose, followed by 50 mg IV q24h) has fungicidal activity against most *Aspergillus* and *Candida* spp., including azole-resistant *Candida* strains. Caspofungin does not have activity against *Cryptococcus, Histoplasma, Blastomyces, Coccidioides*, or *Mucor* spp. It is FDA approved for treatment of candidemia and refractory invasive aspergillosis and as empiric therapy in febrile neutropenia.
  - Metabolism is primarily hepatic, although the cytochrome P450 system is not significantly involved. An increased maintenance dosage is necessary with the use of drugs that induce hepatic metabolism (e.g., efavirenz, nelfinavir, phenytoin, rifampin, carbamazepine, dexamethasone). The maintenance dose should be reduced to 35 mg for patients with moderate hepatic impairment; however, no dose adjustment is necessary for renal failure.

  - In vitro and limited clinical data suggest a synergistic effect when caspofungin is given in conjunction with itraconazole, voriconazole, or amphotericin B for *Aspergillus* infections.
  - **Adverse events:** Fever, rash, nausea, and phlebitis at the injection site are infrequent.
- **Micafungin sodium** is used for candidemia (100 mg IV q24h), esophageal candidiasis (150 mg IV q24h), and as fungal prophylaxis for patients undergoing hematopoietic stem cell transplantation (50 mg IV q24h). The spectrum of activity is similar to that of anidulafungin and caspofungin. There may be clinically insignificant increases in serum concentrations of sirolimus and nifedipine. Micafungin may increase cyclosporine concentrations in about 20% of patients. No change in dosing is necessary in renal or hepatic dysfunction.
  - **Adverse events** include elevated LFTs and rare cases of rash and delirium.
- **Anidulafungin** (200 mg IV loading dose, followed by 100 mg IV q24h) is useful for treatment of candidemia and other systemic *Candida* infections (intra-abdominal abscess and peritonitis) as well as esophageal candidiasis (100-mg loading dose, followed by 50 mg daily). The spectrum of activity is similar to that of caspofungin and micafungin. Anidulafungin is not a substrate inhibitor or inducer of cytochrome P450 isoenzymes and does not have clinically relevant drug interactions. No dosage change is necessary in renal or hepatic insufficiency.
  Adverse events include possible histamine-mediated reactions, elevations in LFTs, and, rarely, hypokalemia.
- Rezafungin was approved by the FDA in 2023 for the treatment of candidemia and invasive candidiasis.

Miscellaneous

- **Flucytosine** (25 mg/kg PO q6h) exerts its fungicidal effects on susceptible *Candida* and *Cryptococcus* spp. by interfering with DNA synthesis.
  - Main clinical uses are in the treatment of cryptococcal meningitis and severe *Candida* infections in combination with amphotericin B. This agent should not be used alone because of risk for rapid emergence of resistance.
  - **Adverse events** include dose-related bone marrow suppression and bloody diarrhea due to intestinal flora conversion of flucytosine to 5-fluorouracil.
  - Peak drug concentrations should be kept between 50 and 100 μg/mL. Close monitoring of serum concentrations and dose adjustments are critical in the setting of renal insufficiency. LFTs should be obtained at least once a week.
- **Terbinafine** (250 mg PO q24h for 6–12 weeks) is an allylamine antifungal agent that kills fungi by inhibiting ergosterol synthesis. It is FDA approved for the treatment of onychomycosis of the fingernails (6 weeks of treatment) or toenails (12 weeks of treatment). It is not generally used for systemic infections.
  - **Adverse events** include headache, GI disturbances, rash, LFT abnormalities, and taste disturbances. This drug should not be used in patients with hepatic cirrhosis or a CrCl of <50 mL/min. It does not significantly inhibit the metabolism of cyclosporine (15% decrease) or warfarin.
- **Griseofulvin** (500–1000 mg/d PO) is an antifungal antibiotic effective against most dermatophytes and has been the drug of choice for chronic infections caused by these fungi (skin and nail infections).
- Brexafemme is used for the treatment of vulvovaginal candidiasis. It is administered 12 hours apart for 1 day, with a total daily dosage of 600 mg.
- Oteseconazole was approved by the FDA to reduce the incidence of recurrent vulvovaginal candidiasis (RVVC) in females with a history of RVVC who are not of reproductive potential.

Common Infections and Presumptive Treatment

TABLE S-1 Respiratory Tract Infections

Infection	Likely Causative Organisms	Empiric Antibiotics (Presumptive Antibiotics)	Alternative Antibiotics
Community acquired Pneumonia	*S. pneumoniae, H.influenzae,* Legionella, *E.coli, Klebsiella sp., S.aureus*	Mild to moderate cases Amoxycillin-500 mg–1 g TDS oral. Severe cases if IV indicated, amoxycillin-clavulanate 1.2 g IV TDS or Ceftriaxone 2 g IV OD + Tab azithromycin 500 mg OD or clarithromycin 500 mg BD (to cover atypical organsims) For 5–7 days	Cefoperazone-Sulbactam 3 g IV 12 hourly OR Meropenem 1 g IV TDS
Lung abscess, Empyema	*S. pneumoniae, E.coli, Klebsiella sp., Pseudomonas aeruginosa, S.aureus,* anaerobes	Amoxycillin- 500 mg–1 g TDS OR Piperacillin-Tazobactam 4.5 g IV 6 hourly	Meropenem 1 g IV TDS
Acute pharyngitis	Viral	None required	
	Group A ß-hemolytic Streptococci (GABHS), Group C, G Streptococcus,	*Oral Penicillin v 500 mg BD or Amoxicillin 500 mg Oral TDS for 10 days*	*In case of penicillin allergy: Azithromycin 500 mg OD for 5 days*

(Continued)

TABLE S-1 Respiratory Tract Infections (Continued)

Ludwig's angina Vincent's angina	Polymicrobial (cover oral anaerobes)	Clindamycin 600 mg IV 8 hourly or Amoxicillin-Clavulanate 1.2 g IV	Piperacillin-Tazobactam 4.5 g IV 6 hourly
Acute bacterial rhinosinusitis	Viral, *S. pneumoniae*, *H. influenzae*, *M. catarrhalis*	Amoxicillin-clavulanate 1 g oral BD for 7 days	
Acute bronchitis	Viral	Antibiotics not required	
Acute bacterial exacerbation of COPD	*S. pneumoniae* *H. influenzae* *M. catarrhalis*	Amoxicillin-clavulanate 1 g oral BD for 7 days	Azithromycin 500 mg oral OD × 3 days

TABLE S-2 Cardiovascular Infections

Condition	Likely Causative Organism	Empiric Antibiotics (Presumptive Antibiotics)	Alternative Antibiotics
Infective Endocarditis: ***Native valve (awaiting cultures) Indolent***	Viridans group Streptococci, other Streptococci, Enterococci	Penicillin G 20MU IV divided doses, 4 hourly Or Ampicillin 2 g IV 4h Or Ceftriaxone 2 g IV OD daily For 4 weeks If additional of: Gentamicin 1 mg/kg IM or IV 8h, duration of treatment can be reduced to 2 weeks.	Vancomycin 20–35 mg/kg loading dose followed by 15–20 mg/kg/dose IV 8 hrly
Infective Endocarditis: In Severe Sepsis	*S.aureus* (MSSA or MRSA) Risk for gram-negative bacilli	Vancomycin 25–30 mg/kg loading followed by 15–20 mg/kg IV 12 hourly (maximum 1 g 12 hourly) AND Meropenem 1 g IV 8h Duration: 4–6 weeks	Daptomycin 6 mg/kg IV once a day AND Meropenem 1 g IV q8h Duration: 4–6 weeks

TABLE S-3 Skin & Soft Tissue Infections

Infection	Likely Causative Organisms	Empiric Antibiotics (Presumptive Antibiotics)	Alternative antibiotics
Cellulitis	*Streptococcus pyogenes* (common), *S.aureus*	Amoxicillin-Clavulanate 1.2 g IV TDS/625 mg oral TDS or Ceftriaxone 2 g IV OD	Clindamycin 600–900 mg IV TDS
Furunculosis	*S.aureus*	Amoxicillin-Clavulanate 1.2 g IV/Oral 625 TDS or Ceftriaxone 2 g IV OD. Duration 5–7 days	Clindamycin 600–900 mg IV TDS
Necrotizing fasciitis	*Streptococcus pyogenes*, *S. aureus*, anaerobes, Enterobacteriaceae (polymicrobial)	Piperacillin-Tazobactam 4.5 g IV 6 hourly or Cefoperazone-Sulbactam 3 g IV 12 hourly AND Clindamycin 600–900 mg IV 8 hourly Duration depends on the progress	Imipenem 1 g IV 8 hourly or Meropenem 1 g IV 8 hourly AND Clindamycin 600–900 mg IV TDS/linezolid 600 mg IV BD/daptomycin 6 mg/kg/day

TABLE S-4 Urinary Tract Infections

Infection	Likely Causative Organisms	Empiric Antibiotics (Presumptive Antibiotics)	Alternative Antibiotics
Acute uncomplicated Cystitis	*E.coli, Staphylococcus saphrophyticus*(in sexually activeyoungwomen), *Klebsiella pneumoniae*	Nitrofurantoin 100 mg BD for 7 days or Cotrimoxazole 960 mg BD for 3–5 days or Ciprofloxacin 500 mg BD for 3–5 days	
Acute uncomplicated Pyelonephritis	*E.coli, Staphylococcus saphrophyticus* (in sexually active young women), *Klebsiella pneumoniae, Proteus mirabilis*	Ceftriaxone 2 g IV OD Complete total duration of 14 days	Piperacillin-Tazobactam 4.5 g IV 6 hourly or Cefoperazone-Sulbactam 3 g IV 12 hourly or Ertapenem 1 g IV OD Or Meropenem 1 g IV TDS
Complicated Pyelonephritis	*Escherichia coli, Klebsiella pneumonia, Proteus mirabilis, Pseudomonas aeruginosa, Enterococcus* sp. Frequently multi-drug resistant organisms are present	Piperacillin-Tazobactam 4.5 g IV 6 hourly or Cefoperazone-Sulbactam 3 g IV 12 hourly	Imipenem 1 g IV 8 hourly or Meropenem 1 g IV 8 hourly
Acute prostatitis	Enterobacteriaceae (*E.coli, Klebsiella sp.*)	Doxycline 100 mg BD or Co-trimoxazole 960 mg BD.	In severe cases, Piperacillin-Tazobactam 4.5 g IV 6 hourly or Cefoperazone-sulbactam 3 g IV 12 hourly or Ertapenem 1 g IV OD or Imipenem 1 g IV 8 hourly or Meropenem 1 g IV 8 hourly

TABLE S-5 Obstetrics and Gynaecological Infections

Infections	Likely Organism	Primary Treatment (Presumptive Antibiotics)	Alternate Treatment
Asymptomatic Bacteriuria during pregnancy > 1,00,000 cfu/mL of bacteria of same species in 2 urine cultures obtained 2–7 days apart.		Nitrofurantoin 100 mg Oral, BD for 7 days or Amoxicillin 500 mg Oral BD × 7–10 days.	Oral cephalosporins, TMP-SMX or TMP alone
Group B streptococcal Disease, Prophylaxis and Treatment	Group B Streptococci	IV Penicillin G 5 million units. (loading dose) then 2.5–3 million units IV QID until delivery. or Ampicillin 2 g IV (Loading dose) then 1 g QID until delivery	Cefazolin 2 g IV (loading dose) and then 1 g TID Clindamycin 900 mg IV TID or vancomycin IV or teicoplanin for penicillin allergy
Septic abortion **Chorioamniotis** **Endomyometritis and Septic Pelvic Vein Phlebitis**	Bacteroides, *Prevotella bivius*, Group B, Group A	Ampicillin 500 mg QID If patient has been partially treated with antibiotics, send blood cultures and start Piperacillin-Tazobactam or Cefoperazone- sulbactam + Metronidazole till the sensitivity report is available.	Ceftriaxone 2 g IV OD
Candidiasis	Candida species	Fluconazole oral 150 mg single dose For milder cases- Intravaginal agents as creams or suppositories clotrimazole, miconazole, nystatin. Intravaginal azoles, single dose to 7–14 days.	
Bacterial vaginosis	Polymicrobial	Metronidazole 500 mg Oral BD × 7 days Or metronidazole vaginal gel 1 HS × 5 days Or Tinidazole 2 g orally ODx 3 days Or 2% Clindamycin Vaginal cream 5 g HS × 5 days	

(Continued)

TABLE S-5 Obstetrics and Gynaecological Infections (Continued)

Infections	Likely Organism	Primary Treatment (Presumptive Antibiotics)	Alternate Treatment
Trichimoniasis	Trichomonas vaginalis	Metronidazole 2 g single dose or 500 mg Oral BD × 7 days or Tinidazole 2 g Oral single dose For treatment failure – retreat with Metronidazole 500 mg Oral BD × 7 Days, if 2nd failure Metronidazole 2 g Oral OD × 3–5 days	
Cervicitis/Urethritis	Polymicrobial/ Gonococcal	Ceftriaxone 250 mg IM Single dose + Azithromycin 1 g single dose OR Doxycycline 100 mg BD × 7 day	
Pelvic Inflammatory Disease	*S. aureus,* Enterobacteriacae, gonococci, gardenella	Outpatient treatment Ceftriaxone 250 mg IM/IV single dose plus +/– Metronidazole 500 mg BD × 14 days Plus Doxycycline 100 mg BD × 14 Days Inpatient Treatment Clindamycin + ceftriaxone till patient admitted then change to OPD treatment	
Mastitis	*S. aureus*	Amoxycillin clavulunate/Cephalexin 500 mg QID/OR Ceftriaxone 2 g OD OR MRSA- Add Clindamycin 300 QID or Vancomycin I g IV 12 hourly /teicoplanin 12 mg/kg IV 12 hourly × 3 doses followed by 6 once daily IV	

TABLE S-6 Bones and Joint Infections

Condition	Likely Causative Organisms	Empiric Antibiotics	Alternative Antibiotics
Acute osteomyelitis OR Septic arthritis	*S.aureus, Streptococcus pyogenes* Enterobacteriaceae	Ceftriaxone 2 g IV OD Followed by Oral therapy by Cloxacillin 500 mg q 8h Or Cephalexin 500 mg q 6h	Piperacillin-tazobactam 4.5 g IV q 6h or Cefoperazone-sulbactam 3 g IV q 12h AND Clindamycin 600–900 mg IV TDS
Chronic Osteomyelitis OR Chronic synovitis		No empiric therapy	Definitive Treatment guided by bone/synovial biopsy culture. Treat for 6 weeks minimum Investigate for TB, Nocardia, fungi. Extensive surgical debridement. Total duration of treatment depends on the joint and the organism.
Prosthetic joint infection	Coagulase negative staphylococci, *Staphylococcus* aureus, Streptococci Gram-negative bacilli, *Enterococcus*, Anaerobes	Ceftriaxone 2 g IV OD. Add Vancomycin1 g IV BD or Teicoplanin 800 mg × 3 doses followed by 400 mg once daily	Preferable not to give empirical therapy till microbiological diagnosis is established. Surgical intervention including removal and replacement of prosthesis maybe required.

TABLE S-7 Gastrointestinal & Intra-Abdominal Infections

Disease	Causative Organisms	Presumptive Antibiotics/First Line	Alternative Antibiotics
Acute Gastroenteritis	Viral, Entero-toxigenic & Entero-pathogenic *E. coli*	None	None
Food poisoning	*S. aureus,* *B. cereus,* *C. botulinum*		
Cholera	*V.cholerae*	Doxycycline 300 mg Oral stat OR Azithromycin Oral in children (20 mg/kg) and pregnant women (1g)	Azithromycin 1 g Oral stat OR Ciprofloxacin 500 mg BD for 3 days
Bacterial dysentery	*Shigella sp.*, Campylobacter, Non-typhoidal salmonellosis Shiga toxin producing *E. coli*	Ceftriaxone 2 g IV OD for 5 days OR oral cefixime 10–15 mg/kg/day × 5 days Antibiotic Treatment not recommended.	Azithromycin 1 g OD × 3 days
Amoebic dysentery	*E. histolytica*	Metronidazole 400 mg Oral TDS for 7–10 days	Tinidazole 2 g Oral OD for 3 days
Giardiasis	*Giardia lamblia*	Metronidazole 250–500 mg oral TID × 7–10 d	Tinidazole 2 g oral × 1 dose
Enteric fever	*Salmonella* Typhi *and* Paratyphi A	Outpatients: Cefixime 20 mg/kg/day for 14 days or Azithromycin 500 mg BD for 7 days. Inpatients: Ceftriaxone 2 g IV BDfor 2 weeks +/–Azithromycin 500 mg BD for 7 days	Cotrimoxazole 960 mg BD for 2 weeks
Cholangitis, cholecystitis	Enterobacteriaceae (*E.coli, Klebsiella sp.*)	Ceftriaxone 2 g IV OD or Piperacillin-Tazobactam 4.5 g IV 8 hourly OR Cefoperazone-Sulbactam 3 g IV 12 hourly For 7–10 days	Imipenem 500 mg IV 6 hourly OR Meropenem 1 g IV 8 hourly For 7–10 days

(Continued)

TABLE S-7 Gastrointestinal & Intra-Abdominal Infections (Continued)

Pseudomem-branous colitis	*C. difficile*	Vancomycin 125 mg orally 4 times daily for 10 days	Metronidazole 500 mg orally 3 times daily for 10–14 days
Spontaneous bacterial Peritonitis	Enterobacteriaceae (*E.coli, Klebsiella sp.*)	Cefotaxime 1–2 g IV TDS or Piperacillin-Tazobactam 4.5 g IV 8 hourly or Cefoperazone-Sulbactam 3 g IV 12h	Imipenem 500 mg IV 6 hourly or Meropenem 1 g IV 8 hourly
Secondary peritonitis, Intra-abdominal abscess/ GI perforation	Enterobacteriaceae (*E.coli, Klebsiella sp.*), Bacteroides (colonic perfora-tion), Anaerobes	Piperacillin-Tazobactam 4.5 g IV 8 hourly or Cefoperazone-Sulbactam 3 g IV 12 hourly in severe infections	Imipenem 1 g IV 8 hourly or Meropenem 1 g IV 8 hourly or Doripenem 500 mg TDS or Ertapenem 1 g IV OD
		In very sick patients, if required, addition of cover for yeast (fluconazole iv 800 mg loading dose day 1, followed by 400 mg day 2 onwards) and for Enterococcus (vancomycin/teicoplanin) may be contemplated	
Pancreatitis Mild-moderate		No antibiotics	
Necrotizing pancreatitis: infected pseudocyst; pancreatic abscess	*Entrobacteriaceae, Enterococci, S. aureus, S. epidermidis, anaerobes, Candida sp.*	Piperacillin-Tazobactam 4.5 g IV 8 hourly empirically or Cefoperazone-Sulbactam 3 g IV 8 hourly in severe infections In very sick patients, if required, addition of cover for yeast (fluconazole iv 800 mg loading dose day 1, followed by 400 mg 2nd day onwards) & and for Enterococcus (vancomy-cin/teicoplanin) may be contemplated For 7–10 days	Imipenem-Cilastatin 500 mg IV 6 hourly or Meropenem 1 g IV 8 hourly or Doripenem 500 mg IV 8h

(*Continued*)

TABLE S-7 Gastrointestinal & Intra-Abdominal Infections (Continued)

Disease	Causative Organisms	Presumptive Antibiotics/First Line	Alternative Antibiotics
Diverticulitis Mild-OPD treatment	*Gram-Negative Bacteria* *Anaerobes*	Amoxycillin-Clavulanate 625 mg TDS for 7 days	Ciprofloxacin + Metronidazole for 7 days
Diverticulitis moderate-severe	*Gram-Negative Bacteria* *Anaerobes*	Ceftriaxone 2 g IV OD + metronidazole 500 mg IV TDS or Piperacillin-Tazobactam 4.5 g IV 8 hourly empirically or Cefoperazoe-Sulbactam 3 g IV 8 Hourly + Metronidazole 500 mg IV TDS or Meropenem 1 g IV 8 hrly or Imipenem Cilastatin 500 mg IV 6 hourly	
Liver Abscess	*Polymicrobial*	Amoxycillin-clavulanate/ 3rd generation cephalosporin + Metronidazole 500 mg I.V.TID / 800 mg oral TID for 6 weeks (Parenteral therapy for at least 2 weeks, and then maybe switched to oral. Total duration: 6 weeks, if incomplete drainage, give parenteral for longer)	Piperacillin-Tazobactam IV

TABLE S-8 Central Nervous System Infections

Condition	Likely Causative Organisms	Empiric Antibiotics (Presumptive Antibiotics)	Alternative Antibiotics
Acute bacterial Meningitis	*S. pneumoniae, H.influenzae, Neisseria meningititidis*	Ceftriaxone 2 g IV 12 hourly +	Chloramphenicol if patient is allergic to penicillin
		Vancomycin 20–35 mg/kg loading dose followed by 15–20 mg/kg/dose IV 8 hrly (TDM is a must) 10–14 days treatment	
Meningitis-Post- neurosur-geryor Penetra-tinghead trauma	*Staphylococcus epidermidis, Staphylococcus aureus, Propioni-bacterium acnes, Pseudomonas aeruginosa, Acinetobacter baumanii*	Meropenem 2 g IV 8 hourly AND Vancomycin 20–35 mg/kg loading dose followed by 15–20 mg/kg/dose IV 8 hrly (TDM is a must) For 14 days.	
Meningitis with basilar skull fractures	*S.pneumoniae, H. influenzae*	Ceftriaxone 2 g IV 12 hourly + Vancomycin 20–35 mg/kg loading dose followed by 15–20 mg/kg/dose IV 8 hrly (TDM is a must) 10–14 days treatment	
Brain abscess, Subdural empyema	Streptococci, Bacteroides, Enterobacteria-ceae, *S.aureus*	Ceftriaxone 2 g IV 12 hourly or Cefotaxime 2 g IV 4–6 hourly AND Metronidazole 1 g IV 12 hourly Duration of treatment to be decided by clinical & radiological response, minimum two months required.	Meropenem 2 g IV 8 hourly

Summary

- Fifth-generation cephalosporin, ceftaroline has coverage against methicillin-resistant *Staphylococcus aureus* (MRSA), *Listeria monocytogenes,* and *Enterococcus faecalis.*
- Beta-lactam/Beta-lactamase inhibitor combinations like tazobactam (partner to ceftolozane), avibactam (to ceftazidime), vaborbactam (to meropenem), and relebactam (to imipenem-cilastatin) are useful against resistant gram-negative bacteria.
- Plazomicin, a synthetic aminoglycoside, is active against >95% of Enterobacterales isolates.
- The addition of vaborbactam improves the activity of carbapenem-nonsusceptible Enterobacterales, including those that harbor KPCs.
- Echinocandins, the first class of fungal cell wall inhibitors to reach clinical use, are an important treatment option for candidemia and invasive candidiasis.

Scan the QR code to access chapter references.

16 Sexually Transmitted Infections, Human Immunodeficiency Virus, and Acquired Immunodeficiency Syndrome

Matthew Hevey, Rachel Presti, Hilary E. L. Reno, Aashna Pankaj Gandhi, Gauri Malavalli Girish, and Jeco Jacob Kuttykandathil

SEXUAL HISTORY AND GENDER AFFIRMING CARE

Taking a Sexual History

- A sexual history should be taken during initial patient visits or preventive exams or when signs or symptoms of a sexually transmitted infection (STI) are present. Patients should be told this is part of the routine medical examination.
- Providers should discuss with their patients: partners, sexual practices, use of protection from STIs, previous STIs, and pregnancy planning or prevention.
- When discussing partners, it is important to determine the number and gender of the patient's partners without making assumptions or using demeaning language. An example opening line is, "Are your sex partners men, women, or both?"

Transgender Medicine

GENERAL PRINCIPLES

Transgender people have a gender identity that differs from the sex that they were assigned at birth. Transgender medicine is aimed at addressing and minimizing disparities in care for transgender and nonbinary people. In the field of HIV and STIs, providing gender affirming care is especially important for the health of transgender and nonbinary persons.

DEFINITION

- Gender, gender identity: A person's internal sense of self from the perspective of gender
- Sex: The sex assigned at birth
- Gender expression: The manner in which an individual expresses his or her gender
- Sexual orientation: The sex (or sexes) that an individual is attracted to
- Nonbinary: Transgender or gender nonconforming people who are not identified as male or female
- Pronouns: Pronouns that individuals preferred to be called; an example of gender-neutral pronouns is ze/zir/zirs instead of he/him/his.

EPIDEMIOLOGY

- It is estimated that transgender people represent 0.6% of the US population.
- In national surveys, as many as one-third of transgender people postpone medical care because of concerns of disrespect, discrimination, or lack of access to knowledgeable providers.
  - The total population of transgenders in India, according to the 2011 Census, is 4.8 lakh. However, estimates suggest that there are 50–60 lakh transgenders in India, but most keep it a secret to avoid discrimination.[1]
  - In India, transgenders (also called Hijras) have been officially recognized as the third gender. The proportion of transgender women who sell sex in India is estimated to be up to 90%.[2]
  - In India, national HIV prevalence is 0.31%, whereas HIV prevalence among the transgender community is estimated to be 8.2%.[3]
  - Transgender people have a much higher prevalence of HIV than the general population, with transgender women having a 49× greater risk of HIV than the adult population globally.

MANAGEMENT

- A safe and welcoming environment should be provided with attention paid to staff training, knowledge of terminology, gender-neutral bathrooms, and changes to medical forms to include gender assessment questions as recommended by the Williams Institute in their Best Practices guide.[1]
- Assumptions about gender, sexual orientation, or pronouns should not be made and each patient should be assessed as an individual for risk for HIV and STIs.
- For providers wanting to learn more about transgender healthcare, the WPATH guidelines are available. Resource guides exist from the UCSF's Center of Excellence for Transgender Health and Fenway Health's National LGBT Health Education Center.
  - WPATH: https://www.wpath.org/publications/soc
  - UCSF Center of Excellence for Transgender Health: http://transhealth.ucsf.edu/protocols
  - National LGBT Health Education Center: https://www.lgbthealtheducation.org

SEXUALLY TRANSMITTED INFECTIONS, ULCERATIVE DISEASES

- Current STI treatment guidelines are found at www.cdc.gov/std.
- Treatment options for each infection can be found in Table 16-1.

Genital Herpes

GENERAL PRINCIPLES

Genital herpes is caused by **herpes simplex virus (HSV)**, types 1 and 2, usually type 2. The proportion of herpes caused by HSV-1 continues to increase among women and MSM (men who have sex with men). HSV-2 is more likely to recur and may require suppressive therapy.

DIAGNOSIS

- Infection is characterized by painful grouped vesicles in the genital and perianal regions that rapidly ulcerate and form shallow tender lesions.

TABLE 16-1 Treatment of Sexually Transmitted Infections

Infection	Recommended Regimen(s)	Alternative Regimens and Notes
Genital ulcer disease		
Herpes simplex		
First episode	• Acyclovir 400 mg PO three times a day × 7–10 d or 200 mg PO five times daily × 7–10 d • Valacyclovir 1 g PO two times a day × 7–10 d • Famciclovir 250 mg PO three times a day × 7–10 d	
Recurrent episodes	• Acyclovir 400 mg PO three times a day × 5 d or 800 mg two times a day × 5 d or 800 mg PO three times a day × 2 d • Valacyclovir 1 g PO once a day × 5 d or 500 mg PO two times a day × 3 d • Famciclovir 1 g PO two times a day × 1 d or 125 mg PO two times a day × 5 d or 500 mg once, then 250 mg two times a day × 2 d	In patients with HIV: • Acyclovir 400 mg PO three times a day × 5–10 d • Valacyclovir 1 g PO twice a day × 5–10 d • Famciclovir 500 mg PO twice a day × 5–10 d
Suppressive therapy	• Acyclovir 400 mg PO twice a day • Valacyclovir 500 mg or 1 g PO once daily • Famciclovir 250 mg PO twice daily	In patients with HIV: • Acyclovir 400–800 mg PO twice to three times a day • Valacyclovir 500 mg PO twice a day • Famciclovir 500 mg PO twice a day
Syphilis		
Primary, secondary, or early latent <1 yr	• Benzathine penicillin G 2.4 million units IM single dose	Penicillin-allergic: • Doxycycline 100 mg PO twice daily × 14 d • Ceftriaxone 1–2 g IM or IV × 14 days • Tetracycline 500 mg PO four times daily × 14 d • Amoxicillin 3 g plus probenecid 500 mg PO twice daily × 14 days
Latent >1 yr, latent unknown duration	• Benzathine penicillin G 2.4 million units IM once weekly × 3 doses	• Doxycycline 100 mg PO twice daily × 28 d • Ceftriaxone 1–2 g IM or IV × 14 days

(Continued)

TABLE 16-1 Treatment of Sexually Transmitted Infections (Continued)

Infection	Recommended Regimen(s)	Alternative Regimens and Notes
Neurosyphilis	• Aqueous crystalline penicillin G 18–24 million U/d (as 3–4 million units every 4 h or continuous infusion) × 10–14 d	• Procaine penicillin 2.4 million units IM once daily + probenecid 500 mg PO four times daily × 10–14 d
In pregnant women	• Penicillin is the recommended treatment—desensitize if necessary	
Chancroid	• Azithromycin 1 g PO single dose • Ceftriaxone 250 mg IM single dose	• Ciprofloxacin 500 mg PO twice daily × 3 d • Erythromycin base 500 mg PO twice daily × 7 d • Some resistance has been reported for these regimens.
Lymphogranuloma venereum	• Doxycycline 100 mg PO twice daily × 21 d • Azithromycin 1 g PO once weekly × 3 weeks	• Erythromycin base 500 mg PO four times a day × 21 d
Vaginitis/vaginosis		
Trichomonas	• Metronidazole 2 g PO single dose • Tinidazole 2 g PO single dose	In patients with HIV (and alternative for HIV-uninfected): • Metronidazole 500 mg PO twice daily × 7 d
In pregnant women	• Metronidazole 2 g PO × 1 (not teratogenic)	
Bacterial vaginosis	• Metronidazole 500 mg PO twice daily × 7 d • Clindamycin cream 2% intravaginal at bedtime × 7 d • Metronidazole gel 0.75% intravaginal once a day for 5 d	• Tinidazole 2 g PO once daily × 2 d or 1 g PO once daily × 5 d • Clindamycin 300 mg PO twice daily × 7 d • Clindamycin ovules 100 mg intravaginal × 3 d
Candidiasis	• Intravaginal azoles in variety of strengths for 1–7 d • Fluconazole 150 mg PO × 1	Ibrexafungerp – 150 mg (2 tabs twice a day) – single day
Severe candidiasis	• Fluconazole 150 mg PO every 72 h × 2–3 doses	• Intravaginal azoles for 7–14 d • Culture and sensitivities maybe helpful
Recurrent candidiasis	• Fluconazole 100, 150, or 200 mg PO once weekly × 6 mo	Culture/sensitivity studies are extremely important due to rising antifungal resistance.

(Continued)

TABLE 16-1 Treatment of Sexually Transmitted Infections (Continued)

Infection	Recommended Regimen(s)	Alternative Regimens and Notes
Urethritis/cervicitis		
Gonorrhea	• Ceftriaxone 250 mg IM once + azithromycin 1 g PO once even if testing for Chlamydia trachomatis is negative. • Given concern for antibiotic resistance, dual treatment is recommended.	• Cefixime 400 mg PO × 1 + Azithromycin 1 g PO × 1 • Oral cephalosporin treatment is not recommended as long as ceftriaxone is available.
Disseminated gonococcal infection	• Ceftriaxone 1 g IM or IV daily + Azithromycin 1 g PO × 1 • Can switch to PO after 24–48 h if substantial improvement, treat for at least 7 d	• Cefotaxime 1 g IV every 8 h • Ceftizoxime 1 g IV every 8 h + Azithromycin 1 g PO × 1
Chlamydia	• Azithromycin 1 g PO single dose • Doxycycline 100 mg PO twice daily × 7 d	• Erythromycin base 500 mg PO or erythromycin ethylsuccinate 800 mg PO four times a day × 7 d • Levofloxacin 500 mg PO daily × 7 d or Ofloxacin 300 mg PO twice daily × 7 d • Amoxicillin 500 mg PO three times daily × 7 d • Retesting is recommended in 3 mo.
Pelvic inflammatory disease		
Outpatient	• Ceftriaxone 500–1000 mg IM once + doxycycline 100 mg PO twice daily × 14 d + consider metronidazole 500 mg orally twice daily × 14 d	• Cefoxitin 2 g IM + probenecid 1 g PO once can be substituted for ceftriaxone
Inpatient	• Ceftriaxone 1 g IV once daily + doxycycline 100 mg IV or PO twice daily × 14 d + metronidazole 500 mg PO or IV twice daily × 14 d + consider metronidazole 500 mg PO twice daily × 14 d	• Clindamycin 900 mg IV every 8 h + gentamicin 2 mg/kg loading dose, then 1.5 mg/kg every 8 h + doxycycline 100 mg PO twice daily × 14 d • Ampicillin-sulbactam 3 g IV every 6 h + doxycycline 100 mg PO twice daily × 14 d

See *cdc.gov/std/* for the current sexually transmitted infection treatment guidelines.

- The initial episode may be associated with inguinal adenopathy, fever, headache, myalgias, and aseptic meningitis; recurrences are usually less severe. Asymptomatic shedding of virus is frequent and leads to transmission.
- Confirmation of HSV infection requires culture or polymerase chain reaction (PCR); however, clinical presentation is often adequate for diagnosis.

TREATMENT

- See Table 16-1 for treatment.

Syphillis

GENERAL PRINCIPLES

- Syphilis is caused by the spirochete *Treponema pallidum.*
- There is a high rate of HIV coinfection in patients with syphilis, from 40% to 70%, and HIV infection should be excluded with appropriate testing.[2]
- Syphilis can have an atypical course in HIV-infected patients; treatment failures and progression to neurosyphilis are more frequent in this population.
- Syphilis rates in the United States are increasing since the year 2000, especially among MSM.
    - In India, syphilis is more commonly reported in men, and secondary followed by latent syphilis are the predominant types seen. Studies have reported the seroprevalence of syphilis in patients attending a sexually transmitted disease clinic in India to be around 6.2%–8% with a decreasing trend in the prevalence.

DIAGNOSIS

Clinical Presentation

- **Primary syphilis** develops within several weeks of exposure and manifests as one or more painless, indurated, superficial ulcerations (chancre).
- **Secondary syphilis** develops 2–10 weeks after the chancre resolves and may produce a rash (usually involves palms and soles), mucocutaneous lesions, adenopathy, and constitutional symptoms.
- **Tertiary syphilis** follows between 1 and 20 years after infection and includes cardiovascular and gummatous disease.
- Neurologic syphilis (general paresis, tabes dorsalis, meningovascular, ocular, or otologic syphilis) is usually a late manifestation, but can occur earlier. Ocular syphilis can occur with any stage of syphilis and is increasingly common. It can lead to blindness. All patients with syphilis should be evaluated for eye complaints. Eye manifestations of syphilis include uveitis and retinitis.[3]
- **Congenital syphilis** occurs by vertical transmission from infected mothers and results in stillbirth in up to 40% of pregnancies. Infected neonates may develop fetal hydrops, rash, hepatomegaly, myocarditis, neurologic disease, and other varied presentations.

Diagnostic Testing

- In **primary syphilis**, dark-field microscopy of lesion exudates, when available, may reveal spirochetes. A nontreponemal serologic test (e.g., rapid plasma reagin [RPR] or Venereal Disease Research Laboratory [VDRL]) should be confirmed with a treponemal-specific test (e.g., fluorescent treponemal antibody absorption or *T. pallidum* particle agglutination).

- Reverse sequence testing (measuring an enzyme-linked immunosorbent assay or chemiluminescence immunoassay before a quantitative RPR) is used by some jurisdictions and may detect early primary syphilis that may otherwise be missed with traditional screening.
- Diagnosis of **secondary syphilis** is made on the basis of positive serologic studies and the presence of a compatible clinical illness.
- **Latent syphilis** is a serologic diagnosis in the absence of symptoms. Nonprimary, nonsecondary syphilis is either early (serologically positive for <1 year) or late (serologically positive for >1 year or for unknown duration).
- To exclude **neurosyphilis**, a lumbar puncture (LP) should be performed in all patients with neurologic, ophthalmic, or auditory signs or symptoms. Additionally, some experts recommend LP in HIV-infected patients with evidence of tertiary disease, treatment failure, or late syphilis.[4] VDRL should be performed on cerebrospinal fluid (CSF).
- Response to treatment should be monitored with nontreponemal serologic tests at 3, 6, and 12 months after treatment. In patients with HIV, tests should be checked every 3 months after treatment for 1 year. A repeat LP should be repeated in 6 months for patients with neurosyphilis to confirm decrease in VDRL titers.

TREATMENT

- See Table 16-1 for treatment.

Chancroid

GENERAL PRINCIPLES

Chancroid is caused by *Haemophilus ducreyi.*

DIAGNOSIS

- Chancroid produces a painful genital ulcer and tender suppurative inguinal lymphadenopathy.
- Identification of the organism is difficult and requires special culture media.

TREATMENT

- See Table 16-1 for treatment.

Lymphogranuloma Venereum

GENERAL PRINCIPLES

Lymphogranuloma venereum is caused by *Chlamydia trachomatis* (serovars L_1, L_2, or L_3).

DIAGNOSIS

- It manifests as a painless genital ulcer, followed by heaped up, matted inguinal lymphadenopathy. Proctocolitis with pain and discharge can occur with anal infection[5] and has been increasingly seen in the United States.[6]
- The diagnosis is based on clinical suspicion and *C. trachomatis* nucleic acid antibody testing (NAAT), if available.

TREATMENT

- See Table 16-1 for treatment.

SEXUALLY TRANSMITTED INFECTIONS, VAGINITIS, AND VAGINOSIS

Trichomoniasis

DIAGNOSIS

Clinical Presentation

- Clinical symptoms of infection by *Trichomonas vaginalis* include malodorous purulent vaginal discharge, dysuria, and genital inflammation.
- Examination reveals profuse frothy discharge and cervical petechiae.
- *T. vaginalis* is often asymptomatic, especially in males.

Diagnostic Testing

- NAATs and antigen detection tests are available to detect *T. vaginalis* and offer improved sensitivity over the traditional visualization of motile trichomonads on a saline wet mount of vaginal discharge.
- Elevated vaginal pH (≥4.5) is usually seen.

TREATMENT

- See Table 16-1 for treatment.

Bacterial Vaginosis

GENERAL PRINCIPLES

The replacement of normal lactobacilli with anaerobic bacteria in the vagina leads to bacterial vaginosis.

DIAGNOSIS

Three of the following criteria are needed to make the diagnosis (Amsel criteria):

- Homogenous, thin, white discharge
- Presence of clue cells on microscopic examination
- Elevated vaginal pH (≥4.5)
- Fishy odor associated with vaginal discharge before or after addition of 10% potassium hydroxide (KOH) (whiff test)

TREATMENT

- See Table 16-1 for treatment.

Vulvovaginal Candidiasis

GENERAL PRINCIPLES

Vulvovaginal candidiasis is not generally considered an STI but commonly develops in the setting of antibiotic therapy. Recurrent infections may be a presenting manifestation of unrecognized HIV infection.

DIAGNOSIS

- Thick, cottage cheese–like vaginal discharge in conjunction with intense vulvar inflammation, pruritus, and dysuria is often present.
- Vaginal pH is normal.
- Definitive diagnosis requires visualization of fungal elements on a KOH preparation of the vaginal discharge.

TREATMENT

- Therapy is often initiated on the basis of the clinical presentation.
- Fluconazole failure may indicate the presence of a **non–*Candida albicans* species**.

Cervicitis/Urethritis

GENERAL PRINCIPLES

Cervicitis and urethritis are frequent presentations of infection with ***Neisseria gonorrhoeae* or *C. trachomatis***, and occasionally *Mycoplasma genitalium*, *Ureaplasma urealyticum*, and *T. vaginalis*. These infections often coexist, and clinical presentations can be identical.

DIAGNOSIS

Clinical Presentation

- Women with urethritis, cervicitis, or both complain of mucopurulent vaginal discharge, dyspareunia, and dysuria.
- Men with urethritis may have dysuria and purulent penile discharge.
- Most infections with these STIs are asymptomatic.
- Disseminated gonococcal infection (DGI) can present with fever, tenosynovitis, vesicopustular skin lesions, and polyarthralgias. DGI may also manifest solely as septic arthritis of the knee, wrist, or ankle (see Chapter 25, Arthritis and Rheumatologic Diseases).

Diagnostic Testing

- A NAAT performed on endocervical, vaginal, urethral (men), urine, or extragenital samples is recommended to make the diagnosis of *C. trachomatis* or *N. gonorrhoeae* infection. In the case of *N. gonorrhoeae*, a Gram stain of endocervical or urethral discharge with gram-negative intracellular diplococci can rapidly establish the diagnosis. Culture can be performed on urethral or endocervical swab specimens.
- Recommendations for testing include NAAT testing at extragenital sites of sexual contact (pharynx, rectum), especially in MSM. Not testing all exposed sites misses the majority of infections in certain populations.

- In addition to NAAT studies, patients with suspected DGI should have blood cultures drawn. In the setting of septic arthritis, synovial fluid analysis and culture is indicated.

TREATMENT

Because of increasing resistance concerns, treatment options for *N. gonorrhoeae* infection are reduced (see Table 16-1).

Pelvic Inflammatory Disease

GENERAL PRINCIPLES

- Pelvic inflammatory disease (PID) is an acute upper genital tract infection in women, involving the uterus, fallopian tubes, and/or ovaries and may involve neighboring pelvic organs. It is usually preceded by cervicitis.
- It is caused by a sexually transmitted agent, and causative organisms include *Neisseria gonorrhoeae, Chlamydia trachomatis,* and *Mycoplasma genitalium.*
- PID is treated as a mixed polymicrobial infection irrespective of the initiating organism.
- Long-term consequences of untreated PID include chronic pain, increased risk of ectopic pregnancy, and infertility.[7]

DIAGNOSIS

Clinical Presentation

Symptoms can range from mild pelvic discomfort and dyspareunia to severe abdominal pain with fever, which may signal complicating perihepatitis (Fitz-Hugh–Curtis syndrome) or tubo-ovarian abscess.

Diagnostic Testing

- Cervical motion tenderness or uterine or adnexal tenderness, vaginal discharge or friability, and the presence of many white blood cells per low-power field on a saline preparation of vaginal or endocervical fluid are consistent with a diagnosis of PID.
- NAATs or culture of endocervical specimens should be obtained to identify *C. trachomatis* or *N. gonorrhoeae* infection.
- All women diagnosed with PID should be screened for HIV infection.
- Differentials include ectopic pregnancy, ovarian cyst rupture/torsion, endometriosis, cystitis, appendicitis, diverticulitis, and irritable bowel syndrome.

TREATMENT

- Patients with severe illness, suspected pelvic abscess, pregnancy, and HIV should be hospitalized. Patients unable to tolerate oral antibiotics also warrant admission.
- Empiric therapy with a second- or third-generation parenteral cephalosporin plus doxycycline along with metronidazole for anaerobic coverage.
- After 24-48 hours of sustained clinical improvement, the patient can be switched to oral antibiotics for a total duration of 14 days.
- Outpatient treatment includes a single IM dose of ceftriaxone (500 mg, maximum of 1g) followed by a 14-day course of doxycycline and metronidazole.
- In the case of patients with IgE-mediated penicillin allergy, clindamycin plus gentamicin can be given as an alternative to cephalosporins.[8]

HUMAN IMMUNODEFICIENCY VIRUS AND ACQUIRED IMMUNODEFICIENCY SYNDROME

HIV Type 1

GENERAL PRINCIPLES

Definition

HIV type 1 is a retrovirus that predominantly infects lymphocytes that bear the CD4 surface protein, as well as co-receptors belonging to the chemokine receptor family (CCR5 or CXCR4), and causes acquired immunodeficiency syndrome (AIDS).

Classification

Diagnosis of AIDS by the Centers for Disease Control and Prevention (CDC) classification is made on the basis of CD4 cell count <200 cells/μL, CD4 percentage <14%, or development of one of the 25 AIDS-defining conditions (Table 16-2).[9]

The WHO classification (Table 16-3) is a clinical classification that classifies patients with HIV into four clinical stages. For adults, adolescents, and children older than 5 years, **advanced HIV disease** is defined as a CD4 of less than 200 cells/μL or a WHO clinical stage 3 or stage 4.[9] All children with HIV younger than 5 years are considered to have **advanced HIV disease.**

Epidemiology

- HIV type 1 is common throughout the world. By the end of 2022, over 39.0 million people worldwide were living with HIV or AIDS, with a significant burden of disease in sub-Saharan Africa.[10,11]
- In the United States, 1.2 million people are estimated to be infected with HIV with 13% of these people unaware of their infection. The CDC recorded 32,100 new infections in the United States in 2021.
- Despite comprising only 14% of the population in the United States, African Americans account for nearly 40% of all new cases of HIV in this country. Hispanics are also disproportionately affected by HIV. Women comprise approximately 24% of the US epidemic.[12,13]
- MSM remain the population most heavily affected by HIV in the United States. Of all new HIV infections in 2021, 70% were MSM.[14,11]

TABLE 16-2 2014 CDC Case Definition of HIV Infection Among Adolescents and Adults

Stage	CD4 Count	CD4 %*	Clinical Evidence
Stage 0	Early HIV infection		
Stage 1	≥500 cells/μL	≥26	No AIDS-defining condition
Stage 2	200–499 cells/μL	14–25	No AIDS-defining condition
Stage 3	<200 cells/μL	<14	*or* Documentation of AIDS-defining condition
Stage unknown	No data	No data	*and* No information on presence of AIDS-defining conditions

*Use CD4 percentage only if no data available for CD4 count

TABLE 16-3	WHO Clinical Staging of HIV Infection
Clinical stage 1	Asymptomatic Persistent generalized lymphadenopathy
Clinical stage 2	• Unexplained moderate weight loss (<10% of body weight) • Recurrent upper respiratory tract infections (sinusitis, tonsillitis, otitis media, and pharyngitis) • Herpes zoster • Angular cheilitis • Recurrent oral ulceration • Papular pruritic eruptions • Seborrheic dermatitis • Fungal nail infections
Clinical stage 3	• Unexplained severe weight loss (>10% of body weight) • Unexplained chronic diarrhea for longer than one month • Unexplained persistent fever (above 37.5°C for >1 month) • Persistent oral candidiasis • Oral hairy leukoplakia • Pulmonary tuberculosis • Severe bacterial infections (e.g., bacteremia, meningitis, pneumonia, empyema, bone or joint infection) • Acute necrotizing ulcerative stomatitis, gingivitis, or periodontitis • Unexplained anemia (<8 g/dL), neutropenia (<500/μL), or HIV-associated immune thrombocytopenia (<50,000/μL) for >1 month
Clinical stage 4	• HIV wasting syndrome • Pneumocystis pneumonia • Tuberculosis—extrapulmonary • Pneumonia, recurrent bacterial • Disseminated nontuberculous mycobacterial infection • Candidiasis of esophagus, trachea, bronchi, or lungs • Disseminated coccidioidomycosis or histoplasmosis • CNS toxoplasmosis • Cryptococcosis—extrapulmonary (including meningitis) • Progressive multifocal leukoencephalopathy • HIV encephalopathy • Cryptosporidiosis, chronic (>1 month) • Isosporiasis, chronic (>1 month) • Chronic herpes simplex (>1 month) infection • Cytomegalovirus disease (retinitis or outside liver, spleen, and nodes) • Recurrent nontyphoidal salmonella bacteremia • Leishmaniasis, atypical disseminated • Lymphoma (cerebral or B-cell non-Hodgkin's) • Kaposi sarcoma • Cervical carcinoma—invasive • Symptomatic HIV-associated nephropathy • Symptomatic HIV-associated cardiomyopathy

- Outside Africa, South Asia constitutes a significant proportion of people living with HIV (PLHIV), although prevalence is 3.9 million South Asian countries. Heterosexual intercourse is the predominant mode of transmission in South Asia.
- An estimated 1.3 million individuals worldwide were infected with HIV in 2022, marking a 38% decline in new HIV infections since 2010.[15] 85.6 million people have become infected with HIV since the start of the epidemic (till the end of 2022).[16]
- Approximately 29.8 million people accessed antiretroviral therapy (ART) globally as of 2022.[17]
- India has the third largest HIV epidemic in the world with 2.4 million people living with HIV as of 2021. Of these, 1.494 million were receiving ART. There were 62,970 new HIV infections and 41,970 AIDS-related deaths reported in India in 2021.
- India has the third largest HIV epidemic in the world with 2.4 million people living with HIV as of 2022. Of these, 72% were receiving ART. There were 66,410 new HIV infections and 39,600 AIDS-related deaths reported in India in 2022.[18]; prevalence in the highest-risk group—female sex workers—is estimated to be about 1.56%.[19]
- There are four main drivers of the HIV epidemic in India: Commercial sex work, heterosexual intercourse, intravenous drug use, and MSM.

- **HIV type 2** is endemic to regions in West Africa. It is characterized by much slower progression to AIDS and resistance to non-nucleoside reverse transcriptase inhibitors (NNRTIs).

Pathophysiology

- After entering the host cell, viral RNA is reverse transcribed into DNA using the HIV **reverse transcriptase**. This viral DNA is inserted into the host genome through the activity of the viral **integrase**. The host cell machinery is then used to produce the relevant viral proteins, which are appropriately truncated by a viral **protease**. Infectious viral particles bud away to infect other CD4 lymphocytes.
- Most infected cells are killed by the host CD8 T-cell response.
- Long-lived latently infected cells persist, especially memory T cells.
- Infection usually leads to CD4 T-cell depletion and **impaired cell-mediated immunity** over a period of 8–10 years.
- Without treatment, >90% of infected patients will progress to AIDS, which is characterized by the development of opportunistic infections (OIs), wasting, and viral-associated malignancies.

Risk Factors

- The virus is primarily transmitted sexually but also via parenteral and perinatal exposure.
- The risk of transmission through blood transfusions from HIV-infected individuals is 93%. Sharing needles and needlestick injuries result in transmission in 63 per 10,000 exposures and 1 in 300, respectively. Since 1985, it is mandatory to screen blood products for HIV, hence, the incidence of acquiring HIV through blood transfusions is very low at present (Table 16-4).
- Among sexual practices, unprotected anal receptive intercourse carries the highest risk of transmission (138 per 10,000 exposures), followed by insertive anal intercourse, vaginal receptive intercourse, and vaginal insertive intercourse. Oral intercourse carries a low risk of transmission.

Prevention

- HIV transmission can be prevented by safe sex practices, which include condom use (male or female) for vaginal, oral, and anal intercourse, decreasing the number of sexual partners, and avoiding needle sharing.

TABLE 16-4 Exposure Route and Percentage of Transmission of HIV

Exposure route	HIV transmission
Blood transfusion	90–95%
Perinatal	15–30%
Sexual intercourse:	
• Vaginal	0.08%–0.19%
• Anal	0.5%–3.38% for receptive anal intercourse; 0.06%–0.16% for insertive anal intercourse
• Oral	0.005–0.01%
Injecting drugs use	0.63–2.14%
Needle stick exposure	0.13%
Mucous membrane splash to eye and oronasal	0.09%

- Postexposure prophylaxis, or the provision of antiretroviral therapy (ART) after needlestick injury or high-risk sexual exposure, can prevent infection.
- Pre-exposure prophylaxis (PrEP), or continuous ART in HIV-negative patients, has proven to decrease the rate of HIV transmission. The current guidelines recommend the use of PrEP for the following high-risk groups[20]
  - MSM
  - Heterosexual HIV-discordant couples
  - Those with multiple sexual partners with inconsistent condom use
  - Commercial sex workers
  - IV drug users
  - A combination of emtricitabine–tenofovir disoproxil fumarate (TDF/FTC) is the approved regimen for PrEP. Other alternatives are TAF/FTC and Cabotegravir (long acting)- IM once a month Before starting PrEP, it is essential to document a negative HIV test, no signs or symptoms of acute HIV infection, hepatitis B status, and normal renal function. These patients should be followed every 3 months for repeat HIV testing as well as STI screening, risk reduction counseling, and every 6 months monitoring of renal function.

DIAGNOSIS

Clinical Presentation

- Acute retroviral syndrome is experienced by up to 75% of patients and is similar to other acute viral illnesses such as infectious mononucleosis due to Epstein–Barr virus (EBV) or cytomegalovirus (CMV) infection. Common presenting symptoms of acute retroviral syndrome are fever, sore throat, nonspecific rash, myalgias, headache, and fatigue.
- As the acute illness resolves spontaneously, many people present to care only after OIs (see later section for clinical presentations) occur late in infection once significant immune compromise has occurred (CD4 count <200 cells/μL). Late presentation can be avoided by routine screening.
- In South Asia, tuberculosis (TB) carries a significant morbidity and mortality in patients with HIV. TB is the most common opportunistic infection in HIV in India, and uncontrolled HIV accelerates the progression of TB. The risk of TB reactivation is 5%–10%

per year in patients with HIV (as opposed to 5%–10% lifetime risk in people with latent tuberculosis infection [LTBI]). Furthermore, the typical manifestations of pulmonary TB are less often seen in advanced HIV and the frequency of extrapulmonary TB increases with lower CD4 counts.

History

Initial evaluation of persons with a confirmed HIV infection should include the following measures:

- Complete history with emphasis on previous OIs, viral coinfections, and other complications.
- Psychological and psychiatric history. Depression and substance use are common and should be identified and treated as necessary.
- Family and social support assessment.
- Assessment of knowledge and perceptions regarding HIV is also crucial to initiate ongoing education regarding the nature and ramifications of HIV infection.

Physical Examination

A complete physical examination is important to evaluate for manifestations of immune compromise. Initial findings may include the following:

- Oral findings: thrush (oral candidiasis), hairy leukoplakia, aphthous ulcers
- Lymphatic system: generalized lymphadenopathy
- Skin: psoriasis, eosinophilic folliculitis, Kaposi sarcoma, molluscum contagiosum, *Cryptococcus*
- Abdominal examination: evidence of hepatosplenomegaly
- Genital examination: presence of ulcers, genital warts, vaginal discharge, and rectal discharge
- Neurologic examination: presence of sensory deficits and cognitive testing

Diagnostic Criteria

- The updated CDC guidelines for screening published in June of 2014 recommend the use of the fourth-generation assay, an antigen/antibody test that involves the detection of the p24 antigen as well as antibodies to HIV-1 and HIV-2. The p24 antigen is a viral capsid protein that can be detected as early as 4–10 days from acute infection, up to 2 weeks earlier than the antibody tests alone. An eclipse phase of infection, during which no testing is positive, still exists for up to 7 days after exposure.
- If the fourth-generation assay is positive, then a differentiation test for HIV-1 and HIV-2 antibodies is performed as a reflex test.
- If the HIV-1 and HIV-2 antibody differentiation test is negative for both HIV-1 and HIV-2, then nucleic acid testing (NAT) of HIV-1 RNA via PCR should be performed (Figure 16-1). If the NAT is positive, this indicates acute infection. Viral loads during acute infection are typically in the range of several million copies per milliliter, so a viral load <1000 copies/mL should be repeated to confirm infection.

NACO GUIDELINES (2021)

All samples reactive in the first test should further undergo confirmatory second/third tests based on different principles/antigens using the same serum/plasma sample as that of the first test. The same blood sample is utilized for performing all the tests for identifying HIV antibodies. For indeterminate results, testing should be repeated on a second sample taken after 14–28 days (Figure 16-2).

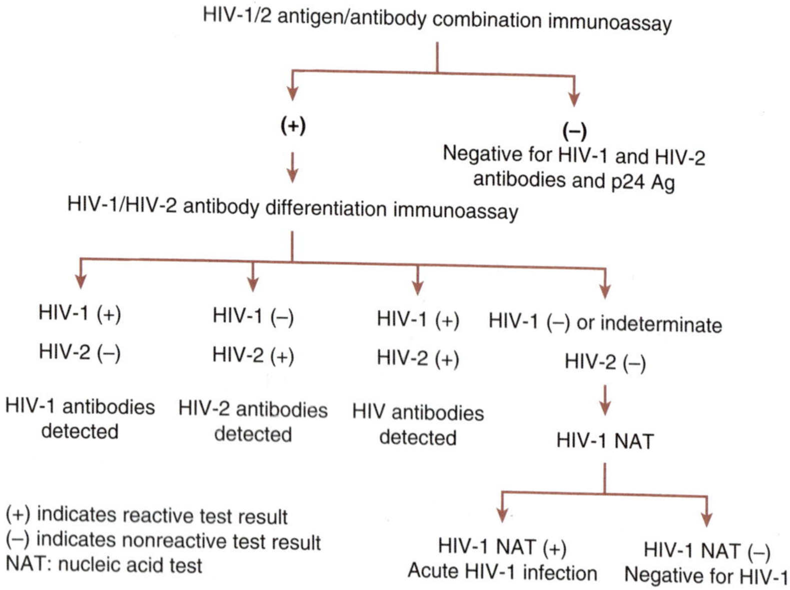

Figure 16-1 Recommended laboratory HIV testing algorithm for serum or plasma specimens. From Centers for Disease Control and Prevention. *Laboratory Testing for the Diagnosis of HIV Infection: Updated Recommendations*. Available at https://stacks.cdc.gov/view/cdc/50872.

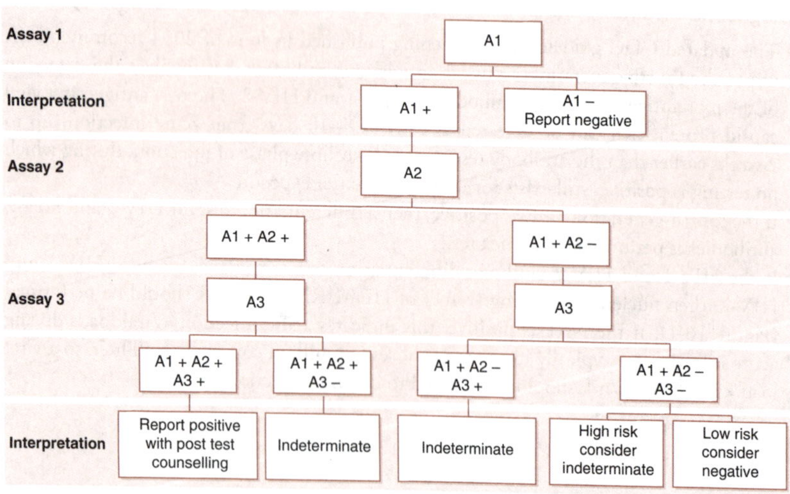

Figure 16-2 Strategy for diagnosis of clinically asymptomatic individuals

Assay A1 should be of high sensitivity and A2 and A3 should be of high specificity. A2 and A3 should also be able to differentiate between HIV 1 and 2 infections.

In case the serological results continue to be indeterminate, then the specimen is to be subjected to a Western blot/viral load.

*A1 is usually a fourth generation ELISA, A2 is a differentiation assay ('tridot' or 'spot' test) and A3 is also a fourth generation ELISA test, using a different method from A1.

Sequence of Appearance of Laboratory Markers of HIV-1 Infection (Table 16-5)

TABLE 16-5 Sequence of Appearance of Laboratory Markers of HIV-1 Infection

Test	Target of Detection	Approximate Time to Positivity (days)
Enzyme-linked immunoassay		
First generation	IgG antibody	35–45
Second generation	IgG antibody	25–35
Third generation	IgM and IgG antibody	20–30
Fourth generation	IgM and IgG antibody and p24 antigen	15–20
Western blot		
Western blot	IgM and IgG antibody	35–50 (indeterminate) 45–60 (positive)
HIV viral load test		
Sensitivity cutoff 50 copies/mL	RNA	10–15
Ultrasensitive cutoff 1–5 copies/mL	RNA	5

Diagnostic Testing

The CDC recommends that **all people aged 13–64 years be offered HIV testing in all health-care settings using an opt-out format.**[21]

- **Persons at high risk should be screened for HIV infection at least annually. High-risk groups include:** IV drug users, MSM, sexual partners of a known HIV patient, persons involved in sex trading and their sexual partners, persons with STIs, persons who have multiple sexual partners or who engage in unprotected intercourse, persons who consider themselves at risk, and persons with findings that are suggestive of HIV infection. More frequent screening (every 3–6 months) is sometimes indicated.
- Other groups for whom HIV testing is indicated are:
  - Pregnant women (opt-out screening)
  - Patients with active TB
  - Donors of blood, semen, and organs
  - Persons with occupational exposures (e.g., needlesticks) and source patients of the exposures

Laboratories

- **Complete blood cell** count and **comprehensive metabolic panel** with assessment of liver and kidney parameters, as well as **urinalysis** to evaluate for proteinuria and glycosuria.
- **CD4 cell count** (normal range, 600–1500 cells/μL) and CD4 percentage. Significant immune deficiency requiring prophylactic antibiotics occurs with CD4 <200 cells/μL.
- **Virologic markers:** Plasma HIV RNA predicts the rate of disease progression.
- **Fasting lipid panel.** HIV is associated with an increased risk of metabolic syndrome and cardiovascular disease. Lipids can be affected by several antiretrovirals.
- **TB testing by interferon-γ release assay (IGRA).**
- **RPR test for syphilis screening, confirmed by fluorescent treponemal antibody assay.**
- ***Toxoplasma* and hepatitis A, B (HBsAg, HBsAb, HBcAb), and C serologies.**

- **Chlamydia/gonococcal urine/cervical probe** for all patients. If patients report receptive anal sex, **rectal probes for gonorrhea and** ***Chlamydia*** are recommended. For those reporting receptive oral sex, **pharyngeal sample for gonorrhea** should be obtained.[22] NAAT is preferred.
- **Cervical Papanicolaou smear** (most commonly using the thin prep method).
- **HIV drug resistance testing** for reverse transcriptase and protease genes at baseline and with treatment failure. Integrase gene resistance testing should be performed for those failing integrase inhibitor–based regimens.
- **HLA B5701** for patients in whom one is considering the use of abacavir.
- **CCR5** tropism testing for patients in whom one is considering the use of maraviroc.
- **Glucose-6-phosphate dehydrogenase (G6PD) level** on initiation of care or before starting therapy with an oxidant drug in those with a predisposing ethnic background.
- In many resource-limited settings in South Asia, performing all the above-mentioned tests may not be feasible and practicable. Tests of higher priority such as a complete blood picture, tests of renal and liver function, and testing for CD4 cell count are mandatory. Plasma HIV RNA is ideally checked, but, in resource-limited settings, this is prioritized to patients with clinical and immunological failure. A tuberculin skin test is a reasonable alternative to TB testing by interferon-γ release assay, with a directive to treat patients for LTBI after active TB is ruled out. The rationale behind this is as follows: in patients, living in endemic areas, without HIV/immunosuppression, the lifetime risk of TB reactivation is 5%–10% but this risk increases to 5%–10% per year with immunosuppression. Similarly, given lower rates of NRTI and NNRTI drug resistance in untreated HIV patients in South Asia, baseline HIV drug resistance testing may be prioritized to patients whose partners have drug-resistant HIV.

TREATMENT

Immunization

- From "Primary Care Guidelines for the Management of Persons Infected with Human Immunodeficiency Virus: 2013 Update by the HIV Medicine Association of the Infectious Diseases Society of America".[23]
- Antibody response to vaccines is improved with undetectable HIV viral load and higher CD4 count.
- **Pneumococcal vaccine:** HIV infection is an indication for both the pneumococcal conjugate (Prevnar) and polysaccharide (Pneumovax) vaccines. If naïve, the conjugate vaccine should be given initially, then the polysaccharide vaccine after at least 8 weeks. Some experts recommend deferring the vaccine until the CD4 cell counts are ≥200 cells/μL because responses are poor when vaccination occurs with low CD4 cell counts. A single booster Pneumovax after 5 years is recommended. If vaccinated with Pneumovax first, then should wait at least 1 year before administering Prevnar.
- **Hepatitis A virus (HAV):** Vaccination for HAV is recommended if seronegative and MSM or have other indications (injection drug use, traveler to endemic country, chronic liver disease, coinfection with Hepatitis B or C.
- **Hepatitis B virus (HBV):** Vaccination for HBV is recommended if seronegative.
- **Influenza:** Annual inactivated influenza vaccination is recommended for all HIV-infected patients regardless of CD4 cell count. Use of the intranasally administered, live, attenuated vaccine is not currently recommended for HIV-infected persons.
- **Varicella:** The live, attenuated varicella vaccine (chickenpox, Varivax) can be safely given to persons with CD4 cell counts ≥200 cells/mL but is contraindicated for persons with CD4 counts <200 cells/mL. There is currently no recommendation to give the zoster vaccine (Zostavax), although it may be considered in HIV-infected adults with CD4 counts ≥200 cells/mL.

- **Measles/mumps/rubella (MMR):** MMR is a vaccine that can be safely given to persons with CD4 cell counts ≥200 cells/µL but is contraindicated for persons with CD4 counts <200 cells/µL.
- **Tetanus/diphtheria/pertussis:** All adults should receive tetanus/diphtheria booster every 10 years with a one-time substitution with tetanus/diphtheria/acellular pertussis vaccine.
- **Human papillomavirus (HPV) vaccine:** HPV-associated malignancies are common in HIV-infected patients. The three-dose vaccine series is safe and effective in HIV-positive subjects and is currently recommended for females aged 9–26 years, males aged 9–21 years, and MSM up to age of 26.

Medication

Antiretroviral therapy (ART) (Table 16-6)

- **Current recommendations from the International AIDS Society-USA**[24] for the initiation of ART are to treat everyone infected with HIV, regardless of CD4 count.
- In the case of patients with TB or cryptococcal meningitis, ART initiation may be slightly delayed to reduce the risk of serious immune reconstitution inflammatory syndrome (IRIS).
- Treatment decisions should be individualized by patient readiness, drug interactions, adherence issues, drug toxicities, comorbidities, and the level of risk indicated by CD4 T-cell counts.
- Women, especially if pregnant, should receive optimal ART to reduce the risk of vertical transmission.
- Maximal and durable suppression of HIV replication is the goal of therapy once it is initiated. **ART** should be individualized and closely monitored by measuring plasma HIV viral load. Reductions in plasma viremia correlate with increased CD4 cell counts and prolonged AIDS-free survival. Isolated viral "blips" (<200 copies/mL) are not indicative of virologic failure, but confirmed virologic rebound should trigger an evaluation of adherence, drug interactions, and viral resistance.
- Any change in ART increases future therapeutic constraints and potential drug resistance.
- **Antiretroviral drugs:** Approved antiretroviral drugs are grouped into five categories. Experts currently recommend using three active drugs from at least two different classes to suppress HIV viremia maximally and durably.
- **Initial therapy:** ART should be started in an outpatient setting by a physician with expertise in the management of HIV infection. Adherence is the key factor for success. Treatment should be individualized and adapted to the patient's lifestyle and comorbidities. Any treatment decision influences future therapeutic options because of the possibility of drug cross-resistance. **Potent initial ART generally consists of a combination of two NRTIs, plus usually an NNRTI, an INSTI, or a boosted PI. INSTI-based regimens are optimal for initial therapy and are preferred. It should be noted that many of the first-line regimens are coformulated as single-tablet daily regimens. Tenofovir alafenamide (TAF) is a new formulation of TDF that is less likely to cause renal toxicity or bone mineral density issues but may have more drug interactions (Table 16-7).**
    - In resource-limited settings in South Asia, treatment is usually initiated with two NRTIs (usually tenofovir-based with either lamivudine [3TC] or emtricitabine [FTC] plus an NNRTI [usually efavirenz in preference to nevirapine]). Boosted PI or INSTI-based regimens are used as second-line therapy in patients intolerant to or failing NNRTI-based therapy.
- **Treatment monitoring:** After starting or changing ART, the viral load should be checked at 4–6 weeks with an expected 10-fold reduction (1.0 $\log_{10}$) and suppression to <50 copies/mL by 24 weeks of therapy. The regimen should then be reassessed if response to treatment is inadequate. When the HIV RNA becomes undetectable and the patient is on a stable regimen, monitoring can be done every 3–6 months.

TABLE 16-6 Antiretroviral Agents

Medication	Mechanism	Dose	Common Side Effects	Monitoring
Nucleoside reverse transcriptase inhibitors (NRTIs)				
Abacavir (Ziagen)	Constrain HIV replication by incorporating into the elongating strand of DNA, causing chain termination.	600 mg orally once daily	Rash, fever—if occur, rechallenge may be fatal	No special monitoring
Emtricitabine (Emtriva)		200 mg orally once daily	Skin discoloration palms/soles (mild)	No special monitoring
Lamivudine (Epivir)		150 mg orally twice daily or 300 mg daily	Rash, peripheral neuropathy	No special monitoring
Zidovudine (AZT) (Retrovir)		600 mg orally daily in two divided doses	Anemia, neutropenia, nausea, malaise, headache, insomnia, myopathy	CBC with differential 4–8 weeks after starting AZT
Nucleotide reverse transcriptase inhibitors (NRTIs)				
Tenofovir alafenamide (TAF)/emtricitabine (Descovy)	Constrain HIV replication by incorporating into the elongating strand of DNA, causing chain termination.	25 mg of TAF with 200 mg of emtricitabine once daily	Weight gain; dyslipidemia; lower but still present risk of nephrotoxicity and bone resorption	Creatinine at baseline, at 2–8 weeks, then every 3–6 months; UA and urine glucose and protein at baseline and repeated as clinically indicated; HBsAg, liver enzymes at baseline, at 2–8 weeks, then every 3–6 months, continue for months after discontinuation; consider bone densitometry
Tenofovir (TDF) (Viread)		300 mg orally once daily	Kidney dysfunction, bone resorption, GI distress	Creatinine at baseline, at 2–8 weeks, then every 3–6 months; UA and urine glucose and protein at baseline and repeated as clinically indicated; consider bone densitometry

(Continued)

TABLE 16-6 Antiretroviral Agents (Continued)

Non-nucleoside reverse transcriptase inhibitors (NNRTIs)				
Doravirine (Pifeltro)	Inhibit HIV by binding noncompetitively to the reverse transcriptase	100 mg daily	Headache, fatigue, abdominal pain	No special monitoring
Efavirenz (Sustiva)		600 mg orally daily	Neurologic disturbances, rash, hepatitis	No special monitoring
Etravirine (Intelence)		200 mg orally twice daily	Rash, peripheral neuropathy	No special monitoring
Nevirapine (Viramune)		200 mg orally daily for 2 weeks, then 200 mg orally twice daily	Rash	No special monitoring
Rilpivirine (Edurant)		25 mg daily	Depression, rash	No special monitoring
Protease inhibitors (PI)				
Atazanavir (Reyataz)	PIs block the action of the viral protease required for protein processing late in the viral cycle	400 mg orally once daily or 300 mg atazanavir with 100 mg ritonavir daily	Hyperbilirubinemia	Bilirubin level every 3–4 months
Atazanavir/cobicistat (Evotaz)		300 mg of atazanavir with 150 mg of cobicistat orally once daily	Hyperbilirubinemia	Bilirubin level every 3–4 months
Darunavir/cobicistat (Prezcobix)		800 mg of darunavir and 150 mg of cobicistat orally once daily	Rash	No special monitoring

(Continued)

TABLE 16-6 Antiretroviral Agents (Continued)

Medication	Mechanism	Dose	Common Side Effects	Monitoring
Darunavir/ritonavir (Prezista/Norvir)		For PI experienced patients: 600 mg of darunavir and 100 mg of ritonavir orally twice daily For PI naïve patients: 800 mg of darunavir and 100 mg of ritonavir orally daily	Rash	No special monitoring
Lopinavir/ritonavir (Kaletra)		400 mg/100 mg orally twice daily	Diarrhea	No special monitoring
Ritonavir (Norvir)		600 mg orally twice daily or in lower doses (e.g., 100 mg orally once or twice daily) for boosting other PIs	GI distress, peripheral paresthesias	No special monitoring
Entry inhibitors				
Enfuvirtide (Fuzeon)	Prevents the fusion of the virus into the host cell	90 mg subcutaneously twice daily	Injection site pain and allergic reaction	No special monitoring

(Continued)

TABLE 16-6 Antiretroviral Agents (Continued)

Integrase Inhibitors (INSTI)				
Bictegravir	Target DNA strand transfer and integration into a human genome.	50 mg orally daily. No longer marketed as a single agent; used in antiretroviral combination	Diarrhea, nausea, headache	No special monitoring
Dolutegravir (Tivicay)		Treatment-naïve or integrase-naïve patients: 50 mg daily When administered with efavirenz, fosamprenavir/ ritonavir, tipranavir/ ritonavir, or rifampin: 50 mg twice daily When administered to integrase-experienced patients with suspected integrase resistance: 50 mg twice daily	Hypersensitivity, insomnia, fatigue, headache, rash	No special monitoring
Elvitegravir		No longer marketed as a single agent; used in antiretroviral combinations	Diarrhea, headache	No special monitoring
Raltegravir (Isentress)		400 mg orally twice daily	Diarrhea, nausea, headache	No special monitoring

(Continued)

TABLE 16-6 Antiretroviral Agents (Continued)

Medication	Mechanism	Dose	Common Side Effects	Monitoring
Cabotegravir		Oral regimen of 30 mg daily with rilpivirine 25 mg daily for 1 month; then intramuscular loading dose of 600 mg with rilpivirine 900 mg intra-muscularly in separate buttock injections; followed by monthly intramuscular injections of 400 mg with 600 mg rilpivirine thereafter	Injection site reactions with intramuscular dose	No special monitoring
Entry and fusion inhibitors				
Maraviroc (Selzentry)	Is a CCR5 receptor blocker	150 mg orally twice daily or 300 mg orally twice daily	Cough, fever, rash	No special monitoring

(Continued)

TABLE 16-6 Antiretroviral Agents (Continued)

Ibalizumab (Trogarzo)	Blocks entry of HIV by blocking CD4 receptor	Loading dose of 2000 mg intravenously over 30 minutes; maintenance dose of 800 mg intravenously every 2 weeks thereafter	Diarrhea, dizziness, nausea, rash, elevated creatinine, lymphopenia	Monthly CBC, creatinine, bilirubin, glucose, lipase
Attachment inhibitor				
Fostemsavir	Binds to gp120 and prevents attachment to CD4 cells.	600 mg orally twice a day	Nausea	No special monitoring

Humanized monoclonal antibody (Ibalizumab) in combination with other antiretroviral agents has been approved for patients with multidrug-resistant HIV-1. Dosage: single loading dose of 2000 mg followed by a maintenance dose of 800 mg every 2 weeks IV.

TABLE 16-7 Preferred and Alternative Antiretroviral Regimens for Nonpregnant Treatment-Naïve Adults and Adolescents with HIV-A1

Preferred regimens (listed alphabetically)
Bictegravir-emtricitabine-tenofovir alafenamide Dolutegravir plus tenofovir alafenamide-emtricitabine
Alternative regimens (agents within class listed alphabetically)
INSTI-based regimens • Dolutegravir-abacavir-lamivudine • Elvitegravir-cobicistat-emtricitabine-tenofovir alafenamide • Raltegravir plus tenofovir alafenamide-emtricitabine
PI-based regimens • Atazanavir (boosted with ritonavir or cobicistat) plus tenofovir alafenamide-emtricitabine • Darunavir (boosted with ritonavir or cobicistat) plus tenofovir alafenamide-emtricitabine
NNRTI-based regimens • Doravirine plus tenofovir alafenamide-emtricitabine • Efavirenz plus tenofovir alafenamide-emtricitabine • Efavirenz-emtricitabine-tenofovir disoproxil fumarate • Rilpivirine-emtricitabine-tenofovir alafenamide
Two-drug regimen • Dolutegravir-lamivudine
Hepatitis B coinfection **TDF or TAF + 3TC or FTC + DTG**
Kidney disease • Avoid TDF in patients with an eGFR <60 mL/min/1.73 m^2 • Avoid TAF in patients with acute kidney injury or eGFR <30 mL/min/1.73 m^2 • ABC can be used instead of TDF/TAF
Osteoporosis: Avoid TDF/TAF
• *Persons of childbearing potential/pregnancy: (Also see section on HIV-pregnancy below)* • *2 NRTIs + integrase inhibitor (small risk of NTDs in early pregnancy but statistically insignificant) or protease inhibitors preferred*

- **Treatment failure** is defined as less than a log (10-fold) reduction of the viral load 4–6 weeks after starting a new antiretroviral regimen, failure to reach an undetectable viral load after 6 months of treatment, detection of the virus after initial complete suppression of viral load (which suggests development of resistance), or persistent decline of CD4 cell count or clinical deterioration. Confirmed treatment failure should prompt changes in ART based on results of genotype testing. In this situation, at least two of the drugs should be substituted with other drugs that have no expected cross-resistance. **HIV resistance testing** at this stage may help determine a salvage regimen in patients with prior ART. The importance of adherence should be stressed. Referral to an HIV specialist is highly recommended in this situation.
- **Drug interactions:** Antiretroviral medications, especially PIs, have multiple drug interactions. **PIs and cobicistat both inhibit and induce the P450 system,** and thus interactions are frequent with other inhibitors of the P450 system, including macrolides (erythromycin,

clarithromycin) and antifungals (ketoconazole, itraconazole), as well as other inducers such as rifamycins (rifampin, rifabutin) and anticonvulsants (phenobarbital, phenytoin, carbamazepine). **Drugs with narrow therapeutic indices that should be avoided or used with extreme caution** include antihistamines (although loratadine is safe), antiarrhythmics (flecainide, encainide, quinidine), long-acting opiates (fentanyl, meperidine), long-acting benzodiazepines (midazolam, triazolam), warfarin, 3-hydroxy-3-methylglutaryl–coenzyme A reductase inhibitors (pitavastatin is the safest), and oral contraceptives. Sildenafil concentrations are increased, whereas methadone and theophylline concentrations are decreased with concomitant administration of certain PIs and NNRTIs.

Complications

Complications of ART: The long-term use of antiretrovirals has been associated with toxicity, the pathogenesis of which is only partially understood at this time.

- **Hyperlipidemia,** especially hypertriglyceridemia, is associated mainly with PIs (especially ritonavir). Improvement has been seen after treatment with atorvastatin, pravastatin, pitavastatin, and/or gemfibrozil.
- **Peripheral insulin resistance, impaired glucose tolerance, and hyperglycemia** have been associated with the use of PI-based regimens, mainly indinavir and ritonavir. Lifestyle changes or changing ART can be considered in these cases.
- **Osteopenia and osteoporosis** are well described in HIV-infected individuals. The pathogenic mechanism of this problem is likely related to the inflammatory milieu of HIV itself, although the use of TDF may contribute. TAF is recommended over TDF in at-risk patients.
- **Osteonecrosis,** particularly of the hip, has been increasingly associated with HIV disease.
- **Lipodystrophy syndrome** is an alteration in body fat distribution and can be stigmatizing to individuals. Changes consist of the accumulation of visceral fat in the abdomen, neck (buffalo hump), and pelvic areas, and/or the depletion of subcutaneous fat, causing facial or peripheral wasting. Lipodystrophy has been associated in particular with older PIs and NRTIs and is uncommon with currently recommended regimens.
- **Lactic acidosis** with liver steatosis is a rare but sometimes fatal complication associated with NRTIs. The mechanism appears to be part of mitochondrial toxicity. Higher rates of lactic acidosis have been reported with the use of the older drugs stavudine and didanosine.

SPECIAL POPULATIONS

Pregnancy

- Mother-to-child transmission (MTCT) accounts for >90% of HIV infection in children.
- Screening
  - All pregnant women should be screened for HIV infection at entry to antenatal care
  - Testing should be repeated in the third trimester for women at high risk
- Antiretroviral therapy
  - Start ARTs as early as possible for all pregnant women with HIV infection regardless of CD4 T-cell count or viral load. ART should be continued even after delivery
  - Starting antiretroviral therapy early in pregnancy is associated with decreased viral loads at the time of delivery
  - 2 NRTIs + integrase inhibitor or protease inhibitors preferred
    - NRTIs
      - ABC + 3TC
      - TAF or TDF + 3TC or FTC

- Integrase inhibitor: DTG (may have an increased risk of neural tube defects in first trimester, but this risk is not statistically significant, risk should be explained to the mother, and adequate folic acid should be provided)
- Protease inhibitor: DRV/r

- Labor and delivery considerations
  - Mode of delivery
    - Cesarean delivery at 38 weeks of gestation is recommended for women with viral loads >1000 copies/mL or unknown viral loads near time of delivery.
    - Scheduled cesarean delivery is not routinely recommended in women with HIV RNA levels ≤1000 copies/mL
    - Avoid invasive labor procedures, such as an artificial rupture of membranes in the setting of viremia, the use of fetal scalp electrodes, and the use of forceps or vacuum extractor when possible. This is to reduce fetal exposure to body fluids.
  - Role of IV zidovudine
    - For women with HIV viral loads >1000 copies/mL, start zidovudine 2 mg/kg IV over 1 hour at labor onset, and then 1 mg/kg/hour IV until delivery.
    - For women with HIV infection receiving combination ART during pregnancy and HIV RNA ≤1,000 copies/mL near delivery, intrapartum zidovudine is not required.
- Following delivery
  - Give postpartum antiretroviral drugs to all **HIV-exposed infants** to reduce perinatal transmission
    - Antiretroviral regimens (at gestational age-appropriate doses) should be given preferably within 6–12 hours of birth
    - Antiretroviral prophylaxis
      - To prevent HIV infection in infants with **low risk of transmission**
      - Options
        - Single-drug regimen: Zidovudine alone for 4 weeks for infants born to mother on regular ART with viral load <50 copies/mL
        - Two-drug regimen: Zidovudine for 6 weeks plus three doses of nevirapine during first week of life for infants at higher risk of transmission but in whom presumptive HIV therapy is not needed.
    - Presumptive HIV therapy
      - For infants with **higher risk of HIV acquisition**, such as those born to mothers who
        - Did not have antepartum or intrapartum antiretroviral drugs
        - Only had intrapartum antiretroviral drugs
        - Had antepartum antiretroviral drugs but did not achieve viral suppression near delivery
        - Acquired HIV infection during pregnancy or breastfeeding.
      - Options include
        - Zidovudine for 6 weeks plus emtricitabine and nevirapine for 2–6 weeks
        - Zidovudine for 6 weeks plus emtricitabine and raltegravir for 2–6 weeks
    - HIV therapy
      - To newborns with confirmed infection
      - Administration of three-drug regimen at treatment doses.
- Breastfeeding recommendations
  - Breastfeeding is not recommended in resource-rich settings due to the availability of safe alternatives
  - However, in resource-limited situations, breastfeeding may be acceptable till safe and adequate diet can be provided
- Other concerns
  - Prevention of secondary transmission to partner
  - Family planning
  - Prophylaxis against opportunistic infection: Similar to nonpregnant adults

Acute HIV Infection

ART given immediately after diagnosing acute infection may provide additional benefits.

- The initiation of early ART in acute infection will suppress the extraordinarily high viral loads seen at this time and reduce further transmission of HIV.
- Early ART may reduce the reservoir of latent virus.
- Early ART maintains immune function and may allow for immunologic control of HIV off ART in resource-limited settings.

Hepatitis

- High rates of coinfection with HBV and hepatitis C virus (HCV) occur in HIV-infected patients.
- Several HIV ART medications (tenofovir, emtricitabine, and lamivudine) also have activity against HBV. Any plan to treat HBV in coinfected patients should ensure that the regimen is fully active against both HIV and HBV. Discontinuation of ART that has been suppressing unrecognized HBV disease can result in reactivation of HBV with resultant acute, and sometimes fatal, HBV infection.
- HCV therapy is rapidly evolving, and a complete delineation of treatment is available in Chapter 19, Liver Diseases.
- Newer directly acting HCV agents appear to be as effective in HIV-infected patients as in monoinfected HCV patients; however, there are significant drug–drug interactions that should be considered, particularly with PI-based therapy, efavirenz, and therapy using the boosting agent cobicistat.

Aging

- With the success of ART, HIV-related mortality is decreasing and HIV-infected persons are experiencing prolonged survival approaching the national survival average.
- In 2015, the CDC estimated that 45% of HIV-infected persons were over the age of 50.
- HIV infection is associated with premature end-organ disease, and thus many of the comorbidities associated with aging may be exacerbated in this growing population, including cardiovascular disease, insulin resistance and diabetes, osteoporosis, neurocognitive impairment, and physical frailty.
- Certain non–AIDS-defining cancers are more common in HIV-infected patients, including anal cancer, lung cancer, and hepatocellular carcinoma. The extent to which this is due to HIV infection versus other risk factors such as smoking, HPV, and HBV/HCV coinfection is unclear.
- The role of long-term HIV infection and ART use in these comorbidities is poorly understood, although the use of NNRTI and PI drug classes is associated with lipid profiles that may exacerbate cardiovascular disease.[25] Higher rates of smoking and alcohol use also exacerbate these comorbidities.

Opportunistic Infections

GENERAL PRINCIPLES

- Potent ART has decreased the incidence, changed the manifestations, and improved the outcome of OIs. However, OIs are still a common presentation of unrecognized HIV infection. Common OIs are listed in Table 16-8.
- A clinical syndrome associated with the immune enhancement induced by potent ART, **IRIS**, generally presents as local inflammatory reactions. Examples include recurrent symptoms of cryptococcal meningitis, paradoxical reactions with TB reactivation, localized *Mycobacterium avium* complex (MAC) adenitis, aggravation of hepatitis viral infection, and CMV vitreitis soon after the initiation of potent ART.

TABLE 16-8 Relation between CD4+ Cell Count and Common Illness in HIV Patients

Opportunistic Infections	Absolute CD4 Count
Asymptomatic Persistent generalized lymphadenopathy Thrombocytopenia	>600
Herpes zoster	500–600
Oral hairy leukoplakia	200–500
Pneumocystis jiroveci pneumonia Miliary TB Esophageal candidiasis Mucocutaneous herpes Cryptosporidiosis/Microsporidia Histoplasmosis	100–200
Toxoplasmosis Cryptococcal meningitis PML (progressive multifocal leukoencephalopathy) HIV-associated dementia	<100
Primary CNS lymphoma	50–100
CMV retinitis MAC infection	<50

Note: Tuberculosis and Kaposi sarcoma can occur at any CD4 count.

- In the case of IRIS, ART is usually continued, and the addition of low-dose steroids might decrease the degree of inflammation. TB and cryptococcal meningitis are the only OIs for which delay of ART is recommended to prevent IRIS.
- Additional details with updates may be found in the Guidelines for the Prevention and Treatment of Opportunistic Infections in HIV-Infected Adults and Adolescents.[26]

TREATMENT

- **Prophylaxis for OIs** can be divided into primary and secondary prophylaxis.
- **Primary prophylaxis** is established before an episode of OI occurs. Institution of primary prophylaxis depends on the level of immunosuppression as judged by the patient's CD4 cell count and percentage (Table 16-9).

TABLE 16-9 Opportunistic Infection Prophylaxis

Opportunistic Infection	Indications for Prophylaxis	Medications
PJP	CD4 <200 cells/μL	• TMP-SMX (1 DS tablet daily) for CD4 <200 or CD4% <15% • Continue prophylaxis until CD4 count >200 × 3 months • Other agents that can be used: Pentamidine, Atovaquone, Dapsone +/– pyrimethamine[a]

(Continued)

TABLE 16-9 Opportunistic Infection Prophylaxis (Continued)

Opportunistic Infection	Indications for Prophylaxis	Medications
Toxoplasmosis[b]	CD4 <100 cells/μL	• Primary prophylaxis: If CD4 <100—TMP-SMX-DS q24h; • Can discontinue if CD4 >200 × 3 months • Secondary prophylaxis: • Sulfadiazine 2–4 g in two to four doses/day + pyrimethamine 25–50 mg Q24h + folinic acid 10–25 mg Q24h Can discontinue if CD4 >200 × 6 months
Mycobacterium avium complex[c]	CD4 <50 cells/μL	• Azithromycin: 1200 mg once weekly or clarithromycin 500 mg twice daily • Alternatives: rifabutin
Coccidioidomycosis	CD4 ≤250 cells/μL	• Secondary prophylaxis until CD4 >250/μL • Fluconazole 400 mg OD or Itraconazole 200 mg BD
Histoplasmosis	CD4 ≤150 cells/μL	Prophylaxis if prior documented disease or CD4 <200 and high-risk Itraconazole 200 mg PO daily
Cryptococcus	CD4 ≤100 cells/μL	Secondary prophylaxis Maintenance phase: Fluconazole 200 mg/day for at least 1 year till CD4 count is >100 and viral load undetectable for at least 3 months

[a]Glucose-6-phosphate dehydrogenase (G6PD) testing should be done for dapsone.
[b]If toxoplasmosis IgG is positive.
[c]May not be required if patient is on effective ART.
DS, double strength; PJP, *Pneumocystis jirovecii* pneumonia; TMP-SMX, trimethoprim-sulfamethoxazole.

- **Secondary prophylaxis** is instituted after an episode of infection has been adequately treated. Most OIs will require extended therapy.
- **Withdrawal of prophylaxis:** Recommendations suggest withdrawing primary and secondary prophylaxis for most OIs if sustained immunologic recovery has occurred (CD4 cell counts consistently >150–200 cells/μL).[27]

PULMONARY SYNDROMES

Pneumocystis jirovecii Pneumonia

GENERAL PRINCIPLES

Pneumocystis jirovecii pneumonia is the most common OI in patients with AIDS characterized by subacute progressive dyspnea.

DIAGNOSIS

Positive direct immunofluorescent stain from induced sputum samples or bronchoalveolar lavage fluid. Alternatively, histopathologic demonstration of organisms in tissue is also adequate for diagnosis. Chest radiography typically shows diffuse, bilateral ground-glass interstitial infiltrates, but it can also have a variety of atypical appearances.

TREATMENT

- Patients must receive 21 days of therapy (Table 16-10).
- **Trimethoprim-sulfamethoxazole** (TMP-SMX) is the treatment of choice. The dosage is 15–20 mg/kg of the TMP component IV daily, divided q6–8h for severe cases, with a switch to oral therapy when the patient's condition improves. Total duration of therapy is 21 days. Prednisone should be added with severe disease as defined below. For patients who cannot receive TMP-SMX, the following alternatives are available:

TABLE 16-10 Treatment of Pneumocystis Pneumonia

Drug	Dose	Major Adverse Reactions
Preferred Regimen		
TMP-SMX	TMP-SMX (15–20 mg/kg/day of trimethoprim component) orally or IV in 3–4 divided doses. IV preferred if PaO_2, 60 mm Hg, respiratory rate >25 or respiratory fatigue, unable to take orally	Rash (SJS/TEN rare), fever, neutropenia, hyperkalemia, transaminase elevations, photosensitivity, increased serum creatinine
Alternative Regimens		
TMP plus dapsone	TMP: 5 mg/kg orally three times a day	Rash, GI distress, transaminase elevation, neutropenia, hyperkalemia
	Dapsone: 100 mg orally once per day	Rash, fever, lymphadenopathy, transaminase elevations (sulfone hypersensitivity syndrome), GI upset, methemoglobinemia, hemolytic anemia
Primaquine plus clindamycin	Primaquine: 30 mg (base) orally once per day	Rash, fever, GI distress, methemoglobinemia, hemolytic anemia, leukopenia, neutropenia
	Clindamycin: 900 mg IV every eight hours OR 600 mg IV every six hours OR 600 mg orally three times daily OR 450 mg orally four times daily	Rash, diarrhea, *Clostridium difficile* colitis, abdominal pain
Atovaquone suspension	750 mg orally twice daily (must be taken with food)	Gastrointestinal distress, fever, transaminase elevation, rash (less frequently than with other regimens)

(Continued)

TABLE 16-10 Treatment of Pneumocystis Pneumonia (Continued)

Drug	Dose	Major Adverse Reactions
Pentamidine (used only in severe disease)	4 mg/kg IV once daily can be reduced to 3 mg/kg IV daily i/v/o toxicity and renal impairment	Nephrotoxicity, infusion reactions, hyperkalemia, hyperglycemia, pancreatitis, cardiac arrhythmias (including TdP), transaminase elevations, hypotension, hypoglycemia, hypokalemia, hypocalcemia Certain adverse effects can be life threatening (e.g., hypoglycemia and hypotension)
Adjunctive Glucocorticoids		
Prednisone Adjunctive glucocorticoids should be given to patients with a room air PaO_2 <70 mm Hg, an alveolar-arterial (A-a) oxygen gradient ≥35 mm Hg, and/or evidence of hypoxemia (e.g., room air O_2 saturation <92%). IV methylprednisolone can be administered as 75% of prednisone dose.	40 mg orally twice daily for five days, followed by 40 mg orally once daily for five days, followed by 20 mg orally once daily for 11 days	

Adapted from Drugs used in the treatment of Pneumocystis pneumonia (PCP) in adults and adolescents. Available at https://www.uptodate.com/contents/image?csi=484065dc-72fc-4b5d-a31a-20990cc5b26a&source=contentShare&imageKey=ID%2F61052

- For mild to moderately severe disease (arterial oxygen tension [PaO_2] >70 mm Hg or alveolar arterial oxygen gradient [$P(A–a)O_2$] <35 mm Hg):
  - TMP, 15 mg/kg PO q8h, and dapsone, 100 mg PO daily. G6PD deficiency should be ruled out before dapsone is used.
  - Clindamycin, 600 mg IV or PO q8h, plus primaquine, 30 mg PO daily. G6PD deficiency should be ruled out before primaquine is used.
  - Atovaquone, 750 mg PO q12h. This drug should be administered with meals to increase absorption.
- For severe disease (PaO_2 <70 mm Hg or $P[A–a]O_2$ ≥35 mm Hg):
  - Prednisone taper should be added. The most frequently prescribed prednisone regimen is 40 mg PO bid on days 1–5 and 40 mg daily on days 6–10, followed by 20 mg on days 11–21.
  - IV pentamidine is used in cases when all other options are exhausted and requires close monitoring for side effects.

- Primary prophylaxis is indicated (see Table 16-2). Secondary PCP prophylaxis can be discontinued if the CD4 count is >200 cells/μL for more than 3 months in patients responding to ART.

Mycobacterium tuberculosis

GENERAL PRINCIPLES

M. tuberculosis is the most frequent opportunistic infection among HIV-infected patients in India and carries significant morbidity and mortality in South Asia. Primary or reactivated disease is common.[28]

DIAGNOSIS

- Clinical manifestations depend on the level of immunosuppression. Patients with higher CD4 cell counts tend to exhibit classic presentations with **apical cavitary disease**.
- Profoundly immunosuppressed patients may demonstrate atypical presentations that can resemble disseminated primary infection, with diffuse or localized pulmonary infiltrates and hilar lymphadenopathy.
- Extrapulmonary dissemination is more common in patients with HIV.

TREATMENT

- For treatment recommendations, see Chapter 14, Treatment of Infectious Diseases.
- Current recommendations suggest the **substitution of rifabutin for rifampin** in patients who are receiving concomitant ART, especially PIs. The dosage for rifabutin needs readjustment due to many significant interactions.[29] In subjects who are ART naïve, ART can be delayed for a few weeks after TB-specific therapy is started.
- The dose of the integrase inhibitors needs to be doubled when administered with rifampin; hence, the dose of DTG is 50 mg twice daily and raltegravir is dosed at 400 mg twice daily.

FEBRILE SYNDROMES

Mycobacterium avium Complex Infection

GENERAL PRINCIPLES

Mycobacterium avium complex (MAC) infection is the most commonly occurring nontuberculous mycobacterial infection in AIDS patients and is responsible for significant morbidity in patients with advanced disease (CD4 cell count <50 cells/μL).

It refers to infections caused by one of two nontuberculous mycobacterial species, either *M. avium* or *M. intracellulare*. They are ubiquitous organisms, occurring in water and soil. Infection occurs via inhalation.

DIAGNOSIS

Clinical Presentation

- There are two principal forms of MAC infection in HIV: disseminated and localized disease
- Disseminated infection with fever, weight loss, night sweats, and GI complaints is the most frequent presentation. Lymphadenopathy and splenomegaly may be present.
- Localized disease occurs in patients with IRIS after initiation of ART. Symptoms include fever and focal lymph node involvement.
- MAC infection can result in bacteremia in AIDS patients.

Diagnostic Testing

- Anemia (occasionally pancytopenia) and elevated alkaline phosphatase and lactate dehydrogenase levels are the usual laboratory abnormalities.
- Mycobacterial blood cultures should be sent in suspected cases of disseminated disease.
- Isolation of organism from the affected lymph nodes confirms localized infection.[30]

TREATMENT

- Initial therapy should include a **macrolide** (i.e., clarithromycin, 500 mg PO bid) and **ethambutol**, 15 mg/kg PO daily.
- Rifabutin, 300 mg PO daily, an aminoglycoside 10–15 mg/kg IV daily, or a fluoroquinolone can be added in severe cases or patients not on effective ART, and based on sensitivities. If rifabutin cannot be used, fluoroquinolones or a parenteral aminoglycoside can be administered.
- Utility of disseminated MAC prophylaxis is currently under debate given prophylaxis toxicity and effectiveness of modern ART. The US Department of Health and Human Services continues to recommend primary prophylaxis, but the International Antiviral Society of USA recommends against primary prophylaxis if effective ART is initiated immediately and viral suppression achieved (AIIa recommendation).
- It is standard of care to offer prophylaxis for MAC to all patients with HIV infection and CD4 count of <50/µL.[31]
- Primary prophylaxis can be stopped in patients who have responded to ART with elevation of CD4 counts to >100/ µL for 3 months.[31]
- Secondary prophylaxis for disseminated MAC can be discontinued if the CD4 count has a sustained increase of >100 cells/µL for 6 months or longer in response to ART, and if 12 months of therapy for MAC is completed and there are no symptoms or signs attributable to MAC.

Histoplasma capsulatum Infections

GENERAL PRINCIPLES

- Histoplasmosis is the most common endemic mycosis in patients with advanced HIV.
- A CD4 count of ≤150 cells/µL is the main risk factor for disease in patients with HIV.
- It often occurs in patients with AIDS who live in endemic areas such as the Mississippi and Ohio River Valleys.
- Histoplasmosis is commonly reported in the Eastern and Northeastern states of India; in Southeast Asia, the highest number of cases is reported in Thailand and Malaysia.
- Transmission occurs via inhalation of spores from the soil of endemic areas. It can lead to acute infection. Some patients develop disease after years of travel to an endemic area due to reactivation of latent foci.
- The severity of infection depends on the degree of the patient's immunosuppression. It can range from asymptomatic infection to life-threatening disseminated disease.

DIAGNOSIS

- Suspect disseminated histoplasmosis in patients with HIV and CD4 counts ≤150 cells/µL who are from an endemic area and have:
  - Fever and weight loss
  - Cough and/or dyspnea
  - Skin and/or mucosal membrane lesions
  - Nausea, vomiting, and abdominal pain

  - Hepatosplenomegaly and/or lymphadenopathy
  - Pancytopenia
  - Organ system-specific symptoms
- Pancytopenia develops because of bone marrow involvement. Elevated transaminases and alkaline phosphatase levels are also seen.
- Pulmonary infiltrates (diffuse interstitial or reticulonodular infiltrates) are seen in 50% of patients with advance HIV and disseminated histoplasmosis.
- In suspected cases, fungal blood cultures are sent, along with serum and urine *Histoplasma* antigen.
- Examination of tissues or body fluids for fungi must be done with special stains and by subjecting the specimens to fungal culture.
- Evidence of granulomas with yeasts resembling *Histoplasma* in extrapulmonary tissue confirms disseminated disease.
- The urine and serum *Histoplasma* antigens can also be used to monitor treatment.[32]

TREATMENT

- Disseminated disease is treated with **liposomal amphotericin B**, 3 mg/kg IV daily for 2 weeks or until the patient clinically improves, followed by **itraconazole**, 200 mg PO bid indefinitely (Table 16-11).

TABLE 16-11 Treatment of Histoplasmosis

Preferred Therapy, Duration of Therapy, Chronic Maintenance	Alternative Therapy	Comments
Induction therapy (for 2 weeks or until clinically improved) ▪ Liposomal amphotericin B at 3 mg/kg IV daily Maintenance therapy ▪ Itraconazole 200 mg orally 3 times daily for 3 days, then twice daily Preferred therapy for less severe disseminated disease Induction and maintenance therapy ▪ Itraconazole 200 mg orally 3 times daily for 3 days, then 200 mg orally twice daily Duration of therapy: At least 12 months	Alternative therapy moderately severe to severe disseminated disease Induction therapy (for 2 weeks or until clinically improved) ▪ Amphotericin B lipid complex 5 mg/kg IV daily ▪ Amphotericin B deoxycholate 0.7 mg/kg IV daily Maintenance therapy Same as "Preferred therapy"	Itraconazole levels should be obtained in all patients to ensure adequate absorption. Serum concentrations of itraconazole + hydroxyitraconazole should be >1 μg/mL Itraconazole oral solution is preferred over capsule by certain specialists because of improved absorption Acute pulmonary histoplasmosis in patients with HIV and CD4+ count >300 cells/μL should be managed as nonimmunocompromised host

(Continued)

TABLE 16-11 Treatment of Histoplasmosis (Continued)

Preferred Therapy, Duration of Therapy, Chronic Maintenance	Alternative Therapy	Comments
Preferred therapy for meningitis Induction therapy (4-6 weeks) ▪ Liposomal amphotericin B 5 mg/kg IV daily Maintenance therapy ▪ Itraconazole 200 mg orally 2-3 times daily for ≥1 year and until resolution of abnormal CSF findings Preferred therapy for long-term suppression therapy In patients with severe disseminated or CNS infection and in patients who relapse despite appropriate therapy (CIII) ▪ Itraconazole 200 mg orally daily		

- CNS disease is initially treated with **liposomal amphotericin B**, 5 mg/kg IV daily for 4–6 weeks, before starting itraconazole.
- Itraconazole absorption should be documented by a serum drug level. Liquid itraconazole is preferred because of improved absorption; however, it can be expensive and difficult to obtain.
- Discontinuation of itraconazole is possible if sustained increase in CD4 count is observed >100–200 cells/μL for more than 6 months.

Coccidioides immitis Infection

GENERAL PRINCIPLES

- Coccidioidomycosis often occurs in AIDS patients who live in endemic areas such as the southwestern United States, Central America, and South America.
- The risk of developing symptomatic infection is increased in patients with HIV who have CD4 counts <250 cells/μL, those who have AIDS and cases where there is a lack of viral suppression.
- Infection may be limited to pneumonia or disseminated with possible involvement of CNS, skin, bones, and joints.

DIAGNOSIS

- Suspect coccidioidomycosis in patients with fever, cough, pleuritic chest pain, night sweats, joint pains, and travel to an endemic area.
- Diagnosis is made by cultures, serology, histology, and clinical picture.
- Culture of organism from specimens or demonstration of spherules on tissue histology confirms diagnosis.
- Elevated coccidioidal antibody titers even in absence of symptoms can indicate the risk of subsequent symptomatic disease in patients with advanced HIV.

TREATMENT

- Management includes antifungals along with improving cell-mediated immunity through ART.
- Mild-to-moderate respiratory involvement like focal pneumonia is treated with oral antifungals – fluconazole 400 mg daily or itraconazole 200 mg bid. Antifungals can be stopped when the CD4 >250 cell/μL, virological suppression on ART, and clinical response is sustained for 3–6 months on therapy, provided the patient can be regularly monitored for recurrence.
- Severe pulmonary or disseminated disease is treated with **liposomal amphotericin B**, 4–6 mg/kg IV daily for 2 weeks or until the patient clinically improves, followed by fluconazole 400 mg daily or itraconazole 200 mg bid for at least 12 months. Discontinuation is dependent on clinical and serological response and should be made in consultation with experts.
- CNS disease is initially treated with **fluconazole** 800–1200 mg daily; liposomal amphotericin may be added to the initial regimen. Treatment with fluconazole is continued lifelong.

Other Endemic Fungi

- Although not listed as AIDS-defining illnesses, patients with advanced HIV are at risk for other endemic fungi depending on which the region they live.
- This includes Blastomycosis in the upper Midwest United States, Paracoccidioidomycosis in Central and South America, and *Talaromyces* (formerly Penicillium) in Southeast Asia, as well as other endemic fungi. **Talaromycosis** has been reported from the Northeastern states of India, particularly Manipur, and the disease is endemic in Southeast Asia and East Asia.

CENTRAL NERVOUS SYSTEM AND RETINAL DISEASE

Cryptococcus Neoformans

GENERAL PRINCIPLES

- Cryptococcosis is an invasive fungal infection caused by *Cryptococcus neoformans*.
- **Cryptococcal meningitis** is the most frequent CNS fungal infection in AIDS patients.
- The severity of infection depends on the degree of the patient's immunosuppression.

DIAGNOSIS

- Patients with CNS infection usually present with symptoms of meningoencephalitis, such as headaches, fever, and possibly mental status changes, but presentation can be more subtle. Cranial neuropathies may also be present.

- Disseminated cryptococcosis can involve lungs and skin, causing cough, breathlessness, and rash.
- Diagnosis is based on **lumbar puncture** results and on the determination of latex cryptococcal antigen, which is usually positive in the serum and the CSF.
- Brain imaging must always be performed prior to lumbar puncture to rule out other space-occupying lesions and raised intracranial pressure.
- **CSF opening pressure** should always be measured to assess the possibility of elevated intracranial pressure.

TREATMENT

- Treatment has three phases: Induction, consolidation, and maintenance (Table 16-12).
- Initial treatment is with liposomal **amphotericin** dosed at 3–4 mg/kg/d IV, and **flucytosine**, 25 mg/kg PO q6h for at least 2 weeks, followed by **fluconazole**, 400 mg PO daily for at least 8 weeks and then 200 mg PO daily, either lifelong or until immune reconstitution occurs. Fluconazole can be discontinued in those who are asymptomatic with regard to signs and symptoms of cryptococcosis and have a sustained increase (>6 months) in their CD4+ counts to ≥200 cells/μL.
- Repeat LPs (removing up to 30 mL CSF until the pressure is <20–25 cm H_2O) may be required to relieve elevated intracranial pressure.
- The 5-flucytosine level should be monitored during therapy to avoid toxicity.
- Alternative initial therapy is with amphotericin B deoxycholate, 0.7 mg/kg/d IV, and flucytosine, 25 mg/kg PO q6h.
- In persons who have persistent elevation of intracranial pressure, a temporary lumbar drain is indicated.

Toxoplasma gondii

GENERAL PRINCIPLES

- Toxoplasmosis, caused by the intracellular protozoan *Toxoplasma gondii*, is the most common CNS infection in patients with AIDS who are not receiving appropriate prophylaxis.
- Patients with the parasite who are immunocompetent are asymptomatic with a latent infection that persists for life.
- In immunosuppressed patients, the parasite reactivates to cause disease, usually with CD4 <100 cells/μL
- Probability of developing the disease is about 30% among AIDS patients with a CD4 <100 who are seropositive for toxoplasma and are not on adequate prophylaxis or ART.

DIAGNOSIS

- It typically causes multiple CNS mass lesions and presents with encephalopathy and focal neurologic findings.
- A presumptive diagnosis can be made when patient has CD4 <100 cells/μL, not on effective prophylaxis for toxoplasma and has the following:
  1. A compatible clinical syndrome
  2. A positive *T. gondii* IgG antibody
  3. Brain imaging (preferably MRI) that demonstrates a typical radiographic appearance (e.g., multiple ring-enhancing lesions)[33]

TABLE 16-12 Treatment of Cryptococcosis

	Preferred Regimens	Alternative Regimens	Comments
• Regimens for induction therapy	• When resources allow: Liposomal amphotericin B (3–4 mg/kg IV once daily) plus flucytosine (100 mg/kg per day orally in 4 divided doses) for a minimum of 2 weeks or Amphotericin B lipid complex (5 mg/kg IV once daily) plus flucytosine (100 mg/kg per day orally in 4 divided doses) for a minimum of 2 weeks • If resources are limited: Liposomal amphotericin B (10 mg/kg IV single dose) plus the combination of flucytosine (100 mg/kg/day orally in 4 divided doses) and fluconazole (1200 mg orally once daily) for a minimum of 2 weeks • If resources are limited and liposomal amphotericin B is not available: Amphotericin B deoxycholate (1 mg/kg IV once daily) plus flucytosine (100 mg/kg per day orally in 4 divided doses) for 7 days, followed by fluconazole monotherapy (1200 mg orally once daily) for a minimum of 7 days	Amphotericin B deoxycholate (0.7 to 1 mg/kg IV once daily) plus flucytosine (100 mg/kg per day orally in 4 divided doses) for a minimum of 2 weeks or Fluconazole (1200 mg orally once daily) plus flucytosine (100 mg/kg orally in 4 divided doses) for a minimum of 2 weeks or Amphotericin B plus fluconazole (800-1200 mg orally once daily) for a minimum of 2 weeks	An LP should be repeated after 2 weeks of induction therapy to confirm CSF sterilization. If a shortened course of polyene therapy is used, we prefer to do a repeat LP earlier in the course (7–14 days) so we can better identify those at risk for treatment failure. During 2-week induction therapy, clinical response should be assessed daily (in a hospital setting if possible).

(Continued)

TABLE 16-12 Treatment of Cryptococcosis (Continued)

CONSOLIDATION THERAPY	Fluconazole (400–800 mg orally or IV once daily) for a minimum of 8 weeks	Itraconazole (200 mg orally twice daily) for a minimum of 8 weeks	• Patients who have had a clear response to therapy can transition to fluconazole pending the results of the repeat CSF culture. • We generally initiate consolidation therapy with the 800 mg/day dosing of fluconazole with adjustment for renal function. • In resource-available settings, the dose can then be reduced to 400 mg/day to complete the 8-week consolidation phase if all of the following criteria are met: 1. The patient received induction therapy with amphotericin B plus flucytosine for 2 weeks. 2. CSF cultures obtained after 2 weeks of induction therapy are negative. 3. ART has been started.
MAINTENANCE THERAPY	Fluconazole (200 mg orally once daily) for a minimum of 1 year	Itraconazole (200 mg orally once daily) for a minimum of 1 year	• The minimum duration of maintenance therapy should be at least 1 year. After that, maintenance therapy can be discontinued in individuals on ART who have a CD4 cell count ≥100 cells/μL and have achieved an undetectable viral load on ART for more than 3 months. • If viral load testing is not available, maintenance therapy should be continued until CD4 is ≥200 cells/μL.

Adapted from Preferred antifungal regimens for cryptococcal meningoencephalitis in nonpregnant patients with HIV. Available at https://www.uptodate.com/contents/image?csi=5a493a81-a72c-45a1-ac57-ac873b2f82da&source=contentShare&imageKey=ID%2F130859

DIAGNOSTIC TESTING

Serology

- In a case of suspected reactivation, a positive IgG assay indicates distant infection, while a negative IgG argues strongly against reactivation toxoplasmosis.
- IgM is negative in reactivation in immunocompromised individuals and those with AIDS.[31]

Imaging

- MRI of the brain is the best radiographic technique for diagnosis.
- Imaging shows multiple ring-enhancing cerebral lesions, most commonly involving corticomedullary junction and basal ganglia.
- Diagnosis is made after a trial of empiric therapy, as seen by a reduction in the size of the mass lesions and clinical improvement in 2–3 weeks.

TREATMENT

- **Sulfadiazine,** 25 mg/kg PO q6h, plus **pyrimethamine**, 200 mg PO on day 1, followed by 50–75 mg PO daily (based on body weight), is the therapy of choice. Co-trimoxazole is an acceptable alternative when sulfadiazine and pyrimethamine are not available.
- **Folinic acid (leucovorin)**, 10–25 mg PO daily, should be added to prevent bone marrow suppression.
- For patients who are allergic to sulfonamides, clindamycin, 600 mg IV or PO q6h, can be used instead of sulfadiazine.[31]
- Doses are reduced after 6 weeks of therapy.
- Secondary prophylaxis can be discontinued among patients with a sustained increase in CD4 count >200 cells/μL for more than 6 months as a result of response to ART and if the initial therapy is complete and there are no symptoms or signs attributable to toxoplasmosis.

Varicella-Zoster Virus

DIAGNOSIS

- Varicella zoster virus (VZV) infection can occur at any CD4 count, but risk of disease is higher at a CD4 count <200 cells/μL.
- It causes two clinically distinct diseases: Varicella (chickenpox) and herpes (shingles).
- HIV viremia and IRIS are also associated with an increased risk of herpes zoster.
- It may cause typical dermatomal lesions or disseminated infection including retinal necrosis.
- It may cause encephalitis, which is more common with ophthalmic distribution of facial nerve.
- Distinct appearance of lesions helps make a clinical diagnosis
- Swabs of vesicular fluid or tissue biopsies can be submitted for viral culture, antigen testing or PCR.

TREATMENT

Acyclovir, 10–15 mg/kg IV q8h for 7–14 days, is the recommended therapy in severe or complicated varicella in HIV. For milder cases, administration of acyclovir (800 mg PO five times a day), famciclovir (500 mg PO tid), or valacyclovir (1 g PO tid) for 1 week is usually effective (Table 16-13).

TABLE 16-13 Treatment of Varicella Zoster

Pre-Exposure Prevention of VZV Primary Infection

Indications

- Adults and adolescents with HIV who have CD4 counts ≥200 cells/μL and who do not have documentation of varicella vaccination, a history or diagnosis of varicella or herpes zoster confirmed by a healthcare provider, or laboratory confirmation of VZV disease; and anyone with HIV who is VZV seronegative should avoid exposure to persons with varicella or herpes zoster.

Vaccination

- Household contacts who are VZV-susceptible should be vaccinated to prevent potential transmission of VZV to at-risk people with HIV.
- In VZV-seronegative persons aged ≥18 years with CD4 counts ≥200 cells/μL, administer primary varicella vaccination (Varivax™) in two doses (0.5 mL SQ) 3 months apart.
- If vaccination results in disease due to live-attenuated vaccine virus, treatment with acyclovir is recommended.
- If post-exposure VariZIG™ has been administered, wait ≥5 months before varicella vaccination.
- If post-exposure acyclovir has been administered, wait ≥3 days before varicella vaccination.
- Administration of varicella vaccine to severely immunocompromised people with HIV (CD4 counts <200 cells/μL) is contraindicated.

Post-Exposure Prophylaxis of VZV Primary Infection

Indications

- Close contact with a person who has active varicella or herpes zoster, and
- Susceptible to VZV (i.e., no history of varicella vaccination, no history of varicella or herpes zoster, or known to be VZV seronegative)

Preferred prophylaxis

- VariZIG 125 IU/10 kg (maximum of 625 IU) IM, administered as soon as possible and within 10 days after exposure to a person with active varicella or herpes zoster
- If post-exposure VariZIG has been administered, wait ≥5 months before varicella vaccination.

Alternative prophylaxis (begin 7–10 days after exposure)

- Acyclovir 800 mg PO 5 times daily for 5–7 days, or
- Valacyclovir 1 g PO 3 times daily for 5–7 days

Preventing Herpes Zoster (Shingles)

Vaccination

- Recombinant zoster vaccine (RZV, Shingrix) is the only available vaccine for prevention of shingles in the United States. As of November 18, 2020, attenuated zoster vaccine live (ZVL, Zostavax) is no longer available for use in the United States.

RZV

- Recommended in adults with HIV aged ≥18 years, regardless of CD4 count:
- RZV 0.5 mL IM injection—2-dose series at 0 and then at 2–6 months.
- RZV should not be given during an acute episode of herpes zoster.
- Following initiation of ART, some experts would delay RZV vaccination until patients are suppressed virologically on ART or until CD4 count recovery to maximize immunologic response to the vaccine.

Source: Adapted from Varicella-Zoster Virus Disease Available at https://clinicalinfo.hiv.gov/

JC Virus

GENERAL PRINCIPLES

- Reactivation of the JC polyomavirus (JCV) in HIV-infected individuals leads to progressive multifocal leukoencephalopathy (PML).
- PML is a rare, fatal demyelinating disease of the central nervous system seen in immunocompromised individuals.
- JCV granule cell neuronopathy, JCV encephalopathy, and meningitis are the other conditions caused by JCV infection.

DIAGNOSIS

- The symptoms of PML include altered mental status, problems in vision (diplopia and hemianopia), weakness (hemi or monoparesis), and disorders of gait (ataxia).
- Neuroimaging shows discrete unilateral or bilateral foci of white matter demyelination that are non-conforming to vascular territories and these areas do not exhibit mass effect or contrast enhancement.
- Lumbar puncture is indicated for CSF analysis and PCR for JCV in those with features suggestive of PML.[34]

TREATMENT

- There is no specific treatment for PML. The main approach is to restore host immune response through effective ART and prolong survival.

CMV Retinitis

GENERAL PRINCIPLES

CMV retinitis is the most common serious ocular complication of AIDS and is associated with reactivation of latent infection. It accounts for 85% of CMV disease in patients with AIDS. It commonly develops in a setting of profound CD4 depletion (CD4 cell count <50 cells/μL), history of prior OI's, high HIV RNA level, and CMV viremia.[35]

DIAGNOSIS

- Patients may report symptoms such as blurred or loss of central vision, floaters, photopsia ("flashing lights"), scotomata ("blind spots"), or peripheral visual field defects. Complications may include retinal detachment leading to complete visual loss.
- The diagnosis of CMV retinitis is made by an experienced ophthalmologist based on characteristic findings during ophthalmoscopic examination. These findings include yellow-white, fluffy retinal lesions with indistinct margins sometimes with a granular appearance. These lesions are often situated near vessels and may be associated with hemorrhage, as observed on indirect ophthalmoscopy.
- CMV viremia can be detected by PCR, and it is usually present in end-organ disease. It can also be seen in the absence of end-organ disease, limiting its diagnostic utility.[35]

TREATMENT

- It can be prevented by initiation of ART early in the course of HIV, but it can still develop in those who not compliant with ART regimen.
- Treatment of CMV retinitis can be local or systemic and is administered in two phases, induction and maintenance.
- **Ganciclovir** is given at an induction dosage of 5 mg/kg IV bid for 14–21 days and a maintenance dosage of 5 mg/kg IV daily indefinitely (unless immune reconstitution occurs). The most common side effect of ganciclovir is **myelotoxicity**, resulting in neutropenia. The neutropenia may respond to granulocyte colony-stimulating factor therapy. An intraocular ganciclovir implant is effective but does not provide systemic CMV therapy.
- **Valganciclovir,** a ganciclovir prodrug, has drug levels equivalent to those of IV ganciclovir. For induction, 900 mg PO bid for 14–21 days is given, followed by 900 mg once a day. **Treatment is indefinite unless immunologic recovery occurs.** Adverse effects are similar to those of ganciclovir.
- Alternatives include **IV foscarnet and IV cidofovir**. These drugs carry a significant risk of **nephrotoxicity**; therefore, adequate hydration and electrolyte monitoring (including calcium) are required.
- For other **invasive CMV diseases**, the optimal therapy is with IV ganciclovir, PO valganciclovir, IV foscarnet, or a combination of two drugs (in persons with prior anti-CMV therapy), for at least 3–6 weeks. Foscarnet has the best CSF penetration and is the drug of choice for CMV encephalitis and myelopathy. Long-term maintenance therapy is indicated.
- After initial therapy and ART, patients may present with visual blurring, floaters, or decreased visual acuity. This may be due to progression, relapse, or immune reconstitution inflammatory syndrome and must be evaluated.[35]

ESOPHAGITIS

Candida

GENERAL PRINCIPLES

- Candida esophagitis is commonly seen in HIV-infected patients with advanced immunosuppression.
- The severity of infection depends on the degree of the patient's immunosuppression.
- Other causes of esophagitis include HSV, CMV, and *Histoplasma*.
- The hallmark of esophageal candidiasis is odynophagia.

DIAGNOSIS

- Most patients have associated oral thrush, but its absence does not exclude esophageal candidiasis.
- Diagnosis requires an endoscopic biopsy of white plaque-like lesions of the esophageal mucosa. Histology shows yeast and hyphae invading mucosal cells with confirmatory fungal cultures.[36]

TREATMENT

- Oral candidiasis usually responds to local therapy with troches or creams (**nystatin** or **clotrimazole**).

- For patients who do not respond or who have esophageal candidiasis, fluconazole, 400 mg PO on day 1 followed by 200–400 mg PO daily for 2–3 weeks is the treatment of choice. Maximum of 800 mg can be given daily, and duration can be extended to 28 days in refractory disease.
- In pregnancy, amphotericin B is the treatment of choice during the first trimester. After the first trimester, the decision must be individualized.
- Liposomal amphotericin B is administered at 3 mg/kg IV daily (if not available, 0.3–0.7 mg/kg IV of amphotericin B deoxycholate is used).[36]

SPECIAL CONSIDERATIONS

Fluconazole-resistant candidiasis is increasing, especially in patients with advanced disease who have been receiving antifungal agents for prolonged periods.

- **Caspofungin or micafungin,** echinocandins, can be considered for refractory cases.
- **Itraconazole** oral suspension (200 mg bid) is occasionally effective, as is posaconazole oral solution (400 mg bid), and posaconazole is generally better tolerated than itraconazole. **Voriconazole** (200 mg bid) may also be useful.
- The duration of therapy is 2–3 weeks and can be extended to 28 days.[36]

DIARRHEA

Cryptosporidium

DIAGNOSIS

- *Cryptosporidium* causes chronic watery diarrhea with malabsorption and wasting in HIV-infected patients.
- Diagnosis is based on the visualization of the parasite in an acid-fast stain or direct immunofluorescence of stool. Polymerase chain reaction testing can also be used. Organisms may be found in stool, biliary secretion, duodenal aspirate, GI tract biopsy, or respiratory tract secretions.[37]

TREATMENT

- No effective specific therapy has been developed. Primary intervention is the initiation of ART.
- **Nitazoxanide,** 500 mg PO bid, for at least 2 weeks may be effective in nonsevere diarrhea. In advanced HIV with severe diarrhea (stool volume >10 L per day) or in cases refractory to initial therapy, combination therapy with azithromycin can be attempted.[37]

Cyclospora, *Cystoisospora*, Microsporidia, and *Campylobacter jejuni*

DIAGNOSIS

These organisms cause chronic diarrhea. Microsporidia can also cause biliary tree disease in patients with advanced infection.

TREATMENT

- *Cyclospora* is treated with **TMP-SMX**, one double-strength (DS) tablet PO bid for 7–10 days. *Cystoisospora* (formerly *Isospora)* is treated with **TMP-SMX**, one DS tablet PO bid for 10 days (increase to qid if diarrhea persists for 48 hours after starting treatment), followed by chronic suppression with TMP-SMX, one DS tablet PO three times a week.[38]
- Microsporidia caused by *Enterocytozoon bieneusi* is treated with optimized ART. For other species, **albendazole**, 400 mg PO bid can be given for 2–4 weeks. Relapses are common when therapy is stopped.
- *Campylobacter jejuni* is treated with either azithromycin, 500 mg PO daily, or ciprofloxacin, 500–750 mg PO bid for 7–14 days.[39]

ASSOCIATED NEOPLASMS

Kaposi Sarcoma

GENERAL PRINCIPLES

Kaposi sarcoma (KS) is caused by coinfection with human herpesvirus-8, also called Kaposi sarcoma–associated herpesvirus.

DIAGNOSIS

In AIDS patients, it commonly presents as localized or widespread mucocutaneous lesions involving skin and oral mucosa, but it can be disseminated. The GI tract and lungs are the usual visceral organs involved. KS can appear even in individuals on HAART with complete suppression of HIV.[40]

TREATMENT

Mild disease is treated with optimization of ART. Severe disease is treated with chemotherapy plus ART. Liposomal doxorubicin is first-line chemotherapy. Cryotherapy or radiation may be useful as well.

Lymphoma

GENERAL PRINCIPLES

- Lymphomas commonly associated with HIV are aggressive B-cell lymphomas, primary CNS lymphoma (PCNSL), primary effusion lymphoma, plasmablastic multicentric Castleman disease, and Hodgkin lymphoma (HL). AIDS-related lymphomas are of the aggressive B-cell type (diffuse large B-cell type, Burkitt, or Burkitt-like).[41]
- **EBV** appears to be the associated pathogen.

DIAGNOSIS

- Primary CNS lymphomas are common and can be multicentric.
- Diagnosis is based on clinical symptoms, the presence of enhancing brain lesions, brain biopsy, and a positive EBV-PCR of the CSF.
- Other OIs need to be ruled out.

- Other potential extranodal sites of involvement, including the bone marrow, GI tract, and liver, require tissue biopsy to confirm the diagnosis.

TREATMENT

- The treatment approach involves integrating therapy appropriate for the stage of malignant lymphoma with limitations imposed by HIV infection.
- Essential components of the treatment strategy must include:
  - Antitumor therapy
  - HAART
  - Prophylaxis for Ois
  - Rapid recognition and treatment of intercurrent infections[42]

  Treatment involves **chemotherapy** and **radiation**. May respond to corticosteroids alone.

Cervical and Perianal Neoplasias

GENERAL PRINCIPLES

- Both HIV-infected men and women are at high risk for HPV-related disease.
- Certain HPV subtypes such as 16 and 18 are oncogenic.
  - CD4 count of <200 cells/mcL, infection with HPV subtypes 16 or 18, and age >34 years are the confirmed risk factors for cervical cancer in women infected with HIV.
  - Cervical cancer in HIV-infected women is more extensive and difficult to cure with a high rate of recurrence.[43]
- Cancer can also arise from perianal condyloma acuminata.

DIAGNOSIS

- Screening for vaginal dysplasia with a Papanicolaou smear is indicated every 6 months during the first year and, if results are normal, annually thereafter.
- Screening for anal intraepithelial neoplasms is currently under evaluation and is recommended by some experts in populations such as MSM, any patient with a history of anogenital condylomas, and women with abnormal vulvar or cervical histology.[44]

TREATMENT

- Management of cervical cancer is not changed by HIV infection.
- ART may result in resolution of HPV infection and CIN, but it has no effects on cancer.
- Unvaccinated males and females ages 9–26 should be given the HPV vaccination series.

Refer to Chapter 22, Cancer, for specific treatments of these neoplasms.

SEXUALLY TRANSMITTED INFECTIONS IN PATIENTS WITH HIV

For treatment, see Table 16-1.

Genital Herpes

HIV-infected individuals are more likely to have prolonged and severe disease as well as treatment failures due to the development of resistance. Treatment guidelines are slightly different for HIV-infected patients. See Table 16-1.

Genital Warts

GENERAL PRINCIPLES

Genital warts are caused by HPV. Different serotypes have been associated with the lesions, notably types 6 and 11. Other common HPV types (16, 18, 31, 33, and 35) are associated with malignant transformation in different anatomic sites.[45] Genital warts in HIV-infected persons are typically more resistant to treatment and have a higher chance of recurrence.[46]

DIAGNOSIS

Diagnosis is made on the basis of physical examination. Biopsy is indicated in the following circumstances:

- Atypical (pigmented, indurated, affixed to underlying tissue, bleeding, or ulcerated)
- Uncertain diagnosis
- Lesions that are unresponsive to standard therapy or worsen during therapy

Differentials include condyloma accuminata and condyloma lata (can be diagnosed through serologic tests).[46]

TREATMENT

- Treatment depends on size, site, and number of lesions; patient preference; cost of therapy; adverse effects; and provider experience.
- Since warts can resolve spontaneously within a year, it is an acceptable alternative for patients to forego treatment and wait for resolution.
- Local therapy is aimed at the removal of the warts. This may reduce but does not eradicate HPV infectivity.
- Treatment modalities are either patient-applied or provider-administered (Table 16-14).
- Lesions usually respond within 3 months of therapy.
- HPV vaccination is recommended for women and men aged 9–26 (see previous section on immunizations) to prevent warts; however, it does not treat existing HPV infection or warts.[45]

TABLE 16-14 Recommended Regimens for External Anogenital Warts

Patient-applied	Provider-administered
Imiquimod 3.75% or 5% cream OR Podofilox (podophyllotoxin) 0.5% solution or gel OR Sinecatechins 15% ointment	Cryotherapy with liquid nitrogen or cryoprobe OR Surgical removal by tangential scissor/shave excision, curettage, laser, or electrosurgery OR Trichloroacetic acid (TCA) or bichloracetic acid (BCA) 80-90% solution

Source: Adapted from Anogenital Warts. Available at https://www.cdc.gov/std/treatment-guidelines/anogenital-warts.htm

Syphilis

See the section on STIs for more complete information.

Additional Resources

- www.aidsinfo.nih.gov
- www.hivmedicationguide.comwww.thebody.com
- www.cdc.gov/hiv
- www.hivinsite.ucsf.edu
- http://naco.gov.in/hiv

Summary

- Routine sexual history assessment is integral during initial patient visits, preventive exams, or when STI symptoms are present. Discussions should cover partners, sexual practices, STI protection, previous STIs, and pregnancy planning.
- Transgender individuals often face disparities in healthcare access and experience, due to discrimination. Higher HIV prevalence among transgender individuals underscores the importance of tailored care. Medical settings should adopt inclusive practices, provide staff training, and follow guidelines.
- Management of STIs includes prompt and accurate diagnosis through clinical examination, laboratory tests, and sometimes imaging. Screening is recommended for high-risk populations.
- Antibiotics or antiviral medications are prescribed based on the specific STI and its sensitivity pattern, along with simultaneous treatment of partners.
- Prevention includes education on safe sexual practices, including consistent and correct condom use, vaccination against certain STIs like HPV and hepatitis B and prompt identification and treatment of asymptomatic infections to reduce transmission rates.
- Acute retroviral syndrome presents with fever, sore throat, rash, myalgias, and fatigue. Opportunistic infections are a common presentation of unrecognized HIV infection.
- ART initiation is recommended for all HIV-infected individuals regardless of CD4 count, with individualized regimens based on patient factors as well as the presence of co-existing opportunistic infections. Monitoring includes viral load, CD4 count, and adjustment of therapy in case of treatment failure or drug resistance. Long-term ART use is associated with toxicity, including hyperlipidemia, insulin resistance, osteoporosis, and lipodystrophy syndrome. Special considerations include management during pregnancy, acute HIV infection, and coinfection with hepatitis.

Scan the QR code to access chapter references.

17

Solid Organ Transplant Medicine and Stem Cell Transplantation

Rowena Delos Santos, Rungwasse Rattanavich, and Hasmukh Jain

Solid Organ Transplant Basics

GENERAL PRINCIPLES

- Solid organ transplantation is a **treatment, not a cure**, for end-stage organ failure of the kidney, liver, pancreas, heart, and lung. Small intestine and vascularized composite allografts are performed in smaller numbers at specialized centers throughout the country. The benefits of organ replacement coexist with the risks of the immediate procedure followed by the risks of chronic immunosuppression. Thus, not all patients with organ failure are transplant candidates.
- Organs from **deceased donors** remain in short supply, with increasing waiting times for potential recipients. **Living donor transplants** are increasingly common in kidney transplantation and are being evaluated in liver and lung transplantations as a partial solution to this shortage. Xenotransplantation is **not** currently a viable option.
- **Immunologic considerations** between donor and recipient prior to the transplant must be fully evaluated including ABO compatibility, HLA typing, cross-matching, and some degree of immune response testing for the proposed donor. Newer protocols using desensitization techniques have had some success in overcoming these immunologic barriers such as a desensitization protocol for ABO incompatibility in living donor kidney transplantations.

DIAGNOSIS

- For indications and contraindications of heart, lung, kidney, and liver transplantations, see sections devoted to cardiology, pulmonology, nephrology, and hepatology.
- **Transplant recipient patient evaluation:** The evaluation of the transplant recipient with general medical or surgical problems should encompass details of the patient's organ transplant and treatment. Thus, the following should always be reviewed when taking a history from an organ transplant recipient:
  - Cause of organ failure
  - Treatment for organ failure prior to transplantation
  - Type and date of transplant
  - Cytomegalovirus (CMV) serology of donor and recipient
  - Induction immunosuppression, particularly use of antibody-based induction therapy
  - Initial allograft function (e.g., nadir creatinine, forced expiratory volume in 1 second [FEV_1], ejection fraction, synthetic function, and transaminases)
  - Current allograft function
  - Complications of transplantation (e.g., surgical problems, acute rejection, delayed graft function, infections, chronic organ dysfunction)
  - Current immunosuppression regimen and recent drug levels

TREATMENT

- **Immunosuppression:** Immunosuppressive medications are used to promote acceptance of a graft (induction therapy), to prevent rejection (maintenance therapy), and to reverse episodes of acute rejection (rejection therapy). These agents are associated with immunosuppressive effects, immunodeficiency toxicities (e.g., infection and malignancy), and nonimmune toxicities (e.g., nephrotoxicity, diabetes mellitus, bone disease, gout, hyperlipidemia, cardiovascular disease, or neurotoxicity).[1,2] Immunosuppressive medications should only be prescribed and administered by physicians and nurses who have appropriate knowledge and expertise. Many variables factor into the choice and dose of drug and the guidelines for each specific organ are different.

- **Glucocorticoids:** Glucocorticoids are immunosuppressive and antiinflammatory. Their mechanisms of action include inhibition of cytokine transcription, induction of lymphocyte apoptosis, downregulation of adhesion molecules and major histocompatibility complex expression, and modification of leukocyte trafficking.
  - Side effects of chronic glucocorticoid therapy are well known.
  - As a result of the associated morbidity, steroids are tapered rapidly in the immediate posttransplant period to achieve maintenance doses of 0.1 mg/kg or less.
  - Steroid-free immunosuppression, rapid steroid tapering, and steroid withdrawal are developed to minimize side effects.
  - Although most long-term transplant recipients have abnormalities in the adrenal axis, increases in glucocorticoid therapy (i.e., stress dosing) are not indicated for routine surgery or illness.[3]
- **Calcineurin inhibitors:** Calcineurin inhibitors (CNIs) inhibit T-lymphocyte activation and proliferation. **They remain the most commonly used immunosuppressant, despite their side effect of nephrotoxicity.** IV calcineurin inhibitors should be avoided because of their extreme toxicity and must never be given as a bolus under any circumstance.
  - **Cyclosporine (CsA)** is a cyclic 11-amino acid peptide derived from a fungus. Its major nonimmune side effect is nephrotoxicity due to glomerular afferent arteriolar vasoconstriction. This action leads to an immediate decline in glomerular filtration rate of up to 30% and a long-term vaso-occlusive fibrotic renal disease that often results in chronic kidney disease in recipients of all organ transplants. Angiotensin-converting enzyme inhibitors, mTOR inhibitors, volume depletion, and nephrotoxins may potentiate this effect. Acute nephrotoxicity is reversible with dose reduction; chronic nephrotoxicity is generally irreversible and nearly universally present in all patients after 8–10 years of therapy.
  - Other **adverse effects** include gingival hyperplasia, hirsutism, tremors, hypertension, glucose intolerance, hyperlipidemia, hyperkalemia, and, rarely, thrombotic microangiopathy. CsA has a narrow therapeutic window, and doses are adjusted based on blood levels (recommended maintenance 12-hour trough levels of 100–300 ng/mL and 2-hour peak levels of 800–1200 ng/mL). Usual doses are 6–8 mg/kg/d in divided doses, with careful attention to levels and toxicities.
  - **Tacrolimus** is a macrolide and, similar to CsA, is nephrotoxic. Tacrolimus is more neurotoxic and diabetogenic than CsA, but it is associated with less hirsutism, hypertension, and gingival hyperplasia. Tacrolimus dosing is based on trough blood levels (recommended maintenance levels of 5–10 ng/mL). Usual starting dose is 0.15 mg/kg/d in divided doses twice daily. Long-acting versions of this medication are also available.
- **Antimetabolites: Inhibition of DNA synthesis**
  - **Azathioprine (AZA)** is a purine analog that is metabolized by the liver to 6-mercaptopurine (active drug), which in turn is catabolized by xanthine oxidase. Azathioprine inhibits DNA synthesis and thereby suppresses lymphocyte proliferation. The major dose-limiting toxicity of this agent is myelosuppression, which is usually reversible after dose reduction or discontinuation of the drug. The usual maintenance dose is 1.5–2.5 mg/kg/d in a single dose. Drug levels are generally not obtained. Azathioprine is generally considered safe in pregnancy.
  - **Mycophenolic acid (MPA)** inhibits inosine monophosphate dehydrogenase (IMPDH) selectively in monocytes. This enzyme is the rate-limiting enzyme of guanine nucleotide

synthesis, which is critical for de novo purine synthesis in both T and B lymphocytes. Two forms are available: mycophenolate mofetil (which is converted to the active metabolite, MPA) and enteric-coated mycophenolate sodium. Adverse effects of MPA commonly include gastrointestinal disturbances (nausea, diarrhea, and abdominal pain) and hematopoetic side effects (leukopenia and thrombocytopenia).

- Antacids that contain magnesium and aluminum interfere with the absorption of MPA and should not be given concurrently.
- Proton pump inhibitors can also interfere with the bioavailability of mycophenolate mofetil, but not enteric-coated MPA, which is absorbed in the small intestine.
- MPA is not used in pregnancy because of its teratogenicity in animal models.
- The usual dose is 1–2 g daily in divided doses, although lesser doses may be used with concomitant tacrolimus compared with cyclosporine (CsA), because of enterohepatic circulation affecting MPA levels. Additionally, the dosage of MPA should be reduced in chronic renal impairment. Drug levels can be obtained to verify absorption or compliance, but the clinical utility of monitoring MPA levels has not been determined.

- **Antiproliferative Agents: mTOR inhibitors**
  - **Sirolimus and everolimus** inhibit the activation of a regulatory kinase, the mammalian target of rapamycin (mTOR), thus prohibiting T-cell progression from the G_1 to the S phase of the cell cycle. mTOR signaling is not isolated to lymphocyte proliferation but also in monocytes/macrophages, dendritic cells, NK cells, and endothelial cells. Thus, inhibition of mTOR may lead to a number of clinical effects related to its antiproliferative, antiviral, antiinflammatory, and antitumor effects.
  - Unlike the calcineurin inhibitors, mTOR inhibitors do not affect cytokine transcription but inhibit cytokine- and growth factor–induced cell proliferation.
  - The major adverse effects include hyperlipidemia (hypertriglyceridemia), anemia, proteinuria, difficulty with wound healing, cytopenias, peripheral edema, oral ulcers, and gastrointestinal symptoms, although other less common side effects have also been described.
  - Although not directly nephrotoxic, mTOR inhibitors may compound the vasoconstriction of calcineurin inhibitors and potentiate their nephrotoxicity. Thus, mTOR inhibitors are best used alone or with steroids and/or other antiproliferative agents.
  - Sirolimus interacts with CsA metabolism, making monitoring of both drugs difficult.
  - The typical dose of sirolimus is 2–5 mg daily in a single dose. Everolimus is administered at 0.75–1.50 mg twice daily. Therapeutic drug monitoring is being perfected, with current trough levels between 5 and 15 ng/mL for sirolimus and 3–8 ng/mL for everolimus most commonly being used.
  - Sirolimus should be avoided in moderate to advanced chronic kidney disease and immediately postoperatively because it is associated with poor wound healing, delayed graft function (kidney transplant), anastomotic bronchial dehiscence (lung transplant), and hepatic artery thrombosis (liver transplant); limited data are available regarding use of everolimus in the immediate postoperative period.
  - Sirolimus is not used in pregnant women because of teratogenicity in animal models.
  - mTOR inhibitors have been effective in reducing intimal proliferation and obliterative vasculopathy in heart transplantation and have been approved as chemotherapy in advanced renal cell, breast, and other malignancies.
- **Biologic agents**
  - **Polyclonal antibodies**
    - Antithymocyte globulin (ATG) is produced by injecting human thymocytes into animals and collecting sera. This process generates antibodies against a wide variety of human immune system antigens. When subsequently infused into human patients, T lymphocytes are depleted as a result of complement-mediated lysis and clearance of antibody-coated cells by the reticuloendothelial system. Lymphocyte function is also disrupted by blocking and modulating the expression of cell surface

molecules by the antibodies. Infusion is through a central vein over 4–6 hours. The most common side effects are fever, chills, and arthralgias.

- Other important **adverse effects** include myelosuppression, serum sickness, and, rarely, anaphylaxis. Two preparations are available: horse ATG (ATGAM) and rabbit ATG (thymoglobulin). Current literature suggests that rabbit ATG is more efficacious. These drugs can be used at the time of transplantation to promote engraftment ("induction") or as a subsequent treatment for acute rejection. The long-term risk of increased malignancy, particularly lymphoma, remains a concern with these agents.
- IV immunoglobulin (IVIG) is an extract pooled from several thousand plasma donors to create a product that is IgG rich. Immunomodulatory and antiinflammatory effects are associated with high dose (1–2 g/kg), but common mechanisms including direct binding to natural antibodies, immunomodulatory proteins, pathogens, inhibition of complement fixation on target tissue, and stimulation of antiinflammatory pathways are also involved. Because of these effects, IVIG is used in the treatment of antibody-mediated rejection, desensitization of preformed HLA, or ABO antibodies. Side effects include flushing, myalgias, chills, headache, and, rarely, anaphylaxis.

◦ **Monoclonal antibodies**

- **Alemtuzumab (Campath 1H)** is a humanized monoclonal antibody against CD52, a molecule with an unclear physiological significance present on B and T cells, which results in depletion of both T and B cells. It can cause significant lymphopenia for up to 6–12 months after dosing, which has led to its use in refractory chronic lymphocytic leukemia. In kidney transplants, it was used off label as an induction agent over the last decade but has seen decreased usage more recently.
- **Basiliximab (Simulect)** is a humanized anti–interleukin-2 receptor (IL-2 receptor or CD 25) monoclonal antibody that competitively inhibits the IL-2 receptor and thereby inhibits proliferation of activated T cells. This drug is administered by a peripheral vein perioperatively as induction therapy at the time of transplantation and is associated with few side effects.
- **Belatacept** is a fusion protein (human IgG bound to CTLA4), which competitively binds to CD80/86 on antigen-presenting cells (APCs). This agent blocks T-cell co-stimulation between CD80/86 on APCs and CD 28 on T cells and downregulates the T cell response. This agent is FDA indicated for use as a substitute for CNIs for long-term use as rejection prophylaxis posttransplant. It is contraindicated for use in liver transplantation and additionally in recipients seronegative for Epstein–Barr virus (EBV) because of increased posttransplant lymphoproliferative disease (PTLD) in EBV-seronegative recipients.
- **Rituximab**, a chimeric monoclonal antibody against the B-cell protein CD20, leads to B cell depletion through complement dependent cytotoxicity, growth arrest and apoptosis. It can induce suppressed B cell counts for up to 6–9 months and occasionally more. Side effects such as fever, bronchospasm, and hypotension are attributed to cytokine release. It also carries the risk of hepatitis B reactivation in patients positive for hepatitis B surface antigen or hepatitis B core antibody. Therefore, prior to starting treatment, patients should be screened for hepatitis B surface antigen and hepatitis B core antibody.
- **Eculizumab**, a humanized monoclonal antibody, is a complement C5 inhibitor that effectively inhibits its cleavage to C5a and C5b, which are required to form the C5-9 or MAC (membrane attack complex) and which result in blockade of proinflammatory prothrombotic and lytic functions of complement. Eculizumab's efficacy is most apparent for atypical HUS and paroxysmal nocturnal hemoglobinuria. Although no strong evidence supports eculizumab use in antibody-mediated rejection, it is used pretransplants for the prevention of antibody-mediated rejection as part of certain off- label desensitization protocols. Risk factors from inhibition of complement

increase the risk of serious infection from encapsulated bacteria; thus, vaccination for *Neisseria meningitis, Streptococcus pneumonia*, and *Haemophilus influenza* type b should be performed before therapy.[4]

- **Infection prophylaxis**
  - **Immunization:** Pneumococcal and hepatitis B vaccination should be given to the recipient at the time of pretransplant evaluation. Influenza A vaccination should be administered yearly. Live vaccines should be avoided after transplantation and also in a live donor if organ donation is imminent. Varicella vaccination in seronegative patients if no contraindication for live vaccine and hepatitis A vaccination (particularly in liver transplant candidates) should be considered before transplant. A newly available inactivated varicella vaccine can now be given both prior to and after transplantation.
  - **Trimethoprim-sulfamethoxazole** prevents urinary tract infections, *Pneumocystis jirovecii* pneumonia, and *Nocardia* infections. The optimal dose and duration of prophylaxis have not been determined, although a minimum of 1 year is generally recommended. In sulfa-allergic patients, dapsone, aerosolized pentamidine, and atovaquone are suitable alternatives.
  - **Acyclovir** prevents reactivation of herpes simplex virus (HSV) and varicella-zoster virus but is ineffective in CMV prophylaxis. HSV can be a serious infection in immunosuppressed individuals, and some form of prophylaxis should be used during the first year. Patients with recurrent HSV infections (oral or genital) should be considered candidates for long-term prophylaxis. Lifetime acyclovir should also be used in EBV-seronegative patients who receive an EBV-positive organ.
  - **Ganciclovir** or **valganciclovir** prevents reactivation of CMV infection when administered to patients who were previously CMV seropositive, received a CMV-positive organ, or both. Typically, they are administered for 3–12 months following transplantation. CMV hyperimmune globulin or IV ganciclovir can also be used for this purpose. Alternatively, patients can be monitored for the presence of CMV replication in the bloodstream by polymerase chain reaction before symptoms develop and can be treated preemptively.
  - **Fluconazole** or **ketoconazole** can be given to patients with a high risk of systemic fungal infections or recurrent localized fungal infections. Both medications increase CsA and tacrolimus levels (see Treatment under the Solid Organ Transplant Basics section).
  - **Nystatin suspension, clotrimazole** troches, or weekly **fluconazole** are used to prevent oropharyngeal candidiasis (thrush).

GRAFT REJECTION

Acute Rejection, Kidney

GENERAL PRINCIPLES

Most episodes of acute rejection occur in the first year after transplantation. The low incidence of acute rejection today usually entails a careful search for inadequate drug levels, nonadherence, or less common forms of rejection (such as antibody-mediated rejection or plasma cell rejection). Late acute rejection (>1 year after transplantation) usually results from inadequate immunosuppression or patient nonadherence.

Definition

An immunologically mediated acute deterioration in renal function associated with specific pathologic changes on renal biopsy including lymphocytic interstitial infiltrates, tubulitis,

TABLE 17-1 Differential Diagnosis of Renal Allograft Dysfunction

>1 wk After Transplant	<3 mo After Transplant	>3 mo After Transplant
Acute tubular necrosis	Acute rejection	Prerenal azotemia
Hyperacute rejection	Calcineurin inhibitor toxicity	Calcineurin inhibitor toxicity
Accelerated rejection	Prerenal azotemia	Acute rejection (nonadherence, low levels)
Obstruction	Obstruction	Obstruction
Urine leak (ureteral necrosis)	Infection	Recurrent renal disease
Arterial or venous thrombosis	Interstitial nephritis	De novo renal disease
Atheroemboli	Recurrent renal disease BK virus nephropathy	Renal artery stenosis (anastomotic or atherosclerotic BK virus nephropathy

and arteritis (cellular rejection) and/or glomerulitis, capillaritis, and positive staining of the peritubular capillaries for the complement component C4d (antibody-mediated rejection).

Epidemiology

Kidney allograft rejection currently occurs in only 10% of patients. Patients who do not receive induction therapy have a 20%–30% incidence of acute rejection.

DIAGNOSIS

Diagnosis of acute renal allograft rejection is made by percutaneous renal biopsy after excluding prerenal azotemia via hydration and repeating laboratory tests. Further workup includes evaluation for calcineurin inhibitor nephrotoxicity (trough and/or peak levels and associated signs), infection (urinalysis and culture), obstruction (renal ultrasound), and surgical complications such as urine leak (renal scan). Newer techniques evaluating early markers of acute rejection in the blood and urine are under investigation.

Clinical Presentation

Manifestations include an elevated serum creatinine, decreased urine output, increased edema, or worsening hypertension. Initial symptoms are often absent except for the rise in creatinine. Constitutional symptoms (fever, malaise, arthralgia, painful or swollen allograft) are uncommon in current practice.

Differential Diagnosis

Differential diagnosis varies with duration after transplantation (Table 17-1).

Acute Rejection, Lung

GENERAL PRINCIPLES

- Of the solid organ transplants, the lung is the most immunogenic organ.
- The majority of patients have at least one episode of acute rejection. Multiple episodes of acute rejection predispose to the development of chronic rejection (bronchiolitis obliterans syndrome).

- **Lung transplant rejection** occurs frequently and most commonly in the first few months after transplantation.

DIAGNOSIS

Diagnosis is generally made by fiberoptic bronchoscopy with bronchoalveolar lavage and transbronchial biopsies.

Clinical Presentation

Manifestations are nonspecific and include fever, dyspnea, and a nonproductive cough. The chest radiograph is usually unchanged and is generally nondiagnostic even when abnormal (perihilar infiltrates, interstitial edema, pleural effusions). Change in pulmonary function testing is not specific for rejection, but a 10% or greater decline in FVC or FEV_1, or both, is usually clinically significant.

Differential Diagnosis

It is important to attempt to distinguish rejection from infection because although the symptoms are similar, the treatments are markedly different.

Acute Rejection, Heart

GENERAL PRINCIPLES

Heart transplant recipients typically have 2–3 episodes of acute rejection in the first year after transplantation with a 50%–80% chance of having at least one rejection episode, most commonly in the first 6 months.

DIAGNOSIS

- Diagnosis is established by endomyocardial biopsy performed during routine surveillance or as prompted by symptoms. None of the noninvasive techniques has demonstrated sufficient sensitivity and specificity to replace the endomyocardial biopsy. Repeated endomyocardial biopsies predispose to severe tricuspid regurgitation.
- **Manifestations** may include symptoms and signs of left ventricular dysfunction, such as dyspnea, paroxysmal nocturnal dyspnea, orthopnea, syncope, palpitations, new gallops, and elevated jugular venous pressure. Many patients are asymptomatic. Acute rejection may also be associated with a variety of tachyarrhythmias (atrial more often than ventricular).

Acute Rejection, Liver

GENERAL PRINCIPLES

- Many liver transplant recipients may be maintained on minimal immunosuppression. Acute rejection typically occurs within the first 3 months after transplant and often in the first 2 weeks after the operation. Acute rejection in the liver is generally reversible and does not portend a potentially serious adverse outcome as in other organs. Recurrent viral hepatitis is a much more frequent and morbid problem.
- **Liver transplant recipients** commonly experience acute allograft rejection, with at least 60% having one episode.

DIAGNOSIS

Diagnosis is made by liver biopsy after technical complications are excluded.

Clinical Presentation

Manifestations may be absent with only a slight elevation in transaminases, or patients may have signs and symptoms of liver failure including fever, malaise, anorexia, abdominal pain, ascites, decreased bile output, elevated bilirubin, and elevated transaminases.

Differential Diagnosis

Differential diagnosis of early liver allograft dysfunction includes primary graft nonfunction, preservation injury, vascular thrombosis, biliary anastomotic leak, or stenosis. These disorders should be excluded clinically or by Doppler ultrasonography. Late allograft dysfunction may be because of rejection, recurrent hepatitis B or C, CMV infection, EBV infection, cholestasis, or drug toxicity.

Acute Rejection, Pancreas

GENERAL PRINCIPLES

- The majority of rejection episodes occur within the first 6 months after transplant. Unlike other organs, clinical findings and biochemical markers correlate poorly with rejection; in particular, if hyperglycemia occurs because of rejection, it is often late, severe, and irreversible. Because 80% of pancreas transplants are performed with a simultaneous kidney transplant with the same immunologic status, renal allograft function and histopathology can be a valuable surrogate for diagnosis of pancreas allograft rejection.
- Most pancreas transplants are done with quadruple immunosuppression, consisting of an induction agent and triple maintenance immunosuppression, including corticosteroids. One-year posttransplant acute rejection rates range between 20% and 30%; this contributes significantly to early and late graft loss.

DIAGNOSIS

At time of surgery, the exocrine (digestive enzymes) secretions of the pancreas can be drained into the recipient's intestine (enteric drainage) or into the bladder (bladder drainage). Serum amylase and lipase are used in both the enteric- and bladder-drained recipient to monitor for rejection, but lack specificity. For the bladder-drained allograft, a fall in urinary amylase correlates with rejection. However, allograft biopsy remains the gold standard, demonstrating septal, ductal, and acinar inflammation and endotheliitis. If a recipient received a simultaneous kidney transplant from the same donor, the creatinine and renal biopsy may also be used to diagnose rejection, although isolated pancreas or kidney rejection may rarely occur.

Clinical Presentation

Manifestations may be absent with only a slight elevation in serum amylase and lipase or fall in urinary amylase (bladder drained). **Hyperglycemia is a late manifestation of rejection.**

Differential Diagnosis

Differential diagnosis of hyperglycemia includes thrombosis (affecting 7% of recipients), islet cell drug toxicity, steroid effect, infection, development of insulin resistance, or recurrent autoimmune disease. Differential diagnosis of elevated serum lipase includes graft pancreatitis, peripancreatic fluid/infection, obstruction, dehydration, and PTLD.

Chronic Allograft Dysfunction

GENERAL PRINCIPLES

- Chronic allograft dysfunction accounts for the vast majority of late graft losses and is the major obstacle to long-term graft survival.
- Chronic allograft dysfunction (formerly chronic rejection) is a slowly progressive, insidious decline in function of the allograft characterized by gradual vascular and ductal obliteration, parenchymal atrophy, and interstitial fibrosis.

DIAGNOSIS

- Diagnosis is often difficult and generally requires a biopsy. The process is mediated by immune and nonimmune factors.
- The manifestations of chronic rejection are unique to each organ system.

TREATMENT

To date, no effective therapy is available for established immune-mediated chronic allograft dysfunction. Some patients, particularly those with renal transplants, will require a second solid organ transplant. Current investigational strategies are aimed at prevention.

BIOMARKERS

- The incidence of acute rejection varies between allograft types. Current recommended routine markers/imaging (i.e., serum creatinine in kidney transplant and echocardiogram in heart transplant) are not sensitive enough to detect graft damage in the early stages of rejection. There are limitations of invasive biopsy for routine surveillance. Noninvasive biomarkers could serve as predictive factors for rejection for early identification of allograft injury and prompt early intervention.
- Unbiased high-throughput gene expression profiling technologies and donor-derived cell-free DNA testing are other tools that can help provide further information into the health of an allograft. These technologies are available in kidney and heart transplant, but not currently available for other organ transplants.[5]
- Allomap: Current heart transplantation guidelines to rule out the presence of a moderate to severe acute rejection in low-risk patients between 6 months and 5 years after transplantation.

Complications

GENERAL PRINCIPLES

- **Infections**
  - Posttransplant infections are a significant cause of morbidity and, in some cases, mortality for transplant recipients. Types of infections vary depending on the time since transplantation (Table 17-2).[6]
  - **CMV infection** from reactivation of CMV in a seropositive recipient or new infection from a CMV-positive organ can lead to a wide range of presentations from a mild viral

TABLE 17-2 Timing and Etiology of Posttransplant Infections

Time Period	Infectious Complication	Etiology
<1 mo after transplant	Nosocomial pneumonia, wound infection, urinary tract infection, catheter-related sepsis, biliary, chest, or other drainage catheter infection	Bacterial or fungal infections
1–6 mo after transplant	Opportunistic infections	Cytomegalovirus *Pneumocystis jirovecii* *Aspergillus* spp. *Toxoplasma gondii* *Listeria monocytogenes* *Strongyloides stercoralis* West Nile virus Varicella-zoster virus (VZV)
	Reactivation of preexisting infections	*Mycobacteria* spp. Endemic mycoses Viral hepatitis
>6 mo after transplant	Community-acquired infections	Bacterial Tick-borne disease Influenza Metapneumovirus Norovirus
	Chronic progressive infection	Reactivated VZV (zoster) Hepatitis B Hepatitis C HIV Cytomegalovirus Epstein–Barr virus Papillomavirus Polyomavirus (BK)
	Opportunistic infections	*P. jirovecii* *L. monocytogenes* *Nocardia asteroides* *Cryptococcus neoformans* *Aspergillus* spp. West Nile virus

syndrome to allograft dysfunction, invasive disease in multiple organ systems, and even death. CMV-seronegative patients who receive a CMV-seropositive organ are at substantial risk, particularly in the first year.

- Because of the potential progression and severity of untreated disease, treatment is usually indicated in viremic transplant patients without tissue diagnosis of invasive disease. Seroconversion with a positive IgM titer or a fourfold increase in IgM or IgG titer suggests acute infection; however, many centers now use polymerase chain reaction–based diagnostic techniques from blood samples, and treatment is usually administered in the patient with evidence of viremia. Common treatment options include oral valganciclovir, 450–900 mg PO bid, or IV ganciclovir, 2.5–5.0 mg/kg bid for 3–4 weeks or until clearance of the virus. Both drugs are adjusted for renal function. Hyperimmune globulin is often used with ganciclovir for patients with organ involvement.

  - Foscarnet and cidofovir are more toxic alternatives and should be reserved for ganciclovir-resistant cases.

- **Hepatitis B and C:** Patients with chronic hepatitis B or hepatitis C or cirrhosis were once considered contraindications to nonhepatic transplant because immunosuppression increases viral replication in organ transplant recipients with either hepatitis B or C. However, advanced medical treatment has created opportunities for a substantial number of patients to be effectively treated before transplantation.[7]
  - **Hepatitis B** can recur as fulminant hepatic failure even in patients with no evidence of viral DNA replication prior to transplantation. In liver transplantation, the risk of recurrent hepatitis B virus infection can be reduced by the administration of hepatitis B immunoglobulin during and after transplantation. Lamivudine therapy initiated before transplantation to lower viral load leads to decreased likelihood of recurrent hepatitis B virus.
  - **Hepatitis C** typically progresses slowly in nonhepatic transplants, and the effect of immunosuppression on mortality because of liver disease remains to be determined. Hepatitis C nearly always recurs in liver transplant recipients whose original disease was due to hepatitis C. Therapy for recurrent hepatitis C virus with directed antiviral therapy can achieve a sustained virologic response and clearance of the virus.
- **EBV** plays a role in the development of PTLD. This life-threatening lymphoma is treated by withdrawal or reduction in immunosuppression and often aggressive chemotherapy.
- **Other viruses:** The role other viruses, such as human herpesvirus (HHV)-6, HHV-7, HHV-8, and polyomavirus (BK and JC), play in causing posttransplant infections is an area of active investigation. Notably, BK virus is known to cause interstitial nephritis, resulting in renal allograft loss and occasionally ureteral stricture, resulting in obstruction. Because BK virus nephropathy results primarily from reactivation of latent BK in the transplanted organ, this is rarely seen in nonrenal transplant recipients.
- **Fungal and parasitic infections**, such as *Cryptococcus, Mucor*, aspergillosis, and *Candida* spp., result in increased mortality after transplantation and should be aggressively diagnosed and treated. The role of prophylaxis with oral fluconazole has not been established.

- **Renal disease:** Chronic allograft dysfunction is the leading cause of allograft loss in renal transplant recipients. Chronic calcineurin inhibitor (CsA or tacrolimus) nephrotoxicity may also lead to chronic renal insufficiency and end-stage renal disease (ESRD), requiring dialysis or transplantation in recipients of lung, heart, liver, or pancreas transplants. The incidence of ESRD secondary to calcineurin inhibitor toxicity in recipients of solid organ transplants is at least 10%, and the incidence of significant chronic kidney disease approaches 50%.
- **Malignancy** occurs in transplant patients with an overall incidence that is three- to fourfold higher than that seen in the general population (age matched). Cancers with an increased risk of fivefold or greater compared with the general population are Kaposi sarcoma, non-Hodgkin lymphoma, and skin, lip, vulvar, anal, and liver cancer, illustrating the oncogenic potential of associated viral infections, as well as the potent role of normal immune function in surveillance and clearance of malignant cells.
  - **Skin and lip cancers** are the most common de novo malignancies (40%–50%) seen in transplant recipients, with an incidence 10–250 times that of the general population. Risk factors include immunosuppression, UV radiation, and human papillomavirus infection. These cancers develop at a younger age, and they are more aggressive in transplant patients. Protective clothing, sunscreens, and avoiding sun exposure are recommended. Examination of the skin is the principal screening test, and early diagnosis

offers the best prognosis. The mTOR inhibitors may be better immunosuppressive choices in patients with recurrent skin cancer as long as no contraindications exist.

 - **PTLD** accounts for one-fifth of all malignancies after transplantation, with an incidence of approximately 1%. This is 30- to 50-fold higher than in the general population, and the risk increases with the use of antilymphocyte therapy for induction or rejection. The majority of these neoplasms are large-cell non-Hodgkin lymphomas of the B-cell type. PTLD results from EBV-induced B-cell proliferation in the setting of chronic immunosuppression. The EBV-seronegative recipient of a seropositive organ is at greatest risk. The presentation is often atypical and should always be considered in the patient with new symptoms. Diagnosis requires a high index of suspicion followed by a tissue biopsy. Treatment includes reduction or withdrawal of immunosuppression and chemotherapy.

SPECIAL CONSIDERATIONS

- **Important drug interactions** are always a concern given the polypharmacy associated with transplant patients. Before prescribing a new medication to a transplant recipient, always investigate drug interactions.
- The combination of **allopurinol and azathioprine** should be avoided because of the risk of profound myelosuppression.
- CsA and tacrolimus are metabolized by cytochrome P450 (3A4). Therefore, CsA and tacrolimus levels are decreased by drugs that induce cytochrome P450 activity, such as rifampin, isoniazid, barbiturates, phenytoin, and carbamazepine. Conversely, CsA and tacrolimus levels are increased by drugs that compete for cytochrome P450, such as verapamil, diltiazem, nicardipine, azole antifungals, erythromycin, and clarithromycin. Similar effects are seen with sirolimus and everolimus.
- **Tacrolimus and CsA** should not be taken together because of the increased risk of severe nephrotoxicity.
- Lower doses of MPA should be used when either tacrolimus or sirolimus is taken concurrently.
- Concomitant administration of CsA and sirolimus may result in a twofold increase in sirolimus levels; to avoid this drug interaction, CsA and sirolimus should be dosed 4 hours apart.

PRINCIPLES OF STEM CELL TRANSPLANTATION

GENERAL PRINCIPLES

- Many malignancies have a steep dose–response curve to cytotoxic chemotherapy or radiotherapy which most often exceeds the tolerance of the bone marrow (BM).
- This necessitates the need to replenish the BM to prevent irreversible and fatal BM aplasia.
- Studies in mice showed that infusion of splenocytes or bone marrow could rescue the animals from the lethal effect of irradiation.[8]
- With hematopoietic stem cell transplant (HSCT) available as a rescue means, dose escalating chemotherapy and irradiation can be administered.
- Hematopoietic stem cell (HPC) transplantation involves the infusion of either allogeneic (different donor) or autologous (patient's own) stem cells following administration of chemotherapy and/or radiation.
- Autologous transplantation involves collection, cryopreservation, and reinfusion of patient's own stem cells. This allows administration of myeloablative doses of chemotherapy with the intent of maximizing the efficacy of the therapy.

- Allogeneic transplantation refers to the infusion of stem cells collected from either HLA-matched or mismatched donors. In addition to facilitating the administration of high doses of chemotherapy, allogeneic transplantation also allows for an immunologic effect mediated by donor T and natural killer cells (graft-versus-tumor effect).

INDICATIONS

- Stem cell transplantation can be considered for patients with high-risk or relapsed disease that is thought to be chemosensitive or susceptible to graft-versus-tumor effect. MM and lymphoma are the most common indications for autotransplantation, whereas MDS and leukemia are the most common indications for allotransplantation.
- Allogeneic transplantations are also considered in nonmalignant disorders, such as congenital immune deficiencies, sickle cell anemia, thalassemia, and inborn errors of metabolism.

Donor Selection

- Initial efforts of allogeneic HPC transplant in the 1950s pioneered by E. Donnall Thomas did not meet with much success due to incomplete understanding of histocompatibility (H) antigens which resulted in either engraftment failure or life-threatening graft-versus-host disease (GVHD).
- With better understanding of human leukocyte antigens during the 1960s, allogeneic HSCT was performed in 100 patients by 1977 in Seattle. In 1990, E. Donnall Thomas was awarded Nobel Prize for his contributions to HSCT.

Appropriate donor selection is crucial and is based on the following factors:

- HLA typing: Major histocompatibility class I and II alleles code for HLA proteins that are expressed on the cell surface and play a major role in immune recognition. High-resolution typing of 10 HLA alleles (e.g., HLA-A, HLA-B, HLA-C, HLA-DRB1, and HLA-DQB1) is the current standard.
- The chance of any given sibling being a full HLA match is only 25%. Patients who lack HLA-identical siblings should have a search for HLA-matched donors through the national registries or National Marrow Donation Program (NMDP), although chances of finding an HLA-matched unrelated donor are significantly influenced by the patient's ethnicity due to disparities in NMDP participation.
- Partial HLA-mismatched transplantations, umbilical cord blood, and haploidentical transplantations (3/6 match) are alternate sources of stem cells for patients without matched sibling or unrelated donors.
- CMV-negative donors are preferred for CMV-negative patients.

Source of Stem Cells

- HLA-matched donors
  - These donors are fully identical with the recipient for specific exons within HLA-A, HLA-B, HLA-C, and HLA-DRB1 genes.
- Unrelated donors
  - Unrelated matched donors can be identified in worldwide registries for patients who do not have an HLA identical sibling donor.
  - Retrospective analyses comparing 8/8 locus-matched unrelated donors with matched related donors have shown comparable overall survival with increased occurrence of acute and chronic GVHD after unrelated transplant.[9,10]
- Umbilical cord blood
  - It is an alternative for stem cell for patients who do not have a readily available HLA-matched sibling or unrelated donor.

- Umbilical cord blood is the blood remaining in the umbilical cord and placenta after the birth of an infant.
- Advantages
  - Rapid availability
  - Low risk of transmitting viruses
  - Decreased requirement of stringent HLA matching (matching at four out of six HLA class I and II molecules is sufficient)
- Disadvantages
  - Low CD34 cell dose per unit
  - Delayed engraftment
  - Delayed immune reconstitution
  - High transplant-related mortality

• Mismatched and haploidentical donors
  - In early studies, mismatched and haploidentical donors, due to the significant bidirectional alloreactive T-cell responses, resulted in a high incidence of graft rejection and severe GVHD.
  - Use of intense myeloablative conditioning regimen would help in overcoming both graft rejection and GVHD but at the risk of prolonged immunosuppression.
  - Absence of KIR inhibitory ligands in the recipient promotes NK cell-mediated graft-versus-leukemia effect.
  - Use of reduced intensity conditioning (RIC) in mismatched and haploidentical transplants
    - High-dose cyclophosphamide can be administered immediately after transplant to selectively eliminate the alloreactive T cells.
    - Double UCB transplant can be used.

• Collection of stem cells—BM
  - BM HPCs are collected by aspirating from the posterior superior iliac spine under general anesthesia or spinal anesthesia.
  - Volume to be collected is 1000 mL (10–15 mL/kg).
  - BM graft is associated with lesser hematopoietic response and lesser GVHD.
  - BM graft is the preferred stem cell source in patients with nonmalignant disorders such as aplastic anemia.
  - BM can be obtained under anesthesia through repeated aspirations from the iliac crest, but this method is rarely used nowadays.

• Collection of stem cells—peripheral blood (PB)
  - This would require mobilization from the BM.
  - Agents used for mobilization include: granulocyte colony-stimulating factor (G-CSF), chemotherapy (cyclophosphamide), or CXCR4 antagonist (plerixafor) or bortezomib (experimental).[11,12]
  - Apheresis: After mobilization, stem cells are collected using specialized apheresis instruments which would process three to four blood volumes over a period of 2–3 hours.
  - PB grafts contain a higher number of CD34 HPCs as well as T lymphocytes in comparison to BM grafts. Thus, PB grafts would result in superior hematopoietic engraftment and lower relapse risk at the cost of increased risk for acute and chronic GVHD.[13,14]

• HPC doses required for transplant
  - Minimum HPC dose for successful HCT: 2×10^6 CD34 cells/kg recipient body weight
  - Optimal HPC dose for HCT: $4–6 \times 10^6$ CD34 cells/kg recipient body weight

Conditioning Regimens

• Conditioning regimens serve two purposes:
  - Suppress the host immune system sufficiently to prevent rejection
  - Eradicate malignant cells

- The use of high-dose chemotherapy ± total body irradiation (TBI) as conditioning regimen was limited to young patients with no serious comorbidities in view of the considerable toxicity to the nonhematopoietic organs.
- The understanding of the contribution of graft-versus-leukemia effect in elimination of leukemic cells and the significant side effects caused by the conditioning regimens led to the development of RIC regimens.
- Thus, conditioning regimens can be classified according to the degree of myelosuppression into the following:
  - Myeloablative conditioning
  - Nonmyeloablative conditioning
  - RIC
  - Radiolabeled monoclonal antibodies
- Myeloablative conditioning regimen
  - Cyclophosphamide 120 mg/kg over 2 days + TBI 12 Gy/2#.
  - Oral busulfan 16 mg/kg over 4 days + cyclophosphamide 120 mg/kg over 2 days.
  - Fludarabine 120–180 mg/m^2 + busulfan 16 mg/kg orally or 12.8 mg/kg intravenously over 4 days.
  - BEAM—carmustine (BCNU) 300 mg/m^2 over 1 day, etoposide 400–800 mg/m^2 over 4 days, cytosine arabinoside 800–1600 mg/m^2 over 4 days, and melphalan 140 mg/m^2 over 1 day.
  - CBV—BCNU 300–500 mg/m^2 followed by etoposide 600–2400 mg/m^2 plus cyclophosphamide 4.8–7.2 g/m^2 over 4 days.
  - Conditioning regimen for multiple myeloma—melphalan 200 mg/m^2 is the preferred regimen. In patients who are elderly with comorbidities, melphalan at a dose of 140 mg/m^2 is used.
  - Other agents which have been combined with melphalan in multiple myeloma are bortezomib, carfilzomib, and bendamustine, but none have been proven to be standard.
- Nonmyeloablative conditioning regimen: Nonmyeloablative regimens cause minimal cytopenia but significant lymphopenia. Engrafting T cells would eliminate the host hematopoietic cells, allowing establishment of donor hematopoiesis.
  - *Flu/TBI*: Fludarabine 90 mg/m^2 over 3 days + low-dose TBI (2 Gy administered on the day of graft infusion)
  - *Total lymphoid irradiation (TLI)/ATG*: TLI (8–12 cGy) over 11 days + ATG 1.25 mg/kg over 5 days
  - *Low-dose TBI*: 1–2 Gy administered on the day of graft infusion
- RIC regimen: These regimens fall in the intermediate category regimens which do not fit the definition of myeloablative or nonmyeloablative regimens.
  - *Flu/Mel*: Fludarabine (125–150 mg/m^2 total dose) × 5 days + melphalan (140 mg/m^2) × 2 days
  - *Flu/Bu2 and Flu/Bu3*: Fludarabine (150–160 mg/m^2 total dose) × 4–5 days + busulfan (8–10 mg/kg orally) × 2–3 days
  - *Flu/Cy*: Fludarabine (150–180 mg/m^2 total dose) × 5–6 days + cyclophosphamide (120–140 mg/kg) × 2 days
  - *Flu/Bu3/TT*: Fludarabine 150 mg/m^2 × 3 days + busulfan (8 mg/kg) × 3 days + thiotepa (5–10 mg/m^2) over 1–2 days
- Radiolabeled monoclonal antibodies: Radiolabeled monoclonal antibodies which bind to cell surface molecules can increase the dose of radiation delivered to the tumor and spare the normal organs such as liver.
  - Anti-CD20 radioimmunoconjugate: Conjugated with yttrium-90
  - Anti-CD45 antibody
  - Anti-CD66 antibody

Graft-Versus-Host Disease Versus Graft-Versus-Leukemia Effect—Balancing the Two Phenomena

- Both GVHD and GVL are mediated by lymphocytes contained and derived from the hematopoietic graft. GVL is closely linked to the development of GVHD. But clinically significant GVHD is not required for the development of GVL.
- GVHD occurs in spite of donor–recipient being HLA matched, due to disparity between them at polymorphic genetic loci outside the MHC. These loci are termed minor histocompatibility antigens.
- GVHD can be acute and chronic.
  - *Acute GVHD:* Conditioning regimen results in the release of molecules (PAMPs and DAMPs) which activate inflammatory cytokines, donor lymphocytes, and recipient antigen-presenting cells leading to proliferation, differentiation, and trafficking of lymphocytes to secondary lymphoid organs and other target organs resulting in organ injury.
  - *Chronic GVHD:* There is a loss of both B- and T-cell immune tolerance.
- GVL
  - GVL is primarily mediated via the donor T lymphocytes and NK cells.
  - Donor T lymphocytes mediate GVL effect by identifying minor histocompatibility antigens in the leukemic cells and also other nonpolymorphic antigens.
  - Alloreactive NK cells are an important mediator of GVL, especially in recipients of HLA-mismatched or haploidentical donors, in whom T-cell depletion is needed to prevent lethal GVHD. KIR locus disparity of the donor and recipient determines the amplitude of NK cell-mediated GVL effect.

Complications

- Hematopoietic transplantation is often preceded by the use of intense chemotherapy and sometimes total body radiation to clear residual disease and immunosuppress the host.
- Toxicities due to conditioning regimens
  - Most common toxicity—nausea, vomiting, and mucositis
  - Cyclophosphamide related—acute hemorrhagic cystitis and acute hemorrhagic cardiomyopathy
  - Serious organ toxicity associated with MAC
    - Diffuse alveolar hemorrhage
    - Idiopathic interstitial pneumonia
    - Hepatic sinusoidal obstruction syndrome: triad of jaundice, tender hepatomegaly, and ascites
- Transient parotitis is related to TBI.
- Opportunistic infection
  - It occurs due to conditioning-related neutropenia, disruption of the oral and gastrointestinal mucosal barriers, indwelling venous catheters, corticosteroid therapy, and alteration of microbiota because of prior antibiotic usage.
  - Bacterial infections: Both gram-negative and gram-positive are more common immediately after transplant during the neutropenic period.
  - Fungal infections: Invasive *Aspergillus* infection and *Candida* infections are the most common fungal infections.
  - Viral infections: Most common viral infection is CMV infection which in most cases is reactivation of a prior infection. Reactivation typically occurs within the first 100 days. Most common manifestation of CMV disease is interstitial pneumonitis followed by enteritis/colitis. Patients post-transplant need CMV viral load monitoring with the patient being initiated on pre-emptive therapy with antivirals when there is CMV reactivation.
  - *P. jirovecii*: All patients post-allogeneic transplantation should be on prophylaxis for PCP with trimethoprim–sulfamethoxazole or other appropriate alternatives.

- **GVHD:** Acute and chronic GVHD are associated with significant morbidity and mortality in allogeneic transplantation patients. The most common tissues affected are the skin, liver, gut, cornea, and lungs. Chronic GVHD can result in diarrhea and sclerodermatous-type skin changes. The prophylaxis and treatment of GVHD include the use of corticosteroids and immunosuppressants, including tacrolimus, cyclosporine, methotrexate, sirolimus, and mycophenolate.

Summary

- Transplantation has transformed into a burgeoning field that is rapidly evolving to optimize organ distribution and survival outcomes.
- Infections remain a risk to the recipients of solid organ transplantation, long after the initial post-transplant period. Factors that affect risk include the recipient's net state of immunosuppression, epidemiologic exposures, and the consequences of the invasive procedures to which the recipient has been subjected.
- Stem cells are cells that have the capacity to self-renew by dividing and to develop into more mature, specialized cells. Stem cells can be unipotent, multipotent, pluripotent, or totipotent, depending on the number of cell types to which they can give rise.
- The influence of stem cells in regenerative medicine and transplantology is immense. Untreatable neurodegenerative diseases have the possibility of becoming treatable with stem cell therapy. Induced pluripotency enables the use of a patient's own cells.

Scan the QR code to access chapter references.

18 Gastrointestinal Diseases

C. Prakash Gyawali, Farhan Quader, and Nikhil Kenny Thomas

Gastrointestinal Bleeding

GENERAL PRINCIPLES

Acute gastrointestinal (GI) bleeding is a common clinical problem that results in substantial morbidity, healthcare resource utilization, and costs, especially when it develops in hospitalized patients.[1]

- **Overt GI bleeding** is the passage of fresh or altered blood in emesis or stool.
- **Occult GI bleeding** refers to a positive fecal occult blood test (stool guaiac or fecal immunochemical test) or iron deficiency anemia without visible blood in the stool.
- **Obscure GI bleeding** consists of GI blood loss of unknown origin that persists or recurs after negative initial endoscopic evaluation.[2]

DIAGNOSIS

Clinical Presentation

History

- Hematemesis, coffee-ground emesis, and/or aspiration of blood or coffee-ground material from a nasogastric (NG) tube indicate an upper GI source of blood loss.
- **Melena**, black sticky stool with a characteristic odor, usually suggests an upper GI source, although small bowel and right-sided colonic bleeds can also result in melena.
- Various shades of **bloody stool (hematochezia)** are seen with distal small bowel or colonic bleeding, depending on the rate of blood loss and colonic transit. Rapid upper GI bleeding can present with hematochezia, typically associated with hemodynamic compromise or circulatory shock.
- **Anorectal bleeding** usually results in bright red blood coating the exterior of formed stool associated with distal colonic symptoms (e.g., rectal urgency, straining, or pain with defecation).
- **Anemia** from blood loss can cause fatigue, weakness, abdominal pain, pallor, or dyspnea.
- Estimation of the amount of blood loss is often inaccurate. If the baseline hematocrit is known, the drop in hematocrit provides a rough estimate of blood loss. In general, lower GI bleeding causes less hemodynamic compromise than upper GI bleeding.
- **Coagulation abnormalities** can propagate bleeding from a preexisting lesion in the GI tract. Disorders of coagulation (e.g., liver disease, von Willebrand disease, vitamin K deficiency, and disseminated intravascular coagulation) can influence the course of GI bleeding (see Chapter 20, Disorders of Hemostasis and Thrombosis).
- **Medications** known to affect the coagulation process or platelet function include warfarin, heparin, low molecular weight heparin, aspirin, nonsteroidal anti-inflammatory drugs (NSAIDs), thienopyridines (clopidogrel [Plavix], prasugrel [Effient], ticlopidine [Ticlid]), thrombolytic agents, glycoprotein IIb/IIIa receptor antagonists (abciximab [ReoPro], eptifibatide [Integrilin], tirofiban [Aggrastat]), direct thrombin inhibitors (argatroban, bivalirudin, dabigatran etexilate), and direct factor Xa inhibitors (rivaroxaban [Xarelto], apixaban).

TABLE 18-1 Causes of Upper Gastrointestinal (UGI) Bleeding

Esophageal causes
- Esophageal varices (e.g., due to portal hypertension)
- Erosive esophagitis
- Esophageal carcinoma
- Mallory–Weiss syndrome

Gastroduodenal causes
- Peptic ulcer (gastric and duodenal) disease
- Erosive gastritis (e.g., after ingestion of NSAIDs, antiplatelets, and alcohol) or duodenitis
- Anticoagulants, SSRI, and bisphosphonates
- Stress ulcers occurring with **shock, sepsis, or severe trauma**
- **Curling ulcers** in the proximal duodenum with **severe burns or trauma**
- Carcinoma stomach
- Dieulafoy lesions
- Angiodysplasia or gastric antral vascular ectasia (GAVE) or vascular malformations
- Rupture of aortic aneurysm or aortic duodenal fistula following aortic graft
- Hematobilia
- Hemosuccus pancreaticus

Other cause
- Coagulation defects
  - Heyde syndrome (aortic stenosis, angiodysplasia, and acquired von Willebrand disease)

- **NSAIDs and aspirin** can result in mucosal damage anywhere in the GI tract. Therefore, dual antiplatelet therapy (e.g., clopidogrel plus aspirin) or concomitant aspirin and anticoagulation with warfarin can escalate the risk for GI bleeding by both initiating and propagating bleeding.
- Causes of UGI bleed are listed in Table 18-1.
- Causes of lower GI bleed are listed in Table 18-2.

Physical Examination

- **Color of stool:** Direct examination of spontaneously passed stool or on **digital rectal examination** (DRE) can help localize the level of bleeding. DRE may also identify anorectal abnormalities, including anal fissures, which induce extreme discomfort during the DRE.

TABLE 18-2 Causes of Lower GI Bleeding

- Diverticulosis
- Hemorrhoids
- Ischemic colitis
- IBD
- Postpolypectomy
- Colon cancer/polyps
- Rectal ulcer
- Vascular ectasia
- Radiation colitis/proctitis
- Others—infections, fistula, and stercoral ulcer

- Fresh blood on an **NG aspirate** may indicate ongoing upper GI bleeding requiring urgent endoscopic attention.[3] The aspirate should be considered positive only if blood or dark particulate matter ("coffee grounds") is seen; **hemoccult testing of NG aspirate has no clinical utility.** A bleeding source in the duodenum can result in a negative NG aspirate. Gastric lavage with water or saline may be useful in assessing the activity and severity of upper GI bleeding and in clearing the stomach of blood and clots before endoscopy. After a diagnosis of upper GI bleeding is made, the NG tube can be removed in a stable patient.
- Constant monitoring or frequent assessment of vital signs is necessary early in the evaluation, as a sudden increase in pulse rate or decrease in blood pressure (BP) may suggest recurrent or ongoing blood loss.
- If the baseline BP and pulse are within normal limits, sitting the patient up and/or having the patient stand may result in **orthostatic hemodynamic changes** (drop in systolic BP of >20 mm Hg, rise in pulse rate of >10 bpm). Orthostatic changes are seen with loss of 10%–20% of the circulatory volume; supine hypotension suggests a >20% loss. Hypotension with a systolic BP of <100 mm Hg or baseline tachycardia >100 bpm suggests significant hemodynamic compromise that requires urgent volume resuscitation.[4]

Diagnostic Testing

Laboratories

- Complete blood cell (CBC) count
- Coagulation parameters (international normalized ratio [INR], partial thromboplastin time)
- Blood group, cross-matching of two to four units of blood
- Comprehensive metabolic profile (creatinine, blood urea nitrogen, liver function tests)

Diagnostic Procedures

- **Endoscopy**
    - **Esophagogastroduodenoscopy (EGD)**, with high diagnostic accuracy and therapeutic capability, is the preferred investigative test in upper GI bleeding. Volume resuscitation or blood transfusion should precede endoscopy in hemodynamically unstable patients. Patients with ongoing bleeding or at risk for an adverse outcome (Table 18-3) benefit most from urgent EGD, whereas stable patients can be endoscoped electively during hospitalization. The Rockall score (RS) and the Glasgow-Blatchford risk score (GBS) stand as the foremost scoring systems utilized in clinical practice. The AIMS65 score is based on albumin levels, prothrombin time (PT), international normalized ratio (INR), altered mental status, systolic blood pressure, and age 65 years or older. One point is assigned to each variable that increases the risk of clinical outcomes. IV erythromycin (infusion of 125–250 mg completed 30 minutes before EGD) empties the stomach of blood and clots and improves visibility for EGD.[5] Second-look EGD after hemostasis has no proven benefit in reducing surgical intervention or overall mortality.[6]
    - **Colonoscopy** can be performed after a rapid bowel purge in clinically stable patients; the purge solution can be infused through an NG tube when not tolerated orally. While diagnostic yield is highest with colonoscopy performed within 24 hours of presentation, patient outcome does not necessarily improve. Therapeutic colonoscopy, however, may reduce transfusion requirements, need for surgery, and length of hospital stay.[7] All patients with acute lower GI bleeding from an unknown source should eventually undergo colonoscopy during the initial hospitalization, regardless of the initial mode of investigation.
    - **Anoscopy** may be useful in the detection of internal hemorrhoids and anal fissures but does not replace the need for colonoscopy.
    - **Push enteroscopy** allows evaluation of the proximal small bowel beyond reach of a standard EGD, especially if no source is found on careful colonoscopy.[8]

TABLE 18-3 Rockall Score for Risk Stratification of Acute Upper Gastrointestinal (GI) Bleeding

		Variable	Points
Complete Rockall Score	Clinical Rockall Score	Age	
		<60 yr	0
		60–79 yr	1
		≥80 yr	2
		Shock	
		Heart rate >100 bpm	1
		Systolic blood pressure <100 mm Hg	2
		Coexisting illness	
		Coronary artery disease, congestive heart failure, other major illness	2
		Renal failure, hepatic failure, metastatic cancer	3
		Endoscopic diagnosis	
		No finding, Mallory–Weiss tear	0
		Peptic ulcer, erosive disease, esophagitis	1
		Cancer of the upper GI tract	2
		Endoscopic stigmata of recent bleeding	
		Clean based ulcer, flat pigmented spot	0
		Blood in upper GI tract, active bleeding, visible vessel, clot	2

From Gralnek et al. Management of acute bleeding from a peptic ulcer. *N Engl J Med.* 2008;359:928 with permission. Copyright © 2008 Massachusetts Medical Society. Reprinted with permission from Massachusetts Medical Society.

A clinical score of 0 or a complete score of 2 or less indicates low risk for rebleeding or death.

- **Capsule endoscopy** is most useful after the upper gut, and the colon has been thoroughly examined and the bleeding source is suspected in the small bowel.[8] In overt obscure GI bleeding, capsule endoscopy has higher diagnostic yield with similar long-term outcomes when compared with angiography.[9]
- **Single- and double-balloon enteroscopy** allows visualization of most of the small bowel through either an oral or anal approach, typically performed when capsule endoscopy localizes bleeding to the small bowel.[8] Balloons at the endoscope tip and overtube can be consecutively inflated and deflated to facilitate deep insertion into the small bowel.
- **Intraoperative enteroscopy** may assist endoscopic therapy or surgical resection of an actively bleeding source in the small bowel.

- **Tagged red blood cell (RBC) scanning** involves labeling RBCs with technetium-99m that may extravasate into the bowel lumen with active bleeding, detected as pooling of the radioactive tracer on gamma camera scanning, to identify the potential bleeding site. **CT angiography** may have similar benefit in localizing bleeding before catheter angiography and has an advantage over CT enterography.[8,1] These tests are particularly useful in unstable active bleeding precluding urgent colonoscopy.

- **Arteriography** demonstrates extravasation of the dye into the intestine when bleeding rates exceed 0.5 mL/min, thereby localizing bleeding. Arteriography is often performed after bleeding is initially localized by other means. Selective cannulation and infusion of vasopressin vasoconstrict the bleeding vessel; alternatively, the bleeding vessel can be embolized.[10]

TREATMENT

- **Restoration of intravascular volume:** Two large-bore (16- to 18-gauge) IV lines or a central venous line should be urgently placed to provide IV fluid resuscitation. Circulatory shock may require volume administration using pressure infusion devices, guided by the patient's condition and degree of volume loss.[4] **Packed RBC transfusion** should be used for volume replacement whenever possible; O-negative blood or simultaneous multiple-unit transfusions may be indicated if bleeding is massive. Transfusion should be continued until hemodynamic stability is achieved and the hematocrit reaches ≥25%–30%. Overcorrection of volume and blood counts does not necessarily improve the outcome and may even be detrimental in variceal bleeding.[11]
- **Oxygen administration:** Supplemental oxygen enhances the oxygen-carrying capacity of blood and should be universally administered in acute GI bleeding.
- **Correction of coagulopathy:** Coagulopathy (INR ≥1.5) increases morbidity and mortality in acute GI bleeding and should be corrected if possible. Platelet infusion may be indicated when the platelet count is <50,000/μL.[12]
- **Endotracheal intubation** protects the airway and prevents aspiration in obtunded patients with massive hematemesis and in active variceal bleeding.
- **Risk stratification:** Validated risk stratification tools, such as the Rockall and Glasgow-Blatchford scores, are available to identify patients at highest risk for an adverse outcome.[13] The Rockall score (see Table 18-3) has a *clinical* component that is rapidly calculated at presentation and a *complete* final score that takes endoscopic findings into account.[14]

Medications

- **Nonvariceal upper GI bleeding:** Pre-endoscopic IV **proton pump inhibitors** (PPIs) (40 mg IV bolus bid or 80 mg IV bolus followed by 8 mg/h continuous infusion) improve outcome in the proportion of patients who have high-risk stigmata of hemorrhage and reduce need for endoscopic therapy in bleeding peptic ulcer disease (PUD).[15] However, meta-analysis does not show benefits in rebleeding, surgical intervention, or mortality between IV PPI infusions and IV bolus therapy in unselected cases.[16] PPI therapy, IV or oral (e.g., omeprazole 40 mg PO bid or equivalent), is more effective than IV histamine-2 receptor antagonist (H_2RA) therapy.[17]
- **Variceal bleeding: Octreotide** (an octapeptide that mimics endogenous somatostatin) infusion acutely reduces portal pressures and controls variceal bleeding, improving the diagnostic yield and therapeutic success of subsequent endoscopy. Octreotide should be initiated immediately (50–100 μg bolus, followed by infusion at 25–50 μg/h) and continued for 3–5 days if variceal hemorrhage is confirmed on EGD.[18] Both **terlipressin** and **octreotide** achieve similar hemostatic effects with comparable safety to octreotide as adjuvants to endoscopic therapy in variceal bleeding.[19,20] A 7-day course of antibiotic prophylaxis with an IV third-generation cephalosporin (ceftriaxone) is recommended (see Chapter 19, Liver Diseases) in any patient with cirrhosis and variceal bleeding; a fluoroquinolone is an alternative.[21]
- **Thalidomide** may be an effective approach for refractory chronic bleeding from GI vascular malformations.[22]

Other Nonpharmacologic Therapies

- **Endoscopic therapy**
  - **Therapeutic endoscopy** offers the advantage of endoscopic hemostasis and should be performed early in acute upper GI bleeding (within 12–24 hours).
  - **Variceal ligation** or **banding** is the endoscopic therapy of choice for esophageal varices, with endotracheal intubation for airway protection if bleeding is massive or the patient is obtunded.[18] Variceal banding can provide both primary and secondary prophylaxis of variceal bleeding, with benefits similar to that from β-blocker therapy alone.[23] Complications include superficial ulceration, dysphagia, and transient chest discomfort.
  - **Sclerotherapy** is also effective but is used mostly when variceal banding is not technically feasible.
  - Endoscopic injection of **cyanoacrylate (glue)** is more effective than β-blocker therapy in primary and secondary prophylaxis of gastric variceal bleeding, but not esophageal variceal bleeding.[24]
- **Transjugular intrahepatic portosystemic shunt** (**TIPS**): An expandable metal stent is deployed between the hepatic veins and the portal vein to reduce portal venous pressure in refractory esophageal and/or gastric variceal bleeding from portal hypertension.[25] Early TIPS reduces treatment failure and mortality in acute variceal bleeding.[26] Encephalopathy may occur in up to 25% of patients and is treated medically (see Chapter 19, Liver Diseases). Duplex Doppler ultrasound assesses for TIPS stenosis if variceal bleeding recurs or if esophageal or gastric varices redevelop.
- **Balloon-occluded retrograde transvenous obliteration** (**BRTO**): Gastric varices are obliterated by interventional radiographic access through a patent gastrorenal shunt.[27] When possible, BRTO is equivalent to TIPS for short-term management of bleeding gastric varices.[28]
- Balloon tamponade may be performed as a temporizing measure for patients with uncontrollable hemorrhage likely due to varices using any of several devices (e.g., Sengstaken-Blakemore tube, Minnesota tube).

Surgical Management

- **Emergent total colectomy** may rarely be required for massive, unlocalized, colonic bleeding; this should be preceded by EGD to rule out a rapidly bleeding upper source whenever possible. Certain lesions (e.g., neoplasia, Meckel diverticulum) require surgical resection for a cure.
- **Total or partial colectomy** may be required for ongoing or recurrent diverticular bleeding.
- **Splenectomy** is curative in bleeding gastric varices from splenic vein thrombosis.
- **Shunt surgery** (portacaval or distal splenorenal shunt) is now rarely performed, but it remains a consideration in patients with good hepatic reserve.

SPECIAL CONSIDERATIONS

Cardiac Patients and Gastrointestinal Bleeding

- In acute coronary syndromes, GI bleeding increases 30-day all-cause mortality rates by a factor of almost 5.[29] Antiplatelet and anticoagulant therapies, especially dual antiplatelet therapy (e.g., aspirin plus clopidogrel), are significant risk factors. Among patients on low-dose aspirin with history of PUD bleeding, continuous aspirin therapy increases the risk for recurrent PUD bleeding.[30]
- **PPI prophylaxis** decreases the risk of GI bleeding, without significant increase in major cardiovascular events in patients on dual antiplatelet therapy.[31]

- Despite concerns that PPIs competitively inhibit the cytochrome P450 enzyme that activates clopidogrel, randomized controlled trials have not substantiated higher vascular events with concurrent use of clopidogrel and PPI.[32,33] Among PPIs, pantoprazole may have the least pharmacodynamic interaction with clopidogrel.[34]
- **Left ventricular assist devices (LVADs)**, used in end-stage heart failure, are associated with GI bleeding rates significantly higher than those seen with dual antiplatelet therapy or anticoagulation.[35] Bleeding is predominantly overt and from upper GI sources, especially angiodysplastic lesions, making EGD or push enteroscopy the initial investigation of choice.[36]

Dysphagia and Odynophagia

GENERAL PRINCIPLES

- **Oropharyngeal dysphagia** (Table 18-4) consists of difficulty in transferring food from the mouth to the esophagus, often associated with nasopharyngeal regurgitation and aspiration. Neuromuscular and less commonly, structural disorders involving the pharynx and proximal esophagus are typical causes.[37]
- **Esophageal dysphagia** (Table 18-5) is the sensation of impairment in passage of food down the tubular esophagus. Etiologies include obstructive processes (such as webs, rings, esophagitis, neoplasia) or esophageal motor disorders.[38]
- **Odynophagia** is pain on swallowing food and fluids and may indicate the presence of esophagitis, particularly infectious esophagitis or pill esophagitis.
- Medications known to cause dysphagia include antibiotics (doxycycline, tetracycline, clindamycin, trimethoprim-sulfamethoxazole) and nonsteroidal anti-inflammatory drugs, such as alendronate, zidovudine, ascorbic acid potassium chloride tablets, theophylline quinidine gluconate, ferrous sulfate, and others.

TABLE 18-4 Causes of Oropharyngeal Dysphagia

Structural	Propulsive	
	Neurogenic	Myogenic
• Zenker diverticulum • Neoplasm	• Cerebrovascular accident • Amyotrophic lateral sclerosis • Guillain-Barré syndrome • Parkinson disease	• Myasthenia gravis • Myotonic dystrophy • Poliomyelitis

TABLE 18-5 Causes of Esophageal Dysphagia

Extraluminal	In the Wall	In the Lumen
• Aortic aneurysm • Thyroid enlargement • Dysphagia lusoria • Rolling hiatus hernia • Mediastinal swelling	• Carcinoma esophagus • Strictures • GERD • Achalasia cardia • Plummer–Vinson syndrome • Schatzki rings	• Atresia • Foreign bodies

DIAGNOSIS

Oropharyngeal Dysphagia

- A detailed neurologic examination is the first diagnostic step. **Barium videofluoroscopy (modified barium swallow)** evaluates the oropharyngeal swallow mechanism and may identify laryngeal penetration.
- Ear, nose, and throat examination; flexible nasal endoscopy; and imaging studies may identify structural etiologies.
- Laboratory tests for polymyositis, myasthenia gravis, and other neuromuscular disorders are performed when neurologic or structural etiologies are not evident.

Esophageal Dysphagia

- **EGD** is the initial test of choice, as it identifies mucosal and structural abnormalities, allows tissue sampling (to evaluate for esophageal eosinophilia, for instance), and offers the option of dilation, which should be performed for most esophageal strictures.[39]
- **Esophageal manometry,** preferably **high-resolution manometry (HRM)**, should be performed when other studies are normal or suggest an esophageal motility disorder. The image-based paradigm of Clouse plots on HRM has simplified testing procedures, allowing for easier analysis, and improved diagnostic utility over conventional manometry.[40]
- **Endoluminal functional lumen imaging probe (EndoFLIP)** evaluates compliance and distensibility of the esophagus and esophagogastric junction, with the potential for higher sensitivity in the detection of esophageal outflow obstruction compared with manometry. EndoFLIP utilizes impedance planimetry during volume-controlled distention of a compliant balloon to measure cross-sectional area, from which a distensibility index is calculated.[41]
- **Barium swallow** defines anatomy and identifies subtle rings and strictures, which may only be seen with a barium pill or a solid barium bolus.
- Acute esophageal obstruction is best investigated with endoscopy. Barium studies should not be performed when esophageal obstruction is expected, as it may take several days for barium to clear, thereby delaying endoscopy. If a contrast study is needed, water-soluble contrast should be used.
- Approach to dysphagia is shown in Figure 18-1.

TREATMENT

- Modification of diet and swallowing maneuvers improves, especially oropharyngeal dysphagia. Patients with dysphagia are advised to chew their food well and eat foods of soft consistencies.
- Enteral feeding through a gastrostomy tube is indicated when frank tracheal aspiration is identified on attempted swallowing.
- Endoscopic retrieval of an obstructing food bolus relieves acute dysphagia.
- Nutrition needs to be addressed in patients with prolonged dysphagia causing weight loss.

Medications

- Mucosal inflammation from reflux disease can be treated with acid suppression.
- Odynophagia generally responds to specific therapy when the cause is identified (e.g., PPIs for reflux disease, antimicrobial agents for infectious esophagitis). Viscous lidocaine swish-and-swallow solutions may afford symptomatic relief.
- Anticholinergic medication (e.g., transdermal scopolamine) helps drooling of saliva.
- **Glucagon** (2–4 mg IV bolus) or sublingual **nitroglycerin** can be attempted in acute food impaction, but meat tenderizer should not be administered.

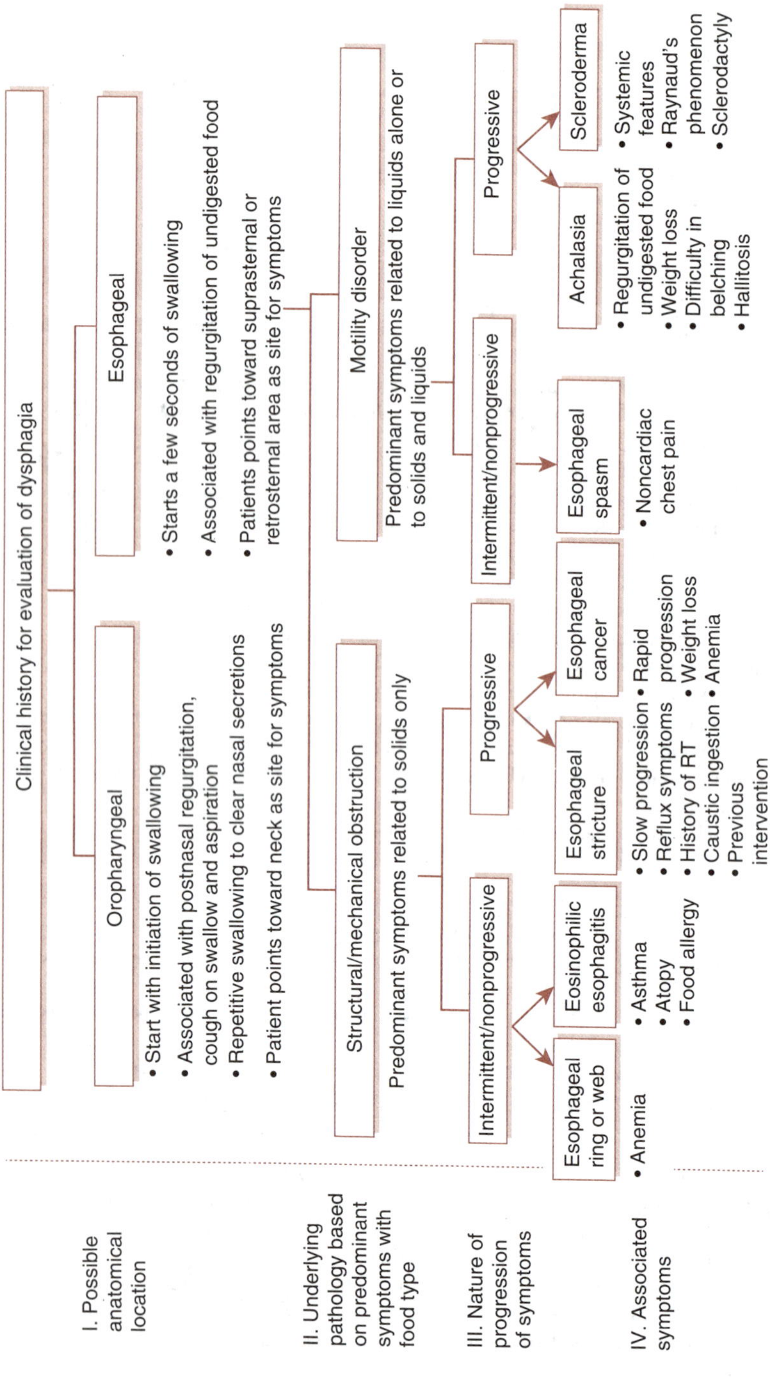

Figure 18-1 Clinical approach to dysphagia.

Other Nonpharmacologic Therapies

- Esophageal dilation is performed for strictures, rings, and webs. Empiric bougie dilation may provide symptomatic benefit even when a defined narrowing is not identified in some settings.
- Pneumatic dilation of the lower esophageal sphincter (LES) and peroral endoscopic myotomy (POEM) are options for achalasia management (see Esophageal Motor Disorders section). Botulinum toxin injection into the LES provides temporary symptom relief in achalasia and esophageal outflow obstruction from motor etiologies.[39]
- Esophageal stent placement can alleviate dysphagia in inoperable neoplasia.

Nausea and Vomiting

GENERAL PRINCIPLES

- Nausea and vomiting may result from side effects of medications, systemic illnesses, central nervous system (CNS) disorders, and primary GI disorders.
- Vomiting that occurs during or immediately after a meal can result from acute pyloric stenosis (e.g., pyloric channel ulcer) or from functional disorders, while vomiting within 30–60 minutes after a meal may suggest gastric or duodenal pathology. Delayed vomiting of undigested food from a previous meal can suggest gastric outlet obstruction or gastroparesis.
- Symptoms of gastroparesis may be indistinguishable from chronic functional nausea and vomiting with normal gastric emptying.[42]

DIAGNOSIS

- **Bowel obstruction and pregnancy should be ruled out.**
- **Medication lists** should be carefully scrutinized for potential offenders, and systemic illnesses (acute and chronic) should be evaluated as etiologies or contributing factors.
- Endoscopy and/or imaging should be considered in the setting of nonresolving or "red flag" symptoms, such as hematemesis or weight loss.

TREATMENT

- Correction of fluid and electrolyte imbalances is an important supportive measure.
- Oral intake should be limited to clear liquids, if tolerated. Many patients with self-limited illnesses require no further therapy.
- NG decompression may be required for patients with bowel obstruction or protracted nausea and vomiting of any etiology.
- Enteral feeding through jejunal tubes or, rarely, total parenteral nutrition (TPN) may be necessary to supplement nutrient intake.

Medications

Empiric pharmacotherapy is often initiated while investigation is in progress or when the etiology is thought to be self-limited.

- **Phenothiazines and related agents.** Prochlorperazine (Compazine), 5–10 mg PO tid–qid, 10 mg IM or IV q6h, or 25 mg PR bid, and promethazine (Phenergan), 12.5–25.0 mg PO, IM, or PR q4–6h may be effective. Drowsiness is a common side effect, and acute dystonic reactions or other extrapyramidal effects may occur.
- **Dopamine antagonists** include metoclopramide (10 mg PO 30 minutes before meals and at bedtime, or 10 mg IV PRN), a prokinetic agent that also has central

antiemetic effects. Drowsiness and extrapyramidal reactions may occur, and a warning has been issued by the US Food and Drug Administration (FDA) regarding the risk of permanent **tardive dyskinesia** with high-dose and/or long-term use.[43] Tachyphylaxis may limit long-term efficacy. Domperidone is an alternate agent that does not cross the blood–brain barrier and therefore has no CNS side effects; however, it is not uniformly available.

- **Antihistaminic agents** are most useful for nausea and vomiting related to motion sickness but may also be useful for other causes. Agents include diphenhydramine (Benadryl, 25–50 mg PO q6–8h or 10–50 mg IV q2–4h), dimenhydrinate (Dramamine, 50–100 mg PO or IV q4–6h), and meclizine (Antivert, 12.5–25.0 mg 1 hour before travel).
- **Serotonin 5-hydroxytryptamine-3 (5-HT$_3$) receptor antagonists. Ondansetron** (Zofran, 0.15 mg/kg IV q4h for three doses or 32 mg IV infused over 15 minutes beginning 30 minutes before chemotherapy) is effective in chemotherapy-associated emesis. It can also be used in emesis that is refractory to other medications (4–8 mg PO or IV up to q8h), especially the sublingual formulation.
- **Neurokinin-1 (NK-1) receptor antagonist. Aprepitant** (Emend, 125 mg PO day 1, 80 mg PO days 2 and 3) is an alternative agent intended for chemotherapy-induced nausea and vomiting.

Diarrhea

GENERAL PRINCIPLES

- **Acute diarrhea** consists of abrupt onset of ≥3 unformed bowel movements in conjunction with associated symptoms such as tenesmus, fecal urgency, increased flatulence, nausea, or vomiting.[44] Infectious agents, toxins, and drugs are the major causes of acute diarrhea. The major causes of acute infectious diarrhea include viruses (norovirus, rotavirus, adenoviruses, astrovirus, etc.), bacteria (*Salmonella, Campylobacter, Shigella,* enterotoxigenic *Escherichia coli, Clostridioides difficile,* etc.), and protozoa (*Cryptosporidium, Giardia, Cyclospora, Entamoeba,* etc.). In hospitalized patients, pseudomembranous colitis, antibiotic- or drug-associated diarrhea, and fecal impaction should be considered.[45]
- Persistent diarrhea: Diarrhea persisting for more than 14 days but fewer than 30 days in duration.
- Chronic diarrhea consists of passage of loose stools with or without increased stool frequency and urgency for more than 4 weeks.[46]
- Etiology and types of diarrhea are listed in Table 18-6.

DIAGNOSIS

- Most acute infectious diarrheal illnesses last less than 24 hours and could be viral in etiology; therefore, stool studies are unnecessary in short-lived episodes without fever, dehydration, or presence of blood or pus in the stool.[47]
- Stool examination is recommended if there is a passage of >6 unformed stools within 24 hours, presence of bloody diarrhea, an immunocompromising condition, or a temperature ≥38.5°C.
- Stool cultures, *Clostridium difficile* toxin assay, ova and parasite examinations, and sigmoidoscopy may be warranted in patients with severe, prolonged, atypical symptoms, or in immunocompromised patients.
- The **fecal osmolar gap** [290 – 2(stool Na$^+$ + stool K$^+$)] can be calculated in patients with chronic diarrhea and voluminous watery stools. The osmotic gap is **<50 mOsm/kg in secretory diarrhea** but **>125 mOsm/kg in osmotic diarrhea.**

TABLE 18-6 Causes of Diarrhea

Watery diarrhea
- **Osmotic diarrhea**
  - Osmotic laxative use (magnesium, phosphate, or sulfate ingestion)
  - Carbohydrate malabsorption (lactose, fructose)
  - Celiac disease
  - Sugar alcohols (mannitol, sorbitol, xylitol)
- **Secretory**
  - Alcoholism
  - Bacterial enterotoxins such as cholera
  - Bile acid malabsorption
  - Hyperthyroidism
  - Medications (quinine, antibiotics, antineoplastics, biguanides, calcitonin, digitalis, colchicine, prostaglandins, ticlopidine)
  - Neuroendocrine tumors (gastrinoma, vipoma, carcinoid tumors, mastocytosis)
  - Nonosmotic laxatives (senna, docusate sodium)
- **Functional**
  - Irritable bowel syndrome

Fatty diarrhea
- *Malabsorption syndromes*
  - Medications (orlistat, acarbose)
  - Celiac sprue
  - Mesenteric ischemia
  - Parasites (*Giardia*)
  - Tropical sprue
  - Whipple disease
- *Maldigestion*
  - Hepatobiliary disorders
  - Pancreatic insufficiency

- **Inflammatory diarrhea**
  - Inflammatory bowel disease
  - Invasive infections (*Clostridium difficile* colitis, tuberculosis, *Entamoeba*, cytomegalovirus, herpes simplex virus)
  - Neoplasms
  - Radiation colitis

- A positive fecal occult blood test or fecal leukocyte test suggests inflammatory diarrhea.
- **Steatorrhea** is traditionally diagnosed by demonstration of fat excretion in stool of >7 g/d in a 72-hour stool collection while the patient is on a 100-g/d fat diet. Sudan staining of a stool specimen is an alternate test; >100 fat globules per high-power field (HPF) is abnormal.
- Laxative screening should be considered when chronic diarrhea remains undiagnosed.

Clinical Presentation

- **Acute diarrhea**
  - **Viral enteritis** and **bacterial infections** with *Escherichia coli* and *Shigella*, *Salmonella*, *Campylobacter*, and *Yersinia* spp. constitute the most common causes.
  - **Pseudomembranous colitis** is usually seen in the setting of antimicrobial therapy and is caused by toxins produced by *C. difficile*.[48]

- **Giardiasis** is confirmed by identification of *Giardia lamblia* trophozoites in the stool, in duodenal aspirate, or in small bowel biopsy specimens. A stool immunofluorescence assay is also available for rapid diagnosis.
- **Amebiasis** may cause acute diarrhea, especially in travelers to areas with poor sanitation and in homosexual men. Stool examination for trophozoites or cysts of *Entamoeba histolytica* or a serum antibody test confirms the diagnosis.
- **Medications** that can cause acute diarrhea include laxatives, antacids, cardiac medications (e.g., digitalis, quinidine), colchicine, and antimicrobial agents; symptoms typically respond to discontinuation.
- **Graft-versus-host disease** should be considered when diarrhea develops after organ transplantation, especially bone marrow transplantation; **sigmoidoscopy with biopsies** should be pursued to confirm this diagnosis.[49]

- **Chronic diarrhea:** After a careful history, a thorough physical examination, and routine laboratory tests, chronic diarrhea can typically be classified into one of the following categories: watery diarrhea (secretory or osmotic), inflammatory diarrhea, or fatty diarrhea (steatorrhea).[50]

TREATMENT

- Adequate hydration, including IV hydration in severe cases, is an essential initial step in managing diarrheal diseases.
- Antibiotic-associated diarrhea and *C. difficile* infections can be prevented by restricting high-risk antibiotic use and prescribing antibiotics based on sensitivity analysis.
- Symptomatic therapy is offered in simple, self-limiting GI infections where diarrhea is frequent or troublesome while diagnostic workup is in progress when specific management fails to improve symptoms and/or when a specific etiology is not identified.
  - **Loperamide, opiates** (tincture of opium, belladonna, and opium capsules), and **anticholinergic agents** (diphenoxylate and atropine [Lomotil]) are the most effective nonspecific antidiarrheal agents.
  - **Pectin** and **kaolin** preparations (bind toxins) and **bismuth subsalicylate** (antibacterial properties) are also useful in symptomatic therapy of acute diarrhea.
  - **Bile acid-binding resins** (e.g., cholestyramine) are beneficial in bile acid-induced diarrhea.
  - **Octreotide** is useful in hormone-mediated secretory diarrhea but can also be of benefit in refractory diarrhea.

Medications

- **Empiric antibiotic therapy** is only recommended in patients with moderate to severe disease and associated systemic symptoms while awaiting stool cultures. Antibiotics can increase the possibility of hemolytic-uremic syndrome associated with Shiga toxin-producing *E. coli* infections (*E. coli* O157:H7), especially in children and the elderly.[51]
- Oral **vancomycin**, **rifaximin**, or **fidaxomicin** are the antibiotics of choice for pseudomembranous colitis. **Metronidazole** can be used intravenously together with **vancomycin** in fulminant disease with hypotension, shock, or ileus. **Fecal microbiota transplant** is a novel treatment option.[52]
- Symptomatic amebiasis is treated with **metronidazole**, followed by **paromomycin** or **iodoquinol** to eliminate cysts.
- Therapy for giardiasis consists of metronidazole or tinidazole, with quinacrine representing an alternative agent.
- Nitazoxanide is the effective first-line treatment for infection by *Blastocystis* species, *Cryptosporidium parvum*, or *Giardia lamblia* in immunocompetent adults and children.

It is also an effective treatment option for *Entamoeba histolytica, Hymenolepis nana, Ascaris lumbricoides*, and *Cyclospora cayetanensis*.

SPECIAL CONSIDERATIONS

- **Opportunistic agents**, including cryptosporidium, microsporidium, cytomegalovirus (CMV), *Mycobacterium avium* complex, and *Mycobacterium tuberculosis*, may cause **diarrhea in patients with advanced HIV** (CD4 counts <50 cells/μL). However, *C. difficile* may be the most commonly identified bacterial pathogen.[53]
- Other causes of diarrhea in this population include venereal infections (syphilis, gonorrhea, chlamydia, herpes simplex virus [HSV]) and nonvenereal infections (amebiasis, giardiasis, salmonellosis, shigellosis). Intestinal lymphoma and Kaposi sarcoma can also cause diarrhea.
- Stool studies (ova and parasites, culture), endoscopic biopsies, and serologic testing may assist in diagnosis. Management consists of specific therapy if pathogens are identified; symptomatic measures may be of benefit in idiopathic cases.[54]

Constipation

GENERAL PRINCIPLES

Definition

Constipation consists of infrequent and incomplete bowel movements, which can be associated with straining, passage of pellet-like stools, bowel movements (<3 per week), a sense of incomplete evacuation, or the use of manual maneuvers to facilitate defecation. Symptoms which last for more than 3 months are considered chronic.

Etiology

- Recent changes in bowel habits may suggest an organic cause, whereas long-standing constipation is more likely to be functional.
- **Medications** (e.g., calcium channel blockers, opiates, anticholinergics, iron supplements, barium sulfate) and systemic diseases (e.g., diabetes mellitus, hypothyroidism, systemic sclerosis, myotonic dystrophy) may contribute.
- Female gender, older age, lack of exercise, low caloric intake, low-fiber diet, and disorders that cause pain on defecation (e.g., anal fissures, thrombosed external hemorrhoids, pelvic floor dyssynergia) are other risk factors.[55]
    - Chronic idiopathic constipation is a normal transit constipation (also known as functional constipation) without identifiable structural or biochemical cause.

  Causes of constipation are listed in Table 18-7.

DIAGNOSIS

- Colonoscopy and barium studies help rule out structural disease and are particularly important in individuals >50 years without prior colorectal cancer screening or with alarm features such as anemia, weight loss, blood in the stool, obstructive symptoms, family history of cancer, or new-onset symptoms.[56]
- Colonic transit studies, radiopaque marker study, anorectal manometry, wireless motility capsule, and defecography are reserved for resistant cases without a structural explanation after initial workup.

TABLE 18-7 Causes of Constipation

Gastrointestinal disorders
1. Dietary: Lack of fiber and/or fluid intake
2. Motility: Irritable bowel syndrome, slow transit constipation
3. Structural: Carcinoma colon, diverticular disease, Hirschsprung disease
4. Defecation: Anorectal disease such as Crohn's, fissures, hemorrhoids
Non-gastrointestinal disorders
1. Drugs: Opiates, anticholinergics, calcium antagonists, iron supplements, aluminium-containing antacids
2. Neurologic: Cerebrovascular accidents, multiple sclerosis, spinal cord lesions, Parkinsonism
3. Psychological: Depression
4. Metabolic/endocrine: Diabetes mellitus, hypercalcemia, hypothyroidism

TREATMENT

- Regular exercise and adequate fluid intake are nonspecific measures.
- Increased **dietary fiber** intake (20–30 g/d) is useful. Fecal impaction should be resolved before fiber supplementation is initiated.
- **Laxatives**
  - **Emollient laxatives** such as docusate sodium, 50–200 mg PO daily, and docusate calcium, 240 mg PO daily, allow water and fat to penetrate the fecal mass. Mineral oil (15–45 mL PO q6–8h) can be given orally or by enema.
  - **Stimulant laxatives** such as castor oil, 15 mL PO, stimulate intestinal secretion and increase intestinal motility. Anthraquinones (cascara, 5 mL PO daily; senna, one tablet PO daily to qid) stimulate the colon by increasing fluid and water accumulation in the proximal colon. Bisacodyl (10–15 mg PO at bedtime, 10 mg rectal suppositories) stimulates colonic peristalsis and is an effective and well-tolerated option for chronic constipation.[57]
  - **Osmotic laxatives** include nonabsorbable salts or carbohydrates that cause water retention in the lumen of the colon. Magnesium salts include milk of magnesia (15–30 mL q8–12h) and magnesium citrate (200 mL PO) to be avoided in renal failure. Lactulose (15–30 mL PO bid–qid) can cause bloating as a side effect.
  - **Lubiprostone** (8–24 µg PO bid), a selective intestinal chloride channel activator, moves fluid into the bowel lumen and stimulates peristalsis.[58]
  - **Linaclotide** (145–290 µg PO qday) and **plecanatide** (3 mg PO qday) are guanylate cyclase C receptor agonists and also move fluid into the intestinal lumen as their mechanism of action.[59,60]
  - **Prucalopride**, a selective serotonin receptor agonist and a prokinetic agent, is approved in Europe and Canada for chronic constipation.[61]
- **Enemas:** Sodium biphosphate (Fleet) enemas can be used for mild to moderate constipation and for bowel cleansing before sigmoidoscopy; these should be avoided in renal failure. Tap water enemas (1 L) are also useful. Oil-based enemas (mineral oil, cottonseed colace, Hypaque) can be used in refractory constipation.
- **Polyethylene glycol** in powder form (MiraLax, 17 g PO daily to bid) can be used regularly or intermittently for the treatment of constipation.
- **Subcutaneous or oral methylnaltrexone, oral alvimopan, oral naloxegol, and oral naldemedine** are peripherally acting µ-opioid receptor antagonists (PAMORAs) that provide rapid relief of opioid-induced constipation.[62]

- **Bowel-cleansing agents:** Patients should be placed on a clear liquid diet the previous day and kept nothing by mouth (NPO) for 6 hours or overnight prior to colonoscopy. Patients may experience mild abdominal discomfort, nausea, and vomiting with the bowel preparation.
  - An iso-osmotic **polyethylene glycol solution** (PEG, GoLYTELY, or NuLYTELY, 1 gallon, administered at a rate of 8 oz every 10 minutes) is commonly used as a bowel-cleansing agent before colonoscopy. Lower volume preparations, such as PEG (2 L or 0.5 gallon) with ascorbic acid or other laxatives, are alternatives.[63]
  - **Nonabsorbable phosphate** (Fleet phosphosoda, 20–45 mL with 10–24 oz liquid, taken the day before and morning of the procedure), a hyperosmotic solution, draws fluid into the gut lumen and produces bowel movements in 0.5–6.0 hours. It is also available in pill form (Visicol or OsmoPrep, 32–40 tablets, taken at the rate of 3–4 tablets every 15 min with 8 oz fluid). Phosphosoda can result in severe dehydration, hyperphosphatemia, hypocalcemia, hypokalemia, hypernatremia, and acidosis. A dreaded rare complication is **acute phosphate nephropathy**, where calcium phosphate deposits cause irreversible dysfunction of renal tubules resulting in renal failure. Consequently, phosphosoda is only used in limited instances.
  - **Split preparations:** Proximity of bowel preparation to procedure time improves effectiveness of cleansing and visualization during the procedure. Splitting bowel preparation into two doses, with one dose administered the evening prior and the second dose administered the morning of the procedure, can improve bowel cleansing.[64]
  - **Two-day bowel preparation** is sometimes indicated in elderly or debilitated individuals when conventional bowel preparation is contraindicated, not tolerated, or ineffective. This consists of magnesium citrate (120–300 mL PO) administered on two consecutive days while the patient remains on a clear liquid diet; bisacodyl (30 mg PO or 10 mg suppository) is administered on both days.
  - **Tap water enemas** (1 L volume) can cleanse the distal colon when colonoscopy is indicated in patients with proximal bowel obstruction.
- Other options: **Biofeedback therapy** and **sacral nerve stimulation** can be effective for idiopathic constipation resistant to medical treatment.[65]

LUMINAL GASTROINTESTINAL DISORDERS

Gastroesophageal Reflux Disease

GENERAL PRINCIPLES

Gastroesophageal reflux disease (GERD) is defined as symptoms and/or complications resulting from reflux of gastric contents into the esophagus and more proximal structures.

DIAGNOSIS

Clinical Presentation

- Typical esophageal symptoms of GERD include **heartburn** and **regurgitation.** GERD can also present as **chest pain**, where an important priority is to exclude a cardiac source before initiating GI evaluation.[66]
- **Extraesophageal manifestations** of GERD can include cough, laryngitis, asthma, and dental erosions.
- Symptom response to a therapeutic trial of PPIs can be diagnostic, but a negative response does not exclude GERD.[67]

Differential Diagnosis

Other disorders that can result in esophagitis include the following:

- **Eosinophilic esophagitis (EoE)**, characterized by eosinophilic infiltration of esophageal mucosa, is increasingly recognized as an etiology for foregut symptoms.
  - Atopy (allergic rhinitis, eczema, asthma) is common, and food allergens may trigger the process.
  - **Dysphagia** is prominent, but symptoms can also mimic GERD.
  - Common EGD findings include corrugated mucosa, longitudinal mucosal furrows, fixed esophageal rings or trachealization, whitish mucosal plaque or exudate, stricture, superficial mucosa tear on passing endoscope, diffusely narrow lumen, and mucosal friability giving the appearance of crepe paper. The following establish a diagnosis of EoE: (1) symptoms related to esophageal dysfunction (such as dysphagia or food impaction), (2) ≥15 eosinophils per HPF on esophageal biopsies, and (3) exclusion of secondary causes of esophageal eosinophilia (such as GERD). Typically, a 2-month course of PPI bid should be given and followed by a repeat EGD with esophageal biopsies to rule out **PPI-responsive esophageal eosinophilia** and confirm the diagnosis of EoE.[68]
  - First-line therapy for EoE consists of PPIs, which also treats concomitant GERD. **Topical steroids** (swallowed fluticasone, 880–1760 μg/d in two to four divided doses, or swallowed budesonide, 1–2 mg/d in two to four divided doses) are options; prednisone is an alternate option if topical steroids are ineffective.[69] Yield of food allergen testing is typically low. Regardless, a six-food elimination diet (SFED) is appropriate when symptoms persist (eggs, milk, soy, gluten, tree nuts, seafood). Patients who do not respond to topical steroids may benefit from longer courses or higher doses of topical steroids, systemic steroids, elimination diet trials, or cautious esophageal dilation.[70]
- **Infectious esophagitis** typically presents with dysphagia or odynophagia and is seen most often in immunocompromised states (AIDS, organ transplant recipients), esophageal stasis (abnormal motility [e.g., achalasia, scleroderma], mechanical obstruction [e.g., strictures]), malignancy, diabetes mellitus, and antibiotic use; however, it can rarely occur in the normal healthy host. The presence of typical oral lesions (thrush, herpetic vesicles) may suggest an etiologic agent. The usual presenting symptoms are dysphagia and odynophagia.
  - ***Candida* esophagitis** is the most common esophageal infection, typically seen in esophageal stasis, impaired cell-mediated immunity from immunosuppressive therapy (e.g., with steroids or cytotoxic agents), malignancies, or AIDS. Endoscopic visualization of typical whitish plaques has near 100% sensitivity for diagnosis. Empiric antifungal agents are appropriate when concurrent oropharyngeal thrush is present, reserving endoscopy for nonresponse to therapy. **Fluconazole** 100–200 mg/d or **itraconazole** 200 mg/d for 14–21 days is recommended as initial therapy for *Candida* esophagitis; nystatin (100,000 units/mL, 5 mL tid for 3 weeks) and clotrimazole troches (10 mg four to five times a day for 2 weeks) are alternatives for oropharyngeal candidiasis. For infections refractory to azoles, a short course of parenteral **amphotericin B** (0.3–0.5 mg/kg/d) can be considered.[71]
  - **HSV esophagitis** is characterized by small vesicles and well-circumscribed ulcers on endoscopy and typical giant cells on histopathology. Viral antigen or DNA can be identified by immunofluorescent antibodies. Treatment consists of **acyclovir** 400–800 mg PO five times a day for 14–21 days or 5 mg/kg IV q8h for 7–14 days. **Famciclovir** and **valacyclovir** are alternate agents. The condition is usually self-limited in immunocompetent hosts.[72]
  - **CMV esophagitis**, which occurs almost exclusively in immunocompromised hosts, can cause erosions or frank ulcerations. **Ganciclovir** 5 mg/kg IV q12h or **foscarnet** 90 mg/kg IV q12h for 3–6 weeks can be used as initial therapy. Oral **valganciclovir** may also be effective.
  - Symptomatic relief can be achieved with 2% viscous **lidocaine** swish and swallow (15 mL PO q3–4h PRN) or **sucralfate** slurry (1 g PO qid).

- **Chemical esophagitis**
  - Ingestion of caustic agents (alkalis, acids) or medications such as oral potassium, doxycycline, quinidine, iron, NSAIDs, aspirin, and bisphosphonates can result in mucosal irritation and damage.
  - With caustic ingestions, cautious early EGD can evaluate the extent and degree of mucosal damage and CT can rule out transmural esophageal necrosis in the setting of mucosal necrosis.[73]
  - The offending medication should be discontinued if possible. Mucosal coating agents (sucralfate) and acid-suppressive agents may help. A second caustic agent to neutralize the first is contraindicated.

Diagnostic Testing

- **Endoscopy** with biopsies is primarily indicated for avoiding misdiagnosis of alternate causes of esophageal symptoms (e.g., EoE), identification of complications, and evaluation of treatment failures. **Alarm symptoms** of dysphagia, odynophagia, early satiety, weight loss, or bleeding should prompt endoscopy.[74]
- **Ambulatory pH or pH impedance monitoring** can be used to quantify esophageal acid exposure and reflux events and/or to assess symptom–reflux correlation in patients with ongoing symptoms despite acid suppression (especially if endoscopy is negative) or those with atypical symptoms. pH impedance testing detects all reflux events regardless of pH and is best performed off PPI therapy to increase yield; abnormal studies can predict symptomatic response to medical or surgical antireflux therapy.[75]
- **Esophageal manometry**, particularly HRM, may identify motor processes contributing to refractory symptoms.

TREATMENT

Medications

- Intermittent or prophylactic over-the-counter **antacids**, **H_2RAs**, and **PPIs** are effective with mild or intermittent symptoms.
- **PPIs** are more effective than standard-dose H_2RA and placebo in symptom relief and endoscopic healing of GERD. Modest gain is achieved by doubling the PPI dose in severe esophagitis or persistent symptoms. Continuous long-term PPI therapy is effective in maintaining remission of GERD symptoms, but the dose should be decreased after 8–12 weeks to the lowest dose that achieves symptom relief.[67] Abdominal pain, headache, and diarrhea are common side effects. Bone demineralization, enteric infections, community-acquired pneumonia, and reduced circulating levels of vitamin B_{12} are reported in observational studies, but conclusive cause-and-effect data are lacking and benefits of PPI therapy continue to outweigh risks.[76]
- Standard doses of **H_2RAs** (Table 18-8) can result in symptomatic benefit and endoscopic healing in up to half of patients. Dosage adjustments are required in renal insufficiency.
- Reflux inhibitors consist of γ-aminobutyric acid (GABA) type B receptor agonists that block transient LES relaxations. **Baclofen**, the prototype agent, reduces reflux events, but central side effects can be limiting.[77] For patients with PPI-refractory GERD, antireflux mucosectomy (ARMS) or antireflux mucosal ablation (ARMA) can be tried.

Surgical Management

- Indications for surgical **fundoplication** include the need for continuous PPIs, noncompliance, or intolerance to medical therapy in patients who are good surgical candidates, ongoing nonacid reflux despite adequate medical therapy, and patient preference for surgery.[67] When symptoms are controlled on PPI therapy, medical therapy and

TABLE 18-8 Dosage of Acid-Suppressive Agents

Medication Therapy	Peptic Ulcer Disease	GERD	Parenteral
Cimetidine[a]	300 mg qid 400 mg bid 800 mg at bedtime	400 mg qid 800 mg bid	300 mg q6h
Ranitidine[a]	150 mg bid 300 mg at bedtime	150–300 mg bid–qid	50 mg q8h
Famotidine[a]	20 mg bid 40 mg at bedtime	20–40 mg bid	20 mg q12h
Nizatidine[a]	150 mg bid 300 mg at bedtime	150 mg bid	
Omeprazole	20 mg daily	20–40 mg daily–bid	
Esomeprazole	40 mg daily	20–40 mg daily–bid	20–40 mg q24h
Lansoprazole	15–30 mg daily	15–30 mg daily–bid	30 mg q12–24h
Dexlansoprazole		30–60 mg daily	
Pantoprazole	20 mg daily	20–40 mg daily–bid	40 mg q12–24h or 80 mg IV, then 8 mg/h infusion

[a]Dosage adjustment required in renal insufficiency.
GERD, gastroesophageal reflux disease.

fundoplication are equally effective. Although fundoplication could provide better symptom control and quality of life in the short term, new postoperative symptoms and surgical failure can also occur.[78]

- Typical GERD symptoms, PPI response, elevated esophageal acid exposure, and correlation of symptoms to reflux events on ambulatory pH monitoring predict a higher likelihood of a successful surgical outcome.
- Patients with medical treatment failures need careful evaluation to determine whether symptoms are indeed related to acid reflux before surgical options are considered; these patients often have other diagnoses, including EoE, esophageal motor disorders, visceral hypersensitivity, and functional heartburn.[67]
- Potential complications of surgery include dysphagia, inability to belch, gas-bloat syndrome, and bowel symptoms, including flatulence, diarrhea, and abdominal pain.

Lifestyle/Risk Modification

- Patients with nocturnal GERD symptoms may benefit from elevating the head of the bed and avoiding meals within 2–3 hours before bedtime.
- Weight loss may benefit certain overweight patients with GERD.
- Lifestyle modifications alone are unlikely to resolve symptoms in the majority of GERD patients and should be recommended in conjunction with medications.

COMPLICATIONS

- **Esophageal erosion and ulceration** (esophagitis) can rarely lead to overt bleeding and iron deficiency anemia.
- **Strictures** can form when esophagitis heals, leading to dysphagia. Endoscopic dilation and maintenance PPI therapy typically resolve dysphagia from strictures.

- **Barrett esophagus (BE)** is a reflux-triggered change from normal squamous esophageal epithelium to specialized intestinal metaplasia and carries a 0.5% per year risk of progression to esophageal adenocarcinoma. Endoscopic screening for BE should be considered for patients with GERD who are at high risk (long duration of GERD symptoms, ≥50 years of age, male gender, Caucasian); patients with BE should undergo periodic surveillance every 3–5 years in the absence of dysplasia.[79] If dysplasia is found in the setting of BE, endoscopic therapy (usually radiofrequency ablation) is preferred to surveillance or surgery.[80]

Esophageal Motor Disorders

GENERAL PRINCIPLES

Definition

- **Achalasia** is the most significant motor disorder of the esophagus, characterized by failure of the LES to relax completely with swallowing and aperistalsis of the esophageal body.[81]
- **Esophagogastric junction outflow obstruction** is a loosely defined spectrum of motor disorder that can present with findings similar to incomplete achalasia.[40]
- **Esophageal hypermotility disorders** consist of **diffuse esophageal spasm**, characterized by premature, nonperistaltic contractions in the esophageal body, and **hypercontractile disorder (Jackhammer esophagus/nutcracker esophagus)** characterized by esophageal body contractions of exaggerated contraction vigor.[40,82]
- **Esophageal hypomotility disorders** are characterized by fragmented, ineffective, or absent esophageal peristalsis, sometimes with LES hypomotility, and are associated with reflux symptoms and increased reflux burden.
- Secondary motility disorders also affect the esophagus, including scleroderma and other connective tissue diseases, diabetes mellitus, Chagas disease, chronic idiopathic intestinal pseudo-obstruction, and neuromuscular disorders of striated muscle.

DIAGNOSIS

Clinical Presentation

- Presenting symptoms in achalasia can include dysphagia, regurgitation, chest pain, weight loss, and aspiration pneumonia.
- Diffuse esophageal spasm and other spastic disorders may have obstructive symptoms (dysphagia, regurgitation) but also perceptive symptoms (chest pain) from heightened esophageal sensitivity.
- LES hypomotility diminishes barrier function, and esophageal body hypomotility affects esophageal clearance of refluxed material, which can lead to prolonged reflux exposure and reflux complications.

Diagnostic Testing

- **Esophageal HRM** represents the gold standard for the diagnosis of esophageal motor disorders.[83] HRM features categorize achalasia into three subtypes that have symptomatic and therapeutic implications.[40]
- **Barium radiographs** may demonstrate a typical appearance of a dilated intrathoracic esophagus with impaired emptying, an air fluid level, absence of gastric air bubble, and tapering of the distal esophagus with a bird's beak appearance in achalasia. A beaded or corkscrew appearance may be seen with diffuse esophageal spasm. A dilated esophagus with an open LES and free gastroesophageal reflux may be seen with severe esophageal hypomotility.
- **Endoscopy** may help exclude a stricture or neoplasia of the distal esophagus in presumed achalasia and spastic disorders. Hypomotility disorders may also manifest a dilated esophagus but with a gaping gastroesophageal junction and evidence of reflux disease.

TREATMENT

Medications

- **Smooth muscle relaxants** such as nitrates or calcium channel blockers administered immediately before meals may provide short-lived symptom relief in spastic disorders and achalasia, but symptom response is suboptimal. Phosphodiesterase inhibitors may provide benefit in hypercontractile disorders but are contraindicated in coronary disease.
- **Botulinum toxin** injection at endoscopy can improve dysphagia for several weeks to months in achalasia and spastic disorders with incomplete LES relaxation.[84] This approach may be useful in elderly and frail patients who are poor surgical risks or as a bridge to more definitive therapy.
- **Neuromodulators** (e.g., low-dose tricyclic antidepressants [TCAs]) may improve perceptive symptoms (such as chest pain) associated with spastic motor disorders and achalasia.
- **Antisecretory therapy** with a PPI is recommended for reflux associated with esophageal hypomotility disorders. No specific promotility therapy exists. Antireflux surgery should be approached with caution in advanced hypomotility disorders.

Surgical Management

Disruption of the circular muscle of the LES using **pneumatic dilation** or surgical incision (**Heller myotomy**) can result in durable symptom relief in achalasia, with comparable symptom outcomes.[85] Gastroesophageal reflux can result when treated with lifelong acid suppression or concurrent partial fundoplication during myotomy. Esophageal perforation occurs in 3%–5% of patients with pneumatic dilation. **POEM** is minimally invasive with similar short-term symptom improvement, but incidence of reflux is higher compared with surgical myotomy.[86,87]

COMPLICATIONS

- Complications of achalasia include aspiration pneumonia and weight loss.
- Achalasia is associated with a 0.15% risk of squamous cell cancer of the distal esophagus, a 33-fold higher risk relative to the nonachalasia population.

Peptic Ulcer Disease

GENERAL PRINCIPLES

Definition

PUD consists of mucosal breaks in the stomach and duodenum when corrosive effects of acid and pepsin overwhelm mucosal defense mechanisms. Other locations include esophagus, small bowel adjacent to gastroenteric anastomoses, and within a Meckel diverticulum.

Etiology

- Risk factors for developing peptic ulcer are *H. pylori* infection, alcohol and tobacco consumption, NSAID use, and Zollinger–Ellison syndrome (ZES).
- ***Helicobacter pylori***, a spiral, Gram-negative, urease-producing bacillus, is responsible for at least half of all PUD and the majority of ulcers that are not due to NSAIDs.
- PUD can develop in 15%–25% of **chronic NSAID and aspirin** users. Past history of PUD, age >60 years, concomitant corticosteroid or anticoagulant therapy, high-dose or multiple NSAID therapy, and presence of serious comorbid medical illnesses increase risk for PUD.[88]
- A gastrin-secreting tumor or **gastrinoma** accounts for <1% of all peptic ulcers.
- Gastric cancer or lymphoma may manifest as a gastric ulcer.

- When none of these etiologies are evident, PUD is designated idiopathic. Most idiopathic PUD could be due to undiagnosed *H. pylori* or undetected NSAID use.
- Cigarette smoking doubles the risk for PUD; it delays healing and promotes recurrence.
- Other causes include stress (acute illness, burns, head injury), viral infection, vascular insufficiency, radiation therapy, Crohn's disease (CD), and chemotherapy.

DIAGNOSIS

Clinical Presentation

- Epigastric pain or dyspepsia may be presenting symptoms; however, symptoms are not always predictive of the presence of ulcers. Epigastric tenderness may be elicited on abdominal palpation. Ten percent may present with a complication (see Complications).
- In the presence of **alarm symptoms** (weight loss, early satiety, bleeding, anemia, persistent vomiting, epigastric mass, and lack of response to PPI), EGD should be performed to assess for complications or alternate diagnoses.

Diagnostic Testing

- **Endoscopy** is the gold standard for diagnosis of peptic ulcers; tissue sampling for *H. pylori* or cancer can also be performed. **Barium studies** also have good sensitivity for diagnosis of ulcers, but smaller ulcers and erosions may be missed.
- **Serum *H. pylori* antibody testing** is the cheapest noninvasive test but has suboptimal diagnostic accuracy.[89] The antibody remains detectable as long as 18 months after successful eradication and cannot be used to document successful eradication of the organism.
- **Stool *H. pylori* antigen testing** has 91% sensitivity and 93% specificity for the diagnosis of *H. pylori* infection and can confirm eradication of *H. pylori* after triple therapy.
- **Rapid urease assay** (e.g., *Campylobacter*-like organism [CLO] test) and histopathologic examination of endoscopic biopsy specimens are commonly used for diagnosis in patients undergoing endoscopy, but may be falsely negative in patients on PPI therapy.
- **Carbon-labeled urea breath testing** is the most accurate noninvasive test for diagnosis, with sensitivity and specificity of 95%; it is often used to document successful eradication after therapy of *H. pylori* infection.[89]
- Endoscopic biopsy and culture for *H. pylori* is not generally recommended as it is expensive, time-consuming, and invasive.
- The current guidelines to diagnose *H. pylori* infection is an upper gastrointestinal endoscopy with gastric biopsies (antrum and corpus) for histology, culture, and RUT. To determine *H. pylori* eradication, both UBT and stool *H. pylori* antigen detection by ELISA are reliable noninvasive tests.

TREATMENT

Medications

- Regardless of etiology, **acid suppression** forms the mainstay of therapy of PUD. Gastric ulcers are typically treated for 12 weeks and duodenal ulcers for 8 weeks.
- Oral PPI or H_2RA therapy will suffice in most instances (see Table 18-9). Dosage adjustment of H_2RAs is necessary in renal insufficiency. Cimetidine can impair metabolism of many drugs, including warfarin anticoagulants, theophylline, and phenytoin.
- Two antibiotics and a PPI-TT (triple therapy) was the mainstay of treatment for ***H. pylori* eradication** but strategy has shifted toward two antibiotics, PPI, and bismuth quadruple therapy because of the rising incidence of clarithromycin resistance. A 10-day course of quadruple therapy was shown to be more effective than a 14-day triple therapy.[90]

TABLE 18-9 Regimens Used for Eradication of *Helicobacter pylori*

Medications and Doses	Comments
Tetracycline (500 mg qid), metronidazole (250 mg qid), bismuth (525 mg qid), and PPI[a]	Bismuth-containing quadruple therapy; first-line therapy
Clarithromycin (500 mg bid), amoxicillin (1 g bid), and PPI[a]	Second-line therapy
Metronidazole (500 mg bid), amoxicillin (1 g bid), and PPI[a]	Second-line therapy in setting of prior macrolide exposure
Clarithromycin (500 mg bid), metronidazole (500 mg bid), and PPI[a]	Therapy for penicillin-allergic patients
Amoxicillin (1 g bid) and PPI[a] for 5 days, followed by clarithromycin (500 mg bid), metronidazole (500 mg bid), and PPI[a] for another 5 days	Sequential therapy
Levofloxacin (250 mg bid), amoxicillin (1 g bid), and PPI[a]	Levofloxacin-based triple therapy; salvage regimen
Two antibiotics selected by sensitivity testing on culture, bismuth (525 mg qid), and PPI[a]	Culture-guided therapy (if failed multiple regimens)

[a]Standard doses for PPI: omeprazole 20 mg, lansoprazole 30 mg, pantoprazole 40 mg, rabeprazole 20 mg, all twice a day. Esomeprazole is used as a single 40 mg dose once a day.
Duration of therapy: 10–14 days. When using salvage regimens after initial treatment failure, choose drugs that have not been used before.
PPI, proton pump inhibitor.

- Several antimicrobial and antisecretory agent regimens are available (Table 18-9). Levofloxacin-based sequential or triple therapy may be superior to standard triple therapy (clarithromycin, amoxicillin, PPI).[91] Other regimens may include LOAD (**l**evofloxacin, **o**meprazole, **n**itazoxanide, and **d**oxycycline) for 7–10 days; ofloxacin, azithromycin, omeprazole, and bismuth for 14 days; and PPI, bismuth, tetracycline, and levofloxacin for 10 days.[92,93] Patients previously exposed to a macrolide antibiotic should be treated with a regimen that does not include clarithromycin.
- Antibiotic resistance is the most important factor in PPI-TT failure. Strategies devised to combat clarithromycin resistance, such as sequential therapy (PPI-dual followed by PPI-TT) and hybrid therapy (PPI plus three antibiotics), have given way to concomitant therapy (simultaneous administration of PPI plus three antibiotics). Quninalones (ciprofloxacin, moxifloxacin, sitafloxacin) and rifabutin-based regimens can be used.
- NSAIDs and aspirin should be avoided when possible; if continued, maintenance PPI therapy or a mucosal protective agent (misoprostol, 400–800 μg/d) is recommended.[94]
- **Sucralfate** coats the eroded mucosal surface without blocking acid secretion and is often used in stress ulcer prophylaxis. Side effects include constipation and reduction of bioavailability of certain drugs (e.g., cimetidine, digoxin, fluoroquinolones, phenytoin, and tetracycline) when administered concomitantly.
- **Antacids** can be useful as supplemental therapy for pain relief in PUD.
- **Vonoprazan,** which is a potassium-competitive acid blocker that inhibits H^+,K^+-ATPase in gastric parietal cell, has been studied for the prevention of peptic ulcer recurrence in Japanese patients during NSAID therapy.
- **Nonpharmacologic measures:** Cessation of cigarette smoking should be encouraged. Alcohol in high concentrations can damage the gastric mucosal barrier, but no evidence exists to link alcohol with ulcer recurrence.

Surgical Management

Surgery is still occasionally required for intractable symptoms, GI bleeding, ZES, and complicated PUD. Surgical options vary depending on the location of the ulcer and the presence of complications.

SPECIAL CONSIDERATIONS

- **ZES** is a group of symptoms consisting of severe peptic ulcer disease, GERD, and chronic diarrhea caused by a gastrin-secreting tumor of the duodenum or pancreas (gastrinoma triangle) that results in increased stimulation of acid-secreting cells of the stomach. Multiple endocrine neoplasia type I can be associated with this syndrome in one-quarter to one-third of patients.[95] The resultant hypersecretion of gastric acid can cause multiple PUD in unusual locations, ulcers that fail to respond to standard medical therapy, or recurrent PUD after surgical therapy. Diarrhea and GERD symptoms are common.
- Gastric acid output is typically >15 mEq/L and gastric pH is <1.0. A fasting serum gastrin level while off acid suppression for at least 5 days serves as a screening test in patients who make gastric acid; a value >1000 pg/mL is seen in 90% of patients with ZES. When serum gastrin is elevated but <1000 pg/mL, a secretin stimulation test may demonstrate a paradoxical 200 pg increment in serum gastrin level after IV secretin in patients with gastrinomas.[96] High-dose PPIs are used for medical management. Specialized nuclear medicine scans (octreotide scans) can be useful in localizing the neoplastic lesion for curative resection. Long-term survival is principally related to underlying comorbidity rather than metastatic gastrinoma.[97]

COMPLICATIONS

- **GI bleeding** (see Gastrointestinal Bleeding section).
- **Gastric outlet obstruction** can occur with ulcers close to the pyloric channel and can manifest as nausea and vomiting, sometimes several hours after meals. Plain abdominal radiographs can show a dilated stomach with an air fluid level. NG suction can decompress the stomach while fluids and electrolytes are repleted intravenously. Recurrence is common, and endoscopic balloon dilation or surgery is often necessary for definitive correction.
- **Perforation** occurs infrequently and usually necessitates emergent surgery. Perforation may occur in the absence of previous symptoms of PUD and may be asymptomatic in patients who are receiving glucocorticoids. A plain upright radiograph of the abdomen may demonstrate free air under the diaphragm.
- **Pancreatitis** can result from penetration into the pancreas from ulcers in the posterior wall of the stomach or duodenal bulb. The pain becomes severe and continuous, radiates to the back, and is no longer relieved by antisecretory therapy. Serum amylase may be elevated. CT scanning may be diagnostic. Surgery is often required for therapy.

MONITORING/FOLLOW-UP

- Repeat EGD or upper GI series should be performed 8–12 weeks after initial diagnosis of all gastric ulcers to document healing; repeat endoscopic biopsy should be considered for nonhealing ulcers to exclude the possibility of a malignant ulcer.
- Duodenal ulcers are almost never malignant; therefore, documentation of healing is unnecessary in the absence of symptoms.

Inflammatory Bowel Disease

GENERAL PRINCIPLES

- Inflammatory bowel disease (IBD) encompasses two types of idiopathic intestinal disease that are differentiated by their location and depth of involvement in the bowel wall.
- The incidence of IBD in Asia is estimated to be less than 5 per 100,000 people.
- **Ulcerative colitis** (UC) is an idiopathic chronic inflammatory disease of the colon and rectum, characterized by mucosal inflammation and typically presenting with bloody diarrhea. Most often, UC affects the rectum (proctitis), but it may extend into the sigmoid (proctosigmoiditis), beyond the sigmoid (distal UC), or include the entire colon into the cecum (pancolitis).
- **CD** results in transmural ulceration of any portion of the GI most often affecting the terminal ileum and colon.

DIAGNOSIS

Clinical Presentation

- Both disorders can present with diarrhea, weight loss, and abdominal pain. UC typically presents with bloody diarrhea. CD can also present with fistula formation, strictures, abscesses, or bowel obstruction.
- **Extracolonic manifestations** of IBD include arthritis, primary sclerosing cholangitis, and ocular and skin lesions (Table 18-10).

Diagnostic Testing

- **Endoscopy** remains the preferred method for diagnosis, especially for UC, where contiguous inflammation is seen starting at the rectum and extending varying distances into the colon. Endoscopy may demonstrate colonic involvement in CD (erosions or ulcers with a patchy distribution and skip lesions); ileoscopy during colonoscopy may demonstrate terminal ileal involvement. **Histopathology** demonstrates chronic mucosal inflammation

TABLE 18-10 Extraintestinal Manifestations of Inflammatory Bowel Disease

Sites	Extraintestinal Manifestations
Musculoskeletal system	Seronegative spondyloarthropathy Hypertrophic osteoarthropathy Osteoporosis, aseptic necrosis, polymyositis
Dermatologic and oral systems	Erythema nodosum, pyoderma gangrenosum, aphthous ulcers Fissures, fistulas
Hepatopancreatobiliary system	Primary sclerosing cholangitis, bile duct carcinoma Autoimmune chronic active hepatitis Gallstones associated with ileal Crohn's disease
Ocular system	Uveitis/iritis, episcleritis, scleromalacia, corneal ulcers, retinal vascular disease
Metabolic system	Growth retardation in children and adolescents, delayed sexual maturation
Renal system	Calcium oxalate stones

with crypt abscesses and cryptitis in UC and may demonstrate multinucleated giant cells and noncaseating granulomas in CD.

- Cross-sectional **imaging studies** (CT and MRI scans) have value in the evaluation of CD, especially when luminal narrowing (stricture) or extraluminal complications (abscess, fistula) are suspected. Although MRI and CT enterography both adequately assess disease activity and bowel involvement in CD, MRI may be superior to CT.[98,99] Contrast radiography (small bowel follow-through series, barium enema) may also be useful, particularly in CD. The abdominal X-ray can assess for the presence of free air, bowel obstruction, or toxic megacolon.
- Fecal calprotectin levels can be used as a marker for intestinal inflammation.
- **Serologic markers** play a limited role as adjuncts for diagnosis. Anti-*Saccharomyces cerevisiae* antibodies are typically seen in CD, and perinuclear antineutrophil cytoplasmic antibodies (p-ANCA) are seen in UC. C-reactive protein (CRP) and erythrocyte sedimentation rate (ESR) represent correlates for disease activity.
- ***C. difficile* colitis** is more frequent in IBD patients compared with non-IBD populations; therefore, **stool studies** are warranted to look for this organism with disease flares.[100] **CMV superinfection** can occur in patients on immunosuppressive agents and can be diagnosed by histopathology during endoscopy.[101]

Severity Scoring

1. Truelove and Witts severity index for UC (Table 18-11)
2. Mayo score for severity of UC (Table 18-12)
3. CD activity index (Table 18-13)

TREATMENT

Medications

Treatment is based on the severity of disease, location, and associated complications.[102] Management aims are to resolve the acute presentation and reduce future recurrences. Both UC and CD can be categorized into three categories of severity for management purposes:

- **Mild to moderate disease:** Patients have little to no weight loss and good functional capacity and are able to maintain adequate oral intake. UC patients have less than four

TABLE 18-11 Truelove and Witts Severity Index for Ulcerative Colitis

	Mild	Moderate	Severe
Bowel movements (no. per day)	Fewer than 4	4–6	Six or more plus at least one of the features of systemic upset (marked with*)
Blood in stools	No more than small amounts of blood	Between mild and severe	Visible blood
Pyrexia (temperature greater than 37.8°C)*	No	No	Yes
Pulse rate greater than 90 bpm*	No	No	Yes
Anemia*	No	No	Yes
Erythrocyte sedimentation rate (mm/h)*	30 or below	30 or below	Above 30

TABLE 18-12 Mayo Score for Severity of Ulcerative Colitis

Measure	Scoring System
Stool frequency (per day)	0: Normal number of stools for patients 1: One to two more stools than normal 2: Three to four more stools than normal 3: >5 more stools than normal
Rectal bleeding	0: No blood seen 1: Streaks of blood with stool less than 50% of the time 2: Obvious blood with stool most of the time 3: Passes blood without stool
Finding on endoscopy	0: Normal or inactive disease 1: Mild disease 2: Moderate disease 3: Severe disease
Physician's global assessment	0: Normal 1: Mild disease 2: Moderate disease 3: Severe disease

TABLE 18-13 Crohn's Disease Activity Index

Clinical or Laboratory Variable	Weighting Factor
Number of liquid or soft stools each day for 7 days	×2
Abdominal pain (graded from 0 to 3 based on severity) each day for 7 days	×5
General well-being, subjectively assessed from 0 (well) to 4 (terrible) each day for 7 days	×7
Complications[a]	×20
Use of diphenoxylate or opiates for diarrhea	×30
An abdominal mass (0 for none; 2 for questionable; 5 for definite)	×10
Absolute deviation of hematocrit from 47% in men and 42% in women	×6
Percentage deviation from standard weight	×1

[a]One point is added for each set of complications: arthralgia of frank arthritis; inflammation of the iris or uvcitis; crythema nodosum, pyoderma gangrenosum, or aphthous ulcers; anal fissures, fistulas, or abseesses; other fistulas; and fever (>100°F) during the previous week.

Remission: CDAI score <150 points.

Moderate-to-severe disease: CDAI score 230–400 points.

bowel movements daily with no rectal bleeding or anemia, normal vital signs, and normal ESR, whereas CD patients have little or no abdominal pain. Treatment typically begins with aminosalicylates but can include antibiotics and glucocorticoids.

- **5-Aminosalicylates (5-ASA):** Various formulations are available, each targeting different parts of the tubular gut, and are useful for both inducing and maintaining remission in mild to moderate disease. Infrequent hypersensitivity reactions include pneumonitis, pancreatitis, hepatitis, and nephritis. **Sulfasalazine** reaches the colon intact, where it is metabolized to 5-ASA and a sulfapyridine moiety. Benefit is seen in UC or CD limited to the colon, either as initial therapy (0.5 g PO bid, increased as tolerated to 0.5–1.5 g PO qid) or to maintain remission (1 g PO bid–qid). The sulfapyridine moiety is responsible for side effects of headache, nausea, vomiting, and abdominal pain, which are treated with dose reduction. Skin rash, fever, agranulocytosis, hepatotoxicity, and paradoxical exacerbation of colitis are rare hypersensitivity reactions. Reversible reduction in sperm counts can be seen in males. Folic acid supplementation is recommended because sulfasalazine can impair folate absorption.

- ◦ **Mesalamine:** Newer 5-ASA preparations lack the sulfa moiety of sulfasalazine and are associated with fewer side effects, but can be expensive.
  - **Asacol** is an oral formulation of 5-ASA released at a pH of 7 in the distal ileum. It is useful in UC and ileocecal/colonic CD at doses of 800–1600 mg PO tid.
  - **Pentasa** has a time- and pH-dependent release mechanism that allows drug availability throughout the small bowel and colon. It is useful in diffuse small bowel involvement with CD but can also be used in UC in doses of 0.5–1.0 g PO qid.
  - **Apriso** also has a pH-dependent release mechanism and distributes mesalamine throughout the colon when administered in doses of 1.5 g PO once daily.
  - **Balsalazide (Colazal)** is cleaved by colonic bacteria to mesalamine and an inert molecule. Therefore, it is only useful for colonic disease, at doses of 2.25 g PO tid for active disease and 1.5 g PO bid for maintenance.
  - **Multimatrix delivery system mesalamine (Lialda)** uses a novel delivery system that allows sustained 5-ASA release throughout the colon while decreasing frequency of administration. It is useful in colonic disease at doses of 1.2–2.4 g PO qday–bid.
- ◦ **Olsalazine (Dipentum)** is a 5-ASA dimer cleaved by colonic bacteria and is useful in colonic disease. Significant diarrhea limits its use.
- ◦ **Antibiotics** are commonly used clinically in mild to moderate CD as well as perianal disease, but not in UC where the role of bacteria has not been established. Their role should be limited to colonic or ileocolonic CD, perianal disease, fistulas, and abscesses. Typical antibiotics used are **metronidazole** (250–500 mg PO tid) and **ciprofloxacin** (500 mg PO bid), usually concurrently, for 2–6 weeks
  - **Budesonide** (Entocort; 6–9 mg PO qday) is a synthetic corticosteroid with first-pass liver metabolism that limits systemic toxicity while retaining local efficacy from high affinity to the glucocorticoid receptor, similar to oral corticosteroids. It is effective and safe for short-term use in mild to moderate ileocolonic CD and can replace mesalamine in inducing remission.[102]
  - **Topical therapy** is useful in IBD limited to distal left colon. Topical mesalamine agents are superior to topical steroids or oral aminosalicylates for mild to moderate distal UC or ulcerative proctitis.[103] Sitz baths, analgesics, hydrocortisone creams, and local heat may provide symptomatic benefit in perianal CD in conjunction with systemic therapy.

- **Moderate to severe disease** refers to CD patients who fail to respond to treatment for mild to moderate disease or those with significant weight loss, anemia, fever, abdominal pain or tenderness, and intermittent nausea and vomiting without bowel obstruction or UC patients with more than six bloody bowel movements daily, fever, mild anemia, and elevated ESR.[104] Predictive factors for moderate- to high-risk disease include age <30 years at initial diagnosis, extensive anatomic involvement, perianal and/or severe rectal disease, deep ulcers, prior surgical resection, and stricturing or penetrating behavior.[102] The goal of therapy is to induce remission rapidly with corticosteroids and to maintain remission with immunosuppressive agents and/or biologic agents as appropriate. Treatment is typically continued until the patient fails to respond to a particular agent or the agent is no longer tolerated.

- **Glucocorticoids** are effective in inducing remission in moderate to severe disease, especially with flares of disease activity.[105]
  - **Prednisone** is started orally (typically 40–60 mg PO daily) and continued until symptom improvement. The dose can then be tapered on a weekly basis because glucocorticoids are not recommended for maintenance therapy, and steroid-sparing alternatives should be sought for patients who appear dependent on these medications.
- **Immunosuppressive agents**
  - **6-Mercaptopurine** (1.0–1.5 mg/kg/d PO), a purine analog, and **azathioprine** (1.5–2.5 mg/kg/d PO), its S-imidazole precursor, cause preferential suppression of T-cell activation and antigen recognition and are useful in maintaining a glucocorticoid-induced remission in both UC and CD. Both azathioprine and 6-mercaptopurine are effective for inducing remission in active CD.[106] Response may be delayed for up to 1–2 months, with optimal response occurring about 4 months after treatment initiation. Side effects include reversible bone marrow suppression, pancreatitis, and allergic reactions.
    - Determination of **thiopurine methyltransferase (TPMT)** enzyme activity prior to initiation of therapy will identify genetic polymorphisms that may predispose to toxicity with the use of these agents.[107]
    - Routine blood cell counts should be performed, initially every 1–2 weeks, to monitor for acute or delayed bone marrow suppression. On stable doses, testing can be performed every 3 months
    - 6-Thioguanine (6-TG) metabolite levels assess adequacy of dosing, whereas high 6-methyl mercaptopurine (6-MMP) levels may predict hepatotoxicity. Addition of allopurinol to the regimen preferentially pushes metabolism toward the active metabolite (6-TG) rather than the toxic metabolite (6-MMP).[108]
  - **Methotrexate** (15–25 mg IM or PO weekly) is effective as a steroid-sparing agent in CD but not UC. Side effects include hepatic fibrosis, bone marrow suppression, alopecia, pneumonitis, allergic reactions, and teratogenicity. In CD patients in remission, methotrexate is not as effective as azathioprine or infliximab for mucosal healing, and methotrexate added to infliximab is no more effective than infliximab monotherapy.[109,110]
    - Baseline CXR and monitoring of CBC and liver function tests should be performed routinely.
    - Patients with abnormal transaminases may require a liver biopsy to assess for hepatic fibrosis prior to treatment, and subsequent biopsies are performed for significant elevations thereafter.

- **Anti–tumor necrosis factor-α (anti–TNF-α) monoclonal antibodies** modify immune system function and are beneficial in moderate to severe CD refractory to other approaches, including immunosuppressives, and indicated both for induction and maintenance of remission. Benefit has also been demonstrated in moderate to severe UC.[111] **Infliximab (Remicade**; 5 mg/kg IV infusions at weeks 0, 2, and 6, followed by maintenance infusions every 8 weeks), **adalimumab (Humira**; 160 mg SC at week 0, then 80 mg SC at week 2, followed by 40 mg SC every 2 weeks), **certolizumab pegol (Cimzia**; 400 mg SC at weeks 0, 2, and 4, followed by maintenance doses every 4 weeks), and **golilimumab (Simponi**, 200 mg SC at week 0, then 100 mg SC at week 2 and every 4 weeks thereafter) are the available anti–TNF-α agents. Combination therapy with infliximab and azathioprine is more effective than monotherapy with either agent in UC.[112] In addition to its role as an option for first-line therapy, adalimumab is also safe and effective for CD patients who have failed infliximab therapy.[113] However, because elective switching from IV infliximab to SC adalimumab is associated with loss of tolerance and efficacy, adherence to the first anti–TNF-α agent is encouraged.[114] Therapeutic drug monitoring can help optimize anti-TNF therapy, especially when symptoms persist.[115]

In moderate to severe CD, infliximab plus azathioprine or infliximab monotherapy is more likely to attain steroid-free clinical remission than azathioprine monotherapy.[116]

- Anti–TNF-α therapy has been associated with reactivation of latent TB; hence, placement of a purified protein derivative skin test and CXR are essential prior to initiation of therapy.[103] Hepatitis B status should also be assessed and vaccination provided prior to therapy. Opportunistic infections as well as infectious complications can develop, and congestive heart failure may worsen during therapy.
- Acute and delayed hypersensitivity reactions, or antibodies to infliximab and anti–double-stranded DNA antibodies, can develop with infliximab infusions. Local injection site reactions have been reported with adalimumab and certolizumab pegol therapy.

- **Vedolizumab** (**Entyvio**; 300-mg infusions at weeks 0 and 2, followed by infusions every 4–8 weeks), an α4β7 integrin antibody, has emerged as an alternative option for induction and maintenance of remission in both CD and UC.[117]
- **Natalizumab** (**Tysabri**; 300 mg infusions at weeks 0, 4, and 8, followed by monthly infusions thereafter) is a humanized monoclonal antibody to α-4 integrin, used for moderate to severe CD refractory to all other approaches, including anti–TNF-α antibodies. This agent may induce reactivation of human JC polyomavirus, causing progressive multifocal leukoencephalopathy, and is now rarely used.
- **Ustekinumab** (**Stelara**; weight-dependent dosing of 260–520 mg infusion at week 1, followed by 90 mg subcutaneous maintenance injections every 8 weeks), a monoclonal antibody to the p40 subunit of interleukin-12 and interleukin-23, has shown promising results in moderate to severely active CD.[118]
- **Tofacitinib** (**Xeljanz**; 5 mg or 10 mg oral twice a day, dosing to be determined) is an oral Janus kinase inhibitor that has shown promise in clinical trials in moderately to severely active ulcerative colitis in induction and maintenance therapy.[119]

- **Severe or fulminant disease** describes patients typically hospitalized because of the severity of their symptoms. Fulminant CD patients have persistent symptoms despite conventional glucocorticoids or anti–TNF-α therapy or have high fevers, persistent vomiting, intestinal obstruction, intra-abdominal abscess, peritoneal signs, or cachexia.[104] Fulminant colitis (both CD and UC) can present with profuse bloody bowel movements, significant anemia, systemic signs of toxicity (fever, sepsis, electrolyte disturbances, dehydration), and elevated laboratory markers of inflammation. **Toxic megacolon** occurs in 1%–2% of UC patients, wherein the colon becomes atonic and modestly dilated, with significant systemic toxicity.
  - Supportive therapy consists of NPO status with NG suction if there is evidence of small bowel ileus. Dehydration and electrolyte disturbances are treated vigorously, and blood is transfused for severe anemia. Anticholinergic and opioid medication should be discontinued in toxic megacolon.
  - Initial investigation includes cross-sectional imaging to evaluate for intra-abdominal abscess. Blood cultures and stool studies to exclude *C. difficile* colitis are performed. Cautious flexible sigmoidoscopy may be done to determine severity of colonic inflammation and for biopsies to exclude CMV colitis.
  - Once infection is excluded, intensive medical therapy with IV **corticosteroids** (methylprednisolone 1 mg/kg body weight or equivalent to 40–60 mg of prednisone) and broad-spectrum antimicrobials should be initiated.
  - If response is not seen, **cyclosporine** infusion (2–4 mg/kg/d to achieve blood levels of 200–400 ng/mL) and tacrolimus infusion represent options in fulminant UC colitis.
  - Nutritional support is administered as appropriate after 5–7 days; TPN is often indicated if enteral nutrition is not tolerated.
  - Clinical deterioration/lack of improvement despite 7–10 days of intensive medical management, evidence of bowel perforation, and peritoneal signs are indications for urgent total colectomy.

Surgical Management

- Surgery is generally reserved for fistulas, obstruction, abscess, perforation, or bleeding; medically refractory disease; and neoplastic transformation.[105] Stricturoplasty is an option for focal tight strictures; biopsies should be obtained to rule out cancer at stricture sites.
- In CD, recurrence close to the resected margins is common after bowel resection. Efforts should be made to avoid multiple resections in CD because of the risk of short bowel syndrome. Immunosuppressive agents should be discontinued before surgery and reinstituted if necessary during the postoperative period.
- **In UC, total colectomy is curative** and may be preferred over long-term immunosuppressive or biologic therapy.

Lifestyle/Risk Modification

- A low-roughage diet often is useful in mild to moderate IBD or in patients with strictures.
- Patients with Crohn's ileitis or ileocolonic resection may need vitamin B_{12} supplementation. Specific oral replacement of calcium, magnesium, folate, iron, vitamins A and D, and other micronutrients may be necessary in patients with small bowel CD.
- **TPN** can be administered in patients with food intolerance for greater than 4 or 5 days. Bowel rest has not been shown to reduce time to remission but can be used for nutritional maintenance and symptom relief while waiting for the effects of medical treatment or as a bridge to surgery.

SPECIAL CONSIDERATIONS

- In patients with both UC and Crohn's colitis lasting longer than 8–10 years, annual or biennial colonoscopic surveillance for neoplasia should be performed ideally using chromoendoscopy. Optimal biopsy technique continues to be studied and includes either four-quadrant mucosal biopsies every 5–10 cm using white light endoscopy or targeted biopsies using chromoendoscopy. Consistent histopathologic evidence of any grade of dysplasia is an indication for total colectomy. Narrow-band imaging during colonoscopy may represent an alternative to chromoendoscopy for targeted biopsies in IBD.[120,121]
- **Smoking cessation** is generally warranted for all patients with IBD. There is epidemiologic evidence of a protective effect on a limited number of patients with UC. However, nicotine has been shown to increase metabolism of many medications routinely used to treat IBD, decreasing their efficacy.
- **Venous thromboembolism:** Patients with IBD are at increased risk for both first and recurrent venous thromboembolism.[122]
- **Family planning** is important in women with active disease as there is an increased association of premature delivery, low birth weight, and congenital abnormalities.[123]
- **Symptom control** is important as adjunct to therapy but must be used cautiously.
  - **Antidiarrheal agents** may be useful as an adjunctive therapy in selected patients with mild exacerbations or postresection diarrhea. They are contraindicated in severe exacerbations and toxic megacolon.
  - **Narcotics** should be used sparingly for pain control because the chronicity of symptoms can lead to potential for dependence.
    - Examples of these experimental agents include thalidomide and interleukin (IL)-11 for Crohn's disease, butyrate enema, nicotine patch, and heparin for ulcerative colitis.

Functional Gastrointestinal Disorders

GENERAL PRINCIPLES

- Functional GI disorders are characterized by the presence of abdominal symptoms in the absence of a demonstrable organic disease process. Symptoms can arise from any part of the luminal gut.
- **Irritable bowel syndrome (IBS)**, primarily characterized by abdominal pain linked to altered bowel habits of at least 3 months in duration, is the best recognized functional bowel disease[124]
- IBS can be of four types: IBS with diarrhea (IBS-D), IBS with constipation (IBS-C), IBS with mixed bowel patterns (IBS-M), and unclassified IBS (IBS-U).

DIAGNOSIS

- Clinical evaluation and investigation should be directed toward prudently excluding organic processes in the involved area of the gut while initiating therapeutic trials when functional symptoms are suspected.[125]
- **Serologic tests for celiac sprue** are recommended in IBS patients. The prevalence of celiac sprue in diarrhea-predominant IBS patients is estimated at 3.6% compared with 0.7% of the general population.[126]
- Patients >50 years old with new-onset bowel symptoms, patients with alarm symptoms (GI bleeding, anemia, weight loss, early satiety), and patients with symptoms not responding to empiric treatment need further workup with endoscopy. Routine cross-sectional imaging is not recommended with typical functional symptoms without alarm features.
- The Rome IV criteria are used to diagnose IBS, which require the presence of at least two or more of the following on an average of at least 1 day/week in the last 3 months: improvement in abdominal pain or discomfort with defecation, onset associated with a change in frequency of stool, and/or an onset accompanied by a change in the form or appearance of stool.

TREATMENT

Patient education, reassurance, and help with diet and lifestyle modification are keys to an effective physician-patient relationship. The psychosocial contribution to symptom exacerbation should be determined, and its management may be sufficient for many patients. Foods such as wheat products, onions, fruits, vegetables, sorbitol, and some dairy products can include short-chain, poorly absorbed, highly fermentable carbohydrates, which are known as fermentable oligosaccharides, disaccharides, monosaccharides, and polyols (FODMAPs), and have been associated with increased gastrointestinal symptoms in IBS patients. Diets low in FODMAPs appear to reduce functional GI symptoms in patients with IBS.[127]

Medications

- **Symptomatic management**
  - **Antiemetic agents** are useful in functional nausea and vomiting syndromes, in addition to neuromodulators.
  - When pain and bloating are the predominant symptoms, **antispasmodic** or **anticholinergic** medications (hyoscyamine, 0.125–0.25 mg PO/sublingual up to qid; dicyclomine, 10–20 mg PO qid) may provide short-term relief.
  - Stool frequency, but not abdominal pain, improves with increased dietary fiber (25 g/d) supplemented with PRN laxatives in constipation-predominant IBS.
  - **Loperamide** (2–4 mg, up to qid/PRN) can reduce stool frequency, urgency, and fecal incontinence.

- Short-term nonabsorbable **antibiotic** therapy (particularly **rifaximin**) may improve bloating and diarrhea in IBS; long-term treatment has not been adequately studied.[128] **Probiotics** (e.g., bifidobacteria) are sometimes beneficial.[126]
- **Lubiprostone** (8 μg bid), a selective chloride channel activator, **linaclotide** (290 μg daily), and **plecanatide** (3 mg daily), guanylate cyclase C agonists, improves constipation-predominant IBS symptoms.[129] Polyethylene glycol 3350 and electrolytes are suitable for use in constipation-predominant IBS.[130]
- **Eluxadoline (Viberzi**, 75–100 mg bid), a μ- and κ-opioid receptor agonist, is approved for the management of diarrhea-predominant IBS.[131] Acute pancreatitis is a potentially serious side effect occurring in 0.4%; history of past pancreatitis, cholecystectomy, alcohol abuse, and hepatic impairment are contraindications.
- **Alosetron** (Lotronex, 1 mg daily to bid), a 5-HT_3 antagonist, is useful in women with diarrhea-predominant IBS.[132] However, its use is restricted to refractory diarrhea because of the rare potential for ischemic colitis.

- **Neuromodulators**
  - Low-dose **TCAs** (e.g., amitriptyline, nortriptyline, imipramine, doxepin: 25–100 mg at bedtime) have neuromodulatory and analgesic properties that are independent of their psychotropic effects. These can be beneficial, especially in pain-predominant functional GI disorders.[125]
  - **Selective serotonin reuptake inhibitors (SSRIs)** (e.g., fluoxetine, 20 mg; paroxetine, 20 mg; sertraline, 50 mg; duloxetine, 20–60 mg) may also have efficacy, sometimes with better side effect profiles compared with TCAs.
  - **Cyclic vomiting syndrome (CVS)** is an increasingly recognized condition with stereotypic episodes of vigorous vomiting and asymptomatic intervals between episodes.[133] Treatment with low-dose TCAs or antiepileptic medications (zonisamide, levetiracetam) has prophylactic benefits.[134] Sumatriptan (25–50 mg PO, 5–10 mg transnasally, or 6 mg SC) or other triptans may abort an episode, especially if administered during a prodrome or early in the episode.[135] Established episodes may require IV hydration, scheduled IV antiemetics (ondansetron, prochlorperazine), benzodiazepines (lorazepam), and pain control with IV narcotics. Before the diagnosis of CVS is made, structural causes and cannabinoid hyperemesis need to be ruled out.

Acute Intestinal Pseudo-Obstruction (Ileus)

GENERAL PRINCIPLES

Definition

- **Acute intestinal pseudo-obstruction or ileus** consists of impaired transit of intestinal contents and obstructive symptoms (nausea, vomiting, abdominal distension, lack of bowel movements) without a mechanical explanation.
- **Acute colonic pseudo-obstruction** or **Ogilvie syndrome** describes massive colonic dilation without mechanical obstruction in the presence of a competent ileocecal valve, resulting from impaired colonic peristalsis.[136]

Etiology

Ileus is frequently seen in the postoperative period (coronary bypass, solid organ transplantation, major orthopedic surgery [hip or knee replacement], spine surgery). Narcotic analgesics administered for postoperative pain control may contribute, as can other medications that slow down intestinal peristalsis (calcium channel blockers, anticholinergic medications, TCAs, antihistamines). Other predisposing causes include virtually any medical insult, particularly life-threatening systemic diseases, infection, vascular insufficiency, and electrolyte abnormalities. Etiology is similar for acute colonic pseudo-obstruction.

DIAGNOSIS

- A careful history and physical examination is essential in the initial evaluation.
- Conventional laboratory studies (CBC, complete metabolic profile, amylase, lipase) help in assessing for a primary intra-abdominal inflammatory process.
- **Obstructive series** (supine and upright abdominal radiograph with a CXR) determines the distribution of intestinal gas and assesses for the presence of free intraperitoneal air.
- **Additional imaging studies** assess for mechanical obstruction and inflammatory processes and include CT, contrast enema, and small bowel series.

TREATMENT

- Basic **supportive measures** consist of NPO, fluid replacement, and correction of electrolyte imbalances. Medications that slow down GI motility (adrenergic agonists, TCAs, sedatives, narcotic analgesics) should be withdrawn or dose reduced. The ambulatory patient is encouraged to remain active and to undertake short walks.
- **Intermittent NG suction** prevents swallowed air from passing distally. In protracted cases, gastric decompression, either using an NG tube or a percutaneous endoscopic gastrostomy (PEG) tube, vents upper GI secretions and decreases vomiting and gastric distension.
- **Rectal tubes** help decompress the distal colon; more proximal colonic distension may necessitate **colonoscopic decompression**, especially when the cecal diameter approaches 12 cm.[136] A flexible decompression tube can be left in the proximal colon during colonoscopy. Turning the patient from side to side may potentiate the benefit of colonoscopic decompression.
- Percutaneous cecostomy tube placement is done under ultrasound and fluoroscopic guidance.

Medications

- **Methylnaltrexone** (**Relistor**; 8–12 mg SC per dose every other day) can be administered in settings where opioid medication use contributes to pseudo-obstruction.
- **Neostigmine** (2 mg IV administered slowly over 3–5 minutes) is beneficial in selected patients with acute colonic distension. This can induce rapid reestablishment of colonic tone and is contraindicated if mechanical obstruction remains in the differential diagnosis. Side effects include abdominal pain, excessive salivation, symptomatic bradycardia, and syncope. A trial of neostigmine may be warranted before colonoscopic decompression in patients without contraindications.[137]
- **Erythromycin** (200 mg IV) acts as a motilin agonist and stimulates upper gut motility; it has been used with some success in refractory postoperative ileus.
- **Alvimopan** is a peripherally acting μ-opioid receptor antagonist that enhances return of bowel function after abdominal surgery but has not been shown to shorten hospital stay.[138]
- **Mosapride citrate** (15 mg PO tid), a 5-HT_4 receptor agonist, may reduce the duration of postoperative ileus when administered postoperatively.[139]
- **Prucalopride**, also a selective 5-HT_4 agonist, can relieve symptoms in patients with chronic intestinal pseudo-obstruction.[140]

Surgical Management

- **Surgical consultation** is required when the clinical picture is suggestive of mechanical obstruction or if peritoneal signs are present. Surgical exploration is reserved for acute cases with peritoneal signs, ischemic bowel, or other evidence for perforation.
- **Cecostomy** treats acute colonic distension when colonoscopic decompression fails.

PANCREATICOBILIARY DISORDERS

Acute Pancreatitis

GENERAL PRINCIPLES

Definition

Acute pancreatitis consists of inflammation of the pancreas and peripancreatic tissue from activation of potent pancreatic enzymes within the pancreas, particularly trypsin.

Etiology

The most common causes are alcohol and gallstone disease, accounting for 75%–80% of all cases (Table 18-14). Less common causes include abdominal trauma, hypercalcemia, hypertriglyceridemia, and a variety of drugs. Post-endoscopic retrograde cholangiopancreatography (ERCP) pancreatitis occurs in 5%–10% of patients undergoing ERCP;

TABLE 18-14 Causes of Pancreatitis
Alcohol use (25%–35%)
Gallstones (40%–70%)
Hypertriglyceridemia (1%–4%)
Idiopathic
Drug-induced pancreatitis • Definite association (azathioprine, sulfonamides, sulindac, tetracycline, valproic acid, didanosine, methyldopa, estrogens, furosemide, 6-mercaptopurine, pentamidine, 5-ASA, steroids, octreotide) • Probable association (thiazides, metronidazole, methandienone, nitrofurantoin, phenformin, piroxicam, procainamide, colaspase, chlorthalidone, asparagine, cimetidine, cisplatin, cytosine arabinoside, diphenoxylate, ethacrynic acid)
Postprocedural (ERCP or abdominal surgery)
Ampullary stenosis, formerly known as sphincter of Oddi dysfunction type I
Autoimmune pancreatitis, type I (systemic IgG4 disease-related) and type II
Viral infection (coxsackie, cytomegalovirus, echovirus, Epstein–Barr virus, hepatitis A/B/C, HIV, mumps, rubella, varicella)
Bacterial infection (*Campylobacter jejuni, Legionella, Leptospirosis, Mycobacterium avium, Mycobacterium tuberculosis, Mycoplasma*)
Trauma (1.5% of cases)
Smoking
Congenital anomalies (annular pancreas)
Genetic disorders (hereditary pancreatitis, cystic fibrosis, alpha-1 antitrypsin deficiency)
Hypercalcemia
Parasitic infections (*Ascaris lumbricoides, Cryptosporidium, Clonorchis sinensis,* microsporidia)
Renal disease (hemodialysis)
Toxins (scorpion bites, organophosphate poisoning)
Vasculitis (polyarteritis nodosa, systemic lupus erythematosus)
Hereditary pancreatitis

prophylaxis with rectal NSAIDs or topical epinephrine and placement of prophylactic pancreatic duct stents can help prevent post-ERCP pancreatitis.[141]

DIAGNOSIS

Clinical Presentation

Typical symptoms consist of acute onset of epigastric abdominal pain, nausea, and vomiting, often exacerbated by food intake. Systemic manifestations can include fever, shortness of breath, altered mental status, anemia, and electrolyte imbalances, especially with severe episodes.

The abdominal exam will typically reveal epigastric tenderness with possible guarding and rigidity and decreased bowel sounds.

In 3% of patients with acute severe pancreatitis, ecchymosis and discoloration may be observed in the periumbilical region (Cullen sign), along the flank (Grey Turner sign), or below inguinal ligament (Fox sign).

Diagnostic Testing

Laboratories

- Serum **lipase** is more specific and sensitive than serum **amylase**, although both are usually elevated beyond three times the upper limits of normal. These values do not correlate with severity or outcome of pancreatitis. Patients with renal insufficiency may have elevated enzymes at baseline from impaired clearance.[142]
- Hepatic function testing may identify biliary obstruction as a possible etiology, and a lipid panel may suggest hypertriglyceridemia as the cause of acute pancreatitis.

Imaging

- **Dual-phase (pancreatic protocol) CT scan** is useful in the initial evaluation of severe acute pancreatitis but should be reserved for patients in whom the diagnosis is unclear, who fail to improve clinically within 48–72 hours, or in whom complications are suspected.[143] CT scan early in presentation may underestimate the severity of acute pancreatitis.
- **MRI with gadolinium** can also be used with at least similar efficacy, especially when CT is contraindicated. Magnetic resonance cholangiopancreatography (MRCP) or endoscopic ultrasound (EUS) is useful to detect a biliary source for pancreatitis before ERCP is performed.[144] These help in identifying local complications too.

TREATMENT

- **Aggressive goal-directed volume repletion** with IV fluids must be undertaken, with careful monitoring of fluid balance, urine output, serum electrolytes (including calcium and glucose), and awareness of the potential for significant fluid sequestration within the abdomen.[145] Intensive care unit monitoring may be necessary. In the setting of mild pancreatitis, Ringer's lactate at a dose of 20 mL/kg bolus followed by 3 mL/kg/h has shown improved outcomes within 36 hours.[146] However, the benefit of Ringer's lactate over normal saline has not been confirmed.
- Early **enteral nutrition** may improve clinical outcomes, and no differences have been found between oral, NG, and nasojejunal administration.[146]
- NG suction is reserved for patients with ileus or protracted emesis. TPN may be necessary when inflammation is slow to resolve (around 7 days) or if an ileus is present. However, enteral feeding is preferred over TPN.
- Acid suppression may be necessary in severely ill patients with risk factors for stress ulcer bleeding, although it has not been shown to decrease symptom duration or severity.[147]

Medications

- **Narcotic analgesics** are usually necessary for pain relief.
- Routine use of prophylactic antibiotics is not recommended in the absence of systemic infection.[145]

Other Nonoperative Therapies

Urgent **ERCP and biliary sphincterotomy** within 72 hours of presentation can improve the outcome of severe gallstone pancreatitis in the presence of cholangitis; benefits are unclear in the absence of cholangitis.[145]

Surgical Management

Cholecystectomy is recommended during the index hospitalization in acute gallstone pancreatitis.[145]

COMPLICATIONS (TABLE 18-15)

TABLE 18-15 Complications of Pancreatitis

Local Complications	Systemic Complications
• Peripancreatic fluid collections • (Peri)Pancreatic necrosis (sterile + infected) • Pancreatic abscess (phlegmon) • Pseudocyst • Pancreatic ascites • Pseudoaneurysm • Involvement of adjacent organs with hemorrhage, thrombosis, bowel infraction, obstructive jaundice, fistula formation, or mechanical obstruction	• Cardiovascular ◦ Shock—hypovolemic and septic—Arrhythmias/pericardial effusion/sudden death • Pulmonary ◦ Respiratory failure/pneumonia/atelectasis/pleural effusion—Acute respiratory distress syndrome (ARDS) • Renal failure ◦ Azotemia ◦ Renal artery/vein thrombosis • Hematological ◦ Hemoconcentation ◦ Disseminated intravascular coagulopathy (DIC) • Metabolic ◦ Hypocalcemia ◦ Hyperglycemia ◦ Hyperlipidemia • Gastrointestinal ◦ Peptic ulcer/erosive gastritis ◦ Ileus ◦ Portal vein or splenic vein thrombosis with varices • Neurological ◦ Visual disturbances—sudden blindness (Purtscher retinopathy) ◦ Confusion, irritability, psychosis ◦ Fat emboli ◦ Encephalopathy • Miscellaneous ◦ Subcutaneous fat necrosis

- **Necrotizing pancreatitis** represents a severe form of acute pancreatitis, usually identified on dynamic dual-phase CT scanning with IV contrast. The presence of radiologically identified pancreatic necrosis increases the morbidity and mortality of acute pancreatitis. Increasing abdominal pain, fever, marked leukocytosis, and bacteremia suggest infected pancreatic necrosis that requires broad-spectrum antibiotics and often surgical debridement. CT-guided percutaneous aspiration for Gram stain and culture can confirm the diagnosis of infected necrosis. **Carbapenems** or a combination of a **fluoroquinolone** and **metronidazole** has good penetration into necrotic tissue.
- The presence of **pseudocysts** is suggested by persistent pain or high amylase levels. Complications include infection, hemorrhage, rupture (pancreatic ascites), and obstruction of adjacent structures. Asymptomatic nonenlarging pseudocysts can be followed clinically with serial imaging studies to resolution. Decompression of symptomatic or infected pseudocysts can be performed by percutaneous, endoscopic, or surgical techniques.[148]
- **Infection:** Potential sources of fever include pancreatic necrosis, abscess, infected pseudocyst, cholangitis, and aspiration pneumonia. Cultures should be obtained and broad-spectrum antimicrobials appropriate for bowel flora should be administered. Antibiotics are only indicated when there is a high clinical suspicion for infection.[146]
- **Pulmonary complications:** Atelectasis, pleural effusion, pneumonia, and acute respiratory distress syndrome can develop in severely ill patients (see Chapter 10, Pulmonary Diseases).
- **Renal failure** can result from intravascular volume depletion or acute tubular necrosis.
- **Other complications:** Metabolic complications include hypocalcemia, hypomagnesemia, and hyperglycemia. GI bleeding can result from stress gastritis, pseudoaneurysm rupture, or gastric varices from splenic vein thrombosis.

Severity Scoring Systems for Acute Pancreatitis

Acute pancreatitis specific scoring systems are the following:

- Ranson score
- Glasgow–Imrie score
- Bedside Index for Severity in Acute Pancreatitis (BISAP) score
- Harmless Acute Pancreatitis Score (HAPS)
- Hong Kong Criteria

Acute pancreatitis nonspecific scoring systems (ICU scoring systems) are the following:

- Acute Physiology and Chronic Health Evaluation (APACHE) II score
- Sequential Organ Failure Assessment (SOFA) score

Chronic Pancreatitis

GENERAL PRINCIPLES

- Chronic pancreatitis represents inflammation, fibrosis, and atrophy of acinar cells resulting from recurrent acute or chronic inflammation of the pancreas.
- Most commonly seen with **chronic alcohol abuse**, it can also result from dyslipidemia, hypercalcemia, autoimmune disease, and exposure to various toxins. An inherited form (**hereditary pancreatitis**) is rarely seen; this can be associated with mutations in genes encoding cationic trypsinogen (*PRSS1*) or pancreatic secretory trypsin inhibitor (*SPINK1*).[149]
- **Autoimmune pancreatitis (AIP)** represents an increasingly recognized subtype of chronic pancreatitis characterized by infiltration of IgG4-positive plasma cells in a classically sausage-shaped pancreas. AIP can be difficult to distinguish from pancreatic cancer on CT, but typically features diffuse narrowing of the main pancreatic duct without dilation.

Initial treatment has traditionally been with high-dose steroids, although low-dose steroids may be similarly effective.[150] Relapses may occur in the pancreas or biliary tree, although retreatment with steroids is effective at inducing remission.[151]

DIAGNOSIS

Clinical Presentation

Chronic abdominal pain, **exocrine insufficiency** from acinar cell injury and fibrosis (manifesting as weight loss and steatorrhea), and **endocrine insufficiency** from the destruction of islet cells (manifesting as brittle diabetes) are the main clinical manifestations.

Diagnostic Testing

Laboratories

- Lipase and amylase may be elevated but are frequently normal and are nonspecific. Bilirubin, alkaline phosphatase, and transaminases may be elevated if there is concomitant biliary obstruction. A lipid panel and serum calcium should also be assessed.
- Indirect pancreatic function testing (such as secretin stimulation, fecal fat, and fecal elastase) can be performed but are not widely available and difficult to perform.

Imaging

- **Calcification** of the pancreas can be seen on imaging. Contrast-enhanced CT has a sensitivity of 75%–90% and a specificity of 85% for the diagnosis of chronic pancreatitis, whereas MRCP is equivalent and a suitable alternative.[149]
- EUS has higher sensitivity for the diagnosis of chronic pancreatitis and is particularly useful for evaluating lesions concerning for neoplasia in the setting of chronic pancreatitis.

TREATMENT

Medications

- **Narcotic analgesics** are frequently required for control of pain, and narcotic dependence is common. **Neuromodulators** (TCAs, SSRIs) and **pregabalin** may improve symptoms and decrease reliance on narcotics.[152] In patients with mild to moderate exocrine insufficiency, the addition of oral pancreatic enzyme supplements may be beneficial for pain control.
- **Pancreatic enzyme supplements** are the mainstay of management of pancreatic exocrine insufficiency in conjunction with a low-fat diet (<50 g fat per day), facilitating weight gain and reduced stool frequency.[153] Enteric-coated preparations (Pancrease, Zenpep or Creon, one to two capsules with meals) are stable at acid pH.
- **Fat-soluble vitamin** supplementation may be necessary.
- **Insulin** therapy is generally required for endocrine insufficiency because the resultant diabetes mellitus is characteristically brittle and thus unresponsive to oral agents.
- When identified, treatment of the underlying disorder (e.g., hyperparathyroidism, dyslipidemia) is indicated. Alcohol cessation should be advised.

Other Nonoperative Therapies

- Patients with pancreatic duct obstruction from stones, strictures, or papillary stenosis may benefit from **ERCP and sphincterotomy.**
- Intractable pain may necessitate **celiac or splanchnic plexus block** (often EUS-guided) for short-term relief in selected patients or even surgery, such as a **Whipple procedure** or lateral pancreaticojejunostomy, in cases of a dilated pancreatic duct.[154]

Tropical Chronic Pancreatitis (TCP)

It is a juvenile form of chronic calcific nonalcoholic pancreatitis, seen almost exclusively in the developing countries of the tropical world.

The classical triad of TCP consists of abdominal pain, steatorrhea, and diabetes. When diabetes is present, the condition is called fibrocalculous pancreatic diabetes (FCPD).

The risk of ductal carcinoma with this disease is accentuated (10% of cases).

Treatment may be frustrating, and may include pancreatic enzymes, duct manipulations at endoscopic retrograde cholangiopancreatography, octreotide, celiac axis blocks for pain control, or surgery via drainage and/or resection.*

Gallstone Disease

GENERAL PRINCIPLES

- **Asymptomatic gallstones (cholelithiasis)** are a common incidental finding for which no specific therapy is generally necessary.[155] Cholesterol stones are the most common type, but pigmented stones can be seen with hemolysis or infection. Risk factors include obesity, female gender, parity, rapid weight loss, ileal disease, and maternal family history.
- **Symptomatic cholelithiasis**, when upper abdominal symptoms are linked to gallstones, is typically treated surgically with cholecystectomy.
- **Acute cholecystitis** is caused most often by obstruction of the cystic duct by gallstones, but acalculous cholecystitis can occur in severely ill or hospitalized patients.

DIAGNOSIS

Clinical Presentation

- Cholelithiasis may present as **biliary colic**, a constant pain lasting for several hours, located in the right upper quadrant, radiating to the back or right shoulder, and sometimes associated with nausea or vomiting.
- These gallstones may go on further to develop complications such as cholecystitis, cholangitis, choledocholithiasis, gallstone pancreatitis, and rarely cholangiocarcinoma.
- Two-thirds of patients with **acute ascending cholangitis** present with right upper quadrant pain, fever with chills and/or rigors, and jaundice (**Charcot triad**), usually in the setting of biliary obstruction (choledocholithiasis, neoplasia, sclerosing cholangitis, biliary stent occlusion). The presence of hypotension and altered mentation defines the **Reynolds pentad**, which is seen less commonly.

Diagnostic Testing

- **Ultrasound scans** have a high degree of accuracy in diagnosis (sensitivity and specificity >95%) and are the preferred initial test.
- **Endoscopic ultrasonography** (EUS) is an excellent method for visualizing the bile duct and gallbladder.
- **Hydroxy iminodiacetic acid** (HIDA) scan can demonstrate nonfilling of the gallbladder in patients with acute cholecystitis, although false-negative results may be seen in acalculous cholecystitis.
- ERCP/MRCP is useful when working up patients with jaundice and dilated CBD or suspected cholangitis.

---

*Rajesh G, Veena AB, Menon S, Balakrishnan V. Clinical profile of early-onset and late-onset idiopathic chronic pancreatitis in South India. *Indian J Gastroenterol.* 2014;33:231–236.

TREATMENT

Medications

- **Supportive measures** include IV fluid resuscitation and broad-spectrum antimicrobial agents, especially in the event of complications such as acute cholecystitis with sepsis, perforation, peritonitis, abscess, or empyema formation.
- **Ursodeoxycholic acid** (8–10 mg/kg/d PO in two to three divided doses for prolonged periods) might be prudent in a select group of patients with small cholesterol stones in normally functioning gallbladders who are at high risk for complications from surgical therapy. Side effects include diarrhea and reversible elevation in serum transaminases.

Other Nonpharmacologic Therapies

Percutaneous cholecystostomy can be performed under fluoroscopy in severely ill patients with acute cholecystitis who are not surgical candidates, especially for acalculous cholecystitis.[156]

Surgical Management

Cholecystectomy is the therapy of choice for symptomatic gallstone disease and acute cholecystitis. Laparoscopic cholecystectomy compares favorably with the open procedure, with lower morbidity, lower cost, shorter hospital stay, and better cosmetic results.[157]

COMPLICATIONS

- **Acute pancreatitis:** See Acute Pancreatitis section.
- **Choledocholithiasis:** Common bile duct obstruction, jaundice, biliary colic, cholangitis, or pancreatitis can result from stones retained in the common bile duct. The diagnosis can be made on ultrasonography, CT, or magnetic resonance cholangiography. ERCP with sphincterotomy and stone extraction is curative.
- **Acute ascending cholangitis** represents a medical emergency with high morbidity and mortality if biliary decompression is not performed urgently. The condition should be stabilized with IV fluids and broad-spectrum antibiotics. Drainage of the biliary tree can be performed through endoscopic (ERCP with sphincterotomy) or percutaneous approaches under fluoroscopic guidance.

OTHER GASTROINTESTINAL DISORDERS

Anorectal Disorders

- **Defecatory disorders** present with difficulty evacuating stool from the rectum or outlet constipation. The diagnosis is ideally made in the setting of compatible symptoms and abnormal testing, including DRE, balloon expulsion testing, barium defecography, MRI, anorectal manometry, and/or pelvic floor electromyography.[158] Management includes biofeedback therapy.[159]
- **Thrombosed external hemorrhoids** present as acutely painful, tense, bluish lumps covered with skin in the anal area. The thrombosed hemorrhoid can be surgically excised under local anesthesia for relief of severe pain. In less severe cases, oral analgesics, sitz baths (sitting in a tub of warm water), stool softeners, and topical ointments may provide symptomatic relief.[160]
- **Internal hemorrhoids** commonly present with either bleeding or a prolapsing mass with straining. Bulk-forming agents such as fiber supplements are useful in preventing straining

at defecation. Sitz baths and Tucks pads may provide symptomatic relief. Ointments and suppositories that contain topical analgesics, emollients, astringents, and hydrocortisone (e.g., Anusol-HC Suppositories, one per rectum bid for 7–10 days) may decrease edema but do not reduce bleeding. Hemorrhoidectomy or band ligation can be curative and is indicated in patients with recurrent or constant bleeding.[160]

- **Anal fissures** present with acute onset of pain during defecation and are often caused by hard stool. Anoscopy reveals an elliptical tear in the skin of the anus, usually in the posterior midline. Acute fissures heal in 2–3 weeks with the use of stool softeners, oral or topical analgesics, and sitz baths. The addition of oral or topical nifedipine to these conservative measures can improve pain relief and healing rates.[161]
- **Perirectal abscess** commonly presents as a painful induration in the perianal area. Patients with IBD and immunocompromised states are particularly susceptible. Prompt drainage is essential to avoid the serious morbidity associated with delayed treatment. Antimicrobials directed against bowel flora (metronidazole, 500 mg PO tid, and ciprofloxacin, 500 mg PO bid) should be administered in patients with significant inflammation, systemic toxicity, or immunocompromised states.

Celiac Sprue

GENERAL PRINCIPLES

- Celiac sprue consists of chronic inflammation of proximal small bowel mucosa from an immunologic sensitivity to **gluten** (protein found in wheat, barley, and rye), resulting in malabsorption of dietary nutrients. The condition remains incompletely recognized and underdiagnosed.[162]
- Clinical presentation can vary greatly from asymptomatic iron deficiency anemia to significant diarrhea and weight loss. Other presenting features can include osteoporosis, dermatitis herpetiformis, abnormal liver enzymes, and abdominal pain; incidental recognition at endoscopy can also occur.[163]
- More than 7% of patients with nonconstipated IBS have celiac-associated antibodies, suggesting that gluten sensitivity may trigger symptoms resembling IBS.[164]
- Celiac sprue is associated with dermatitis herpetiformis, type 1 diabetes, autoimmune thyroid disease, and Down syndrome.

DIAGNOSIS

- Noninvasive serologic tests are highly sensitive and specific and should be checked while the patient is on a gluten-containing diet. Both **IgA anti-tissue transglutaminase (TTG) and antiendomysial antibodies** have accuracies close to 100%. Quantitative IgA levels should also be checked; IgG antibodies against TTG are checked if the patient is IgA deficient.[165]
- EGD with small bowel biopsies is performed to confirm diagnosis with positive serologic testing or if suspicion remains high despite negative noninvasive testing. Classic biopsy findings include blunting or absence of villi and prominent intraepithelial lymphocytosis.
- Almost all patients with celiac sprue carry HLA-DQ2 and HLA-DQ8 molecules, so absence of these alleles has high negative predictive value when the diagnosis is in question or if patients are on a gluten-free diet.
- Nonceliac gluten sensitivity should only be considered after exclusion of celiac disease with appropriate testing; differentiation is important for risk identification for nutrient deficiency, complications, and family member risk.

TREATMENT

Medications

- Patients may require iron, folate, vitamin D, and vitamin B_{12} supplements.
- **Corticosteroids** (prednisone, 10–20 mg/d) may be required in refractory cases once inadvertent gluten ingestion has been excluded; immunosuppressive drugs have also been used.[166]

Lifestyle/Risk Modification

- A **gluten-free diet** is first-line therapy and results in prompt improvement in symptoms. Dietary nonadherence is the most frequent cause for persistent symptoms.
- If symptoms persist despite a strict gluten-free diet, radiologic and endoscopic evaluation of the small bowel should be performed to rule out complications, including collagenous colitis and **small bowel lymphoma.** However, the prognosis of adults with unrecognized celiac disease is good despite positive celiac antibodies; therefore, mass screening appears unnecessary.[167]

TROPICAL SPRUE

- It is an acquired chronic diarrheal disorder of unclear etiology affecting residents of and visitors to tropical regions. It is common in India and Pakistan; less common in Burma, Indonesia, Borneo, Singapore, Malaysia, and Vietnam; and uncommon in China, Middle East, and Africa.
- Patients usually present with profuse diarrhea, weight loss, and malabsorption, notably of vitamin B_{12} and folate.
- Histologic findings suggesting tropical sprue in the appropriate clinical context include incomplete duodenal villous blunting without development of flat mucosa, frequent involvement of the terminal ileum with more marked inflammation and villous blunting than in the duodenum, and a conspicuous eosinophil infiltrate in the lamina propria.
- Differences between tropical and celiac sprue are tabulated in Table 18-16.

ABDOMINAL TB

Abdominal tuberculosis can involve the peritoneum, gastrointestinal tract, lymph nodes, and/or solid organs.

TABLE 18-16 Differences Between Celiac Sprue and Tropical Sprue

	Celiac Sprue	Tropical Sprue
Etiology	Immune mediated	Infectious
Family history	Positive	Negative
Residence/travel to tropics	No	Yes
Gender affected	Females > males	Males = females
Part of intestine involved	Proximal	Proximal and distal
Iron deficiency anemia	Common	Rare
Severe folic acid deficiency	Rare	Common
Anti-tissue transglutaminase (TTG) and antiendomysial antibodies	Positive	Negative
Treatment	Gluten-free diet	Oral tetracycline and folic acid

Approximately 15%–25% of cases with abdominal TB have concomitant pulmonary TB.

Patients present with weight loss, abdominal pain, ascites, diarrhea, hepatomegaly, bowel obstruction, and abdominal mass.

The gross pathology is characterized by transverse ulcers, fibrosis, thickening and stricturing of the bowel wall, enlarged and matted mesenteric lymph nodes, omental thickening, and peritoneal tubercles. The most common site of involvement of the gastrointestinal tuberculosis is the ileocecal region.

Peritoneal tuberculosis occurs in three forms: wet type with ascitis, dry type with adhesions, and fibrotic type with omental thickening and loculated ascites.

The patient can contract the disease via ingestion of unpasteurized milk or undercooked meat, reactivation of latent TB, or hematogenous spread.

Diagnosis of peritoneal TB may be done by demonstration of *M. tuberculosis* in peritoneal fluid or a biopsy specimen of an infected site via culture and/or CB-NAAT.

Imaging of the abdomen, preferably CT scan, can help in the diagnosis.

Ascitic fluid examination reveals straw-colored fluid with high protein, serum ascites albumin gradient less than 1.1 g/dL, predominantly lymphocytic cells, and adenosine deaminase levels above 36 units/L.

Management is with conventional antitubercular therapy for at least 6 months. Post treatment complications such as strictures can be seen in some patients.[*,†]

AMEBIASIS

Intestinal amebiasis is caused by the protozoan *E. histolytica*. The prevalence of the disease is more in developing countries due to the socioeconomic status and poor sanitation. The majority of infections are asymptomatic. Symptoms range from mild abdominal cramps and watery diarrhea to severe colitis producing bloody diarrhea with mucus.

The most common extraintestinal manifestations are an amebic liver abscess. Rarely, amebiasis may affect the heart, brain, kidneys, spleen, and skin. Other complications include proctocolitis, toxic megacolon, peritonitis, brain abscess, and pericarditis.

Diagnosis of intestinal amebiasis is by stool microscopy, stool antigen testing, or stool PCR.

Invasive colitis is managed by metronidazole/tinidazole. Luminal agents such as paromomycin and diloxanide furoate are also used. An amebic liver abscess can be managed by aspiration using CT guidance in combination with metronidazole and chloroquine.[‡,§]

Diverticulosis and Diverticulitis

GENERAL PRINCIPLES

Definition

- **Diverticula** consist of outpouchings in the bowel, most commonly in the colon, but can also be seen elsewhere in the gut.

---

[*] McGuinness FE, Hamilton D, Al Nabulsi J. Tuberculosis of the gastrointestinal tract and peritoneum. In: McGuinness FE, editor. Clinical Imaging of Non-Pulmonary Tuberculosis. Berlin: Springer; 2000. p. 107–138.

[†] Sood R, Sethu Madhavan M. Diagnostic approach to abdominal tuberculosis. In: Agarwal AK, Jain DG, editors. Clinical Medicine: A Practical Manual for Students and Practitioners. India: Jaypee Brothers Medical Publishers (P) Ltd; 2007. p. 249.

[‡] Saidin S, Othman N, Noordin R. Update on laboratory diagnosis of amoebiasis. *Eur J Clin Microbiol Infect Dis.* 2019;38(1):15–38.

[§] Shirley DT, Farr L, Watanabe K, Moonah S. A review of the global burden, new diagnostics, and current therapeutics for amebiasis. *Open Forum Infect Dis.* 2018;5(7):ofy161.

- **Diverticular bleeding** can occur from an artery at the mouth of the diverticulum.
- **Diverticulitis** results from microperforation of a diverticulum and resultant extracolonic or intramural inflammation.
- In Asia, the prevalence is approximately 13%–25%. Here, predominantly right-sided colonic diverticula are common (unlike the Western world where left-sided diverticula are much more common).

DIAGNOSIS

Clinical Presentation

- Diverticulosis is most frequently asymptomatic. Although diverticulosis may be found in patients being investigated for symptoms of abdominal pain and altered bowel habits, a causal link is difficult to establish.
- Typical symptoms of diverticulitis include left lower quadrant abdominal pain, fevers and chills, and alteration of bowel habits. Localized left lower quadrant abdominal tenderness may be elicited on physical examination.
- Diverticular bleed is the most common cause of lower GI bleed.

Diagnostic Testing

Laboratories

Diverticulitis may be associated with an elevated white blood cell count with a left shift.

Imaging

- Diverticula are frequently seen on screening colonoscopy.
- Imaging studies, most commonly CT scans, can be useful in the diagnosis of diverticulitis.
- **Colonoscopy is contraindicated for 4–6 weeks after an episode of acute diverticulitis**, but it should be performed after that interval to exclude a perforated neoplasm.

TREATMENT

- Increased dietary fiber is generally recommended in patients with diverticulosis, although no hard data exist to support its benefit.[168]
- A low-residue diet is recommended for mild diverticulitis, although no evidence exists to support this practice.[169]

Medications

- Oral **antibiotics** (e.g., ciprofloxacin, 500 mg PO bid, and metronidazole, 500 mg PO tid, for 10–14 days) may suffice for mild diverticulitis.
- Despite optimistic initial reports, mesalamine does not appear to be effective in preventing recurrence of diverticulitis in phase III controlled trials; no therapy has been proven to prevent recurrent diverticulitis.[170]
- Hospital admission, bowel rest, IV fluids, and broad-spectrum IV antimicrobial agents are typically required in moderate to severe cases.

Surgical Management

- Surgical consultation should be obtained early in moderate to severe diverticulitis because operative intervention may be necessary should complications arise.
- Elective surgical resection is not recommended following acute uncomplicated diverticulitis, but may be necessary in recurrent diverticulitis; surgical decisions need to be individualized to each patient's unique presentation.[171]

Gastroparesis

GENERAL PRINCIPLES

Definition

Gastroparesis consists of abnormally delayed emptying of stomach contents into the small bowel in the absence of gastric outlet obstruction or ulceration, usually as a result of damage to the nerves or smooth muscle involved in gastric emptying.

Etiology

- **Mechanical obstruction should always be excluded.**
- In addition to evaluating acute metabolic derangements and potential offending medications (narcotics, anticholinergic agents, chemotherapeutic agents, glucagon-like peptide-1, and amylin analogs), patients with gastroparesis should be screened for **diabetes mellitus**, thyroid dysfunction, neurologic disease, prior gastric or bariatric surgery, and autoimmune disorders (e.g., scleroderma).
- If no predisposing cause is identified, gastroparesis is designated **idiopathic**.

DIAGNOSIS

Clinical Presentation

Gastroparesis presents with clinical symptoms of early satiety, bloating, nausea, vomiting, and abdominal pain.

Diagnostic Testing

- A **gastric-emptying study** (gamma camera scan after a radiolabeled meal) can confirm the diagnosis; medications that can delay gastric emptying (i.e., opioids and anticholinergics) should be stopped at least 48 hours prior to testing.
- Endoscopic evidence of retained food debris in the stomach after an overnight fast may be an indirect indicator of delayed gastric emptying.

TREATMENT

- First steps in management include fluid restoration, correction of electrolytes, nutritional support, and optimization of glucose control for diabetic patients. Indications for enteral feeding, preferably postpyloric, include unintentional loss of >10% of usual body weight and/or refractory symptoms requiring repeated hospitalizations prolongation. Domperidone is not available in the United States.
- **Erythromycin** (125–250 mg PO tid or 200 mg IV).[172]
- Nutritional consultation can help address nutritional deficiencies and optimize diet, especially to decrease dietary fat and insoluble fiber.[173] Small particle size diets reduce symptoms in patients with diabetic gastroparesis.[174]

Medications

- **Metoclopramide** (10 mg PO qid half an hour before meals) often represents the first line of prokinetic therapy, but has variable efficacy and side effects (drowsiness, tardive dyskinesia, parkinsonism) may be limiting.
- **Domperidone** (20 mg PO qid before meals and at bedtime) does not cross the blood–brain barrier, but hyperprolactinemia can result. ECGs should be checked at baseline and on follow-up given the risk of QT prolongation.
- **Antiemetics** may improve associated nausea and vomiting but will not improve gastric emptying.

Surgical Management

- **Enteral feeding** through a jejunostomy feeding tube may be required for supplemental nutrition and is favored over TPN.
- **Gastric electrical stimulation** using a surgically implanted stimulator (Enterra) may reduce symptoms of nausea and vomiting in half of medically refractory patients, but gastric emptying is typically not enhanced by this approach.[175]

Ischemic Intestinal Injury

GENERAL PRINCIPLES

- **Acute mesenteric ischemia (AMI)** results from arterial (or rarely venous) compromise to the superior mesenteric circulation.
- AMI is classified as either occlusive or nonocclusive mesenteric ischemia (NOMI). Occlusive mesenteric arterial ischemia (OMI) is subdivided into acute thromboembolism and acute thrombosis.
- **Ischemic colitis** results from mucosal ischemia in the inferior mesenteric circulation during a low-flow state (hypotension, arrhythmias, sepsis, vasopressors, ergotamine, aortic vascular surgery) in patients with atherosclerotic disease.[176] Vasculitis, sickle cell disease, vasospasm, and marathon running can also predispose to ischemic colitis.
- Chronic mesenteric ischemia is rare, generally characterized by postprandial abdominal pain.

DIAGNOSIS

Clinical Presentation

- Patients with AMI may present with abdominal pain, but physical examination and imaging studies can be unremarkable until infarction has occurred. As a result, diagnosis is late and mortality is high.
- Ischemic colitis may manifest as transient bleeding or diarrhea; severe insults can lead to stricture formation, gangrene, and perforation. The heterogeneity of clinical presentation of ischemic colitis helps explain why clinical suspicion is often low. Although recurrences of ischemic colitis are infrequent (<10% at 5 years), mortality is high (one-third at 5 years) and driven by unrelated causes.[177]
- Classic symptoms of chronic mesenteric ischemia include postprandial abdominal pain associated with significant weight loss, food fear, nausea, vomiting, or diarrhea.

Diagnostic Testing

- **Urgent angiography** is indicated if the suspicion for AMI is high.
- CT with contrast has high sensitivity and specificity for the diagnosis of primary AMI, whereas Doppler EUS may help exclude chronic mesenteric ischemia.[178,179]
- In patients with ischemic colitis, characteristic "**thumb-printing**" of the involved colon may be seen on plain radiographs of the abdomen.
- Colonoscopy may reveal mucosal erythema, edema, and ulceration, sometimes in a linear configuration; evidence of gangrene or necrosis is an indication for surgical intervention.

TREATMENT

- Treatment of AMI is essentially surgical and increasingly **endovascular**, whereas both arterial bypass and percutaneous angioplasty represent options for chronic mesenteric ischemia.[180]

- In patients with ischemic colitis, in the absence of peritoneal signs or evidence of gangrene or perforation, expectant management with fluid and electrolyte repletion, broad-spectrum antimicrobials, and maintenance of stable hemodynamics usually suffices.
- Evidence of gangrene or necrosis in the setting of ischemic colitis represents an indication for surgery.

Summary

- Regardless of the etiology of UGIB, resuscitative interventions are most important initial measures to improve the outcome for patients including hemodynamic stabilization, an appropriate blood transfusion strategy, with or without acid-lowering agents, while also providing subsequent urgent endoscopic assessment and intervention.
- Establishing an accurate diagnosis of the underlying dysphagia-causing pathology is important in determining the probable natural evolution of dysphagia, the ultimate aim of treatment, and which treatment modality is best placed to address the underlying deficit.
- Infection commonly causes acute diarrhea. Noninfectious etiologies become more common as the duration of diarrhea becomes chronic.
- As *Helicobacter pylori* infection leads to a number of gastric pathologies, including inflammation, gastroduodenal ulcers, and malignancies, early detection and treatment are crucial to preventing the spread of the infection.
- First-line treatment for *H. pylori*-induced PUD is a triple regimen comprising two antibiotics and a proton pump inhibitor.
- Besides the GI tract, both Crohn disease and ulcerative colitis have many extraintestinal manifestations, which need to be evaluated and managed.

Scan the QR code to access chapter references.

19 Liver Diseases

Saad Alghamdi, Tina Zhu, Avegail Flores, and Nikhil Kenny Thomas

Evaluation of Liver Disease

GENERAL PRINCIPLES

- Liver disease presents as a spectrum of clinical conditions that ranges from asymptomatic disease to end-stage liver disease (ESLD).
- A comprehensive investigation combining thorough history and physical examination with diagnostic tests, liver histology, and imaging can often establish a precise diagnosis.

DIAGNOSIS

Clinical Presentation

History

History taking should focus on the following:

- History of present illnesses
- Medication history: prescription, herbal medicine, and dietary supplements
- Toxin exposures: alcohol, illicit, and recreational drugs
- Common signs and symptoms of liver disease: icterus, ascites and edema, pruritus, encephalopathy, gastrointestinal (GI) bleeding
- Family history of liver disease
- Comorbid conditions: obesity, diabetes, hyperlipidemia, inflammatory bowel disease (IBD), systemic hypotension, human immunodeficiency virus (HIV)
- Risk factors for infection: intravenous/intranasal drug use, body piercings, tattooing, sexual history, travel to foreign countries, occupation

Physical Examination

A detailed physical examination is necessary. Physical stigmata of acute and chronic liver disease include the following:

- Jaundice ascites, peripheral edema, pleural effusions
- Splenomegaly, dilated abdominal veins, hepatomegaly/shrunken liver
- Gynecomastia and testicular hypotrophy, amenorrhea and breast atrophy in females
- Muscle wasting, white nails, Dupuytren contracture
- Telangiectasias, palmar erythema, pubic hair changes

Specific liver disorders may be associated with distinctive physical abnormalities: arthritis, acne, skin color changes (pigmentation), Kayser–Fleischer rings, parotid gland enlargement, clubbing, platypnea, orthodeoxia, or S_3 gallop.

Diagnostic Testing

Laboratories

- **Serum enzymes:** Hepatic disorders with predominant elevations in aminotransferases are referred to as hepatocellular; hepatic disorders with predominant elevation in alkaline phosphatase (ALP) are referred to as cholestatic.
  - Elevations in **aspartate aminotransferase (AST) and alanine aminotransferase (ALT)** suggest hepatocellular injury. Some caution should be taken with interpreting AST and

TABLE 19-1 Causes of Elevated Serum Aminotransferases

ALT > AST		AST > ALT	
Hepatic	**Nonhepatic**	**Hepatic**	**Nonhepatic**
Chronic mild elevations (<150 units/L)			
Chronic viral hepatitis (B, C, D) α_1-Antitrypsin deficiency Autoimmune hepatitis Hemochromatosis Medications and toxins Steatosis and steatohepatitis	Celiac disease Hyperthyroidism	Alcohol-related liver injury Cirrhosis Wilson disease	Hypothyroidism Macro-AST Myopathy Strenuous exercise
Acute severe elevations (>1000 units/L)			
Acute viral hepatitis Autoimmune hepatitis Acute bile duct obstruction Acute Budd–Chiari syndrome Hepatic artery ligation Ischemic hepatitis Medications/toxins Wilson disease	None	Medications or toxins in a patient with underlying alcoholic liver injury	Acute rhabdomyolysis

ALT elevations, as they may also be elevated in the setting of muscle or blood breakdown, e.g., rhabdomyolysis, myocardial infarction, or hemolysis (Table 19-1).

- AST:ALT ratio >2:1 is suggestive, while a ratio >3:1 is highly suggestive of alcoholic liver disease. A low level of ALT in the serum in alcoholic patients is due to an alcohol-induced deficiency of pyridoxal phosphate.
- ALT/LDH ratio <1.5 suggests ischemic hepatitis while a ratio >1.5 is seen with paracetamol toxicity or viral hepatitis.
- **ALP** is an enzyme found in a variety of tissues (bone, intestine, kidney, leukocytes, liver, and placenta). The concomitant elevation of other hepatic enzymes (e.g., **γ-glutamyl transpeptidase** [GGT] **or 5′-nucleotidase**) helps to confirm that a hepatic process is causing the ALP elevation. ALP is often elevated in biliary obstruction, space-occupying lesions or infiltrative disorders of the liver, and conditions that cause intrahepatic cholestasis (primary biliary cholangitis [PBC], primary sclerosing cholangitis [PSC], drug-induced cholestasis). *Nonhepatic causes of elevated alkaline phosphatase* are the following: bone disease, pregnancy, chronic renal failure, lymphoma or other malignancies, congestive heart failure, childhood growth, infection, or inflammation.
- If ALP is normal, raised serum γ-GT is a good guide to alcohol intake of more than 60 g/d.

- **Excretory products**
  - **Bilirubin** is a degradation product of hemoglobin and nonerythroid hemoproteins (e.g., cytochromes, myoglobin, catalases, and endothelial nitric oxide synthase). Total serum bilirubin is composed of conjugated (direct) and unconjugated (indirect) fractions. Unconjugated hyperbilirubinemia occurs as a result of excessive bilirubin production (hemolysis, hemolytic anemias, ineffective erythropoiesis, and resorption of hematomas), reduced hepatic bilirubin uptake (Gilbert syndrome and drugs such as rifampin and probenecid), or impaired bilirubin conjugation (Gilbert or Crigler-Najjar syndrome). Elevation of conjugated and unconjugated fractions occurs in

TABLE 19-2 Types of Bilirubinemia and Etiology

Predominantly Unconjugated Hyperbilirubinemia	Predominantly Conjugated Hyperbilirubinemia
1. Increased production of bilirubin	**1. Decreased hepatocellular excretion**
Hemolytic anemias	Liver damage or toxicity (e.g., hepatitis)
Resorption internal hemorrhage (e.g., GI bleeding, hematomas)	Deficiency of membrane transporters—Dubin–Johnson syndrome, Rotor syndrome
Ineffective erythropoiesis	
2. Reduced hepatic uptake	**2. Impaired intra/extrahepatic bile flow**
Drugs that interfere with membrane carrier systems	Inflammatory destruction of bile ducts (e.g., primary biliary cirrhosis)
Diffuse liver disease (hepatitis, cirrhosis)	Gallstones
Some cases of Gilbert syndrome	Carcinoma: Head of pancreas, periampullary carcinoma, cholangiocarcinoma
3. Impaired bilirubin conjugation	
Physiologic jaundice of the newborn	
Crigler–Najjar syndrome types I and II	
Gilbert syndrome	
Diffuse liver disease (hepatitis, cirrhosis)	

Dubin–Johnson and Rotor syndromes and in conditions associated with intrahepatic (i.e., hepatocellular, canalicular, or ductular damage) and extrahepatic (i.e., mechanical obstruction) cholestasis. Causes for hyperbilirubinemia are listed in Table 19-2.

- Algorithm for approach to jaundice is given in Figure 19-1.
  - **α-Fetoprotein (AFP)** is normally produced by fetal liver cells. Its production falls to normal adult levels of <10 ng/mL within 1 year of life. AFP is an insensitive and nonspecific biomarker for hepatocellular carcinoma (HCC), with a sensitivity and specificity of 61% and 81%, respectively, at a cutoff of 20 ng/mL and 22% and 100%, respectively, at a cutoff of 200 ng/mL.[1] Levels of >400 ng/mL or a rapid doubling time are suggestive of HCC; mild to moderate elevations can also be seen in acute and chronic liver inflammation. Increased concentrations in pregnancy indicate neural tube defects of the fetus.
- **Synthetic function**
  - **Serum albumin levels** and **prothrombin time.** This is mainly because hepatic synthesis of albumin tends to decrease in ESLD, and an increase in prothrombin time depends on the decreased synthesis of liver-derived coagulation factors (early liver disease).

Imaging

- **Ultrasonography** is a relatively nonexpensive, low-risk imaging test that uses sound waves to identify changes in the liver surface and parenchyma, biliary tree, and gallbladder. It is frequently used as a first-line imaging for the evaluation of right-sided abdominal pain, meal-related epigastric discomfort, and abnormal liver function tests (LFTs). It can reveal and characterize liver masses, abscesses, and cysts. Color flow Doppler ultrasonography

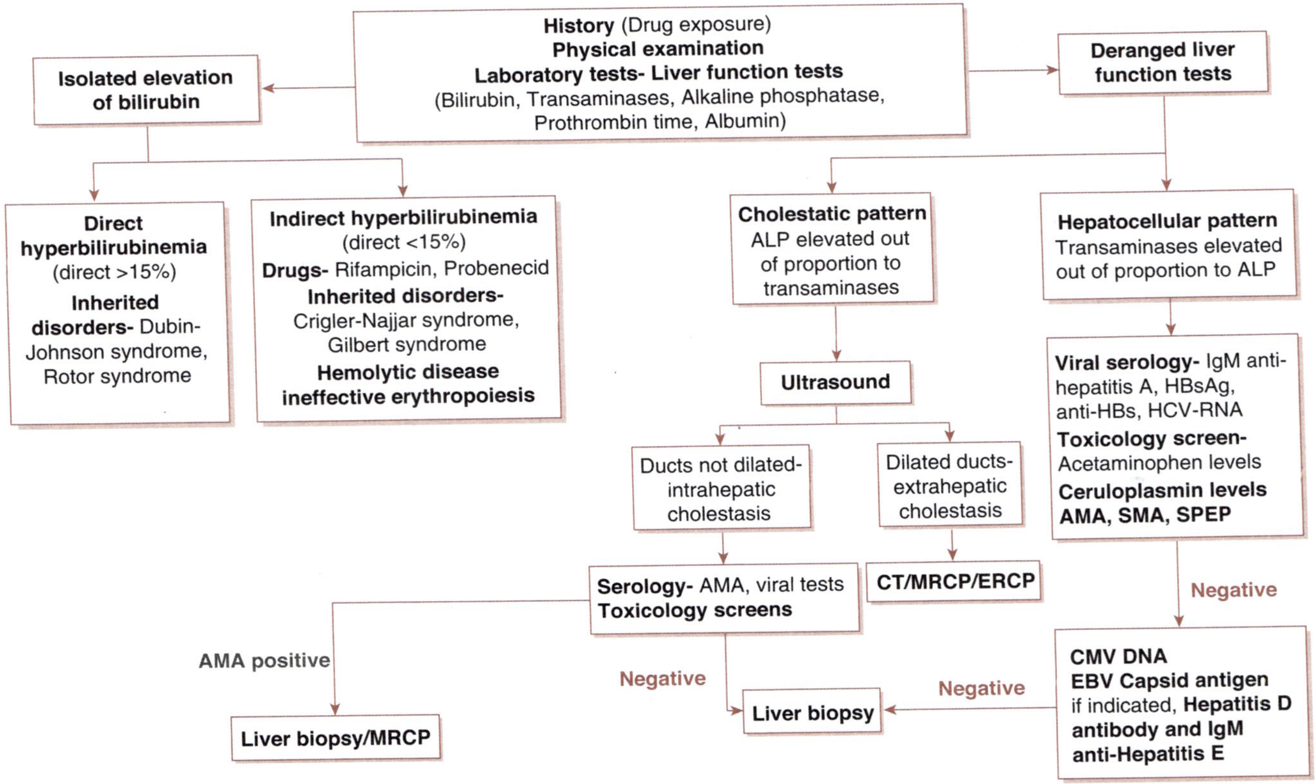

Figure 19-1 Algorithmic approach to a patient with jaundice. AMA, antimitochondrial antibody; SMA, smooth muscle antibodies; SPEP, serum protein electrophoresis.

can assess patency and direction of blood flow in the portal and hepatic veins and may be useful in the assessment of portal hypertension, which often occurs in cirrhosis. Ultrasonography is recommended for HCC screening in patients with cirrhosis. However, ultrasonography is less sensitive for detecting small or infiltrative tumors in comparison to CT or magnetic resonance imaging (MRI). Body habitus and central adiposity can limit the usefulness of the examination. The sensitivity is also operator-dependent.

- **Endoscopic ultrasound** (EUS) aids in diagnostic and therapeutic aspects of liver disease including diagnosis and management of focal hepatic lesions, simple hepatic cysts, hepatic abscesses, and portal hypertension. EUS-guided ethanol and EUS-guided neodymium-doped yttrium aluminum garnet (Nd:YAG; $Nd:Y_3Al_5O_{12}$) laser ablation are also used to treat focal hepatic lesions.
- **Helical CT scan** with IV contrast is useful to evaluate liver parenchyma. It uses iodinated contrast enhancement to define space-occupying lesions (e.g., abscess or tumor) and can calculate liver volume. Triple-phase CT (arterial, venous, and delayed phases) or quadruple-phase CT (noncontrast, arterial, venous, and delayed phase) is indicated for liver mass evaluation. A delayed phase is useful when hepatocellular carcinoma is suspected.
- **MRI** with contrast offers information similar to that provided by CT, with the additional advantage of better characterization of liver lesions, fatty infiltration, and iron deposition. It is the modality of choice in patients with an iodinated contrast allergy. However, MRI cannot be used in patients with renal failure (glomerular filtration rate [GFR] <30 mL/min/1.73 m^2) because of the very low risk of gadolinium-associated nephrogenic systemic fibrosis. Of all the cross-sectional imaging techniques, MRI provides the highest tissue contrast. This, in conjunction with various contrast agents (especially hepatobiliary contrast agents), allows for definitive noninvasive characterization of liver lesions.
- **Magnetic resonance cholangiopancreatography (MRCP)** is a specialized MRI that provides an alternative noninvasive diagnostic modality to visualize the intrahepatic and extrahepatic bile ducts. MRCP does not require contrast administration into the ductal system.
- **Elastography** uses the principle of Hook's law to measure liver stiffness as a surrogate for fibrosis. Noninvasive tools for fibrosis staging are increasingly used in the evaluation of chronic liver disease, especially in chronic hepatitis C and nonalcoholic steatohepatitis. Vibration-controlled transient elastography (VCTE or TE) was approved by the Food and Drug Administration (FDA) in 2013 and is considered the most studied noninvasive tool. Other emerging tools for noninvasive fibrosis evaluation include magnetic resonance elastography (MRE), two-dimensional and point shear wave elastography, or acoustic radiation force impulse elastography.

Diagnostic Procedures

- **Percutaneous transhepatic cholangiography (PTC) and endoscopic retrograde cholangiopancreatography (ERCP)** are invasive explorations of the biliary tree that involve injection of contrast into the tree itself. They are most effectively used to investigate abnormalities that have been detected on ultrasonography, CT, or MRI/MRCP. PTC and ERCP allow for diagnostic and therapeutic maneuvers including biopsy, brushings, stenting, and drain placement.
- **Transjugular assessment of portal pressure** is an invasive procedure to measure the hepatic venous pressure gradient (HVPG), which is the difference between the wedged (representing the portal venous pressure) and the free hepatic venous pressures. The normal HVPG pressure is <6 mm Hg. HVPG >6 mm Hg is considered portal hypertension. Complications of portal hypertension such as ascites and esophageal varices (EV) usually manifest with HVPG >10 mm Hg. EV form when HVPG is greater than 10 mm Hg and the chance of EV bleeding occurs when HVPG exceeds 12 mm Hg.

- **Liver biopsy** is an invasive procedure that is typically performed percutaneously. Suspicious liver lesions are usually biopsied with ultrasound or CT guidance, although imaging is not absolutely required. If coagulopathy, thrombocytopenia, and/or ascites are of concern, a transjugular liver biopsy can be performed instead. Finally, surgical laparoscopy is also an alternative, invasive way to obtain liver tissue. Bleeding, pain, infection, injury to nearby organs, and (rarely) death are potential complications.
- Additional noninvastive tests to assess fibrosis and cirrhosis are available. These include serum direct and indirect biomarkers of fibrosis, proprietary and nonproprietary serum biomarkers, and noninvasive imaging tools. They are being considered as alternative options to biopsy, although precise guidelines for their use are not yet defined.

VIRAL HEPATITIS

The hepatotropic viruses include hepatitis A virus (HAV), hepatitis B virus (HBV), hepatitis C virus (HCV), hepatitis D virus (HDV), and hepatitis E virus (HEV) (Tables 19-3 and 19-4). Nonhepatotropic viruses, which indirectly affect the liver, include Epstein–Barr virus (EBV), cytomegalovirus (CMV), herpesvirus (HSV), measles, Ebola, and others. Other causes and complications of acute hepatitis are listed in Tables 19-5 and 19-6.

Acute viral hepatitis is defined by an array of symptoms that may vary from mild, nonspecific symptoms to acute or fulminant hepatic failure. This condition may resolve or progress to chronic hepatitis, in certain cases, or to liver failure as a consequence of diffuse necroinflammatory liver injury.

TABLE 19-3 Clinical and Epidemiologic Features of Hepatotropic Viruses

Organism	Hepatitis A	Hepatitis B	Hepatitis C	Hepatitis D	Hepatitis E
Incubation	15–45 d	30–180 d	15–150 d	30–150 d	30–60 d
Transmission	Fecal–oral	Blood Sexual Perinatal	Blood Sexual (rare) Perinatal (rare)	Blood Sexual (rare)	Fecal–oral Organ transplantation
Risk groups	Residents of and travelers to endemic regions Children and caregivers in daycare centers	Injection drug users Multiple sexual partners Men who have sex with men Infants born to infected mothers Healthcare workers	Injection drug users Transfusion recipients	Any person with hepatitis B virus Injection drug users	Residents of and travelers to endemic regions Zoonosis: workers in pig farms
Fatality rate	1.0%	1.0%	<0.1%	2%–10%	1%
Carrier state	No	Yes	Yes	Yes	No
Chronic hepatitis	None	2%–10% in adults; 90% in children <5 yr	70%–85%	Variable	Rare
Cirrhosis	No	Yes	Yes	Yes	No

TABLE 19-4 Viral Hepatitis Serologies[a]

Hepatitis	Acute	Chronic	Recovered/Latent	Vaccinated
HAV	IgM anti-HAV+	NA	IgG anti-HAV+	IgG anti-HAV+
HCV	All tests possibly negative HCV NAT+ HCV RNA+ Anti-HCV Ab+	Anti-HCV Ab+ HCV RNA+	Anti-HCV Ab+ HCV RNA–[b]	NA
HDV	IgM anti-HDV+[c] HDV Ag+[c]	IgG anti-HDV+[c]	IgG anti-HDV+[c]	Vaccination against HBV
HEV	IgM anti-HEV	NA	IgG anti-HEV	NA

[a]For hepatitis B virus serologies, see Table 19-7.
[b]Negative HCV RNA results should be interpreted with caution. Differences are found in thresholds for detection among assays and among laboratories.
[c]Markers of HBV infection are also present because HDV cannot replicate in the absence of HBV.
Ab, antibody; HAV, hepatitis A virus; HCV, hepatitis C virus; HDV, hepatitis D virus; HEV, hepatitis E virus; NA, not applicable.

TABLE 19-5 Causes for Acute Hepatitis

Infectious: Viruses (Described Earlier), Bacteria, Parasites, Fungi	Toxin/Drugs: Alcohol (Described Later)	Immunologic: Autoimmune Hepatitis, Primary Sclerosing Cholangitis
Metabolic or hereditary • Nonalcoholic fatty liver disease • Hemochromatosis • Wilson disease	**Pregnancy-related** • Preeclampsia • Acute fatty liver of pregnancy • HELLP syndrome	**Ischemic and vascular** • Cardiogenic shock • Hypotension • Cocaine, methamphetamine, ephedrine • Acute Budd–Chiari syndrome

TABLE 19-6 Complications of Acute Viral Hepatitis

Hepatic Complications	Extrahepatic Complications
Fulminant hepatic failure	Aplastic anemia
Cholestatic viral hepatitis	Renal failure
Relapsing hepatitis	Polyarteritis nodosa
Post-hepatitis syndrome	Henoch–Schoenlein purpura
Chronic hepatitis	Myocarditis
Cirrhosis	Transverse myelitis
Hepatocellular carcinoma	Peripheral neuropathy

Acute or fulminant hepatic failure (FHF) is defined as a clinical syndrome characterized by evidence of coagulopathy (INR >1.5) and any degree of altered mental status in a patient without preexisting liver disease and duration of illness <26 weeks.

Chronic viral hepatitis is defined as the presence of persistent (>6 months) virologic replication, as determined by serologic and molecular studies, with necroinflammatory and fibrotic injury. Symptoms and biochemical abnormalities may vary from none to moderate. Histopathologic classification of chronic viral hepatitis is based on etiology, grade, and stage. Grading and staging are measures of the severity of inflammation and fibrosis, respectively. Chronic viral hepatitis may lead to cirrhosis and HCC.

Hepatitis A Virus

GENERAL PRINCIPLES

- HAV is an **RNA virus** in the **picornavirus family.** It is transmitted via the fecal–oral route and is the most common cause of acute viral hepatitis worldwide.
- Large-scale outbreaks because of contamination of food and drinking water can occur.
- A vaccine is available, with two doses given at least 6 months apart.
- The period of greatest infectivity is 2 weeks before the onset of clinical illness.
- Viral shedding in infected patients' feces continues for 2–3 weeks after the onset of symptoms.

DIAGNOSIS

- HAV can be silent (subclinical), especially in children and young adults. Symptoms vary from mild illness to FHF and commonly include malaise, fatigue, pruritus, headache, abdominal pain, myalgias, arthralgias, nausea, vomiting, anorexia, and fever.
- **Physical examination** may reveal jaundice, hepatomegaly, and, in rare cases, lymphadenopathy, splenomegaly, or a vascular rash.
- **Aminotransferase** elevations range from 10 to 100 times the upper limit of normal.
- The diagnosis of acute HAV is made by the detection of **IgM anti-HAV antibodies.**
- The **recovery phase** and **immunity phase** are characterized by the presence of **IgG anti-HAV antibodies and the decline of IgM anti-HAV antibodies.**
- Liver biopsy is rarely needed.
- **FHF** is rare, but the risk increases with age: 0.1% in patients younger than 15 years to >1% in patients older than 40 years.

TREATMENT

- Supportive symptomatic treatment.
- Liver transplantation should be considered for FHF.

OUTCOME AND PROGNOSIS

- Symptoms of acute HAV hepatitis may last from weeks to months (median 8 weeks). HAV does not progress to chronic viral hepatitis (and therefore neither cirrhosis nor HCC).
- A prolonged cholestatic disease, characterized by persistent jaundice and waxing and waning of liver enzymes, is more frequently seen in adults.

Hepatitis B Virus

GENERAL PRINCIPLES

- **HBV** is a **DNA virus** in the **hepadnavirus family.** The United States is considered an area of low prevalence for the infection. Eight genotypes of HBV have been identified (A through H). The prevalence of HBV genotypes varies depending on the geographic location. Genotypes A, B, and C are the most prevalent in the United States.
- Modes of transmission include vertical (mother to infant) and horizontal (person to person) via the following routes: parenteral or percutaneous (e.g., injection drug use, needlestick injuries), direct contact with the blood or open sores of an infected person, and sexual contact with an infected individual.
- The rate of progression from acute to chronic HBV is approximately 90% for a perinatal-acquired infection, 20%–50% for infections acquired between the age of 1–5 years, and <5% for an adult-acquired infection.
- The course of HBV infection is affected by factors including coinfections with hepatitis C and D viruses and the HIV as well as hepatotoxic factors (primarily alcohol consumption).
- Acute hepatitis B treatment is rarely needed unless there is severe hepatic dysfunction (prolonged jaundice, coagulopathy, or encephalopathy).

DIAGNOSIS

Clinical Presentation

- According to the natural history of chronic HBV infection, four different **clinical phases** have been defined (Table 19-7). Some persons will not fit the phases when the ALT and HBV DNA do not fall in the same phase and are considered to be in an indeterminate phase.
  - **High replicative phase with HBeAg positivity**/immune tolerant
  - **HBeAg-positive immune-reactive phase**
  - **Inactive HBV carrier phase**
  - Immune reactivation phase (HBeAg-negative chronic hepatitis)
- **Occult infection (HBsAg-negative)** is most commonly associated with undetectable or periodically very low serum concentrations of HBV-DNA accompanied by its presence in the liver.
- **Extrahepatic manifestations** include polyarteritis nodosa, glomerulonephritis, cryoglobulinemia, serum sickness–like illness, membranous nephropathy, membranoproliferative glomerulonephritis, and papular acrodermatitis (predominantly in children).

Diagnostic Testing

- HBV antigens (hepatitis B surface antigen [HBsAg] and HBeAg) can be detected in the serum. In the liver tissue, **HBsAg** stains in the hepatocyte cytoplasm and **hepatitis B core antigen (HBcAg)** stains in the hepatocyte nuclei.
- **HBV DNA** is the most accurate marker of viral replication. It is detected by polymerase chain reaction (PCR).
- For use of HBV markers in clinical practice, see Table 19-7.
- **Liver biopsy** is useful to assess the degree of inflammation (grade) and fibrosis (stage) as well as other potential histologic abnormalities in patients with chronic hepatitis. Liver histology is an important adjuvant diagnostic test in guiding treatment decisions.

TABLE 19-7 Use of Hepatitis B Virus (HBV) Markers in Clinical Practice

Test	Acute HBV	Resolved Acute HBV	Immune-Tolerant Chronic HBV	Immune-Active Chronic HBV (Wild-Type)	Immune-Active Chronic HBV (Precore or Basal Core Promoter Mutant)	Low-Replication Chronic HBV	Vaccine Immunity
HBsAg	+	–	+	+	+	+	–
HBeAg	+	–	+	+	–	–	–
Anti-HBs	–	+	–	–	–	–	+
Anti-HBe	–	+	–	–	+	+	–
IgM anti-HBc	+	–	–	–	–	–	–
IgG anti-HBc	–	+	–	+	+	+	–
HBV DNA	$>10^6$ IU/mL	Neg	$>10^{6-10}$ IU/mL	$>10^6$ IU/mL	$>10^{3-4}$ IU/mL	$<10^2$ IU/mL	Neg
ALT/AST	++++	Normal	Normal	+++	++	Normal	Normal

ALT, alanine aminotransferase; AST, aspartate aminotransferase; HBc, hepatitis B core antigen; HBeAg, hepatitis B e antigen; HBsAg, hepatitis B surface antigen; Neg, negative.

TREATMENT

The treatment goal is viral eradication or suppression to prevent progression to end-stage liver disease (ESLD) and HCC. End points of treatment include the following:

- Normalization of serum ALT
- Maintained suppression of serum HBV DNA levels to undetectable levels
- HBeAg clearance and seroconversion to antibody anti-HBe
- HBsAg clearance and seroconversion to antibody anti-HBs
- Improvement in liver histology

Chronic HBV treatment is only recommended in immune active phase, immune reactivation phase, cirrhosis, or when extrahepatic manifestations are present (see Table 19-8).

TABLE 19-8 AASLD Treatment Guidelines for Chronic Hepatitis B

	ALT	HBV DNA	Treatment?	Fibroscan	Biopsy?[a]
HBeAg positive	<ULN	Any	No. If HBV DNA > 20,000, monitor ALT and HBV DNA levels every 3–6 mo and HBeAg every 6–12 mo.		
	>ULN but <2× ULN	2000–20,000 IU/mL	Treat if lab abnormalities persist for >6 mo. Treat if ALT elevation persists and patient is over age 40 or if there is at least F2 fibrosis or A3 inflammation.	Recommended	Consider
		>20,000	Treat if ALT elevation persists and patient is over age 40 or if there is at least F2 fibrosis or A3 inflammation.	Recommended	Consider
	>2× ULN	2000–20,000 IU/mL	Treat if lab abnormalities persist for >6 mo. Treat if ALT elevation persists and patient is over age 40 or if there is at least F2 fibrosis or A3 inflammation.	Recommended	Consider
		>20,000	**Treat**	Recommended	

(Continued)

TABLE 19-8 AASLD Treatment Guidelines for Chronic Hepatitis B (Continued)

	ALT	HBV DNA	Treatment?	Fibroscan	Biopsy?[a]
HBeAg negative	<ULN	>2000 IU/mL	No. Monitor ALT and HBV DNA every 3 mo for 1 yr and then every 6 mo.		
		<2000	No. Monitor ALT and HBV DNA levels every 3–6 mo and and HBsAg annually.	Recommended	
	>ULN but <2× ULN	>2000 IU/mL	Treat if staging of liver disease is a least F2 fibrosis or A3 inflammation or age >40	Recommended	Consider
		<2000	Treat if staging of liver disease is a least F2 fibrosis or A3 inflammation or age >40	Recommended	Consider
	>2× ULN	>2000 IU/mL	**Treat**		
		<2000	Treat if staging of liver disease is a least F2 fibrosis or A3 inflammation or age >40		Consider

[a]Biopsy indicated for >40 years of age, ALT persistently 1–2× ULN, and family history of hepatocellular carcinoma. Alternative methods of noninvasive fibrosis testing may be used. AALSD, American Association for the Study of Liver Diseases; ALT, alanine aminotransferase; HBeAg, hepatitis B e antigen; HBV, hepatitis B virus; ULN, upper limit of normal (ULN for AALSD: 35 units/L for males, 25 units/L for females).

Medications

Medications for the treatment of hepatitis B are divided into three main groups: nucleoside analogs (entecavir, lamivudine, telbivudine), nucleotide analogs (tenofovir, adefovir), and the interferons (IFNs). Current practices recommend entecavir, tenofovir, and interferon.

- **Entecavir** is a potent anti-HBV oral nucleoside (guanosine) analog and is well tolerated. The dose is 0.5–1.0 mg daily in naïve and lamivudine (LAM)-resistant patients. Entecavir has a high genetic barrier for resistance (1.2%) over several years. However, in patients resistant to LAM, the resistance to entecavir could be as high as 40%. In patients with renal impairment, dose adjustment is needed. Entecavir is pregnancy category C.
- **Tenofovir disoproxil fumarate** (TDF) is a potent anti-HBV oral nucleotide (acyclic) analog and is well tolerated. The dose is 300 mg daily. Tenofovir has a high genetic barrier for resistance; no clinical resistance has been identified thus far. It is rarely reported to

induce renal failure and Fanconi syndrome and may also lead to decreased bone density. Tenofovir is pregnancy category B.

- **Tenofovir alafenamide** (TAF) is preferred over TDF for patients with renal or bone disease (or risk of) and appears to have comparable efficacy with TDF. Consider TAF for patients with GFR < 60, chronic steroid use, osteoporosis, or history of fragility fractures. For patients who cannot tolerate TDF and who have previously been exposed to lamivudine, switching to TAF is preferred over switching to entecavir.
- **Pegylated IFNs** (α2a and α2b, in their pegylated form) are antiviral, immunomodulatory, and antiproliferative glycoproteins that have been used in the treatment of chronic HBV for several years. IFNs are parenteral agents and associated with a poor tolerability profile, especially in patients with advanced liver disease. Long-term studies have shown a durable benefit in responders. Neither IFN nor pegylated IFN-α induces antiviral resistance. The IFNs are pregnancy category C.

Treatment Algorithm

See Table 19-9.

Treatment Responses

- **Complete response:** Undetectable HBV-DNA and seroconversion to anti-HBs
- **Virologic response:** Undetectable HBV-DNA with HBsAg presence

TABLE 19-9 Guideline-Based Treatment of HBV

	HBeAg+		HBeAg–		Cirrhosis (HBeAg±)	
	HBV DNA (IU/mL)	ALT (units/L)	HBV DNA (IU/mL)	ALT (units/L)	HBV DNA (IU/mL)	ALT (units/L)
AASLD, 2018	>20,000	≥2x ULN or significant liver disease	≥2000	≥2x ULN or significant liver disease	Detectable	Any
AATA, 2018	>2000	>ULN	>2000	>ULN	Detectable	Any
EASL, 2017	>2000	>ULN and/or at least moderate liver necroinflammation or fibrosis	>2000	>ULN and/or at least moderate liver necroinflammation or fibrosis	Detectable	Any
	>20,000	>2x ULN	>20,000	>2x ULN	Detectable	Any

ULN for ALT is defined by the AASLD as 35 units/L for men and 25 units/L for women, and defined by the EASL as approximately 40 units/L for both men and women. ULN is defined by the AATA based on the physician's local laboratory.

AASLD, American Association for the Study of Liver Diseases; AATA, Asian American Treatment Algorithm; ALT, alanine aminotransferase; EASL, European Association for the Study of the Liver; HBeAg, hepatitis B e-antigen; HBV, hepatitis B virus; HBV DNA, hepatitis B virus deoxyribonucleic acid; ULN, upper limit of normal.

- **Partial virologic response:** Decrease in HBV-DNA level by more than 1 $\log_{10}$ IU/mL in relation to the baseline value and its maintenance above the detection threshold over the 6-month course of drug therapy (treatment with drugs with a high genetic barrier should be continued)
- **Virologic breakthrough:** Increase in HBV-DNA level by at least 1 $\log_{10}$ IU/mL in patients with previously undetectable viremia during the course of therapy
- **Primary drug resistance:** No reduction in viremia by at least 1 $\log_{10}$ IU/mL in relation to the baseline value during a 3-month period of drug therapy

PREVENTION

- **Preexposure prophylaxis**
  - **Consider HBV vaccination** in all patients, especially those from high-risk groups. HBV vaccines are made of inactivated viruses and are safe for immunocompromised patients.
  - The vaccination schedule is three IM injections at 0, 1, and 6 months in infants or healthy adults. Protective antibody response (anti-HBs positive) is observed in >90% after the third dose.
- **Postexposure prophylaxis**
  - **Infants born to HBsAg-positive mothers should receive HBV vaccine and hepatitis B immunoglobulin (HBIg), 0.5 mL, within 12 hours of birth.** Immunized infants should be tested at approximately 12 months of age for HBsAg, anti-HBs, and anti-HBc.
  - Persons **who are unvaccinated or do not demonstrate anti-HBs, and have had sexual contact or needlestick with an individual with HBV,** should receive HBIg (0.04–0.07 mL/kg) and the first dose of HBV vaccine at different sites. This should be done as soon as possible, preferably within 48 hours but no more than 7 days after exposure. A second dose of HBIg should be administered 30 days after exposure, and the vaccination series should be completed.
  - Persons who have received all three doses of a hepatitis B vaccination series and have confirmed anti-HBs positivity require no further treatment.
  - Postexposure prophylaxis with HBIg plus a nucleotide or nucleoside analog should be used initially after liver transplantation to prevent HBV recurrence in certain patients.

OUTCOME AND PROGNOSIS

Chronic hepatitis B

- Morbidity and mortality in chronic HBV are linked to the level and persistence of viral replication. Spontaneous clearance of HBsAg occurs in 0.5% of patients annually.
- For HCV/HBV coinfected individuals, there is a risk of HBV reactivation during HCV treatment with direct-acting antivirals (DAAs).
- Once the diagnosis of chronic HBV is established, the 5-year cumulative incidence of developing cirrhosis ranges from 15% to 40%.
- 5%–10% cases of chronic HBV progress to HCC **with or without preceding cirrhosis.**

Hepatitis C Virus

GENERAL PRINCIPLES

- HCV is an RNA virus in the **flavivirus** family. There are six genotypes with multiple subtypes. Genotype 1 accounts for about 75% and genotypes 2 and 3 account for about 20% of HCV infections in the United States.

- **HCV** is the most common chronic bloodborne infection and is a global health problem, with approximately **180 million carriers worldwide**.
- The most frequent mode of transmission is parenteral. Less common modes of transmission include high-risk sexual practices and perinatal transmission. Transmission by transfusion of blood products (and their derivatives) and organ transplantation has been reduced to near zero in developed countries because of screening.

DIAGNOSIS

Clinical Presentation

- The incubation period varies from 15 to 150 days.
- **Acute HCV hepatitis** is defined as presenting within 6 months of exposure to HCV. During this time, there is a 20%–50% chance of spontaneous resolution of infection.[2] Symptoms can be nonspecific and include malaise, fatigue, pruritus, headache, abdominal pain, myalgias, arthralgias, nausea, vomiting, anorexia, and fever.
- **Chronic HCV hepatitis** runs an indolent course, sometimes for decades, with fatigue as the only symptom. It may only become clinically apparent late in the natural course, when symptoms associated with advanced liver disease develop.
- **Extrahepatic manifestations** include mixed cryoglobulinemia (10%–25% of patients with HCV), glomerular diseases (mixed cryoglobulinemia syndrome, membranous nephropathy, polyarteritis nodosa), porphyria cutanea tarda, cutaneous necrotizing vasculitis, lichen planus, lymphoma, diabetes mellitus, and other autoimmune disorders.

Diagnostic Testing

- **Antibodies against HCV (anti-HCV)** can be detectable within 2 weeks of infection with third-generation enzyme immunoassay (EIA). **Antibodies do not confer immunity.** The third-generation assays have a sensitivity of 97% and specificity of 99%. Anti-HCV testing is now available as point-of-care assay with equivalent performance as laboratory-based testing. A false-positive test (anti-HCV positive with HCV RNA negative) may be detected in the setting of autoimmune hepatitis (AIH) or hypergammaglobulinemia. A false-negative test (anti-HCV negative with HCV RNA positive) may be seen in HIV immunosuppressed individuals and in patients on hemodialysis.
- **HCV RNA** detected by PCR is the gold standard for confirming the diagnosis if HCV infection and monitoring treatment response with detection limits of 12–43 IU/mL. **HCV nucleic acid testing (NAT)** can detect infection in as early as 3–5 days and may be used as a confirmatory test.
- **HCV genotypes and subtypes** can be detected by commercially available serologic and molecular assays. HCV genotype, at the present time, guides direct-acting antiviral treatment (DAAT) choice. In the future, HCV genotype may no longer be needed pretreatment as pangenotypic regimen become more frequently available.
- **Liver biopsy** is rarely used to guide HCV treatment because of the availability of highly effective DAAT.

TREATMENT

- Treatment is recommended for all patients with chronic HCV infection.
- Patients with limited life expectancy that cannot be remediated by HCV treatment, liver transplantation, or another directed therapy should not be treated.
- The **goal of treatment** is eradication of HCV, as determined by sustained virologic response (SVR). SVR is defined as the absence of detectable HCV RNA 12 weeks after

completion of therapy. SVR reduces morbidity and end-stage complications of HCV infection including cirrhosis, HCC, and death.

Medications

Current treatment regimens for chronic HCV are all **oral and IFN-free** and may include the following:

- **Ribavirin** is a guanosine analog antiviral agent (nucleoside inhibitor). It is generally not effective when used alone but plays an important role in combination treatment.
- **Direct-acting antivirals** (DAAs) target specific nonstructural proteins of the virus, resulting in disruption of viral replication. Current treatment regimens for HCV include the combination of more than one DAA with or without ribavirin (Table 19-10).
  - **Nonstructural proteins 3/4A (NS3/4A) protease inhibitors (PIs)** include glecaprevir, asunaprevir, grazoprevir, voxilaprevir, and paritaprevir.
  - **NS5A inhibitors** include ledipasvir, daclatasvir, elbasvir, velpatasvir, pibrentasvir, and ombitasvir.
  - **NS5B polymerase inhibitors (NPIs)** include sofosbuvir and dasabuvir.
  - Availability of DAA pangenotypic (effective on all HCV genotypes) regimens will likely be favored in the market.

The selection of a particular treatment regimen is based on several factors, most notably:

- Treatment-naïve (never-treated) or treatment-experienced (previously failed treatment)
- HCV genotype and subtype
- Cirrhosis
- Decompensated cirrhosis
- Potential drug interactions, especially the use of acid-blocking medications
- Severe chronic renal disease or end-stage renal disease
- Comorbid conditions (e.g., posttransplant state and HIV coinfection)

For chronic infection, all treatment regimens have similar efficacy.

TABLE 19-10 First-line Recommended DAA Therapies for Patients with and without Cirrhosis

Genotype	GT1	GT2	GT3	GT4	GT5/6
First-line DAA regime for patients without cirrhosis	Sofosbuvir/ Ledipasvir*	Sofosbuvir/ Ledipasvir**	Sofosbuvir/ Ledipasvir***	Sofosbuvir/ Ledipasvir*	Sofosbuvir/ Ledipasvir*
Duration	8–12 weeks	12 weeks	12 weeks	12 weeks	12 weeks
First-line DAA regime for patients with cirrhosis	Sofosbuvir/ Ledipasvir*	Sofosbuvir/ Ledipasvir**	Glecaprevir/ Pibrentasvir	Sofosbuvir/ Ledipasvir*	Sofosbuvir/ Ledipasvir*
Duration	24 weeks	24 weeks	16 weeks	24 weeks	24 weeks

*GLEC/PIB (8 weeks) or SOF/VEL (12 weeks) may be used depending on patient-specific factors or drug-drug interactions (DDIs)

**GLEC/PIB (8 weeks) may be used depending on patient-specific factors or DDIs

***GLEC/PIB (8–12 weeks) may be used depending on patient-specific factors or DDIs

PREVENTION

No pre- or postexposure prophylaxis or vaccine exists. Prevention of high-risk behaviors and lifestyle modifications should be encouraged.

OUTCOME AND PROGNOSIS

HCC develops in approximately **2%–4% of patients per year.**

Hepatitis D Virus

HDV is a circular RNA virus and is the only member of the genus *Delta virus*. It is found throughout the world and is endemic to the Mediterranean basin, the Middle East, and the Amazon basin of South America. Outside these areas, infections occur primarily in individuals who have received transfusions or inject drugs. **HDV requires the presence of HBV for infection and replication.** In countries such as the United States where HDV infection is rare, testing for HDV coinfection is not necessary in all patients with HBV. In patients with coinfection (acute hepatitis B and D), the course is transient and self-limited. The rate of progression to chronicity is similar to the one reported for acute HBV. **IFN-α** is the **treatment of choice** for chronic hepatitis D.

Hepatitis E Virus

HEV is an **RNA virus** from the Hepeviridae family. It is considered a zoonotic disease with reservoirs in pigs, wild boar, and deer. Transmission is **fecal-oral**, such as that of HAV, and HEV can occur in outbreaks. Acute hepatitis E is clinically indistinguishable from other acute viral hepatitis and is usually self-limited, with the exception of pregnancy (mortality can be as high as 10%–30% in the third trimester), preexisting chronic liver disease, and organ transplantation. Hepatitis E can rarely progress to chronic infection (HEV RNA for >6 months). Most cases have occurred in solid organ transplant recipients or immunosuppressed individuals (e.g., HIV). In a retrospective multicenter study of 59 transplant recipients with chronic hepatitis E, ribavirin monotherapy for 3 months achieved an SVR of 78%.[3]

DRUG-INDUCED LIVER INJURY

GENERAL PRINCIPLES

- The National Institutes of Health (NIH) maintains a searchable database of over 1000 drugs, herbal medications, and dietary supplements that have been associated with drug-induced liver injury (DILI) at http://livertox.nih.gov/.
- There are three major classifications of DILI that occur as a result of both intrinsic and idiosyncratic hepatotoxicity:
    - Hepatocellular injury refers to injury to the liver cell.
    - Cholestatic injury refers to injury to the biliary system or to hepatocytes with resulting intrahepatic cholestasis.
    - Mixed hepatocellular and cholestatic injury refers to injury to both.
- DILI is associated with approximately 50% of all cases of FHF in the United States, with acetaminophen being the most common causative agent. Acute DILI progresses to chronic injury in 5%–10% of cases.[4]

- Besides acute DILI, other less common types of DILI include chronic hepatitis, chronic cholestasis, granulomatous hepatitis, fibrosis or cirrhosis, and carcinogenesis. Patients with chronic DILI who develop fibrosis or cirrhosis may show signs of hepatic decompensation comparable with fibrosis or cirrhosis from other etiologies. Common causes for DILI and examples are mentioned in Table 19-11.

DIAGNOSIS

Clinical Presentation

- The acute presentation can be clinically silent. Symptoms are nonspecific and include nausea/vomiting, malaise, fatigue, jaundice, pruritus, and abdominal pain. In the acute setting, the majority of patients will recover after cessation of the offending drug.
- Fever and rash may also be seen in association with hypersensitivity reactions.

Diagnostic Criteria

- Clinical suspicion
- Temporal relation of liver injury to drug usage

TABLE 19-11 Clinicopathologic Classification of Drug-Induced Liver Disease

Category	Drugs
Hepatic adaptation	Phenytoin, warfarin Rifampin, flavaspidic acid
Dose-dependent hepatotoxicity	Acetaminophen, nicotinic acid, amodiaquine, hycanthone
Other cytopathic toxicity, acute steatosis	Valproic acid, didanosine, HAART agents, fialuridine, L-asparaginase, some herbal medicines
Acute hepatitis	Isoniazid, dantrolene, nitrofurantoin, halothane, sulfonamides, phenytoin, disulfiram, acebutolol, etretinate, ketoconazole, terbinafine, troglitazone
Chronic hepatitis	Nitrofurantoin, etretinate, diclofenac, minocycline, nefazodone
Granulomatous hepatitis	Allopurinol, carbamazepine, hydralazine, quinidine, quinine
Cholestasis without hepatitis	Oral contraceptives, androgens
Cholestatic hepatitis	Chlorpromazine, tricyclic antidepressants, erythromycins, amoxicillin–clavulanic acid
Cholestasis with bile duct injury	Chlorpromazine, flucloxacillin, dextropropoxyphene
Chronic cholestasis	Chlorpromazine, haloperidol, erythromycin, cimetidine/ranitidine, nitrofurantoin, imipramine, azathioprine
Vanishing bile duct syndrome	Chlorpromazine, flucloxacillin, trimethoprim–sulfamethoxazole
Sclerosing cholangitis	Intra-arterial floxuridine, intralesional scolicidals
Steatohepatitis	Perhexiline, amiodarone
Vascular disorders	Contraceptive drugs, anabolic steroids, azathioprine
Tumors	Contraceptive pill, danazol

- Resolution of liver injury after the suspected agent has been discontinued (except in cases of chronic DILI)

Diagnostic Testing

Biochemical Abnormalities

- The R-ratio is calculated by dividing ALT by ALP, using multiples of ULN for both values. The R-ratios of >5 define hepatocellular, <2 define cholestatic, and between 2 and 5 define a mixed pattern of enzymes.
- **Hepatocellular injury:** AST and ALT elevation more than two times the upper limit of normal.
- **Cholestatic injury:** ALP and conjugated bilirubin elevation more than two times the upper limit of normal.
- **Mixed injury:** Increases in all of the mentioned biochemical abnormalities to more than two times the upper limit of normal.

Diagnostic Procedures

Liver biopsy may be indicated if the diagnosis is unclear.

TREATMENT

- Treatment includes cessation of offending drug and institution of supportive measures.
- An attempt to remove the agent from the GI tract should be made in most cases of acute toxic ingestion using lavage or cathartics (see Chapter 28, Toxicology).
- Management of acetaminophen overdose is a medical emergency (see Chapter 28, Toxicology).

Surgical Management

Liver transplantation may be an option for patients with drug-induced FHF.

OUTCOME AND PROGNOSIS

Prognosis of DILI is often unique to the offending medication.

ALCOHOLIC LIVER DISEASE

GENERAL PRINCIPLES

- Alcohol use disorder is a significant medical and socioeconomic problem.
- Patients may underestimate or minimize their reported alcohol abuse.
- The spectrum of alcoholic liver disease includes fatty liver, alcoholic steatohepatitis, severe alcoholic hepatitis, and cirrhosis. Fatty liver is the most common and occurs in up to 90% of alcoholics.
- Of all excessive alcohol users, between 10% and 20% will develop cirrhosis and 35% will develop alcoholic hepatitis. More than half of the latter will progress to cirrhosis.
- Alcoholic cirrhosis is a common cause of ESLD and HCC.

DIAGNOSIS

Clinical Presentation

- **Fatty liver**
  - Patients are usually asymptomatic.
  - Clinical findings include hepatomegaly and mild liver enzyme abnormalities.

- **Alcoholic hepatitis**
  - Alcoholic hepatitis may be clinically silent or severe enough to lead to rapid development of hepatic failure and death.
  - Symptoms include fever, abdominal pain, anorexia, nausea, vomiting, weight loss, and jaundice.
  - In severe cases, patients may develop transient portal hypertension.
- **Alcoholic cirrhosis**
  - The presentation is variable, from clinically silent disease to decompensated cirrhosis.
  - Patients frequently give a history of drinking until the onset of symptoms.

Diagnostic Testing

Laboratories

- In alcoholic fatty liver, LFTs may be normal or demonstrate **mild elevation in serum aminotransferases** (AST greater than ALT) and ALP.
- In alcoholic hepatitis, LFTs typically demonstrate elevation in serum aminotransferases (AST greater than ALT with a 3:1 or 2:1 ratio) and ALP. Hyperbilirubinemia (conjugated) and elevated prothrombin time (PT)/international normalized ratio (INR) may also be observed.
- Laboratory abnormalities associated with a poor prognosis include renal failure, leukocytosis, a markedly elevated total bilirubin, and elevation of PT/INR that does not normalize with subcutaneous or IV vitamin K. Administration of oral vitamin K is not recommended because of poor gut absorption in patients with jaundice.
- A number of classification systems have been developed to risk-stratify patients with alcoholic hepatitis and assess response to treatment:
  - **Maddrey's Discriminant Function (DF)** = $4.6 \times (PT_{patient} - PT_{control})$ + serum bilirubin. Scores <32 and >32 have 93% and 68% 1-month survival, respectively.
  - **The Glasgow Alcoholic Hepatitis Score (GAHS)** incorporates patient age, white blood cell count, blood urea, PT/INR, and serum bilirubin. A score <9 has no difference in survival between untreated and steroid-treated patients. A score >9 has a difference in 1-month survival between untreated (52% 1-month survival) and steroid-treated (78% 1-month survival) patients.[5]
  - The **Lille model** incorporates age, renal insufficiency, albumin, PT, bilirubin, and the evolution of bilirubin at day 7 (bilirubin on day 7–bilirubin on day 0) to predict 6-month mortality in patients with severe alcoholic hepatitis who have received steroids. In a prospective study, a score of ≥0.45 was associated with a lower 6-month survival compared with a score <0.45 (25% vs. 85%). A score >0.45 suggests that a patient is not responding to steroid therapy.[6]
  - **Age, serum bilirubin, INR, and serum creatinine (ABIC) score:** (Age × 0.1) + (serum bilirubin × 0.08) + (serum creatinine × 0.3) + (INR × 0.8) was validated in an independent prospective cohort. Using cutoff values of 6.71 and 9, the score identified patients with AH who have a low (100% survival), intermediate (70% survival), and high (25% survival) risk of death at 90 days.

Diagnostic Procedures

- Liver biopsy may be indicated if the diagnosis of alcoholic hepatitis is unclear.
- Typical histopathologic findings in alcoholic liver disease include hepatocyte ballooning with and without Mallory-Denk bodies, lobular inflammation with neutrophilic infiltrates, hepatocyte necrosis, periportal fibrosis, perivenular and pericellular fibrosis, ductal proliferation, and fatty changes.

TREATMENT

- Encourage alcohol abstinence.
- Referral to programs or counselors for alcohol rehabilitation.
- Evaluate and correct nutrient deficiencies. Nutrition support can be given orally via a small-bore feeding tube or via peripheral parenteral nutrition (PPN) or total parenteral nutrition (TPN). Good nutrition improves nitrogen balance, may improve LFTs, and may decrease hepatic fat accumulation, but it generally does not enhance survival.
- Baclofen may be considered to decrease or suppress alcohol cravings.

Medications

Treatment of acute alcoholic hepatitis with corticosteroids is controversial. However, there is evidence that patients with a DF >32 and GAHS >9 may have a short-term benefit from steroid therapy. An early decrease in bilirubin levels after 1 week of steroids portends a better prognosis (Lille score).

- **Oral prednisolone** (40 mg/d PO for 4 weeks, followed by a taper over 2–4 weeks) is a steroid treatment for patients with severe alcoholic hepatitis. Prednisolone is preferred (but not demonstrated to be better) over prednisone as the latter requires conversion to its active form, prednisolone, within the liver. It has been tried in severe cases (discriminant function >32) in the absence of any infection. Prednisolone demonstrated a reduction on short-term mortality (28 days), which did not reach significance. There was no benefit on medium- or long-term mortality (90 days and 1 year, respectively).[7]
- **Pentoxifylline** (400 mg PO tid for 4 weeks) is a nonselective phosphodiesterase inhibitor that, in a recent trial, did not show improved outcomes in this patient group.

Surgical Management

Patients with cirrhosis and ESLD can be evaluated for liver transplantation but are required to abstain from alcohol for 6 months prior to evaluation, maintain abstinence, and be part of a rehabilitation program.

Outcome and Prognosis

- Fatty liver may be reversible with abstinence.
- In alcoholic hepatitis, prognosis depends on the severity of presentation and alcohol abstinence. The in-hospital mortality for severe cases is high because of complications including sepsis and renal failure. Liver transplantation may be offered in highly selected patients with severe disease at initial presentation and excellent social support.[8]
- In alcoholic cirrhosis, prognosis is variable and depends on the degree of liver decompensation. Abstinence from alcohol may promote significant liver chemistry improvement.

IMMUNE-MEDIATED LIVER DISEASES

Autoimmune Hepatitis

GENERAL PRINCIPLES

AIH is a chronic inflammation of the liver of unknown cause, associated with circulating autoantibodies and hyperglobulinemia.

- Women are affected more than men (gender ratio 3.6:1).
- Extrahepatic manifestations may be found in 30%–50% of patients and include synovitis, celiac disease, Coombs-positive hemolytic anemia, autoimmune thyroiditis, Graves' disease,

rheumatoid arthritis, ulcerative colitis (UC), type I diabetes, immune thrombocytopenia, autoimmune polyendocrine syndrome type 1, and other immune-mediated processes. Two types of AIH have been proposed based on differences in their immunologic markers. They have a good response to corticosteroid therapy.

- **Type I AIH** is the most common form of the disease and constitutes 80% of AIH cases. It is associated with antinuclear antibodies (ANAs) and anti–smooth muscle antibodies (SMAs).
- **Type 2 AIH** is characterized by antibodies to liver/kidney microsome type 1 (anti-LKM1) and/or liver cytosol type 1 (anti-LC1). This type is predominately seen in children and young adults.
- Autoantibody-negative phenotype AIH is common in Japanese population.

DIAGNOSIS

Clinical Presentation

- AST and ALT elevations are usually more marked than those of bilirubin and ALP, although a cholestatic pattern with high levels of conjugated bilirubin and ALP can occur.
- Elevated serum globulins, particularly γ-globulins (IgG), are characteristic of AIH. Hyperglobulinemia is generally associated with circulating autoantibodies, which are helpful in identifying AIH.
- In approximately 30%–40% of cases, the clinical presentation is similar to acute viral hepatitis. A smaller percentage of patients may present in FHF or with asymptomatic elevation of serum ALT. It presents with cirrhosis in at least 25% of patients.
- The most common symptoms at presentation include fatigue, jaundice, myalgias, anorexia, diarrhea, acne, abnormal menses, and right upper quadrant abdominal discomfort.
- Patients with AIH may overlap with clinical and histologic findings consistent with other liver diseases (e.g., PBC, PSC, Wilson disease, and autoimmune cholangitis).
- The International Autoimmune Hepatitis Group released a diagnostic scoring system in 1993. The scoring system accounts for sex, LFTs, elevated IgG, antibodies such as ANA/SMA, HLA genetic variants and history of other autoimmune disease, histologic features, treatment response, and likelihood of an etiology other than AIH.[9]

Diagnostic Testing

Liver biopsy is recommended for definitive diagnosis.

- **"Piecemeal necrosis" or interface hepatitis** with lobular or panacinar inflammation (lymphocytic and plasmacytic infiltration) are the histologic hallmarks of AIH.
- Histologic changes, such as ductopenia or destructive cholangitis, may indicate overlap syndromes with AIH and PSC, PBC, or autoimmune cholangitis.

TREATMENT

Begin treatment in patients with serum AST and ALT levels >5 times the upper limit of normal, hyperglobulinemia, and histologic features of interface hepatitis, bridging, or multiacinar necrosis.

Medications

- Therapy consists of prednisone (50–60 mg/d PO) monotherapy or prednisone at a lower dose (30 mg/d PO) with azathioprine (AZA; 50 mg or up to 1–2 mg/kg). The dose of prednisone is tapered down every 10–15 days to 10–20 mg, whereas the dose of AZA remains unchanged. Continue combination therapy for at least a year while biochemical abnormalities improve. The prednisone is then tapered and discontinued during the second year, while AZA monotherapy continues.

- The combination of prednisone and AZA decreases corticosteroid-associated side effects; however, AZA should be used with caution in patients with pretreatment cytopenias or thiopurine methyltransferase (TPMT) deficiency.
- **Budesonide** (6–9 mg/d PO), in combination with AZA (1–2 mg/kg/d PO), may also result in normalization of AST and ALT, with fewer steroid-specific side effects, in **noncirrhotic** adults with AIH.[10]
- Second-line treatments for suboptimal response or treatment failures include mycophenolate mofetil, tacrolimus, cyclosporine, and budesonide.
- Rapamycin, rituximab, and infliximab are emerging as rescue drugs.

Surgical Management

- Consider liver transplantation in patients with ESLD and those with AIH-mediated FHF.
- After transplantation, recurrent AIH is seen in approximately 15% of patients. De novo AIH or immunologically mediated hepatitis, defined as hepatitis with histologic features similar to AIH in patients transplanted for nonautoimmune diseases, has been described in about 5% of transplant recipients.[11]

Monitoring and Follow-Up

- About 90% of adults have improvements in the serum aminotransferase, bilirubin, and γ-globulin levels within the first 2 weeks of treatment.
- Histologic improvement lags behind clinical and laboratory improvement by 3–8 months.

OUTCOME AND PROGNOSIS

- The overall goal of treatment is normalization of aminotransferases, hyperglobulinemia (IgG), and liver histology.
- Remission is achieved in 65% and 80% of patients within 1.5–3 years of treatment, respectively.
- Relapses occur in at least 20%–50% of patients after cessation of therapy and require retreatment.

Primary Biliary Cholangitis

GENERAL PRINCIPLES

Primary biliary cholangitis (PBC) is a cholestatic hepatic disorder of unknown etiology with autoimmune features. It is formerly known as primary biliary cirrhosis

- It most often affects middle-aged women (>90%) and is more commonly described in Caucasians. It is caused by granulomatous destruction of the interlobular bile ducts, which leads to progressive ductopenia and cholestasis.
- Cholestasis is generally slowly progressive and can lead to cirrhosis and liver failure.
- Extrahepatic manifestations include keratoconjunctivitis sicca (Sjögren), renal tubular acidosis, gallstones, thyroid disease (Hashimoto), lichen planus, scleroderma, Raynaud phenomenon, CREST syndrome (calcinosis, Raynaud phenomenon, esophageal dysmotility, sclerodactyly, and telangiectasia), and celiac disease.

DIAGNOSIS

Clinical Presentation

- Fatigue, jaundice, pruritus, and dermatographism are often the most troublesome symptoms.
- Patients may present de novo with manifestations of ESLD.
- Although there are no examination findings that are specific for PBC, xanthomata and xanthelasma can be a clue to underlying cholestasis.

Diagnostic Testing

- Antimitochondrial (AMA) antibodies are present in >90% of patients.
- Typical features include elevated levels of ALP, total bilirubin, cholesterol, and IgM.

Diagnostic Procedures

Liver biopsy is helpful for both diagnosis and staging.

TREATMENT

Medications

- No curative therapy is available; treatment aims to slow down the progression of disease.
- **Ursodeoxycholic acid (UDCA)** (13–15 mg/kg/d PO) is a bile acid derivative with hepatocyte cytoprotective properties that stimulate hepatocellular and ductular secretions. Traditionally, UDCA has been suggested to reduce mortality when given long term.
- **Obeticholic acid** (OCA; 10–50 mg/d PO) is a derivative of the primary bile acid chenodeoxycholic acid and affects bile acid homeostasis. In a trial of patients with PBC who had an inadequate response to UDCA, a 3-month treatment with OCA plus UDCA significantly reduced levels of ALP, GGT, and ALT when compared with UDCA plus placebo.[12]

Surgical Management

- Liver transplantation is an option in advanced disease.
- Recurrent PBC after transplantation has been documented at a rate of 20% over 10 years.

PROGNOSIS AND OUTCOME

- PBC progresses along a path of increasingly severe histologic damage (florid bile duct lesions, ductular proliferation, fibrosis, and cirrhosis).
- Progression to cirrhosis and liver failure may occur years from diagnosis.

Primary Sclerosing Cholangitis

GENERAL PRINCIPLES

PSC is a cholestatic liver disorder characterized by inflammation, fibrosis, and obliteration of the extrahepatic and/or intrahepatic bile ducts.

- PSC can be subdivided into **small duct** and **large duct disease**. Small duct disease is defined as typical histologic features of PSC with a normal cholangiogram. In classic PSC, typical "beads on a string" strictures of the biliary tree can be detected by cholangiography. Small duct disease carries a more favorable prognosis.[13] There is the third type which is *associated with autoimmune hepatitis* and it affects both small and large bile ducts.
- The peak incidence is at about age 40 years. Most patients are middle-aged men, and the male-to-female ratio is 2:1.

- PSC is frequently associated with IBD (80% of patients have concomitant UC). The clinical course of these conditions is not correlated.
- PSC increases the risk of colon cancer, in addition to the risk conferred by IBD alone.

DIAGNOSIS

Clinical Presentation

- Clinical manifestations include intermittent episodes of jaundice, hepatomegaly, pruritus, weight loss, and fatigue. Patients may also present with acute cholangitis.
- Acute cholangitis is defined as an infection of the biliary ductal system usually caused by bacteria ascending from its junction with the duodenum and is a frequent complication in patients with strictures of the biliary ducts. Symptoms of acute cholangitis include fever, chills, rigors, pruritis, jaundice, right upper quadrant pain, and hepatosplenomegaly.
- Cholangiocarcinoma is the most frequent neoplasm associated with PSC. Patients with PSC have a significant lifetime risk of developing cholangiocarcinoma.

Diagnostic Testing

- The diagnosis of PSC should be considered in individuals with IBD who have increased levels of ALP even in the absence of symptoms of hepatobiliary disease.
- **ANA** is positive in up to 50% of cases, and perinuclear antineutrophil cytoplasmic antibody (p-ANCA) is positive in 80% of cases.
- MRCP is the preferred diagnostic study of choice.

Diagnostic Procedures

- ERCP is a therapeutic procedure in patients with PSC when acute cholangitis is suspected. It is also performed when a dominant (severe) stricture is seen on MRCP to obtain duct brushings and biopsies to evaluate for cholangiocarcinoma. Sending brushings for fluoresence in situ hybridization (FISH) may aid in the diagnosis of cholangiocarcinoma. Intraductal endoscopy, specifically cholangioscopy, can provide direct visualization of the biliary ducts with the advantage of direct tissue sampling.
- Liver biopsy is helpful in the diagnosis of small-duct PSC, in the exclusion of other diseases, and in staging. Characteristic histologic findings include concentric periductal fibrosis ("onion skinning"), degeneration of bile duct epithelium, ductular proliferation, ductopenia, and cholestasis.

TREATMENT

Medications

- At this time, there is no established medical treatment for PSC.
- Several randomized, placebo-controlled trials comparing the use of UDCA (13–23 mg/kg/d) showed improvement of LFTs in the UDCA group compared with placebo. However, there was no difference in long-term survival or time to liver transplantation. UDCA (>28 mg/kg/d) was associated with a higher risk of serious adverse events including death and transplantation and is **not** currently recommended for **PSC.**[14]
- Episodes of cholangitis should be managed with IV antibiotics and endoscopic therapy.

Other Nonpharmacologic Therapies

- ERCP can dilate and stent dominant strictures but does not slow down the disease progression.
- Surgical management
  - Colectomy for UC does not affect the course of PSC.

- Patients with decompensated cirrhosis or recurrent cholangitis should be referred for liver transplantation. Recurrent PSC after liver transplantation has been documented.
- Selected hilar cholangiocarcinomas may be considered for liver transplantation.
- Gallbladder polyps follow-up should be comanaged with a liver or GI specialist.

COMPLICATIONS OF CHOLESTASIS

Nutritional Deficiencies

GENERAL PRINCIPLES

Any condition that blocks bile excretion (at the level of the liver cell or the biliary ducts) is defined as cholestasis. Laboratory evidence of cholestasis includes elevated ALP and bilirubin.

- **Nutritional deficiencies** result from fat malabsorption.
- **Fat-soluble vitamin deficiency** (vitamins A, D, E, and K) is often present in advanced cholestasis and is particularly common in patients with steatorrhea.

DIAGNOSIS

Clinical Presentation

- Characteristic manifestations of vitamin deficiencies are discussed in Chapter 2, Nutrition Support.
- Patients with steatorrhea may give a history of oily, foul-smelling diarrhea that sticks to the toilet bowl or is difficult to flush.

Diagnostic Testing

- 25-Hydroxyvitamin D serum concentrations reflect the total body stores of vitamin D. Vitamin D deficiency in the setting of malabsorption and steatorrhea is a good surrogate clinical marker for total body concentrations of other fat-soluble vitamins.
- Stool can be tested for fecal fat. Both spot tests and 24-hour collections can be done.

TREATMENT

Medications

Vitamin supplements, given orally or parenterally, are given to correct deficiencies.

Osteoporosis

GENERAL PRINCIPLES

- Osteoporosis is defined as a decrease in the amount of bone (mainly trabecular bone), leading to a decrease in its structural integrity and increase in the risk of fractures.
- The relative risk of osteopenia in cholestasis is 4.4 times greater than the general population, matched for age and gender. It is particularly common in cholestasis because of PBC.[15]

DIAGNOSIS

Bone mineral density should be measured by dual-energy X-ray absorptiometry (DEXA) in all patients at the time of diagnosis and during follow-up (every 1–2 years).

TREATMENT

Treatment of bone disease includes weight-bearing exercise, oral calcium supplementation (1.0–1.5 g/d), bisphosphonate therapy, and vitamin D supplementation.

Pruritis

GENERAL PRINCIPLES

The pathophysiology is debated and may be due to the accumulation of bile acid compounds or endogenous opioid agonists.

DIAGNOSIS

Patients with cholestasis can develop itching with either a normal or elevated bilirubin level.

Serum bile acids level may aid the diagnosis when ALP or bilirubin is normal.

TREATMENT

Medications

First Line

- Pruritus is best treated with cholestyramine, a basic anion exchange resin. It binds bile acids and other anionic compounds in the intestine and inhibits their absorption. The dose is 4 g mixed with water before and after the morning meal, with additional doses before lunch and dinner, up to a maximum of 16 g/d. Administer cholestyramine apart from other medicines or vitamins as cholestyramine will impair absorption.
- Colestipol, another similar resin, is also available.

Second Line

- Antihistamines (hydroxyzine, diphenhydramine, or doxepin, 25 mg PO at bedtime) and petrolatum may provide relief from pruritis.
- Rifampin (150–600 mg/d) and naltrexone (25–50 mg/d) are reserved for intractable pruritus. Long-term therapy with rifampin is associated with minor, transient elevations in serum aminotransferase levels in 10%–20% of patients—abnormalities that usually do not require dose adjustment or discontinuation. In rare instances, it can induce severe DILI.

METABOLIC LIVER DISEASES

Wilson Disease

GENERAL PRINCIPLES

Wilson disease (WD) is an autosomal recessive disorder (*ATP7B* gene on chromosome 13) that results in progressive copper overload.

- Female-to-male ratio is 2:1.
- Absent or reduced function of ATP7B protein leads to decreased hepatocellular excretion (protein transporter) of copper into bile. The protein transporter is located in the trans-Golgi network of the liver and brain. This results in hepatic copper accumulation and injury. Eventually, copper is released into the bloodstream and deposited in other organs,

notably the brain (basal ganglia, putamen, and globus pallidus [i.e., lenticular nucleus]), kidneys, and cornea.

- Extrahepatic manifestations include Kayser–Fleischer rings in the Descemet membrane in the periphery of the cornea because of copper deposition (diagnosed on slit-lamp examination), Coombs-negative hemolytic anemia, renal tubular acidosis, arthritis, osteopenia, and cardiomyopathy.

DIAGNOSIS

Clinical Presentation

- The average age at presentation of liver dysfunction is 6–20 years, but it can manifest later in life. Liver disease can be highly variable, ranging from asymptomatic with only mild biochemical abnormalities to FHF.
- Most patients with the FHF presentation of WD have a characteristic pattern of clinical findings including Coombs-negative hemolytic anemia with features of acute intravascular hemolysis, rapid progression to renal failure, a rise in serum aminotransferases from the beginning of clinical illness (typically <2000 IU/L), and normal or markedly subnormal serum ALP (typically <40 IU/L).
- The diagnosis of WD should be considered in patients with unexplained liver disease with or without neuropsychiatric symptoms, first-degree relatives with WD, or individuals with FHF (with or without hemolysis).
- Neuropsychiatric disorders usually occur later, most of the time in association with cirrhosis. The manifestations include asymmetric tremor (wing-beating tremor), dysarthria, ataxia, parkinsonism, choreoathetosis, and psychiatric features.
- Dermatological findings include lunulae ceruleae (bluish discoloration at the base of fingernails). Other manifestations include cardiomyopathy, osteoarthritis, and chondrocalcinosis.

Diagnostic Testing

- Low serum ceruloplasmin level (<20 mg/dL), elevated serum free copper level (>25 μg/dL), and elevated 24-hour urinary copper level (>100 μg) are seen in patients with WD.
- Urinary copper excretion >1600 μg copper per 24 hours following the administration of 500 mg of D-penicillamine at the beginning and again 12 hours later during the 24-hour urine collection is seen in patients with Wilson disease.[16]
- The liver histology (massive necrosis, steatosis, glycogenated nuclei, chronic hepatitis, fibrosis, cirrhosis) findings are nonspecific and depend on the presentation and stage of the disease. Elevated hepatic copper levels of >250 μg/g dry weight (normal <40 μg/g) on biopsy are highly suggestive of WD. MRI of the brain may show hyperintensities in the basal ganglia in the T2 sequence—characteristic "face of the giant panda" pattern.
- Mutation analysis by whole-gene sequencing is possible and should be performed on individuals in whom the diagnosis is difficult to establish by clinical and biochemical testing. Many patients are compound heterozygotes for mutations in the *ATP7B* gene, making identification of mutations difficult.

TREATMENT

Medications

Treatment is with the copper-chelating agents penicillamine and trientine. Zinc salts that block the intestinal absorption of copper are also used.

- **Penicillamine** 1–1.5 g/d (in divided doses bid or qid) and pyridoxine 25 mg/d (to avoid vitamin B_6 deficiency during treatment) are indicated in patients with hepatic failure.

Use may be limited by side effects (e.g., hypersensitivity, bone marrow suppression, proteinuria, systemic lupus erythematosus, Goodpasture syndrome). Penicillamine should never be given as initial treatment to patients with neurologic symptoms.

- **Trientine** 1–1.5 g/d (in divided doses bid or qid) may also be used in hepatic failure. This has similar side effects as penicillamine but at a lower frequency. The risk of neurologic worsening with trientine is less than with penicillamine.
- **Zinc salts** 50 mg tid are indicated in patients with chronic hepatitis and cirrhosis in the absence of hepatic failure. Other than gastric irritation, zinc has an excellent safety profile.
- Other agents tried include ammonium tetrathiomolybdate, potassium sulfide, Carbarylamine resins, and dimercaprol.

Surgical Management

Liver transplantation is the only therapeutic option in FHF or in patients with progressive dysfunction despite chelation therapy.

MONITORING AND FOLLOW-UP

- For monitoring, serum copper and ceruloplasmin, liver biochemistries, INR, complete blood cell count, urinalysis (especially for those on chelation therapy), and physical examination should be performed regularly, at least twice annually.
- The 24-hour urinary excretion of copper should be measured annually while on medication. More frequent monitoring may be needed if there is suspicion of noncompliance or if dose adjustment is required. The estimated serum free copper may be elevated or low in situations of nonadherence and overtreatment, respectively.
- First-degree relatives of any newly diagnosed patient with WD should be screened for WD.

OUTCOME AND PROGNOSIS

After liver transplantation, in the absence of neurologic symptoms, patients require no further medical treatment.

Hereditary Hemochromatosis

GENERAL PRINCIPLES

Hereditary hemochromatosis (HH) is an autosomal recessive disorder of iron overload.

- This is the most common inherited form of iron overload affecting Caucasian populations. One in 200–400 Caucasian individuals is homozygous for hemochromatosis (*HFE*) gene mutations. It rarely manifests clinically before middle age (40–60 years).
- HH is most frequently caused by a missense mutation (C282Y) in the *HFE* gene located on chromosome 6. **Approximately 90% of patients with HH are homozygote for the C282Y mutation.** Less frequent mutations that lead to HH include H63D and S65C and the compound heterozygous C282Y/H63D and C282Y/S65C mutations.
- Secondary iron overload states include thalassemia major, sideroblastic anemia, chronic hemolytic anemias, iatrogenic parenteral iron overload, chronic hepatitis B and C, alcohol-induced liver disease, porphyria cutanea tarda, and aceruloplasminemia.

DIAGNOSIS

Clinical Presentation

- Presentation varies from **asymptomatic disease** to **cirrhosis** and HCC.
- Clinical findings include increased pigmentation (bronze skin), porphyria cutanea tarda, diabetes, cardiomyopathy, arthritis, hypopituitarism, hypothyroidism, hypogonadism, and hepatic dysfunction.
- There is susceptibility to infection due to siderophilic bacteria such as *Yersinia enterocolitica*, *Vibrio vulnificus*, and *Listeria monocytogenes*.

Diagnostic Testing

Diagnosis is based on laboratory testing, imaging, and liver biopsy.

- The diagnosis is suggested by **high fasting transferrin saturation** (TSAT; **>45% for men or >55% for women**) (**serum iron divided by the total iron-binding capacity**). Other nonspecific laboratory tests include elevated serum iron and ferritin levels. **Ferritin level >1000 ng/mL is an accurate predictor of the degree of fibrosis in patients with HH.**
- If TSAT is >45% and ferritin is elevated, then check for HFE genotype homozygosity. If patient is a C282Y homozygote, then
  - If ferritin <1000 ng/mL and liver enzymes are normal, proceed to therapeutic phlebotomy.
  - If ferritin >1000 ng/mL or liver enzymes are elevated, proceed to liver biopsy for histology and hepatic iron concentration (HIC).
- The normal content of iron in the liver ranges from 300 to 1500 μg/g dry weight. In patients with HH, HIC ranges from 2000 to 30,000 μg/g dry weight.
- In patients with elevated TSAT and heterozygosity of the C282Y mutation, exclude other liver or hematologic diseases and consider liver biopsy.
- **MRI** is the modality of choice for noninvasive quantification of iron storage in the liver and for noninvasive surveillance of HCC. It allows for repeated measures and minimizes sampling error.

TREATMENT

Therapy consists of **phlebotomy** every 7–14 days (500 mL blood) until iron depletion is confirmed by a ferritin level of 50–100 ng/mL and a TSAT of <40%. Maintenance phlebotomy of one or two units of blood three to four times a year is continued for life, unless there are contraindications for rapid mobilization of iron stores (i.e., heart failure).

Erythrocytapheresis and iron chelation have been tried.

Patients with HH should avoid excess alcohol consumption. Vitamin C and iron supplementation should be avoided.

Medications

- **Iron chelation with deferoxamine** is an alternative to phlebotomy, but it is often more expensive and has side effects such as GI distress, visual and auditory impairments, and muscle cramps. Deferoxamine binds free iron, facilitates urinary excretion, and is recommended only when phlebotomy is contraindicated. Deferoxamine is only given IV, IM, or SC.
- Deferasirox is an oral iron chelator that selectively binds iron, forming a complex that is excreted through the feces.

Surgical Management

Liver transplantation may be considered in cases of HH with cirrhosis.

OUTCOME AND PROGNOSIS

- The survival rate in appropriately treated noncirrhotic patients is identical to that of the general population.
- Patients who undergo liver transplantation for hemochromatosis have better survival rates if they are iron depleted via phlebotomy prior to transplantation compared with patients who are iron overloaded prior to transplantation.
- The relative risk for HCC is approximately 20, with an annual incidence of 3%–4%. Patients with HH and advanced fibrosis or cirrhosis should be screened annually for HCC.[17]

α_1-Antitrypsin Deficiency

GENERAL PRINCIPLES

- α_1-Antitrypsin (α_1AT) deficiency is an autosomal recessive disease associated with accumulation of misfolded α_1AT in the endoplasmic reticulum of hepatocytes. The most common allele is protease inhibitor M (PiM—normal), followed by PiS and PiZ (deficient variants). African Americans have a lower frequency of these alleles.
- The most prevalent deficiency alleles Z and S are derived from European ancestry.[18]
- α_1AT deficiency can also be associated with emphysema in early adulthood, as well as other extrahepatic manifestations including panniculitis, pancreatic fibrosis, ANCA-positive vasculitis, and membranoproliferative glomerulonephritis.

DIAGNOSIS

Clinical Presentation

- The disease may present as neonatal cholestasis or, later in life, as chronic hepatitis, cirrhosis, or HCC.
- The presence of significant pulmonary and hepatic disease in the same patient is rare (1%–2%).

Diagnostic Testing

- Low serum α_1AT level (10%–15% of normal) will flatten the α_1-globulin curve on serum electrophoresis.
- Deficient α_1AT phenotype (PiSS, PiSZ, and PiZZ).
- Elevated AST and ALT.

Diagnostic Procedures

Liver biopsy shows characteristic periodic acid–Schiff–positive diastase-resistant globules in the periportal hepatocytes.

TREATMENT

Currently, there is no specific medical treatment for liver disease associated with α_1AT deficiency. Gene therapy for α_1AT deficiency is a potential future alternative.

Surgical Management

Liver transplantation is an option for those with cirrhosis and is curative, with survival rates of 90% at 1 year and 80% at 5 years.

OUTCOME AND PROGNOSIS

- Chronic hepatitis, cirrhosis, or HCC may develop in 10%–15% of patients with the PiZZ phenotype during the first 20 years of life.
- Controversy exists as to whether liver disease develops in heterozygotes (PiMZ, PiSZ, PiFZ).

MISCELLANEOUS LIVER DISORDERS

Metabolic-associated Fatty Liver Disease (MAFLD)

GENERAL PRINCIPLES

- Nonalcoholic fatty liver disease (NAFLD) is a clinicopathologic syndrome that encompasses several clinical entities that range from simple steatosis to steatohepatitis, fibrosis, ESLD, and HCC in the absence of significant alcohol consumption. Its global prevalence is estimated at 25%, placing a significant burden on the healthcare system.
- The terminology of metabolic (dysfunction)-associated fatty liver disease (MAFLD) is defined as hepatic steatosis entity in addition to the presence of overweight or obesity, diabetes mellitus, or evidence of metabolic dysfunction.
- It is defined as the presence of liver steatosis (diagnosed histologically through blood biomarkers or scores or through imaging studies) along with the presence of either one of the following conditions: overweight or obesity (body mass index, BMI > 25 kg/m^2), metabolic dysfunction (which covers hypertriglyceridemia or hypercholesterolemia, increased waist circumference, insulin resistance, and systemic hypertension).
- NAFLD is characterized by excessive hepatic fat accumulation, associated with insulin resistance (IR), and defined by the presence of steatosis in >5% of hepatocytes according to histologic analysis or by a proton density fat fraction >5.6% assessed by proton magnetic resonance spectroscopy (1H-MRS) or quantitative fat/water-selective MRI.
- Nonalcoholic steatohepatitis (NASH) is part of the spectrum of NAFLD and is defined as the presence of hepatic steatosis and inflammation with hepatocyte injury (ballooning) with or without fibrosis.
- The prevalence of MAFLD is 80%–90% in obese adults, 30%–50% in patients with diabetes mellitus, 90% or more in patients with hyperlipidemia, 3%–10% in children, and as high as 40%–70% among obese children. Other risk factors include jejunoileal bypass surgery and drugs (amiodarone, tamoxifen, estrogen, methotrexate, ART).

In June 20023, AASLD announced new nomenclature, as follows:

- Steatotic liver disease (SLD) was chosen as an overarching term to encompass the various etiologies of steatosis.
- Nonalcoholic fatty liver disease (NAFLD) has been redefined as metabolic dysfunction-associated SLD (MASLD). MASLD encompasses patients who have hepatic steatosis and have at least one of five cardiometabolic risk factors.
- A new category, outside pure MASLD, termed MetALD (pronunciation: Met A-L-D) was selected to describe those with MASLD who consume greater amounts of alcohol per week (140 g/week and 210 g/week for females and males, respectively).
- Metabolic dysfunction-associated steatohepatitis (MASH) is the replacement term for NASH.
- Those with no metabolic parameters and no known cause have cryptogenic SLD.

DIAGNOSIS

Clinical Presentation

The disease may vary from asymptomatic liver fatty infiltration to advanced fibrosis, cirrhosis, and HCC. Clinically, hepatomegaly can be seen in 5%–11% of patients.

The disease is associated with metabolic syndrome, OSA, PCOS, vitamin D deficiency, and hyperuricemia.

Diagnostic Testing

- When hepatic steatosis is detected on imaging and patients have symptoms or signs attributable to liver disease or have abnormal liver biochemistries, they should be evaluated for MAFLD and worked up accordingly.
- In patients with hepatic steatosis detected on imaging who lack any liver-related symptoms or signs and have normal liver biochemistries, it is reasonable to assess for metabolic risk factors (e.g., obesity, IR, dyslipidemia) and alternate causes for hepatic steatosis such as significant alcohol consumption or medications.
- Clinical diagnosis can be made based on adequate history, physical examination, laboratory tests, and typical imaging findings after excluding other causes of hepatic steatosis.
  - Noninvasive predictive models, serum biomarkers (cytokeratin-18 [CK-18] fragments, generated during cell death [M65 fragment], or apoptosis [M30 fragment]), and imaging studies are increasingly used as surrogate measures of liver fibrosis, inflammation, and steatosis, without replacing liver biopsy.
- Vibration-controlled transient elastography or magnetic resonance elastography are useful noninvasive tools to assess liver fibrosis in NAFLD patients.
- Liver biopsy should be considered in patients at high risk for steatohepatitis or advanced fibrosis or if the diagnosis remains unclear. It remains the gold standard test for the diagnosis of NASH.

TREATMENT

Nonpharmacologic Therapies

- Therapies to correct or control associated conditions are warranted (weight loss through diet and exercise, tight control of diabetes and IR, appropriate treatment of hyperlipidemia, and discontinuation of possible offending agents).
- All patients with NAFLD should be encouraged to lose at least 7%–10% of their body weight. Weight loss may lead to improvement of liver enzymes and histology.

Medications

Medications with long-term efficacy and safety are lacking in NAFLD. Vitamin E and/or pioglitazone may be used but treatment should be given only in **biopsy-proven** NASH in patients without contraindications with ample discussions of risks and benefits. Metformin, vitamin C, betaine, cytoprotective agents (UDCA, pentoxifylline), and statins have been tried.

Newer agents in trials are the following: farnesoid X receptor agonists (obeticholic acid), dual PPARα and PPARγ agonists (saroglitazar), caspase inhibitor (Emricasan), dual inhibitor of CCR2 and CCR5 (cenicriviroc), and lysyl oxidase–like-2 antibody (simtuzumab).

Surgical Management

Liver transplantation should be considered in patients with NASH-related end-stage liver disease.

OUTCOME AND PROGNOSIS

- Approximately 25% of patients with simple steatosis will progress to NASH.
- Progression to NASH cirrhosis has been reported at a rate of 11% over a 15-year period.
- NASH with cirrhosis requires hepatocellular carcinoma surveillance with an ultrasound every 6 months.
- Cardiovascular disease is the most common cause of death in NAFLD patients.[19]

Ischemic Hepatitis

GENERAL PRINCIPLES

Ischemic hepatitis results from acute liver hypoperfusion. Clinical circumstances associated with acute hypotension or hemodynamic instability include severe blood loss, substantial burns, cardiac failure, heat stroke, sepsis, toxemia of pregnancy, sickle cell crisis, antiphospholipid antibody syndrome, cocaine toxicity, and aortic dissection.

DIAGNOSIS

Clinical Presentation

Ischemic hepatitis presents with an acute and frequently transient and severe rise of aminotransferases during or following an episode of liver hypoperfusion.

Diagnostic Testing

- Laboratory studies show a rapid rise in levels of serum AST, ALT (>1000 mg/dL), and lactate dehydrogenase (LDH) within 1–3 days of the insult.
- Total bilirubin, ALP, and INR may initially be normal but subsequently rise as a result of reperfusion injury.

Diagnostic Procedures

Liver biopsy is not routinely needed because the diagnosis can usually be made with clinical history. Classic histologic features include variable degrees of zone 3 (centrilobular) necrosis with collapse around the central vein. Coexistent features may include passive congestion, sinusoidal distortion, fatty change, and cholestasis. Inflammatory infiltrates are rare.

TREATMENT

Treatment consists of supportive care and correction of the underlying condition that caused the circulatory collapse.

OUTCOME AND PROGNOSIS

Prognosis is dependent on rapid and effective treatment of the underlying condition.

Hepatic Vein Thrombosis

GENERAL PRINCIPLES

Hepatic vein thrombosis (HVT), also known as Budd–Chiari syndrome, causes hepatic venous outflow obstruction. It has multiple etiologies and a variety of clinical consequences.

- Thrombosis is the main factor leading to obstruction of the hepatic venous system, frequently in association with myeloproliferative disorders, antiphospholipid antibody syndrome, paroxysmal nocturnal hemoglobinuria, factor V Leiden, protein C and S deficiency, Jak-2 mutation, and contraceptive use.
- Membranous obstruction of the inferior vena cava (IVC) and stenosis of the IVC anastomosis after liver transplantation are conditions that present clinically similar to HVT.
- Some cases are idiopathic.

DIAGNOSIS

Clinical Presentation

Patients may present with fulminant, acute, subacute, or chronic illness characterized by ascites, hepatomegaly, and right upper quadrant abdominal pain. Other symptoms may include jaundice, encephalopathy, GI bleeding, and lower extremity edema.

Diagnostic Testing

- Serum-to-ascites albumin gradient (SAAG) is >1.1 g/dL. Serum albumin, bilirubin, AST, ALT, and PT/INR are usually abnormal.
- Laboratory evaluation to identify a hypercoagulable state should be performed (see Chapter 20, Disorders of Hemostasis and Thrombosis).
- The diagnosis can be established with Doppler ultrasound. Other diagnostic tools include magnetic resonance venography, hepatic venography, or cavography.
- Consider cross-sectional imaging to exclude space-occupying lesion leading to external compression and subsequently hepatic venous outflow obstruction.

TREATMENT

- Correct underlying cause when possible.
- To prevent propagation of the clot, initiate anticoagulation immediately, if there are no contraindications.
- Thrombolysis can be considered for well-defined clots and angioplasty if the venous obstruction is amenable to intervention for highly selected patients.
- Manage portal hypertension complications per guidelines.
- Consider transjugular intrahepatic portosystemic shunt (TIPS) if there is minimal improvement despite anticoagulation and maximal medical therapy.[20]

Surgical Management

Liver transplantation is an option in selected patients.

Portal Vein Thrombosis

GENERAL PRINCIPLES

Portal vein thrombosis (**PVT**) is seen in a variety of clinical settings, including abdominal trauma, cirrhosis, malignancy, hypercoagulable states, intra-abdominal infections, pancreatitis, and after portocaval shunt surgery and splenectomy.

DIAGNOSIS

Clinical Presentation

- PVT can present as an acute or chronic condition.

- The acute phase may go unrecognized. Symptoms include abdominal pain/distension, nausea, anorexia, weight loss, diarrhea, or features of the underlying disorder. Bowel ischemia may result from extensive PVT with extension to the superior mesenteric vein.
- Chronic PVT may present with variceal hemorrhage or other manifestations of portal hypertension.

Diagnostic Testing

- In patients with no obvious etiology, a hypercoagulable workup should be performed.
- **Ultrasonographic Doppler** examination is sensitive and specific for establishing the diagnosis. Portal venography, CT, or magnetic resonance venography can also be used.

TREATMENT

Medications

- In patients with acute PVT with or without cirrhosis, anticoagulation is recommended in the absence of any obvious contraindications. Treatment is aimed to prevent further thrombosis and recanalization, to treat complications and concurrent disease, and to identify underlying risk factors.
- In patients with chronic PVT, anticoagulation is recommended for patients with hypercoagulable conditions without cirrhosis. Anticoagulation in cirrhotic patients with chronic PVT remains controversial.[21]

Nonpharmacologic Therapies

In the setting of chronic PVT, treatment should focus on the complications of portal hypertension and include nonselective β-blockers, endoscopic band ligation, and diuretics for ascites.

Surgical Management

Portosystemic derivative surgery carries a high morbidity and mortality, especially in patients with cirrhosis. In some instances where surgery is precluded or the thrombus expands despite adequate anticoagulation, interventional radiology may be able to deploy TIPS. This may theoretically resolve symptomatic portal hypertension and prevent the thrombus recurrence or extension by the creation of a portosystemic shunt.[22]

FULMINANT HEPATIC FAILURE

GENERAL PRINCIPLES

- FHF is a condition that includes evidence of a combination of coagulation abnormalities and any degree of mental alteration (encephalopathy) in a patient without pre existing liver disease and with an illness of <26 weeks in duration.
- In 20% of cases, no clear cause is identified. Acetaminophen hepatotoxicity and viral hepatitis are the most common causes of FHF. Other causes include AIH, drug and toxin exposure, ischemia, hemophagocytic lymphohistiocytosis, acute fatty liver of pregnancy, WD, Reye syndrome, HELLP syndrome, and Budd–Chiari syndrome. Other drugs (paracetamol, monoamine oxidase inhibitors, isoniazid, carbamazepine, valproate, halogenated anesthetics) and toxins (*Amanita phalloides*, alcohol, "Ecstasy") also cause FHF.
- Acute inflammation with varying degrees of necrosis and collapse of the liver's architectural framework are the typical histologic changes seen in FHF.

DIAGNOSIS

Clinical Presentation

- Patients may present with mild to severe mental status changes (hepatic encephalopathy [HE]) in the setting of moderate to severe acute hepatitis, jaundice, and coagulopathy.
- Patients may develop cardiovascular collapse, acute renal failure, cerebral edema, features of raised ICT, and sepsis.

Diagnostic Testing

- Aminotransferases are typically elevated and, in many cases, are >1000 IU/L.
- INR >1.5 that does not correct with the administration of vitamin K is characteristic.
- Thrombocytopenia and leukocytosis, azotemia, hypoglycemia, hyponatremia, acidosis or alkalosis, and hyperammonemia may be present.
- Workup to determine the etiology of FHF should include acute viral hepatitis panel, serum drug screen (including acetaminophen level), ceruloplasmin, AIH serologies, and pregnancy test.
- Right upper quadrant ultrasound with Doppler should be obtained to evaluate obstruction of hepatic venous inflow or outflow.
- CT of the head may be obtained to evaluate and track progression of cerebral edema; however, the radiologic findings may lag behind its development and do not substitute for serial bedside assessments of neurologic status.
- Liver biopsy is seldom used to establish etiology or prognosis. Given the presence of coagulopathy, a transjugular approach to liver biopsy may be attempted if necessary.

TREATMENT

- Supportive therapy (quiet dark room, avoid patient stimulation, maintain head of bed elevation to 30 degrees) in the intensive care unit (ICU) setting with liver transplant capabilities is essential.
- Precipitating factors, such as infection, should be identified and treated. Blood glucose, electrolytes, acid–base balance, coagulation parameters, and fluid status should be serially monitored.
- Antiencephalopathy measures should be initiated.
- Sedatives should be avoided to appropriately gauge the patient's mental status.
- *N*-acetylcysteine (NAC) may be used in cases of FHF in which acetaminophen ingestion is suspected or when circumstances surrounding admission is inadequate. NAC also appears to improve spontaneous survival when given during early HE stages (grades I and II) even in the setting of nonacetaminophen FHF.[23]
- Fresh frozen plasma and the use of recombinant activated factor VIIa should only be considered in the setting of active bleeding or when invasive procedures are required.
- Infection surveillance and prevention should be done.
- Antiviral therapy is done if the underlying cause is herpes or hepatitis B. Glucocorticoids are helpful only in the case of AIH.
- Cerebral edema and intracranial hypertension are related to the severity of encephalopathy. In patients with grade III or IV encephalopathy, intracranial pressure monitoring may be considered if local expertise is available (intracranial pressure should be maintained below 20–25 mm Hg and cerebral perfusion pressure should be maintained above 50–60 mm Hg). Management of cerebral edema, when identified by CT imaging, includes intubation with sedation to avoid overstimulation, elevation of the head of the bed, use of mannitol (0.5–1 g/kg), and/or use of hypertonic saline (30% hypertonic saline at a rate of 5–20 mL/h to maintain a serum sodium of 145–155 mmol/L).

Lactulose is not indicated for encephalopathy in this setting. Its use may result in increased bowel gas that can interfere with the surgical approach for liver transplantation.[24]

- Liver transplantation should be urgently considered in cases of severe FHF. Poor prognostic indicators in acetaminophen-induced FHF include arterial pH <7.3, INR >6.5, creatinine >3.4 mg/dL, and encephalopathy grades III through IV (King's College Criteria).

OUTCOME AND PROGNOSIS

- In the United States, 45% of adults with FHF have a spontaneous recovery, 25% undergo liver transplantation, and 30% die without liver transplantation.[25]
- Death often results from progressive liver failure, GI bleeding, cerebral edema, sepsis, or arrhythmia.
- A rapid decline in aminotransferases correlates poorly with prognosis and does not always indicate an improved response to therapy.

CIRRHOSIS

- Cirrhosis is a chronic condition characterized by diffuse replacement of liver cells by fibrotic tissue, which creates a nodular-appearing distortion of the normal liver architecture. Advanced fibrosis represents the end result of many etiologies of liver injury.
- In the GBD Study 2017, the estimated number of people with compensated cirrhosis was 112 million worldwide, corresponding to an age-standardized global prevalence of compensated cirrhosis of 1395 cases per 100,000 population.[26]
- Globally, among individuals with cirrhosis, 42% had HBV infection and 21% had HCV infection. The proportion of patients with cirrhosis and heavy alcohol use was high in Europe (16%–78%) and the Americas (17%–52%) and was generally lower in Asia (0%–41%).[27] Other etiologies are listed in Table 19-12.
- Main complications of cirrhosis (Table 19-13) include portal hypertension with various clinical manifestations (ascites, esophageal and gastric varices, portal hypertensive gastropathy and colopathy, hypersplenism, gastric antral vascular ectasia, spontaneous bacterial peritonitis [SBP], hepatorenal syndrome [HRS], HE, and HCC). Frequent laboratory abnormalities encountered in a patient with cirrhosis include anemia, leukopenia, thrombocytopenia, hypoalbuminemia, coagulopathy, and hyperbilirubinemia.

TABLE 19-12 Etiology of Cirrhosis

Alcohol	**Nonalcoholic Fatty Liver Disease**
Chronic viral hepatitis: Hepatitis B, hepatitis C, delta hepatitis (hepatitis D) + hepatitis B	**Intrahepatic/extrahepatic biliary obstruction:** Recurrent biliary obstruction (e.g., gallstones)
Autoimmune hepatitis	**Cryptogenic or idiopathic**
Biliary cirrhosis: Primary biliary cirrhosis, secondary biliary cirrhosis, primary sclerosing cholangitis, autoimmune cholangiopathy	**Inherited metabolic liver disease:** Hemochromatosis, Wilson disease, α_1-antitrypsin deficiency, cystic fibrosis, glycogen storage disease
Drug-induced cirrhosis: Methotrexate, methyldopa, isoniazid, phenylbutazone, sulfonamides	**Others:** Indian childhood cirrhosis, cardiac cirrhosis, chronic venous outflow obstruction

Modified Child–Pugh classification of the severity of liver disease according to the degree of ascites, the serum concentrations of bilirubin and albumin, the prothrombin time, and the degree of encephalopathy is shown in Table 19-14.

Portal Hypertension

GENERAL PRINCIPLES

- Portal hypertension is the main complication of cirrhosis and is characterized by increased resistance to portal flow and increased portal venous inflow. Portal hypertension is established by measuring the pressure gradient between the hepatic vein and the portal vein (normal portosystemic pressure gradient is approximately <5 mm Hg).
- Direct and indirect clinical consequences of portal hypertension appear when the portosystemic pressure gradient exceeds 10 mm Hg.
- Causes of portal hypertension (Table 19-15) in patients without cirrhosis include idiopathic portal hypertension, schistosomiasis, congenital hepatic fibrosis, noncirrhotic portal fibrosis (NCPF), sarcoidosis, cystic fibrosis, arteriovenous fistulas, splenic and portal vein thrombosis, HVT (Budd–Chiari syndrome), myeloproliferative diseases, nodular regenerative hyperplasia, and focal nodular hyperplasia.

TABLE 19-13 Complications of Cirrhosis

• Portal hypertension and sequelae	• Portal gastropathy	• Bleeding manifestations and coagulopathy
• Ascites	• Hepatopulmonary syndrome	• Cirrhotic cardiomyopathy
• Spontaneous bacterial peritonitis	• Hepatocellular carcinoma	• Portopulmonary hypertension
• Hepatic encephalopathy	• Hepatic hydrothorax	• Hepatic osteodystrophy
• Hepatorenal syndrome		• Portal cholangiopathy

TABLE 19-14 Child–Pugh Classification of Severity of Cirrhosis

	Points Assigned		
Parameter	**1**	**2**	**3**
Ascites	Absent	Slight	Moderate
Bilirubin	<2 mg/dL (<34.2 μmol/L)	2–3 mg/dL (34.2–51.3 μmol/L)	>3 mg/dL (>51.3 μmol/L)
Albumin	>3.5 g/dL (35 g/L)	2.8–3.5 g/dL (28–35 g/L)	<2.8 g/dL (<28 g/L)
Prothrombin time			
Seconds over control	<4	4–6	>6
INR	<1.7	1.7–2.3	>2.3
Encephalopathy	None	Grade 1–2	Grade 3–4

Score of 5–6 is considered Child–Pugh class A (well-compensated disease), 7–9 is class B (significant functional compromise), and 10–15 is class C (decompensated disease). These classes correlate with 1- and 2-year patient survival: class A, 100% and 85%; class B, 80% and 60%; and class C, 45% and 35%.

TABLE 19-15 Causes of Portal Hypertension

Prehepatic Causes	Intrahepatic Causes	Posthepatic Causes
Portal vein thrombosis, splenic vein thrombosis, massive splenomegaly (Banti syndrome, Gaucher disease)	Presinusoidal (schistosomiasis, sarcoidosis, NCPF), sinusoidal (cirrhosis, amyloid), postsinusoidal (veno-occlusive syndrome	Severe right-sided heart failure, Budd–Chiari syndrome, constrictive pericarditis, restrictive cardiomyopathy, and hepatic vein outflow obstruction

DIAGNOSIS

Portal hypertension frequently complicates cirrhosis and presents with ascites, splenomegaly, and GI bleeding from varices (esophageal or gastric), portal hypertensive gastropathy (PHG), gastric antrum vascular ectasia (GAVE), or portal hypertensive colopathy.

- Ultrasonography, CT, and MRI showing cirrhosis, splenomegaly, collateral venous circulation, and ascites are suggestive of portal hypertension.
- Upper endoscopy may show varices (esophageal or gastric), PHG, or GAVE.
- Transjugular portal pressure measurements are uncommonly needed except when clinical diagnosis cannot be made.

TREATMENT

Treatment of GI bleeding because of portal hypertension is covered in Chapter 18, Gastrointestinal Diseases.

Ascites

GENERAL PRINCIPLES

Ascites is the abnormal (>25 mL) accumulation of fluid within the peritoneal cavity. Other causes of ascites, unrelated to portal hypertension, include cancer (peritoneal carcinomatosis), heart failure, tuberculosis, myxedema, pancreatic disease, hypoalbuminemia (nephrotic syndrome, protein-losing enteropathy), dialysis, surgery or trauma to the lymphatic system (chylous) or ureters, and serositis.

DIAGNOSIS

- Presentation ranges from ascites detected only by imaging methods to a distended, bulging, and sometimes tender abdomen. Percussion of the abdomen may reveal shifting dullness.
- **SAAG** is calculated as serum albumin minus the ascites albumin; a gradient ≥1.1 indicates portal hypertension–related ascites (97% specificity).[28] A SAAG of <1.1 is found in nephrotic syndrome, peritoneal carcinomatosis, serositis, TB, and biliary or pancreatic ascites.
- Ultrasonography, CT, and MRI are sensitive methods to detect ascites.
- **Diagnostic paracentesis** (60 mL) should be performed in the setting of new-onset ascites, suspicion of malignant ascites, or to rule out SBP. **Therapeutic paracentesis** (large volume) should be performed when tense ascites causes significant discomfort or respiratory compromise or when suspecting abdominal compartment syndrome.

- Routine diagnostic testing should include SAAG calculation, red and white blood cell counts and differential, total protein, and culture. Amylase and triglyceride measurement, cytology, adenosine deaminase levels, and mycobacterial smear/culture can be performed to confirm specific diagnoses.
- Bleeding, infection, persistent ascites leak, and intestinal perforation are possible complications.
- Large-volume paracentesis (>5 L) may lead to circulatory collapse, encephalopathy, and renal failure. Concomitant administration of IV albumin (6–8 g/L ascites removed) can be used to mitigate the risks of paracentesis-induced circulatory dysfunction and hepatorenal syndrome.
- Approach to ascites is shown in Figure 19-2.

TREATMENT

- Alcohol abstinence
- Dietary sodium restriction to 88 mEq (2000 mg) of sodium per day

Medications

- **Diuretic therapy** is initiated along with **salt restriction** (<2 g sodium or 88 mmol Na^+/d). Diuretics should be used with caution.
- **Spironolactone** 100 mg PO daily is a reasonable starting dose. The daily dose can be increased by 50–100 mg every 7–10 days to a maximum dose of 400 mg until satisfactory weight loss or side effects occur. Hyperkalemia and gynecomastia are common side effects. Other potassium-sparing diuretics such as amiloride, triamterene, or eplerenone are substitutes that can be used in patients in whom painful gynecomastia develops.
- **Loop diuretics**, such as furosemide (20–40 mg, increasing to a maximum dose of 160 mg PO daily), can be added to spironolactone. Torsemide or bumetanide may be considered in patients with unresponsiveness to furosemide.
- Patients should be observed closely for signs of dehydration, electrolyte disturbances, encephalopathy, muscle cramps, and renal insufficiency. Nonsteroidal anti-inflammatory agents may blunt the effect of diuretics and increase the risk of renal dysfunction.

Other Alternative Therapies

- TIPS is effective in the management of recurrent or refractory ascites.
- Complications of TIPS include shunt occlusion, bleeding, infection, cardiopulmonary compromise, HE, hepatic failure, and death.

Spontaneous Bacterial Peritonitis

GENERAL PRINCIPLES

- SBP is an infectious complication of portal hypertension–related ascites defined as >250 neutrophils/µL in the ascites fluid.
- Bacterascites is defined as culture-positive ascites in the presence of normal neutrophil counts (<250 neutrophils/µL) in the ascites fluid. This condition may be spontaneously reversible or the first step in the development of SBP. In the presence of signs or symptoms of infection, bacterascites should be treated like SBP.
- Risk factors for SBP include ascites fluid protein concentration <1.5 mg/dL, acute GI bleeding, and a prior episode of SBP.

Gross Appearance of Fluid (special tests)	PMN Count (cells/mm^3)	SAAG (g/dL)	Other Testing	Working Diagnosis	Confirmatory Testing
1. Transparent Yellow/ Crystal Clear/Cloudy Yellow	<250 (Total WBC count <500)	≥1.1	Total Protein <2.5 g/dL	Uncomplicated Cirrhotic Ascites	Ultrasound and/or Liver Biopsy
			Total Protein ≥2.5 g/dL	Cardiac Ascites	Chest Films, ECG
		<1.1	Total Protein <2.5 g/dL	Nephrotic Ascites	24-hour Urine protein
2. Bloody (Subtract 1 WBC/750 RBCs. Subtract 1 PMN/250 RBCs)		≥1.1	Monomicrobial infection, Total Protein <1 g/dL, Glucose >50 mg/dL, LDH <225 U/L	Spontaneous Bacterial Peritonitis	Clinical response to antibiotics
		<1.1	Polymicrobial infection, Total Protein >1 g/dL, Glucose <50 mg/dL, LDH ≥225 U/L	Secondary Bacterial Peritonitis	Upright abdominal film, Abdominal CT with water soluble contrast
		<1.1	Ascitic Fluid Amylase >100 U/L	Pancreatic ascites	Abdominal CT
3. Milky (TG concentration)	≥250 (Total WBC count <500 or ≥500)	≥1.1	Positive Cytology	Peritoneal Carcinomatosis and Portal Hypertension	Search for primary tumor
			TB testing	Tuberculous Peritonitis and underlying cirrhosis	Culture of laparo-scopic specimen of peritoneum
4. Dark Brown (bilirubin concentration)		<1.1	Positive Cytology	Peritoneal Carcinomatosis and Portal Hypertension	Search for primary tumor
			TB testing	Tuberculous Peritonitis	Culture of laparo-scopic specimen of peritoneum

Figure 19-2 Abdominal paracentesis.

DIAGNOSIS

Clinical Presentation

SBP may be asymptomatic. Clinical manifestations include abdominal pain and distention, fever, decreased bowel sounds, and worsening HE. Cirrhotic patients with ascites and evidence of any clinical deterioration should undergo diagnostic paracentesis to exclude SBP.

Diagnostic Testing

The diagnosis is confirmed when >250 neutrophils/μL are found in the ascites fluid. Gram stain reveals the organism in only 10%–20% of samples.

- Ascites cultures are more likely to be positive when 10 mL of the fluid is inoculated into two blood culture bottles at the bedside.
- The most common organisms are *Escherichia coli*, *Klebsiella*, and *Streptococcus pneumoniae*. Polymicrobial infection is uncommon and should lead to the suspicion of secondary bacterial peritonitis. Checking total protein, LDH, and glucose on ascites fluid is helpful in distinguishing secondary bacterial peritonitis from SBP.

TREATMENT

Medications

- Patients with SBP should receive empiric antibiotic therapy with IV third-generation cephalosporins (ceftriaxone, 2 g IV daily, or cefotaxime, 2 g IV q6–8h, depending on renal function). Therapy should be tailored based on culture results and antibiotic susceptibility. Paracentesis should be repeated if no clinical improvement occurs in 48–72 hours, especially if the initial fluid culture was negative.[29]
- Oral quinolones can be considered a substitute for IV third-generation cephalosporins in the absence of vomiting, shock, grade II (or higher) HE, or serum creatinine >3 mg/dL.
- Patients with <250 neutrophils/μL in the ascites fluid and signs or symptoms of infection (fever or abdominal pain or tenderness) should also receive empiric antibiotic therapy.
- Concomitant use of albumin 1.5 g/kg body weight at time of diagnosis and 1.0 g/kg body weight on day 3 improves survival and prevents renal failure in SBP.[29]

Primary Prophylaxis (No Prior History of SBP)

Patients with severe liver disease with ascitic fluid protein <1.5 mg/dL along with impaired renal function (creatinine ≥1.2, blood urea nitrogen ≥25, or serum Na ≤130) or liver failure (Child score ≥9 and bilirubin ≥3) should be treated with long-term norfloxacin 400 mg PO daily.

Secondary Prophylaxis (After the First Episode of SBP)

Norfloxacin 400 mg PO daily or Ciprofloxacin 500 mg PO daily, or trimethoprim-sulfamethoxazole single strength 1 tab PO daily is the treatment of choice for prevention of recurrent SBP to be continued lifelong or till liver transplant.[30]

Acute Kidney Injury in Patients with Cirrhosis and Hepatorenal Syndrome

GENERAL PRINCIPLES

Acute kidney injury (AKI) in decompensated cirrhosis is a common complication. Revised consensus recommendations define AKI as an increase in serum creatinine ≥0.3 mg/dL within 48 hours or a percentage increase of serum creatinine ≥50% from a known or presumed baseline within the prior 7 days. Hepatorenal syndrome (HRS) results from severe peripheral vasodilatation, which leads to renal vasoconstriction. The definition of HRS-AKI (type I HRS) is provided in Table 19-16. Common precipitating factors include systemic bacterial infections, SBP, GI hemorrhage, and large-volume paracentesis without volume expansion. HRS is a diagnosis of exclusion.[31]

DIAGNOSIS

HRS is observed in cirrhotic patients with ascites, with and without hyponatremia. HRS has been divided into two types.

- **Type I** HRS (HRS -AKI) is characterized by the acute onset of rapidly progressive renal failure (<2 weeks) unresponsive to volume expansion.
- **Type II** HRS (HRS-non-AKI) progresses more slowly but relentlessly and often clinically manifests as diuretic-resistant ascites.

TREATMENT

Medications

Specific medical therapy is only recommended for type I HRS.

- 25% IV albumin at 1 g/kg body weight (max 100 g) for two consecutive days should be given if the cause of AKI is unidentifiable.
- Terlipressin (vasopressin analog) intravenous bolus (1–2 mg every 4–6 hours) with albumin is not FDA approved for use in the United States. In a placebo-controlled trial, 34% of patients who received terlipressin had a reversal of their HRS in comparison with 13% who received placebo.[32]

TABLE 19-16 Diagnostic Criteria of HRS-AKI

- Diagnosis of cirrhosis and ascites
- Diagnosis of AKI (an increase in serum creatinine ≥0.3 mg/dL within 48 h or a percentage increase of serum creatinine ≥50% from a known or presumed baseline within the prior 7 d)
  - Stage 1: increase in serum creatinine ≥0.3 mg/dL or an increase ≥1.5- to 2-fold from baseline
  - Stage 2: increase in serum creatinine >2- to 3-fold from baseline
  - Stage 3: increase in serum creatinine >3-fold from baseline, >4 mg/dL with an acute increase ≥0.3 mg/dL, or initiation of renal replacement therapy
- No response after 2 consecutive days of diuretic withdrawal and plasma volume expansion with albumin 1 g/kg
- Absence of shock
- No current or recent use of nephrotoxic drugs (NSAIDs, aminoglycosides, iodinated contrast media, etc.)
- No macroscopic signs of structural kidney injury, defined as
  - Absence of proteinuria (>500 mg/d)
  - Absence of microhematuria (>50 RBCs per high-power field)
  - Normal findings on renal ultrasonography

Adapted from AngeliP, GinesP, WongF, et al. Diagnosis and management of acute kidney injury in patients with cirrhosis: revised consensus recommendations of the International Club of Ascites. *J Hepatol.* 2015;62:968-974.

AKI, acute kidney injury; HRS, hepatorenal syndrome; RBC, red blood cell.

- Midodrine is given orally (starting at 7.5 mg and increasing the dose at 8-hour intervals up to a maximum of 15 mg by mouth three times daily), and octreotide is given either as a continuous intravenous infusion (50 μg/h) or subcutaneously (100–200 μg three times daily), with IV albumin are commonly used regimens for the management of HRS in the United States.
- Norepinephrine can be an alternative to terlipressin.
- Renal replacement therapy may be used when liver transplantation is an option.

Other Nonpharmacologic Therapies

Hemodialysis may be indicated in patients listed for liver transplantation.

Surgical Management

Liver transplantation may be curative. Patients receiving hemodialysis for more than 6 weeks should be considered for liver and kidney transplantation.

OUTCOME AND PROGNOSIS

Without treatment, patients with type I HRS have a poor prognosis, with death occurring within 1–3 months of onset. Patients with type II HRS have a longer median survival.

Hepatic Encephalopathy

GENERAL PRINCIPLES

- HE is the syndrome of disordered consciousness and altered neuromuscular activity that is seen in patients with acute or chronic hepatocellular failure or portosystemic shunting.
- Minimal hepatic encephalopathy (MHE): It is a form of HE that is not associated with any grossly evident signs of cognitive dysfunction but with cognitive deficits that can be demonstrated with neuropsychological testing.
- According to national guidelines, HE is classified using four main axes: The underlying cause, the severity of the disease manifestation, the time course of the disease, and the existence of precipitating factors.
- HE is classified according to the underlying disease into the following:
  - Type A: Resulting from acute liver failure
  - Type B: Resulting from portosystemic bypass or shunting
  - Type C: Resulting from cirrhosis[33] (type C HE can be minimal HE, episodic HE, or persistent HE)
- The grades of HE are dynamic and can rapidly change (Table 19-17).
- Timing is further subclassified into episodic, recurrent, or persistent. To classify as recurrent, episodes of HE occur within intervals of less than 6 months, whereas persistent HE involves altered behavior that is always present in the setting of recurrent HE.
- **Precipitating factors** include medication noncompliance to lactulose, azotemia, FHF, opioids or sedative-hypnotic medications, acute GI bleeding, hypokalemia and alkalosis (diuretics and diarrhea), constipation, infection, high-protein diet, progressive hepatocellular dysfunction, HCC, and portosystemic shunts (surgical or TIPS). Treating precipitating factors can resolve HE in 90% of all patients.

DIAGNOSIS

- Asterixis (flapping tremor) is present in stage I through III encephalopathy. This motor disturbance is not specific to HE.

TABLE 19-17 Grading of Hepatic Encephalopathy

WHC Including MHE	ISHEN	Description	HESA	CHESS
Unimpaired		• No encephalopathy at all, no history of HE		
Minimal	**Covert**	• Psychometric or neuropsychological alterations of tests exploring psychomotor speed/executive functions or neurophysiological alterations without clinical evidence of mental change	Grade 0	0–1
Grade I		• Trivial lack of awareness • Euphoria or anxiety • Shortened attention span • Impairment of addition or subtraction • Altered sleep rhythm	Grade 1	0–3
Grade II	**Overt**	• Lethargy or apathy • Disorientation for time • Obvious personality change • Inappropriate behavior • Dyspraxia • Asterixis	Grade II	1–6
Grade III		• Somnolence to semistupor • Responsive to stimuli • Confused • Gross disorientation • Bizarre behavior	Grade III	3–6
Grade IV		• Coma	Grade IV	9

CHESS, clinical HE staging scale; HE, hepatic encephalopathy; HESA, HE scoring algorithm; ISHEN, International Society for Hepatic Encephalopathy and Nitrogen Metabolism; MHE, minimal hepatic encephalopathy; WHC, West Haven criteria.

- The electroencephalogram shows slow, high-amplitude, and triphasic waves.
- Determination of blood ammonia level is not a sensitive or specific test for HE.
- Psychometric tests such as Reitan number connection test can used to detect early encephalopathy.

TREATMENT

- **Protein restriction and nutritional support**—maintaining an energy intake of 35–40 kcal/kg/day, with a protein intake of 1.2–1.5 g/kg/day
- Treatment of the precipitating cause

Medications include nonabsorbable disaccharides (lactulose, lactitol, and lactose in lactase-deficient patients) and antibiotics (neomycin, metronidazole, and rifaximin).

- **Lactulose**, 15–45 mL PO (or via nasogastric tube) bid–qid, is the first choice for treatment of HE. Lactulose dosing should be adjusted to produce three to five soft stools per day. Oral lactulose should not be given to patients with ileus or possible bowel obstruction. In the acute phase, a starting dose of 30 mL every 1–2 hours is recommended. This can then be transitioned to every 4 hours, 6 hours, and then 8 hours once the patient starts having bowel movements.
- **Lactulose enemas** (prepared by the addition of 300 mL lactulose to 700 mL distilled water) may also be administered in patients who cannot tolerate oral intake.
- **Rifaximin** is an oral nonsystemic broad-spectrum antibiotic that is used at a dose of 550 mg PO bid with no serious adverse events. In a placebo-controlled trial, rifaximin reduced the risk of HE and the time to first hospitalization over a 6-month period.
- **L-Ornithine-L-aspartate** (LOLA), branched-chain amino acids, prebiotics, probiotics, sodium benzoate, PEG, flumazenil, zinc, and melatonin have been tried for HE.
- The use of liver support systems, such as the molecular adsorbent recirculating system (MARS®) and Prometheus® device, have shown some promise in the acute setting.

Hepatocellular Carcinoma

GENERAL PRINCIPLES

HCC frequently occurs in patients with cirrhosis, especially when associated with viral hepatitis (HBV or HCV), alcoholic cirrhosis, α_1AT deficiency, and hemochromatosis.

DIAGNOSIS

Clinical Presentation

- Clinical presentation is directly proportional to the stage of disease. HCC may present with right upper quadrant abdominal pain, weight loss, and hepatomegaly.
- Suspect HCC in a cirrhotic patient who develops manifestations of liver decompensation.
- Surveillance for HCC should be performed every 6 months with a sensitive imaging study. The combination of imaging with AFP is not recommended because it is unlikely to provide a gain in the detection rate. In patients with hepatitis B, surveillance should begin after age 40 years even in the absence of cirrhosis.

Diagnostic Testing

- AFP (see Section Evaluation of Liver Disease).
- Investigational serum markers for HCC include lens culinaris agglutinin-reactive AFP, des-γ-carboxyprothrombin (DCP), **prothrombin** induced by vitamin K absence or antagonist-II (PIVKA-II), α-L-fucosidase, and glypican-3 (GPC3).
- Liver ultrasound, triple-phase CT, and MRI with contrast are sensitive and often used for detection of HCC. Liver biopsy should be considered for patients at risk for HCC with suspicious liver lesions >1 cm with noncharacteristic imaging features (absence of arterial hypervascularity and venous or delayed phase washout). The CT/MRI findings are interpreted using imaging diagnostic algorithms, namely Liver Imaging Reporting and Data System (LI-RADS), for HCC diagnosis (Table 19-18).

TREATMENT

Surgical Management

- Hepatic resection is the treatment of choice in noncirrhotic patients.
- Liver transplantation is the treatment of choice for select cirrhotic patients who fall within Milan criteria (single HCC <5 cm or up to three nodules <3 cm).

TABLE 19-18 LI-RADS Criteria for HCC Diagnosis

Diagnostic Category	CT/MRI Criteria	Management Recommendation
LR-NC: *Noncategorizable*	Cannot be categorized because of image degradation or omission	Repeat or alternative diagnostic imaging in ≤3 months
LR-1: *Definitely benign* • 0% HCC • 0% malignancy	Simple cyst, solid nodule with characteristics features of hemangioma	Return to surveillance in 6 months
LR-2: *Probably benign* • 13% HCC • 14% malignancy	<20 mm with no major features, LR-M features, or ancillary features favoring malignancy	Return to surveillance in 6 months *OR* Consider repeat diagnostic imaging in ≤6 months
LR-3: *Intermediate probability of HCC* • 38% HCC • 40% malignancy	Nonrim APHE *AND*: • <20 mm with no additional major features No APHE *AND*: • <20 mm with ≤1 additional major feature *OR* • ≥20 mm with no additional major features	Repeat or alternative diagnostic imaging in 3–6 months
LR-4: *Probably HCC* • 74% HCC • 80% malignancy	Nonrim APHE *AND*: • <10 mm with ≥1 additional major feature OR • 10–19 mm with enhancing capsule appearance and no other major features *OR* • ≥20 mm with no additional major features	Multidisciplinary discussion for tailored workup • May include biopsy
	No APHE *AND*: • <20 mm with ≥2 additional major features *OR* • ≥20 mm with ≥1 additional major feature	
LR-5: *Definitely HCC* • 94% HCC • 97% malignancy	Nonrim APHE *AND*: • 10–19 mm with nonperipheral washout *OR* • 10–19 mm with threshold growths *OR* • ≥20 mm with ≥1 additional major feature	HCC confirmed • Multidisciplinary discussion for consensus management
LR-M: *Probably or definitely malignant, not specific for HCC* • 36% HCC • 93% malignancy	Targetoid mass: • Rim APHE • Peripheral washout • Delayed central enhancement • Targetoid diffusion restriction • Targetoid transitional phase or hepatobiliary phase signal intensity	Multidisciplinary discussion for tailored workup • Often includes biopsy

(Continued)

TABLE 19-18 LI-RADS Criteria for HCC Diagnosis (Continued)

Diagnostic Category	CT/MRI Criteria	Management Recommendation
	Nontargetoid mass not meeting LR-5 criteria *AND* no TIV, with ≥1 of the following: • Infiltrative appearance • Marked diffusion restriction • Necrosis or severe ischemia • Other feature suggesting non-HCC malignancy	
LR-TIV: *Malignancy with TIV* • 79% HCC • 92% malignancy	Unequivocal enhancing soft tissue in vein, regardless of visualization of parenchymal mass	Multidisciplinary discussion for tailored workup • May include biopsy

APHE, arterial phase hyperenhancement; HCC, TIV, tumor in vein.

- Milan criteria are used by the United Network for Organ Sharing (UNOS) for priority status (exception points) for liver transplantation candidacy in patients with HCC.

Locoregional Therapy

- Radiofrequency ablation (RFA) is a percutaneous ablation treatment using radiofrequency energy to produce a 3 cm area of necrosis. Sustained complete response and low complication rates were shown in very early HCC in patients with cirrhosis.
- Comparative effectiveness of other ablative techniques such as stereotactic body radiation and microwave ablation remains unclear.
- There are two transarterial embolization approaches available.
  - Transarterial chemoembolization with conventional approach (cTACE) or doxorubicin-eluting beads (DEB-TACE) improves survival in selected nonsurgical patients with large or multifocal HCC who do not have vascular invasion or metastatic disease.
  - Transarterial radioembolization (TARE) with Ytrrium-90 may be considered in patients with HCC who are not candidates for resection or transplantation but data are still emerging.
- Selected patients with tumors beyond Milan criteria HCC can be bridged or downstaged to meet Milan criteria with TACE, radiofrequency ablation (RFA), and transarterial radioembolization (TARE) prior to liver transplantation.
- The risk of hepatic decompensation because of locoregional therapy must be considered when selecting patients for bridging or downstaging.[34]

Medications

- **Sorafenib** is a small molecule that inhibits tumor cell proliferation and angiogenesis. In patients with advanced HCC and Child A cirrhosis, median survival and radiologic progression were 3 months longer for patients treated with sorafenib compared with placebo. The benefits of sorafenib in Child B cirrhosis with advanced HCC have not been established.[35]
- Phase 3 trials comparing **lenvatinib** (multikinase inhibitor against VEGFR1, VEGFR2 and VEGFR3) or nivolumab (human IgG4 anti-PD-1 monoclonal ab) with sorafenib in advanced HCC with metastatic disease are ongoing.
- **Chemotherapy.** There are no consistently effective combination cytotoxic agents for the management of HCC.
- Treatment of HCC based on Barcelona-Clínic Liver Cancer (BCLC) staging system is depicted in Figure 19-3.

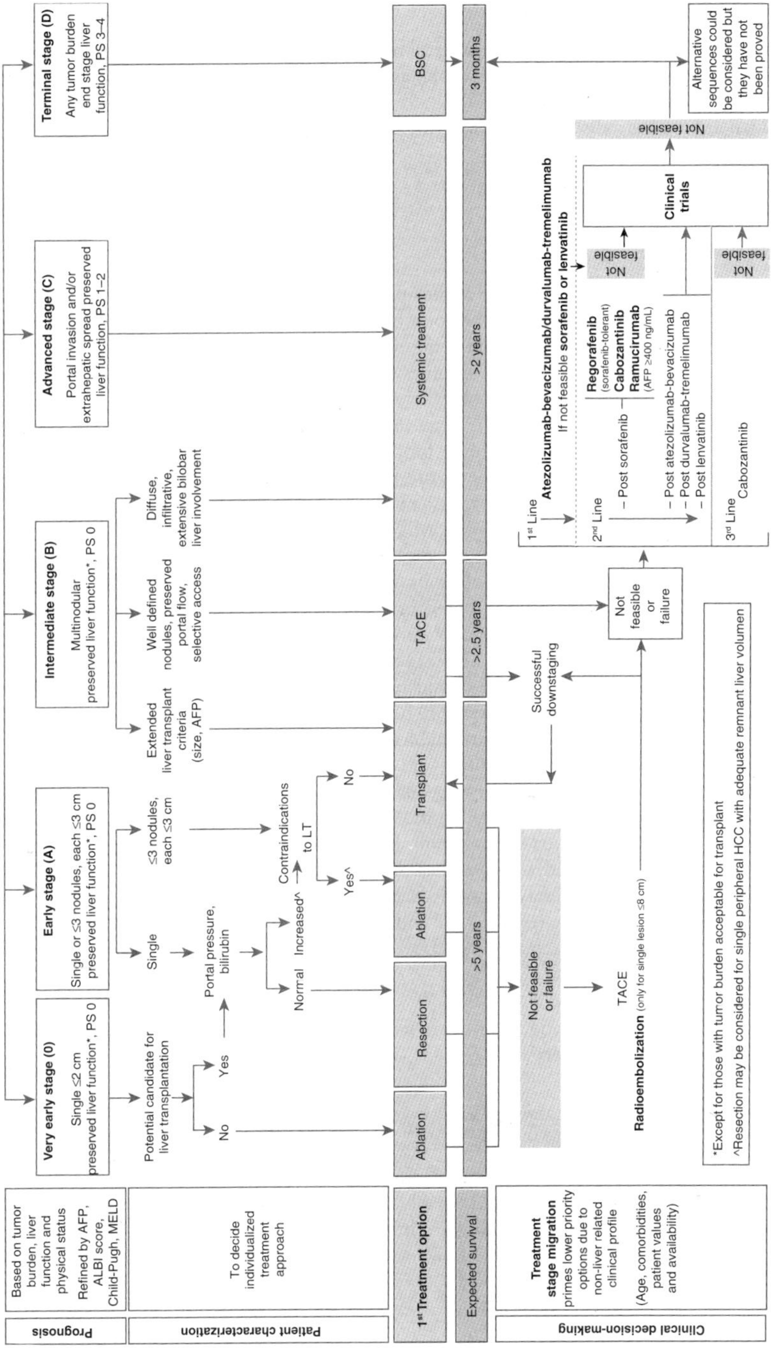

Figure 19-3 Barcelona-Clínic Liver Cancer (BCLC) staging system and management of HCC. PS, performance status.

OUTCOME AND PROGNOSIS

Early diagnosis is essential because surgical resection and liver transplantation can improve long-term survival. Liver transplantation has demonstrated, in patients meeting Milan criteria, a recurrence-free survival of 80%–90% at 3–4 years. Advanced HCC that is beyond Milan criteria has a dismal prognosis, with a 5-year survival of approximately 10%.[34]

LIVER TRANSPLANTATION

GENERAL PRINCIPLES

- Liver transplantation is an effective therapeutic option for irreversible acute liver disease and ESLD for which available therapies have failed. Whole cadaveric livers and partial livers (split-liver, reduced-size, and living-related) are used in the United States as sources for liver transplantation. There continues to be a disparity between supply and demand of suitable livers for transplantation.
- The Model for End-Stage Liver Disease (MELD) score allows for prioritization for liver transplantation. It is calculated by a formula that takes into account serum bilirubin, serum creatinine, and INR. Patients are regularly evaluated for a liver transplantation when they achieve a MELD of 15. Patients are considered for "exception MELD points" for conditions such as HCC within Milan criteria, hepatopulmonary syndrome, portopulmonary hypertension, hepatic hydrothorax, polycystic liver disease, familial amyloidosis, small unresectable hilar cholangiocarcinoma, and unusual tumors. Also, metabolic diseases such as primary oxaluria, hemochromatosis, alpha-1 antitrypsin deficiency, cystic fibrosis, WD, and tyrosinemia qualify for standard MELD exception points.
- Sodium has been incorporated to MELD to increase priority for organ allocation.
- Patients with cirrhosis should be considered for transplant evaluation when they have a decline in hepatic synthetic or excretory functions, ascites, HE, or complications such as HRS, HCC, recurrent SBP, or variceal bleeding.
- Candidates for liver transplantation are evaluated by a multidisciplinary team that includes hepatologists, transplant surgeons, transplant nurse coordinators, social workers, psychologists, and financial coordinators.
- General **contraindications** to liver transplant include severe and uncontrolled extrahepatic infection, AIDS, advanced cardiac or pulmonary disease, extrahepatic malignancy, multiorgan failure, unresolved psychosocial issues, medical noncompliance issues, and ongoing substance abuse (e.g., alcohol and illegal drugs).

TREATMENT

Immunosuppressive, infectious, and long-term complications are discussed in Chapter 17, Solid Organ Transplant Medicine.

Summary

- The crucial step in the evaluation of jaundice is history and physical examination to classify jaundice by etiology and type: hepatocellular, cholestatic, or hemolytic.
- Viral hepatitis is a global public health concern that affects millions of people and causes thousands of deaths due to acute and chronic infections, cirrhosis, and liver cancer.

- Drug-induced hepatotoxicity or drug-induced liver injury (DILI) could be intrinsic, which is predictable and idiosyncratic, which could be immune or nonimmune mediated.
- Metabolic (dysfunction)-associated fatty liver disease (MAFLD) is defined as hepatic steatosis entity in addition to the presence of overweight or obesity, diabetes mellitus, or evidence of metabolic dysfunction.
- The most common causes of cirrhosis are hepatitis C virus (HCV), alcoholic liver disease, and nonalcoholic steatohepatitis (NASH), while hepatitis B virus (HBV) and HCV are the most common causes in the developing world.
- Novel tools for the surveillance and diagnosis of HCC include protein-, genomics-, and composite algorithm-based clinical/biomarker panels. Magnetic resonance imaging-based novel techniques have improved HCC diagnosis.

Scan the QR code to access chapter references.

20 Disorders of Hemostasis and Thrombosis

Kristen M. Sanfilippo, Brian F. Gage, Tzu-Fei Wang, Roger D. Yusen, and Sohan M.

HEMOSTASIS DISORDERS

Hemostatic Disorders

GENERAL PRINCIPLES

Normal hemostasis involves a sequence of interrelated reactions that lead to platelet aggregation (primary hemostasis) and activation of coagulation factors (secondary hemostasis) to produce a durable vascular seal.

- **Primary hemostasis** consists of an immediate but temporary response to vessel injury, where platelets and von Willebrand factor (**vWF**) interact to form a primary hemostatic plug.
- **Secondary hemostasis** results in formation of a fibrin clot (Figure 20-1). Injury exposes extravascular tissue factor to blood, which initiates activation of factors VII and X and prothrombin. Subsequent activation of factors XI, VIII, and V leads to generation of thrombin, conversion of fibrinogen to fibrin, and formation of a durable clot.[1]

DIAGNOSIS

Clinical Presentation

History

A detailed history can assess bleeding risk or severity, determine congenital or acquired etiologies, and evaluate for primary or secondary hemostatic defects.

- Prolonged bleeding after dental extractions, circumcision, menstruation, labor and delivery, trauma, or surgery may suggest an underlying bleeding disorder.
- Family history may suggest an inherited bleeding disorder.

Physical Examination

- Primary hemostasis defects often cause mucosal bleeding and excessive bruising.
    - Petechiae: <2 mm subcutaneous bleeding, do not blanch with pressure, typically present in areas subject to increased hydrostatic force (the lower legs and periorbital area)
    - Ecchymoses: >3 mm black-and-blue patches due to rupture of small vessels from trauma
- Secondary hemostasis defects can result in **hematomas**, hemarthroses, or prolonged bleeding after trauma or surgery.

Diagnostic Testing

Laboratories

The history and physical examination guide the initial diagnostic work-up. Initial studies should include a complete blood count (**CBC**) with platelet count, as well as prothrombin time (**PT**), activated partial thromboplastin time (**aPTT**), and a blood smear.

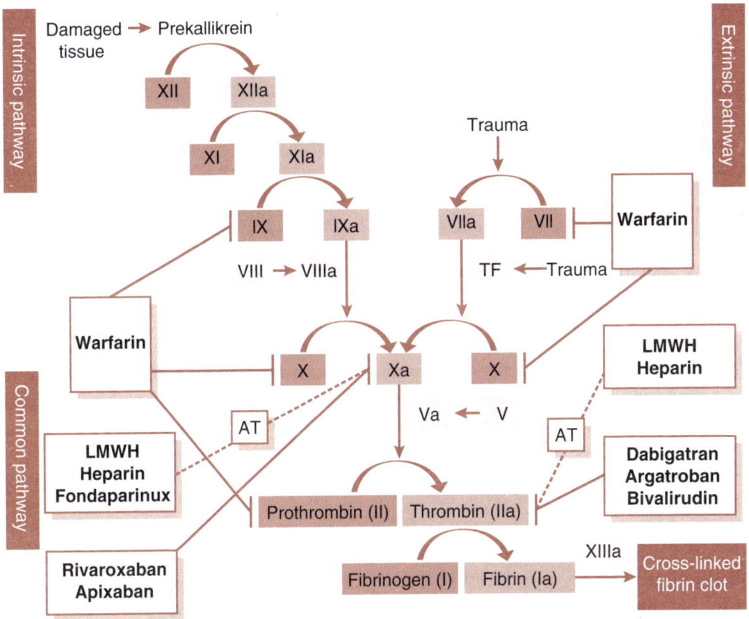

Figure 20-1 Coagulation cascade. *Solid arrows* indicate activation. *Solid* or *dashed lines* that run into a vertical line are associated with drugs represent a point of inhibition. Extrinsic pathway includes the right upper portion of cascade above factor X. Intrinsic pathway includes the left upper portion of the cascade above factor X. Common pathway includes the lower portion of the cascade from factor X and below. AT, antithrombin; LMWH, low-molecular-weight heparin; TF, tissue factor.

- **Primary hemostasis tests**
  - A low **platelet count** requires review of the peripheral blood smear to rule out platelet clumping artifact or giant platelets.
  - The **platelet function assay-100 (PFA-100)** instrument assesses vWF-dependent platelet activation in flowing citrated whole blood. Patients with von Willebrand disease (vWD) and qualitative platelet disorders can have prolonged PFA-100 closure times, often with normal platelet counts. However, anemia (hematocrit <30%) and/or thrombocytopenia (platelet $<100 \times 10^9$/L) can cause prolonged closure times without underlying bleeding disorders.
  - **In vitro platelet aggregation** studies measure platelet secretion and aggregation in response to platelet agonists (see Qualitative Platelet Disorders section).
  - Laboratory evaluation of vWD includes measurement of vWF antigen (**vWF:Ag**) and **vWF activity** and **vWF multimer analysis.**
- **Secondary hemostasis** (Figure 20-1)
  - **PT:** Measures time to form a fibrin clot after adding thromboplastin (tissue factor and phospholipid) and calcium to citrated plasma. An elevated PT is a sensitive test to deficiencies of **extrinsic pathway** (factor VII), **common pathway** (factors X and V and prothrombin), and **fibrinogen** and to use of vitamin K antagonists and direct factor Xa and thrombin (IIa) inhibitors. Reporting a PT ratio as an international normalized ratio (INR) reduces interlaboratory variation in monitoring warfarin use.[2]

TABLE 20-1 Factor Deficiencies That Cause Prolonged Prothrombin Time and/or Activated Partial Thromboplastin Time and Correct With 50:50 Mix

Assay Result	Suspected Factor Deficiencies
↑ aPTT; normal PT	XII, XI, IX, VIII, HMWK, PK
↑ PT; normal aPTT	VII
↑ PT and ↑ aPTT	II, V, X, or fibrinogen

aPTT, activated partial thromboplastin time; HMWK, high-molecular weight kininogen; PK, prekallikrein; PT, prothrombin time.

- **aPTT:** Measures the time to form a fibrin clot after activation of citrated plasma by calcium, phospholipid, and negatively charged particles. Besides heparin, low-molecular weight heparin (**LMWH**), fondaparinux, and direct anti-Xa and thrombin (IIa) inhibitors, deficiencies and inhibitors of coagulation factors of the **intrinsic pathway** (e.g., high-molecular weight kininogen, prekallikrein, factor XII, factor XI, factor IX, and factor VIII), **common pathway** (e.g., factor V, factor X, prothrombin), and **fibrinogen prolong the aPTT**.
- **Thrombin time:** Measures time to form a fibrin clot after addition of thrombin to citrated plasma. Quantitative and qualitative deficiencies of fibrinogen, fibrin degradation products, heparin, LMWH, fondaparinux, and direct thrombin (IIa) inhibitors prolong thrombin time.
- **Fibrinogen:** Measured by adding thrombin to dilute plasma and measuring clotting time. Conditions causing hypofibrinogenemia include decreased hepatic synthesis, massive hemorrhage, and disseminated intravascular coagulation (**DIC**).
- **D-dimers** result from plasmin digestion of fibrin (i.e., fibrin degradation products). Elevated D-dimer concentrations occur in many disease states (i.e., venous thromboembolism [**VTE**], DIC, trauma, and cancer).
- **Mixing studies** determine whether a factor deficiency or an inhibitor has prolonged the PT and/or aPTT. In a patient with factor deficiency, mixing patient plasma 1:1 with normal pooled plasma (all factor activities = 100%) restores deficient factors sufficiently to normalize or nearly normalize the PT or aPTT (Table 20-1). If mixing fails to correct the PT or aPTT, a specific factor inhibitor, a nonspecific inhibitor (e.g., lupus anticoagulant [**LA**]), or an anticoagulant drug may have caused the prolongation.

PLATELET DISORDERS

Thrombocytopenia

- **Thrombocytopenia** is defined as a platelet count of $<150 \times 10^9$/L (reference range varies depending on local laboratory standard).
- Thrombocytopenia occurs from decreased production, increased destruction, or sequestration of platelets (Table 20-2).

Immune Thrombocytopenia

GENERAL PRINCIPLES

Immune thrombocytopenia (ITP) is an acquired immune disorder in which antiplatelet antibodies cause shortened platelet survival and suppress megakaryopoiesis leading to

TABLE 20-2 Classification of Thrombocytopenia

Decreased Platelet Production	Increased Platelet Clearance
Marrow failure syndromes Congenital Acquired: Aplastic anemia, paroxysmal nocturnal hemoglobinuria *Hematologic malignancies* *Marrow infiltration:* Cancer, granuloma *Myelofibrosis:* Primary or secondary *Nutritional:* Vitamin B_{12} and folate deficiencies *Physical damage to the bone marrow:* Radiation, alcohol, chemotherapy	*Immune-mediated mechanisms* Immune thrombocytopenic Thrombotic thrombocytopenic purpura/hemolytic-uremic syndrome Post-transfusion purpura Heparin-induced thrombocytopenia *Non–immune-mediated mechanisms* DIC Local consumption (aortic aneurysm) Acute hemorrhage
Increased Splenic Sequestration	**Infections Associated With Thrombocytopenia**
Portal hypertension Felty syndrome Lysosomal storage disorders Infiltrative hematologic malignancies Extramedullary hematopoiesis	HIV, HHV-6, ehrlichiosis, rickettsia, malaria, hepatitis C, CMV, Epstein-Barr, *Helicobacter pylori, Escherichia coli* O157, dengue

CMV, cytomegalovirus; DIC, disseminated intravascular coagulation; HHV-6, human herpesvirus 6.

thrombocytopenia and increased bleeding risk.[3] Etiologies of ITP include idiopathic (primary), associated with coexisting conditions (secondary), or drug induced.

Epidemiology

Adult primary ITP has an incidence of 3.3 cases per 10^5 persons.[4]

Etiology

- In **primary ITP**, autoantibodies bind to platelet surface antigens and cause premature clearance by the reticuloendothelial system in addition to immune-mediated suppression of platelet production.
- **Secondary ITP** occurs in the setting of systemic lupus erythematosus (**SLE**), antiphospholipid antibody syndrome (**APS**), HIV, hepatitis C virus (**HCV**), *Helicobacter pylori*, and lymphoproliferative disorders.[3]
- **Drug-dependent ITP** results from drug–platelet interactions prompting antibody binding.[5] Medications linked to thrombocytopenia include quinidine and quinine; platelet inhibitors abciximab, eptifibatide, tirofiban, and ticlopidine; beta-lactam antibiotics such as penicillins and cephalosporins, piperacillin, daptomycin, rifampin, ethambutol, sulfonamides, and vancomycin; anticonvulsants phenytoin, valproic acid, and carbamazepine; analgesics acetaminophen, naproxen, ibuprofen, and diclofenac; cimetidine; and chlorothiazide and gold compounds.[6]

DIAGNOSIS

Clinical Presentation

- **ITP** typically presents as mild mucocutaneous bleeding and petechiae or incidental thrombocytopenia. Occasionally, ITP can present as major bleeding.

- Physical examination is focused on signs of bleeding on skin and oral mucosa—wet purpura—and any presence of lymphadenopathy or hepatosplenomegaly which could suggest an underlying condition for thrombocytopenia.
- Risk of bleeding is highest with platelet counts $<30 \times 10^9$/L.[7]
- The time elapsed since diagnosis determines whether ITP is referred to as *newly diagnosed* (up to 3 months since diagnosis), *persistent* (3–12 months since diagnosis), and *chronic* (>12 months since diagnosis).

Diagnostic Testing

Diagnosis by Exclusion

Normalization of platelet counts with discontinuation of suspected drug and confirmation if thrombocytopenia recurs when rechallenged support the diagnosis of **drug-induced ITP**.

Laboratories

- Review a peripheral blood smear to confirm automated platelet count, assess for platelet clumping (artifactual pseudothrombocytopenia) and to determine platelet, red cell, and white cell morphologies.
- Laboratory tests do not confirm the diagnosis of primary ITP, although they help to exclude secondary causes. Primary **ITP** often has the scenario of isolated thrombocytopenia in the absence of a likely underlying causative disease or medication.
- Test for infection-associated causes (e.g., HIV, HCV).[7]
- In case of bleeding disproportionate to the platelet count, it is advisable to get PT and aPTT done to rule out secondary causes.
- Rule out causes for secondary ITP by doing appropriate testing, namely, antinuclear antibodies (ANA), *H. pylori* testing, and thyroid function testing. In suspected cases, it is advisable to test for vitamin B_{12} and folate deficiency and liver disease.
- Serologic tests for antiplatelet antibodies generally do not help diagnose **ITP** because of poor sensitivity and low negative predictive value (**NPV**).[8]

Diagnostic Procedures

Diagnosis of ITP does not typically require bone marrow examination, although it can help to exclude other causes in select patients with additional CBC abnormalities, unresponsiveness to immune suppression therapy, or atypical signs or symptoms.[7]

TREATMENT

- The decision to treat primary ITP depends on the severity of thrombocytopenia and bleeding risk. The therapeutic goal is to achieve a safe platelet count to prevent major bleeding (typically $\geq 30 \times 10^9$/L) and minimize treatment-related toxicities.
- Initial therapy (Fig. 20-2). Based on severity of bleeding, critical bleeding (bleed into critical anatomical sites causing hemodynamic instability or respiratory compromise) should be treated with platelet transfusion along with corticosteroids (dexamethasone 40 mg IV once daily for 4 days or methylprednisolone 1 g once daily IV for 3 days) and IVIG (1 g/kg single dose). Severe bleeding (bleeding that results in a fall in hemoglobin of 2 or more g/dL or requires transfusion of 2 or more units of pRBCs but does not meet the definition of critical bleeding) is treated with glucocorticoids and IVIG. Minor bleeding (bleeding that do not meet criteria of critical or severe bleeding) and severe thrombocytopenia with no bleed (<20,000 cells/mcL) is treated with oral glucocorticoids (dexamethasone 40 mg once daily for 4 days or prednisone 1 mg/kg for 1–2 weeks followed by tapering over 6 weeks). Other hemostatic therapies include tranexamic acid (1–1.5 g three to four times daily or 10 mg/kg IV three times daily) or aminocaproic acid (4–12 g/day IV or oral) administration. When indicated, it consists of glucocorticoids (e.g., prednisolone

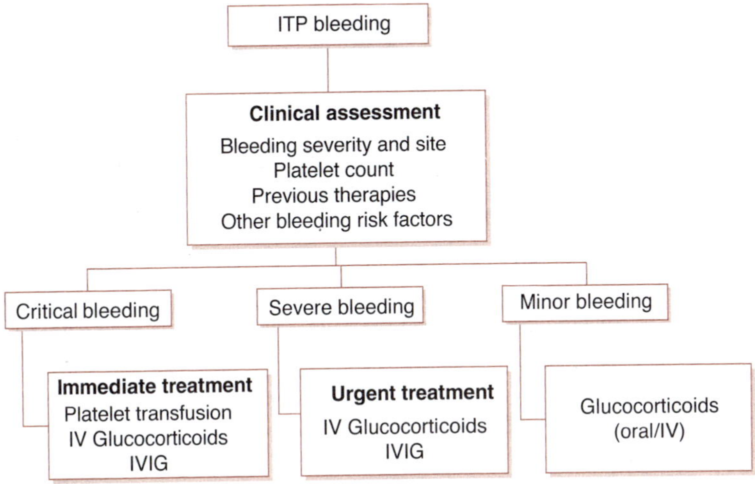

Figure 20-2 Treatment of ITP.

1–2 mg/kg/d for 2–3 weeks followed by taper or dexamethasone 40 mg orally for 4 days, or injection methylprednisolone 30 mg/kg daily [maximum 1000 mg] for 3–4 days).[9] Nonresponders to glucocorticoids or patients with active bleeding may also receive IV immunoglobulin (IVIG; 1 g/kg for one to two doses). Rh-positive patients may also receive anti-D immunoglobulin (WinRho) (ineffective postsplenectomy) as an alternative to IVIG. WinRho works by forming anti-D-coated red blood cell (RBC) complexes, which bind to splenic macrophages, saturate the reticuloendothelial system, and prevent platelet destruction. WinRho may cause severe hemolysis and requires postinfusion monitoring of hemoglobin and reticulocyte count. Reduce WinRho dose if hemoglobin (Hgb) is <10 g/dL and avoid when the Hgb is <8 g/dL. Most primary ITP cases respond to therapy within 1–3 weeks.

- Around 30%–40% of patients will relapse during a steroid taper (relapsed/refractory ITP).
- **Second-line therapies.** Indicated when the initial treatment fails to increase the platelet count to safe level (<20,000/mcL for >3 months after initial diagnosis) or decrease in platelet count below safe level on tapering the first-line drugs. They include splenectomy, TPO-RA (thrombopoeitin receptor agonist), and rituximab.
- Two-thirds of patients with refractory ITP will obtain a durable complete response following splenectomy. To be considered after a span of at least 1 year of diagnosis to wait for late spontaneous remission. Administer pneumococcal, meningococcal, and *Haemophilus influenzae* type B vaccines before (preferred) or after splenectomy.
- Treatment options for those who fail splenectomy include single or combined therapies with prednisone, IVIG, androgen therapy with danazol, dapsone, other immunosuppressive agents, azathioprine, rituximab (anti-CD20 monoclonal antibody), and/or thrombopoietin receptor (TPO-R) agonists.[7]
- There are two TPO-R agonists for treatment of refractory primary ITP patients with increased bleeding risk: romiplostim, dosed SC weekly, and eltrombopag, taken orally once a day. TPO-R agonists produce durable platelet count improvements in a majority of refractory ITP patients beginning 5–7 days after initiation. Potential complications include thromboembolic events and bone marrow fibrosis.[10,11]

- Management of secondary ITP may include a combination of treatment for the underlying disease and therapies similar to those used for primary ITP.
- Platelet transfusion for severe drug-induced thrombocytopenia may decrease risk of bleeding. IVIG, steroids, and plasmapheresis have uncertain benefit.

Thrombotic Thrombocytopenic Purpura and Hemolytic-Uremic Syndrome

GENERAL PRINCIPLES

Definition

Thrombotic thrombocytopenic purpura (TTP) and **hemolytic-uremic syndrome** (HUS) are thrombotic microangiopathies (**TMAs**) caused by platelet–vWF aggregates and platelet–fibrin aggregates, respectively, resulting in thrombocytopenia, microangiopathic hemolytic anemia (**MAHA**), and organ ischemia. Usually, clinical and laboratory features permit differentiation of TTP from HUS. TMA may occur in association with DIC, HIV infection, malignant hypertension, vasculitis, organ and stem cell transplant–related toxicity, adverse drug reactions, and pregnancy-related complications of pre-eclampsia/eclampsia and **HELLP** (**h**emolysis, **e**levated **l**iver enzymes, **l**ow **p**latelets) syndrome.

Epidemiology

Sporadic TTP has an incidence of approximately 11.3 cases per 10^6 persons, occurring more frequently in women and African Americans.[12] **Typical HUS** usually occurs in gastroenteritis outbreaks affecting children. Adults may present with both **typical** and **atypical** (non–gastroenteritis-associated) variants of HUS.

Etiology

- Autoantibody-mediated removal of plasma vWF-cleaving protease: A disintegrin and metalloproteinase with a thrombo spondin type 1 motif, member 13 (ADAMTS13), leading to elevated levels of abnormally large vWF multimers, typically causes **sporadic TTP**.[13] The abnormal vWF multimers spontaneously adhere to platelets and may produce occlusive vWF–platelet aggregates in the microcirculation and subsequent microangiopathy. Second-hit events may involve endothelial dysfunction or injury.
- Severe ADAMTS13 deficiency does not cause HUS and other types of TMA, with the exception of some cases associated with HIV and pregnancy.
- **Typical or enteropathic HUS** has an association with *Escherichia coli* (O157:H7) production of Shiga-like toxins in Shiga toxigenic *E. coli* HUS (**STEC-HUS**).
- **HUS** can also be associated with transplantation, endothelial-damaging drugs, and pregnancy.[14]
- Inherited or acquired defects in regulation of the alternative complement pathway are present in 30%–50% of atypical HUS cases.[15]

DIAGNOSIS

Clinical Presentation

- The complete clinical pentad of TTP, present in <30% of cases, includes consumptive thrombocytopenia, MAHA, fever, renal dysfunction, and fluctuating neurologic deficits. Abdominal complaints are more common—pain, nausea, vomiting, or diarrhea. Neurological symptoms can range from mild (headache and confusion) to severe (seizures, focal deficits, coma). Renal involvement manifesting as decreased kidney function can be seen, but anuria/AKI is rare in TTP, whereas it is seen in HUS.

- The findings of thrombocytopenia and MAHA should raise suspicion for **TTP-HUS** in the absence of other identifiable causes.
- Patients with autosomal recessive inherited ADAMTS13 deficiencies have relapsing TTP (Upshaw–Schulman syndrome).
- Diarrhea, usually bloody, and abdominal pain often precede STEC-HUS.
- Marked renal dysfunction usually occurs in HUS.

Diagnostic Testing

- TMAs produce schistocytes (fragmented red cells) and thrombocytopenia on blood smears. The findings of anemia, elevated reticulocyte count, low or undetectable haptoglobin, markedly elevated lactate dehydrogenase (**LDH**), elevated indirect bilirubin, and negative Coombs test support the presence of nonimmune hemolysis.
- Sporadic TTP has TMA findings, normal PT and aPTT, mild-to-moderate azotemia, very low or undetectable ADAMTS13 enzyme activity (<10%), and often detectable ADAMTS13 inhibitory antibody.
- Typical HUS has TMA and acute renal failure. *E. coli* O157 stool culture has a higher sensitivity than Shiga toxin assays. However, stool samples obtained after diarrhea has resolved reduce the sensitivity of both tests.[16]
- In the absence of precipitating risk factors, testing for **atypical HUS** should include molecular and serologic tests for complement regulator factor H and I mutations (complement-mediated TMA) or autoantibodies through reference laboratories. Approach to thrombotic microangiopathy is described in Figure 20-3.

TREATMENT

- The mainstay of therapy for **TTP** consists of rapid treatment with plasma exchange (**PEX**) of 1.0–1.5 plasma volumes daily. PEX is continued for several days after normalization of platelet count and LDH.
    - If PEX is not available or will be delayed, infuse **fresh frozen plasma** (**FFP**) immediately to replace ADAMTS13.
    - Common practice includes the administration of **glucocorticoids**: prednisone 1 mg/kg PO per day. Consider a brief course of high-dose corticosteroids (methylprednisolone 0.5–1.0 g/d IV) in critically ill or PEX nonresponding patients.[17]
    - Platelet transfusion in the absence of severe bleeding is relatively contraindicated owing to potential risk of additional microvascular occlusions.
    - 90% of treated patients have a remission; however, relapses may occur days to years later.
    - Therapy with **rituximab** can achieve durable remissions following TTP relapses and is being studied in the upfront treatment setting.[18,19]
    - **Immunosuppression** with cyclophosphamide, azathioprine, or vincristine and splenectomy may have success in the treatment of refractory or relapsing TTP.[20,21]
- **STEC-HUS** does not usually improve with PEX, and treatment remains supportive, mainly hydration. Antibiotic therapy does not hasten recovery or minimize toxicity for STEC-HUS and is used only for extrarenal Shiga toxin-induced sequelae such as pneumonia.
- **TMA associated with calcineurin inhibitors** (cyclosporine, tacrolimus), typically given in the transplant setting, usually responds to drug dose reduction or discontinuation of the offending agent.
- **Atypical HUS** often leads to chronic renal failure necessitating dialysis.
- In 2011, the US Food and Drug Administration (**FDA**) approved eculizumab for treatment of **atypical HUS**. Eculizumab is a humanized monoclonal antibody that binds to complement protein C5, blocking its cleavage into C5a and the cytotoxic membrane attack complex C5b-9, thus inhibiting complement activation.[22]

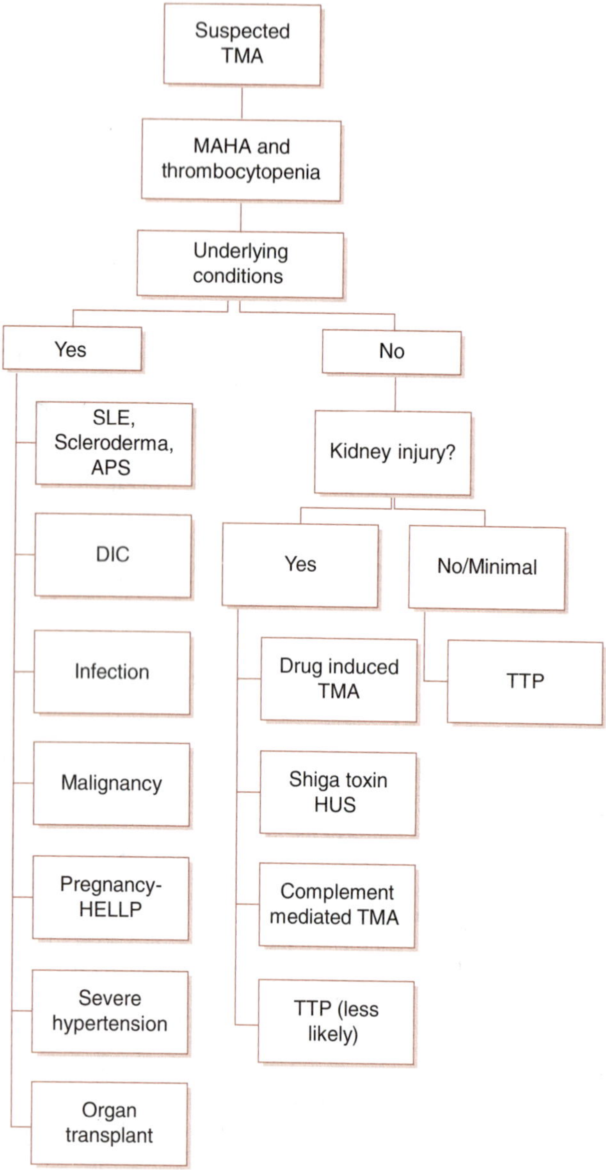

Figure 20-3 Approach to thrombotic microangiopathy.

- *Neisseria meningitides* vaccination is recommended 2 weeks before starting eculizumab; however, in **atypical** HUS, this grace period is typically not possible, thus prophylactic antibiotics should be given for 2 weeks.

Heparin-Induced Thrombocytopenia

GENERAL PRINCIPLES

Definition

Heparin-induced thrombocytopenia (HIT) is an acquired hypercoagulable disorder associated with the use of heparin or heparin-like products and due to autoantibodies targeting the anticoagulant and platelet factor 4 (**PF4**) complexes. HIT typically presents with thrombocytopenia or a decrease in platelet count by at least 50% from pre-exposure baseline after exposure to heparin products. Major complications of HIT consist of arterial and venous thromboembolic events.

Epidemiology

The incidence of **HIT** ranges from 0.1% to 1.0% in medical and obstetric patients receiving prophylactic and therapeutic unfractionated heparin (**UFH**) to >1%–5% in patients receiving prophylactic UFH after cardiothoracic surgery.[23] Patients exposed only to LMWH have a low incidence of HIT.[24] HIT rarely occurs in association with the synthetic pentasaccharide fondaparinux.[25]

Etiology

Immune-responsive patients produce autoantibodies that bind to PF4/heparin complexes, which can activate platelets, cause thrombocytopenia, and lead to clot formation through increased thrombin generation.[26]

DIAGNOSIS

Clinical Presentation

- **HIT** usually develops within 5–10 days of heparin exposure (**typical-onset HIT**). Exceptions include **delayed-onset HIT**, which occurs after stopping heparin, and **early-onset HIT**, which starts within the first 24 hours of heparin administration in patients with recent exposure to heparin.[23]
- Suspect HIT when thrombocytopenia occurs during heparin exposure by any route in the absence of other causes of thrombocytopenia.
- The **4T scoring system** (Table 20-3) determines HIT pretest probability and has an NPV of >95% (Fig. 20-4).[27]
- HIT rarely causes severe thrombocytopenia (platelet count $<20 \times 10^9$/L) and bleeding.
- **Thromboembolic complications** occur in 30%–75% of HIT patients (i.e., heparin-induced thrombocytopenia and thrombosis [HITT]). Thrombosis can precede, be concurrent with, or follow thrombocytopenia.
- HIT causing venous thrombi at heparin injection sites produces full-thickness skin infarctions, sometimes in the absence of thrombocytopenia.
- HIT can cause systemic allergic responses following an IV bolus of heparin characterized by fever, hypotension, dyspnea, and cardiac arrest.
- HIT can cause thrombosis at catheter sites, thrombosis at unusual sites (venous limb gangrene, skin necrosis, spinal ischemia, cerebral venous thrombosis), and bilateral adrenal hemorrhage secondary to adrenal thrombosis.

Diagnostic Testing

- Obtain surveillance platelet counts every 2–3 days during heparin exposure in patients with >1% risk of HIT.[23]
- For suspected HIT, laboratory tests for PF4 antibodies improve diagnostic accuracy.

TABLE 20-3 4T Scoring System for Pretest Probability of Heparin-Induced Thrombocytopenia

T Category	0 Points	1 Point	2 Points
Thrombocytopenia	PLT fall <30% or nadir <10 × 10⁹/L	PLT fall 30%–50% or nadir 10–19 × 10⁹/L	PLT fall >50% and nadir ≥20 × 10⁹/L
Timing of thrombocytopenia	≤4 d without prior exposure	Likely within 5–10 d, not clear; >10 d; ≤1 d (with exposure 31–100 d)	Within 5–10 d of exposure or ≤1 d (with exposure in last 30 d)
Thrombotic event	No thrombus	Thrombus recurrence or progression; erythematous skin lesion; suspected thrombus	Confirmed thrombus; skin necrosis; acute reaction after UFH bolus
Other causes for thrombocytopenia	Definite	Possible	None apparent

Data from *J Thromb Haemost*. 2006;4:759-765; *J Thromb Haemost*. 2010;8:1483–1485.
Sum the points for each of the four categories to determine the clinical probability: high (6–8 points), intermediate (4–5 points), low (0–3 points).
PLT, platelets; UFH, unfractionated heparin.

  - The test for PF4 antibodies in patients' serum is a sensitive screening test but lacks specificity.
  - Specificity improves when a positive enzyme-linked immunosorbent assay (**ELISA**) is quantified in optical density (**OD**) units. The higher the OD, the more likely it is that the patient has HIT.
- There are two functional assays for HIT: serotonin release assay (**SRA**) and heparin-induced platelet activation (**HIPA**; more common in Europe).
  - Both tests detect PF4 antibodies in patients' serum capable of activating control platelets in the presence of heparin.
  - Both tests have high specificity for HIT but lower sensitivity than ELISA.
  - Testing in reference laboratories typically delays results for days.
- For a low clinical probability of HIT, testing for HIT antibodies is *not* indicated.
  - For a moderate to high clinical probability of HIT, PF4 ELISA testing is indicated. A negative PF4 ELISA effectively rules out HIT.
  - A functional test (SRA or HIPA) should confirm a positive PF4 ELISA to improve testing specificity.

TREATMENT

- Because HIT test results are not often immediately available, clinical assessment should determine initial management.
- When HIT is strongly suspected or confirmed, **eliminate all heparin exposure.**
- Patients with HIT are at high risk for VTE and require alternative anticoagulation with a parenteral direct thrombin inhibitor (**DTI**)[28] (i.e., **argatroban or bivalirudin**), although fondaparinux also has been used.[29] Do not use LMWH in patients with HIT.
- Assess for symptomatic VTE, and screen (e.g., lower extremity venous compression ultrasound) to assess for asymptomatic VTE, as VTE warrants a full course of anticoagulation.[26]

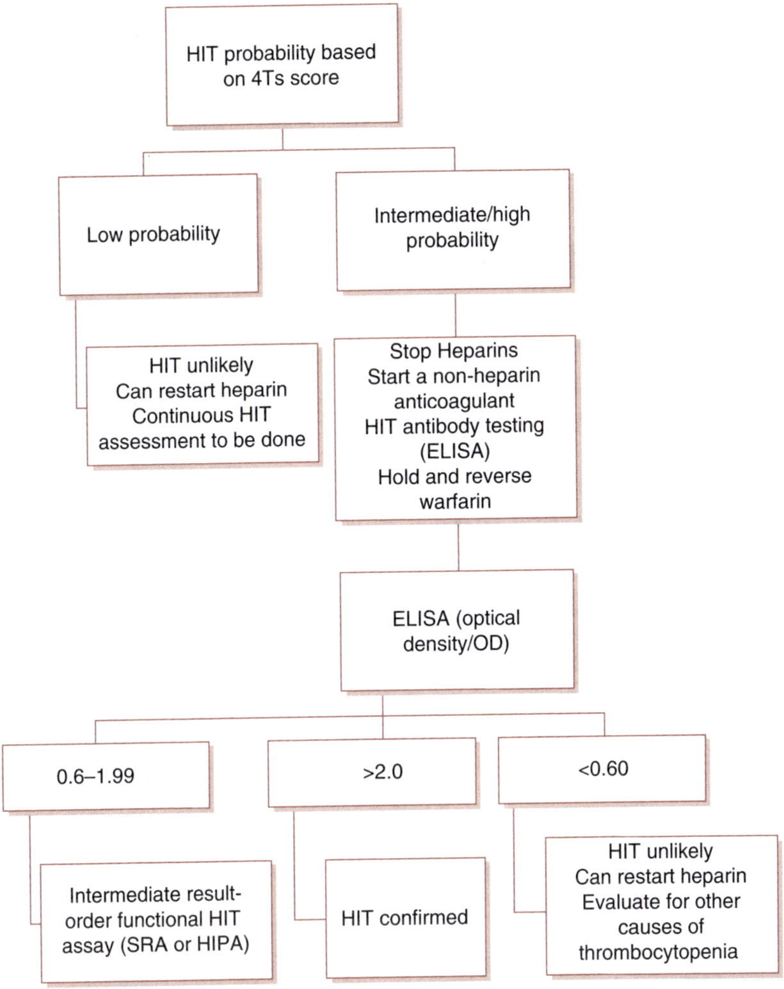

Figure 20-4 Approach to a patient with HIT.

- Start warfarin only after the platelet count normalizes to $>150 \times 10^9$/L, at an initial dose no greater than 5 mg daily, overlapping with a DTI for 5 days, to reduce the risk of limb gangrene due to ongoing hypercoagulable conditions and depletion of proteins C and S.
- DTIs prolong the INR and require careful monitoring when transitioning from DTI to warfarin (see Medications under Approach to Venous Thromboembolism).
- Avoid using oral DTI and anti-Xa inhibitors because they have not been adequately evaluated for safety and efficacy in HIT patients with or without thrombosis.
- The recommended duration of anticoagulation therapy for HIT depends on the clinical scenario: 4–6 weeks for **isolated HIT** (without thrombosis) and 3 months

for **HIT-associated thrombosis** (see treatment duration in Approach to Venous Thromboembolism section).[23]

- Warfarin must not be started until the individual is stably anticoagulated with a non-heparin agent and his/her platelet count has recovered.
- Immunoassay ELISA is ordered first since its turnaround time is faster compared to that of functional assays.
- Options for initial anticoagulation include parenteral direct thrombin inhibitors such as argatroban, bivalirudin, danaparoid, and fondaparinux.

Post-transfusion Purpura

GENERAL PRINCIPLES

Definition

Post-transfusion purpura (PTP), a rare syndrome characterized by the formation of alloantibodies against platelet antigens, most commonly HPA-1a, follows blood component transfusion and causes severe thrombocytopenia.

Epidemiology

PTP has an incidence of 1 in 50,000 to 100,000 blood transfusions, although approximately 2% of the population has a potential risk for PTP based on the frequency of HPA-1b/1b.

Etiology

Glycoprotein (GP) IIIa has a polymorphic epitope called HPA-1a/b, the antigen most commonly involved in PTP. **PTP** typically occurs in HPA-1a/1b–negative multiparous women or previously transfused patients when re-exposed to HPA-1a by transfusion. An amnestic response produces alloantibodies to the HPA-1a, which appear to also recognize the patient's HPA-1a–negative platelets and cause thrombocytopenia via platelet destruction.

DIAGNOSIS

- In **PTP**, severe thrombocytopenia ($<15 \times 10^9$/L) usually occurs within 7–10 days of transfusion.
- Confirmation of suspected **PTP** requires detection of platelet alloantibodies.

TREATMENT

Although spontaneous platelet recovery eventually occurs, bleeding may require treatment. Effective therapies include IVIG and plasmapheresis. Transfusion with platelets from a donor who lacks the causative epitope (typically HPA-1a) does not clearly have higher efficacy than random platelet transfusion. Reserve transfusion for patients with PTP and severe bleeding.[30]

Gestational Thrombocytopenia

GENERAL PRINCIPLES

Definition

Gestational thrombocytopenia (platelet counts $\geq 70 \times 10^9$/L) is a benign, mild thrombocytopenia associated with pregnancy.

Epidemiology

Gestational thrombocytopenia spontaneously occurs in approximately 5%–7% of otherwise uncomplicated pregnancies.[31]

Etiology

The mechanism of gestational thrombocytopenia remains unknown.

DIAGNOSIS

Clinical Presentation

Gestational thrombocytopenia most commonly occurs in the third trimester of pregnancy but can occur anytime during pregnancy. The mother has no symptoms or signs on physical examination and the fetus remains unaffected (no neonatal thrombocytopenia). There are no abnormalities on CBC other than thrombocytopenia.

Differential Diagnosis

Other causes of thrombocytopenia during pregnancy include **ITP, pre-eclampsia, eclampsia, HELLP syndrome, acute fatty liver of pregnancy, TTP, and DIC.**

Diagnostic Testing

To distinguish between gestational thrombocytopenia and other syndromes, diagnostic testing includes an evaluation for infection and hypertension and laboratory testing for hemolysis and liver dysfunction.

OUTCOME/PROGNOSIS

Gestational thrombocytopenia and thrombocytopenia associated with pre-eclampsia and eclampsia usually resolve promptly after delivery.

Thrombocytosis

GENERAL PRINCIPLES

Definition

Thrombocytosis is defined as a platelet count of >450 × 10^9/L by the World Health Organization (WHO).

Etiology

Thrombocytosis has reactive and clonal etiologies that may coexist.

- **Reactive thrombocytosis** may occur during recovery from thrombocytopenia; after splenectomy; or in response to iron deficiency, acute infectious or chronic inflammatory states, trauma, and malignancies.
  - Low risks of thrombosis or bleeding.
  - Platelets normalize after improvement of the underlying disorder.
  - If accompanied by thrombotic complications, evaluate for an underlying myeloproliferative disorder.
- **Essential thrombocytosis** (ET) is a chronic myeloproliferative disorder. Eventual progression to myelofibrosis, acute myeloid leukemia, or myelodysplastic syndrome occurs in a minority of ET patients.[32]

DIAGNOSIS

Clinical Presentation

History

ET may present as an incidental discovery or present with thrombotic or hemorrhagic symptoms. The risk of thrombosis increases with age, prior thrombosis, duration of disease, and other comorbidities.[33] Erythromelalgia, due to microvascular occlusive platelet thrombi, presents as intense burning or throbbing of the extremities, typically involving the feet. Cold exposure usually relieves symptoms. Hemorrhage can occur with platelet counts >1000 × 10^9/L, and acquired deficiencies of large vWF multimers often accompany hemorrhage patients with ET.[34]

Physical Examination

Approximately 50% of ET patients develop mild splenomegaly. Typical signs of erythromelalgia include erythema and warmth of affected digits.

Diagnostic Criteria

In 2016, the **WHO** revised criteria (requires all four) included:[35]

- Sustained platelet count ≥450 × 10^9/L peripheral blood smear.
- Bone marrow biopsy showing increased mature megakaryocytes and no increase in erythropoiesis or granulopoiesis or reticulin fiber deposition (greater than grade I).
- Exclusion of BCR-ABL1 positive chronic myelogenous leukemia (**CML**), polycythemia vera, primary myelofibrosis, myelodysplastic syndrome, or other myeloid neoplasm
- Presence of *JAK2 V617F*, *CALR*, or *MPL* mutation **or**, if clonal marker not present, no evidence for reactive thrombocytosis.[36]

TREATMENT

Patients with high or intermediate risk of thrombosis based on the International Prognostic Score for Thrombosis in Essental Thrombocythemia (IPSET)[37] (high: age >60 years with a *JAK2 V617F* mutation and/or a history of thrombosis at any age, intermediate: age >60, no *JAK2* mutation, no history of thrombosis) require cytoreduction therapy. Platelet-lowering drugs include **hydroxyurea** and **anagrelide** or **interferon-α** in pregnant patients or females in their childbearing years.[38] The majority of thrombotic complications occur at modest platelet count elevations. Treatment typically aims for a platelet count of ≤400 × 10^9/L.

Low-dose aspirin (40–100 mg/d given in two divided doses) orally can help alleviate vasomotor symptoms and thrombo-hemorrhagic complication in ET.

- Administer hydroxyurea orally at a dosage of 15 mg/kg with a target platelet count range of 4–10 lakhs/mcL. CBC and liver function tests to be done once in 2 weeks to monitor adverse events such as anemia and neutropenia. For anagrelide, start with a dosage of 0.5 mg two to four times daily, subsequently titrating to 1–4 mg/d to maintain a platelet count within the range of 4–10 lakhs/mcL. However, it's important to note that while anagrelide provides equivalent platelet count control, it is associated with a higher incidence of complications.[39]
- Anagrelide side effects include palpitations, atrial fibrillation, fluid retention, and headache.
- Plateletpheresis rapidly lowers platelet counts, although it is reserved for patients who have acute arterial thromboses.

Qualitative Platelet Disorders

GENERAL PRINCIPLES

Qualitative platelet disorders present with mucocutaneous bleeding and excessive bruising with an adequate platelet count, PT, and aPTT and normal screening tests for vWD. Most potent platelet defects produce prolonged PFA-100 closure times. However, a normal PFA-100 does not exclude qualitative platelet disorders, and high clinical suspicion of a disorder should lead to further testing (Fig. 20-5).

Classification

- **Inherited disorders** of platelet function include receptor, signal transduction, cyclooxygenase (COX), secretory (e.g., storage pool disease), adhesion, or aggregation defects. In vitro platelet aggregation studies can identify patterns of agonist responses consistent with a particular defect, such as the rare autosomal recessive disorders of adhesion

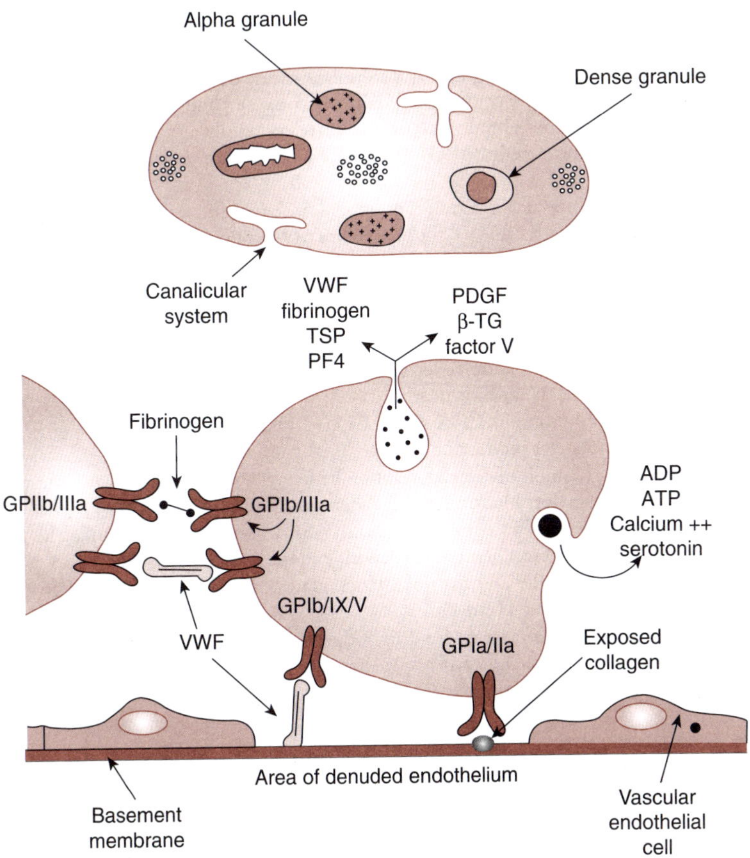

Figure 20-5 Qualitative platelet defects.

in **Bernard–Soulier syndrome** (lack of GP Ib/IX [vWF receptor]) and aggregation in **Glanzmann thrombasthenia** (lack of GP IIb/IIIa [fibrinogen receptor]).

- **Acquired** platelet defects are more common than hereditary platelet qualitative disorders.
  - Conditions associated with acquired qualitative defects include metabolic disorders (uremia, liver failure), myeloproliferative diseases, myelodysplasia, acute leukemia, monoclonal gammopathy, and cardiopulmonary bypass platelet trauma.
  - **Drug-induced** platelet dysfunction is a side effect of many drugs, including high-dose penicillin, aspirin (ASA) and other **NSAIDs**, and ethanol. Other drug classes, such as β-lactam antibiotics, β-blockers, calcium channel blockers, nitrates, antihistamines, psychotropic drugs, tricyclic antidepressants, and selective serotonin reuptake inhibitors, cause platelet dysfunction in vitro, but they rarely cause bleeding.
  - Certain **foods and herbal products** may affect platelet function including omega-3 fatty acids, garlic and onion extracts, ginger, gingko, ginseng, and black tree fungus. Patients should stop using herbal medications and dietary supplements ≥1 week before major surgery.[40,41]

TREATMENT

- Treatment of **uremic platelet dysfunction** can include dialysis to improve uremia; desmopressin (**DDAVP**) 0.3 μg/kg IV to stimulate release of vWF from endothelial cells; or conjugated estrogens (0.6 mg/kg IV daily for 5 days)[42] and platelet transfusions in actively bleeding patients, although transfused platelets rapidly acquire the uremic defect. Transfusion or erythropoietin (**EPO**) to increase a hematocrit toward 30% might assist in hemostasis.[43,44]
- Antifibrinolytic agents such as aminocaproic acid or tranexamic acid are commonly used as adjunct therapies with DDAVP for procedures or bleeding complications.
- Reserve platelet transfusions for major bleeding episodes. Anecdotal reports have described successful control of severe bleeding with recombinant factor VIIa (**rFVIIa**).
- **Reversal of drug-induced platelet dysfunction**
  - **NSAIDs** other than ASA reversibly inhibit **COX**. Their effects only last several days. **COX-2 inhibitors** have antiplatelet activity in large doses, but they have a minimal effect on platelets at therapeutic doses.
  - **Aspirin** irreversibly inhibits COX-1 and COX-2. Its effects diminish over 7–10 days because of new platelet production.
  - **Thienopyridines** inhibit platelet aggregation by irreversibly (clopidogrel and prasugrel) or reversibly (ticagrelor) blocking platelet adenosine diphosphate receptor P2Y12.
  - **Dipyridamole,** alone or in combination with ASA (Aggrenox), inhibits platelet function by increasing intracellular cyclic adenosine monophosphate (**cAMP**).
  - **Abciximab, eptifibatide, and tirofiban** block platelet IIb/IIIa–dependent aggregation (see Chapter 4, Ischemic Heart Disease).
  - Platelet transfusion compensates for drug-induced platelet dysfunction, except immediately following tirofiban and eptifibatide therapy.
  - Hold antiplatelet agents for 7 days before elective invasive procedures.

Inherited Macrothrombocytopenia (Bengal Macrothrombocytopenia in Indian Context)

- These are a subgroup of thrombocytopenias characterized by the presence of giant platelets and decreased platelet count with variable bleeding manifestation. They constitute a heterogeneous group of platelet disorders sometimes associated with syndromes such as renal failure, hearing loss, and presenile cataracts.

- Bengal macrothrombocytopenia, previously called asymptomatic constitutional macrothrombocytopenia (ACMT), is prevalent in the eastern region of India characterized by low platelet count during routine blood tests in patients with variable bleeding tendencies and sometimes no history of bleeding at all, no significant drug history causing thrombocytopenia, normal coagulation parameters, mean platelet volume (MPV) greater than 10 fL, and confirmation of the presence of giant platelets on peripheral smear by light microscopy.*

INHERITED BLEEDING DISORDERS

Hemophilia A

GENERAL PRINCIPLES

Definition

Hemophilia A is an X-linked recessive coagulation disorder due to mutations in the gene encoding factor VIII.

Epidemiology

Hemophilia A affects ~1 in 5000 live male births. Approximately 40% of cases occur in families with no prior history of hemophilia, reflecting the high rate of spontaneous germline mutations in the factor VIII gene.[45]

DIAGNOSIS

Clinical Presentation

- Patients with severe hemophilia experience frequent spontaneous hemarthroses and hematomas, hematuria, and delayed post-traumatic and postoperative bleeding. Repeated bleeding into a "target" joint causes chronic synovitis and hemophilic arthropathy.
- Moderate hemophiliacs have fewer spontaneous bleeding episodes, and mild hemophiliacs may only bleed excessively after trauma or surgery.

Diagnostic Testing

The severity of hemophilia is based on baseline factor VIII activity: Severe (<1%), moderate (1%–5%), and mild (>5%–<40%).

Mild hemophiliacs with factor VIII ≥30% may not have a prolonged aPTT.

TREATMENT

Medications

First Line

- Mild-to-moderate hemophilia A with minor bleeding:
  - **DDAVP** (0.3 μg/kg IV infused over 30 minutes, or 150 μg intranasal) increases factor VIII activity three- to fivefold. Because not all patients have an expected response to DDAVP, they should undergo a DDAVP challenge to assess responsiveness before use. To avoid tachyphylaxis, no more than 3 consecutive doses should be given per week.[46]
- Mild-to-moderate hemophilia A with major bleeding OR severe hemophilia A with any bleeding:

---

*Ali S, Shetty S, Ghosh K. Bengal macrothrombocytopaenia is not totally an innocuous condition. *Blood Cells Mol Dis*. 2016;60:3–6.

- ◦ **Factor VIII replacement** is the mainstay of therapy with many hemophiliac patients able to do home infusion.
- ◦ **Factor VIII concentrate** increases factor VIII activity by 2% for every 1 IU/kg infused, thus a 50 IU/kg IV bolus raises factor VIII activity by 100% over baseline. Extended treatment should follow with 25–30 IU/kg IV bolus q12h and adjust dose based on peak and trough factor VIII levels to maintain sufficient levels.
- ◦ One to three doses of **factor VIII** concentrates targeting peak plasma activities of 30%–50% typically stop mild hemorrhages.
- ◦ Major traumas and surgery require maintenance of levels >80%.
- ◦ Adjust doses based on peak and trough factor VIII levels to achieve individualized targets based on bleeding risk.
- ◦ Continuous infusion of factor VIII provides a safe and effective alternative to intermittent infusion.[47,48]

Second Line

Second-line factor VIII sources include **cryoprecipitate** and **FFP**.

Hemophilia B

GENERAL PRINCIPLES

Definition

Hemophilia B is an X-linked recessive coagulation disorder secondary to mutations in the gene encoding factor IX.

Epidemiology

Hemophilia B affects ~1 in 30,000 male births.

DIAGNOSIS

Clinical Presentation

Hemophilia B remains clinically indistinguishable from hemophilia A.

Diagnostic Testing

Factor IX activity. Hemophilia A (Factor VIII) and B (Factor IX) use the same severity scale based on degree of decreased factor activity.

TREATMENT

Therapy of hemophilia B consists of **factor IX replacement** with either **plasma-derived factor IX** or **recombinant factor IX** (BeneFIX).

- DDAVP lacks efficacy because it does **not** increase factor IX levels.
- Postinfusion peak targets, duration of therapy, and laboratory monitoring for treatment of hemophilia B–related bleeding are similar to those for hemophilia A.
- Every 1 IU/kg of factor IX replacement typically raises plasma factor IX activity by 1%. Factor IX has a half-life of 18 to 24 hours, hence once-a-day dosing.

COMPLICATIONS OF HEMOPHILIA A AND B THERAPY

Inhibitors

- Alloantibodies to factors VIII and IX in response to replacement therapy develop in approximately 20% and 12% of severe hemophilia A and B patients, respectively. These alloantibodies neutralize infused factor VIII or IX.

- Determining the titer of a factor VIII or IX inhibitor, using a laboratory assay that reports inhibitor strength in Bethesda units (**BUs**), predicts inhibitor behavior and guides therapy.
- Treatment options for factor VIII or IX inhibitors include[49]:
  - Large doses of factor VIII or IX concentrates overcome inhibitors for patients with low titer (BU <5).
  - Because factor VIII or IX concentrates will not overcome inhibitors in patients with high titers (BU >5), bypassing agents such as rFVII or activated prothrombin complex concentrate (aPCC) are used.[50]
    - **rFVIIa** (NovoSeven®) is dosed at 90 μg/kg every 2 hours until hemostasis occurs.
    - **aPCC** (most commonly used-Factor Eight Inhibitor Bypassing Activity [FEIBA®]), dosed at 75–100 IU/kg q12h. FEIBA® contains activated factors VII, VIII, XI, X, and thrombin, and it can cause thrombosis or DIC.
- Emicizumab (Hemlibra®) is a humanized monoclonal antibody that bridges activated factor IX and X to restore the function of missing activated factor VIII. It is given as weekly subcutaneous injections and reduces annualized bleeding rate by 80%–90% in hemophilia A patients with inhibitors.[51] Thrombotic microangiopathy is a rare complication in patients receiving concurrent aPCC. It is FDA approved for routine prophylaxis in hemophilia A with inhibitors. Ongoing clinical trials have also shown promising results in hemophilia A without inhibitors.

von Willebrand Disease

GENERAL PRINCIPLES

Classification

vWD has three main types[52]:

- **Type 1 vWD,** due to a quantitative deficiency of vWF (70%–80% of cases)
- **Type 2 vWD,** due to a qualitative defect of vWF, includes four subtypes (2A, 2B, 2M, 2N):
  - Type 2A: reduced vWF high molecular weight multimer
  - Type 2B: pathologically enhanced platelet affinity to vWF
  - Type 2M: reduced platelet affinity to vWF
  - Type 2N: defective FVIII binding to vWF
- **Type 3 vWD,** due to a near complete lack of vWF.[53]

Epidemiology

vWD, the most common inherited bleeding disorder, affects around 0.1%–1% of the population.

Etiology

Most forms of **vWD** have an autosomal dominant inheritance with variable penetrance, although autosomal recessive forms (types 2N and 3) exist. vWF circulates as multimers of variable size and facilitate adherence of platelets to injured vessel walls and stabilize FVIII in plasma.

DIAGNOSIS

Clinical Presentation

- Clinical findings consist of mucocutaneous bleeding (epistaxis, menorrhagia, gastrointestinal bleeding), easy bruising, and bleeding from trauma or surgery.

Diagnostic Testing

Testing for suspected vWD should include vWF:Ag, vWF:RCo and FVIII activity. See American Society of Hematology pocket guide on vWD.

TREATMENT

Goal of therapy is to raise vWF:RCo and factor VIII activity to ensure adequate hemostasis. vWF:RCo activities >50% control most hemorrhages.

- **DDAVP** 0.3 μg/kg IV can be used to treat type 1 vWD. Because only two-thirds of patients will respond, a test dose should assess for a response. For responders undergoing **minor invasive procedures**, infuse 1 hour before, followed by q12–24h for 3 more doses postoperatively as needed, with or without oral antifibrinolytic drugs (i.e., aminocaproic acid or tranexamic acid).
  - DDAVP does not effectively treat most type 2 or type 3 vWD patients.
  - DDAVP is contraindicated in type 2B vWD because of the risk of thrombocytopenia.
  - Common side effects of DDAVP include hyponatremia, nausea, and flushing. Patients should limit fluid intake to 1200 mL/d within 24 hours of any dose.
- **vWF plasma-derived concentrate transfusions** (Alphanate, Humate-P, and Wilate) and **recombinant vWF** (Vonvendi®) should aim to raise vWF:RCo activity to ~100% and maintain it between 50% and 100% until sufficient hemostasis occurs (typically 5 to 10 days). Cryoprecipitate is a second-line vWF source. Indications for concentrate transfusions:
  - type 1 vWD-DDAVP nonresponders
  - type 1 vWD-major bleeding or surgery
  - all other vWD types requiring hemostasis treatment

ACQUIRED COAGULATION DISORDERS

Vitamin K Deficiency

GENERAL PRINCIPLES

Vitamin K deficiency is usually caused by malabsorption states or poor dietary intake, especially when combined with antibiotic-associated loss of intestinal bacterial colonization. Hepatocytes require vitamin K to complete the γ-carboxylation-mediated synthesis of clotting factors (X, IX, VII, prothrombin) and the natural anticoagulant proteins C and S.

DIAGNOSIS

A **prolonged PT that corrects after a 1:1 mix with normal pooled plasma** suggests that a patient has Vitamin K deficiency.

TREATMENT

Oral **Vitamin K replacement** (e.g., phytonadione 5 mg PO daily) typically has good absorption in patients who have had poor dietary intake. IV Vitamin K repletion has excellent bioavailability in patients who have malabsorption, and its more reliable absorption make it the preferred parenteral route when compared to SC.

Liver Disease

GENERAL PRINCIPLES

Liver disease can impair hemostasis (**see** Figure 20-1) due to a reduction in coagulation factor production by hepatocytes, with the exception of vWF and factor VIII. Cholestasis, which leads to impaired vitamin K absorption, can also contribute because of decreased production of Factors II, VII, IX, and X. Patients who have stable liver disease typically only have a mild coagulopathy, though decompensated liver disease will worsen the coagulopathy severity. Liver disease may produce other hemostatic complications that include thrombocytopenia due to splenic sequestration, DIC, hyperfibrinolysis. Infection, renal insufficiency, and vasomotor dysfunction may also disrupt the fragile balance of procoagulant and anticoagulant activities.[54] Although PT/INR and aPTT prolongations imply an increased risk of bleeding, they do not reflect concurrent reductions in protein C and protein S.

TREATMENT

- **Vitamin K** replacement may shorten a prolonged PT/INR caused by a vitamin K antagonist, dietary deficiency, or cholestasis.
- **For patients who have an elevated INR, aPTT, or both, FFP** may decrease active bleeding or prevent/lessen bleeding in those undergoing an invasive procedure, but it may cause volume overload and does not work immediately. In these clinical settings, clinicians often use a threshold of PT >1.5 control for determining when to use FFP, despite limited supportive evidence.
- **Cryoprecipitate,** 1.5 units/10 kg body weight, corrects hypofibrinogenemia (<100 mg/dL), while FFP does not provide a significant amount of Factor II replacement.
- **Prothrombin complex concentrate** (PCC) will work more rapidly than FFP in normalizing an elevated INR for the indications of active bleeding or upcoming invasive procedure, and it requires less volume administration, but it has not undergone extensive safety and efficacy testing in patients who have liver disease.
- Randomized controlled trials failed to show a hemostasis benefit for **recombinant factor VIIa** in GI bleeding, and it may cause thrombosis.[55]
- **Platelet transfusion** may decrease active bleeding or prevent/lessen bleeding in those undergoing an invasive procedure in patients who have severe thrombocytopenia ($<50 \times 10^9$/L), and it may prevent bleeding in patients who have severe thrombocytopenia ($<10 \times 10^9$/L).

Disseminated Intravascular Coagulation

GENERAL PRINCIPLES

Etiology

DIC occurs in a variety of systemic illnesses that include sepsis, trauma, burns, shock, obstetric complications, and malignancies (notably, acute promyelocytic leukemia).

Pathophysiology

Exposure of tissue factor to the circulation generates excess thrombin, leading to platelet activation, consumption of coagulation factors (including fibrinogen) and regulators (antithrombin [AT] and proteins C and S), fibrin generation, generalized microthrombi, and reactive fibrinolysis.

TABLE 20-4 International Society on Thrombosis and Haemostasis Disseminated Intravascular Coagulation Scoring System

Use Only in Patients With an Underlying Condition Known to be Associated With DIC.

	0 Points	1 Point	2 Points
Thrombocytopenia	>100 × 10^9/L	≤100 × 10^9/L	≤50 × 10^9/L
D-dimer	Normal	<10 × upper limit of normal	≥10 × upper limit of normal
PT Prolongation	<3 s	3–6 s	>6 s
Fibrinogen	>100 mg/dL	≤100 mg/dL	

Data from *Thromb Haemost.* 2001;86:132; *Crit Care Med.* 2004;32:24167.
Sum the points for each of the four categories to determine the clinical probability of having DIC: compatible with overt DIC ≥5 points, and suggestive of nonovert DIC <5 points.
DIC, disseminated intravascular coagulation.

DIAGNOSIS

Clinical Presentation

Consequences of **DIC** include bleeding, organ dysfunction secondary to microvascular thrombi and ischemia, and less often, large arterial and venous thrombosis.[56]

Diagnostic Testing

No test confirms diagnosis of DIC. The International Society on Thrombosis and Haemostasis (**ISTH**) devised a clinical scoring system for objective detection of DIC (Table 20-4). Serial "DIC panels" help assess clinical management and prognosis.

TREATMENT

Treatment of DIC consists of supportive care and correction of the underlying disorder if possible. **FFP**, **cryoprecipitate**, and **platelets** can be administered when needed clinically (e.g., bleeding or surgery), rather than strictly based on a laboratory threshold. Despite the coagulopathy, patients who have large-vessel venous or arterial thrombi should undergo anticoagulation if they do not have other contraindications. Nonbleeding patients who have DIC should receive thromboprophylaxis with heparin.

Acquired Inhibitors of Coagulation Factors

GENERAL PRINCIPLES

Acquired inhibitors of coagulation factors may occur de novo (autoantibodies) or may develop in hemophiliacs (alloantibodies) following factor VIII or IX infusions. Of the acquired **inhibitors, those directed against factor VIII occur most commonly.** De novo inhibitors often arise in patients who have underlying lymphoproliferative or autoimmune disorders.

DIAGNOSIS

Patients who have a factor VIII inhibitor typically present with an abrupt onset of bleeding or bruising, a prolonged aPTT that does not correct after 1:1 mixing with normal plasma, a markedly decreased factor VIII activity, and a normal PT. Patients rarely develop autoantibodies that inhibit other factors (II, V, X) and subsequently prolong aPTT and PT, which do not correct after mixing studies.

TREATMENT

- **rFVIIa (NovoSeven®) or aPCC,** used in a similar manner as for hemophiliacs who have alloantibodies to factor VIII (see Inherited Bleeding Disorders section), treats bleeding problems.
- **Recombinant porcine factor VIII (OBI-1)** lacks the B domain allowing low cross-reactivity to anti-Factor VIII antibodies. In addition, efficacy can be monitored with Factor VIII activity levels in conjunction with clinical evaluation. In an initial trial of patients with acquired hemophilia A, bleeding control was achieved in 86% of patients.[57]
- **Immunosuppression** with rituximab,[58] prednisone, or prednisolone ± cyclophosphamide[59] can eradicate inhibitors.

VENOUS THROMBOEMBOLIC DISORDERS

Approach to Venous Thromboembolism

GENERAL PRINCIPLES

Definition

- **Thrombosis** refers to a blood clot that occur in veins, arteries, or chambers of the heart.
- VTE refers to **deep vein thrombosis** (DVT) and associated **pulmonary embolism** (PE).
- **Thrombophlebitis** consists of inflammation in a vein due to a blood clot.
- **Superficial venous thrombophlebitis** refers to thrombosis and inflammation in a nondeep axial vein (e.g., great saphenous vein, small saphenous vein).

Classification

The anatomic location of DVT/PE, clot burden, and sequelae may affect prognosis and treatment recommendations.

- DVT can be **deep** or **superficial** and **proximal** or **distal.**
  - **Proximal lower extremity DVTs** occur in deep veins from the common femoral vein to the popliteal vein (or the confluence of tibial and peroneal veins); distal lower extremity DVTs occur in the **tibial and peroneal veins.**
  - **Proximal upper extremity DVTs** occur in the subclavian, brachiocephalic, axillary, and brachial veins, whereas **distal upper extremity DVTs** occur in the cephalic and basilic veins.
  - **Other** important venous thromboses sites include the vena cava (superior and inferior), abdominal veins (hepatic, portal, superior mesenteric, and splenic), pelvic veins (iliac, ovarian, penile), retinal veins, and cerebral veins, and cavernous sinus.
- PE anatomic location in the pulmonary arterial system characterizes **PE** as **central/proximal** (main pulmonary artery, lobar, or segmental) or **distal** (subsegmental).
- Chest imaging may also classify PE severity based on **clot burden.**
- PE severity classification may refer to **cardiovascular dysfunction** variables that define **submassive PE** (e.g., right ventricular [RV] strain, RV dysfunction, elevated troponin, elevated NT-proBNP) or **massive PE** (systemic hypotension). (Table 20-5)

TABLE 20-5 European Society of Cardiology Morality Risk Classification of Patients Who Have Acute Pulmonary Embolism

Early Mortality Risk		Risk Parameters and Scores			
		Shock or Hypotension	**PESI Class III V or sPESI ≥1**	**Signs of RV Dysfunction on an Imaging Test[a]**	**Cardiac Laboratory Biomarkers[b]**
High		+	(+)[c]	+	(+)[c]
Intermediate	**Intermediate-high**	–	+	Both positive	
	Intermediate-low	–	+	Either one (or none) positive[d]	
Low		–	–	Assessment optional; if assessed, both negative[d]	

Reprinted from Konstantinides SV, Torbicki A, Agnelli G, et al. 2014 ESC Guidelines on the diagnosis and management of acute pulmonary embolism: the task force for the diagnosis and management of acute pulmonary embolism of the European Society of Cardiology (ESC) Endorsed by the European Respiratory Society (ERS). *Eur Heart J.* 2014;35:3033-3073 with permission from Oxford University Press.

[a]Echocardiographic criteria of RV dysfunction include RV dilation and/or an increased end-diastolic RV–LV diameter ratio (e.g., ≥1), hypokinesia of the free RV wall, or increased velocity of the tricuspid regurgitation jet. Computed tomographic (CT) angiography criterion for RV dysfunction is an increased end-diastolic RV/LV diameter ratio (e.g., ≥1.0).

[b]Markers of myocardial injury or of heart failure as a result of right ventricular dysfunction.

[c]Classify shock or hypotension as high risk, despite any PESI or sPESI score.

[d]Classify low-risk PESI (Class I–II) or sPESI patients (score of 0) who have elevated cardiac biomarkers or signs of RV dysfunction on imaging tests.

LV, left ventricular; PESI, pulmonary embolism severity index; RV, right ventricular; sPESI, simplified PESI.

Epidemiology

- Without treatment, half of patients with proximal lower extremity DVT develop PE.
- DVTs in the upper extremities often occur with an indwelling catheter and may cause PE.
- DVT may occur concomitantly with superficial thrombophlebitis.
- Untreated acute symptomatic PE has a 10%–30% short-term mortality.[60,61]
- Patients who have hemodynamic instability associated with acute PE have a >15% risk of death in the subsequent 30 days, despite treatment.
- Patients who have acute PE without shock or hypotension but with signs of right ventricular dysfunction or myocardial injury have a 3%–15% 30-day mortality risk.
- Patients who have acute symptomatic PE with normal blood pressure and RV function have a 30-day mortality risk of <1%.
- The 3-month mortality after the initiation of anticoagulant therapy in low-risk patients averages around 2%.[62]

Etiology

- Venous thromboemboli arise under conditions of **blood stasis**, **hypercoagulability** (changes in the soluble and formed elements of the blood), or venous **endothelial dysfunction/injury (Virchow's triad)**.
- Hypercoagulable states may have an **inherited** or **acquired** etiology (see Risk Factors section).
- VTEs are classified as **provoked or unprovoked**, where provoked are attributed to an identifiable risk factor (e.g., surgery) and unprovoked have no identifiable cause.
- **Superficial thrombophlebitis** occurs in association with varicose veins, trauma, infection, and hypercoagulable disorders.
- Causes of **pulmonary arterial occlusion** not due to thromboemboli include embolism of marrow/fat, amniotic fluid, and foreign substances that enter the venous system, in situ thrombi (e.g., sickle cell disease), malignancy (e.g., pulmonary artery sarcoma), and inflammation/fibrosis (e.g., fibrosing mediastinitis).

Risk Factors

- Risk factors for VTE can be categorized as **inherited, acquired, or unknown (idiopathic)**.
- **Inherited thrombophilia** are suggested by spontaneous VTE at a young age (<50 years), recurrent VTE, VTE in first-degree relatives, thrombosis in unusual anatomic locations (i.e., abdominal), and recurrent fetal loss.
- The most common inherited risk factors for VTE include gene mutations (**factor V Leiden and prothrombin gene G20210A**) and deficiencies of the natural anticoagulants **protein C, protein S, and AT.**
- **Homocystinuria**, a rare autosomal recessive disorder caused by deficiency of cystathionine-β-synthase, leads to extremely high plasma homocysteine and causes early-onset arterial and venous thromboembolic events. However, mild elevation of homocysteine may be caused by a mutation in methylenetetrahydrofolate reductase (**MTHFR**) but does not cause VTE.[63,64] Therefore, thrombophilia testing should not include *MTHFR* mutation testing.
- Spontaneous VTE in unusual locations, such as cavernous sinus, mesenteric vein, or portal vein, may be the initial presentation of paroxysmal nocturnal hemoglobinuria (**PNH**) or myeloproliferative disorders (JAK2 mutation).
- **Spontaneous (idiopathic) VTEs** have a high risk of recurrence (8%–10% per year) after stopping anticoagulant therapy, regardless of the presence of an inherited thrombophilia.[65]
- **Acquired hypercoagulable** states may arise secondary to malignancy, immobilization, infection, trauma, surgery, collagen vascular diseases, nephrotic syndrome, HIT, DIC, medications (e.g., estrogen), and pregnancy.

- Acquired **autoantibodies** associated with HIT and antiphospholipid syndrome (**APS**) can cause arterial or venous thrombi.
- **APS** is a hypercoagulable disorder that requires the presence of at least one clinical **and** one laboratory criterion.[66]
    - **APS clinical criteria:**
        - **Unprovoked** arterial or venous thrombosis in any tissue or organ *or*
        - **Pregnancy** morbidities (unexplained late fetal death; premature birth complicated by eclampsia, pre-eclampsia, placental insufficiency; or ≥ three unexplained consecutive spontaneous abortions at <10 weeks of gestation or one at ≥10 weeks).
    - **APS laboratory criteria:**
        - Presence of autoantibodies such as **LA**, anticardiolipin, or β_2-glycoprotein-1 antibodies
        - Approximately 10% of patients with SLE have an LA; however, most patients with an LA do not have SLE
        - Confirmation of positive autoantibody tests (must be done at least 12 weeks apart)
    - APS may include **other features**, such as thrombocytopenia, valvular heart disease, livedo reticularis, neurologic manifestations, and nephropathy.

Prevention

Identifying patients at high risk for VTE and instituting prophylactic measures should remain a high priority (see **Chapter 1, Inpatient Care in Internal Medicine**).

DIAGNOSIS

Clinical Presentation

- **Lower or upper extremity** DVT **symptoms** commonly include **pain, edema, redness, and warmth.**
- **Superficial thrombophlebitis** presents as a tender, warm, erythematous, and often palpable thrombosed vein. Accompanying DVT may produce additional symptoms and signs.
- **PE** may produce shortness of breath, chest pain (pleuritic), hypoxemia, hemoptysis, pleural rub, new right-sided heart failure, and tachycardia.[67]

Differential Diagnosis

- The **differential diagnoses of lower extremity DVT** include cellulitis, Baker cyst (behind knee), hematoma, venous insufficiency, postphlebitic syndrome, lymphedema, sarcoma, arterial aneurysm, myositis, rupture of the gastrocnemius, and abscess.
- **Symmetric, bilateral lower extremity edema** suggests heart, renal, or liver failure as the cause of the signs and symptoms, but it does not exclude the presence of DVT.
- The **differential diagnosis of PE** includes dissecting aortic aneurysm, pneumonia, acute bronchitis, pericardial or pleural disease, heart failure, costochondritis, rib fracture, and myocardial ischemia.

Diagnostic Testing

Clinical Probability Assessment

Clinical decision rules help to exclude VTE when used in combination with other diagnostic tests (such as normal D-dimer).

- **Clinical predictors of DVT** from **Wells criteria** include: history of DVT, paralysis/paresis/immobilization of the leg, recently bedridden, major surgery within 4 weeks, active cancer, leg vein tenderness, swelling of entire leg, calf diameter > 3 cm larger than other calf, pitting edema confined to symptomatic leg, dilated collateral superficial leg veins, and alternative diagnoses less likely than DVT. **Outpatients** who have one or fewer of these predictors (i.e., low Wells score) are unlikely to have a DVT.[68] However, since the Wells criteria for DVT in **inpatients** performs only slightly better than chance, clinicians should not use it in hospitalized patients.[69]

- **Pretest assessment of the probability of a DVT** provides useful information when combined with the results of a **venous compression ultrasound, a D-dimer test**, or both, in determining whether to exclude or accept the diagnosis of DVT or perform additional imaging studies.[68]

  Validated clinical risk factors for a PE in outpatients who present to an emergency department include signs and symptoms of DVT, high clinical suspicion of PE, tachycardia, immobility in the past 4 weeks, history of VTE, active cancer, hemoptysis,[70] and lack of an alternative diagnosis that is at least as likely as PE. Patients who have one or fewer of these predictors (i.e., a low **simplified Wells score**) are unlikely to have a PE.
- The combination of a **low (simplified) Wells score and a normal D-dimer** essentially rules out a PE.[71]
- A normal D-dimer and a negative chest CT essentially rule out PE, and a lower extremity compression ultrasound does not typically assist further with the diagnostic testing.[72]

Laboratories

- **D-dimer** and fibrin degradation products may increase during VTE and after surgery.
  - D-dimer testing for VTE has a low positive predictive value (**PPV**) and specificity; **patients with a positive test require further evaluation.**
  - A **sensitive quantitative D-dimer assay** has a high enough NPV to exclude a **DVT** when the **objectively defined clinical probability** is low and/or a **noninvasive test** is negative.[73,74] In the setting of a moderate to high clinical pretest probability (e.g., patients with cancer), a negative D-dimer does not have sufficient NPV for excluding the presence of DVT or PE.[75,76]
  - Compared to a **fixed D-dimer cutoff of 500 μg/L, upward age adjustment of the cutoff (age × 10 in patients at least age 50 years)** will increase the number of patients who can have PE excluded based on the combination of nonelevated D-dimer and objective clinical probability assessment (i.e., low-intermediate or unlikely pretest probability).[77]
- Signs and symptoms of the **APS** should lead to laboratory evaluation.
  - Serologic tests (e.g., IgG and IgM **β_2-glycoprotein-1 antibodies**, and IgG and IgM **cardiolipin antibodies**) and clotting assays (e.g., **LA**) detect APS, and performing both improves sensitivity.
  - LAs may prolong the aPTT or PT/INR, although this prolongation does not predispose to bleeding.
- In the setting of **spontaneous VTE in unusual sites and hemolytic anemia**, use peripheral blood flow cytometry to assess for missing antigens on red cells and leukocytes and detect **PNH.**

Imaging

- **DVT-specific testing.**[78] Initial diagnostic imaging for suspected acute DVT almost exclusively consists of **compression ultrasound**, called **duplex examination** when performed with Doppler testing, of the veins,[79] although some other diagnostic options include magnetic resonance venography, **CT** venography, and venography.
  - In addition to assessing for DVT, imaging may detect other pathology (**see** Differential Diagnosis **section**).
  - Compression ultrasound has a high sensitivity in **symptomatic** patients and a low sensitivity in **asymptomatic** patients.
  - Compression ultrasound has a low sensitivity for detecting **calf** DVT and may fail to visualize parts of the iliac vein, the upper extremity venous system, and the pelvic veins.
  - Compression ultrasound may have difficulty distinguishing between acute and **chronic** DVT.

- **Lower extremity venous compression ultrasound** may help diagnose or exclude VTE in patients who have suspected PE and a nondiagnostic ventilation/perfusion (**V/Q**) scan, a nondiagnostic or negative chest CT with high suspicion of PE, or a contraindications to or difficulty completing imaging for PE (see PE-specific testing section).
- **Serial testing** can improve the diagnostic yield of compression ultrasound. If a patient with a clinically suspected lower extremity DVT has a negative initial noninvasive test and no satisfactory alternative explanation, one can withhold anticoagulant therapy and **repeat testing** at least once 3–14 days later.
- **Ultrasound is recommended to exclude DVT in the setting of superficial venous thrombosis.**[80]

- **PE-specific testing**
  - **Contrast-enhanced spiral (helical) chest CT**
    - PE-protocol chest CT (pulmonary angiography) requires IV administration of iodinated contrast.
    - Contraindications to spiral CT include renal dysfunction and dye allergy.
    - Used according to standardized protocols in conjunction with expert interpretation, spiral CT has good accuracy for detection of large (proximal) PEs, but it has lower sensitivity for detecting small (distal) emboli.[81]
    - The sensitivity of CT for PE improves by combining the CT pulmonary angiography results with objective grading of clinical suspicion.
    - **Clinical suspicion discordant with the objective test finding** (e.g., high suspicion with a negative CT scan or low suspicion with a positive CT scan) **should lead to further testing.**
    - Advantages of CT scan over V/Q scan include an unambiguous grade in many cases (positive or negative) with fewer indeterminate or inadequate studies and the detection of alternative or concomitant diagnoses, such as dissecting aortic aneurysm, pneumonia, and malignancy.[82]
    - For patients who have a contraindication to CT, alternative testing options include (1) V/Q scan and/or (2) leg venous compression ultrasound, which uses proximal DVT as a surrogate for PE.[72]
  - **V/Q scan**
    - V/Q scans administer radioactive material (via inhaled and IV routes).
    - V/Q scans are classified as **normal, nondiagnostic** (i.e., very low probability, low probability, intermediate probability), or **high probability** for PE.
    - V/Q scans are most useful in patients who have a normal CXR because nondiagnostic V/Q scans commonly occur in the setting of an abnormal CXR.
    - Use of **clinical suspicion** improves the accuracy of V/Q scanning. In patients with normal or high-probability V/Q scans and matching pretest clinical suspicion, the testing has a PPV of 96%.[83]
  - **Pulmonary angiography**
    - Angiography requires placement of a pulmonary artery catheter, infusion of IV contrast, and exposure to radiation.
    - Contraindications to angiography include renal dysfunction and dye allergy.
    - Less invasive tests (i.e., CT angiography) with similar or better diagnostic accuracy have mostly replaced pulmonary angiography for the assessment of acute PE.
  - **Electrocardiogram, troponin and brain natriuretic peptide (BNP) levels, arterial blood gas, CXR, and echocardiogram** may to help assess clinical probability of PE, cardiopulmonary reserve, and potential benefit of thrombolysis (**see** thrombolytic therapy **in Medications section**), but these tests do not rule out or rule in PE, with the exception of seeing an intracardiac clot with echo. Common ECG abnormalities in PTE include **sinus tachycardia**, and T-wave inversions in precordial leads, ventricular fibrillation (VF), right bundle branch block pattern, **S1Q3T3** pattern, QR pattern in

V1, QS pattern in precordial leads, ST elevation in precordial leads, and low voltage in limb leads. The chest X-ray signs in pulmonary embolism includes Westermark sign, Hampton hump, and Palla sign.
  - **Studies do not support extensive screening for an associated occult malignancy** in patients with a first, unprovoked VTE.[84] However, such patients should undergo a comprehensive history and physical examination, routine blood work, age- and gender-appropriate cancer screening (e.g., colonoscopy, mammography, Papanicolaou smear, prostate-specific antigen), and specific cancer screening tests indicated for distinct populations (e.g., chest CT to search for lung cancer in smokers of advanced age).

TREATMENT

- **VTE therapy** should aim to prevent recurrent VTE, consequences of VTE (i.e., postphlebitic syndrome [i.e., pain, edema, and ulceration], pulmonary arterial hypertension, and death), and complications of therapy (e.g., bleeding and HIT/HITT).
- Clinicians should perform standard laboratory tests (i.e., CBC, PT/INR, and aPTT) and assess bleeding risk before starting anticoagulants.
- Unless contraindications exist, **initial treatment of VTE should consist of anticoagulation** with IV or SC UFH, SC LMWH, SC pentasaccharide (fondaparinux), or a rapid-onset direct oral anticoagulant (**see** Medications).

Medications

- **Anticoagulants, oral**
  - **Warfarin, an oral anticoagulant,** inhibits reduction of vitamin K to its active form and leads to depletion of the vitamin K–dependent clotting factors II, VII, IX, and X, and proteins C, S, and Z.
    - Warfarin rapidly depletes factor VII and protein C, while the depletion of factor II takes several days because of its relatively long half-life.
    - Because of the rapid depletion of the anticoagulant protein C and a slower depletion of factor II, despite the rise of the INR due to factor VII depletion, patients might develop increased hypercoagulability during the first few days of warfarin therapy if warfarin is not combined with a parenteral anticoagulant.[85]
    - The **starting dose** of warfarin depends on many factors and ranges from 2 to 4 mg in older or petite patients to 10 mg in young, robust patients (www.warfarindosing.org). Patients with polymorphisms in genes for cytochrome P450 2C9 or vitamin K epoxide reductase (*VKORC1*) may benefit from lower-dose warfarin initiation.
    - Warfarin dosing adjustments depend on INR results.
    - **Treatment of DVT/PE with warfarin requires overlap therapy with a parenteral anticoagulant** (UFH, LMWH, or pentasaccharide) for at least 4–5 days and until the INR reaches at least 2.0.
      - For most indications, **target INR** is 2.5 with a therapeutic range of 2–3.
    - **INR monitoring should occur frequently during the first month of warfarin therapy (e.g., twice weekly for 1–2 weeks, then weekly for 2 weeks, then less frequently).**
      - Patients receiving a stable warfarin dose should have INR monitoring performed approximately monthly, although patients with labile INRs should have more frequent monitoring (e.g., weekly).
    - Typical **warfarin dose adjustments** after the first couple of weeks of therapy change the weekly dose by 10%–25%.
      - Starting or discontinuing **medications that affect warfarin metabolism or binding,** especially amiodarone, certain antibiotics (e.g., rifampin, sulfamethoxazole), or antifungal drugs (e.g., fluconazole), should trigger more frequent INR monitoring and may require dose adjustments >25%.

    - In eligible patients, home INR monitoring may improve INR control and patient satisfaction.[86]
    - Compliant patients with VTE or Afib who have unacceptable INR lability likely benefit from an oral anticoagulant other than warfarin.
  - Warfarin is teratogenic, at least during the first trimester.
- **Direct oral anticoagulants** (DOACs) (Table 20-6) currently have one of two primary mechanisms of action: **direct thrombin inhibitor** (dabigatran) and **direct Xa inhibitors** (rivaroxaban, apixaban, edoxaban, and betrixaban)
  - As compared to warfarin, DAOCs have a more rapid onset, shorter half-life, wider therapeutic window, and more predictable pharmacokinetics. These features allow patients with a new VTE to begin apixaban or rivaroxaban immediately, without the need for an overlapping parenteral agent. Dabigatran and edoxaban still need at least 5 days of initial parenteral agents if prescribed for a new VTE. None of the DOACs need INR monitoring or dose adjustments in patients with normal renal function, but the initial dose of a DOAC for a new VTE is higher than the maintenance dose.
  - Betrixaban is only FDA approved as prophylaxis of VTE in adult hospitalized medically ill patients; it is not approved for treatment of VTE.
  - Compared to warfarin, the DOACs have a lower risk of intracranial hemorrhage.[87]
  - Issues of concern include the lack of validated antidotes for some DOACs, risk of thrombosis due to missed doses, and drug level effects based on renal function.
- **Anticoagulants, parenteral**
  - **UFH** inactivates thrombin and factor Xa via AT.
    - At usual doses, UFH prolongs aPTT and thrombin time, although it has variable effect on the PT and INR.
    - Because the anticoagulant effects of UFH normalize within hours of discontinuation, and **protamine sulfate** reverses it even faster, UFH is the anticoagulant of choice during initial therapy for patients with a high risk of bleeding.
    - Abnormal renal function does not typically affect UFH dosing.
    - For **therapeutic anticoagulation**, UFH is usually administered IV with a bolus (e.g., 80 units/kg) followed by continuous infusion (e.g., 18 units/kg/h) that has a dose titration based on standard protocols (i.e., heparin nomogram), usually to a goal aPTT of 2- to 2.5-fold of normal range (Table 20-6).
    - Because of its short half-life, minimal renal clearance, and lack of drug interactions, UFH is often the preferred anticoagulant to use in **ICU patients** who have VTE and either a planned invasive procedures or high risk of bleeding.
    - UFH is the anticoagulant of choice for inpatients with a mechanical heart valve who need **bridging** of anticoagulation.
  - **LMWHs,** produced by chemical or enzymatic cleavage of UFH, indirectly inactivate thrombin and factor Xa via AT.
    - Because LMWH inactivates factor Xa to a greater extent than it does thrombin (IIa), LMWH minimally prolongs the aPTT.
    - Factor Xa monitoring is not needed, except in special circumstances: renal dysfunction, morbid obesity, or pregnancy. For therapeutic anticoagulation, peak factor Xa levels, measured 4 hours after an SC dose, should be 0.6–1.0 IU/mL for q12h dosing and 1–2 IU/mL for q24h dosing.[88]
    - Different LMWH preparations have different dosing recommendations (Table 20-6).
    - Given the renal clearance of LMWHs, they are generally contraindicated in patients with creatinine clearance (**CrCl**) <10 mL/min, and patients with a CrCl of 10–30 mL/min require dose adjustments (e.g., enoxaparin 1 mg/kg daily).
    - **LMWH** used to be the first choice long-term anticoagulant in patients who have **cancer and VTE**. LMWH and vitamin K antagonists (e.g., warfarin) have similar mortality and bleeding among patients with cancer and VTE, but LMWH

TABLE 20-6 Anticoagulant Dosing for Treatment of Venous Thromboembolism

Anticoagulant	Mechanism of Action	Initial Treatment Dose(s)	Subsequent Dose	Contraindications[a]
Warfarin	Vitamin K antagonist	2–10 mg; overlapped for 4–5 d with a faster-acting anticoagulant; goal INR 2–3 (see www.warfarindosing.org)	Adjusted per INR	Pregnancy
Apixaban	Direct FXa inhibitor	10 mg PO bid × 7 d	5 mg PO bid	
Edoxaban	Direct FXa inhibitor	Initially treat with parenteral anticoagulant for 5–10 d	60 mg PO daily, *or* 30 mg PO daily (if CrCl 30–50 mL/min, body weight ≤60 kg, or using strong P-gp inhibitor)	
Rivaroxaban	Direct FXa inhibitor	15 mg PO bid × 21 d	20 mg PO daily	CrCl <30 mL/min
Dabigatran	Direct thrombin (FIIa) inhibitor	Initially treat with parenteral anticoagulant for 5–10 d	150 mg bid (CrCl >30 mL/min)	CrCl <15 mL/min
Dalteparin	FXa > FIIa inhibition	200 IU/kg SC daily	Transition to oral agent *or*, for cancer patients, after 30 d of initial therapy, reduce dose to 150 IU/kg SC daily	HIT; hypersensitivity to pork
Enoxaparin	FXa > FIIa inhibition	1 mg/kg SC q12h or 1.5 mg/kg SC q24h; lower dose if CrCl <30 mL/min	Transition to long-term oral agent[b]	HIT; hypersensitivity to pork
Fondaparinux	Binds to antithrombin, primarily inhibiting FXa	Weight <50 kg: 5 mg SC daily Weight 50–100 kg: 7.5 mg SC daily Weight >100 kg: 10 mg SC daily	Transition to long-term oral agent[b]	CrCl <30 mL/min
Tinzaparin	FXa > FIIa inhibition	175 IU/kg SC daily	Transition to long-term oral agent[b]	HIT
Unfractionated heparin	Binds to antithrombin	Continuous IV: Goal aPTT 2.0–2.5× normal range	Transition to long-term oral agent[b]	HIT; hypersensitivity to pork

Low-molecular weight heparin can be prescribed long term for VTE (e.g., in setting of cancer).

[a]Invasive procedures (e.g., neuraxial anesthesia), bleeding, and bleeding diathesis (e.g., liver disease, thrombocytopenia) are contraindications to all anticoagulants.

[b]For venous thromboembolism (VTE) treatment, overlap therapy of warfarin and parenteral agent should be at least 5 days, until the INR is at least 2.

aPTT, activated partial thromboplastin time; CrCl, creatinine clearance; FIIa, factor IIa; FXa, factor Xa HIT, heparin-induced thrombocytopenia; INR, international normalized ratio; P-gp, P-glycoprotein.

is more effective.[89] The Hokusai VTE Cancer study found that compared with dalteparin (200 IU/kg SC daily × 1 month, then 150 IU/kg SC daily), edoxaban (60 mg p.o. daily) reduced recurrent VTE but increased major bleeding, especially in patients who enrolled with an upper GI malignancy.[90]

- DOACs are increasingly used in cancer patients.
- **LMWH** is the first choice in **pregnant** women (without artificial heart valves) who have VTE.

◦ **Fondaparinux,** a synthetic pentasaccharide structurally similar to the region of the heparin molecule that binds AT, functions as a selective indirect factor Xa inhibitor.
  - Because fondaparinux inhibits factor Xa, it does not prolong the aPTT.
  - Dosing of fondaparinux is weight based (Table 20-6).
  - Similar to the LMWHs, factor Xa monitoring is not used routinely.
  - Fondaparinux is not recommended for patients with CrCl <30 mL/min.
  - Though not FDA approved for use with suspected immunologic HIT, fondaparinux has been used in this setting.[91]

◦ **Argatroban** is a synthetic direct thrombin inhibitor used for immunologic **HIT** therapy.
  - Argatroban has a half-life of <1 hour, and a reversal agent is not available.
  - Argatroban is infused IV at an initial rate of ≤2 µg/kg/min. Special patient populations require lower initial infusion rates: patients with recent cardiac surgery, heart failure, hepatic dysfunction, or anasarca.[23]
  - aPTT monitoring should occur 2 hours after beginning the infusion, and the infusion rate should undergo adjustment to achieve a therapeutic aPTT (1.5–3.0 times the patient's baseline aPTT).
  - Once the platelet count has recovered, before conversion to warfarin, argatroban therapy should be overlapped with warfarin therapy for at least 5 days and until a therapeutic INR due to warfarin is achieved.
  - INR monitoring during argatroban and warfarin coadministration may cause confusion; for an INR >4, discontinue argatroban, remeasure the INR within 4–6 hours, and then restart the argatroban.

◦ **Bivalirudin** is a direct thrombin inhibitor with an indication for treatment of immunologic **HIT** in the setting of percutaneous coronary intervention in patients receiving ASA.
  - Bivalirudin has a half-life of 25 minutes in patients with normal renal function.
  - Because of its renal clearance, bivalirudin requires dose adjustment of the infusion rate in patients with renal insufficiency.
  - Bivalirudin dosing for HIT should start at a rate of 0.15–0.20 mg/kg/h IV with titration to a target aPTT 1.5–2.5 times baseline. An initial bolus dose is not recommended.[23,92] Lower rates should be initiated for patients with renal insufficiency.[93]
  - aPTT monitoring during bivalirudin therapy should occur 2 hours after a dose change.
  - The interpretation of the INRs in patients receiving warfarin must take into account the increased PT/INR caused by bivalirudin.

◦ **AT concentrate** may assist with the treatment of VTE associated with **congenital AT deficiency.**[94]

- **Thrombolytic therapy**
  ◦ In the life-threatening situation of an acute PE associated with shock or persistent hypotension from RV overload, rapid reperfusion treatment and cardiorespiratory support can relieve the RV overload and prevent hemodynamic deterioration.
  ◦ Thrombolytic therapy (e.g., alteplase or recombinant tissue plasminogen activator [rtPA] as a 100-mg IV infusion over 2 hours) is indicated for patients who have **hemodynamically unstable ("massive") PE** who do not have a contraindication (e.g., a high risk of bleeding).[95–97]

- Decompensation of hemodynamically stable treated acute PE may benefit from thrombolytic therapy,[97] such as a non-FDA approved 50 mg IV bolus dose of rtPA,[98] with other non-approved doses of rtPA sometimes used for PE-associated cardiac arrest including 10 mg IV bolus followed by drip of 40 mg IV over 15–30 minutes.
- In patients who have intermediate-risk/submassive PE, fibrinolytic therapy prevents hemodynamic decompensation but increases the risk of intracranial hemorrhage/stroke.[96,99,100]
- Thrombolytic therapy (administered either IV or by catheter-directed thrombolysis) for DVT **increases hemorrhage** and does not prevent post-thrombotic syndrome,[101] with the possible exception of patients who have massive iliofemoral DVT.[102]
- Thrombolysis may salvage a limb with a DVT that compromises arterial supply (phlegmasia cerulea dolens).[103]

- **Duration of anticoagulation for DVT or PE**
  - An individual's risk of recurrent VTE, risk of hemorrhage, risk of adverse outcomes, and preferences should determine the duration of anticoagulation, and these characteristics may change over time.[95,97]
  - Guidelines recommend 3 months of anticoagulation for treatment of provoked, proximal DVT or PE occurring in the setting of a surgical or nonsurgical (e.g., immobility, pregnancy, etc) transient risk factor as these events have low recurrence risk (≤2% per year).[97,104,105]
  - Guidelines recommend at least 3 months of anticoagulant therapy for patients with a **first episode of VTE** associated with **less compelling and transient risk factors**, such as prolonged travel, oral contraceptive pills/hormone replacement therapy, or minor injury.[95,97]
  - For **unprovoked PE**, many experts anticoagulate for >3 months in patients with low to moderate risk of bleeding.[97] Some experts recommend long-term anticoagulation for men with low to moderate risk of bleeding and an unprovoked PE.[106]
  - Patients with **cancer and VTE** should continue anticoagulation until cancer resolution or development of a contraindication.[97,107]
  - For patients with a **first VTE and an inherited hypercoagulable risk factor**, consider an extended anticoagulation duration:
    - **Heterozygous factor V Leiden or heterozygous prothrombin 20210A** modestly increases the odds of recurrence (relative risk, 1.6 and 1.4, respectively); prolonged anticoagulation is not recommended.
    - **Deficiency of protein S, protein C, or AT** carries a significant risk of recurrence (JAMA. 2009;301:2472); long-term anticoagulation is recommended.
    - **APS or two inherited risk factors** have a high risk of recurrence so indefinite anticoagulation is recommended (if not contraindicated).
  - Patients with **recurrent idiopathic VTE** should receive extended-duration anticoagulation, unless a contraindication develops or patient preferences or high bleeding risk dictate otherwise.[97]
  - **Extended anticoagulation after an idiopathic VTE** reduces the risk of recurrence but may cause hemorrhage.
    - The relative risk reduction of VTE depends on the thromboprophylaxis: it is only 32% with low-dose ASA but greater with rivaroxaban, apixaban, warfarin, or LMWH.[108]
    - Once daily oral rivaroxaban 20 mg or 10 mg is more effective than ASA.[109]
    - Twice-daily oral **apixaban** 5 or 2.5 mg[110] or **dabigatran** 150 mg is more effective than placebo.[111]
    - When **warfarin** is used for extended prophylaxis, a target INR of 2–3 is more effective than a target INR < 2.[112]
  - Effective LMWHs for extended prophylaxis include **enoxaparin** (1.5 mg/kg qd or 1 mg/kg bid) and **dalteparin** 150 IU/kg qd. Because extended use of LMWH can lead

to osteoporosis, we prefer them only among patients with a prior VTE and cancer. **During periods of increased VTE risk** patients with a history of VTE, especially those with additional risk factors, should receive prophylactic anticoagulation (e.g., low-dose LMWH).

- **Other Nonpharmacologic Therapies**
    - **Leg elevation** reduces edema associated with DVT.
    - **Ambulation** is encouraged for patients with DVT, especially after improvement of pain and edema, although strenuous lower extremity activity should initially be avoided.
    - **Fitted below-the-knee graduated compression stockings** can reduce swelling after DVT, but does not prevent DVT recurrence, and the reduction of post-thrombotic syndrome is controversial.[113]
    - **Inferior vena cava (IVC) filters** are mainly indicated for acute DVTs when there are absolute contraindications to anticoagulation (e.g., bleeding).
    - Prophylactic IVC filters in patients with acute DVT/PE halve the risk of recurrent PE; however, they do not decrease mortality, and they increase DVT recurrence.[114]
        - Several types of **temporary/retrievable IVC filters** exist and provide a physical barrier against emboli from the lower extremities. To reduce the risks from retrievable IVC filters, they should be removed when they are no longer indicated. However, if an IVC filter placed for VTE is left in place after a bleeding contraindication has resolved, guidelines recommend a full course of anticoagulation.[115]

Surgical Management

Surgical embolectomy

- Surgical embolectomy has a role in patients who have massive/high-risk PE and a contraindication to thrombolytic therapy or who failed thrombolytic therapy. Depending on center expertise, catheter-based interventions should be considered as a potential alternative option to surgical embolectomy.[97]
- Patients who have a **right heart thrombus that straddles the interatrial septum** via a patent foramen ovale/atrial septal defect should be considered for surgical embolectomy.[115]
- Embolectomy for **free-floating right heart thrombus** remains controversial.[116]

SPECIAL CONSIDERATIONS

Anticoagulant Bridging

- **Perioperative management of anticoagulation** requires close coordination with the surgical service (see Perioperative Medicine in Chapter 1) to address timing of interventions and therapeutic changes with the aim of VTE prevention and avoidance of bleeding.
- **Invasive procedures** usually require discontinuation of anticoagulation.
    - For patients receiving warfarin who need a preoperative INR ≤1.4, stop the warfarin therapy 4–5 days before the invasive procedure.
    - To achieve an INR around 1.7, halve the warfarin dose for 4 days before surgery.[117]
    - In situations where a clinician aims to minimize the patient's time off therapeutic anticoagulation, initiate parenteral anticoagulation when the INR becomes subtherapeutic (approximately 3 days after the last warfarin dose) and stop the parenteral anticoagulation 6–48 hours before the procedure (depending on the half-life of the parenteral drug).
    - In some instances, IV UFH is the preferred bridging therapy (e.g., pregnant woman with a mechanical heart valve).
    - After the procedure, resume warfarin, and/or parenteral anticoagulation as soon as hemostasis and bleeding risk reach an acceptable level, typically within 24 hours.[118]

- Studies are needed to address the risks and benefits of anticoagulation for **isolated subsegmental PE.**
- **Upper extremity acute DVT** that involves axillary or more proximal vein(s) should receive standard-duration (e.g., 3 months) anticoagulation.[119] DVT associated with a functioning central venous catheter does not require catheter removal, but anticoagulation should continue past the 3-months duration as long as the catheter remains in place.[95]
- **Isolated calf acute DVT** without severe symptoms or risk factors for extension may undergo serial imaging in 1–2 weeks instead of anticoagulation. Alternatively, treat with 6–12 weeks of anticoagulation in patients at low risk of bleeding. However, patients who have severe DVT symptoms, significant risk factors for extension, or documented clot extension should get full-dose anticoagulation.
- **Superficial vein thrombophlebitis (SVT)**
  - **Small SVTs (<5 cm in length)** and SVT associated with IV infusion therapy do not require anticoagulation; the treatment consists of oral NSAIDs and warm compresses.
  - Treatment of **extensive SVT (e.g., >5 cm in length)** with a short course of prophylactic doses of fondaparinux (2.5 mg SC daily for 45 days) (N Engl J Med. 2010;363:1222) or LMWH (e.g., enoxaparin 40 mg SC daily for 10 days)[120] decreases the incidence of SVT recurrence, SVT extension, and VTE but increases the risk of bleeding.[95]
  - **Recurrent SVT** may be treated with anticoagulation or vein stripping.[94]
- **Chronic PE** occurs in 2%–4% of patients with PE,[121] and patients with this disorder should undergo evaluation for chronic thromboembolic pulmonary hypertension (**CTEPH**). Additionally, patients who have PH associated with acute PE should undergo evaluation for resolution of PH. Continued PH should lead to further testing (e.g., V/Q scan). Those diagnosed with CTEPH should undergo extended-duration anticoagulation, consideration of **riociguat** therapy,[122] and evaluation for possible pulmonary **thromboendarterectomy**.

COMPLICATIONS

- **Bleeding** is the major complication of anticoagulation.
  - Up to 2% of patients who receive anticoagulation for VTE therapy experience major bleeding.
  - Patients taking anticoagulants have a major bleeding rate of 1%–3% per year.
  - Concomitant use of **antiplatelet agents** increases the risk of bleeding.
  - Major bleeding after an acute VTE should lead to the discontinuation of anticoagulation and consideration of a temporary or permanent IVC filter. If the bleeding risk is resolved, the anticoagulant should be resumed and any temporary IVC filter can be retrieved.
- **Warfarin-associated INR elevation in asymptomatic patients**
  - For an asymptomatic minor INR elevation (INR<5), hold or reduce the warfarin dose until the INR returns to a safe range, and then resume warfarin at a reduced dose.
  - For an asymptomatic moderate INR elevation 5 ≤ INR <9 in an asymptomatic patient, hold one or more warfarin doses. Oral vitamin K_1 is not needed for the INR to decline.[123]
  - For an asymptomatic severe INR elevation (INR ≥9), consider checking for a spurious test result (recheck the INR), or treat with vitamin K (e.g., oral vitamin K_1 2–10 mg).[124]
- **Bleeding with warfarin**
  - **For patients who have warfarin-associated bleeding and an elevated INR, give Vitamin K replacement** PO or IV. (Vitamin K has variable absorption when administered SC.) IV vitamin K carries the risk of anaphylactoid reactions, so the oral route is preferred unless more rapid INR correction is deemed necessary. With adequate replacement therapy, the INR will fall within 12 hours and normalize completely

in 24–48 hours.[125] Treat serious hemorrhage with IV vitamin K (10 mg) by slow infusion and with IV 4-factor PCC. When 4-factor PCC is not available, use three-factor PCC and/or FFP (two or three units) Because of the long half-life of warfarin (approximately 36 hours), repeat the vitamin K treatment (e.g., oral Vit K) every 8–12 hours to prevent INR rebound.

- Although expensive and potentially thrombogenic,[126] **rFVIIa** may stop life-threatening warfarin-associated (elevated INR) bleeding.

- **Bleeding with UFH, LMWH, and pentasaccharide**
  - Discontinuation usually sufficiently restores normal hemostasis.
  - With moderate to severe bleeding, **FFP** may reduce bleeding.
  - For patients receiving **UFH** who develop major bleeding, heparin can be completely reversed by infusion of **protamine sulfate** in situations where the potential benefits outweigh the risks (e.g., intracranial bleed, epidural hematoma, retinal bleed).
  - Approximately 1 mg of protamine sulfate IV neutralizes 100 units of heparin, up to a maximum dose of 250 mg. The dose can be given as a loading dose of 25–50 mg by slow IV injection over 10 minutes, with the rest of the dose over 12 hours.
  - Heparin serum concentrations decline rapidly owing to a short half-life after IV administration, and the amount of protamine required decreases based on time since heparin treatment.
  - For major bleeding associated with **LMWH**, protamine sulfate neutralizes only approximately 60% of LMWH.[127] Protamine does not reverse **pentasaccharide** (e.g., **fondaparinux**).
  - For patients with serious bleeding on fondaparinux, **andexanet alfa** (see below) may be used.
- **Bleeding with direct oral anticoagulants** (DOACs)
  - **Reversal of dabigatran: Idarucizumab** (5 g IV) is a monoclonal antibody that binds to dabigatran with >350-fold affinity compared to thrombin and neutralizes its activity in minutes.[128,129] Because the majority of dabigatran remains unbound in plasma, hemodialysis can also decrease dabigatran concentration.
  - **Reversal of factor Xa inhibitors: Andexanet alfa** is a recombinant, modified human factor Xa decoy protein that binds all factor Xa inhibitors inactivating them; in addition, it also inhibits tissue factor pathway inhibitor (TFPI), thus increasing tissue factor–associated thrombin generation. The inhibition of TFPI is thought to be the mechanism behind the 18% rate of thrombosis within 30-days of andexanet administration. Dosing includes an 800 mg bolus at 30 mg/min followed by 960 mg infused at 8 mg/min in patients who received a full Xa dose (e.g., rivaroxaban >10 mg, apixaban >5 mg) within the prior 8 hours. Four-factor PCC also can reverse direct factor Xa inhibitors, but evidence is limited.[130]
- **Occult gastrointestinal or genitourinary bleeding** is a relative but not absolute contraindication to anticoagulation, although its presence before or during anticoagulation warrants an investigation for underlying disease.
- **Warfarin-induced skin necrosis**, associated with rapid depletion of protein C, may rarely occur (incidence <0.1%) during initiation of warfarin therapy.
  - Necrosis occurs most often in areas with a high percentage of adipose tissue, such as breast tissue, flank, hips, and thighs, and it can be life-threatening.
  - Therapeutic anticoagulation with an immediate-acting anticoagulant (e.g., UFH, LMWH) and/or avoiding "loading doses" of warfarin prevents warfarin-induced skin necrosis.
- **Warfarin is absolutely contraindicated in early** (i.e., first-trimester) **pregnancy** because of the **risk of teratogenicity**, and it is often avoided during the entire **pregnancy** because of the **risk of fetal bleeding**, although it is safe for infants of nursing mothers.
- **Osteoporosis** may occur with long-term heparin or warfarin use.[131]

MONITORING/FOLLOW-UP

- For a suspicious clinical presentation, **testing for intrinsic hypercoagulable risk factors** ideally should wait until the patient is in stable health and off anticoagulation therapy for at least 2 weeks (e.g., at the end of a standard course of treatment) **to avoid false-positive results** for nongenetic testing.
    - Although uncommon, if reasons exist to screen for hypercoagulable risk factors around the time of diagnosis, collect blood for **factor V Leiden and prothrombin gene mutations and LA.**
    - If done, blood collection for **protein C, protein S, and AT activity and antigen level** testing should occur while patients are not on anticoagulation and should be avoided in the setting of acute thrombosis. If testing occurs near the time of the acute VTE, normal protein C, protein S, and AT tests rule out congenital deficiencies, and abnormally low results require confirmation through repeat testing (or screening first-degree relatives) to rule out a temporary deficiency related to the acute thrombosis.
- Although **testing for PE in patients with DVT and testing for DVT in patients with PE** will produce many positive findings, such testing rarely affects therapy.
- **Outpatient therapy** is appropriate for most DVTs and for selected (low-risk) PEs.[132]
- Decisions regarding the **prolongation of anticoagulation duration** remain controversial in patients with residual thrombosis on compression ultrasonography at the end of standard-duration anticoagulation for proximal DVT[133] or in those with a positive D-dimer weeks after completing a standard duration of therapy for VTE.[134] Prolonged-duration anticoagulation reduces VTE recurrence but increases bleeding.
- After completion of anticoagulation for an unprovoked VTE, **low-dose ASA** reduces the risk of arterial and venous thrombosis.[135]
- After completion of anticoagulation for an unprovoked VTE, **apixaban** (5 or 2.5 mg orally twice daily) or **rivaroxaban** (20 or 10 mg orally once daily) reduce the risk of recurrent VTE and rivaroxaban is more effective than low-dose ASA.[109,110]

Summary

- The underlying pathophysiology of ITP is better understood today and has led to the development of new treatments, including TPO-RAs, syk inhibitor, Fcγ receptor (FcγR) inhibition, and other treatments.
- The absence of fever and neurologic symptoms, the prevalence of acute kidney failure (uremia), and the incidence in children separate HUS from TTP.
- Platelet transfusions are contraindicated during the acute phase of HIT, as transfused platelets can bind to IgG and become activated and release PF4, thus worsening the hypercoagulable state.
- A new era of prevention of bleeding in hemophilia began with the introduction of a bispecific monoclonal antibody emicizumab that mimics the effects of FVIII in the tenase complex.
- von Willebrand disease in females is often a more clinically severe disease due to menorrhagia.
- In patients with DVT who do not get pulmonary emboli, recurrent thrombosis and "post-thrombotic syndrome" are major causes of morbidity.

Scan the QR code to access chapter references.

21 Hematologic Disorders and Transfusion Therapy

Amy Zhou, Francesca Ferraro, Ronald Jackups, Morey Blinder, and Mounika R.N

ANEMIA

GENERAL PRINCIPLES

Definition

Anemia is defined as a decrease in circulating red blood cell (RBC) mass; the usual criteria in adults being hemoglobin (Hgb) <12 g/dL or hematocrit (Hct) <36% for nonpregnant women and Hgb <13 g/dL or Hct <39% in men.

It can be further categorized as:

	Mild	Moderate	Severe
Nonpregnant women (≥15 years)	11–11.9 g/dL	8–10.9 g/dL	<8 g/dL
Pregnant women	10–11 g/dL	7–9.9 g/dL	<7 g/dL
Men (≥15 years)	11–12.9 g/dL	8–10.9 g/dL	<8 g/dL

Classification

Anemia can be broadly classified into three etiologic groups: **blood loss (acute or chronic), decreased RBC production, and increased RBC destruction (hemolysis)**. Anemia can also be categorized by RBC size as microcytic, normocytic, or macrocytic.

DIAGNOSIS

Anemia is always caused by an underlying disorder; thus, a careful evaluation to determine the etiology is required in each case.

Clinical Presentation

Based on the history, one can often discern the duration of the illness (acute or chronic), the severity, and the underlying etiology.

- Acute anemia: Patients with abrupt onset of anemia tolerate diminished RBC mass poorly. Patients may have symptoms of fatigue, malaise, dyspnea, syncope/presyncope, or angina.
- Chronic anemia: In contrast to acute anemia, patients with chronic anemia are less symptomatic, at times only presenting with fatigue or dyspnea with increased activity or exertion. However, patients usually have symptoms when Hgb <7 g/dL.
- The following history will aid in the evaluation and management of anemia:
  - Gastrointestinal (GI) hemorrhage
  - Obstetric and menstrual history
  - Comorbidities associated with anemia such as GI surgery or malabsorption, renal disease, rheumatologic disease, or other chronic inflammatory conditions

- ∘ Comorbid conditions that may be exacerbated by anemia, such as cardiovascular disease
- ∘ Family history of anemia
- ∘ History of blood donation or prior RBC transfusions
- ∘ Prescribed and over-the-counter medicines including supplements, alcohol consumption, diet, ethnic background, and religious beliefs pertaining to blood transfusions
- ∘ Symptoms suggestive of other cytopenias such as bruising (thrombocytopenia) or severe or recurrent infections (neutropenia)

Physical Examination

Common signs and symptoms of anemia include pallor, tachycardia, hypotension, dizziness, tinnitus, headaches, decreased cognitive ability, fatigue, and weakness. Atrophic glossitis, angular cheilosis, koilonychia (spoon nails), and brittle nails are more common in severe, long-standing anemia. Patients may also experience reduced exercise tolerance, dyspnea on exertion, and heart failure. High-output heart failure and hypovolemic shock may be seen in acute, severe cases.

Diagnostic Testing

Laboratories

- The complete blood count (CBC), reticulocyte count, and inspection of the peripheral smear will guide further laboratory testing because they provide a morphologic classification and assessment of RBC production.
- The Hgb level is a measure of the concentration of Hgb in blood as expressed in grams per deciliter (g/dL), whereas the Hct is the percentage of the blood that is RBCs. Hgb and Hct are unreliable indicators of red cell mass in the setting of rapid shifts of intravascular volume (i.e., an acute bleed).
- The most useful red cell indices are:
  - ∘ Mean corpuscular volume (MCV): Measures the mean volume of the RBCs. Reference range: 80–96 fL.
    - ▪ **Microcytic: MCV <80 fL**
    - ▪ **Normocytic: MCV 80–96 fL**
    - ▪ **Macrocytic: MCV >96 fL**
  - ∘ Red cell distribution width (RDW): Reflects the variability in the volume of the RBCs and is proportional to the standard deviation of the MCV. An elevated RDW indicates an increased variability in RBC size, which is a nonspecific but important finding in anemic patients.
  - ∘ Mean corpuscular Hgb: Defines the concentration of Hgb in each cell, which is expressed in picograms, and an elevated level is often indicative of spherocytes or a hemoglobinopathy.
- **The relative reticulocyte count** measures the percentage of immature (juvenile red cells with RNA remnants) red cells in the blood and reflects production of RBCs in the bone marrow (BM).
  - ∘ A normal RBC has a life span of approximately 120 days, and the reticulocytes circulate for about 1 day; therefore, the normal reticulocyte count is 0.4%–2.9%.
  - ∘ In the setting of anemia from blood loss, the BM should increase its production of RBCs in response to the blood loss, and thus a reticulocyte count of 1% in this setting is inappropriately low. Therefore, RPI needs to be calculated.
  - ∘ **The reticulocyte production index** (RPI) is a determination of the BM's ability to respond to anemia and is calculated by % reticulocytes/maturation correction × actual Hct/normal Hct (normally 45). The maturation correction factor is nothing but reticulocyte maturation time = 1 day for Hct ≥40%; 1.5 days for Hct 30%–40%; 2.0 days for Hct 20%–30%; and 2.5 days for Hct <20%.

- When anemia is severe, the reticulocyte count should be corrected for anemia, expressed as Reticulocyte Index (RI):

$$\text{Reticulocyte Index (RI)} = \text{Observed reticulocyte } \% \times (\text{Measured Hb or PCV/Appropriate normal Hb or PCV})$$

RI <2 with anemia indicates decreased production of RBCs (hypoproliferative anemia). RI >2 with anemia may indicate a compensatory increase in RBC production caused by hemolysis or bleeding (hyperproliferative anemia).

- The absolute reticulocyte count (relative reticulocyte count × RBCs) may provide a more accurate reflection of a patient's response to anemia than the relative reticulocyte count.
- Automated reticulocyte counting allows the evaluation of other parameters, such as **reticulocyte hemoglobin content** (CHr) and the proportion of immature reticulocytes (**immature reticulocyte fraction** [IRF]). A CHr <29 pg suggests iron deficiency (ID), while a reduced IRF (<0.23) suggests underproduction.

- The **peripheral smear** should be reviewed to assess the morphologic characteristics of RBCs including the shape, size, presence of inclusions, and orientation of cells in relation to each other. RBCs assume many abnormal forms, such as acanthocytes, schistocytes, spherocytes, or tear drop cells, and abnormal orientation such as agglutination or Rouleaux formation. Each is associated with several specific disease processes that may warrant additional evaluation.

Diagnostic Procedures

A **BM biopsy** is often indicated in cases of unexplained anemia with a low reticulocyte count or with anemia associated with other cytopenias. The severity of anemia that should trigger a BM biopsy is not well defined, but it should be strongly considered if the diagnosis is uncertain and RBC transfusions are required. It is useful in identifying MDS with single lineage dysplasia causing unexplained anemia.

ANEMIAS ASSOCIATED WITH DECREASED RED BLOOD CELL PRODUCTION

Iron Deficiency Anemia

GENERAL PRINCIPLES

- **Iron deficiency** is the most common cause of anemia in the ambulatory setting and is usually a chronic microcytic anemia with a low reticulocyte count (the count rises with treatment).
- The most common causes of ID anemia are blood loss (e.g., menses, GI blood loss, hookworm infection, malaria), decreased absorption (e.g., achlorhydria, celiac disease, bariatric surgery, *Helicobacter pylori* infection), and increased iron requirement (e.g., pregnancy).
- It is important to determine the cause of ID, and in the absence of menstrual bleeding, evaluation of the GI tract should be performed to identify a potential cause including the possibility of an occult malignancy.

DIAGNOSIS

Clinical Presentation

- Patients often present with cold intolerance along with fatigue or malaise that is typically worsened with activity.

- Pica (consumption of substances of no nutritional value such as ice, starch, or clay) occurs in about 25% of patients with chronic ID anemia and rarely occurs in other clinical settings.
- Koilonychia, that is, spoon-shaped (concave) nails, is primarily recognized as a manifestation of chronic ID.
- Restless leg syndrome is a common but a nonspecific finding in patients with ID anemia.
- Pallor is a common physical finding in patients with ID anemia but is not specific.

Diagnostic Testing

Peripheral blood smear may show hypochromia (increased central pallor of RBCs), microcytosis, pencil-shaped cells, few tear drops, and target cells may be seen. The reticulocyte count is inappropriately low in ID anemia, and there is high RDW.

Laboratories

- **Ferritin** is the primary storage form for iron in the liver and is a specific marker of an absolute ID. The reference range is 30–400 ng/mL.
  - A ferritin level of <10 ng/mL in women or <20 ng/mL in men almost always reflects low iron stores.
  - Ferritin is an acute-phase reactant, so normal levels may be seen in inflammatory states despite low iron stores. **A serum ferritin level of >200 ng/mL generally excludes an** ID; however, in renal dialysis patients, a functional ID may be seen with a ferritin up to 500 ng/mL.
- **Iron, total iron binding capacity (TIBC), and transferrin saturation** are often used in combination with ferritin to diagnose ID anemia. Serum iron level alone is an unreliable indicator given its significant fluctuation after a meal.
- Mean corpuscular hemoglobin/RBC index, or **Mentzer index**, can help differentiate between the two causes of microcytic/hypochromic anemia. These causes are an ID and thalassemia minor. An index greater than 15 suggests ID, while an index less than 11 suggests thalassemia minor.
  - An earlier marker of ID is the reticulocyte/reticulated hemoglobin content (CHr), which is decreased (<29 pg) in ID (reticulated Hb equivalent is provided instead of reticulated Hb content on certain analyzers and the normal range may vary).

Diagnostic Procedures

- A **BM biopsy** that shows absent staining for iron. It is graded using Perls Prussian Blue stain: Grade 0 represents decreased iron stores, Grades 1–3 represent normal, and Grades 4–6 represent increased iron stores. It is the definitive test to diagnose ID anemia and is helpful when the serum tests do not clearly demonstrate the diagnosis.
- **An iron challenge** can be performed in the absence of response to oral iron replacement to differentiate poor absorption from other causes (e.g., nonadherence or occult blood loss). After an 8-hour fast, a baseline iron is measured immediately followed by oral intake of liquid ferrous sulfate 5 mg/kg given with orange juice or vitamin C-containing beverage. Serum iron is measured again after 90 minutes. Normal iron absorption will result in an increase of serum iron of at least 50 μg/dL and a lower level is indicative of poor absorption.
- **ID is not a final diagnosis**; rather, it is indicative of an underlying etiology that is decreasing iron availability and/or increasing iron needs which must be identified and, if possible, treated. In a woman of reproductive age, vaginal blood loss must be considered and explored with a detailed bleeding history. GI blood loss or malabsorptive states must be considered in all patients. Although it is especially important in men and in all patients older than 50 years, it is important to remember that celiac disease and GI malignancy can occur in both sexes at any age. Blood donors are at risk of ID, and thus current or previous blood donation is an important element to obtain from the patient history.

Additional considerations include detailed medication history (e.g., oral anticoagulants, antacids, proton pump inhibitors) and dietary history.

TREATMENT

- **Oral iron therapy.** Given in stable patients with mild symptoms. Several different preparations are available (Table 21-1).
  - Iron is best absorbed on an empty stomach, and 3–10 mg of elemental iron can be absorbed daily.
  - Oral iron ingestion may induce a number of GI side effects, including epigastric distress, bloating, and constipation. As a result, nonadherence is a common problem. These side effects can be decreased by initially administering the drug with meals or every other day and increasing the dosage as indicated/tolerated. Concomitant treatment with a stool softener can also alleviate some of these symptoms.
  - Ferrous sulfate is the most commonly prescribed formulation. If there are unacceptable side effects, consider using a lower dose or an alternative formulation such as ferrous gluconate or ferrous fumarate, which contain lower amounts of elemental iron and may be better tolerated.
  - Ferrous sulfate 325 mg (containing 65 mg elemental iron) given in the morning on an empty stomach has proven to be as effective as higher doses under some circumstances, as has every other day dosing.[1,2]
  - In general, patients responding to oral iron therapy should see an increase in reticulocyte count within 1 week of therapy; an increase in Hgb of 2 g/dL every 3 weeks is expected. Treatment should be continued until the total iron deficit is replete.
- **Parenteral iron therapy** (Table 21-2). There are several formulations of IV iron, and indications for parenteral iron over oral iron include:
  - Poor absorption (e.g., inflammatory bowel disease, malabsorption).
  - Very high iron requirements that cannot be met with oral supplementation (e.g., ongoing bleeding)
  - Intolerance to oral preparations
  - Functional ID in chronic kidney disease (CKD)

Specific Considerations

- IV iron infusion **should not be given** in patients with an active infection (i.e., fever) owing to concern for increased adverse reactions.
- The total iron replacement dose may be estimated using the patient's baseline Hgb and body weight (https://reference.medscape.com/calculator/iron-replacement-parenteral-dosing). The modified Ganzoni formula (subject weight [kg] × [15 – current

TABLE 21-1 Oral Iron Preparations

Preparation	Common Dosing Regimen	Elemental Iron (mg per dose)
Ferrous sulfate	325 mg qd–tid	65
Ferrous gluconate	300 mg tid	36
Ferrous fumarate	100 mg tid	33
Iron polysaccharide complex	150 mg bid	150
Carbonyl iron	50 mg bid–tid	50
Ferric maltol	30 mg bid-tid	30 (complexed with 201.5 mg trimaltol) per capsule

TABLE 21-2 IV Iron Preparations

Preparation	IV Administration	Caution
Iron dextran (INFeD)	The entire dose may be diluted and infused in one setting; 1000 mg can be given over 1 h.	A 0.5-mL test dose should be given; observe patient for at least 1 h before full dose.
Iron sucrose (Venofer)	Administered undiluted as slow IV injection or infusion in diluted solution: Injection: 100 mg over 2–5 min 200 mg over 2–5 min Infusion: 100 mg/100 mL over 15 min 300 mg/250 mL over 1.5 h 400 mg/250 mL over 2.5 h >500 mg/250 mL over 3.5 h	
Ferric gluconate (Ferrlecit)	Injection: 125 mg over 10 min Infusion: 125 mg/100 mL over 1 h	
Ferric deriso-maltose (iron isomaltoside)	Weight ≥50 kg: Single dose of 1000 mg	
Ferumoxytol (Feraheme)	510 mg over 20 min; given as 2 doses 7 d apart	Observe patient for at least 30 min after administration. Serious hypersensitivity reactions have been observed with rapid IV injection (<1 min).
Ferric carboxy-maltose (Injectafer)	750 mg over 15–30 min; given as 2 doses 7 d apart	

Hb (g/dL)] × 2.4 + 500) can also be used to calculate the patient's total body iron deficit to guide dosing.

- **Iron dextran** (INFeD) **is a less-expensive agent and allows for high-dose repletion in a single dose**; however, infusion can be complicated by serious side effects including **anaphylaxis.**
  - An IV **test dose** of 0.5 mL should be administered over 5–10 minutes at 30–60 minutes before the full dose. Methylprednisolone, diphenhydramine, and 1:1000 epinephrine 1-mg ampule (for SC administration) should be immediately available at all times during the infusion.
  - A dose of 1000 mg can be administered over 1 hour.[3]
  - Delayed reactions to IV iron, such as arthralgia, myalgia, fever, pruritus, and lymphadenopathy, may be seen within several days of therapy and usually resolve spontaneously or with NSAIDs.
- **Second-generation iron products** include **ferric gluconate** (Ferrlecit) and **iron sucrose** (Venofer) and can be given at a faster infusion rate than INFeD. Anaphylaxis is rare, and a test dose is not needed; however, a single infusion is typically insufficient to replenish

the entire iron deficit, so multiple doses are required. Higher doses of iron sucrose (i.e., >400 mg/250 mL doses) are associated with a higher adverse event rate.

- **Third-generation iron products** include **ferumoxytol** (Feraheme), iron isomaltoside, and **ferric carboxymaltose** (Injectafer) and allow for administration of a high dose with a rapid infusion. A rare complication is severe hypotension, which can be related to the rapidity of the injection. Of note, ferumoxytol is also available as an MRI contrast agent and will transiently show a significant increase in iron stores in the liver.

Thalassemia

GENERAL PRINCIPLES

Definition

The **thalassemia syndromes** are inherited disorders characterized by reduced Hgb synthesis associated with mutations in either the α- or β-gene of the molecule (Table 21-3).

Etiology

- **β-Thalassemia** results in a decreased production of β-globin and a resultant excess of α-globin, forming insoluble α-tetramers and leading to ineffective erythropoiesis.
    - **β-Thalassemia** minor (trait) occurs with one gene abnormality with underproduction of β-chain globin. Patients are asymptomatic and present with microcytic, hypochromic RBCs and Hgb levels >10 g/dL.
    - **β-Thalassemia** intermedia occurs with dysfunction in both β-globin genes so that anemia is more severe (Hgb 7–10 g/dL).
    - **β-Thalassemia** major (Cooley anemia) is caused by mutations of both β-globin genes that fail to produce significant amounts of β-globin and generally requires lifelong RBC transfusion support.

TABLE 21-3 Thalassemias

	Genotype	Hemoglobin (g/dL)	Mean Cellular Volume (fL)	Transfusion Dependent
α-Thalassemia				
Silent carrier	α α/α–	Normal	None	No
Trait	α–/α– or α α/––	>10	<80	No
Hemoglobin H	α–/––	7–10	<70	+/–
Hydrops fetalis	––/––	Incompatible with life		
β-Thalassemia (Thal)				
Silent carrier	β/β^+	>10	<80	No
β-Thal minor (trait)	β/β^0	>10	<80	No
β-Thal intermedia	β^+/β^+	7–10	65–75	+/–
β-Thal major	β^+/β^0 or β^0/β^0	<7	<70	Yes

β^+, β-thalassemia genes produce some β-globin chains but with impaired synthesis; β^0, β-thalassemia genes produce no β-globin chains.

- **α-Thalassemia** occurs with a deletion of one or more of the four α-globin genes, leading to a β-globin excess.
  - Mild microcytosis and mild hypochromic anemia (Hgb >10 g/dL) are seen with the loss of one or two α-globin genes (silent carrier and α-thal trait).
  - Deletion of three α-globin genes (Hgb H disease) results in splenomegaly and hemolytic anemia. In patients with Hgb H disease, transfusion or splenectomy is often not necessary until after the second or third decade of life. In addition, oxidant drugs similar to those that exacerbate glucose-6-phosphate dehydrogenase (G6PD) deficiency should be avoided because increased hemolysis may occur.
  - Hydrops fetalis occurs with the loss of all four α-globin genes and is incompatible with life.

DIAGNOSIS

- Peripheral smear may show microcytic hypochromic RBCs, along with marked anisopoikilocytosis, few spherocytes, and polychromatophils-nucleated RBCs.
- Hgb electrophoresis is often diagnostic for β-thalassemia showing an increased percentage of Hgb A_2 and Hgb F. (Hgb electrophoresis is preferably done before blood transfusion when the patient presents with anemia for the first time or done 4–6 weeks after the last transfusion. In case of not being able to perform the test due to requirements of frequent transfusions, Hgb electrophoresis of parents can be done for diagnosis and this parental study is also helpful in diagnosing thalassemia in children younger than 1 year. Gene analysis is another option for the diagnosis with widespread availability of next-generation sequencing [NGS].)
- Silent carriers with a single α-chain loss generally have a normal electrophoresis. Adults with Hgb H disease demonstrate Hgb H (β-tetramers) on electrophoresis. The diagnosis of α-thalassemia is confirmed by α-globin gene analysis.

TREATMENT

- Patients with either α- or β-thalassemia trait require no specific treatment. However, in areas where the incidence of thalassemia is high and in certain ethnic groups, premarital counseling and testing for thalassemia traits should be mandatory.
- In patients with more severe forms of the disease, RBC transfusions to maintain an Hgb level of 9–10 g/dL are needed to prevent the skeletal deformities that result from accelerated erythropoiesis.
- In severe forms of thalassemia, repeated transfusions result in tissue iron overload, which may cause congestive heart failure (CHF), hepatic dysfunction, glucose intolerance, and secondary hypogonadism. **Iron chelation therapy** delays or prevents these complications. Once clinical organ deterioration has begun, it may not be reversible.
- **Chelation therapy** is indicated for transfusion-associated iron overload from any cause. It is indicated in patients with a ferritin consistently >1000 ng/mL, which may occur after a transfusion burden of >20 units of packed RBCs.
  - Deferoxamine, 40 mg/kg SC or IV over 8–12 hours of continuous infusion.[4]
  - Deferasirox dispersible tablet 20–40 mg/kg/d (Exjade) is an effective oral chelating agent, but GI disturbances often limit adherence to therapy. Deferasirox film-coated tablet (Jadenu) is available and dosed at 70% of Exjade (7–21 mg/kg/d). This formulation is often better tolerated. Dose can be titrated every 3–6 months based on ferritin level. Efficacy is similar to that of deferoxamine.
  - Chelation therapy should be continued until ferritin levels of <1000 ng/mL are achieved and maintenance therapy is often needed when RBC transfusions are ongoing.

- Hydroxyurea (15–35 mg/kg/d) to increase Hgb F may reduce transfusion requirements in some patients with β-thalassemia.
- Stem cell transplantation (SCT) is the only curative therapy and should be considered in young patients with thalassemia major who have HLA-identical donors. Gene therapy is the subject of ongoing research and holds promise.[5]
- Splenectomy should be considered in patients with accelerated (more than two units/month) transfusion requirements. To decrease the risk of postsplenectomy sepsis, immunization against pneumococcus, *Haemophilus influenzae*, and *Neisseria meningitidis* should be administered at least 2 weeks before surgery if not previously vaccinated (see Appendix A, Immunizations and Postexposure Therapies). Splenectomy is rarely recommended in patients who are younger than 5–6 years because of the increased risk of sepsis.

Sideroblastic Anemias

GENERAL PRINCIPLES

Definition

Sideroblastic anemias are hereditary or acquired RBC disorders characterized by abnormal iron metabolism associated with the presence of ring sideroblasts in the developing RBCs in the BM which represent abnormal mitochondrial iron accumulation.

Etiology

- Acquired
  - Primary sideroblastic anemia (myelodysplastic syndrome [MDS])
  - Secondary sideroblastic anemia is caused by drugs (i.e., chloramphenicol, cycloserine, ethanol, isoniazid, pyrazinamide), lead or zinc toxicity, chronic ethanol use, or copper deficiency
- Hereditary
  - X-linked
  - Autosomal: Defects in *SCL25A38* (mitochondrial transporter protein) or PSU1 mutations
  - Mitochondrial: Pearson marrow-pancreas syndrome

DIAGNOSIS

A BM examination including cytogenetics is needed to evaluate for the presence of the hallmark ring sideroblasts using Perls Prussian Blue stain, or other abnormal marrow forms with abnormally increased number and size of cytoplasmic siderotic granules.

TREATMENT

- Remove any possible offending agent.
- Pyridoxine 50–200 mg daily may be effective to treat hereditary sideroblastic anemias.

Macrocytic/Megaloblastic Anemia

GENERAL PRINCIPLES

Definition

Megaloblastic anemia is a term used to describe disorders of impaired DNA synthesis in hematopoietic cells, but this also affects other normally proliferating cells such as in the GI tract.

Etiology

- **Vitamin B_{12} deficiency** occurs insidiously over several years because daily vitamin B_{12} requirements are low compared to total body stores.
  - Most cases of megaloblastic anemia are due to vitamin B_{12} deficiency.
  - Vitamin B_{12} deficiency occurs in up to 20% of untreated patients within 8 years of partial gastrectomy and in almost all patients with total gastrectomy or pernicious anemia (PA). Older patients with gastric atrophy may develop a food-bound vitamin B_{12} deficiency in which vitamin B_{12} absorption is impaired. In nonvegan adults, vitamin B_{12} deficiency is almost always due to malabsorption.
  - PA usually occurs in individuals older than 40 years (mean age of onset, 60 years). Up to 30% of patients have a positive family history. PA is an immune-mediated disorder associated with other autoimmune disorders (Graves disease 30%, Hashimoto thyroiditis 11%, and Addison disease 5%–10%). In patients with PA, 90% have anti-parietal cell antibodies, and 60% have anti-intrinsic factor antibodies.
  - Other etiologies of vitamin B_{12} deficiency include pancreatic insufficiency, bacterial overgrowth, and intestinal parasites (*Diphyllobothrium latum*).
- **Folate deficiency** results from a negative folate balance arising from malnutrition, malabsorption, or increased requirement (pregnancy, hemolytic anemia).
  - Folate deficiency is now rare in the United States because of fortification of grains with folic acid.
  - Patients on weight-losing diets, alcoholics, the elderly, and psychiatric patients are particularly at risk for nutritional folate deficiency.
  - Folate deficiency may be seen in several settings:
    - **Pregnancy and lactation** in which there is a three- to fourfold increased daily folate requirements.
    - Folate malabsorption secondary to celiac disease or bariatric surgery.
    - Drugs that can interfere with folate absorption include ethanol, trimethoprim, pyrimethamine, diphenylhydantoin, barbiturates, and sulfasalazine.
    - Dialysis-dependent patients require more folate intake because of increased folate losses.
    - Patients with hemolytic anemia, such as sickle cell anemia, require increased folate for accelerated erythropoiesis and can present with aplastic crisis (rapidly falling RBC counts) with folate deficiency.
- **Thiamine-responsive megaloblastic anemia syndrome:** It is an autosomal recessive disease characterized by megaloblastic anemia associated with deafness and diabetes mellitus.

DIAGNOSIS

Clinical Presentation

- In addition to symptoms of anemia, vitamin B_{12} deficiency may demonstrate neurologic symptoms, such as peripheral neuropathy, paresthesias, lethargy, hypotonia, and seizures.
- Important physical findings include signs of poor nutrition, pigmentation of skin creases and nail beds, or glossitis. Jaundice or splenomegaly may indicate ineffective and extramedullary hematopoiesis.
- Vitamin B_{12} deficiency may cause decreased vibratory and positional sense, ataxia, paresthesias, confusion, and dementia. Neurologic complications may occur in the absence of anemia and may not fully resolve despite adequate treatment. **Folic acid deficiency does not result in neurologic disease.**

Diagnostic Testing

Laboratories

- Macrocytic anemia is usually present unless there is also a coincident cause of microcytic anemia, and leukopenia and thrombocytopenia may occur.
- The peripheral smear shows macro-ovalocytes; hypersegmented neutrophils or macropolycyte (>5% of neutrophils containing six or more nuclear lobes) are common.
- Lactate dehydrogenase (LDH) and indirect bilirubin are typically elevated, reflecting ineffective erythropoiesis and premature destruction of RBCs (intramedullary hemolysis).
- Serum vitamin B_{12} and folate levels should be measured.
- RBC folate is a more accurate indicator of body folate stores than serum folate, particularly if measured after folate therapy or improved nutrition has been initiated.
- **Serum methylmalonic acid (MMA) and homocysteine (HC)** may be useful when the vitamin B_{12} is 100–400 pg/mL (or borderline low as defined by the laboratory reference range). MMA and HC are elevated in vitamin B_{12} deficiency; only HC is elevated in folate deficiency.
- Detecting **antibodies to intrinsic factor** is specific for the diagnosis of PA. Anti parietal cell antibodies may be present in many patients.

Diagnostic Procedures

BM biopsy may be necessary to rule out MDS or acute myeloid leukemia because these disorders may present with findings similar to those of megaloblastic anemia including a hypercellular marrow with an accumulation of immature cells.

TREATMENT

- Potassium supplementation may be necessary when treatment is initiated to avoid potentially serious arrhythmias due to transient hypokalemia induced by enhanced hematopoiesis.
- Reticulocytosis should begin within 1 week of therapy, followed by a rising of Hgb over 6–8 weeks.
- Coexisting ID is present in one-third of patients and is a common cause for an incomplete response to therapy.
- Folic acid 1 mg PO daily is given until the deficiency is corrected. High doses of folic acid (5 mg daily) may be needed in patients with malabsorption syndromes.
- Vitamin B_{12} deficiency is corrected by administering cyanocobalamin. Initial treatment (1000 μg/d intramuscular cyanocobalamin) is typically administered in the setting of severe anemia, neurologic dysfunction, or chronic malabsorption. After 1 week of daily therapy, a commonly employed regimen is 1000 μg/wk given for 4 weeks and then 1000 μg/month for life.
- High-dose enteral therapy (1000–2000 μg/d PO) may be considered after initial repletion in those without neurologic involvement or for convenience or cost.[6]

NONMEGALOBLASTIC MACROCYTOSIS

Alcoholism, with or without liver disease, is the most common cause for nonmegaloblastic macrocytosis. The other causes include hypothyroidism, aplastic anemia, and certain drugs (pyrimethamine, sulfonamides, metformin, phenytoin).

Anemia of Chronic Renal Insufficiency

GENERAL PRINCIPLES

Anemia of chronic renal insufficiency is attributed primarily to decreased endogenous erythropoietin (EPO) production and may occur as the creatinine clearance declines to below 50 mL/min. Other causes including a functional ID may contribute to the etiology (see the previous description).

DIAGNOSIS

- RBCs are often normocytic and normochromic; however, with increasing severity of the condition, they may become hypochromic and eventually microcytic, with the occasional presence of echinocytes (burr cells). If the patient's creatinine level is >1.8 mg/dL, the primary cause of the anemia can be assumed to be EPO deficiency and/or ID, and an EPO level is unnecessary.
- Iron status should be evaluated in patients undergoing dialysis by obtaining levels of ferritin and transferrin saturation, which show hypoferremia and decreased transferrin saturation. Oral iron supplementation is not considered effective in CKD; therefore, parenteral iron is recommended to maintain a ferritin level of >500 ng/mL.[7]

TREATMENT

- Treatment has been revolutionized by erythropoiesis-stimulating agents (ESAs) including EPO and darbepoetin alfa (Table 21-4).

TABLE 21-4 Erythropoietin Dosing

	Agent and Initial Dose (SC or IV)	
Indication	**Erythropoietin[a] (Procrit, Epogen)**	**Darbepoetin[b] (Aranesp)**
Chemotherapy-induced anemia from nonmyeloid malignancy, multiple myeloma, lymphoma; anemia secondary to malignancy or myelodysplastic syndrome	40,000 units/wk or 150 units/kg 3 times a week	2.25 μg/kg/wk or 100 μg/wk or 200 μg/2 wk or 500 μg/3 wk
Anemia associated with renal failure	50–150 units/kg 3 times a week	0.45 μg/kg/wk
Anemia associated with HIV infection	100–200 units/kg 3 times a week	Not approved
Anemia of chronic disease	150–300 units/kg 3 times a week	Not approved
Anemia in patients unwilling or unable to receive RBCs; anemic patients undergoing major surgery	600 units/kg/wk × 3 300 units/kg/d × 1–2 wk	Not recommended

[a] Dose increase after 48 weeks up to 900 units/kg/wk or 60,000 units/wk; discontinue if hematocrit (Hct) is >40%; resume when Hct is <36% at 75% of previous dose.
[b] Dose increase after 6 weeks up to 4.5 mg/kg/wk or 150 mg/wk or 300 mg/2 wk; hold dose if Hct is >36%, then resume when Hct is <36% at 75% of previous dose.
RBC, red blood cell.

- Therapy is initiated in predialysis patients who are symptomatic.
- Objective benefits of reversing anemia include enhanced exercise capacity, improved cognitive function, elimination of RBC transfusions, and reduction of iron overload. Subjective benefits include increased energy, enhanced appetite, better sleep patterns, and improved sexual activity.
- Administration of ESAs can be IV (hemodialysis patients) or SC (predialysis or peritoneal dialysis patients). In dialysis and predialysis patients with CKD, **the target Hgb should be between 11–12 g/dL and should not exceed 12 g/dL.** Hgb and Hct should be measured at least monthly while receiving an ESA. Dose adjustments should be made to maintain the target Hgb.
- Side effects of ESAs: Targeting higher Hgb levels and/or exposure to high doses of ESAs is associated with a greater risk of cardiovascular complications and mortality. In addition, a higher Hct level from ESAs increases the risk of stroke, heart failure, hypertension, and deep vein thrombosis.[8]
- **Suboptimal responses to ESA therapy** are most often due to ID, inflammation, bleeding, infection, malignancy, malnutrition, and aluminum toxicity.
  - Because anemia is a powerful determinant of life expectancy in patients on chronic dialysis, IV iron administration has become first-line therapy for individuals with transferrin saturation <20% and/or ferritin <500 ng/mL. It has also been shown to reduce the ESA dosage required to correct anemia.
  - A ferritin level and transferrin saturation should be tested at least monthly during the initiation of ESA therapy with a goal ferritin level of >200 ng/mL and a transferrin saturation of >20% in dialysis-dependent patients and a ferritin level of >100 ng/mL and a transferrin saturation of >20% in predialysis or peritoneal dialysis patients.
  - Iron therapy is unlikely to be useful if the ferritin level is >500 ng/mL.
  - Secondary hyperparathyroidism that causes BM fibrosis and relative ESA resistance may also occur.

Anemia of Chronic Disease

GENERAL PRINCIPLES

- Anemia of chronic disease (ACD) often develops in patients with long-standing inflammatory diseases, malignancy, autoimmune disorders, and chronic infection.
- Etiology is multifactorial, including defective iron mobilization during erythropoiesis, inflammatory cytokine-mediated suppression of erythropoiesis, and impaired EPO response to anemia. Hepcidin is a critical regulator of iron homeostasis and is normally low when iron is deficient, allowing for increased iron absorption and utilization. Chronic inflammation increases hepcidin levels and causes a functional ID due to impaired iron recycling and utilization. Hepcidin is renally cleared, suggesting a role in anemia of chronic renal disease.[9]

DIAGNOSIS

- Anemia is normocytic and normochromic; however, with increasing severity, it may become hypochromic and eventually microcytic.
- The soluble transferrin receptor level is helpful in differentiating ACD (normal) and ID (elevated) when the ferritin is indeterminate. Measurement of serum hepcidin may become part of the standard evaluation of anemia when the assay becomes widely available.
- Iron studies may show low serum iron and TIBC.

- Ferritin level below 30 ng/mL suggests coexisting ID and should be treated with supplemental iron. Clinical responses to IV iron therapy may occur in patients with ferritin levels up to 100 ng/mL.

TREATMENT

- Therapy for ACD is directed toward the underlying disease and eliminating exacerbating factors such as nutritional deficiencies and marrow-suppressive drugs.
- Enteral iron is typically ineffective in ACD because of reduced intestinal absorption of iron.
- ESA therapy should be considered if the patient is transfusion dependent or has symptomatic anemia. ESA therapy is discontinued when the Hgb is >11 g/dL to reduce risk of cardiovascular adverse events. Suboptimal (<1 g/dL) increase in Hgb 2 weeks after ESA dose prompts a re-evaluation of iron stores.
  - Effective doses of ESA are higher than those reported in anemia from renal insufficiency.
  - If no responses have been observed at 900 units/kg/wk, further dose escalation is unlikely to be effective.

Anemia in Cancer Patients

Although ESA therapy has been shown to reduce transfusion requirements in chemotherapy-related anemia, their use remains controversial because of evidence of increased mortality risk in cancer patients.[10] In addition, ESAs are ineffective in patients who are not receiving chemotherapy and have not been shown to increase quality of life.[11] They confer an elevated risk of thrombosis regardless of baseline Hgb level. Current guidelines recommend ESA therapy should only be considered in transfusion-dependent cancer patients with Hgb level <10 g/dL who are receiving myelosuppressive chemotherapy.

Anemia Associated With HIV Disease

- Anemia is the most common cytopenia in patients with HIV; the prevalence increases as the disease progresses and the CD4 count declines.[12]
- *Mycobacterium avium* complex infections are frequently associated with severe anemia. Diagnosis is established on BM examination or culture. Treatment of *M. avium* complex is described in Chapter 16, Sexually Transmitted Infections, Human Immunodeficiency Virus, and Acquired Immunodeficiency Syndrome.
- Parvovirus B19 should be considered in HIV-infected patients with transfusion-dependent anemia and a low reticulocyte count.
  - Laboratory studies: Parvovirus by polymerase chain reaction from serum or BM.
  - Treatment with IV immunoglobulin (IVIG) 0.4 g/kg daily for 5–10 days results in erythropoietic recovery. Relapses have occurred between 2 and 6 months and can be successfully managed with maintenance IVIG at a dose of 0.4 g/kg IV every 4 weeks.[13]

Aplastic Anemia

GENERAL PRINCIPLES

- Aplastic anemia (AA) is a disorder of hematopoietic stem cells that usually presents with pancytopenia.
- Most cases are acquired and idiopathic, but AA can also arise from an inherited BM failure syndrome such as Fanconi anemia, dyskeratosis congenita, and Shwachman–Diamond syndrome.
- Approximately 20% of cases may be associated with drug or chemical exposure (Table 21-5).

TABLE 21-5 Commonly Used Drugs That Can Induce Red Blood Cell Disorders

Sideroblastic Anemia	Aplastic Anemia[a]	G6PD Deficiency	Immune Hemolytic Anemia
Chloramphenicol	Acetazolamide	Dapsone	Cephalosporins (cefotetan, ceftriaxone)
Cycloserine	Antineoplastic drugs	Doxorubicin	Penicillins (piperacillin)
Ethanol	Carbamazepine	Methylene blue	Purine nucleoside analogues (fludarabine, cladribine)
Isoniazid	Chloramphenicol	Nalidixic acid	NSAIDs (diclofenac, ibuprofen)
Pyrazinamide	Gold salts	Nitrofurantoin	Quinidine
	Hydantoins	Pegloticase	Quinine
	Penicillamine	Phenazopyridine	Rifampin
	Sulfonamides	Primaquine	Sulfonamides (trimethoprim/sulfamethoxazole)
	Phenylbutazone	Rasburicase	
	Quinacrine	Sulfacetamide	
		Sulfamethoxazole	
		Sulfanilamide	
		Sulfapyridine	

Data compiled from multiple sources. Agents listed are available in the United States.
[a]Drugs with ≥30 cases reported; many other drugs rarely are associated with aplastic anemia and are considered low risk.
G6PD, glucose-6-phosphate dehydrogenase.

- Approximately 10% of cases are associated with viral illnesses (e.g., viral hepatitis, Epstein–Barr virus, cytomegalovirus [CMV], and HIV).
- Clonal hematopoiesis is a feature of AA, with MDS and acute myeloid leukemia (AML) developing in ~15% of patients.

DIAGNOSIS

Diagnostic Criteria

AA is a diagnosis of exclusion, and other causes of pancytopenia should be ruled out.

Prognosis in AA is dependent on disease severity and patient age:[14]

- Moderate or nonsevere AA
  - BM cellularity <30%
  - Absence of criteria for severe AA
  - At least two of three blood lines are lower than normal
- Severe AA
  - BM cellularity <25% with normal cytogenetics, OR
  - BM cellularity <50% with normal cytogenetics, and <30% residual hematopoietic cells, AND two of three peripheral blood criteria:
    - Absolute neutrophil count (ANC) <500/μL
    - Platelet count <20,000/μL
    - Absolute reticulocyte count <20,000/μL
  - No other hematologic disease
- Very severe AA
  - The criteria of severe AA are met, AND
  - ANC <200/μL

Diagnostic Testing

BM biopsy is required for diagnosis. The BM results in a patient with AA may be difficult to distinguish from hypocellular MDS and paroxysmal nocturnal hemoglobinuria (PNH). Evidence of dysplasia or abnormal cytogenetics is indicative of MDS. PNH clones can be detected by flow cytometry of the blood or BM.

TREATMENT

- Suspected offending drugs should be discontinued and exacerbating factors corrected. Rarely, spontaneous recovery of normal hematopoiesis can occur, usually within 1–2 months of discontinuing the offending drug.
- Once the diagnosis is established, care should be provided in a center experienced with AA.
- Therapy is optional in moderate AA unless there is transfusion dependence; however, severe or very severe AA requires urgent treatment given the high risk of infectious and hemorrhagic complications.
- Patients younger than the age of 50 with severe AA, should be evaluated for eligibility for allogeneic SCT.
- Patients over the age of 50 with severe AA or younger patients without SCT donor are treated with eltrombopag 75–150 mg/d along with cyclosporine and antithymocyte globulin (ATG).[15] Overall response rates at 6 months were 94% and the 2-year survival rate was 97%.
- AA typically does not respond to ESAs. Granulocyte colony-stimulating factor may be effective in some patients and can be used while awaiting definitive therapy; however, there is no clear evidence of survival benefit with the use of these agents.
- Immunosuppressive treatment with cyclosporine and ATG should be considered in patients with severe AA who do not undergo an SCT.[16] Overall response rates at 3 months were between 60% and 80%, and most responses occur by 6 months.
- Corticosteroids alone have not been shown to be effective and can increase the risk of infections and **should not** be used in the treatment of AA.
- **Transfusions in AA.** RBC transfusions should be kept to a minimum to avoid alloimmunization. Prophylactic platelet transfusions are generally recommended if the platelet count is <10,000/μL. Transfusion of irradiated, leukocyte-depleted blood products is preferred to decrease the risk of alloimmunization.

ANEMIAS ASSOCIATED WITH INCREASED RED BLOOD CELL DESTRUCTION

Anemias Associated With Increased Erythropoiesis

GENERAL PRINCIPLES

Definition

Anemias associated with increased erythropoiesis (i.e., an elevated reticulocyte count) are caused by bleeding or hemolysis and may exceed the capacity of normal BM to correct the Hgb. Bleeding is much more common than hemolysis.

Etiology

- **Blood loss.** If no obvious source, suspect occult loss into GI tract, retroperitoneum, thorax, or deep compartments of thigh depending on history (recent instrumentation, trauma, hip fracture, coagulopathy).
- **Hemolysis** can be categorized into two broad groups based on the cause of destruction: intrinsic (caused by deficits inherit to the RBC) and extrinsic (caused by factors external to the RBC).
  - In general, intrinsic causes are inherited, whereas extrinsic causes tend to be acquired. Intrinsic disorders are a result of defects of the red cell membrane (i.e., hereditary spherocytosis), Hgb composition (i.e., sickle cell disease [SCD]), or enzyme deficiency (i.e., G6PD deficiency).
  - Extrinsic disorders can result from antibodies (i.e., cold or warm reactive immunoglobulin), infectious agents (i.e., malaria), trauma, chemical agents (i.e., venom), or liver disease.
  - Hemolytic disorders are also commonly categorized by the location of RBC destruction: intravascular (within the circulation) or extravascular (within the macrophage in the liver or spleen).

DIAGNOSIS

Laboratory findings of patients with suspected hemolysis typically include:

- **Normocytic or macrocytic anemia (higher MCV due to increased reticulocytes which are slightly larger than mature RBCs) with an elevated reticulocyte count.**
- **Elevated LDH** and **indirect hyperbilirubinemia** reflect increased RBC turnover.
- **Decreased haptoglobin** due to binding of intravascular Hgb.
- The **direct Coombs test** (direct antiglobulin testing [DAT]) is an indicator of the presence of antibodies or complement bound to RBC.
- The **indirect Coombs test** indicates the presence of antibody in the plasma.
- A peripheral blood smear is essential and can aid in determining the etiology of hemolysis. Intravascular hemolysis may reveal red cell fragmentation (i.e., schistocytes, helmet cells), whereas spherocytes often occur in extravascular hemolysis. Polychromasia and nucleated RBCs are indicators of increased erythropoiesis.

Sickle Cell Disease

GENERAL PRINCIPLES

- SCD is a group of hereditary Hgb disorders in which Hgb undergoes a sickle shape transformation under conditions of deoxygenation.
- The most common are homozygous sickle cell anemia (Hgb SS) or other double-heterozygous conditions (Hgb SC, Hgb S–β°, or Hgb S–β+ thalassemia).
- Newborn-screening programs for hemoglobinopathies are available throughout the United States and identify most patients in infancy.
- In the United States, the incidence of SCD is approximately 1 in 625 births.
- **Sickle cell trait** is present in 7%–8% of African Americans. It is generally considered to be a benign carrier state, but high-altitude hypoxia is associated with splenic infarction, whereas intense physical exertion has been associated with sudden death and rhabdomyolysis.[17]
- Sickle cell trait has been associated with an increased risk of pulmonary embolism, proteinuria, and CKD. Minimizing other risk factors for kidney disease is likely to benefit patients at risk.[18]

DIAGNOSIS

Diagnostic Testing

- Hgb analysis by high-pressure liquid chromatography is commonly used and distinguishes most hemoglobinopathies.
- Laboratory abnormalities include anemia (mean Hgb in SCD, 8 g/dL), reticulocytosis (3%–15%), indirect hyperbilirubinemia, elevated LDH, and decreased or absent haptoglobin. Leukocytosis (10,000–20,000/µL) and thrombocytosis (>450,000/µL) are common, because of enhanced stimulation of the marrow compartment and autosplenectomy.
- Peripheral smear shows sickle-shaped RBCs, target cells (particularly in double heterozygous states like Hgb SC and Hgb S–β thalassemia), and Howell–Jolly bodies, indicative of functional asplenism. Other features of hemolysis such as polychromasia (reticulocytosis) and nucleated RBCs can be seen.
- In cases that are less evident, such as sickle cell trait, the peripheral smear may show elliptocyte-like cells. To confirm the suspicion, a sickling test using sodium metabisulphite can be done, though it is less reliable than Hb high performance liquid chromatography (HPLC).

Clinical Presentation

- Clinical presentation of SCD is heterogeneous and is dependent on type and degree of hemoglobinopathy. The most common clinical manifestations of SCD result from hemolysis and/or vascular occlusions.
- Vascular occlusions include pain crises, avascular necrosis (AVN), priapism, and acute chest syndrome (ACS), whereas hemolytic complications include pulmonary hypertension, cholelithiasis, and leg ulcers. Strokes and renal medullary infarctions are complications of both.
- **Vaso-occlusive complications** (**VOCs**) result from polymerization of deoxygenated Hgb S. These polymerized RBCs assume the classic sickle shape and develop a marked loss of deformability, leading to vaso-occlusion. These are triggered by dehydration, infection, hypoxia, pregnancy, stress, acidosis, and cold weather.
    - **Acute painful episodes ("sickle cell pain crisis")**
        - Sickle cell pain crisis is the most common VOC and manifestation of SCD.
        - Pain is typically in the long bones, back, chest, and abdomen.
        - Precipitating factors can include stress, infection, dehydration, alcohol, and weather. However, a majority of cases have no identifiable trigger.
        - Typical duration of the episode is 2–6 days.
        - Higher levels of Hgb F seem to be protective against VOC.
    - **ACS** is a life-threatening emergency that occurs when there is irreversible occlusion of the pulmonary microvasculature. The diagnosis is based on a pulmonary infiltrate involving at least one complete segment and one of the following: fever, hypoxemia, tachypnea, respiratory failure, chest pain, or wheezing. ACS precipitated by pulmonary fat emboli as the inciting event may be more severe and associated with other organ dysfunction, including stroke.
    - **Priapism** often presents in adolescence and may result in impotence.
    - **Retinopathy** is caused by chronic vaso-occlusion of the retina, which causes proliferative retinopathy and may lead to complications including vitreous hemorrhage and retinal detachment.
    - **Functional asplenia** results from recurrent splenic infarcts due to sickling and eventually results in the loss of splenic function. The majority of cases occur before the age of 1. Functional asplenia places patients at higher risk of infection, especially with encapsulated organisms.

- **AVN** is the result of infarction of bone trabeculae and occurs most commonly in the femoral and humeral heads. Up to 50% of adults affected by SCD can manifest AVN, which is a leading cause of pain and disability.

- **Hemolytic complications**
  - **Cholelithiasis** is present in >80% of patients and is primarily due to bilirubin stones. It may lead to acute cholecystitis or biliary colic.
  - **Leg ulceration** occurring at the ankle is often chronic and recurring.
  - **Pulmonary hypertension** has been linked to several hemolytic disorders and can occur in up to 60% of patients with SCD. The diagnosis is best established by a right-sided heart catheterization.[19] The pathophysiology is unclear but may be the result of nitric oxide depletion.
- **Renal medulla infarction** is the result of repeated occlusion of renal medullary capillaries, resulting in CKD in many patients. This can lead to isosthenuria (inability to concentrate urine) and hematuria, predisposing patients to dehydration and thus increasing the risk of VOC.
- **Neurologic complications** occur in up to 25% of patients with SCD by the age of 45 and include cerebrovascular events (transient ischemic attacks, ischemic stroke, cerebral hemorrhage), seizure, and sensory hearing loss.[20] Ischemic stroke is felt to result from recurrent endothelial injury from hemolysis and vaso-occlusion, resulting in intimal hyperplasia with large-artery vasculopathy.[21] High cerebral flow rate (>200 cm/s) detected by transcranial Doppler has been associated with increased risk of stroke in children. This risk is greatly reduced by routine transfusion or exchange therapy.[22] Current recommendations for adults include evaluation for known additional stroke risk factors with management accordingly.[23]
- **Infections** typically occur in tissues susceptible to vaso-occlusive infarcts (i.e., lungs, bone, kidney). The most common infectious organisms include *Streptococcus pneumoniae, Staphylococcus aureus, Salmonella* spp., *Mycoplasma pneumoniae*, or *H. influenzae*. Vaccinations are a key mechanism in prevention.
- **Aplastic "crisis"** occurs when there is a transient interruption of erythropoiesis due to an inciting event causing a sudden decrease in Hgb with a very low reticulocyte count. The most common etiology in children with SCD is parvovirus B19 infection. Folate deficiency and ingestion of toxins such as phenylbutazone can precipitate aplastic crisis.
- **Pregnancy** in a patient with sickle cell anemia should be considered high risk and is associated with an increase in both maternal and fetal complications. Maternal complications include an increased risk of VOC, ACS, and infections.[24] Fetal complications include preterm delivery, low birth weight, and increased risk of stillbirth.

TREATMENT

- Evidence-based management of SCD has been recently updated and is available online at http://www.nhlbi.nih.gov/health-pro/guidelines/sickle-cell-disease-guidelines.
- **Acute painful episodes.** Management of **acute painful episodes** consists of rehydration (3–4 L/d), evaluation for and management of infections, analgesia, and if needed, antipyretic and empiric antibiotic therapy.
  - **Opioids** are typically used and are effectively administered by a **patient-controlled analgesia (PCA) pump**, allowing the patient to self-administer medication within a set limit of infusions (lockout interval) and basal rate. Morphine or hydromorphone are the commonly used opioids for moderate or severe pain and the doses vary considerably from patient to patient. If a PCA pump is not used, morphine (0.1–0.2 mg/kg IV q2–3h) or hydromorphone (0.02–0.04 mg/kg IV q2–3h) may be used.

  - Transfusion therapy has no proven role in the treatment of uncomplicated vaso-occlusive crises unless a symptomatic anemia is present or other complications occur.
  - Supplemental oxygen does not benefit an acute pain crisis unless hypoxia is present.
- **ACS.** Multimodal treatment includes adequate analgesia, volume resuscitation, supplemental oxygen and incentive spirometry, and blood transfusion. It is unclear whether exchange transfusion is superior to simple RBC transfusion; however, it is standard practice to perform exchange transfusion for moderate to severe cases, whereas simple transfusion to >10 g/dL for mild cases may be sufficient. The presentation of ACS is clinically indistinguishable from pneumonia; thus, empiric broad-spectrum antibiotics should also be administered.
- **Priapism** is initially treated with hydration and analgesia. Persistent erections for more than 24 hours may require transfusion therapy or surgical drainage.
- **AVN** management consists of local heat, analgesics, and avoidance of weight bearing. Hip and shoulder arthroplasty are often effective at decreasing symptoms and improving function.
- **Cholelithiasis.** Induced acute cholecystitis should be treated medically with antibiotics followed by cholecystectomy when the attack subsides. Elective cholecystectomy for asymptomatic gallstones is controversial.
- **Leg ulcers** should be treated with rest, leg elevation, and intensive local care. Wet to dry dressings should be applied three to four times per day. A zinc oxide–impregnated bandage (Unna boot), changed weekly for 3–4 weeks, can be used for nonhealing or more extensive ulcers.
- There is no standard therapy for treatment of **pulmonary hypertension** in SCD and clinically effective therapy remains elusive.[25]
- **Acute stroke** should be managed based on current standards. Long-term transfusions to maintain the Hgb S concentration to <50% for at least 5 years significantly reduce the incidence of recurrence. Patients with suspected **aplastic crisis** require hospitalization. Therapy includes folic acid, 5 mg/d, as well as RBC transfusions until recovery. **Iron chelation therapy** can be used to treat iron overload in patients with transfusion-related iron overload similar to that described for thalassemia. Emerging therapies for SCD include additional disease modifying agents such as crizanlizumab and voxelotor to decrease the frequency of VOC and improve the anemia, respectively.
- Hematopoietic SCT is potentially curative, although its use is restricted by the high cost, toxicity, and limited availability of suitable donors. Less-toxic conditioning regimens and the use of alternative sources of donor cells has improved transplant success. However SCT may be superseded by investigational gene therapy and gene editing approaches or SCT may be augmented by gene therapies allowing autologous SCT of modified cellular products.

Risk Modification

- **Dehydration and hypoxia** should be avoided because they may precipitate or exacerbate irreversible sickling.
- **Folic acid** (1 mg PO daily) is administered to patients with SCD because of chronic hemolysis.
- **Hydroxyurea** (15–35 mg/kg PO daily) has been shown to increase levels of Hgb F and significantly decreases the frequency of VOC and ACS in adults with SCD.[26] In practice, the dose is increased until the ANCs are between 2000 and 4000/μL.
- **L-glutamine** (0.3 g/kg PO twice daily) recently became available for the prevention of VOC and may be incorporated into preventative care with or without concomitant hydroxyurea.[27]

- **Antimicrobial prophylaxis** with penicillin VK, 125 mg PO bid to age 3 and then 250 mg PO bid until age 5, is effective at reducing risk of infection.[28] Patients who are allergic to penicillin should receive erythromycin 10 mg/kg PO bid. Prophylaxis should be stopped at age 5 to avoid development of resistant organisms.[29]
- **Immunizations** against the usual childhood illnesses should be given to children with SCD, including hepatitis B vaccine. After 2 years of age, a polyvalent pneumococcal vaccine should be administered. Yearly influenza vaccine is recommended.
- **Ophthalmologic examinations** are recommended yearly in adults because of the high incidence of proliferative retinopathy.
- Local and regional anesthesia can be used without special precautions. Care should be taken to avoid volume depletion, hypoxia, and hypernatremia. For surgery with general anesthesia, RBC transfusions to increase the Hgb to 10 g/dL is as effective as more aggressive thresholds to decrease postoperative complications and more effective than withholding preoperative transfusions.[30]

Glucose-6-Phosphate Dehydrogenase Deficiency

GENERAL PRINCIPLES

G6PD deficiency represents the most common disorder of RBC metabolism worldwide. Deficiency of G6PD renders RBCs more susceptible to oxidative damage through decreased glutathione reduction, leading to chronic or acute episodic hemolysis in the presence of oxidative stress.

Classification

More than 400 variants of G6PD are recognized. The severity of hemolysis depends on the degree of deficiency present.[31]

- Milder forms, such as those seen in men of African heritage in the United States, result in self-limiting acute hemolytic episodes.
- More severe forms, such as the Mediterranean variant, can result in severe hemolysis.
- The most severe type causes a chronic, hereditary, nonspherocytic hemolytic anemia in the absence of an inciting cause.

Epidemiology

- X-linked inheritance; thus degree of involvement in females is dependent on lyonization.
- G6PD is felt to be protective against malaria, thus accounting for its prevalence in malaria-endemic areas.
- Hemolysis is triggered by exposure to mediators of oxidative stress (i.e., drugs [see Table 21-5]), infections, and fava beans. Patients being considered for medications that trigger G6PD-dependent hemolysis should be tested for a deficiency before starting the drug.

DIAGNOSIS

- Varying degrees of anemia and reticulocytosis are the most significant features. Peripheral smear in the absence of hemolysis red cell morphology appears normal. Patients undergoing drug-induced hemolysis may show Heinz bodies (precipitated denatured hemoglobin) and bite cells.
- Diagnosis is determined by measuring G6PD activity in RBCs from a peripheral blood sample.
- False-negative results may occur in patients with a recent episode of hemolysis or in patients recently transfused because these cells have higher levels of G6PD.

TREATMENT

- In the most common form of G6PD deficiency, hemolytic episodes tend to be self-limiting; the mainstay of treatment is supportive.
- The underlying cause of oxidative stress should be addressed (i.e., treatment of infection, removal of drug).

Autoimmune Hemolytic Anemia

GENERAL PRINCIPLES

Definition

Autoimmune hemolytic anemia (AIHA) results from autoantibodies targeted to antigens on the patient's RBCs, resulting in either extravascular hemolysis (removal of RBC by tissue macrophages in the liver or spleen) or complement-mediated intravascular hemolysis.

Classification

There are two main types of AIHA: warm and cold AIHA. Warm AIHA antibodies interact best with RBCs at 37°C, whereas cold antibodies (or cold agglutinins) are most active at temperatures below 37°C and almost always fix complement.

Etiology

- Warm AIHA (70%–80%) is usually caused by an IgG autoantibody. It may be idiopathic or secondary to an underlying process (i.e., lymphoma, chronic lymphocytic leukemia [CLL], Kaposi sarcoma, collagen vascular disorder, Hepatitis C, HIV, or drugs [see Table 21-5]).
- Cold AIHA (or cold agglutinin disease [CAD], 10%–15%) is typically caused by an IgM autoantibody.
    - The acute form of CAD is often secondary to an infection (*Mycoplasma*, Epstein–Barr virus).
    - The chronic form is due to a paraprotein associated with lymphoma, CLL, or Waldenström macroglobulinemia (WM) in approximately one-half of cases and is primary (idiopathic) in the others.
    - Paroxysmal cold hemoglobinuria
- Combined warm and cold autoantibodies (6%–8%)
- Drug-induced hemolytic anemia

DIAGNOSIS

- Laboratory data usually identify hemolysis with anemia, reticulocytosis, elevated LDH, decreased haptoglobin, and indirect hyperbilirubinemia.
- Peripheral blood smear may show spherocytes, occasional fragmented RBCs in warm AIHA, and RBC agglutination in CAD. Polychromasia and nucleated RBCs may be seen in either form.
- The hallmark of diagnosis is by a positive **DAT (also known as a direct Coombs test)**. The DAT detects the presence of IgG or complement in the form of C3 bound to the RBC surface. The typical results for the DAT are shown here:
    - Warm AIHA: IgG positive and C3 positive or negative
    - Cold AIHA: IgG negative and C3 positive
- The indirect antiglobulin test (indirect Coombs) detects the presence of autoantibodies in the serum but also detects alloantibodies in the serum from alternate causes, including from transfusion or maternal–fetal incompatibility.

- An elevated cold agglutinin titer is seen with cold AIHA.
- If secondary AIHA is suspected, a workup for the underlying cause should be performed.

TREATMENT

- Initial therapy should be aimed at correcting complications from the hemolytic anemia. Definitive therapy should include identification and treatment of any underlying cause.
- RBC transfusions may result in the hemolysis of transfused cells, but they are still indicated in severe or life-threatening anemia.
- **If a complete crossmatch cannot be completed in a timely manner, transfusion of universal donor (O-negative) or type-matched blood is appropriate.**
- Warm AIHA
    - First-line treatment involves **glucocorticoids**, such as oral prednisone 1 mg/kg/d, which is effective in 70%–80% of patients. Response is typically seen in 7–10 days. When hemolysis has abated, glucocorticoids can be tapered over 2–3 months. Rapid steroid taper can result in relapse.
    - Second-line treatments include **splenectomy**, which should be considered for steroid-resistant AIHA, and **rituximab**, a monoclonal antibody directed against CD20 antigen expressed on B cells. Rituximab 375 mg/m^2 weekly for four doses has been shown to be effective in 80%–90% of cases, and responses to treatment are observed with monotherapy or in combination with corticosteroids.[32] Low-dose rituximab, 100 mg weekly for four doses, has also demonstrated efficacy in AIHA.[33]
    - Additional immunosuppressive therapies such as azathioprine, cyclophosphamide, cyclosporine, and mycophenolate mofetil have also been used.
    - Treatment for relapsed/refractory cases is not well defined and includes azathioprine, cyclophosphamide, cyclosporine, and mycophenolate mofetil.[34]
- Primary CAD
    - Avoidance of cold exposure can minimize exacerbations. RBC transfusions at 37°C and keeping the room warm can prevent exacerbation of hemolysis.
    - Glucocorticoids and splenectomy are not effective and should not be used.
    - Plasma exchange removes 60%–70% of IgM, thus offering effective, temporary control of the disease.
    - Rituximab as a single agent or in combination with other agents (fludarabine or bendamustine) has shown to be effective in some cases and may be used as first-line therapy.[35]

Drug-Induced Hemolytic Anemia

GENERAL PRINCIPLES

- **Drug-induced hemolytic anemia** is anemia resulting from exposure to a medication. Table 21-5 lists common offending medications.
- Hemolysis occurs by several mechanisms such as drug-induced antibodies, hapten formation, and immune complexes. The most commonly implicated agents are cephalosporins, penicillins, NSAIDs, and quinine or quinidines.

TREATMENT

The initial treatment may be similar to treatment of warm AIHA with corticosteroids if the etiology is unclear, but if drug-induced hemolytic anemia is suspected, **the most important treatment is discontinuation of the offending agent.**

Microangiopathic Hemolytic Anemia

GENERAL PRINCIPLES

Definition

Microangiopathic or mechanical hemolytic anemia (MAHA) is a syndrome of traumatic intravascular hemolysis causing fragmentation of the RBCs that are seen on peripheral blood smear (schistocytes). It is not a specific diagnosis but suggests a limited differential diagnosis.

Etiology

Possible causes of MAHA include **mechanical heart valve, malignant hypertension, vasculitis, adenocarcinoma, preeclampsia/eclampsia, disseminated intravascular coagulation (DIC), thrombotic thrombocytopenic purpura (TTP), and hemolytic-uremic syndrome (HUS)/atypical HUS** (see Chapter 20, Disorders of Hemostasis and Thrombosis, for a discussion of DIC, TTP, and HUS/atypical HUS).

DIAGNOSIS

MAHA is established by confirming the presence of hemolysis through laboratory data (LDH, haptoglobin, indirect bilirubin) and peripheral blood smear findings. Examination of the blood film is the most important laboratory procedure in making this diagnosis which shows a combination of red cell fragments (schistocytes), thrombocytopenia, and polychromasia.

TREATMENT

The treatment depends on the underlying etiology of microangiopathy (see Chapter 20).

WHITE BLOOD CELL DISORDERS

Leukocytosis and Leukopenia

GENERAL PRINCIPLES

Definition

- Leukocytosis is an elevation in the absolute WBC count (>10,000 cells/μL).
- Leukopenia is a reduction in the WBC count (<3500 cells/μL).

Etiology

- **Leukocytosis**
  - An elevated WBC can be the normal BM response to an infectious or inflammatory process, corticosteroids, β-agonist or lithium therapy, or splenectomy, and is usually associated with an **absolute neutrophilia**.
  - Occasionally, leukocytosis is due to a primary BM disorder with an increase in WBC production and/or delayed maturation. This may occur in the setting of hematologic malignancies such as leukemias or myeloproliferative neoplasms (MPNs) and can affect any cell in the leukocyte lineage.
  - Stressors capable of causing an acute leukocytosis include surgery, exercise, trauma, and emotional stress. Other nonmalignant etiologies of leukocytosis include certain medications, asplenia, smoking, obesity, and chronic inflammatory conditions.
  - A "**leukemoid reaction**" is defined as an excessive WBC response usually reserved for neutrophilia (>50,000/μL) due to a reactive cause.
  - Lymphocytosis is less commonly encountered and is typically associated with atypical infections (i.e., viral), medication use, or leukemia/lymphoma.

- Eosinophilia could be seen with allergic rhinitis, asthma, ABPA, Churg–Strauss syndrome, parasitic infection (helminths, filaria, flukes), and drug allergy (drug rash with eosinophilia and systemic symptoms [DRESS] syndrome).

- **Leukopenia**
  - Leukopenia can occur in response to infection (i.e., HIV), inflammation, primary BM disorders (i.e., malignancy), autoimmune disorders, medications, environmental exposure (i.e., heavy metals or radiation), and vitamin deficiencies.
  - Many cases are medication induced (i.e., chemotherapeutic or immunosuppressive drugs).
  - Idiopathic chronic benign neutropenia may be caused by an antineutrophil antibody or an inherited disorder.
  - Large granular lymphocytic leukemia can be a cause of neutropenia, especially in patients with rheumatoid arthritis.

DIAGNOSIS

Diagnostic Testing

Laboratories

- Review of the peripheral smear is very helpful in the evaluation of WBC disorders. The presence of blasts is concerning for acute leukemia and warrants emergent evaluation or a shift to left in neutrophilic series suggests sepsis or chronic myeloid leukemia when it is significant.
- Flow cytometry of the blood may help determine if there is an underlying clonal process in lymphocytosis (i.e., CLL).
- A BCR-ABL molecular study may be warranted in cases of unexplained neutrophilia to diagnose chronic myeloid leukemia (CML), especially if there is associated eosinophilia or basophilia.
- Additional laboratory abnormalities are related to the underlying disorder and may include elevation in LDH and uric acid from high cell turnover in acute leukemia.
- An infectious workup should be performed as indicated, including assessment for HIV.
- Prothrombin time, international normalized ratio (INR), partial thromboplastin time, and fibrinogen should also be considered, especially if acute promyelocytic leukemia is suspected, because this can be associated with DIC.

Diagnostic Procedures

A BM biopsy with ancillary studies such as cytogenetics, special stains, and flow cytometry may be required to establish the diagnosis.

TREATMENT

- The primary goal of therapy is treatment of the underlying cause.
- See Chapter 22, Cancer, for the treatment of acute and chronic leukemia.
- If symptoms of **leukostasis** are present (neurologic symptoms, dyspnea, or hypoxia), emergent leukopheresis should be performed to decrease WBC burden, relieve symptoms, and prevent long-term sequelae.
- Growth factor support should be considered in patients with chronic neutropenia and ongoing infections until the neutropenia resolves (see Oncologic Emergencies in Chapter 22, Cancer).

PLATELET DISORDERS

Discussed in Chapter 20, Disorders of Hemostasis and Thrombosis

BONE MARROW DISORDERS

Myelodysplastic Syndrome

Discussed in Chapter 22, Cancer.

Myeloproliferative Neoplasms

GENERAL PRINCIPLES

MPNs are a group of disorders characterized by clonal expansion of a hematopoietic stem cell resulting in overproduction of mature, largely functional cells. The 2022 World Health Organization (WHO) designated eight conditions as MPNs, including polycythemia vera (PV), essential thrombocythemia (ET) (discussed in Chapter 22, Cancer), CML (discussed in Chapter 22, Cancer), primary myelofibrosis (PMF), chronic neutrophilic leukemia (CNL), chronic eosinophilic leukemia (CEL), juvenile myelomonocytic leukemia (JMML), MPN, and not otherwise specified (NOS).[36] The most common MPNs include PV, ET, CML, and PMF.

DIAGNOSIS

Diagnostic Criteria

- PV
  Criteria for the diagnosis of PV have been updated in the WHO 2022 classification and major criteria include Hgb >16.5 g/dL in men or Hgb > 16 g/dL in women, a BM biopsy showing hypercellularity for age with panmyelosis, and presence of *JAK2 V617F or JAK2 exon 12* mutation. Minor criterion includes a subnormal serum EPO level. The diagnosis of PV requires meeting either all three major criteria, or the first two major criteria and the minor criterion.[36] (Table 21-6).

TABLE 21-6 WHO 2022 Diagnostic Criteria for Polycythemia Vera

Major Criteria
1. Hgb >16.5 g/dL in men and Hgb >16.0 g/dL in women Or Hct >49% in men and Hct >48% in women 2. BM biopsy showing hypercellularity for age with trilineage growth (panmyelosis) including prominent erythroid, granulocytic, and megakaryocytic proliferation with pleomorphic, mature megakaryocytes (differences in size) 3. Presence of *JAK2 V617F* mutation or *JAK2* exon 12 mutation
Minor Criteria
Subnormal serum erythropoietin level
Diagnosis of PV requires meeting either all three major criteria or the first two major criteria and the minor criterion

Adapted from Tefferi A, Barbui T. Polycythemia vera: 2024 update on diagnosis, risk-stratification, and management. *Am J Hematol.* 2023 Sep;98(9):1465–1487.
BM, bone marrow; Hct, hematocrit; Hgb, hemoglobin; WHO, World Health Organization.

- **PMF**

  The WHO 2022 diagnostic criteria for PMF are listed in Table 21-7.[36] The updated classification has divided PMF into prePMF and overt PMF. For both prePMF and overt PMF, all three major criteria and at least one minor criteria need to be met for the diagnosis.
- **ET**

  Peripheral smear reveals thrombocytosis (450 × 10^9/L or higher) with platelet anisocytosis.
- **CNL**

  Peripheral smear is characterized by leukocytosis (WBC ≥25 × 10^9/L) with segmented or band neutrophils (80% or higher), few neutrophil precursors (less than 10%), and rare myeloblasts.
- **CEL**

  It is characterized by peripheral eosinophilia (≥1500/μL or higher) on at least two occasions over an interval of at least 4 weeks, evidence of clonality, BM with abnormal BM morphology, and not meeting WHO criteria for other myeloid neoplasms.

Diagnostic Testing

Laboratories

- Patients with PV typically present with an elevated Hct but may also have elevations in WBC or platelet count. The *JAK2*V617F mutation is present in >95% of patients. A low EPO level is often present.
- Patients with PMF may present with leukocytosis or cytopenias, depending on the stage of the disease, and may have mutations in *JAK2* (50%), *MPL* (10%), or calreticulin (*CALR*) (40%). Immature granulocytes, tear drop cells, and nucleated RBCs may be seen on the peripheral blood smear (leukoerythroblastic smear).
- About 10%–15% of ET and PMF patients lack all three driver mutations (*JAK2* V617F, *MPL W515L/K*, and *CALR* exon 9), which are also known as triple-negative MPN.

Diagnostic Procedures

A BM biopsy should be included in the diagnostic workup of PMF, including reticulin stain to evaluate for fibrosis. A BM biopsy may not be required for PV in cases with sustained absolute erythrocytosis defined as a Hgb >18.5 g/dL in men or >16.5 g/dL in women. Cytogenetic studies should be performed and have a significant impact on prognosis in PMF.[37]

TREATMENT

- **PV:** The main goal of treatment is to decrease the risk of thrombotic complications. Treatment includes serial phlebotomy along with aspirin 81 mg/d. Hydroxyurea may be added depending on the risk for thrombosis.
  - In patients with low risk for thrombosis (age <60 years, no history of thrombosis): serial phlebotomy to keep goal Hct <45% in men and <42% in women.
  - Patients with high risk for thrombosis (age >60 years, prior thrombosis) should be treated with serial phlebotomy and hydroxyurea.
  - Ruxolitinib 10 mg twice a day, a JAK inhibitor first approved for treatment of myelofibrosis, was recently approved by the Food and Drug Administration (FDA) for the treatment of PV in patients who fail hydroxyurea therapy. It improves the Hct and improves pruritus.[38]
- **PMF:** Patients are risk stratified based on several prognostic scoring systems and treatment depends on the risk category. Treatment may not be needed for low-risk patients.

TABLE 21-7 WHO 2022 Diagnostic Criteria for Primary Myelofibrosis (PMF)

Pre-PMF Criteria
Major Criteria
1. Megakaryocytic proliferation and atypia, without reticulin fibrosis > grade 1, accompanied by increased age-adjusted BM cellularity, granulocytic proliferation, and often decreased erythropoiesis 2. Not meeting the WHO criteria for *BCR-ABL1 CML, PV, ET*, MDS, or other myeloid neoplasms 3. Presence of *JAK2, CALR*, or *MPL* mutation or in the absence of these mutations, presence of another clonal marker, or absence of minor reactive BM reticulin fibrosis
Minor Criteria
Presence of at least one of the following, confirmed in two consecutive determinations: a. Anemia not attributed to a comorbid condition b. Leukocytosis $\geq 11 \times 10^9$/L c. Splenomegaly detected clinically and/or by imaging d. LDH increased to above upper normal limit of institutional reference range e. Leukoerythroblastosis
Diagnosis of pre-PMF requires meeting all three major criteria and at least one minor criterion
Overt PMF criteria
Major Criteria
1. Presence of megakaryocytic proliferation and atypia, accompanied by either reticulin and/or collagen fibrosis grades 2 or 3 2. Not meeting WHO criteria for ET, PV, *BCR-ABL1* CML, MDS, or other myeloid neoplasms 3. Presence of *JAK2, CALR*, or *MPL* mutation or in the absence of these mutations, presence of another clonal marker, or absence of reactive myelofibrosis
Minor Criteria
Presence of at least one of the following, confirmed in two consecutive determinations: a. Anemia not attributed to a comorbid condition b. Leukocytosis $\geq 11 \times 10^9$/L c. Splenomegaly detected clinically and/or by imaging d. LDH increased to above upper normal limit of institutional reference range e. Leukoerythroblastosis
Diagnosis of overt PMF requires meeting all 3 major criteria and at least 1 minor criterion

Adapted from Tefferi A. Primary myelofibrosis: 2023 update on diagnosis, risk-stratification, and management. Am J Hematol. 2023 May;98(5):801–821.

CML, chronic myelogenous leukemia; ET, essential thrombocythemia; LDH, lactate dehydrogenase; MDS, myelodysplastic syndrome; PV, polycythemia vera; WHO, World Health Organization.

- Low-dose aspirin should be started to decrease the risk of thrombosis in the absence of significant thrombocytopenia.
- Cytoreductive agents such as hydroxyurea have been used historically to improve leukocytosis but do not significantly improve constitutional symptoms or splenomegaly and can cause myelosuppression.
- Allogeneic hematopoietic SCT is the only curative therapy and should be considered for high-risk patients.
- Ruxolitinib is approved for the treatment of patients with intermediate and high-risk myelofibrosis. It is effective in improving constitutional symptoms and splenomegaly. The main side effect is myelosuppression, and initial dosing is dependent on the platelet count.[39,40]
- Splenectomy may be considered for painful splenomegaly in patients intolerant to or not responsive to the JAK inhibitor.
- Involved-field radiotherapy may also offer symptomatic relief for drug-refractory splenomegaly or sites of extramedullary hematopoiesis; however, the effects are usually transient.

MONOCLONAL GAMMOPATHIES

Monoclonal Gammopathy of Unknown Significance

GENERAL PRINCIPLES

Definition

Monoclonal gammopathy of unknown significance (MGUS) is a commonly occurring premalignant condition characterized by the presence of a small (<10%) population of neoplastic, clonal plasma cells or lymphoplasmacytic cells in the BM that occurs in the absence of any end-organ damage. For non-IgM MGUS, progression to a more serious disorder including multiple myeloma, WM, or primary amyloidosis (AL) occurs at a rate of approximately 1% per year. For IgM MGUS, progression to WM or primary AL amyloidosis occurs at a rate of 1%–5% per year.

DIAGNOSIS

- Patients with MGUS are asymptomatic and diagnosed when a monoclonal protein is detected on serum protein electrophoresis (SPEP) during workup of an elevated serum protein or other unrelated clinical finding. Most of the gammopathies are identified as IgG, but gammopathies in all immunoglobulin classes occur.
- Serum free light chain assay is used in both prognosis of MGUS and in the diagnosis of multiple myeloma.
- The Multiple Myeloma International Working Group updated diagnostic criteria for non-IgM MGUS 2014 requiring all three criteria:
  - Presence of a serum monoclonal protein (non-IgM type) <3 g/dL
  - Presence of clonal BM plasma cells comprising <10% of the total nucleated cells in the marrow.
  - Absence of end-organ damage attributed to the underlying plasma cell disorder, such as hypercalcemia, renal insufficiency, anemia, or lytic bone lesions
- The Multiple Myeloma International Working Group updated diagnostic criteria for IgM MGUS in 2014 requiring the following diagnostic criteria:
  - Serum IgM monoclonal protein <3 g/dL
  - BM lymphoplasmacytic infiltration <10%
  - No evidence of anemia, constitutional symptoms, hyperviscosity, lymphadenopathy, hepatosplenomegaly, or other end-organ damage that can be attributed to the underlying lymphoproliferative disorder

TREATMENT

There is no treatment recommended for MGUS. The vast majority of patients will not progress to a malignant disease. Yearly surveillance with a CBC, serum creatinine and calcium, SPEP, urine protein electrophoresis (UPEP), and serum free light chains. If a patient develops an anemia, hypercalcemia, renal dysfunction, or bone pain, additional evaluation including a BM biopsy and imaging (i.e., skeletal survey, PET CT scan or MRI) are recommended.

PROGNOSIS

MGUS can evolve into a malignant lymphoproliferative disorder. Factors for higher risk of progression include an M protein >1.5 g/dL, non-IgG monoclonal gammopathy, and abnormal serum free light chain ratio (<0.26 or >1.65).

Multiple Myeloma

Discussed in Chapter 22, Cancer.

Waldenström Macroglobulinemia

WM is an uncommon IgM monoclonal disorder also known as lymphoplasmacytic lymphoma, characterized by mild hematologic abnormalities, and accompanied by tissue infiltration including lymphadenopathy, splenomegaly, or hepatomegaly. Because of its high molecular weight and concentration, IgM gammopathy can lead to hyperviscosity (central nervous system, visual, cardiac) manifestations. Presence of IgM monoclonal protein associated with ≥10% clonal lymphoplasmacytic cells in bone marrow confirms the diagnosis. In these cases, emergent plasmapheresis to decrease IgM concentration is indicated. The L265P mutation in MYD88 L265P is a commonly (>90%) recurring mutation in patients with WM and can be useful in differentiating WM from B-cell disorders that have similar features.[41] Asymptomatic patients may be observed initially, whereas durable responses have been observed in those requiring chemotherapy.[42] The Bruton tyrosine kinase inhibitor **ibrutinib** received FDA approval in January 2015 for treatment of WM based on an overall response rate of 62% in a study of 63 patients with WM.[43]

Amyloidosis

GENERAL PRINCIPLES

Primary (AL) amyloidosis is an infiltrative disorder due to monoclonal, light chain deposition in various tissues most often involving the kidney (renal failure, nephrotic syndrome), heart (nonischemic cardiomyopathy), peripheral nervous system (neuropathy, especially autonomic neuropathy), and GI tract/liver (macroglossia, diarrhea, nausea, vomiting, hepatosplenomegaly). Carpal tunnel syndrome, jaw claudication, and articular deposits of amyloid can also be a manifestation of systemic amyloidosis. Unexplained findings in any of these organ systems should prompt evaluation for amyloidosis. Primary amyloidosis must be distinguished from nonclonal secondary systemic amyloidosis.[44] Other physical examination findings that can lead to suspicion of amyloidosis diagnoses such as shoulder pads from amyloid deposition, amyloid purpura, and raccoon eyes secondary to factor X deficiency can be seen.

DIAGNOSIS AND TREATMENT

- SPEP, UPEP, and serum free light chains may detect an M protein or an abnormal free light chain ratio that is found in >90% of patients with AL amyloidosis. In the absence of a measurable M protein, consider other types of secondary systemic amyloidosis. In addition to Congo red staining for amyloid in the BM or other affected tissue, mass spectroscopy to identify the presence of light chains establish the diagnosis of AL amyloidosis. An NT-proBNP, troponin T or I, and 24-hour urinary protein are important in assessing organ involvement and staging.
- Several effective chemotherapy regimens have been developed during the last decade, including bortezomib-based regimens such as CyBorD (cyclophosphamide, bortezomib, dexamethasone).[45,46] Melphalan has been substituted for cyclophosphamide with disease activity.[47] Additionally, those with adequate organ function and a good performance status should be considered for autologous stem cell transplant (auto-SCT).
- Various monoclonal antibodies have also shown activity in patients with relapsed and refractory disease in clinical trials and are investigational.
- However, treatment of amyloidosis remains difficult, and progressive organ failure is frequent. Cardiac involvement generally portends the worst prognosis.
- Transthyretin-related hereditary amyloidosis may be cured by liver transplantation.

Transfusion Medicine

GENERAL PRINCIPLES

Transfusion is a commonly used therapy for a variety of hematologic and hemostatic disturbances. The benefits and risks must be carefully weighed in each situation because blood products are a limited resource with potentially life-threatening side effects.

TREATMENT

- **Packed RBCs (pRBCs).** RBC transfusion is indicated to increase the oxygen-carrying capacity of blood in anemic or bleeding patients.
  - Hgb threshold for transfusion has been extensively studied and current recommendations are shown.[48]
    - Stable patient, no cardiac risk factors: Hgb ≤7 g/dL.[49]
    - Septic shock: Hgb ≤7 g/dL.[50]
    - Cardiac risk factors: Hgb ≤8 g/dL.[51]
    - Active acute coronary syndrome: Thresholds have not been established; higher Hgb thresholds (8–10 g/dL) may be considered.
    - The new AABB international guidelines 2023 recommend restrictive transfusion strategies for RBC transfusion:
      - **Recommendation 1:** For hospitalized adult patients who are hemodynamically stable, transfusion is considered when the hemoglobin concentration is <7 g/dL. For patients undergoing cardiac surgery, a threshold of 7.5 g/dL may be chosen, and for those undergoing orthopedic surgery, 8 g/dL.
      - **Recommendation 2:** For hospitalized adult patients, transfusion is considered when the hemoglobin concentration is <7 g/dL in those with hematologic and oncologic disorders.
  - One unit of pRBCs increases the Hgb level by approximately 1 g/dL or Hct by 3% in the average adult.
  - If the cause of anemia is easily treatable (e.g., iron or vitamin B_{12} deficiency) and no cerebrovascular or cardiopulmonary compromise is present, it is preferable to avoid transfusion.

- **Fresh frozen plasma (FFP):** Plasma transfusion is used to replace certain plasma proteins, usually coagulation factors, to treat bleeding or as bleeding prophylaxis for patients undergoing invasive procedures.
  - Common indications include:
    - Acquired coagulopathy in a patient with serious or massive bleeding
    - Warfarin overdose with major bleeding: consider using four-factor (II, VII, IX, X) prothrombin complex concentrates instead of FFP
    - Factor deficiencies for which specific factor concentrates are unavailable
  - The usual dose of FFP is 10–20 mL/kg. One unit of FFP contains approximately 250 mL of plasma and 250 units of factor activity for each factor.
  - FFP should not be used as a volume expander and is usually not indicated in patients who are not currently bleeding, even those with an abnormal PT or activated PTT. In the case of warfarin overdose with a very prolonged PT but no bleeding, vitamin K should be used instead.
  - FFP has been used in patients undergoing high-risk surgery (e.g., neurosurgery) with a high INR (>1.5–2.0); however, there is no evidence supporting a clear INR threshold as FFP is often ineffective in decreasing a slightly elevated INR.
- **Platelets:** Platelet transfusion is indicated to prevent or treat bleeding in a thrombocytopenic patient or patients with dysfunctional platelets (e.g., due to aspirin).
  - Platelet count threshold for transfusion[52]
    - Nonbleeding, stable inpatients: $\leq 10 \times 10^9$/L.[53]
    - Nonbleeding, stable outpatients: $\leq 20 \times 10^9$/L.
    - Central line placement in a stable patient: $\leq 20 \times 10^9$/L.
    - Major invasive procedures or bleeding: $\leq 50 \times 10^9$/L.
    - High-risk surgery (e.g., neurosurgery) or life-threatening bleeding may require a higher threshold.
  - Most platelet infusions in the United States are from a single donor collected by platelet pheresis rather than pooled platelets from a number of individuals.
  - One unit of single donor platelets increases the platelet count by $30–50 \times 10^9$/L, but this response may be blunted in patients with platelet refractoriness (see below).
  - Platelets have a short shelf life (<5 days) and are stored at room temperature; they must never be placed on ice or refrigerated, which can cause platelet activation.
  - **Platelet refractoriness** (poor platelet recovery after transfusion) may be due to immunologic causes (anti-ABO, anti-HLA, or antiplatelet antibodies) or nonimmunologic causes (e.g., sepsis, DIC, fever, active bleeding, splenic sequestration, certain drugs). Immunologic causes are likely if a 10- to 60-minute post-transfusion platelet count shows little increment and may be prevented in future transfusions by the use of ABO- and/or HLA-compatible platelets.[54]
- **Cryoprecipitate**
  - Cryoprecipitate contains the cold-precipitated portion of plasma and is enriched in the following factors:
    - Fibrinogen
    - von Willebrand factor (vWF)
    - Factor VIII
    - Factor XIII
  - It is most commonly indicated to replace **fibrinogen** in patients with hypofibrinogenemia or DIC, and it should not be used to replace vWF or factor VIII, for which specific products exist.
  - One unit increases fibrinogen concentration by approximately 7–8 mg/dL. Doses are frequently ordered in pools of 5 or 10 units.
- **Granulocyte transfusion** is indicated in neutropenia from chemotherapy and hematopoietic cell transplantation (absolute neutrophil count <500 cells/μL; evidence of bacterial or

fungal infection; and unresponsiveness to antimicrobial treatment, generally for at least 48 hours).

SPECIAL CONSIDERATIONS

- **Pretransfusion testing**
  - The **type and screen** procedure tests the recipient's RBCs for the A, B, and D (Rh) antigens and also screens the recipient's serum for antibodies against other RBC antigens.
  - The **crossmatch** tests the recipient's serum for antibodies against antigens on a specific donor's RBCs and is performed for each unit of blood that is dispensed for a patient. If a patient has no history of RBC antibodies, the serologic crossmatch may be replaced by an instantaneous computer crossmatch. Plasma and platelets do not require a crossmatch.
- **Modifications of blood products**
  - **Leukoreduction** is performed by the use of filters to eliminate WBC contamination before storage or at the bedside. Indicated for all patients to reduce the risk of the following transfusion complications:
    - Nonhemolytic febrile transfusion reactions
    - Transfusion-transmitted CMV infection
    - Formation of HLA alloantibodies
  - **CMV-seronegative** blood products may be indicated for immunocompromised patients who are CMV-seronegative to reduce the risk of CMV transmission. However, prestorage leukoreduced products are considered equivalently "CMV-reduced risk" and can be used in place of CMV-seronegative products.
  - **Irradiation** eliminates immunologically competent lymphocytes to prevent transfusion-associated graft-versus-host disease and is indicated for certain immunocompromised patients, SCT recipients, and patients who receive directed donations from HLA-matched donors or relatives.
  - **Washing** of pRBCs is rarely indicated but should be considered for patients in whom plasma proteins may cause a serious reaction (e.g., recipients with IgA deficiency or a history of anaphylactic reactions).
  - **Pathogen reduction** uses UV light to inactivate replicating pathogens such as bacteria and most viruses, as well as donor leukocytes, replacing CMV-reduced-risk blood and irradiation. It is currently only approved for platelets and plasma and is not in widespread use.
- **Blood administration**
  - Patient and blood product identification procedures must be carefully followed to avoid any transfusion-related errors including ABO-incompatible transfusion.
  - The IV catheter should be at least 18 gauge to allow adequate flow.
  - All blood products should be administered through a 170- to 260-μm "standard" filter to prevent infusion of macroaggregates, fibrin, and debris.
  - No fluids other than saline may be infused into the same line during transfusion.
  - Patients should be observed with vital signs for the first 10–15 minutes of each transfusion for adverse effects and at regular intervals thereafter.
  - RBC infusion is typically administered over 1–2 hours, with a maximum of 4 hours.
- **Emergency transfusion** may be considered in situations in which massive blood loss has resulted in cardiovascular compromise.
  - Before the patient's ABO type can be confirmed, "emergency release" blood may be used, consisting of uncrossmatched group O pRBCs and group AB or A plasma.
  - If **massive transfusion** (replacement of ≥10 units of pRBCs in <24 hours) is indicated, hemostatic components (plasma, platelets, and cryoprecipitate) should be included to correct the loss and dilution of hemostatic factors. In addition, care must be taken to manage the potential iatrogenic complications of massive transfusion,

such as hypothermia, hypocalcemia (due to the citrated preservative solution), and hyperkalemia.

COMPLICATIONS

- **Transfusion-transmitted infections**
  - Donors and blood products are screened for HIV-1/2, human T-lymphotropic virus 1/2, hepatitis B, hepatitis C, West Nile virus, Zika virus, syphilis, *Trypanosoma cruzi* (Chagas), and bacteremia (platelets only).
  - Viral transmission may occur when donors are in the "window period" (i.e., undetectable to testing).
    - The risk of hepatitis B transmission is approximately 1 in 1,000,000; other tested viruses have a transmission risk of <1 in 1,000,000 (human immunodeficiency virus infection: 1 in 1,467,000).
    - CMV transmission risk may be reduced in immunocompromised patients by the use of CMV-seronegative or prestorage leukoreduced products, as well as pathogen reduction.
  - Bacterial transmission may occur from either a donor infection or a contaminant at the time of collection or processing.
    - Platelet transfusions are more likely than RBCs to have bacterial contamination because they are stored at room temperature. This risk may be mitigated by pathogen reduction.
    - The most common organisms identified are *Yersinia enterocolitica* in RBCs and *Staphylococcus* spp. in platelets.
- **Noninfectious hazards of transfusion**
  - **Acute hemolytic transfusion reactions** are usually caused by **preformed antibodies** in the recipient and are characterized by intravascular hemolysis of the transfused RBCs soon after the administration of ABO-incompatible blood.
    - **Fever, chills, back pain, chest pain, nausea, vomiting, anxiety, and hypotension** may develop. Acute renal failure with hemoglobinuria may occur. In the unconscious patient, hypotension or hemoglobinuria may be the only manifestation.
    - If a hemolytic transfusion reaction is suspected, **the transfusion should be stopped immediately and all IV tubing should be replaced**. Samples of the patient's blood should be delivered to the blood bank along with the remainder of the suspected unit for repeat of the crossmatch. Direct and indirect Coombs tests should be performed, and the plasma and freshly voided urine should be examined for free Hgb.
    - Management includes preservation of intravascular volume and protection of renal function. Urine output should be maintained at ≥100 mL/h with the use of IV fluids and diuretics or mannitol, if necessary. The excretion of free Hgb can be aided by alkalinization of the urine. Sodium bicarbonate can be added to IV fluids to increase the urinary pH to ≥7.5.
  - **Delayed hemolytic transfusion reactions** typically occur 3–10 days after transfusion and are caused by either a primary or an anamnestic antibody response to specific RBC antigens on donor RBCs.
    - Hgb and Hct levels may fall.
    - The DAT is usually positive, depending on when follow-up testing is conducted.
    - Reactions may at times be severe; these cases should be treated similarly to acute hemolytic reactions.
  - **Nonhemolytic febrile transfusion reactions** are characterized by fevers and chills.
    - Cytokines released from white cells are thought to be the cause.
    - Treatment and future prophylaxis may include acetaminophen and prestorage leukoreduced blood products.

- **Allergic reactions** are characterized by urticaria and, in severe cases, bronchospasm and hypotension.
    - The reactions are due to plasma proteins that elicit an IgE-mediated response. The reaction may be specific to the plasma proteins of a particular donor and therefore may occur infrequently or never again.
    - Treatment and future prophylaxis may include antihistamines such as diphenhydramine or corticosteroids.
    - **Anaphylactic reactions** may require the addition of corticosteroids and washed or plasma-reduced products. Additionally, check serum immunoglobulins because patients with IgA deficiency who receive IgA-containing blood products may experience anaphylaxis with small exposure to donor plasma.
- **Transfusion-associated circulatory overload** (TACO) is a relatively common yet under-recognized complication of blood transfusion. Volume overload with pulmonary edema and signs of CHF may be seen when patients with cardiovascular compromise are transfused. The clinical and radiographic features may be difficult to distinguish from that of transfusion-related acute lung injury (TRALI).[55] Slowing the rate of transfusion and judicious use of diuretics help prevent this complication, as well as avoidance of unnecessary transfusion.
- **TRALI** is indistinguishable from acute respiratory distress syndrome and occurs within 6 hours of a transfusion.
    - Symptoms include dyspnea, hypoxemia, and possibly fever.
    - New or worsening pulmonary edema is typically seen on CXR, as with TACO, but without evidence of volume overload.
    - Anti-HLA or antineutrophil antibodies in the donor's serum directed against the recipient's WBCs are thought to cause the disorder.
    - On recognition, transfusions must be stopped and the blood bank notified so that other products from the donor(s) in question may be quarantined.
    - Hypoxemia resolves rapidly, typically in about 24 hours, but ventilatory assistance may be required during that time.
    - Despite clinical or radiographic findings that suggest pulmonary edema, data indicate that diuretics have no role and may be detrimental.[56]
- **Transfusion-associated graft-versus-host disease** is a rare but serious complication usually seen in immunocompromised patients (and immunocompetent patients receiving blood from a relative) and is thought to result from the infusion of immunocompetent donor T lymphocytes.
    - Symptoms include rash, elevated liver function tests, and severe pancytopenia.
    - Mortality is >80%.
    - **Irradiation** or pathogen reduction of blood products for at-risk patients prevents this disease.
- **Post-transfusion purpura** is a rare syndrome of severe thrombocytopenia and purpura or bleeding that starts 7–10 days after exposure to blood products. This disorder is described in Chapter 20, Disorders of Hemostasis and Thrombosis, in the Platelet Disorders section.
- **Electrolyte abnormalities:** These include hypocalcemia (as citrate, an anticoagulant in blood products), hyperkalemia (release of potassium from cells during storage), and hypokalemia (alkalinization of the blood as citrate is converted to bicarbonate by the liver in patients with normal hepatic function).

Summary

- Iron deficiency anemia (IDA) is the most common nutritional deficiency in the world. The most common causes of IDA are gastrointestinal (GI) bleeding and menstruation in women, decreased dietary iron intake, and absorption are also culpable causes.
- Patients with transfusion-dependent β-thalassemia (TDT) primarily rely on regular transfusion and iron chelation therapy, which can be associated with considerable treatment burden and cost.
- All patients with clinical features suspicious for pernicious anemia should be tested for anti-IF antibodies regardless of cobalamin levels.
- In severe warm-antibody AIHA, there is evidence for the upfront addition of rituximab to prednisolone in the first line. In cold agglutinin disease, the development of complement inhibitors and B-cell targeting agents makes it possible to individualize therapy.
- Primary myelofibrosis (PMF) is often but not always accompanied by JAK2, CALR, or MPL mutations; additional features include bone marrow reticulin/collagen fibrosis, aberrant inflammatory cytokine expression, anemia, hepatosplenomegaly, extramedullary hematopoiesis (EMH), constitutional symptoms, cachexia, risk of leukemic progression, and shortened survival.
- The diagnosis of multiple myeloma requires the presence of one or more myeloma defining events in addition to evidence of either 10% or more clonal plasma cells on bone marrow examination or a biopsy-proven plasmacytoma.

Scan the QR code to access chapter references.

22

Cancer

Siddhartha Devarakonda, Amanda Cashen, Daniel Morgensztern, Ramaswamy Govindan, and Anudeep Padakanti

Introduction

Cancer is one of the leading causes of mortality both worldwide and in the South Central Asia, where approximately 9.9 million deaths excluding nonmelanoma skin cancer are estimated for 2020.[1,2] In South Central Asia, the most common malignancy is breast cancer followed by lip-oral cavity, cervix uteri, and lung (Table 22-1). Cancer death rates have declined over the past decade owing to better uptake of screening strategies, advances in drug development, and availability of better supportive care. Improved understanding of the molecular pathways operative in cancer cells has led to the development of targeted agents, immunotherapy, and personalized treatment approaches associated with meaningful clinical benefit.

Approach to the Cancer Patient

GENERAL PRINCIPLES

Risk Factors

- The lifetime probability of being diagnosed with cancer is approximately 40% in men and 38% in women.
- Tobacco use is the most common cause of cancer and is associated with lung, head and neck, esophageal, gastric, pancreatic, kidney, and bladder cancers.
- Diet, obesity, inactivity, alcohol abuse, and height have also been shown to be associated with increased risk of developing selected cancers.

TABLE 22-1 Estimated New Cancer Cases and Rates of Death for Most Common Cancer Diagnoses for 2020

United States				
Sites	New Cases			Deaths
	Both Sexes	Male	Female	Total
Breast	253,465	2550	253,465	42,617
Lung	227,875	116,335	111,540	138,225
Prostate	209,512	209,512		32,438
Colorectum	155,008	81,654	73,354	54,443

South Central Asia region		
Site	New Cases (Total)	Deaths (Total)
Breast	254,881	124,975
Lip-oral cavity	174,448	98,015
Cervix uteri	148,128	91,985
Lung	121,369	109,356

- Chronic inflammatory states such as ulcerative colitis and infections such as HIV, hepatitis, Epstein–Barr virus (EBV), human papillomavirus (HPV), and *Helicobacter pylori* are also associated with increased cancer risk.
- Several familial cancer syndromes have been described and have important implications for cancer screening (Table 22-2).
- Prior exposure to cytotoxic chemotherapy or radiation therapy is associated with an increased risk of developing secondary cancers. For instance, exposure to alkylating agents or topoisomerase II inhibitors increases the risk of developing treatment-related leukemia, and exposure to radiation therapy increases the risk for developing cancers such as breast cancer, angiosarcoma, and osteosarcoma.

DIAGNOSIS

- Obtaining tissue is crucial for a definitive tissue diagnosis, examining molecular features, and treatment planning.
- **Cytology** specimens often consist of only a few malignant cells that are obtained either invasively through fine-needle aspiration (FNA), brushings (Pap smear or endoscopic), or aspiration of body fluids (blood, cerebrospinal fluid [CSF], pleural, pericardial, or peritoneal) or noninvasively through collection of fluids such as sputum and urine. Although these approaches are relatively less invasive compared to surgical approaches and easier to pursue, cytologic samples may be inadequate for molecular testing. Furthermore, the absence of information about tissue architecture may preclude the precise diagnosis of certain malignancies such as lymphomas.
- **Histology** specimens are obtained through large-core needle biopsies, excisional biopsies, or surgical resection. These specimens are ideal for diagnoses and provide enough tissue for molecular testing.

STAGING

- Once a tissue diagnosis is obtained, most cancer patients will require additional imaging, procedures, and laboratory testing for determining the disease burden and stage. This workup is cancer and patient specific, and it also varies by local and institutional patterns of practice. Organizations such as the American Society of Clinical Oncology, National Comprehensive Cancer Network, and European Society of Medical Oncology review available evidence and issue periodic recommendations to guide appropriate staging workup and management.
- Cancer stage provides an assessment of the extent of tumor dissemination, which is crucial for treatment.
    - Most malignancies are staged according to the tumor, lymph node, and metastasis (TNM) system from stages I to IV. The T classification is based on the size and extent of local invasion. The N classification describes the extent of lymph node involvement, and the M classification is based on the presence or absence of distant metastasis.
    - Performance status provides a quantitative measure of a patient's generalized well-being and quality of life. It has important implications for treatment planning (Table 22-3).

TREATMENT

Surgical Management

- Surgical resection is often performed with curative intent, although selected patients may benefit from palliative surgery that is performed for debulking large tumor masses (e.g., ovarian cancer), increasing the efficacy of immunotherapy (e.g., renal cell carcinoma

TABLE 22-2 List of Selected Familial Cancer Syndromes With High Penetrance

Syndrome	Defect	Associated Cancer Type
Ataxia-telangiectasia	*ATM*	Multiple; predominantly leukemia and lymphoma
Birt-Hogg-Dube	*BHD*	Chromophobe RCC
Bloom syndrome	*BLM*	Multiple
Cowden syndrome	*PTEN*	Multiple; predominantly breast, thyroid, RCC, endometrial
Familial adenomatous polyposis	*APC*	Colorectal, desmoid
Fanconi anemia	*DNA* repair complex	Multiple; predominantly MDS and AML
Hereditary breast–ovarian cancer	*BRCA1* and *BRCA2*	Multiple; predominantly breast, ovarian
Hereditary diffuse gastric cancer	*CDH1*	Gastric, lobular breast cancer
Hereditary leiomyomatosis and RCC	*FH*	Papillary RCC
Lynch syndrome (HNPCC)	Mismatch repair	Multiple; predominantly colorectal
Hereditary papillary RCC	*MET*	Papillary RCC
Juvenile polyposis syndrome	*MADH4 (SMAD4), BMPR1A*	Digestive tract and pancreas
Li-Fraumeni syndrome	*TP53*	Multiple
MEN type 1	*MEN1*	Islet cell tumors
MEN type 2	*RET*	Medullary thyroid cancer
Neurofibromatosis type 1	*NF1*	MPNST, glioma
Neurofibromatosis type 2	*NF2*	Meningioma, glioma, schwannoma
Nijmegen breakage syndrome	*NBS1*	Predominantly lymphoma
Peutz–Jeghers syndrome	*LKB1 (STK11)*	Multiple; predominantly breast, GI, pancreas
Retinoblastoma, hereditary	*RB*	Retinoblastoma, primitive neuroectodermal tumor
Rothmund–Thomson syndrome	*RECQL4*	Osteosarcoma
Tuberous sclerosis (TS)	*TSC1, TSC2*	RCC, giant cell astrocytoma
von Hippel-Lindau	*VHL*	Clear cell RCC
Xeroderma pigmentosum	Nucleotide excision repair	Multiple, cutaneous

AML, acute myeloid leukemia; GI, gastrointestinal; HNPCC, hereditary nonpolyposis colorectal cancer; MDS, myelodysplastic syndrome; MEN, multiple endocrine neoplasia; MPNST, malignant peripheral nerve sheath tumor; RCC, renal cell carcinoma.

TABLE 22-3 Eastern Cooperative Oncology Group (ECOG) and Karnofsky Score

ECOG	Karnofsky Score Correlate	Description
0	100	Fully active, able to carry on all predisease performance without restriction.
1	80–90	Restricted in physically strenuous activity but ambulatory and able to carry out work of a light or sedentary nature (e.g., light housework, office work).
2	60–70	Ambulatory and capable of all self-care but unable to carry out any work activities. Up and about >50% of waking hours.
3	40–50	Capable of only limited self-care, confined to bed or chair >50% of waking hours.
4	20–30	Completely disabled. Cannot carry on any self-care. Totally confined to bed or chair.
5	0	Dead.

Reprinted from Oken MM, Creech RH, Tormey DC, et al. Toxicity and response criteria of the Eastern Cooperative Oncology Group. *Am J Clin Oncol.* 1982;5:649; with permission from Wolters Kluwer Health.

[RCC]), or relieving symptoms (e.g., mastectomy for local control in a patient with metastatic disease).

- Surgery can facilitate staging and guide subsequent therapeutic decisions (adjuvant treatment), including chemotherapy or radiation therapy.
- Surgical resection of isolated or oligometastatic sites in selected patients can improve survival. Examples include solitary brain metastases, pulmonary metastases from sarcomas, and liver metastases from colorectal cancer.

Principles of Radiation Therapy

- Radiation is used for treatment of benign and malignant diseases. Commonly used forms of radiation include external-beam photons and electrons.
- Brachytherapy is an alternative method of radiation therapy, where radioactive sources are placed close to or in contact with their target tissue. Brachytherapy sources can be temporary or permanent.
- Radioactive substances can also be administered systemically. For instance, iodine-131 is administered orally for treating thyroid cancer, yttrium-90 microspheres are injected into the liver vasculature in hepatocellular cancer, and radium-223 is dosed intravenously in patients with prostate cancer and skeletal metastases.
- Radiation planning is designed to optimize precision doses of radiation to a tumor while sparing surrounding tissues.
- **Curative** intent radiotherapy is used in several settings.
    - **Neoadjuvant:** Preoperative therapy intended to reduce both the extent of surgery and the risk of local relapse. Radiation in this setting is commonly administered in combination with chemotherapy.
    - **Adjuvant:** Postoperative therapy intended to reduce the risk of local relapse.
    - **Definitive:** High dose with curative intent.

- **Concurrent chemoradiation:** Chemotherapy with definitive radiation is associated with increased efficacy but at a cost of increased toxicity compared to either chemotherapy or radiation alone.

- **Palliative** radiotherapy is used in lower dosing to reduce symptoms, including bone pain, obstruction, bleeding, and neurologic symptoms.
- The total dose of radiation administered is usually divided over several days (fractionated). This allows time for normal tissue repair and increases the probability of delivering radiation to tumor cells in a radiosensitive phase of cell cycle. Radiation treatments are usually delivered either through conventional fractionation, hypofractionation, hyperfractionation, or accelerated fractionation schedules.
  - **Conventional fractionation** consists of daily fractions typically of 1.8–2.0 Gy, usually delivered 5 days per week.
  - **Hypofractionation** refers to the delivery of radiation divided into larger doses, with treatment once a day or less often.
  - **Hyperfractionation** refers to the delivery of radiation divided into smaller doses per fraction, with treatments more than once per day.

Other Local Ablative Therapies

- Local ablative therapy with modalities such as lasers, cryoablation, microwave, radiofrequency, and high intensity–focused ultrasound are increasingly being pursued in patients with cancer for pain palliation or attempting local disease control.

Principles of Chemotherapy

- Cytotoxic chemotherapy targets all dividing cells and has broad toxicities.
- In patients with resectable disease, chemotherapy may be used before the surgery (neoadjuvant) or following complete resection (adjuvant).
- Chemotherapy is typically given in cycles of 2–4 weeks. In most regimens, IV treatment is given on the first few days of the cycle, with no further treatment until the next cycle. In other regimens, treatments are administered weekly for 2–3 weeks, with 1 week off between cycles.
- **Curative** intent chemotherapy includes neoadjuvant, adjuvant, and chemoradiation regimens in solid tumors. Chemotherapy alone is curative in many lymphomas, leukemias, and germ cell tumors.
- **Palliative** chemotherapy is used in advanced solid tumors and relapsed hematologic malignancies, with a focus on prolonging survival and improving the quality of life.
- Most agents have a very narrow therapeutic index, and dosing is based on body surface area (mg/m^2). Chemotherapy toxicities are variable and can be life threatening.

Principles of Targeted Therapy

- The advent of molecularly targeted agents has led to marked advances in the treatment of selected malignancies.
- The most common classes of drugs are monoclonal antibodies and receptor tyrosine kinase inhibitors (TKIs). Monoclonal antibodies are administered IV and by standard nomenclature have names that end with the stem -mab. Substems indicate the source and target of the antibody. The most common source substems in oncology include -xi- indicating a chimeric antibody (e.g., cetuximab), -zu- indicating humanized antibody (e.g., bevacizumab), and -u- indicating fully human antibodies (e.g., ipilimumab). The most common target substems include -ci- indicating circulatory system (e.g., bevacizumab), -tu- indicating tumor (e.g., cetuximab), and -li- indicating immune system (e.g., ipilimumab).
- TKIs are administered orally and have names that end with -ib. The most common substem is -ti- indicating tyrosine kinase inhibition (e.g., imatinib).
- Most antibodies are used in combination with chemotherapy or radiation, whereas TKIs are mostly used as single agents.

- Toxicities of targeted therapies are unique to each agent, although specific classes of drugs can be associated with characteristic side effects.
  - Inhibitors of the epidermal growth factor receptor (EGFR) frequently cause an acne-like rash on the face and upper chest, which can be severe. Treatment is typically with topical corticosteroids or oral minocycline.
  - Inhibitors of human epidermal growth factor receptor 2 (HER2) are associated with a reversible decline in cardiac systolic function, which should be monitored in these patients periodically.
  - Inhibitors of angiogenesis are associated with endothelial toxicity, leading to hypertension, proteinuria, delayed wound healing, mild cardiac toxicity, increased risk of bleeding, thromboembolism, and gastrointestinal (GI) perforation/fistula. All antiangiogenics should be held in the perioperative period.

Principles of Immunotherapy

- Under normal physiological conditions, the immune checkpoint molecules maintain self-tolerance by preventing autoimmunity and limiting collateral damage to tissues during response to infections.
- Programmed cell death 1 (PD-1) is a receptor expressed primarily on the surface of activated T cells. Binding of PD-1 to one of its ligands, PD-L1 or PD-L2, inhibits the cytotoxic T cell response.
- Tumor cells may co-opt this pathway to escape T cell-induced antitumor activity.
- The interaction between PD-1 and PD-L1 may be blocked by monoclonal antibodies against PD-1 (nivolumab, pembrolizumab) or PD-L1 (atezolizumab, durvalumab, avelumab).
- These immune checkpoint blockers have been approved for the treatment of multiple tumors including melanoma, lung cancer, bladder cancer, kidney cancer, head and neck cancer, and lymphomas.
- PD-L1 expression by immunohistochemistry (IHC) has been associated with response to anti-PD-1 or PD-L1 antibodies in some cancers.
- Other modalities of immunotherapy include bispecific antibodies such as blinatumomab, which engage T cells to recognize cancer cells, and chimeric antigen receptor–T cells (CAR-Ts) such as tisagenlecleucel and axicabtageneciloleucel, which are specially engineered T cells capable of attacking tumor cells. Blinatumomab, axicabtageneciloleucel, and tisagenlecleucel are currently approved in the United States for the management of hematological malignancies.[3–5]
- Natural killer (NK) cell-based immunotherapy represents one of the novel immunotherapeutic strategies, unleashing immune suppression of NK cells to attack various cancers. It includes adoptive NK cell transfer, chimeric antigen receptor (CAR)-modified NK cells, antibodies, cytokines, and drug treatment.

Assessing Response to Therapy

Objective assessment of changes in tumor burden is crucial for planning cancer treatment and evaluating the efficacy of experimental interventions. Criteria such as the Response Evaluation Criteria in Solid Tumors are commonly used for this purpose (Table 22-4).[6]

Lung Cancer

EPIDEMIOLOGY AND ETIOLOGY

Lung cancer is the second most common cause of cancer deaths in South Central Asia, with estimated deaths of 109,356 in 2020. Smoking is the strongest risk factor for lung cancer, with over 90% of cases being tobacco related. The risk of smoking-related lung cancer persists for 20–30 years after quitting smoking. Other environmental risks include exposure to asbestos and possibly, gases such as radon.

TABLE 22-4	Summary of Selected Response Evaluation Criteria in Solid Tumors (RECIST) 1.1 Criteria
Measurable lesions	Tumor: >10 mm in longest diameter (LD) on axial CT or MRI
	Lymph node: >15 mm in short axis on CT
Method	Sum of longest diameter (SLD) of the lesions in axial plane. Up to five target lesions (two per organ).
Response	
Complete response (CR)	Disappearance of all non-nodal target lesions. All target lymph nodes must be <10 mm in short axis.
Partial response (PR)	At least 30% decrease in the SLD of target lesions, with baseline sum of diameters as reference.
Progressive disease (PD)	New lesions or SLD increased by ≥20%.
Stable disease (SD)	Neither PR nor PD.

PATHOLOGY

Non–small-cell lung cancer (NSCLC) accounts for over 85% of cases. The most common histologic subtypes are adenocarcinoma and squamous cell carcinoma. Small-cell lung cancer (SCLC) is associated with a rapid tumor growth and early development of metastases compared to NSCLC.

SCREENING

- In 2011, the National Lung Screening Trial (NLST) showed a 20% relative reduction in lung cancer mortality and a 6.7% relative reduction in all-cause mortality.[7] The NLST included more than 50,000 asymptomatic current and former smokers at high risk for developing lung cancer. Participants were randomly assigned to screening with baseline low-dose chest CT (LDCT) or CXR, followed by annual scans at years 1 and 2.
- The number needed to screen to prevent one lung cancer death was 320 in the NLST.
- Based on these data, the US Preventive Services Task Force (USPSTF) currently recommends annual screening for lung cancer with LDCT in current smokers or former smokers who quit within the past 15 years, are between 55 and 80 years old, and have a ≥30-pack-year smoking history.

DIAGNOSIS

Clinical Presentation

- Patients with early stage disease are often asymptomatic. However, when present, symptoms may be related to local disease (cough, dyspnea, wheezing, hemoptysis), intrathoracic extension (hoarseness from recurrent laryngeal nerve involvement, dysphagia, chest wall pain, Horner syndrome, symptoms related to brachial plexus involvement, superior vena cava [SVC] syndrome), systemic metastases (fever, jaundice, bone pain, headaches, back pain), or paraneoplastic syndromes.
- Paraneoplastic syndromes in lung cancer typically include hypercalcemia, hyponatremia from syndrome of inappropriate antidiuretic hormone secretion, and hypertrophic pulmonary osteoarthropathy.

Diagnostic Testing

- Any patient with a smoking history and concerning pulmonary symptoms should undergo a chest CT scan. A normal CXR does not exclude lung cancer. Diagnosis can be made from bronchoscopy with biopsy, brushings or washings, ultrasound or CT-guided needle biopsy, and pleural fluid cytology if an effusion is present. Biopsy is preferable to FNA and helps acquire adequate tissue for molecular testing, which plays an important role in treatment decision-making.
- Staging evaluation in all patients should include a CT scan of the chest and abdomen. Additional imaging depends on the initial findings. In potentially curable patients, evaluation typically includes a brain MRI, positron emission tomography (PET)/CT scan, and mediastinoscopy.

TREATMENT

Non–Small-Cell Lung Cancer

- **Stages I and II:** Surgery is the preferred therapy. Radiation therapy, with or without chemotherapy, is an option for those who are not candidates for surgical resection. Postoperative platinum doublet chemotherapy improves overall survival in patients with surgically resected stage IB with >4-cm tumor, and II and III NSCLC.
- **Stage III:** The standard therapy is concurrent radiation and chemotherapy. Surgery is indicated for selected patients.
    - Consolidation immunotherapy with durvalumab for 1 year following completion of chemoradiation is indicated in selected patients with stage III NSCLC.[8]
- **Stage IV:** Therapy is administered with palliative intent and choice of therapy is guided by presence of targetable alterations[9] (*EGFR, ALK, ROS1, ERBB2, BRAF,* and *MET*), PDL1 expression of the tumor as measured by IHC, histology, and patient performance status.
    - Frontline therapy with platinum-based doublet chemotherapy is the standard of care for patients without actionable gene alterations and PD-L1 lower than 50%.
    - More recently, therapy with pembrolizumab, has been shown to be superior to chemotherapy in patients whose tumors show >50% PD-L1 expression.[10]
    - Combining pembrolizumab with platinum and pemetrexed chemotherapy has been shown to be superior to chemotherapy alone in patients with nonsquamous NSCLC, regardless of tumor PD-L1 status.[11]
    - Chemotherapy is the preferred option for patients with squamous NSCLC whose tumors show <50% PD-L1 expression.
    - EGFR TKIs, such as osimertinib, erlotinib, or afatinib, should be considered as frontline therapy in patients whose tumors harbor activating mutations in *EGFR.*
    - Alectinib, crizotinib, ceritinib, and brigatinib are TKIs effective in patients with tumor harboring the *EML4-ALK* fusion gene.
    - Crizotinib is also associated with marked clinical activity in tumors harboring *ROS1* rearrangements and exon 14 skipping mutations in *MET.*
    - Dabrafenib and trametinib are active in NSCLCs harboring *BRAF V600E* mutations.
    - Selpercatinib and prasetinib are effective in *RET* fusion mutation.
    - Sotorasib and adagrasib are orally useful in *K-Ras G12C* mutation.
    - Trastuzumab deruxtecan can be used in *HER2* mutated NSCLC.
    - Nivolumab, pembrolizumab, and atezolizumab are approved in patients previously treated with platinum-based doublets.

Small-Cell Lung Cancer

- **Limited stage (stages I to III):** The standard therapy is concurrent radiation and chemotherapy with a platinum agent (carboplatin or cisplatin) plus etoposide.
- **Extensive stage (stage IV):** The treatment of choice is with chemotherapy, usually with a platinum agent (cisplatin or carboplatin) plus etoposide.
- Prophylactic cranial irradiation is recommended for all patients with limited stage and can be considered in extensive stage patients after completion of initial therapy. Selected patients with extensive stage may also benefit from consolidation thoracic radiotherapy in combination with prophylactic cranial irradiation.

Breast Cancer

EPIDEMIOLOGY AND ETIOLOGY

Overall, breast cancer is the most common cancer in South Central Asia. Also, it is the most common cancer among women while less than 1% are reported in men. According to Globocan 2020, number of new cases registered were 254,881 while the number of deaths reported were 124,975. *BRCA1* and *BRCA2* mutations are associated with a 57% and 49% cumulative risk of breast cancer by age 70, respectively.[12] However, less than 10% of all breast cancers are attributable to mutations involving susceptibility genes. Alcohol consumption, early menarche, late menopause, nulliparity, obesity, hormone replacement therapy, and delayed first pregnancy are all risk factors for breast cancer. Women receiving mantle field radiation for Hodgkin disease also carry a higher lifetime risk.

PATHOLOGY

- Noninvasive: Ductal carcinoma in situ (DCIS) and lobular carcinoma in situ (LCIS).
- Invasive: Ductal carcinoma is more common than lobular carcinoma.
- Estrogen receptor (ER) is expressed in nearly 75% of all cases. ER positivity (ER+) is associated with good prognosis and responsiveness to endocrine therapies.
- Progesterone receptor expression (PR+) usually correlates with ER expression.
- Approximately 20% of tumors are HER2 positive (HER2+) by IHC or fluorescent in situ hybridization (FISH). HER2 positivity is associated with higher grade cancers and patients may benefit from HER2-directed targeted therapies (e.g., trastuzumab).
- 10%–15% of breast cancers are triple negative (lack expression of hormone receptors and are HER2 negative). These cancers are more aggressive and do not benefit from hormone receptor or HER2-targeted therapies.

SCREENING AND PREVENTION

- The American Cancer Society (ACS) recommends a clinical breast examination every 3 years between 20 and 39 years of age and annually thereafter. Meanwhile, the USPSTF currently does not recommend the use of the breast examination for routine screening. The role of self-breast examination is controversial and should only be performed as an adjunct to clinical examination and mammography.
- The ideal age to begin screening mammography and optimal screening intervals are unknown, and recommendations vary among organizations and clinicians.
- The ACS recommends annual mammography from age 45, for as long as the person does not have serious illnesses that shorten life expectancy. MRI along with mammography is indicated in select individuals with a strong family history of breast cancer. The USPSTF recommends biennial mammography from age 50 to 74.

- Prophylactic mastectomy and oophorectomy are offered to carriers of *BRCA1* or *BRCA2* mutations after discussion regarding the patients reproductive wishes.
- Chemoprevention with tamoxifen or raloxifene is an option in women who are at high risk for developing breast cancer (family history and LCIS).

DIAGNOSIS

Clinical Presentation

Most breast cancers are identified by screening tests, but patients can present with a palpable mass in the breast or axilla. Some patients may have nipple discharge, pain, nipple retraction, and/or skin changes associated with the mass. Patients with inflammatory breast cancer complain of a "heavy" warm breast with an associated erythematous rash on the breast. Inflammatory breast cancer is rare, but patients with these symptoms should be promptly evaluated by a clinician experienced with this diagnosis.

Diagnostic Testing

- Patients with palpable breast masses require diagnostic mammograms and ultrasonography. Patients with axillary mass and no detectable breast mass by routine imaging and examination should receive an MRI to identify occult cancer. Any clinically concerning mass needs to be biopsied irrespective of its radiographic appearance.
- Bone scan and CT imaging are indicated in patients with stage III or higher disease. Patients with stage I or II disease should undergo staging imaging if there are new symptoms such as pain or signs of abnormal lab tests (complete blood count, complete metabolic panel).

TREATMENT

Surgery

- Lumpectomy (breast conservation therapy) with adjuvant radiation is equivalent to mastectomy.[13]
- Sentinel lymph node biopsy is done to pathologically stage the axilla unless there are clinical or radiologic signs of lymph node involvement. In the case of clinically positive lymph nodes, an axillary lymph node dissection is done at the time of surgery.
- Whole-breast radiation therapy with radiotherapy boost to the tumor bed is recommended for patients following breast conservation surgery (BCS). Postmastectomy radiation is recommended in selected patients with T3/T4 tumor, positive margin, large tumor, or positive lymph nodes.

Endocrine Therapies

- These are recommended only for ER and/or PR positive breast cancers in adjuvant or metastatic disease.
  - Tamoxifen is an estrogen antagonist used in ER+ breast cancer.
  - Fulvestrant is an ER antagonist that is approved for use in postmenopausal women.
  - Luteinizing hormone–releasing hormone (LHRH) agonists (goserelin, leuprolide) can be used for ovarian suppression in premenopausal women, as an alternative to oophorectomy.
- Aromatase inhibitors (AIs) decrease the production of estrogen by blocking androgen to estrogen conversion in peripheral tissues. AIs are the most commonly used endocrine drugs in postmenopausal patients. Letrozole, anastrozole, and exemestane are the three AIs used in practice.

Treatment by Stage

- **DCIS and LCIS (stage 0):** Mastectomy or lumpectomy with negative margins followed by adjuvant radiation. Repeat resections for positive margins may be necessary. Tamoxifen is typically used if the tumor is ER+.
- **Resectable breast cancer (stages I–III):**
  - Surgical approach depends on the size of the tumor, patient preference, and the presence or absence of contraindications to BCS. Contraindications for BCS include multicentric disease, extensive microcalcifications, and previous irradiation. Neoadjuvant (preoperative) chemotherapy or hormonal therapy can be used to shrink larger tumors to facilitate BCS.
  - For ER+ and/or PR+ cancers, adjuvant endocrine therapy with tamoxifen or a combination of AI and ovarian suppression is recommended in premenopausal women.[14] AI with ovarian suppression is the preferred adjuvant endocrine therapy for women ≤35 years old diagnosed with breast cancer and women at higher risk of recurrence. For postmenopausal women, an AI is standard of care. The treatment duration is 5–10 years.
  - Adjuvant chemotherapy is generally recommended based on biomarkers (ER, PR, HER2 status), stage, and prognostic multigene assay (Oncotype Dx, Mammaprint, etc) in ER/PR positive stage I/II cancers. For instance, chemotherapy does not offer significant survival benefit in patients with favorable (0–10) or midrange (11–25) Oncotype Dx scores.[15,16]
  - Adjuvant treatment with the HER2 monoclonal antibody trastuzumab dramatically reduces rate of relapse and improves survival in HER2+ breast cancer.[17]
  - Pertuzumab is another HER2 monoclonal antibody that may be used in combination with trastuzumab for the treatment of HER2+ cancer in the neoadjuvant, adjuvant, and metastatic settings.[18]
- **Treatment of metastatic breast cancer**
  - Radiation therapy may be used for brain and bone metastases.
  - Endocrine therapy is usually preferred in ER/PR+ patients with low tumor burden. CDK4/6 inhibitors (palbociclib, ribociclib, abemaciclib) are an important first or second-line therapy. Everolimus (mammalian target of rapamycin [mTOR] inhibitor) with endocrine therapy is a helpful therapy in the second-line setting.
  - Chemotherapy is used in patients with negative hormone receptors and high visceral tumor burden or when endocrine therapy is no longer effective.
  - Triple negative (ER/PR/HER2–) metastatic breast cancer requires chemotherapy. Patients with a *BRCA* mutation have the option of a poly-ADP-ribose phosphorylase (PARP) inhibitor (olaparib) in second-line or beyond.
    - Sacituzumab govitecan is an antibody conjugate with irinotecan used in metastatic triple-negative breast cancer.
  - HER2+ metastatic breast cancer may be treated with HER2-directed targeted drugs, such as trastuzumab, pertuzumab, or lapatinib, usually in combination with chemotherapy.
    - Trastuzumab deruxtecan is an antibody drug conjugate consisting of trastuzumab with the topoisomerase I inhibitor deruxtecan. It has shown remarkable activity in patients who have previously used anti-HER2 therapy and has also shown activity in HER2 low breast cancers.
  - Bone-protecting agents, such as bisphosphonates or denosumab (an anti-RANKL antibody), are recommended for patients with bone metastases to reduce risks of fracture or other bone complications.

Head and Neck Cancer

EPIDEMIOLOGY AND ETIOLOGY

Head and neck squamous cell cancer (HNSCC) includes carcinoma of the lip, oral cavity, pharynx, nasopharynx, and larynx. It is the most common cancer among males and overall it is the second most common cancer in South Central Asia. Tobacco use and alcohol consumption are associated with increased risk of developing HNSCC. HPV infection is implicated in oropharyngeal squamous cell carcinomas, and the incidence of HPV-associated HNSCC has quadrupled since the 1980s. EBV infection is associated with nasopharyngeal cancers.

- **Field cancerization** is an important concept in HNSCC. Given the diffuse nature of mucosal exposure to tobacco smoke, the primary cancer site is often surrounded by areas of premalignant lesions (carcinoma in situ and dysplasia). For this reason, patients with tobacco-associated HNSCC are at increased risk for developing secondary cancers.
- **Leukoplakia and erythroplakia** are premalignant lesions of the oral mucosa. Leukoplakia refers to a white mucosal patch that cannot be scraped out, whereas erythroplakia appears red and velvety. Erythroplakias are associated with a higher risk of malignant transformation.

DIAGNOSIS

Clinical Presentation

Patients with HNSCC can present with a variety of symptoms depending on the primary tumor site: oral mass, nonhealing ulcers, trismus from invasion of pterygoid muscles, dysphagia, odynophagia, otitis media from eustachian tube blockage, hoarseness, neck mass, weight loss, and cranial nerve palsies. Nasopharyngeal tumors can invade the cavernous sinus and frequently affect the abducens and trigeminal nerves. Salivary gland tumors, which can have nonsquamous pathology, can invade the facial nerve and cause facial nerve-related symptoms.

Diagnostic Testing

- Comprehensive ear, nose, and throat evaluation with fiberoptic endoscopy or mirror examination is required. Particular attention should be paid to dentition. Functional evaluation that includes assessment of swallowing, biting, chewing, and speech should be performed.
- Examination under anesthesia is a critical component of staging. Imaging should include a panorex to evaluate dentition and mandibular involvement. A CT of the neck and chest should be obtained to evaluate lymph node involvement and rule out pulmonary metastases, respectively. Whole-body PET can be considered in select patients.
- p16 positivity on IHC is used as a surrogate for HPV infection and is an independent favorable prognostic factor for survival.[19]
- **Stage classification:** Stage I to II disease does not show lymph node involvement. Stage III tumors are larger (defined as >4 cm for most sites) or have isolated lymph node involvement. Stage IVA and IVB tumors are locally advanced or show bilateral or bulky cervical lymph node involvement. Stage IVC tumors are associated with distant metastasis.

TREATMENT

- *Early stage (I–II):* Either surgery or definitive radiation.
- *Locally advanced (stage III–IVA/B):* Treatment approaches include:
    - Surgical resection followed by adjuvant radiation with or without chemotherapy

  - Concurrent chemotherapy with radiation
  - Induction chemotherapy followed by concurrent chemotherapy and radiation, or radiation alone
- *Metastatic (stage IVC):* Palliative chemotherapy and immunotherapy.
- **Chemotherapy:** Cisplatin is the chemotherapy agent commonly used in combination with radiation for definitive treatment. Induction regimens usually involve a platinum combination with drugs such as 5-fluorouracil (5FU) and a taxane (paclitaxel or docetaxel).
- **Immunotherapy:** Nivolumab and pembrolizumab are antibodies directed against PD-1, with both approved in patients with metastatic disease progressing on chemotherapy.[20,21]
- **Targeted therapy:** Cetuximab, a monoclonal antibody against EGFR, can be used in combination with definitive radiation in patients who cannot tolerate traditional chemotherapeutic regimens or in combination with cisplatin and 5FU for the treatment of metastatic disease.[22]
- **Surgery:** Nodal neck dissection is an important part of surgical management. Radical neck dissection refers to surgical removal of lymph nodes from all five neck stations unilaterally, along with excision of the internal jugular vein, spinal accessory nerve, and sternocleidomastoid. Modified neck dissections spare some of these structures.
- **Organ sparing:** Chemoradiation or induction chemotherapy followed by radiation can potentially spare patients from undergoing a total laryngectomy and improve quality of life.
- **Supportive care:** Dental evaluation is indicated before radiation. Patients undergoing definitive radiation or adjuvant radiation may develop severe mucositis requiring the placement of gastric feeding tube for nutrition. Surgery may lead to loss of speech, swallowing dysfunction, permanent tracheostomy, and disfigurement. Swallowing impairment can lead to aspiration. Radiation can result in severe xerostomia.

GASTROINTESTINAL MALIGNANCIES

Esophageal Cancer

EPIDEMIOLOGY AND ETIOLOGY

According to Globocan 2020, in South Central Asia the incidence of esophageal cancer is 105,034 with a deaths of 97,436. Esophageal cancer is three to four times more common in men than in women. Risk factors include tobacco, alcohol, obesity, gastroesophageal reflux disease, Barrett esophagus, achalasia, and caustic injury.

PATHOLOGY

Adenocarcinomas are most common in the lower third of the esophagus and at the gastroesophageal junction and have had a sharp increase in incidence over the last few decades. Squamous cell carcinomas are more common in the upper and middle esophagus.

DIAGNOSIS

Clinical Presentation

Patients usually present with progressive dysphagia and weight loss. Other symptoms include odynophagia, cough, regurgitation, and hoarseness.

Diagnostic Testing

- The diagnosis is usually established through upper endoscopy with biopsy.
- Staging workup includes CT of the chest and abdomen (with or without PET) to determine the presence of distant metastases. For patients without distant metastases, endoscopic ultrasonography (EUS) is required for the definition of tumor depth and lymph node status.
- Tumors located above the carina increase the risk of tracheoesophageal (TE) fistula formation and should be evaluated with bronchoscopy. Patients with TE fistulas often present with postprandial cough and aspiration pneumonia.

TREATMENT

- **Resectable disease:** Patients with resectable disease are candidates for esophagectomy with or without preoperative chemotherapy and radiation, depending on the extent of disease.[23]
- **Unresectable primary disease:** Patients diagnosed with locally advanced disease are usually managed by concurrent chemoradiation.
- **Metastatic disease** is treated with palliative chemotherapy, usually with regimens including 5FU, platinum, and a taxane or anthracycline agent. Ramucirumab, an antibody against vascular endothelial growth factor (VEGF) receptor-2, is approved for use in the second-line setting in combination with paclitaxel or as a single agent.[24]
- **Trastuzumab** can be used in combination with chemotherapy in patients with *HER2*-amplified esophageal or gastroesophageal junction metastatic adenocarcinomas.
- **Pembrolizumab** can be used in gastric and gastroesophageal junction tumors that have progressed on chemotherapy.[25]

Gastric Cancer

EPIDEMIOLOGY AND ETIOLOGY

The highest incidence rates for gastric cancer are in Eastern Asia, South-Central Asia, Central and Eastern Europe, South America, South-Eastern Asia. Gastric cancer accounts for an estimated 11,413 deaths in 2020 in the United States and 89,595 deaths in South Central Asia. Risk factors include *H. pylori* infection, previous partial gastrectomy for benign ulcer, achlorhydria associated with pernicious anemia, cigarette smoking, and blood group A. Hereditary diffuse gastric cancer is an inherited type of gastric cancer in families with germline *CDH1* (E-cadherin) mutations.

PATHOLOGY

More than 90% are adenocarcinomas. Tumors may be subdivided according to the Lauren classification into intestinal or diffuse types. Intestinal type is more common in older patients and has a better prognosis. Diffuse type, the most common subtype in the United States, is more prevalent in younger patients and is associated with a worse prognosis. Linitis plastica (leather bottle stomach) refers to a diffusely infiltrating type of gastric adenocarcinoma. Nearly 15%–20% of patients with gastric cancer have *HER2* amplification or overexpression.

DIAGNOSIS

Clinical Presentation

The most common symptoms are weight loss, decreased appetite, and abdominal discomfort. Dysphagia may occur with gastroesophageal junction tumors, and persistent vomiting may occur if there is pyloric obstruction. Physical examination may show metastases to the left supraclavicular node (Virchow node) or periumbilical node (Sister Mary Joseph node).

Diagnostic Testing

Diagnosis is established by upper endoscopy. CT of the chest and abdomen should be obtained in all patients, and CT of the pelvis should be performed in women to exclude ovarian involvement (Krukenberg tumor). Other tests include *H. pylori* testing, EUS, and PET scan. Staging laparoscopy may be indicated before surgery in select patients for assessing peritoneal involvement.

TREATMENT

- Medically fit patients with resectable disease should undergo surgery. Chemotherapy or chemoradiation is commonly used, either before or after the resection, except in patients with very early stage disease.
- Patients with unresectable disease are treated with palliative chemotherapy. Trastuzumab can be used in combination with chemotherapy in patients with HER2-positive gastric cancers. Trastuzumab deruxtecan can be used in metastatic colorectal cancers in patients who have previously received anti-HER2 therapy. Trastuzumab and anthracyclines should not be administered concurrently owing to increased cardiotoxicity. Immune checkpoint blockers are approved for use in patients for gastric cancer progressing on chemotherapy.
- Genetic counseling is recommended for all members in a high-risk family (defined by criteria such as the presence of *CDH1* germline mutation in a family, or diffuse gastric cancer under age of 40 in a family member, etc.). Prophylactic total gastrectomy is recommended in carriers of *CDH1* germline mutations.

Colorectal Cancer

EPIDEMIOLOGY AND ETIOLOGY

Colorectal cancer is the third most common malignancy worldwide. The incidence is higher in Western industrialized countries, with 155,008 cases estimated to be diagnosed in the United States in 2020. According to Globocan 2020, incidence of colorectal cancer is 102,987 among countries in South Central Asia. Although the incidence of colorectal cancer in adults aged 50 or older is declining, largely because of screening colonoscopy, the incidence among young adults (aged 20–49) has increased over the last few decades. Risk factors include age >50, physical inactivity, obesity, diet with increased red meat and decreased fiber, personal history of polyps or colorectal cancer, inflammatory bowel disease, and hereditary syndromes such as Lynch syndrome and familial adenomatous polyposis.

DIAGNOSIS

Clinical Presentation

The most common symptoms include lower GI bleeding, abdominal pain, change in bowel habits, and obstruction. Patients can also rarely present with perforation, peritonitis, and fever. Any unexplained iron deficiency anemia should be evaluated with upper and lower endoscopy to evaluate for a GI malignancy. Colorectal carcinomas are also identified through screening colonoscopies.

Diagnostic Testing

- A thorough family history must be obtained to rule out a hereditary cancer syndrome, especially in younger (<50 years) patients.
- Diagnosis is typically made through colonoscopy with biopsy.
- Imaging studies include CT scan of the chest, abdomen, and pelvis. PET scan is not routinely indicated but is useful in patients being considered for definitive resection of oligometastatic disease.

TREATMENT

- **Localized disease** should be treated with surgical resection. Adjuvant chemotherapy is indicated in patients with stage III disease and may also be beneficial in selected patients with stage II disease. The preferred regimen in the adjuvant setting includes 5FU (or capecitabine), leucovorin, and oxaliplatin (FOLFOX). The duration of adjuvant chemotherapy is about 3–6 months.
- **Metastatic disease**
  - Combination chemotherapy, usually including 5FU plus leucovorin, capecitabine, oxaliplatin, and/or irinotecan (FOLFOX, FOLFIRI, XELOX, and FOLFOXIRI).
  - The combination of bevacizumab, a VEGF monoclonal antibody, and chemotherapy improves survival compared with chemotherapy alone.
  - EGFR-targeting antibodies, cetuximab and panitumumab, are associated with improved outcomes when combined with chemotherapy in tumors lacking *KRAS*, *NRAS*, and *BRAF* gene mutations.[26]
  - Immune checkpoint blockers pembrolizumab and nivolumab are active and approved for use in patients with mismatch repair deficient colon cancers.[27]
  - The TKI regorafenib and chemotherapy drug trifluridine/tipiracil are approved for use in treatment refractory colon cancer.
  - **Surgical resection of metastatic disease**, with a curative intent, can be attempted in patients with a limited number of liver or lung metastases. Aggressive chemotherapy can be employed in selected patients initially presenting with unresectable liver metastases to achieve maximal response and make them eligible for resection.
  - Local and regional therapies such as chemoembolization or radioembolization can be considered in patients with metastatic disease limited to the liver.

Treatment of Rectal Cancer

Patients without metastatic disease should undergo endorectal ultrasound or pelvic MRI for the evaluation of tumor depth and lymph node status.

- **Early stage disease:** The treatment of choice is resection. Low anterior resection (LAR) is suitable for tumors located in the middle and upper third of the rectum, whereas abdominoperineal resection (APR) might be warranted in low-lying cancers. Preoperative radiation can be considered in low-lying cancers with an attempt to convert APR to a sphincter-preserving LAR.
- **Locally advanced disease:** These patients are usually treated with 5FU (or capecitabine)-based neoadjuvant chemoradiation followed by surgery and adjuvant chemotherapy (FOLFOX). The radiation and chemotherapy dosing schedule for these patients is an area of active investigation.
- **Metastatic disease:** The standard of care is palliative chemotherapy with the same drugs used in colon cancer.

Pancreatic Cancer

EPIDEMIOLOGY AND ETIOLOGY

Pancreatic cancer is the third most common cause of cancer-related death in the United States, estimated to result in 47,683 deaths in 2020. According to Globocan 2020, number of deaths among countries in South Central Asia is 21,144. Incidence increases with age, with median age at diagnosis between 60 and 80 years. Risk factors include cigarette smoking, obesity, inactivity, diabetes, chronic nonhereditary, and hereditary pancreatitis, and inherited syndromes such as hereditary breast and ovarian cancers, ataxia telangiectasia, hereditary intestinal polyposis syndrome, and familial atypical multiple mole and melanoma syndrome.

PATHOLOGY

Pancreatic adenocarcinoma is the most common subtype. *KRAS* is mutated in nearly 90% of pancreatic adenocarcinomas and is an oncogenic driver for this disease. Pancreatic neuroendocrine tumors are less common, associated with a better prognosis, and managed differently.

DIAGNOSIS

Clinical Presentation

Common symptoms include painless jaundice, anorexia, weight loss, and back and abdominal pain. Pancreatic cancer should be suspected when diabetes mellitus develops suddenly in patients older than 50 years.

Diagnostic Testing

Diagnosis is usually suspected by the presence of a pancreatic mass or dilated biliary duct on CT scan or ultrasound. Those without metastatic disease will require endoscopic retrograde cholangiopancreatography or EUS-guided FNA. Pancreatic protocol CT (triple-phase, contrast-enhanced, helical CT) with thin slices is often recommended to evaluate tumorresectability.

- Resectability is defined, based on the absence of distant metastases and the extent to which the superior mesenteric artery, superior mesenteric vein, portal vein, hepatic artery, and celiac axis are involved.
- CA19-9 is not a reliable diagnostic marker because it can be elevated in patients with benign biliary obstruction and falsely low in 10% of patients who are Lewis-negative phenotypes.

STAGING

Based on imaging, pancreatic cancer is classified as resectable, borderline resectable, locally advanced, or metastatic disease. The definition of borderline resectability can be variable but usually involves focal abutment of vasculature by the pancreatic tumor.

TREATMENT

- **Resectable disease:** Surgical resection is currently the only cure for this disease. Pancreaticoduodenectomy (Whipple procedure) is indicated for tumors located in the head of pancreas, whereas distal pancreatectomy is pursued for tumors in the distal pancreas. Only 10%–15% of patients present with resectable disease at diagnosis. Patients who have adequately recovered from surgery may benefit from adjuvant chemotherapy (usually mFOLFIRINOX or gemcitabine and capecitabine) plus/minus radiation, as nearly 70% of patients eventually relapse at a distant site.

- **Borderline resectable and locally advanced disease:** For borderline resectable disease, induction chemotherapy and chemoradiotherapy are often used in an attempt to decrease the tumor size and increase the probability of resection with negative margins. For locally advanced disease, chemotherapy with or without radiation is used for disease control.
- **Metastatic disease** is treated with palliative chemotherapy.
  - FOLFIRINOX, a combination chemotherapy regimen consisting of oxaliplatin, irinotecan, 5FU, and leucovorin,[28] and the combination of gemcitabine with albumin-bound paclitaxel (nab-paclitaxel) are the most commonly used regimens in patients with good performance status. Patients who are unable to tolerate these regimens can be treated with single-agent gemcitabine.
  - Nanoliposomal irinotecan is active and approved for use in patients with pancreatic cancer progressing after first-line chemotherapy incorporating gemcitabine.

Hepatocellular Carcinoma

EPIDEMIOLOGY AND ETIOLOGY

A total of 42,284 patients were diagnosed with HCC in 2020 in the United States. According to Globocan 2020, among South Central Asian countries, the incidence of liver cancer is 54,698 and number of deaths were 52,769. Risk factors include chronic viral hepatitis B or C, autoimmune hepatitis, nonalcoholic steatohepatitis, hemochromatosis, and cirrhosis. Most patients with hepatocellular carcinoma (HCC) have cirrhosis.

SCREENING

Patients with chronic hepatitis B and family history of HCC or cirrhosis, irrespective of etiology, are candidates for screening. Ultrasonography every 6–12 months is the preferred screening modality. Addition of α-fetoprotein (AFP) monitoring to ultrasound screening can increase detection rates but may also increase false positive rates. Use of AFP alone is not recommended owing to poor sensitivity and specificity.

DIAGNOSIS

Clinical Presentation

Common symptoms include abdominal pain, anorexia with weight loss, jaundice, and vomiting. Invasion of the hepatic veins may cause Budd–Chiari syndrome, characterized by tender hepatomegaly and tense ascites. HCC should be suspected in patients with stable cirrhosis who decompensate rapidly. The most common paraneoplastic syndromes include hypoglycemia, hypercalcemia, dysfibrinogenemia, and erythrocytosis.

Diagnostic Testing

- The classic feature of HCC in CT is rapid enhancement during the arterial phase of contrast administration, followed by "washout" during the later venous phases. Lesions <1 cm have low probability of being HCC and should be followed with repeated imaging to detect growth suspicious of malignancy. MRI is also commonly used in the diagnostic setting.
- Tumors that do not show the radiologic hallmarks for HCC may need biopsy for diagnosis.
- Serum AFP is commonly used as a biomarker in conjunction with imaging to improve the diagnostic accuracy.

- It is important to assess liver function in patients with HCC through scoring systems such as the Child–Pugh classification.

TREATMENT

- **Surgery** is currently the only curative option. Liver transplant should be considered in patients ineligible for surgery. To be deemed eligible for transplantation, patients are required to fulfill the Milan criteria, which include: single tumor ≤5 cm or up to three tumors <3 cm, absence of macrovascular invasion, and absence of extrahepatic disease.
- **Other local therapies** such as percutaneous ethanol injection, radiofrequency ablation, cryoablation, transarterial chemoembolization, and radiation can be considered in select patients for palliation or to control tumor growth.
- **Chemotherapy** has minimal efficacy in HCC.
- **TKIs**, sorafenib, lenvatinib, and regorafenib are active and approved in HCC.[29]
- Nivolumab is approved for use in patients with HCC progressing on sorafenib.[30]

GENITOURINARY MALIGNANCIES

Renal Cancer

EPIDEMIOLOGY AND ETIOLOGY

RCC is estimated to result in approximately 69,569 deaths in the United States in 2020. Among South Central Asian countries, the incidence of kidney cancer was 25,855 and the number of deaths were 14,966 in 2020. It is more commonly diagnosed in men, and the risk increases with age. Other risk factors include tobacco smoking, obesity, and hypertension.

PATHOLOGY

RCC is a malignancy of the renal parenchyma. Clear cell RCC is the most common subtype (80%–85%), followed by papillary (15%) and chromophobe (5%) RCCs. Transitional cell (urothelial) carcinoma of the renal pelvis is treated as bladder cancer.

DIAGNOSIS

Clinical Presentation

Most patients are diagnosed by incidental findings on CT scan. The most common symptoms are anemia, hematuria, cachexia, and fever. The classic triad of flank pain, hematuria, and a palpable mass is uncommonly seen. Hypercalcemia is the most common paraneoplastic manifestation of RCC. Although erythrocytosis from erythropoietin production can be seen in RCC, anemia is more common. Stauffer syndrome refers to a paraneoplastic syndrome characterized by nonmetastatic hepatic dysfunction seen in RCC.

Diagnostic Testing

CT is usually sufficient for staging. MRI and magnetic resonance angiography may be useful for further evaluation of the collecting system and inferior vena cava for involvement. The role of PET imaging is limited because normal renal tissue excretes fluorodeoxyglucose in the urine and has a high background activity. A biopsy should be performed in metastatic disease to discern RCC from metastatic transitional cell carcinoma of the renal pelvis, as this will impact treatment decisions. Biopsies of localized tumors are not contraindicated, as tumor seeding is a rare occurrence with modern interventional techniques. RCC often metastasize to brain and bone. In patients without metastatic disease, resection can be both diagnostic and therapeutic.

TREATMENT

- **Localized disease:** The treatment of choice is surgery. A nephron-sparing approach (partial nephrectomy) can be considered if feasible.
- **Locally advanced disease:** The treatment of choice is radical nephrectomy, which involves removal of the Gerota's fascia, perirenal fat, regional lymph nodes, and ipsilateral adrenal gland.
  - Adjuvant therapy with the TKI, sunitinib, can be considered in patients at high-risk for disease recurrence following nephrectomy; however, this has not been shown to improve overall survival and thus the benefit in progression-free survival must be weighed against drug toxicities and cost.[31]
- **Metastatic disease**
  - Surgery is an option in patients with oligometastatic disease. Cytoreductive nephrectomy followed by immunotherapy with interferon-α was considered in patients with resectable primary tumors and good performance status. However, recent data suggest a lack of benefit with cytoreductive surgery in patients treated with VEGF-targeted therapies.[32] There is a small subset of patients with relatively indolent oligometastatic disease for whom delayed systemic therapy may be appropriate, and resection of limited disease alone is preferred. However, there is no specific diagnostic test to identify this subset *a priori.*
  - Targeted agents approved for metastatic RCC include the VEGF inhibitors sunitinib, sorafenib, pazopanib, lenvatinib, cabozantinib, and axitinib, and the mTOR inhibitors temsirolimus and everolimus. The choice of therapy depends on the histology, patient risk category, and adverse effect profile of targeted therapies.
  - **Immunotherapy** with high-dose IL-2 should be considered in select patients with good performance status given the potential for durable cures in a small subset (approximately 5%–15%) of patients.
    - The combination of nivolumab and ipilimumab is active and approved for use in high-risk patients with untreated metastatic RCC.[33]
    - Nivolumab is also approved for use as a single agent in patients progressing after targeted therapies.

Bladder Cancer

EPIDEMIOLOGY AND ETIOLOGY

Bladder cancer is one of the most commonly diagnosed malignancies in the United States, with 80,617 cases in 2020. Among South Central Asian countries, the incidence of bladder cancer was 35,949 and the number of deaths were 18,243 in 2020. Transitional cell or urothelial carcinoma is the most common histology. Tobacco smoking, chronic cystitis from long-term indwelling catheters, previous pelvic radiation or prolonged cyclophosphamide use, and exposure to benzene and other industrial chemicals are all risk factors. Bladder cancer is three times more common in men than in women and has a median age of 65 at diagnosis. *Schistosoma haematobium* infection is linked to squamous cell bladder cancer.

DIAGNOSIS

Clinical Presentation

Most patients present with hematuria (microscopic or macroscopic). Lower urinary tract symptoms such as increased frequency, urgency, and dysuria can be seen in patients with bladder neck tumors.

Diagnostic Testing

The presence of >3 red blood cells per high-power field is considered significant hematuria. Hematuria should be evaluated with urine cytology, upper tract imaging (IV pyelogram or CT), and cystoscopy with transurethral resection of bladder tumor (TURBT).

STAGING

Bladder cancers are broadly divided into non–muscle-invasive, muscle-invasive, and metastatic cancers. Cystoscopy with biopsies or TURBT determines the depth of invasion; imaging is not reliable to distinguish noninvasive from muscle-invasive disease in the majority of cases. To diagnose muscle-invasive bladder cancer, the biopsy specimen must have muscle fibers present; if none are seen, repeat biopsy is recommended as treatment differs significantly between noninvasive and invasive disease.

TREATMENT

The following describes treatment options by stage:

- **Superficial tumors** (no muscle invasion, stages 0–I) are treated with TURBT. Intravesicular bacille Calmette-Guérin (BCG) instillation reduces recurrence, and both induction and maintenance courses can be used. Intravesicular chemotherapy (typically mitomycin C) can be used in cases of BCG failure.
- **Muscle-invasive disease** is defined by the invasion of muscle or adjacent tissue (stages II and III). The treatment of choice is radical cystectomy with urinary diversion by creating an ileal conduit. Neoadjuvant chemotherapy has been shown to provide a survival benefit and should be considered in appropriate patients. For patients who cannot get neoadjuvant treatment, adjuvant chemotherapy can help reduce recurrences. Radiation, often with concurrent chemotherapy, is an alternative to surgery if resection cannot be performed.
- **Metastatic disease**, including node-positive or distant disease, is managed with chemotherapy, most commonly the combination of gemcitabine and cisplatin or methotrexate, vinblastine, doxorubicin, and cisplatin.
    - **Immune checkpoint blockers** pembrolizumab, nivolumab, avelumab, durvalumab, and atezolizumab are active and approved for use in patients with urothelial cancers.[34]
    - Erdafitinib is an oral drug used in advanced or metastatic urothelial carcinoma with susceptible FGFR genetic alteration.

Prostate Cancer

EPIDEMIOLOGY AND ETIOLOGY

Prostate cancer is the most common cancer in men in the United States, with an estimated 209,512 new cases and 32,438 deaths in 2020. Among South Central Asian countries, the incidence of prostate cancer was 54,451 and the number of deaths were 26,537 in 2020. African American ethnicity, family history, age, and a high-fat/low-vegetable diet are common predisposing risk factors.

SCREENING

The absolute risk reduction in mortality from annual prostate-specific antigen (PSA) is modest and should be discussed with patients older than 50 years of age with known risk factors. The USPSTF currently recommends selective PSA-based screening for men aged 55–69, after a thorough conversation of the potential risks and benefits of screening. There are conflicting data from American and European trials looking at the benefit of prostate cancer screening.

DIAGNOSIS

Clinical Presentation

The most common presentation in the United States is asymptomatic elevation in PSA. Digital rectal examination (DRE) findings of asymmetric induration or nodules are suggestive, and any palpable nodule should be biopsied. Less common symptoms are obstructive symptoms, new-onset erectile dysfunction, hematuria, or hematospermia. Bone is the most common site of metastatic involvement, and patients with skeletal metastases can present with pain, fractures, and nerve root compression.

Diagnostic Testing

DRE supplemented by transrectal ultrasound-guided biopsy helps in assessing T stage. PSA testing and Gleason scoring in the initial biopsy are important in staging and risk category assessment. Although patients with high-risk disease are likely to benefit from routine imaging (CT, MRI, or bone scan) for detection of metastatic disease, symptom-directed imaging is appropriate in patients with low-risk disease.

- Gleason grades range from 1 to 5. Typically, clinically relevant cancers are scored from grade 3 (well-differentiated) to grade 5 (poorly differentiated) gland pattern. **Gleason score** is the sum of the grades for the primary and secondary patterns seen on the biopsy. Overall scores of 6 indicate low-risk, 7 indicate intermediate-risk, and 8+ indicate high-risk histologies.
- Risk categorization: Based on these characteristics, tumors are classified as low (PSA ≤10 ng/mL, Gleason score <7, and stage up to T2a), intermediate (PSA >10 to ≤20 ng/mL, Gleason score 7, and stage T2b), or high (PSA >20 ng/mL, Gleason score >7, and stage T2c) risk.

STAGING

Early stage disease (T1–T2) is confined to the prostate, and locally advanced disease (T3–T4) is defined by local invasion. Stage IV disease is defined by nodal involvement (N1) and metastatic disease (M1).

TREATMENT

The most important predictors of outcome are pretreatment PSA levels, Gleason score, and clinical TNM stage.

- **Early stage disease:** Outcomes are equivalent between radical prostatectomy, external-beam radiation, or brachytherapy, although brachytherapy alone is not recommended in higher-risk disease. Late toxicities are variable but usually include incontinence and erectile dysfunction. Active surveillance is a suitable option for men with low-risk disease.
- **Locally advanced disease** is often treated with different combinations of surgical, radiation, and hormonal therapy. Surgery (if previous radiation), radiation (if previous prostatectomy), brachytherapy, and sometimes systemic hormonal therapy can be considered in patients who show an asymptomatic increase in PSA levels after surgery or radiation.

The question of adjuvant (soon after surgery) or "salvage" (at time of PSA recurrence) radiation superiority is currently being studied in randomized, prospective trials.

- **Metastatic disease** is incurable and is initially treated with surgical or medical castration with an LHRH receptor agonist or antagonist, termed androgen deprivation therapy (ADT), because testosterone/androgens play a major role in tumor growth. The antiandrogens flutamide or bicalutamide may be added for combined androgen blockade, which has shown marginal improvements in overall survival compared with LHRH monotherapy in meta-analyses.
  - ADT in combination with chemotherapy or abiraterone is active and useful in treating select patients with high-risk/high-volume metastatic prostate cancer that is castration sensitive.[35–37]
  - **Castration-resistant disease** is diagnosed in patients who experience disease progression on ADT therapy. Chemotherapy with docetaxel, cabazitaxel, or therapy with abiraterone, enzalutamide, radium-223, and sipuleucel-T are effective options for these patients. Sipuleucel-T is an autologous cell-based vaccine targeting prostatic acid phosphatase.[38]

Testicular Cancer and Germ Cell Tumors

EPIDEMIOLOGY AND ETIOLOGY

Testicular cancers are relatively rare tumors with about 9407 cases diagnosed in 2020 in the United States. Among South Central Asian countries, the incidence of testicular cancer was 7197 and the number of deaths were 1896 in 2020. However, they are the most common tumors diagnosed in men aged 15–35. Nonseminomatous tumors are more common in younger men, whereas seminomas are more common after the age of 30. Incidence is higher in Caucasians than in patients of other ethnicities. Other risk factors include cryptorchidism and Klinefelter syndrome.

PATHOLOGY

Fifty percent of testicular cancers are seminomas, and the remainder are nonseminomas or of mixed histology. Nonseminomas include embryonal carcinoma, teratoma, choriocarcinoma, and yolk sac tumors. Pure seminomas carry a better prognosis compared to nonseminomas or mixed histology tumors.

DIAGNOSIS

Clinical Presentation

The most common presentation is that of a painless testicular mass, but patients can also present with testicular pain, hydrocele, or gynecomastia. Advanced testicular cancer can present with back or flank pain, fevers, night sweats, and weight loss.

Diagnostic Testing

Trans-scrotal biopsies of testicular masses should not be pursued and an inguinal orchiectomy is necessary for establishing a diagnosis. Tumor markers, including AFP, β-human chorionic gonadotropin (β-hCG), and lactate dehydrogenase (LDH), should be ordered. In patients with pure seminomas, AFP is not elevated; thus, elevated AFP suggests a focus of undetected nonseminoma. Preoperative CT of the abdomen and pelvis and CXR should be performed.

STAGING

Staging is based on TNM status and serum markers (S). In general, stage I represents disease confined to the scrotum, stage II indicates lymph node involvement, and stage III is defined by the presence of visceral metastases.

TREATMENT

- **Stage I:** The treatment of choice is high-inguinal orchiectomy. Adjuvant radiation to retroperitoneal nodes, retroperitoneal nodal dissection, chemotherapy with carboplatin, and active surveillance are possible adjuvant management approaches based on histology and other risk features such as lymphatic or vascular involvement.
- **Stages II–III:** Chemotherapy with BEP (bleomycin, etoposide, and cisplatin) or EP regimen results in high rates of cure.
  - Second-line chemotherapy regimens include VeIP (vinblastine, ifosfamide, cisplatin) and TIP (paclitaxel, ifosfamide, cisplatin). High-dose chemotherapy with stem cell therapy may be used in more advanced cases refractory to initial treatment or as part of clinical trials.
  - Sperm banking should be discussed with all patients before beginning treatment.

GYNECOLOGIC MALIGNANCIES

Cervical Cancer

EPIDEMIOLOGY AND ETIOLOGY

Cervical cancer death rates have declined by almost 80% between 1930 and 2010 because of the widespread implementation of screening programs. In countries that lack a cervical cancer screening and prevention program, cervical cancer is the second most common cancer seen in women. Among South Central Asian countries, the incidence of cervix uteri cancer was 148,128 and the number of deaths were 91,985 in 2020. The most important risk factor is persistent HPV infection, detected in >99% of tumors, usually HPV-16 and -18. Other risk factors include early onset of sexual activity, multiple sexual partners, high-risk partner, history of sexually transmitted disease, and chronic immunosuppression (HIV infection).

The prophylactic quadrivalent HPV vaccine protects against types 6, 11, 16, and 18 (Gardasil), whereas the bivalent vaccine protects against HPV-16 and -18. Vaccinated women should continue routine Pap smears because the vaccine is not effective against all HPV subtypes. Cervical cancer screening should begin at age 21, with use of cytology (age 21–29) or cytology plus HPV cotesting (age 30–65) every 3–5 years based on the modality of testing used, per the USPSTF guidelines. Visual inspection with acetic acid is a simple tool for screening that can be used by healthcare workers and has shown to reduce the cervical cancer mortality.[39]

PATHOLOGY

The most common histology seen is squamous cell carcinoma followed by adenocarcinoma.

DIAGNOSIS

Clinical Presentation

Patients with early stage lesions are commonly asymptomatic and diagnosed incidentally on Pap smear, which underscores the importance of screening. Symptoms observed at presentation include irregular or heavy vaginal bleeding or postcoital bleeding. Patients with advanced disease may present with back pain, hematochezia, or vaginal passage of urine or stool.

Diagnostic Testing

Diagnosis is obtained through cervical cytology and biopsy. A large cone biopsy is recommended in women without gross cervical lesions or with microinvasive disease to define depth of lesion. Clinical examination, CXR, IV pyelogram, proctosigmoidoscopy, and cystoscopy are required to assess International Federation of Gynecology and Obstetrics stage. CT, MRI, and PET imaging are used to guide treatment.

TREATMENT

Patients with early stage disease are treated with hysterectomy and/or pelvic radiation. Chemoradiation can be used in locally advanced tumors and as adjuvant therapy in high-risk patients following hysterectomy. Metastatic disease is treated with chemotherapy.

Endometrial Cancer

EPIDEMIOLOGY

Endometrial cancer is the most common gynecologic cancer in the United States, estimated to account for ~61,738 new cases in 2020. Among South Central Asian countries, the incidence of corpus uteri cancer was 25,573 and the number of deaths were 9478 in 2020. Risk factors include obesity, unopposed estrogen, early menarche, late menopause, nulliparity, chronic anovulation, and tamoxifen use. Patients with hereditary cancer syndromes, such as Lynch syndrome, have increased incidence of endometrial cancer.

PATHOLOGY

There are two molecularly and morphologically distinct histologic subtypes:

- Type I: These are associated with exposure to unopposed estrogen (exogenous use, chronic anovulation, obesity, diabetes, nulliparity, and late menopause).
- Type II: These are more sporadic and not associated with the same risk factors as type I. These tumors show non-endometrioid histologies (serous, clear cell) and are associated with an aggressive behavior.

DIAGNOSIS

Clinical Presentation

The most common presentation is abnormal vaginal bleeding. Any vaginal bleeding in a postmenopausal woman, including spotting and staining, should be evaluated.

Diagnostic Testing

Tissue diagnosis is obtained through endometrial biopsy or through dilation and curettage. Cystoscopy, proctoscopy, and radiologic imaging might be necessary following clinical evaluation. Surgical exploration and staging are indicated in medically fit patients.

TREATMENT

- Surgery is indicated for staging and treatment.
- Patients with cervical extension (stage II) may benefit from adjuvant radiotherapy.
- Patients with extrauterine disease extension and those with distant metastases are treated with chemotherapy. Surgical cytoreduction before chemotherapy is a treatment option in selected women with metastatic disease.
- Chemotherapy, radiation, and hormone therapy are considered for patients in whom surgical staging and debulking is not feasible.

Ovarian Cancer

EPIDEMIOLOGY

Ovarian cancer is the leading cause of gynecologic mortality in the United States, with 14,359 deaths estimated in 2018. Among South Central Asian countries, the incidence of ovarian cancer was 59,730 and the number of deaths were 41,407 in 2020. Risk factors include early menarche, late menopause, nulligravidity, family history, and familial syndromes including patients with *BRCA1* and *BRCA2* mutations and Lynch syndrome. Oral contraception use and pregnancy are associated with a low risk of ovarian cancer, suggesting a role for ovulation in malignant transformation.

PATHOLOGY

Most tumors are seen in patients between the ages of 40 and 65, and the majority of tumors are epithelial. Nonepithelial ovarian malignancies (germ cell, sex cord-stromal, and mixed) are seen in younger patients.

DIAGNOSIS

Clinical Presentation

Patients with early-stage disease have nonspecific symptoms including bloating and abdominal discomfort. Patients usually have advanced disease at presentation and may have increasing abdominal girth, ascites, and abdominal pain.

Diagnostic Testing

- Cancer antigen 125 is elevated in most patients but is not specific.
- Surgical staging is an important aspect of management and is usually performed without prior histologic diagnosis for tumor debulking.

TREATMENT

- **Stage I** (without pelvic extension): Surgery is the preferred treatment.
- **Stage II** (extension to uterus, fallopian tubes, or other pelvic tissues): Treatment includes surgery and adjuvant chemotherapy.
- **Stage III** (peritoneal or lymph node involvement) **and IV** (distant metastasis): The treatment of choice is cytoreductive surgery and systemic chemotherapy with platinum and taxane agents administered intravenously (with or without intraperitoneal chemotherapy). In inoperable patients, neoadjuvant chemotherapy followed by surgery leads to equivalent results.

- PARP inhibitors are associated with activity in patients with ovarian cancer carrying *BRCA* mutations. Olaparib is the first PARP inhibitor to be approved for use in ovarian cancer.
    - PARP inhibitors such as rucaparib, olaparib, and niraparib are also approved for maintenance therapy in ovarian cancer.
- **Germ cell ovarian cancers** are rare, typically occur in younger women, and are curable with fertility-preserving surgery and chemotherapy.
- **Stromal tumors** usually present in early stages and are commonly cured with resection alone.

Cancer of Unknown Primary

Cancer of unknown primary site is defined as biopsy-proven malignancy for which the primary site of origin cannot be identified after a thorough history and physical examination, blood tests, and routine imaging studies.

PATHOLOGY

These malignancies are classified using light microscopy into adenocarcinoma (60%), poorly differentiated carcinoma/poorly differentiated adenocarcinoma (29%), squamous cell carcinoma (5%), poorly differentiated malignant neoplasm (5%), and neuroendocrine carcinoma (1%). Further identification usually requires specialized tests including IHC staining, molecular studies, electron microscopy, and genetic analysis.

DIAGNOSIS

- In most cases, it is required to perform several studies to facilitate a diagnosis.
- Routine tests include pelvic and rectal examination, urinalysis, stool occult blood testing, and tumor marker testing in select patients (e.g., PSA in older men and β-hCG and AFP in younger men).
- CT of the chest, abdomen, and pelvis and symptom-oriented endoscopy are often warranted depending on the suspected site of origin. PET scans are particularly useful in identifying the primary site in squamous cell carcinomas involving the cervical lymph nodes.
- IHC, electron microscopy, cytogenetic analysis for identifying characteristic abnormalities, and molecular profiling can yield important diagnostic clues and guide treatment.

TREATMENT

Treatment for favorable subgroups of patients with cancer of unknown primary is tailored to the likely primary site of origin (Table 22-5). Most patients who have unfavorable disease with good performance status are treated with an empiric combination chemotherapy regimen, such as carboplatin and paclitaxel.

Melanoma

EPIDEMIOLOGY AND ETIOLOGY

It is estimated that nearly 96,445 new cases of cutaneous melanoma were diagnosed in 2020 in the United States. Among South Central Asian countries, the incidence of melanoma was 6232 and the number of deaths were 3579 in 2020. Lifetime risk of melanoma is

TABLE 22-5 Treatment Recommendations for Selected Favorable Subgroups of Cancer of Unknown Primary

Subgroup	Treat for
Women with adenocarcinoma involving the axillary nodes	Stage II or III breast cancer
Women with papillary serous adenocarcinoma in the peritoneal cavity	Stage III ovarian carcinoma
Men with blastic bone metastases and elevated prostate-specific antigen	Prostate cancer
Men with poorly differentiated midline carcinoma	Extragonadal germ cell tumor
Squamous cell carcinoma of the cervical lymph nodes	Locally advanced head and neck cancer
Single metastasis	Local treatment with surgery or radiation therapy

higher among Caucasians (1 in 50) compared to African Americans (1 in 1000). Exposure to UV radiation, increased number of nevi (>50), history of >5 atypical nevi, large congenital nevi, immune suppression, and familial risk (*CDKN2A* mutations) are known risk factors. Uveal (5%) and mucosal (1%) melanomas are rare.

PATHOLOGY

The most common types are superficial spreading (most common), nodular, lentigo maligna, acral lentiginous, and rare variants such as nevoid and desmoplastic. In most instances, histologic subtype does not influence staging or management (with the exception of desmoplastic melanoma, in which sentinel node biopsy may not be required). Breslow thickness, mitotic rate, ulceration, and presence or absence of disease at resection margins are important elements of histology that influence management and prognosis.

DIAGNOSIS

Clinical Presentation

Melanoma should be suspected in persons with pigmented skin lesions with asymmetry, border irregularity, color variegation, diameter >6 mm, or evolution (change in characteristics) (ABCDEs of melanoma). Patients can present with pigmented lesions that itch, bleed, or show ulceration at diagnosis. Desmoplastic melanoma can present as a firm cutaneous mass.

Diagnostic Testing

The workup often involves adequate sampling of the lesion, IHC for markers of melanocytic origin (e.g., S100, MART1, HMB45), and genotype testing for detection of mutations in the *BRAF* gene. Primary lesions >0.75 mm in Breslow thickness, with ulceration, ≥1 mitoses/mm^2, or lymphovascular invasion, require a sentinel lymph node biopsy. CT imaging of chest, abdomen, and pelvis with or without PET can be considered in patients with node-positive disease. Patients with metastatic disease require brain MRI.

TREATMENT

- **Localized disease:** The treatment of choice is resection with wide margins (0.5–2 cm depending on Breslow thickness).
  - **Adjuvant therapy** with TKIs dabrafenib and trametinib, or immune checkpoint blockers can be considered in selected patients.[40–42]
- **Metastatic disease:** There has been substantial progress in the management of metastatic melanoma.
  - ***BRAF* mutant:** About 50% of patients harbor the V600E mutation. These patients benefit from therapy with the BRAF inhibitors vemurafenib or dabrafenib, either alone or in combination with MEK inhibitors such as trametinib.[43]
  - **Immunotherapy:** Ipilimumab, nivolumab, and pembrolizumab, are active and currently approved for use in patients with metastatic melanoma.[44,45]

Central Nervous System Tumors

EPIDEMIOLOGY AND ETIOLOGY

Brain and other central nervous system (CNS) tumors are estimated to be diagnosed in 23,880 patients in 2020. Among South Central Asian countries, the incidence of brain and nervous system tumors was 48,322 and the number of deaths were 41,043 in 2020. Ionizing radiation and familial cancer syndromes such as neurofibromatosis types 1 and 2, Li-Fraumeni syndrome, and Von Hippel-Lindau syndrome are known risk factors.

PATHOLOGY

Meningiomas, gliomas, pituitary tumors, and embryonal tumors are the predominantly encountered primary CNS tumors in adults. The World Health Organization (WHO) classification further classifies gliomas based on the histology (e.g., astrocytoma, oligodendroglioma) and grade (I–IV).

DIAGNOSIS

Clinical Presentation

Patients with brain tumors typically present with a variety of symptoms ranging from headache, nausea, vomiting, seizures, and focal deficits to global neurologic dysfunction, based on the extent of mass effect and location of the tumor.

Diagnostic Testing

Workup includes MRI of the brain and molecular testing of the surgical biopsy or resected tumor specimen for *MGMT* methylation, 1p/19q codeletion, and *IDH1* mutation, which may help guide therapy.

TREATMENT

- Gross total resection should be attempted in all patients, when possible. If resection is not feasible, a biopsy should be obtained for diagnosis and molecular testing.
- **Grade I tumors:** The treatment of choice is surgical excision.
- **Grade II tumors:** The treatment of choice is surgical excision. Recent data seem to favor treatment with adjuvant PCV (procarbazine, lomustine, and vincristine) and radiation in selected patients undergoing subtotal resection.

- **Grade III tumors:** The standard treatment is surgical excision followed by radiation and chemotherapy with either temozolomide or PCV.
- **Grade IV tumors/glioblastoma multiforme (GBM):** The treatment of choice is surgical excision or maximal debulking followed by concurrent chemoradiation with temozolomide and adjuvant temozolomide on completion of chemoradiation. Bevacizumab is approved for recurrent GBM. Treatment is often individualized for elderly patients.
- A portable device that generates low-intensity alternating electric fields (TTFields) through electrodes applied on the scalp is approved for use and can be considered in patients with recurrent GBM.
- **Meningioma:** It can be observed in asymptomatic patients for lesions that do not seem to be expanding. Surgical excision can be curative. Radiation is an option for inoperable tumors and in the adjuvant setting.

Sarcoma

EPIDEMIOLOGY AND ETIOLOGY

In the United States, approximately 17,000 patients were diagnosed with sarcomas in the year 2020. Risk increases with age. Predisposing factors include prior radiation, chemical and chemotherapy exposure, genetic syndromes, Paget disease of the bone, HIV/human herpesvirus 8 (HHV8) infection (Kaposi sarcoma), and chronic lymphedema (lymphangiosarcoma, also known as Stewart–Treves syndrome).

PATHOLOGY

Soft tissue sarcomas consist of at least 70 different types of histologies. Review by a pathologist who has expertise in the diagnosis of sarcoma is recommended.

DIAGNOSIS

Clinical Presentation

Symptoms depend on the site of disease. Sarcomas arising in extremities can present as a painless soft tissue mass. Visceral sarcomas can be associated with GI bleeding, early satiety, dysphagia, dyspepsia, or vaginal bleeding. Retroperitoneal tumors can result in early satiety, nausea, paresthesias, or abdominal mass and pain.

Diagnostic Testing

Initial imaging studies include MRI for sarcomas involving the extremities or pelvis and CT for retroperitoneal and visceral sarcomas. PET/CT maybe helpful in high-grade sarcomas. Chest imaging with CT is important because the majority of sarcomas first metastasize to the lungs.

TREATMENT

- **Early stage (stages I–III):**
  - Surgical excision is the mainstay of therapy. Adjuvant radiotherapy is often indicated in patients with large (>5 cm) tumors and positive or equivocal margins when re-excision is not feasible.
  - Although the role of neoadjuvant and adjuvant chemotherapy is controversial, patients should be evaluated by medical oncology at a center that has extensive experience in the treatment of sarcoma.

- **Metastatic disease:**
  - Palliative chemotherapy is the primary mode of treatment. Doxorubicin, ifosfamide, gemcitabine, docetaxel, dacarbazine, eribulin, and trabectidin are commonly used.
  - Olaratumab, an antibody targeting the platelet derived growth factor receptor, PDGFRA in combination with doxorubicin, and the TKI pazopanib are also active in certain subtypes of sarcoma.
  - Metastasectomy can be considered in patients with oligometastatic disease.
  - The use of immune checkpoint blockers in sarcoma currently remains investigational.
  - **GI stromal tumor** (GIST): The most common site is stomach, followed by small bowel. Surgery should be performed if feasible. Most GISTs demonstrate mutations in *KIT* and are highly responsive to imatinib. Adjuvant and/or neoadjuvant imatinib is often utilized in select patients.
  - **Ewing sarcoma:** Unlike many soft tissue sarcomas, this tumor has a high cure rate and is almost always responsive to multiagent chemotherapy and radiation. Metastatic disease can be potentially cured with chemotherapy in a few cases.

HEMATOLOGIC MALIGNANCIES

Myelodysplastic Syndrome

EPIDEMIOLOGY AND ETIOLOGY

- Myelodysplastic syndromes (MDSs) comprise a heterogeneous group of myeoid neoplasms that are broadly characterized by cytopenias associated with a dysmorphic and usually cellular bone marrow and an increased risk of leukemic transformation. The median age at diagnosis is ≥65 years for de novo MDS. Cytopenias in MDS are due to clonal abnormalities of marrow cells affecting one or more cell lines, ultimately leading to reduced hematopoiesis. Therapy-related myeloid neoplasms, including acute myeloid leukemia (AML) and MDS, account for 10%–20% of all myeloid neoplasms.
- Environmental factors such as exposure to chemicals, radiation, and chemotherapy, as well as genetic syndromes and benign hematologic disorders (such as paroxysmal nocturnal hemoglobinuria), have been associated with an increased risk of MDS.
- Chromosome abnormalities occur in up to 80% of cases, leading to accumulation of multiple genetic lesions, loss of tumor suppressor genes, and/or activating oncogene mutations.

PATHOLOGY

The current WHO classification system[46] includes the following subclasses of MDS: MDS with unilineage dysplasia (anemia, neutropenia, or thrombocytopenia); MDS with multilineage dysplasia; MDS with ring sideroblasts; MDS with excess blasts (5%–20%); MDS with isolated deletion of 5q; and MDS unclassifiable.

DIAGNOSIS

Clinical Presentation

Symptoms can be related to bone marrow failure including fatigue, fever, bruising, or bleeding. Some cases are discovered incidentally through routine blood work. Leukopenia can cause frequent infections. Sweet syndrome (acute febrile neutrophilic dermatosis) during the course of MDS may herald leukemic transformation.

Diagnostic Testing

Complete blood counts usually show single or multilineage cytopenia. Macrocytosis is common. Peripheral blood smear can show dimorphic erythrocytes and large platelets. Neutrophils can be hypogranulated and have abnormally segmented nuclei (pseudo–Pelger-Huet cells). Obtaining a bone marrow aspirate and biopsy is important. The bone marrow is usually hypercellular. Cytogenetic analyses and next-generation sequencing are required to identify abnormalities, which aid in prognostication and therapeutic planning.

TREATMENT

- Therapy for MDS is generally unsatisfactory, and stem cell transplantation is the only curative option. A prognostic scoring system such as the Revised International Prognostic Scoring System (Table 22-6) is often used to determine patient risk category and treatment approach.

TABLE 22-6 Revised International Prognostic Scoring System (IPSS-R) for Myelodysplastic Syndromes

Score	Cytogenetics	Marrow Blasts (%)	Hemoglobin (g/dL)	Neutrophils ($\times 10^9$/L)	Platelets ($\times 10^9$/L)
0	Very good: –Y, del(11q)	≤2	≥10	≥0.8	≥100
0.5				<0.8	50–99
1	Good: normal, del(5q), del(12p), del(20q), double including del(5q)	2.1–4.9	8–9.9		<50
1.5			<8		
2	Intermediate: del(7q), +8, +19, i(17q), any other single or double independent clones	5–10			
3	Poor: –7, inv(3)/t(3q)/del(3q), double including –7/del(7q), complex with 3 abnormalities	>10			
4	Very poor: complex with >3 abnormalities				

Total Score	Risk Category	Median Overall Survival (years)	Median Time to 25% Acute Myeloid Leukemia Risk (years)
≤1.5	Very low	8.8	NR
2.0–3.0	Low	5.3	10.8
3.5–4.5	Intermediate	3	3.2
5.0–6.0	High	1.6	1.4
>6.0	Very high	0.8	0.73

- Asymptomatic patients with low risk disease can be followed with supportive care (transfusions, etc.) but otherwise without specific therapy.
- Patients with very–low-risk or low-risk MDS with symptomatic anemia, low erythropoietin level (<500 mU/mL), and low transfusion requirement can be treated with erythropoiesis-stimulating agents.
- Treatment with immunosuppressive agents such as antithymocyte globulin and cyclosporine can be considered in patients who have hypocellular MDS and/or demonstrate a paroxysmal nocturnal hemoglobinuria clone.
- Treatment with hypomethylating agents such as 5-azacytidine or decitabine should be considered in patients with intermediate or high-risk MDS. These agents can improve blood counts and quality of life, and delay transformation to AML.
- 5q-deleted MDS is associated with a good prognosis and higher probability of response to treatment with lenalidomide.
- Patients with high- and very–high-risk MDS are candidates for stem cell transplantation if eligible.

Acute Myeloid Leukemia

EPIDEMIOLOGY AND ETIOLOGY

AML is the most common type of acute leukemia in adults. Median age at presentation is around 65 years. Risk factors are similar to those of MDS. Antecedent MDS increases the risk of AML.

PATHOLOGY

The current WHO classification (Table 22-7) includes the following categories: AML with recurrent genetic abnormalities; AML with MDS-related changes; therapy-related AML; AML, not otherwise specified (NOS); myeloid sarcoma; myeloid proliferations related to Down syndrome; and blastic plasmacytoid dendritic neoplasms.

The AML NOS category includes the French–American–British (FAB) subtypes M0 (AML minimally differentiated), M1 (AML without maturation), M2 (AML with maturation), M4 (acute myelomonocytic leukemia), M5 (acute monocytic leukemia), M6 (acute erythroleukemia), and M7 (acute megakaryoblasticleukemia). FAB subtype M3

TABLE 22-7 Acute Leukemias With Recurrent Genetic Abnormalities

Acute Myeloid Leukemia	Acute Lymphoblastic Leukemia (ALL)
Recurrent genetic abnormalities	**Recurrent genetic abnormalities**
t(8;21); *RUNX1-RUNX1T1*	t(9;22); *BCR1-ABL*
inv(16) or t(16;16); *CEFB-MYH11*	t(V;11); *V/MLL* (*MLL* rearranged)
t(15;17); *PML-RARA*	t(12;21); *TEL/AML1* (*ETV6-RUNX1*)
t(9;11); *MLLT3-MLL*	t(1;19); *E2A-PBX1*
t(6;9); *DEK-NUP214*	t(5;14); *IL3-IGH*
inv(3) or t(3;3); *RPN1-EVI1*	ALL with hyperdiploidy
t(1;22); *RBM15-MKL1*	ALL with hypodiploid
Provisional entities at molecular level	
NPM1 mutated	
CEBPA mutated	

(acute promyelocytic leukemia [APL]) is classified as AML with recurrent genetic abnormalities due to the presence of t(15;17).

DIAGNOSIS

Clinical Presentation

Symptoms are related to bone marrow failure, including fatigue, fever, bruising, or bleeding. Most patients present with pancytopenia and circulating blasts. Patients with a high blast count are at risk for leukostasis, manifested by dyspnea, chest pain, headaches, confusion, and cranial nerve palsies. Extramedullary tissue invasion by leukemic cells (most commonly with AML-M5) can result in hepatomegaly, splenomegaly, lymphadenopathy, rashes (leukemia cutis), gingival hypertrophy, CNS dysfunction, cranial neuropathies, or infiltrative masses (granulocytic sarcomas or chloromas).

Diagnostic Testing

AML is defined by the presence of ≥20% blasts in the bone marrow and/or in the peripheral blood. AML with t(8;21), inv(16), and t(15;17) can be diagnosed irrespective of the blast percentage. Bone marrow specimens should be submitted for flow cytometry, molecular testing, and cytogenetics. This information is used to classify AML into prognostic groups and guide treatment.[47]

TREATMENT

- **Remission induction:** Induction chemotherapy consists of a 7 + 3 regimen that includes administration of cytarabine over 7 days in combination with an anthracycline (daunorubicin or idarubicin) on the first 3 days. Approximately 60%–80% of AML patients achieve remission with induction chemotherapy. However, patients achieving remission eventually relapse without additional consolidation therapy.
- **Consolidation:** Options include high-dose cytarabine with or without subsequent stem cell transplantation. Optimal consolidation strategy is dependent on disease risk category (Table 22-8).

TABLE 22-8 Cytogenetic Abnormalities in Acute Myeloid Leukemia and Associated Prognosis

Risk Group	Cytogenetic and Molecular Features	Preferred Consolidation Strategy
Favorable	t(15;17), t(8;21), inv(16). Mutated *NPM1* without mutated *FLT3*-ITD, or mutated *CEBPA*	Chemotherapy
Intermediate	Normal cytogenetics. Mutated *FLT3*-ITD, t(9,11), cytogenetic abnormalities not classified under favorable or unfavorable risk groups	Allogeneic hematopoietic cell transplantation
Unfavorable	Complex karyotype (defined as ≥3 abnormalities, excluding the favorable-risk cytogenetics), monosomal karyotype, inv(3), t(6;9), *MLL* rearranged, del(5q), −5, −7, +8 t(9,22), mutated RUNX, mutated TP53, mutated ASXL1	Allogeneic hematopoietic cell transplantation

- APL (AML-M3) is characterized by high cure rates. Treatment includes the use of all-*trans*-retinoic acid and arsenic trioxide.
- Recent studies have shown drugs such as enasidinib and decitabine to be active in patients with high-risk AML harboring mutations in *IDH2* and *TP53*, respectively.[48,49]

Acute Lymphoblastic Leukemia

EPIDEMIOLOGY AND ETIOLOGY

Acute lymphoblastic leukemia (ALL) is the most common childhood leukemia. The median age at presentation is 35 years with a bimodal distribution including one peak at 4–5 years and a second gradual increase after the age of 50. Advanced age is a poor prognostic factor.

PATHOLOGY

ALL can arise from B- or T-lymphocyte progenitors. The WHO classifies ALL into three categories: B cell with recurrent genetic abnormalities, T cell, and B cell, NOS (see Table 22-7).

DIAGNOSIS

Clinical Presentation

Symptoms include fatigue, fever, and bleeding. Leukostasis is uncommon, even with high white blood cell counts. Lymphadenopathy and splenomegaly are present in approximately 20% of cases. CNS may be involved at presentation, manifesting as headache or cranial nerve palsies.

Diagnostic Testing

Basic workup is similar to that required in AML. Immunophenotyping is often necessary to distinguish ALL from AML.

TREATMENT

- Several complex regimens such as the Berlin-Frankfurt-Munster (comprising induction, consolidation, delayed intensification, and maintenance schedule with the drugs such as vincristine, daunorubicin, methotrexate, L-asparginase, cytarabine, cyclophosphamide, etoposide, and steroids), hyperfractionated cyclophosphamide, vincristine, doxorubicin, and dexamethasone (Hyper-CVAD), Cancer and Leukemia Group B 8811, and the German Multicenter ALL regimen have been used for the treatment of ALL. Treatment is subdivided into induction, consolidation, and maintenance phases, usually administered over a course of 2–3 years.
- Because of the high risk of CNS relapse, prophylactic intrathecal therapy and high-dose methotrexate or cytarabine are administered during the intensive phase.
- Allogeneic stem cell transplantation is an option in relapsed ALL and in patients with high-risk disease.

Chronic Myeloid Leukemia

EPIDEMIOLOGY AND ETIOLOGY

Chronic myeloid leukemia (CML) accounts for nearly 14% of leukemias diagnosed in the United States, with a median age at diagnosis of 65 years.

PATHOLOGY

- CML is associated with the fusion of two genes, *BCR* on chromosome 22 and *ABL1* on chromosome 9, resulting in the *BCR-ABL1* fusion gene (Philadelphia chromosome). The fusion protein is associated with deregulated kinase activity.
- The natural history of CML is a triphasic process with a chronic phase, an accelerated phase, and a blast phase. Chronic phase is associated with an asymptomatic accumulation of differentiated myeloid cells in the marrow, spleen, and circulation. CML patients will invariably progress to accelerated and blast phases without treatment.

DIAGNOSIS

Clinical Presentation

Patients can present in any of three phases, although the majority present in the chronic phase of their illness. Symptoms are usually related to splenomegaly (pain, left abdominal mass, early satiety) or anemia. Peripheral blood counts show increased white blood cells with all levels of granulocytic differentiation, from myeloblasts to segmented neutrophils. Transformation from chronic phase to blast phase can be insidious through the accelerated phase or abrupt.

Diagnostic Testing

The presence of the *BCR-ABL1* rearrangement by cytogenetics, FISH, or polymerase chain reaction (PCR) in the peripheral blood or bone marrow confirms the diagnosis of CML. Cytogenetics and quantitative PCR (qPCR) of BCR-ABL1 are performed at regular intervals to monitor response to treatment.

TREATMENT

- Patients are treated with oral TKIs such as imatinib, dasatinib, and nilotinib. The choice of agent typically depends on treatment-related adverse effects and patient preference. Phase III trials comparing second-generation TKIs (dasatinib or nilotinib) to imatinib as initial therapy for CML in chronic phase have demonstrated faster and deeper responses with the former with similar overall survival.
- Complete hematologic remission (CHR) is defined as normalization of peripheral blood counts and absence of splenomegaly, whereas complete cytogenetic response (CCyR) is defined by the absence of Philadelphia chromosome metaphases on bone marrow cytogenetic analysis; major molecular remission is defined by qPCR when *BCR-ABL1* transcripts in the peripheral blood are ≤0.1% on the International Scale (IS). CHR and/or *BCR-ABL1* transcripts in the marrow ≤10% (IS) by 3 months, CCyR and/or *BCR-ABL1* transcripts in the marrow ≤1% (IS) by 6 months, and *BCR-ABL1* transcripts in the marrow ≤0.1% (IS) by 12 months after starting a TKI constitute an optimal response to therapy.[50]
- Failure to achieve treatment milestones often requires switching therapies.
- For patients with mutations such as T315I or those who fail second-generation TKI, ponatinib and omacetaxine are available as third-line therapy.
- Stem cell transplantation can be considered in patients who fail second-line therapy or those who present with accelerated/blast crisis phase.
- Blast crises are more challenging to manage, and treatment often involves TKIs, chemotherapy, and stem cell transplantation with dismal outcomes.

Chronic Lymphocytic Leukemia

EPIDEMIOLOGY AND ETIOLOGY

Chronic lymphocytic leukemia (CLL) is the most common form of leukemia in Western countries. CLL carries the highest familial risk of all hematologic malignancies.

PATHOLOGY

The diagnosis of CLL requires the presence of more than 5000 lymphocytes/μL and characteristic cell surface markers including the B-cell antigens CD19, CD20, and CD23. Of note, CD5, a T-cell antigen, is expressed in virtually all cases of CLL.

STAGING

The classification of CLL, based on the extent of systemic infiltration of lymphocytes, is used to determine the prognosis and initiation of treatment (Table 22-9). Molecular and cytogenetic markers have become increasingly useful for prognostication.

DIAGNOSIS

Clinical Presentation

Most patients are diagnosed while asymptomatic. When present, symptoms include fatigue, weight loss, lymphadenopathy, anemia, thrombocytopenia, and infections. Patients can also present with a hemolytic anemia, immune thrombocytopenia, or Richter syndrome, which is a transformation of CLL to diffuse large B-cell lymphoma.

Diagnostic Testing

Flow cytometry aids in the identification of CLL surface markers on B cells. FISH of the peripheral blood for evaluating 17p, 11q, and 13q deletion, and trisomy 12, mutation status of Ig heavy chain variable region, and assessing the expression of ZAP70 and CD38 are of prognostic importance.

TREATMENT

- Many patients do not require treatment at the time of initial diagnosis if asymptomatic.
- **Active disease** as defined by the International Workshop on CLL is an indication for treatment. Active disease is characterized by progressive marrow failure, massive or symptomatic splenomegaly (>6 cm below costal margin) or lymphadenopathy (>10 cm in longest diameter), progressive lymphocytosis (>50% increase in 2 months or

TABLE 22-9 Chronic Lymphocytic Leukemia Clinical Staging

Rai	Binet
Stage 0: Lymphocytosis	Stage A: Lymphocytosis
Stage 1: Lymphadenopathy	Stage B: Lymphadenopathy in ≥3 areas
Stage 2: Splenomegaly	Stage C: Hgb <10 g/dL or platelets <100,000/μL
Stage 3: Hgb <11 g/dL	
Stage 4: Platelets <100,000/μL	

Hgb, hemoglobin.

doubling time of <6 months), autoimmune anemia and/or thrombocytopenia that is poorly responsive to standard therapy, and the presence of constitutional symptoms.[51]

- Treatment options include alkylating agents (chlorambucil, cyclophosphamide, bendamustine), purine analogues (fludarabine), and anti-CD20 monoclonal antibodies such as rituximab, ofatumumab, and obinutuzumab (anti-CD20). Oral targeted agents have shown significant efficacy in CLL and are particularly helpful in patients with high-risk cytogenetics, such as 17p and 11q deletions: ibrutinib (BTK inhibitor), idelalisib (PI3K inhibitor), and venetoclax (BCL-2 inhibitor).[52–54]

Hairy Cell Leukemia

EPIDEMIOLOGY AND ETIOLOGY

Hairy cell leukemia is a rare disorder, most commonly seen in elderly men.

DIAGNOSIS

Clinical Presentation

Most patients present with malaise and fatigue. Splenomegaly and hepatomegaly may be evident on examination. With more advanced disease, pancytopenia develops, and patients may present with bleeding or recurrent infections.

Diagnostic Testing

Peripheral blood leukocytes have the characteristic "hairy" appearance and are tartrate-resistant acid phosphatase positive. Flow cytometry is positive for CD20, CD11c, CD103, CD123, cyclin D1, and annexin A1. The majority of patients with hairy cell leukemia harbor the *BRAF* V600E mutation.

TREATMENT

- The decision to treat is based on the development of cytopenias, symptomatic splenomegaly, constitutional symptoms, and recurrent infections.
- Cladribine and pentostatin are typically used for treatment and have high cure rates. These agents can induce significant and prolonged immunosuppression.

Hodgkin Lymphoma

EPIDEMIOLOGY AND ETIOLOGY

EBV and HIV infections, autoimmune conditions, and immunosuppressant use have been described as risk factors for HL.

PATHOLOGY

- HL is subdivided into nodular lymphocyte predominant (NLPHL) and classical HL subtypes.
- The Reed–Sternberg (RS) cells consistently express the CD30 and CD15 antigens. In contrast to the other histologic subtypes, RS cells are infrequent in NLPHL. Instead, "popcorn cells" are seen within a background of inflammatory cells in NLPHL.

DIAGNOSIS

Clinical Presentation

Most patients present with painless lymphadenopathy. B symptoms are more common in advanced stages.

Diagnostic Testing

FNA is often inadequate to make a diagnosis, and therefore a minimum of a core needle biopsy is necessary. If initial biopsy is nondiagnostic, excisional biopsy may be required. Additional workup includes history and physical, complete blood cell counts, chemistry, LDH, erythrocyte sedimentation rate (ESR), and whole-body PET scan.

STAGING

The Lugano classification derived from Ann Arbor staging system classifies lymphomas into four stages (Table 22-10). Patients with early stage disease (stages I–II) are further stratified into favorable- and unfavorable-risk categories. Favorable risk is defined by the presence of two or less sites of disease, mediastinal width less than one-third of maximal thoracic diameter, ESR <50 mm/h (<30 mm/h with B symptoms), and absence of extranodal extension.[55]

TABLE 22-10 Lugano Classification for Staging of Lymphomas
Stage I: Involvement of a single lymph node region (e.g., cervical, axillary, inguinal, mediastinal) or lymphoid structure such as the spleen, thymus, or Waldeyer's ring
Stage II: Involvement of two or more lymph node regions or lymph node structures on the same side of the diaphragm. Hilar nodes should be considered to be "lateralized" and, when involved on both sides, constitute stage II disease[a]
Stage III: Involvement of lymph node regions or lymphoid structures on both sides of the diaphragm[b]
Stage IV: Diffuse or disseminated involvement of one or more extranodal organs or tissue beyond that designated E, with or without associated lymph node involvement[c]
Bulky disease: A single nodal mass, in contrast to multiple smaller nodes, of 10 cm or ≥1/3 of the transthoracic diameter at any level of thoracic vertebrae as determined by CT; record the longest measurement by CT scan

The term "X" (used in the Ann Arbor staging system) is no longer necessary. This classification is derived from Ann Arbor staging with Cotswolds modifications.

[a]For the purpose of defining the number of anatomic regions, all nodal diseases within the mediastinum are considered to be a single lymph node region, and hilar involvement constitutes an additional site of involvement. The number of anatomic regions should be indicated by a subscript (e.g., II-3).

[b]This may be subdivided into stage III-1 or III-2: stage III-1 is used for patients with involvement of the spleen or splenic hilar, celiac, or portal nodes; and stage III-2 is used for patients with involvement of the para-aortic, iliac, inguinal, or mesenteric nodes.

[c]All cases are subclassified to indicate the absence (A) or presence (B) of the systemic symptoms of significant unexplained fever, night sweats, or unexplained weight loss exceeding 10% of body weight during the 6 months prior to diagnosis. The designation "E" refers to extranodal contiguous extension (i.e., proximal or contiguous extranodal disease) that can be encompassed within an irradiation field appropriate for nodal disease of the same anatomic extent. More extensive extranodal disease is designated stage IV.

TREATMENT

- The treatment of choice for HL is chemotherapy with ABVD (doxorubicin, bleomycin, vinblastine, dacarbazine), with or without radiation, depending on the stage and risk category.
- Interim PET-CT findings play an important role in guiding treatment in selected patients with HL.[56]
- Relapsed disease is treated with salvage chemotherapy with or without stem cell transplantation. Brentuximab vedotin, a CD30-directed antibody–drug conjugate, and the PD-1 inhibitors pembrolizumab and nivolumab are effective treatments for relapsed HL.[57–59]

Non-Hodgkin Lymphoma

EPIDEMIOLOGY AND ETIOLOGY

Non-Hodgkin lymphoma (NHL) is the sixth most common malignancy in the United States. Risk factors include immunodeficiency, autoimmune disorders, bacterial infections (*H. pylori*, *Borrelia burgdorferi*, and *Chlamydia psittaci*), viral infections (HIV, EBV, HHV8, and human T-lymphotropic virus-1), and immunosuppression in the setting of previous transplantation.

PATHOLOGY

NHL may be broadly divided into indolent (e.g., follicular, marginal, small lymphocytic), aggressive (e.g., diffuse large B cell, mantle cell, peripheral T cell), and very aggressive (Burkitt, lymphoblastic) subtypes. Several recurrent chromosomal abnormalities have been described in patients with NHL (Table 22-11).

DIAGNOSIS

Clinical Presentation

Clinical manifestations depend on the histologic subtype and can be characteristic in some rare subtypes of NHL. For instance, pruritic plaques can be seen in mycosis fungoides (a primary cutaneous T-cell NHL) and isolated splenomegaly in splenic marginal zone lymphomas.

TABLE 22-11 Selected Chromosomal Abnormalities in B-Cell Non-Hodgkin Lymphomas

Cytogenetic Abnormality	Histology	Oncogene
t(14;18)	Follicular, DLBCL	**BCL2**
t(11;14)	Mantle cell	Cyclin D1
t(1;14)	MALT lymphoma	**BCL10**
t(11;18)	Marginal zone/extranodal marginal zone	
t(2;5)	ALK-positive anaplastic large-cell lymphoma	**ALK**
t(9;14)	Lymphoplasmacytic lymphoma	
8q24 translocations	Burkitt lymphoma	**MYC**

DLBCL, diffuse large B-cell lymphoma; MALT, mucosa-associated lymphoid tissue.

Diagnostic Testing

Essential workup often includes history, physical examination, complete blood cell count, chemistry, PET/CT, and bone marrow biopsy. The CSF evaluation is indicated in patients with high-grade lymphomas, HIV-related lymphomas, and involvement of the epidural space, nasopharynx, and paranasal sinuses. Patients suspected to have primary CNS lymphomas require an ophthalmologic examination. Occasionally, patients with aggressive lymphomas can present with a spontaneous tumor lysis syndrome (TLS) (Table 22-12).

STAGING

Patients are staged by the Ann Arbor classification. Patients with diffuse large B-cell lymphoma are usually stratified according to the International Prognostic Index, which uses five adverse prognostic factors: age >60 years, Ann Arbor stage III or IV, abnormal serum LDH, two or more extranodal sites involved, and Eastern Cooperative Oncology Group performance status of ≥2.

TREATMENT

Indolent Lymphomas

- **Stage I–II:**
  - Observation, involved-field radiotherapy (IFRT), single-agent rituximab, rituximab with chemotherapy, and combined-modality therapy with rituximab, chemotherapy, and IFRT are all options.
  - Gastric mucosa-associated lymphoid tissue (MALT) lymphomas are related to *H. pylori* infection and respond well to *H. pylori*–directed therapy. Gastric MALT lymphomas that do not respond to or relapse after *H. pylori* therapy, and other isolated extranodal lymphomas (salivary gland, breast, conjunctiva) may be treated with IFRT.
- **Stage III–IV**
  - There is no convincing evidence to support early intervention versus "watchful waiting" in asymptomatic patients.[60] A combination of an anti-CD20 antibody (rituximab or obinutuzumab) and chemotherapy or single-agent rituximab can be used for treatment.
- **Relapsed disease**
  - First-line therapy can be repeated in patients who were in first remission for >2 years. Radioimmunotherapy with ibritumomab (anti-CD20 antibody conjugated with yttrium-90), idelalisib, lenalidomide, and stem cell transplant are all effective options.

TABLE 22-12 Defining Features of Tumor Lysis Syndrome (Cairo–Bishop)

Manifestation	Features
Laboratory	1. Uric acid ≥8 mg/dL or 25% increase from baseline 2. Potassium ≥6 mEq/dL or 25% increase from baseline 3. Phosphorus ≥6.5 mg/dL in children and >4.5 mg/dL in adults or 25% increase from baseline 4. Calcium ≤7 mg/dL or 25% decrease from baseline
Clinical	1. Creatinine ≥1.5 × upper normal limit 2. Cardiac arrhythmia or sudden death 3. Seizure

Aggressive Lymphomas

Diffuse Large B-Cell Lymphoma

- **Stage I–II:** Limited-stage disease is managed with chemotherapy (rituximab, cyclophosphamide, doxorubicin, vincristine, and prednisone [R-CHOP]) with or without IFRT.
- **Stage III–IV:**
  - Patients beginning therapy for aggressive lymphomas should be monitored closely for signs of TLS and should receive adequate IV hydration and appropriate prophylaxis with allopurinol and/or rasburicase.
  - Chemotherapy with R-CHOP is the standard. Patients with *MYC* translocations, especially those with "double-hit" lymphomas (combined translocations of *MYC* and either *BCL2* or *BCL6*), have significantly worse outcomes and are often treated with the infusional chemotherapy regimen dose-adjusted R-EPOCH.
  - **CNS prophylaxis** with intrathecal chemotherapy or high-dose methotrexate should be considered for patients with testicular, orbital, epidural, paranasal sinus, or extensive bone marrow involvement with elevated LDH.
  - Primary CNS lymphoma is treated with complex regimens that usually incorporate high-dose methotrexate, cytarabine, and rituximab with consideration of consolidation with stem cell transplantation. Whole-brain radiation is an effective therapy, but it should be avoided if possible because of the high rate of late neurotoxicity.

Burkitt Lymphoma

- Burkitt lymphomas are usually treated with complex multidrug protocols and CNS prophylaxis.

Mantle Cell Lymphoma

- Chemotherapy regimens incorporating rituximab, cytarabine, and bendamustine are often used. Consolidation with stem cell transplantation can be considered in first remission. Maintenance rituximab is considered in all patients.

Relapsed Non-Hodgkin Lymphoma

- Younger patients without significant comorbidities are candidates for stem cell transplantation at relapse. Several effective salvage regimens such as ICE (ifosfamide, carboplatin, etoposide), DHAP (dexamethasone, cisplatin, cytarabine), and ESHAP (etoposide, methylprednisone, cytarabine, cisplatin) are available. Rituximab is added to the salvage regimens for B-cell lymphomas.
- Allogeneic transplantation can be considered in patients with relapsed lymphoblastic lymphoma, refractory disease at relapse, or a duration of remission of <1 year after initial therapy.
- CAR-T cell therapies, such as axicabtageneciloleucel and tisagenlecleucel, are novel immunotherapeutic approaches that are currently approved for use in patients with refractory diffuse large B-cell lymphomas.[3,5]

Multiple Myeloma

EPIDEMIOLOGY AND ETIOLOGY

Multiple myeloma (MM) is the second most frequent hematologic malignancy after NHL. The median age at diagnosis is 66 years. A small percentage of cases are familial.

DIAGNOSIS

Clinical Presentation

The most common presentation is anemia. Patients can also have bone pain, renal failure, fatigue, weight loss, and hypercalcemia. Patients with extramedullary plasmacytomas can present with radiculopathy, cord compression, or CNS involvement.

Diagnostic Testing

Initial evaluation includes routine blood work, β_2-microglobulin (B2M), serum and urine protein electrophoresis, serum free light chain estimation, skeletal survey, and bone marrow examination. The diagnosis is confirmed by the presence of 10% or more clonal plasma cells in the bone marrow or a biopsy-proven plasmacytoma, with evidence of end-organ damage (hypercalcemia, renal dysfunction, anemia, or bone lesions). A clonal marrow plasma cell percentage of ≥60%, κ or λ free light chain ratio of ≥100, and the presence of one or more focal lesions on MRI are also criteria for diagnosis of myeloma because they are associated with a high risk of progression to end-organ damage.[61] Revised International Myeloma Working Group diagnostic criteria for multiple myeloma and smoldering multiple myeloma are summarized in Table 22-13.

STAGING

- The International Staging System for MM uses B2M and albumin to stratify patients into: stage I (B2M <3.5 mg/dL and albumin ≥3.5 g/dL), stage II (B2M 3.5–5.5 mg/dL

TABLE 22-13 Revised International Myeloma Working Group Diagnostic Criteria for Multiple Myeloma and Smoldering Multiple Myeloma
Definition of multiple myeloma
Clonal bone marrow plasma cells ≥10% or biopsy-proven bony or extramedullary plasmacytoma and any one or more of the following myeloma-defining events:
• Evidence of end-organ damage that can be attributed to the underlying plasma cell proliferative disorder, specifically: • Hypercalcemia: Serum calcium >0.25 mmol/L (>1 mg/dL) higher than the upper limit of normal or >2.75 mmol/L (>11 mg/dL) • Renal insufficiency: Creatinine clearance <40 mL/min or serum creatinine >177 μmol/L (>2 mg/dL) • Anemia: Hemoglobin value of >20 g/L below the lower limit of normal, or a hemoglobin value <100 g/L • Bone lesions: One or more osteolytic lesions on skeletal radiography, CT, or PET-CT
• Any one or more of the following biomarkers of malignancy: • Clonal bone marrow plasma cell percentage ≥60 • Involved:uninvolved serum free light chain ratio ≥100 • >1 focal lesions on MRI studies
Definition of smoldering multiple myeloma
Both of the following criteria must be met:
• Serum monoclonal protein (IgG or IgA) ≥30 g/L or urinary monoclonal protein ≥500 mg per 24 h and/or clonal bone marrow plasma cells 10%–60% • Absence of myeloma-defining events or amyloidosis
Definition of monoclonal gammopathy of undetermined significance
All of the following three criteria must be met:
• Serum monoclonal protein <30 g/L • Bone marrow plasma cells <10% • Absence of myeloma-defining events or amyloidosis (or Waldenström macroglobulinemia in the case of IgM MGUS)

TABLE 22-14 Risk Stratification in Myeloma Based on mSMART (Mayo Stratification for Myeloma and Risk-Adapted Therapy) Model[64]

Standard Risk	Intermediate Risk	High Risk
Trisomies, t(11;14), and t(6;14)	t(4;14), 1q gain, deletion 13, hypodiploidy, complex karyotype	17p del, t(14;16), and t(14;20)
		High-risk gene expression profile signature

From Mikhael JR, et al. Management of newly diagnosed symptomatic multiple myeloma: updated Mayo Stratification of Myeloma and Risk-Adapted Therapy (mSMART) consensus guidelines 2013. Mayo Clin Proc. 2013;88:360376.

irrespective of albumin levels or B2M <3.5 mg/dL with albumin <3.5 g/dL), and stage III (B2M ≥5.5 mg/dL).

- Cytogenetic features (Table 22-14) can be used for risk stratification and guiding treatment.

TREATMENT

- Transplant-eligible patients are offered autologous stem cell transplantation following approximately 4 months of treatment with a regimen that includes dexamethasone, a proteasome inhibitor (e.g., bortezomib), and/or an immunomodulatory agent (e.g., lenalidomide), whereas initial therapy is continued for 12–18 months in transplant-ineligible patients.
- Maintenance therapy with either lenalidomide or bortezomib is considered following initial therapy based on the patient's risk category.
- Several drugs including newer proteasome inhibitors (carfilzomib), IMiDs (pomalidomide), monoclonal antibodies targeting CD38 (daratumumab) and SLAMF7 (elotuzumab), and selinexor are active in relapsed myeloma.[62,63]
- CAR-T therapies for MM are investigational.

ONCOLOGIC EMERGENCIES

The most common oncology emergencies are febrile neutropenia (FN), TLS, malignant hypercalcemia, spinal cord compression, SVC syndrome, and brain metastases with increased intracranial pressure (Table 22-15).

Febrile Neutropenia

- FN is defined as an absolute neutrophil count (ANC) of <500/μL, with a single core temperature of >38.3°C or a persistent temperature (>1 hour) of >38.0°C.
- Risk of FN is proportional to the duration of neutropenia.
- Although most solid tumor chemotherapy regimens are associated with a brief (<5 days) duration of neutropenia, neutropenia with leukemia and transplantation regimens can be more persistent.
- Risk is also increased with regimens that cause mucositis (inflammation and ulceration of the oral and GI mucosa).

TABLE 22-15 Oncologic Emergencies

Emergency	Etiology	Presentation	Management
Neutropenic fever	Infectious	Temperature >38.3°C or >38°C two times 1 h apart	1. Antibiotic coverage: gram-negative with pseudomonal activity, and gram-positive if risk factors (catheters, pneumonia, mucositis, Staphylococcus colonization, sepsis), and also fungal if unstable 2. IV hydration and supportive care as appropriate
Tumor lysis syndrome (TLS)	Massive lysis of cancer cells (mostly with chemotherapy)	Hyperuricemia, hyperkalemia, hyperphosphatemia, hypocalcemia, AKI, cardiac arrhythmias, and/or seizures	1. Prevention with IV fluids and prophylactic allopurinol or rasburicase based on estimated risk of TLS 2. Treatment: Aggressive hydration, rasburicase, dialysis
Hypercalcemia	Humoral, PTHrP, bone metastasis, calcitriol mediated (lymphomas)	Dehydration, CNS symptoms, constipation, ileus, weakness, cardiac (bradycardia, short QT, prolonged PR, etc.)	1. IV hydration 2. Bisphosphonates or denosumab (if low creatinine clearance) 3. Calcitonin (if symptomatic, rapid onset) 4. Steroids can be useful
Spinal cord compression (SCC)	Metastatic or involvement of spine in SCC	Pain, weakness, sensory loss, incontinence, ataxia	1. Steroids 2. Neurosurgery consultation 3. RT 4. Chemotherapy can be considered in few cases of SCC
Superior vena cava (SVC) syndrome	Obstruction of SVC by primary or metastatic cancer (mostly intrathoracic)	Dyspnea, stridor (laryngeal edema), facial and upper extremity swelling, risk of cerebral edema and herniation	1. Histologic diagnosis is important 2. Consider upfront endovascular stent and RT if comatose or respiratory compromise 3. Treatment depends on tumor type: SCLC, lymphoma, germ cell: chemotherapy; NSCLC: RT; thymic tumors: surgery

(Continued)

TABLE 22-15 Oncologic Emergencies (Continued)

Emergency	Etiology	Presentation	Management
Hyperleukocytosis with leukostasis	Intravascular accumulation of blasts, with or without DIC	Chest pain, respiratory distress, stupor, TLS, DIC	1. Leukapheresis: symptomatic patients (count threshold AML >50 × 10^3/μL, ALL and CML >150 × 10^3/μL, CLL >500 × 10^3/μL); asymptomatic patients (AML >100 × 10^3/μL, ALL >200 × 10^3/μL) 2. Hydroxyurea for cytoreduction

AKI, acute kidney injury; ALL, acute lymphoblastic leukemia; AML, acute myeloid leukemia; CLL, chronic lymphocytic leukemia; CML, chronic myeloid leukemia; CNS, central nervous system; DIC, disseminated intravascular coagulation; NSCLC, non–small-cell lung cancer; PTHrP, parathyroid hormone-related protein; RT, radiotherapy; SCLC, small-cell lung cancer.

DIAGNOSIS

- Evaluation should include a complete physical examination including assessment of catheter sites, perianal region, and dentition and mucosal surfaces. DRE should not be performed, considering the potential risk for bacterial translocation.
- Cultures of blood (bacterial and fungal), along with stool and sputum cultures in symptomatic patients, should be obtained. Chest imaging is considered in symptomatic patients. Viral PCR studies may also be considered when indicated, as a viral etiology may alter management.

TREATMENT

- Emergent IV antibiotic therapy is critical to prevent life-threatening sepsis.
  - Antibiotics with coverage of gram-negative bacilli (including *Pseudomonas aeruginosa*) must be used.
  - Empiric coverage of methicillin-resistant *Staphylococcus aureus* (MRSA) with vancomycin or linezolid is not recommended unless patients are hemodynamically unstable or have severe oral mucositis, pneumonia, evidence of a catheter-related infection, or a recent infection with MRSA.
  - Antimicrobial regimens should be tailored to treat the source of infection, if one is identified.
  - Pre-emptive antifungal therapy should be considered if fever persists for >72 hours in the presence of lung infiltrates or positive serologic tests (galactomannan, beta-D-glucan).
  - Gram-negative coverage should continue until ANC is >500/μL.
  - Low-risk patients (afebrile for 24 hours after antibiotics, negative culture results, and expected duration of myelosuppression for <1 week) can be treated as outpatients with oral, broad-spectrum antibiotics such as fluoroquinolone, amoxicillin/clavulanic acid, or clindamycin.
  - Consuming raw fruits and vegetables is not associated with excessive risk for infection in neutropenic patients.
- Growth factors
  - G-CSF is the most commonly used growth factor and is usually given SC in doses of 5 μg/kg/d.

- ◦ Although growth factors can reduce the duration of hospitalization for FN, they have not been shown to improve survival.
- ◦ Growth factors should not be given within 24 hours after chemotherapy or during radiation because of the potential for increased myelosuppression.
- ◦ Prophylactic growth factors are used when the predicted risk of FN is high and the neutropenia is predicted to result in chemotherapy delays.

Tumor Lysis Syndrome

- TLS is a group of metabolic disturbances resulting from significant tumor breakdown with release of intracellular products into circulation.
- TLS occurs in tumors that grow rapidly and are sensitive to cytotoxic chemotherapy. The risk of TLS is high in patients with acute leukemias and high-grade lymphomas, bulky tumors, elevated pretreatment LDH and uric acid levels, and renal dysfunction.
- TLS can also be spontaneous (not treatment related).

DIAGNOSIS

TLS is characterized by the presence of certain laboratory and clinical criteria (see Table 22-15).

TREATMENT

- The most important intervention to prevent TLS is aggressive hydration to maintain a urine output of at least 100 mL/m^2/h.
- Prophylactic strategies include the use of the xanthine oxidase inhibitor, allopurinol/febuxostat, or rasburicase depending on the risk, before treatment initiation.
- Rasburicase is a recombinant enzyme that degrades uric acid that can be used for the prophylaxis and treatment of hyperuricemia. It is indicated in patients with an elevated uric acid level before treatment initiation and those at a high risk for developing hyperuricemia (predicted based on tumor type, tumor burden, and pretreatment LDH level).
- Hyperkalemia is an immediate threat and should be treated aggressively.
- Calcium administration should be restricted in asymptomatic patients with hypocalcemia or hyperkalemia to prevent risk of metastatic calcification in the setting of hyperphosphatemia.
- Hyperphosphatemia should be treated with phosphate binders and hydration.
- Patients with persistent electrolyte abnormalities (hyperkalemia, hyperphosphatemia, and high calcium-phosphate products) and a pronounced decrease in urine output may require renal replacement therapy.

Malignant Hypercalcemia

- Malignant hypercalcemia is a common paraneoplastic syndrome and occurs in nearly 10%–20% of cancer patients.
- A serum total calcium level of >10.5 mg/dL is generally considered elevated. Measuring ionized calcium can be necessary and helpful in patients with abnormal serum albumin levels.
- Osteolysis and humoral hypercalcemia through tumor production of parathyroid hormone (PTH), PTH-related protein (PTHrP), or vitamin D analogues are the predominant mechanisms of hypercalcemia.

DIAGNOSIS

Classic symptoms usually develop with total calcium levels above 12 mg/dL and include polyuria, polydipsia, anorexia, constipation, nausea, vomiting, and confusion. Patients are usually severely hypovolemic because of excessive fluid losses and limited intake.

TREATMENT

- Aggressive hydration with normal saline is important. Diuretics should not be used unless volume overload is present.
- IV bisphosphonates, pamidronate 90 mg or zoledronic acid 4 mg, inhibit bone resorption and are used in the management of severe or symptomatic hypercalcemia. Zoledronic acid is contraindicated in patients with severe renal dysfunction.
- Calcitonin can be used in patients with severe symptomatic hypercalcemia for short-term and immediate control of calcium levels.
- Hypercalcemia caused by tumor production of vitamin D analogues may respond to corticosteroids.

Spinal Cord Compression

Malignant spinal cord compression (MSCC) affects approximately 5%–10% of patients with cancer and is commonly seen in patients with lung, breast, prostate, and lymphoid malignancies.

DIAGNOSIS

- The study of choice for MSCC is MRI of the entire spine.
- Most patients present with back pain and local tenderness in the involved region, before onset of neurologic deficits. Therefore, attention to the complaint of new back pain in a patient with a history of cancer is paramount. Pain is worse in a recumbent position and aggravated by sneezing, coughing, or bearing down (Valsalva maneuver). Other symptoms include weakness, sensory loss, and bladder or bowel incontinence.
- Timely diagnosis and intervention are crucial to prevent permanent neurologic damage.

TREATMENT

- Patients suspected of having MSCC should be started on glucocorticoids. Treatment should not be delayed for imaging. The most commonly used corticosteroid regimen is a 10-mg dexamethasone loading dose, followed by 4 mg every 4–6 hours.
- Consultation from surgical and radiation oncology services should be obtained in a timely fashion. Outcomes are better with surgery compared to radiation therapy in patients who are surgical candidates.
- Systemic chemotherapy can be used to treat patients with chemosensitive tumors.

Superior Vena Cava Syndrome

- Cancer-related SVC syndrome results from obstruction of blood flow through the SVC through invasion, external compression, or thrombosis in the setting of a malignancy.
- The severity and rapidity of symptom onset depends on the rate at which the SVC is occluded and if there has been enough time for collateral venous drainage to develop.

- Lung cancer, lymphomas, thymic neoplasms, germ cell tumors, mesothelioma, and other solid tumors that cause mediastinal involvement are the cancers that are commonly associated with SVC syndrome.

DIAGNOSIS

- Symptoms can range from asymptomatic interstitial edema of the head and neck to life-threatening complications, such as airway narrowing from upper airway or laryngeal edema and cerebral herniation and ischemia secondary to cerebral edema, as a consequence of venous outflow obstruction.
- Facial plethora, cyanosis, and arm edema are often observed. Physical examination can show presence of venous collaterals on the chest and neck. Close attention should be paid to detect stridor, headaches, or confusion.
- Contrast-enhanced CT scan of the chest allows identification of the underlying cause and level of obstruction.

TREATMENT

- Management of SVC syndrome depends on the presentation and underlying malignancy. Patients presenting with stridor from laryngeal edema and stupor from cerebral edema need emergent management with stent placement and/or radiation. Upfront radiation before obtaining a histologic diagnosis in patients who are stable can obscure a pathologic diagnosis and should not be pursued.
- Steroids have a role in the management of patients with steroid-responsive tumors such as lymphomas and thymomas. Their role in the management of other cancers is unclear and not recommended. Although steroids have anecdotally been used to control edema in patients with airway obstruction, they have not been systematically studied for use in this setting.
- Avoid upper limb cannulation as it may aggravate symptoms.
- Every effort should be made to obtain a pathologic diagnosis in a timely fashion because this information is crucial to plan management. Chemotherapy is the treatment of choice for patients with cancers such as SCLC, lymphomas, and germ cell tumors that tend to be chemosensitive.
- Stent placement and radiotherapy may be required for management and symptom relief of SVC syndrome in patients with less chemoresponsive tumors such as NSCLC.
- Anticoagulation is indicated in patients with SVC thrombosis.

Hyperleukocytosis With Leukostasis

Hyperleukocytosis refers to an elevated white blood cell count (often $>100 \times 10^9$/L) as a result of leukemic proliferation. Leukostasis is a medical emergency as a result of hypoperfusion due to the elevated blast count. The clinical features and emergent management of leukostasis have been summarized in Table 22-15.

Brain Metastases With Increased Intracranial Pressure

- Brain metastases are common in patients with malignancies. Patients with lung cancer, breast cancer, and melanoma have the highest incidence of brain metastases.
- Most lesions are supratentorial and located at the junction of gray and white matter.

DIAGNOSIS

- Headache, confusion, and focal neurologic deficits are the most common symptoms. However, nearly a third of these patients can be asymptomatic.
- CT scan of the head with IV contrast or a brain MRI is required for diagnosis.

TREATMENT

- Increased intracranial pressure from peritumoral edema or hemorrhage can lead to cerebral herniation and death in untreated patients.
- Symptomatic treatment with dexamethasone at an initial dose of 10 mg, followed by 4 mg every 6 hours, usually relieves symptoms.
- Treatment approach depends on several factors including the type of malignancy, its treatment responsiveness, location, number, and size.
- Neurosurgery, stereotactic radiosurgery or whole-brain radiation, and occasionally treatment with chemotherapy or targeted therapies are the commonly employed modalities of treatment.
- Anticonvulsants are indicated only in patients with seizures.

MANAGEMENT OF TREATMENT TOXICITIES

Nausea

- Historically, nausea was one of the most debilitating side effects of chemotherapy. The advent and use of effective antiemetic therapies have made chemotherapy much more tolerable for cancer patients.
- Incidence of chemotherapy-induced nausea and vomiting (CINV) is widely variable and depends on both drug and dose used.
- CINV can be categorized as acute (<24 hours) or delayed (>24 hours). Acute CINV is an important predictor of delayed CINV.
- Based on emetic risk, intravenous chemotherapeutic agents are grouped as high risk (>90%), moderate risk (30%–90%), low risk (10%–30%), and minimal risk groups (<10%), while oral antineoplastic agents are grouped as moderate/high-risk groups (>30%) and minimal- and low-risk groups (<30%).
- **Prevention** of CINV is more effective than treatment. Commonly used prophylactic agents which are used either single or in combination, depending on the emetogenicity of the specific chemotherapy regimen, include:
  - Dexamethasone, which has active antiemetic properties. It is frequently administered via IV before chemotherapy (premedication) and continued orally for 2–3 days with certain chemotherapy regimens.
  - 5-Hydroxytryptamine-3 (5-HT_3) receptor antagonists (ondansetron, granisetron, dolasetron, palonosetron), which are highly effective and widely used as premedications.
  - Aprepitant, NK-1 receptor antagonist, which is used with moderate and highly emetogenic regimens.
  - Olanzapine, an antipsychotic agent, is also effective in preventing and managing CINV associated with highly emetogenic regimens.

TREATMENT

- Post-treatment nausea should not be immediately assumed to be secondary to chemotherapy. Secondary causes, including bowel obstruction, brain metastasis with cerebral edema, constipation, narcotics, and gastroenteritis, should all be considered.

- Initial treatment with prochlorperazine is often effective. Lorazepam and other anxiolytics also have antiemetic properties. 5-HT_3 antagonists are less effective in treatment than in prevention but are frequently used. Olanzapine has also been studied and found to be active in treating CINV.

Diarrhea

- Diarrhea is a common side effect of many chemotherapies (irinotecan, 5FU, capecitabine), targeted agents (erlotinib, cetuximab, sunitinib, lapatinib), and newer immunotherapies (ipilimumab, nivolumab, pembrolizumab).
- Diarrhea can also be a symptomatic manifestation of the underlying cancer (such as carcinoid syndrome in neuroendocrine tumors).
- Imaging of the abdomen, *Clostridium difficile* testing, and even obtaining a colonoscopy might be required in selected patients (e.g., ipilimumab-related colitis).
- Special attention should be paid to transplant patients because testing serum levels of immunosuppressants and testing for opportunistic infections constitute an important part of workup.

TREATMENT

- Hydration to avoid volume depletion is critical.
- Patients who test positive for *C. difficile* should be appropriately managed with suitable antibiotics such as oral vancomycin or metronidazole.
- Empiric and aggressive treatment with loperamide can be considered in patients with chemotherapy-related diarrhea. When loperamide is ineffective, diphenoxylate, atropine, or other similar agents can be used.
- Timely initiation of steroid therapy is important in immunotherapy and GVHD-related diarrhea.

Extravasation Injuries

- Extravasation refers to the escape of a drug into the extravascular space, either by leakage from a vessel or by direct infiltration.
- Based on the severity of local toxicity of extravasated cytotoxic chemotherapy, drugs have been classified as irritants which cause inflammation at the administration site and along the vein; and vesicants which cause tissue necrosis (blistering, sloughing of tissue, and varying degrees of deep tissue damage) with a more severe and/or lasting injury.
- The treatment of extravasation injuries involves immediately stopping the infusion, avoiding flushing the cannula, and making maximal effort to aspirate the remaining drug in the cannula. Topical application of heat (vinca alkaloids, etoposide) or cold (anthracyclines, mitomycin) should be done accordingly. Specific antidotes such as hyaluronidase, corticosteroids, sodium thiosulfate, dexrazoxane, and dimethyl sulfoxide can also be used, depending on the chemotherapeutic agent.

SUPPORTIVE CARE: COMPLICATIONS OF CANCER

Cancer Pain

- The two main mechanisms for pain are nociceptive (somatic or visceral) and neuropathic.
    - Nociceptive pain is caused by stimulation of pain receptors and neuropathic pain by direct injury to the peripheral nervous system or CNS.

  - Somatic pain typically occurs with bone metastases, musculoskeletal inflammation, or after surgery and is characterized by a well-localized, dull, or aching pain.
  - Visceral pain results from tumor infiltration and compression or distention of viscera and is described as diffuse, deep, squeezing, and pressure-like sensation.
  - Neuropathic pain occurs because of tumor infiltration of peripheral nerves, roots, or spinal cord, as well as chemical injury caused by chemotherapy, radiotherapy, or surgery. This pain is described as a sharp or burning sensation.
- These three types of pain may occur alone or in combination in the same patient.
- Cancer pain in adults may be classified into three levels on the basis of a 0–10 numerical scale: mild pain (1–3), moderate pain (4–6), and severe pain (7–10).

TREATMENT

- Cancer pain is usually managed through a stepwise approach (the "WHO ladder"), according to the level of pain.
  - Step 1: Patients with mild pain and not taking opioids may be treated with nonopioid analgesics including NSAIDs or acetaminophen.
  - Step 2: Patients with no response to nonopioids or moderate pain are treated with weak opioids such as codeine, hydrocodone, and oxycodone, either alone or in combination with acetaminophen.
  - Step 3: Severe pain is treated with opioids such as morphine, hydromorphone, methadone, or transdermal fentanyl.
- Tramadol, which has weak affinity to μ-opioid receptors and is considered a nonopioid drug, can be used in patients with mild to moderate pain not responding to NSAIDs and those who wish to defer opioid treatment.
- Co-analgesics should be considered in specific cases.
  - Systemic corticosteroids may be useful in pain caused by bone metastases, increased cranial pressure, spinal cord compression, and nerve compression or infiltration.
  - Tricyclic antidepressants, such as nortriptyline, and anticonvulsants, such as gabapentin, are commonly indicated in neuropathic pain.
  - Bisphosphonates (zoledronic acid and pamidronate) and radiolabeled agents (strontium-89 and samarium-153) may help in treating bone metastases–related pain.
- Patients who experience inadequate pain control despite aggressive opioid therapy or who cannot tolerate opioid titration owing to side effects may benefit from interventional therapies, such as regional infusion of analgesics and neuroablative or neurostimulatory procedures.
- Uncontrolled pain should be treated as a medical emergency. Patients in acute pain may often require opioids dosed through a patient-controlled analgesia delivery system. These patients require close monitoring.

Bone Metastasis

- Commonly seen in patients with prostate, breast, lung, kidney, and bladder cancers and myeloma.
- Bone scan (nuclear imaging with technetium-99m) is sensitive for blastic lesions but not lytic lesions). Concerning lesions on bone scan should be evaluated with plain radiograph films or CT to identify lesions at risk for pathologic fracture.

TREATMENT

- Pain should be managed aggressively with opioids. NSAIDs may offer additional relief.
- Lesions at risk for fracture should be treated surgically or with radiation therapy.
- Bisphosphonates and RANK ligand inhibitors may reduce the risk of fracture and reduce pain.

Fatigue

- Common symptom in cancer, occurring in an estimated 80% of patients with advanced disease.
- Close attention should be paid to any signs of underlying depression, which should be managed appropriately.

TREATMENT

- The first step in the treatment is the identification of treatable contributing factors such as pain, poor nutrition, emotional distress, sleep disturbance, and comorbidities (anemia, infection, organ dysfunction). Appropriate pain management, nutrition support, sleep therapy, exercise, and necessary supportive care can help address some of these issues.
- Transfusion support and erythropoietin may be helpful in selective patients with anemia.
- Psychostimulants such as methylphenidate or modafinil can prove helpful in some patients with severe symptoms.

Anorexia and Cachexia

- Anorexia is defined as loss of appetite with associated weight loss.
- Cachexia is a metabolic syndrome characterized by profound involuntary weight loss.

TREATMENT

- In addition to caloric supplementation, patients may benefit from pharmacologic therapy.
- Megestrol acetate is active, with symptomatic improvement in <1 week. Despite the quick increase in the appetite, it may take several weeks to achieve weight gain. Megestrol is also associated with an increased risk of thromboembolism and should be used with caution in patients with a prior history of such.
- Dexamethasone provides a short-lived improvement, usually without significant weight gain.
- Dronabinol has limited benefits in anorexia and is associated with sedation.

Paraneoplastic Syndromes

Malignant tumors invade local tissue, produce metastasis, and can produce a variety of products that can stimulate hormonal, hematologic, dermatologic, and neurologic responses. Paraneoplastic syndromes are symptom complexes in cancer patients which are not directly related to mass effects, invasion, metastasis, or the secretion of hormones indigenous to the tissue of origin. Common manifestations include cutaneous endocrine, hematologic, neurologic, and others (Table 22-16).

Tumor Markers

Tumor markers are substances present in, or produced by, a tumor itself or produced by the host in response to a tumor that can be used in the diagnosis of cancers or monitoring its prognosis (Table 22-17).

TABLE 22-16 Paraneoplastic Syndrome	
Cutaneous	
Acanthosis nigricans	Carcinoma of stomach, lung, and uterus
Paraneoplastic pemphigus	B-cell lymphoproliferative disorders, CLL, thymoma
Dermatomyositis	Bronchogenic, breast carcinoma
Sign of Leser–Trelat (rapid increase in number and size of seborrheic keratosis)	Adenocarcinoma (stomach, rectum, breast, lungs, colon)
Exfoliative dermatitis	Lymphoma
Acquired diffuse palmoplantar keratoderma	Breast, lung, gastric cancers, leukemia
Bazex syndrome (acrokeratosis paraneoplastica)	Squamous cell carcinoma of the upper aerodigestive tract
Pityriasis rotunda	Hepatocellular ca, gastric ca, leukemia, lymphoma, prostate ca
Paget disease	Invasive breast carcinoma
Erythema gyratum repens	Transitional carcinoma of the kidney, lung adenocarcinoma, breast adenocarcinoma, esophageal adenocarcinoma
Sweet syndrome	Leukemia
Pyoderma gangrenosum	AML, CML, myeloma
Necrolytic migratory erythema	Glucagonoma
Hypertrophic osteoarthropathy and clubbing of the fingers	Bronchogenic carcinoma
Endocrine	
Cushing syndrome	Small-cell carcinoma of lung
Syndrome due to inappropriate antidiuretic hormone secretion	Small-cell carcinoma of lung
Hypercalcemia	Squamous cell carcinoma of lung Renal carcinoma
Carcinoid syndrome	Bronchial carcinoid
Hypoglycemia	Fibrosarcoma
Hematologic	
Polycythemia	Renal carcinoma, hepatocellular carcinoma
Venous thrombosis (Trousseau syndrome)	Pancreatic carcinoma
Disseminated intravascular coagulation	Acute promyelocytic leukemia, prostatic adenocarcinomas
Neurologic	
LEMS, cerebellar degeneration	SCLC, ovary, breast, uterus, Hodgkin disease, and others
Opsomyoclonus	Neuroblastoma, lung, breast
Sensory neuronopathy	SCLC

(Continued)

TABLE 22-16 Paraneoplastic Syndrome (Continued)

Limbic encephalitis	SCLC, testicular, breast
Encephalomyelitis	SCLC, others
Dermatopolymyositis	Lung, uterus, ovary
Multifocal encephalomyelitis/ sensory neuronopathy	SCLC, breast cancer
Stiff-man syndrome	Breast, SCLC
Retinal degeneration	SCLC, melanoma
Neuromyotonia	Thymoma
Others	
Nonbacterial thrombotic endocarditis	Advanced mucus-secreting adenocarcinomas
Nephrotic syndrome	Various cancers
Primary amyloidosis	Multiple myeloma
Secondary amyloidosis	Renal cell carcinoma and other solid tumors
Gastrointestinal dysmotility syndrome	Small-cell carcinoma of lung, lymphoma, ovarian cancer

TABLE 22-17 Tumor Markers

Tumor Markers	Associated Cancer
Placental alkaline phosphatase	Seminoma
Neuron-specific enolase (NSE)	Small-cell carcinoma of lung, neuroblastoma
Tartrate-resistant acid phosphatase (TRAP)	Hairy cell leukemia
Human chorionic gonadotropin (hCG)	Trophoblastic tumors, nonseminomatous tumors of testis
Calcitonin	Medullary carcinoma of thyroid
Catecholamine	Pheochromocytoma
α-Fetoprotein	Hepatocellular carcinoma, nonseminomatous germ cell tumors of testis
Carcinoembryonic antigen (CEA)	Carcinomas of the colon, pancreas, lung, and stomach May also be elevated in cigarette smoking, peptic ulcer disease, inflammatory bowel disease, pancreatitis, hypothyroidism, cirrhosis, and biliary obstruction
CA-125	Malignant conditions—epithelial ovarian carcinoma (including fallopian tube and primary serous peritoneal carcinoma), endometrial carcinoma, endocervical adenocarcinoma, pancreatic carcinoma, etc. Benign conditions—endometriosis, cirrhosis, acute peritonitis, acute pancreatitis, acute pelvic inflammatory disease, first trimester of pregnancy, etc.

(Continued)

TABLE 22-17 Tumor Markers (Continued)

Tumor Markers	Associated Cancer
Human epididymis protein 4 (HE4)	Ovarian tumors
CA 15-3	Breast carcinoma, pancreatic, lung, ovarian, colorectal, and liver cancer In some benign breast and liver diseases
CA 27-29	Breast cancer
CA 19-9	Pancreatic and colorectal cancer
Prostate-specific antigen (PSA)	Prostate carcinoma Other conditions include prostatitis, benign prostatic hypertrophy, prostatic trauma, and after ejaculation
Prostatic acid phosphatase (PAP)	Prostate carcinoma
Thyroglobulin	Thyroid cancer
S-100	Melanoma
Inhibin A and B	Granulosa cell tumor
BCR–ABL mutation	Chronic myeloid leukemia
Beta-2 microglobulin	Multiple myeloma
Bladder tumor-associated antigen	Bladder cancer
Nuclear mitotic apparatus protein (NuMA, NMP22)	Bladder cancer

Targeted Agents in Oncology

Optimization of treatment using targeted therapy (molecules targeting specific enzymes, growth factor receptors, and signal transducers), thereby interfering with a variety of oncogenic cellular processes, is the future of therapy in various cancers (Table 22-18).

TABLE 22-18 Targeted Agents

Molecule Expressed	Targeted Agent
Breast cancer	
Her2/neu receptor	Trastuzumab Lapatinib Neratinib Emtansine Pertuzumab
BRCA 1/2	Olaparib Talazoparib
PDL1	Atezolizumab
PIK3CA	Alpelisib
Ovarian cancer	
BRCA 1/2	Olaparib Rucaparib

(Continued)

TABLE 22-18 Targeted Agents (Continued)

Molecule Expressed	Targeted Agent
Colorectal cancers	
K-RAS wild (absence mutations in exons 2, 3, 4)	Cetuximab
K-RAS and N-RAS (absence mutations in exons 2, 3, 4)	Panitumumab
MSI-H/dMMR	Nivolumab ± ipilimumab or pembrolizumab
Melanomas	
BRAF V600E	Dabrafenib Vemurafenib
BRAF V600E/V600K	Trametinib/cobimetinib + vemurafenib
Solid tumors	
MTRK	Entrectinib/larotrectinib
MSI-H/dMMR	Pembrolizumab
Urothelial carcinoma	
FGFR2/FGFR3	Erdafitinib
PDL1	Pembrolizumab
Lung cancer (non–small-cell lung cancer)	
EGFR (exon 19 DEL)	Osimertinib (third-generation TKI) Afatinib (second-generation TKI) Gefitinib (first-generation TKI)
EGFR (exon 20 insertions)	Amivantamab
EGFR (exon 20-point mutation T790M)	Osimertinib
EGFR (exon 21 SUBS)	Erlotinib Dacomitinib
ALK	Alectinib Brigatinib Crizotinib Ceritinib Lorlatinib
ROS	Crizotinib Ceritinib Lorlatinib
PDL1	Pembrolizumab Nivolumab
T790M	Osimertinib
MET exon 14 skipping mutations	Capmatinib
BRAF V600E	Dabrafenib Trametinib
KRAS-G12C	Sotorasib Adagrasib
RET fusion mutation	Selpercatinib Pralsetinib

Summary

- Cigarette smoking is the most prevalent lung cancer risk factor, although environmental exposures, such as biomass fuels, asbestos, arsenic, and radon, are all important lung factor risk factors with levels of exposure that vary widely across the globe.
- The main known risk factors for gastric cancer are *Helicobacter pylori* infection, tobacco smoking, a high intake of meat, obesity, and alcohol consumption.
- As the third most common malignancy and the second most deadly cancer, colorectal cancer has been increasing in prevalence in South Asia.
- Various types of structural chromosomal abnormalities and intragenetic aberrations occur in AML, as well as epigenetic changes. These are targets of therapy and research.
- Tumor lysis syndrome is an emergency that can occur spontaneously or after the initiation of chemotherapy associated with the following metabolic disorders: hyperkalemia, hyperphosphatemia, hypocalcemia, and hyperuricemia leading to end-organ damage.

Scan the QR code to access chapter references.

23 Diabetes Mellitus and Related Disorders

Cynthia J. Herrick, Janet B. McGill, and Anudeep Gaddam

Diabetes Mellitus

GENERAL PRINCIPLES

- **Diabetes mellitus** is a group of metabolic diseases characterized by hyperglycemia resulting from defects in insulin secretion, insulin action, or both. Diabetes affects an estimated 537 million adults worldwide between the age of 20 and 79 (10.5% of all adults in this age range). By 2030, 643 million people will have diabetes globally, increasing to 783 million by 2045. Among the IDF regions, the Western Pacific has the highest number of people with diabetes (163 million), followed by the South east Asian region (88 million), Europe (59 million), Middle East and North Africa (55 million), and North America and the Caribbean (47.6 million). Currently, the lowest numbers are found in South and Central America (36.1 million) and Africa (19.4 million). Beta-cell dysfunction may play a more prominent role in the pathogenesis of type 2 diabetes in population or subgroups in whom low BMI coexists with a high prevalence of the disease, as seen in Southeast Asia, the type 2B, or the Asian-Indian phenotype.[1] A substantial percentage of affected persons are not diagnosed. Type 2 diabetes mellitus (T2DM) represents 90%–95% of all cases of diabetes, with type 1 diabetes mellitus (T1DM) and other causes representing the remaining 5%–10%.[2,3]
- Persons with diabetes are at risk for microvascular complications, including retinopathy, nephropathy, and neuropathy, and are at increased risk for macrovascular disease.
- T2DM is accompanied by hypertension (approximately 75%) and hyperlipidemia (>50%) in adult patients and is considered a "cardiac risk equivalent" because of the excess risk for macrovascular disease, cardiovascular disease (CVD) events, and mortality.[4]

Classification

Diabetes mellitus is classified into four clinical classes[3]:

1. T1DM accounts for <10% of all cases of diabetes and results from a cellular-mediated autoimmune destruction of the beta (β) cells of the pancreas.
2. T2DM accounts for >90% of all cases of diabetes. Insulin resistance followed by reduced insulin secretion from β cells that are unable to compensate for the increased insulin requirements characterizes T2DM.
3. **Other specific types of diabetes** include those that result from genetic defects in insulin secretion or action (known as monogenic diabetes), pancreatic surgery or disease of the exocrine pancreas (cystic fibrosis), endocrinopathies (e.g., Cushing syndrome, acromegaly), or drugs (corticosteroids, antiretroviral, atypical antipsychotics), and diabetes associated with other syndromes.
4. **Gestational diabetes** (GDM) is glucose intolerance with onset or diagnosis during pregnancy. The prevalence of GDM depends on the criteria used for diagnosis and varies by age and ethnic group (generally from 5%–6% of pregnancies to 15%–20% of pregnancies). Diagnostic criteria for GDM vary based on practice location with a two-step method (50-g, 1-hour screen followed by 100-g, 3-h oral glucose tolerance test [OGTT]) used in the United States and a one-step method (75-g, 2-hour OGTT) more common internationally.[5] About 60% of women with GDM will develop T2DM in the

ensuing 5–10 years, and all remain at an increased risk for the development of T2DM later in life.

- All patients with GDM should undergo diagnostic testing 4–12 weeks postpartum with a 2-h OGTT or fasting plasma glucose and every 1–3 years thereafter with either test or an A1C to determine whether abnormal carbohydrate metabolism has persisted or is recurrent.[5]
- Weight loss and exercise are encouraged to decrease the risk of persistent prediabetes or T2DM after delivery.
- **Maturity-onset diabetes of the young** (**MODY**): Mutations in islet cell transcription factors/glucokinase genes affect 2%–3% of the population, although it often goes unrecognized. Its unique features are as follows: (1) monogenic defect of insulin secretion, (2) autosomal dominant mode of inheritance with glucose intolerance present in at least three successive generations with only one parent affected, and (3) occurrence of onset before the age of 25 years in at least one and ideally two family members. People with MODY usually have a normal BMI. Eleven different genes have been identified so far, mutations in which lead to MODY. Most types can be managed well with diet, exercise, and OHAs. Insulin is very rarely required for management (Table 23-1).[6]
- **Latent autoimmune diabetes in adults** (**LADA**) is a disorder in which, despite the presence of islet cell antibodies (ICA) at the diagnosis of diabetes, the progression of autoimmune beta-cell failure is slow, not usually requiring insulin at least in the first 6 months after diagnosis up to usually 5 years, and sometimes longer.
- **Fibrocalculous pancreatic diabetes** (**FCPD**): Seen almost exclusively in developing countries, FCPD is characterized by a triad of abdominal pain, steatorrhea, and diabetes. Some genes implicated are SPINK-1, cathepsin B, and CTFR genes. Seventy percent of patients with FCPD are males in their second and third decades. Classically, patients are malnourished with low BMI, but very high insulin requirements. While the presence of microvascular complications is similar as in other types of diabetes, the presence of macrovascular complications is rare, believed to be due to young age, lean body, and low lipid levels. Risk of pancreatic cancer is very high in this population.[6]

Drugs Causing Hyperglycemia

- **Drugs interfering with insulin secretion and synthesis:** Phenytoin, beta-blockers, calcium channel blockers, L-asparaginase, tacrolimus
- **Drugs interfering with insulin action:** Glucocorticoids, OCPs, antipsychotics
- **Drugs interfering with insulin secretion and action:** Thiazide diuretics, cyclosporine

DIAGNOSIS

- Progression from impaired fasting glucose or impaired glucose tolerance to T2DM occurs at the rate of 2%–22% (average, about 12%) per year depending on the population studied.
- Lifestyle modification, including a balanced hypocaloric diet to achieve 7% weight loss in overweight patients and regular exercise of ≥150 minutes per week, is recommended for persons with prediabetes to prevent progression to T2DM.[7]
- Metformin may be considered in patients with prior GDM, those with body mass index (BMI) ≥35, age <60 years, or those with progressive hyperglycemia.[7]
- Diagnostic criteria for prediabetes and diabetes are listed in Table 23-2.

TREATMENT

- **Goals of therapy** are alleviation of symptoms; achievement of glycemic, blood pressure, and lipid targets; and prevention of acute and chronic complications of diabetes.

TABLE 23-1 Comparison of the Clinical and Biochemical Features of the Most Common Types of Diabetes

Features	Type I Diabetes	Type 2 Diabetes	GCK-MODY	HNF1A-/HNF4A-MODY
Age of diagnosis (yrs)	10–30	>25	Present from birth, diagnosis at any age	<25 (15–45)
Diabetic ketoacidosis	Common	Rare	Rare	Rare
Insulin dependent	Yes	No	No	No
Parental history of diabetes	<15%	>50% (in young onset)	95%–100%, if tested	60%–90%
Obesity	Uncommon	Common	Uncommon	Uncommon
Insulin resistance	Uncommon	Common	Uncommon	Uncommon
Presence of β-cell antibodies	>90%	Negative	Rare	Rare
C-peptide concentrations	Undetectable/low	Normal/high	Normal	Normal
Optimal first-line treatment	Insulin	Metformin	None/diet	Sulfonylurea derivative/meglitinide

GCK, glucokinase; HNF, hepatocyte nuclear factor; MODY, maturity-onset diabetes of the young.

TABLE 23-2 Diagnosis of Diabetes

Prediabetes Diagnosis (Increased Risk for Developing Diabetes)	Diabetes Diagnosis
A1C 5.7%–6.4% (39–46 mmol/mol)	A1C ≥6.5% (48 mmol/mol)[a]
Fasting plasma glucose (FPG) 100–125 mg/dL (5.6–6.9 mmol/L) (impaired fasting glucose)	FPG ≥126 mg/dL (7.0 mmol/L)[a]
Oral glucose tolerance test (OGTT): Glucose 140–199 mg/dL (7.8–11.0 mmol/L) 2 h after 75-g glucose load (impaired glucose tolerance)	OGTT: Glucose ≥200 mg/dL (11.1 mmol/L) 2 h after 75-g glucose load[a]
	Symptoms of diabetes (polyuria, polydipsia, fatigue, weight loss) and random plasma glucose level ≥200 mg/dL (11.1 mmol/L)

[a]Should be repeated unless unequivocal hyperglycemia is present.

- Glycemic control recommendations are the same for T1DM and T2DM: Fasting and preprandial capillary blood glucose (BG) 80–130 mg/dL (3.9–7.2 mmol/L), postprandial capillary BG <180 mg/dL (<10 mmol/L), and A1C <7% (<53 mmol/mol) or as close to normal as possible while avoiding significant hypoglycemia.[8] The American Association of Clinical Endocrinologists (AACE) recommends an A1C target of <6.5% (<48 mmol/mol) for most adults.[9] This degree of glycemic control has been associated with the lowest risk for microvascular complications in patients with T1DM and T2DM.[10,11]
- Intensive diabetes therapy leading to very tight glycemic control in patients with risk factors for CVD has been associated with increased mortality in two studies,[12,13] but not in others.[14] Hypoglycemia was implicated as the cause of higher mortality in one of the studies.[13] Less tight glycemic goals may be appropriate for patients with a history of cardiovascular disease (CVD) or those at high risk for CV events.[8]
- The blood pressure target for patients with diabetes is <140/90 mm Hg, but a lower goal of <130/80 mm Hg may be considered for younger patients or those at high risk of CVD.[9,15] The use of either an angiotensin-converting enzyme (ACE) inhibitor or an angiotensin receptor blocker (ARB) is recommended as first-line therapy. For patients not at goal, a thiazide diuretic should be added if the glomerular filtration rate (GFR) is >30 mL/min/1.73 m^2 and a loop diuretic added if the GFR is <30 mL/min/1.73 m^2.[2,9,15]
- High-intensity statin therapy (atorvastatin 40–80 mg daily or rosuvastatin 20–40 mg daily) is recommended in all patients with diabetes and CVD as well as in patients age 40–75 with CVD risk factors.[9,15] Moderate-intensity statin therapy can be considered in patients age 40–75 with no other CVD risk factors and in patients with age <40 or >75 with CVD risk factors.
- The low-density lipoprotein (LDL) goal for patients with diabetes and CVD is <70 mg/dL (3.9 mmol/L). If that goal is not achieved with statin therapy, the addition of either ezetimibe or a PCSK9 inhibitor is advised.[9,15]
- Aspirin therapy should be advised in patients with diabetes who are older than 50 years (both men and women) with any one additional risk factor (family history of premature ASCVD, systemic HTN, dyslipidemia, smoking, CKD/albuminuria) and not at increased risk of bleeding. Low doses (75–162 mg) are appropriate for primary prevention.[15]
- **Assessment of glycemic control** consists of the following:
  - **Self-monitoring of blood glucose (SMBG)** is recommended for all patients who take insulin and provides useful information for those on noninsulin therapies. Patients using multiple daily injections or insulin pumps should test their blood glucose three or more times daily. Less frequent testing may be appropriate for those on noninsulin therapies. Although most SMBG is done before meals and at bedtime, periodic testing 1–2 hours after eating may be necessary to achieve postprandial glucose targets.[8]
  - **Continuous glucose monitoring (CGM)** has been shown to reduce A1C in adults older than 25 years and reduce hypoglycemia in patients of all ages on intensive insulin therapy. CGM measures interstitial glucose, which provides a close approximation of BG values. Hypoglycemia and hyperglycemia alarms may help patients with widely fluctuating BG levels or hypoglycemia unawareness. Some of the CGM devices are approved for insulin dosing and may supplant the need for SMBG.
  - **A1C** provides an integrated measure of BG values over the preceding 2–3 months. A1C should be obtained every 3 months in patients not at goal or when either diabetes therapy or clinical condition changes and twice yearly in well-controlled patients. A1C should confirm results of SMBG or CGM, and discordant values should be investigated. An A1C level that is higher than expected should be evaluated by a diabetes educator to ensure meter accuracy, appropriate technique, and frequency of testing. When the A1C is lower than expected, blood loss, transfusion, hemolysis, and hemoglobin variants should be considered. The correlation between A1C and mean plasma

glucose is sufficiently strong that laboratory reports may include both the A1C result and the estimated average glucose.[8]

- Fructosamine and glycated albumin are becoming HbA1c surrogates, especially in select patients in whom the measurement of HbA1c may be biased or even unreliable. These especially include patients with rapid changes of glucose homeostasis and larger glycemic excursions (i.e., temporarily high blood glucose spikes), red blood cell disorders, and CKD.
- **Ketones** can be detected in a fingerstick blood sample by measuring β-hydroxybutyrate with a handheld meter. Urine ketones can be qualitatively identified, using Ketostix or Acetest tablets. Patients with T1DM should test for ketones during febrile illness, for persistent elevation of glucose (>300 mg/dL [16.7 mmol/L]), or if signs of impending diabetic ketoacidosis (e.g., nausea, vomiting, abdominal pain) develop. Testing for β-hydroxybutyrate is useful in emergency departments to determine whether a patient with hyperglycemia has ketonemia.[16]
- **Autoantibodies:** These include antibodies to cytoplasmic proteins in the beta cell/ICA, antibodies to glutamic acid decarboxylase (GAD-65), insulin autoantibodies (IAA), and antibodies to protein tyrosine phosphatase (IA-2A).

Autoantibodies against GAD-65 are found in 80% of type 1 diabetics at clinical presentation. Presence of ICA and IA-2A at diagnosis for type 1 diabetes ranges from 69%–90% to 54%–75%, respectively.

MANAGEMENT

Comprehensive diabetes management includes coordinated diet, exercise, and medication plans. **Patient education** in medical nutrition therapy, exercise, SMBG, medication use, and insulin dosing and administration is integral to the successful management of diabetes.

Medical Nutrition Therapy

- Medical nutrition therapy includes dietary recommendations for a healthy, balanced diet to achieve adequate nutrition and maintain an ideal body weight.[17]
- Caloric restriction is recommended for overweight individuals, with individualized targets that may be as low as 1000–1500 kcal/d for women and 1200–1800 kcal/d for men depending on activity level and starting body weight.
- Caloric intake is usually distributed as follows: 45%–65% of total calories as carbohydrates, 10%–30% as protein, and <30% as total fat (<7% saturated fat) with <300 mg/d of cholesterol.
- In patients with LDL cholesterol >100 mg/dL (2.6 mmol/L), total fat should be restricted to <25% of total calories, saturated fat to <7% of calories, and cholesterol to <200 mg/d.
- Patients with progressive kidney disease may benefit from restriction of protein intake to 0.8 g/kg/d. Patients with severe chronic kidney disease (CKD) will need additional restrictions of potassium- and phosphorus-containing foods.
- "Carbohydrate counting" is a useful skill for patients on intensified insulin therapy who adjust insulin doses based on the carbohydrate content of meals and snacks.

Exercise

Exercise improves insulin sensitivity, reduces fasting and postprandial BG levels, and offers numerous metabolic, CV, and psychological benefits in patients with diabetes.

- In general, 150 minutes per week is recommended as part of a healthy lifestyle and has been shown to assist with the prevention and management of T2DM in adults.[17]
- Patients may need individualized guidance regarding exercise, and they are more likely to exercise when counseled by their physician to do so.

Diabetes Mellitus in Hospitalized Patients

GENERAL PRINCIPLES

Diabetes-specific indications for hospitalization

- **Diabetic ketoacidosis (DKA)** is characterized by a plasma glucose level of >250 mg/dL (13.9 mmol/L) in association with an arterial pH <7.30 or serum bicarbonate level of <15 mEq/L and moderate ketonemia or ketonuria; however, patients may present with ketoacidosis and lower glucose levels.[18,19]
- **Hyperosmolar hyperglycemic state (HHS)** includes marked hyperglycemia (≥600 mg/dL [33.3 mmol/L]) and elevated serum osmolality (>320 mOsm/kg), often accompanied by impaired mental status.[20]
- **Hypoglycemia** is an indication for hospitalization if it is induced by a sulfonylurea (SFU) medication, is due to a deliberate drug overdose, or results in coma, seizure, injury, or persistent neurologic change.
- **Newly diagnosed T1DM** or newly recognized GDM can be indications for hospitalization, even in the absence of ketoacidosis.
- **Patients with T2DM** are rarely admitted to the hospital for initiation or change in insulin therapy unless hyperglycemia is severe and associated with mental status change or other organ dysfunction.

Management of diabetes in hospitalized patients

Hyperglycemia (BG ≥140 mg/dL [7.8 mmol/L]) is a common finding in hospitalized patients and may be due to previously diagnosed diabetes, undiagnosed diabetes, medications, or stress-induced hyperglycemia. Up to 40% of general medical and surgical patients exhibit hyperglycemia, and approximately 80% of intensive care unit (ICU) patients will demonstrate transient or persistent hyperglycemia.[18]

- Patients with T1DM should be clearly identified as such at the time of admission.
- A1C can help identify previously undiagnosed diabetes in hospitalized patients and may assist with the evaluation of prior glucose control. A1C is not accurate in patients who are severely anemic, experience bleeding, undergoing hemolysis, or have been transfused.[18]
- Data regarding use of noninsulin therapies in inpatients are increasing. Dipeptidyl peptidase 4 inhibitor use alone or with basal insulin may provide adequate glucose control with less hypoglycemia than basal-bolus insulin regimens.[18]
- Medication reconciliation on admission should include a careful assessment of home diabetes medications, level of glucose control, kidney function, expected diagnostic studies and treatments, and the possible need for insulin treatment.
- Patients who are required to fast for diagnostic testing or treatments should have all noninsulin therapies stopped.
- **Patients hospitalized for reasons other than diabetes and who are eating normally** may continue or restart outpatient diabetes treatments, unless specifically contraindicated.
- Use of noninsulin therapies may be appropriate in psychiatric units, rehabilitation settings, or stable patients preparing for discharge.
- **Glucose targets for inpatients** aim to reduce morbidity and mortality, while minimizing hypoglycemia.
  - In critical care settings, the glucose target is 140–180 mg/dL (7.8–10.0 mmol/L) with frequent monitoring recommended to avoid hypoglycemia.[18]
  - In noncritical care settings, the glucose target is <140 mg/dL (7.8 mmol/L) fasting and premeal and <180 mg/dL (10.0 mmol/L) postmeal or on a random glucose check with reassessment of the insulin regimen if glucose falls below 100 mg/dL (5.6 mmol/L).[18,19,21]

Management of hyperglycemia in critical care settings

- Variable IV insulin infusion is recommended for critical illness, emergency surgery, or major surgery. Numerous algorithms have been published that direct insulin dose adjustments based on capillary BG values performed hourly at the bedside.
- An IV infusion of a dextrose-containing solution or other caloric source should be provided to prevent hypoglycemia and ketosis. For fluid-restricted patients, 10% dextrose in water (D10W) can be infused at a rate of 10–25 mL/h to provide a steady, consistent source of calories.
- An intermediate- or long-acting insulin should be given 2 hours prior to insulin infusion discontinuation.

Management of hyperglycemia in non–critical care hospital settings

- BG should be checked on admission in all patients and monitored four times per day in hyperglycemic patients, especially in patients treated with insulin.
- Scheduled insulin with basal, nutritional, and correction components provides superior glycemic control compared with correction or "sliding scale" insulin alone.[18,19,21]
- For patients who are naïve to insulin, the starting dose of basal insulin should equal 0.1–0.2 units/kg. Scheduled premeal insulin should be 0.1–0.2 units/kg divided by three meals. **Example:** Your patient weighs 80 kg. The starting insulin dose should be 8–16 units of long-acting insulin plus 3–5 units of rapid-acting insulin before each meal. A correction dose of 1–2 units per 50 mg/dL (2.8 mmol/L) of BG, beginning at 140 mg/dL (7.8 mmol/L), can be added to the premeal doses.
- Patients with T1DM should continue their home insulin doses and may continue the use of an insulin pump if there is a hospital policy in place to do so. Insulin doses in patients with T2DM should be reduced by 20%–40% on admission. If their home insulin dose is excessive compared with a weight-based dose of 0.4–0.5 units/kg or distribution between basal and premeal insulin is uneven, further reductions and adjustments may be necessary.
- Meal-time insulin doses should be given shortly before or immediately after meals, and the correction factor or sliding scale dose should be added to the premeal dose.
- The glucose threshold for sliding scale (corrective) insulin should be higher at bedtime, or corrective insulin should not be given at bedtime. Adjustments in the next-day basal or premeal insulin doses are indicated if correction doses of insulin are frequently required or if clinical status or medications change.
- Extreme hyperglycemia (≥300 mg/dL [16.7 mmol/L]) on one or more consecutive tests should prompt testing for ketoacidosis with electrolytes and ketone measurements.
- Hypoglycemia should be treated promptly with oral or IV glucose, and the capillary BG should be repeated every 10 minutes until >100 mg/dL (5.5 mmol/L) and stable.

  Reevaluation of scheduled doses and assessment of risk factors for hypoglycemia (declining renal function, hepatic impairment, poor intake) should be undertaken for any BG <70 mg/dL (3.9 mmol/L).[18]
- **Enteral nutrition:** Intermittent tube feeds should be matched by either short-acting (human regular) insulin or intermediate-acting (human NPH [neutral protamine Hagedorn]) insulin. Patients with baseline hyperglycemia may need a basal insulin dose in addition to the doses given to cover tube feeds. For example, nighttime enteral feeding lasting 6–8 hours should be managed with NPH, with or without a basal insulin dose. NPH can be given three to four times daily for continuous tube feeds, allowing a change in insulin dose if the feeding is interrupted.[18,19,21]
- **Total parenteral nutrition (TPN):** Patients supported with TPN are likely to develop hyperglycemia, and some require large amounts of insulin. See Chapter 2, Nutrition Support, for insulin management of patients on TPN.

Diabetic Ketoacidosis

GENERAL PRINCIPLES

Epidemiology

DKA, a potentially fatal complication of diabetes, occurs in up to 5% of patients with T1DM annually and can occur in insulin-deficient patients with T2DM.

Pathophysiology

DKA is a catabolic condition that results from severe insulin deficiency, often in association with stress and activation of counterregulatory hormones (e.g., catecholamines, glucagon).

Risk Factors

Precipitating factors for DKA include inadvertent or deliberate interruption of insulin therapy, sepsis, trauma, myocardial infarction (MI), and pregnancy. DKA may be the first presentation of T1DM and, rarely, T2DM. DKA with euglycemia or lower-than-expected glucoses can occur with the use of antidiabetes drugs like the sodium glucose cotransport inhibitor 2 (SGLT-2), with atypical antipsychotic agents and with some cancer chemotherapy.

Prevention

DKA can be prevented in many cases, and its occurrence suggests a breakdown in education, communication, and problem solving. Therefore, diabetes education should be reinforced at every opportunity, with special emphasis on (1) self-management skills during sick days; (2) the body's need for more, rather than less, insulin during such illnesses; (3) testing of blood or urine for ketones; and (4) procedures for obtaining timely and preventive medical advice.

DIAGNOSIS

History

- Patients may describe a variety of symptoms including polyuria, polydipsia, weight loss, nausea, vomiting, and vaguely localized abdominal pain generally in the setting of persistent hyperglycemia. A high index of suspicion is warranted because clinical presentation may be nonspecific.
- Tachycardia; decrease of capillary filling; rapid, deep, and labored breathing (Kussmaul respiration); and fruity breath odor are common physical findings.
- Prominent gastrointestinal (GI) symptoms and abdominal tenderness on examination may give rise to suspicion for intra-abdominal pathology.
- Dehydration is invariable, and respiratory distress, shock, and coma can occur.

Diagnostic Testing

- High anion gap metabolic acidosis.
- Positive serum β-hydroxybutyrate or ketones (a semiquantitative measurement of acetone, acetoacetate, and β-hydroxybutyrate) and positive urine ketones.
- Plasma glucose ≥250 mg/dL (13.9 mmol/L). Euglycemic DKA (plasma glucose <200 mg/dL [11.1 mmol/L]) has been described in pregnancy, alcohol ingestion, fasting or starvation, during hospitalization, and in patients with both T1DM and T2DM treated with SGLT-2 inhibitors.[22] Hyponatremia, hyperkalemia, azotemia, and hyperosmolality are other possible findings.
- A focused search for a precipitating infection is recommended if clinically indicated.
- An ECG should be obtained to evaluate electrolyte abnormalities and for unsuspected myocardial ischemia.

TREATMENT

Management of DKA should preferably be conducted in an ICU (Table 23-3). **If treatment is conducted in a non-ICU setting, close monitoring is mandatory until ketoacidosis resolves and the patient's condition is stabilized.** The therapeutic priorities are fluid replacement, adequate insulin administration, and potassium repletion. Administration of bicarbonate, phosphate, magnesium, or other therapies is not routinely advised but may be appropriate in selected patients.[19]

- **Monitoring of therapy**
  - BG levels should be monitored hourly, serum electrolyte levels every 2–4 hours, and arterial blood gas values as often as necessary for a severely acidotic or hypoxic patient.
  - Serum sodium tends to rise as hyperglycemia is corrected; failure to observe this trend suggests that the patient is being overhydrated with free water.
  - Dextrose should be initiated when the blood glucose is <250 mg/dL (13.9 mmol/L) or is predicted to fall to <200 mg/dL (11.1 mmol/L) in 1 hour. Use of a separate dextrose-containing fluid bag allows the fluid resuscitation and glucose infusion to be titrated separately (two-bag approach) and has been shown to result in shorter duration of treatment.[23]
  - Serial measurements of β-hydroxybutyrate in addition to electrolytes may provide additional information about recovery. Restoration of renal buffering capacity by normalization of the serum bicarbonate level is the most reliable index of metabolic recovery. Note that hyperchloremia may cause closure of the anion gap before the serum bicarbonate level has normalized, making anion gap closure a less reliable indicator of recovery of DKA than serum bicarbonate.[19]
  - Use of a flowchart is an efficient method of tracking clinical data (e.g., weight, fluid balance, mental status) and laboratory results during the management of DKA.
  - Telemetry is recommended given the propensity to electrolyte abnormalities.
- **IV antimicrobial therapy** should be started promptly for documented or suspected bacterial, fungal, and other treatable infections. Empiric broad-spectrum antibiotics can be started in septic patients pending results of blood cultures. Note that DKA is not typically accompanied by fever, so infection must be considered in a febrile patient.

COMPLICATIONS

Complications of DKA include life-threatening conditions that must be recognized and treated promptly.

- **Lactic acidosis** may result from prolonged dehydration, shock, infection, and tissue hypoxia in DKA patients. Lactic acidosis should be suspected in patients with refractory metabolic acidosis and a persistent anion gap despite optimal therapy for DKA. Management includes adequate volume replacement, control of sepsis, and judicious use of bicarbonate.
- **Arterial thrombosis** manifesting as stroke, MI, or an ischemic limb occurs with increased frequency in DKA. However, routine anticoagulation is not indicated except as part of the specific therapy for a thrombotic event.
- **Cerebral edema** is observed more frequently in children than in adults.[19]
  - Symptoms of increased intracranial pressure (e.g., headache, altered mental status, papilledema) or a sudden deterioration in mental status after initial improvement in a patient with DKA should raise suspicion for cerebral edema.
  - Overhydration with free water and excessively rapid correction of hyperglycemia are known risk factors. Watch for a decrease in serum sodium level or failure to rise during therapy.

TABLE 23-3 Treatment of Diabetic Ketoacidosis

IV Fluids	**Replete Circulating Volume**
Goals: First, replete circulating volume and then replenish total-body water deficit	0.9% saline: 1 L bolus and then 500–1000 mL/h if cardiac and renal function normal
Estimate fluid deficit by subtracting current weight from recent dry weight	**Replenish total-body water deficit** 0.45% saline (0.9% saline if hyponatremic): 150–500 mL/h
Usually 7%–9% of body weight Hypotension → >10% loss of body fluids (Diabetes Care. 2004;27:S94)	Adjust repletion according to BP and UOP examinations; no faster than 3 mOsm/kg/h; aim for positive fluid balance over 12–24 h
Insulin	**Do not start until K >3.5 mmol/L**
Goals: Turn off ketogenesis; correct hyperglycemia	**Bolus: 0.1 units/kg**
	Infusion: 0.1 units/kg/h
	(Regular insulin 100 units in 100 mL 0.9% saline at 10 mL/h = 10 units/h)
	Goal decrease in BG = 50–75 mg/dL/h (2.8–4.2 mmol/L/h)
	Avoid correcting >100 mg/dL/h (5.6 mmol/L/h) to reduce risk of osmotic encephalopathy
	Continue at 1–2 units per hour until HCO_3 >15 mEq/L, clinical improvement, and anion gap closed
	Administer SC basal insulin 2 h prior to stopping insulin infusion
Dextrose (5%)	Add when BG <250 mg/dL (13.9 mmol/L)
Goal: Prevent hypoglycemia	Consider giving glucose as a separate infusion of 50–100 mL/h (two-bag approach). Concurrently reduce insulin infusion to 0.05 units/kg/h
Potassium as KCl	Add to fluids at 10–20 mEq/h
Goal: Prevent hypokalemia as insulin shifts potassium into the cell	
Bicarbonate	Not routinely recommended
	May consider if (1) shock/coma; (2) pH <6.9; (3) HCO_3 <5 mEq/L; (4) cardiac/respiratory dysfunction; or (5) severe hyperkalemia
	50–100 mEq in 1 L 0.45% saline over 30–60 min; follow arterial pH
	Avoid hypokalemia by adding 10 mEq KCl
Phosphate and magnesium	Not routinely recommended
	May give KPhos IV fluids if not eating
	May give 10–20 mEq of magnesium sulfate IV with ventricular arrhythmias

BG, blood glucose; BP, blood pressure; HCO_3, bicarbonate; K, potassium; KCl, potassium chloride; KPhos, potassium phosphate; UOP, urine output.

  - Neuroimaging with a CT scan can establish the diagnosis. Prompt recognition and treatment with IV mannitol is essential and may prevent neurologic sequelae in patients who survive cerebral edema.
- **Rebound ketoacidosis** can occur because of premature cessation of IV insulin infusion or inadequate doses of subcutaneous (SC) insulin after the insulin infusion has been discontinued. All patients with T1DM and patients with T2DM who develop DKA (indicating severe insulin deficiency) require both basal and premeal insulin in adequate doses to avoid recurrence of metabolic decompensation.

Hyperosmolar Hyperglycemic State

GENERAL PRINCIPLES

HHS is one of the most serious life-threatening complications of T2DM.[24]

Epidemiology

- HHS occurs primarily in patients with T2DM, and in 30%–40% of cases, it is the initial presentation of a patient's diabetes.[24]
- HHS is significantly less common than DKA, with an incidence of <1 case per 1000 person-years.

Pathophysiology

- Ketoacidosis is absent because the ambient insulin level may effectively prevent lipolysis and subsequent ketogenesis while being inadequate to facilitate peripheral glucose uptake and to prevent hepatic residual gluconeogenesis and glucose output.
- Precipitating factors for HHS include dehydration, stress, infection, stroke, noncompliance with medications, dietary indiscretion, and alcohol and cocaine abuse. Impaired glucose excretion is a contributory factor in patients with renal insufficiency or prerenal azotemia.

DIAGNOSIS

Clinical Presentation

In contrast to DKA, the onset of HHS is usually insidious. Several days of deteriorating glycemic control are followed by increasing lethargy. Clinical evidence of severe dehydration is the rule. Some alterations in consciousness and focal neurologic deficits may be found at presentation or may develop during therapy. Therefore, repeated neurologic assessment is recommended.

Differential Diagnosis

The differential diagnosis of HHS includes any cause of altered level of consciousness, including hypoglycemia, hyponatremia, severe dehydration, uremia, hyperammonemia, drug overdose, and sepsis. Seizures and acute stroke-like syndromes are common presentations.

Diagnostic Testing

Clinical findings include (1) hyperglycemia, often >600 mg/dL (33.3 mmol/L); (2) plasma osmolality >320 mOsm/L; (3) absence of ketonemia; and (4) pH >7.3 and serum bicarbonate level of >20 mEq/L (>15 mmol/L in UK guidelines). Prerenal azotemia and lactic acidosis can develop. Although some patients will have detectable urine ketones, most patients do not have a metabolic acidosis. Lactic acidosis may develop from an underlying ischemia, infection, or other cause.[19,24]

TREATMENT

- See Table 23-4 for detailed treatment recommendations.
- **Underlying illness:** Detection and treatment of any underlying predisposing illness are critical in the treatment of HHS. Antibiotics should be administered early, after appropriate cultures, in patients in whom infection is known or suspected as a precipitant to HHS. A high index of suspicion should be maintained for underlying pancreatitis, GI bleeding, renal failure, and thromboembolic events, especially acute MI.

COMPLICATIONS

Complications of HHS include thromboembolic events (cerebral and MI, mesenteric thrombosis, pulmonary embolism, and disseminated intravascular coagulation), cerebral edema, acute respiratory distress syndrome, and rhabdomyolysis.

TABLE 23-4 Treatment of Hyperosmolar Hyperglycemic State

IV Fluids Goals: Restore hemodynamic stability and intravascular volume by fluid replacement; this is the primary treatment and supersedes insulin; patients often require much more fluid than with diabetic ketoacidosis	**Replete Circulating Volume** 0.9% saline × 1–1.5 L **Replenish total-body water deficit** 0.45% Saline if Na is elevated Aim for positive fluid balance over 24–72 h; may require 10–12 L
Potassium as KCl Goal: Prevent hypokalemia as insulin shifts potassium into the cell	Add to fluids at 10–20 mEq/h; begin as soon as urine output confirmed
Insulin Goals: Plays a secondary role; slowly corrects hyperglycemia	**Do not start until K >3.5 mmol/L** **Bolus: 5–10 units (if BG >600 mg/dL); smaller bolus if BG <600 mg/dL (33.3 mmol/L)** **Infusion: 0.10–0.15 units/kg/h** Avoid correcting >100 mg/dL/h (5.6 mmol/L/h) to reduce risk of osmotic encephalopathy **Administer SC basal insulin 2 h prior to stopping insulin infusion**
Dextrose (5%)	Add when BG 250–300 mg/dL (13.9–16.7 mmol/L)
Goal: Prevent hypoglycemia	Can give as a separate infusion of 50–100 mL/h (two-bag approach) Concurrently reduce insulin infusion to 1–2 units/h
Bicarbonate	Not routinely recommended
	May be required if concurrent lactic acidosis

BG, blood glucose; K, potassium; KCl, potassium chloride.

MONITORING/FOLLOW-UP

- **Monitoring of therapy:** Use of a flowchart is helpful for tracking clinical data and laboratory results.
- Initially, BG levels should be monitored every 30–60 minutes and serum electrolyte levels every 2–4 hours; frequency of monitoring can be decreased during recovery.
- Neurologic status must be reassessed frequently; persistent lethargy or altered mentation indicates inadequate therapy. On the other hand, relapse after initial improvement in mental status suggests too rapid correction of serum osmolarity.

Type 1 Diabetes

GENERAL PRINCIPLES

A comprehensive approach is necessary for successful management of T1DM. A team approach that includes the expertise of physicians, diabetes educators, dietitians, and other members of the diabetes care team offers the best chance of success.

DIAGNOSIS

T1DM can present at any age, and because of the variable time course and severity of hyperglycemia, the diagnosis can be challenging in adults.

- The rate of destruction of β cells is rapid in infants and children and slower in adults. Therefore, ketoacidosis as an initial presentation is more common in young patients.
- T1DM is characterized by severe insulin deficiency. Exogenous insulin is required to control BGs, prevent DKA, and preserve life. Ketosis develops in 8–16 hours and ketoacidosis in 12–24 hours without insulin.
- Early in the course of T1DM, some insulin secretory capacity remains, and the insulin requirement may be lower than expected (0.3–0.4 units/kg). Tight control of BG level from the onset has been shown to preserve the residual β-cell function and prevent or delay later complications.
- LADA is characterized by mild to moderate hyperglycemia at presentation that often responds to noninsulin therapies, initially in the first 6 months after diagnosis. Adults with LADA will have one or more β cell–specific autoantibodies and tend to require insulin therapy sooner than patients with classic T2DM (months to years).
- T1DM should be suspected when there is a family history of T1DM, thyroid disease, or other autoimmune disease. Presentation with ketoacidosis suggests T1DM, but confirmatory tests may be useful to guide therapy.
- Autoantibodies include islet cell autoantibodies, antibodies to insulin, antibodies to GAD (anti-GAD), antibodies to zinc transporter 8 (ZnT8), and antibodies to tyrosine phosphatases IA-2 and IA-2β. Measuring one or more of these autoantibodies along with a C-peptide can help to confirm the diagnosis of T1DM; however, 20% of insulin-deficient adults are antibody negative.[3]

TREATMENT

Treatment of T1DM requires lifelong insulin replacement and careful coordination of insulin doses with food intake and activity.[25]

- A regimen of **multiple daily insulin injections** that include basal, premeal, and correction doses is preferred to obtain optimal control in both hospitalized patients and outpatients. This regimen implies that capillary glucose monitoring will occur four times daily, 10–30 minutes before meals and at bedtime or that a patient is using a CGM device.

- The **insulin requirement** for optimal glycemic control is approximately 0.5–0.8 units/kg/d for the average nonobese patient. A conservative total daily dose (TDD) of 0.4 units/kg/d is given initially to a newly diagnosed patient; the dose is then adjusted, using SMBG values. Higher doses may be required in obese or insulin-resistant patients, in adolescents, and in the latter part of pregnancy.
- **Basal insulin** (administered as NPH twice daily, detemir once or twice daily, glargine once or twice daily, or insulin degludec once daily) should provide 40%–50% of the TDD of insulin and should be adjusted by 5%–10% daily until the fasting glucose is consistently <130 mg/dL (7.2 mmol/L). In general, basal insulin is given regardless of nothing by mouth (NPO) or dietary status and should not be held without a direct order.
- **Premeal insulin** doses of insulin are given to cover caloric intake at meals or with snacks. Bolus doses are adjusted according to the BG, the anticipated carbohydrate intake, and the anticipated activity level. The total premeal complement should roughly equal the total basal dose, with one-third given before or after each meal. Rapid-acting insulins (lispro, aspart, glulisine, or inhaled technosphere insulin) are preferred, but regular human insulin can be used.
- The third component of a comprehensive insulin regimen is "**correction factor**" insulin, which is similar to sliding scale, adjusted according to the premeal fingerstick glucose testing and the patient's estimated insulin sensitivity. In general, patients with lower BMI should use a less aggressive scale than patients with higher BMI or more insulin-resistant patients. Correction factor and premeal doses should use the same insulin and be given together in the same syringe. At times, a correction dose of rapid-acting insulin may be needed to treat hyperglycemia in the absence of food intake.

- **Insulin preparations:** After SC injection, there is individual variability in the duration and peak activity of insulin preparations and day-to-day variability in the same subject (Table 23-5).
- **SC insulin administration:** The abdomen, thighs, buttocks, and upper arms are the preferred sites for SC insulin injection. Absorption is fastest from the abdomen, followed by the arm, buttocks, and thigh, probably as a result of differences in blood flow. Injection sites should be rotated within the regions, rather than randomly across separate regions, to minimize erratic absorption. Exercise or massage over the injection site may accelerate insulin absorption.
    - Regular human insulin is now available in an inhaled form as technosphere insulin. This comes in 4-, 8- and 12-unit cartridges for bolus dose insulin administration. Onset occurs at 0.2–0.25 hour with peak effect within the first hour and a duration of action of 3 hours. It is contraindicated in patients with asthma or chronic obstructive pulmonary disease because of risk of bronchospasm. Pulmonary function tests are required prior to starting and at regular intervals during therapy.
- **Continuous SC insulin infusion** using an insulin pump is widely used for insulin delivery in patients with T1DM and increasingly in T2DM. Use of an insulin pump integrated with CGM, known as a sensor-augmented pump (SAP), adds additional features such as suspension of insulin delivery on reaching a preset low threshold or above the threshold if glucose is declining and predicted to reach a hypoglycemic value within a specified period. Progress in insulin delivery devices and continuous monitoring show promise for reliable hybrid closed loop systems (the patient inputs bolus dose information) or fully closed loop systems.
    - A typical regimen provides 50% of total daily insulin as basal insulin and the remainder as multiple preprandial boluses of insulin, using a programmable insulin pump. A rapid-acting insulin (aspart, lispro, or glulisine) is used to fill the pump and is infused continuously to provide basal insulin.
    - Insulin pumps have advanced features that allow patients to fine-tune their basal and bolus doses but require diabetes education to use the pump to its full potential.

TABLE 23-5 Approximate Kinetics of Insulin Preparations

Insulin Type	Onset of Action (h)	Peak Effect (h)	Duration of Activity (h)
Rapid-acting			
Lispro, aspart, glulisine	0.25–0.50	0.50–1.50	3–5
Regular	0.50–1.00	2–4	6–8
Technosphere insulin	0.25–0.5	1.0–1.5	2–3
Intermediate-acting			
NPH	1–2	6–12	16–20
Lente[a]	1–2	6–12	16–20
Long-acting[b]			
Detemir	3–4	8–12	18–24
Glargine	4–6	Possible[c]	20–24
Ultralente[a]	3–4	Variable	18–24
PZI[a]	3–4	Unclear	18–24
Degludec	3–4	Flat	24–40

[a]Not available in the United States; possibly generic manufacturers.
[b]Some patients with type 1 diabetes have improved control when the long-acting basal insulin is given twice a day rather than once daily.
[c]Insulin dosage and individual variability in absorption and clearance rates affect pharmacokinetic data. Duration of insulin activity is prolonged in renal failure. After a lag time of approximately 5 hours, insulin glargine generally has a mostly flat peakless effect over a 22- to 24-hour period; however, broad peaks can occur. Insulin degludec has the longest duration of action, allowing administration at any time of the day.
NPH, neutral protamine Hagedorn; PZI, protamine zinc insulin.

Patients must check their blood sugars regularly because DKA can occur rapidly if the insulin infusion is disrupted (i.e., faulty infusion set).

- SAPs integrated with CGM offer additional protection from hypoglycemia by suspending the pump on reaching a low glucose threshold or prior to the low being reached.
- Hybrid closed loop systems, whereby the patient inputs bolus dose information and calibrates the system regularly, are currently available. Fully closed loop systems, whereby the patient will not manually enter information, are in development.

Type 2 Diabetes

GENERAL PRINCIPLES

- T2DM results from defective insulin secretion followed by loss of β-cell mass in response to increased demand as a result of insulin resistance.[26]
- T2DM is usually diagnosed in adults, with both incidence and prevalence increasing with age; however, T2DM now accounts for up to one-third of new cases of diabetes diagnosed between the ages of 5 and 15 years.

- T2DM is associated with obesity, family history of diabetes, history of GDM or prediabetes, hypertension, physical inactivity, and race/ethnicity. African Americans, Latinos, Asian Indians, Native Americans, Pacific Islanders, and some groups of Asians have a greater risk of developing T2DM than Caucasians.[3,7]
- T2DM may be asymptomatic and, therefore, can remain undiagnosed for months to years.
- The loss of pancreatic β cells is progressive. Insulin secretion is usually sufficient to prevent ketosis, but DKA or HHS can develop during severe stress. T2DM in patients who present with or later develop ketosis or DKA, but who do not require insulin between episodes, is termed ketosis-prone T2DM.[3]
- The mechanisms underlying the β-cell loss in T2DM are unknown, but programmed cell death in response to genetic and environmental factors has been demonstrated in animal models.[27]

TREATMENT

Medications

- The achievement of glycemic control requires individualized therapy and a comprehensive approach that incorporates lifestyle and pharmacologic interventions. Guidelines have been published by several professional organizations regarding the choice and sequence of antidiabetic therapy.[9,28]
- Considerations for selecting noninsulin therapy (Table 23-6) in patients with T2DM include the following:
  - Oral therapy should be initiated early in conjunction with diet and exercise.
  - Metformin is the recommended first-line therapy if tolerated.
  - The glucose-lowering effects of metformin, insulin secretagogues, DPP-4 inhibitors glucagon-like peptide-1 (GLP-1) receptor analogs, and SGLT-2 inhibitors are observed within days to weeks, whereas the maximum effect of thiazolidinediones may not be observed for several weeks to months.
  - Combination therapy with two or more oral or injectable agents may be needed at the time of diagnosis to achieve A1C and glucose targets in patients presenting with significant hyperglycemia and will likely be needed as β-cell function deteriorates over time. The AACE recommends dual therapy for initial A1C ≥7.5% (>58 mmol/mol) and triple therapy or insulin for initial A1C >9% (>75 mmol/mol). A preference for medications with lower risk of hypoglycemia (metformin, GLP-1 receptor agonists, DPP-4 inhibitors, SGLT-2 inhibitors) reduces the risk of hypoglycemia.[9] The American Diabetes Association (ADA) recommends proceeding to two-drug, three-drug, and injectable combinations if the A1C goal is not achieved in 3-month increments. Dual therapy is recommended at the time of diagnosis if the A1C is >9% (>75 mmol/mol).[28] About 60% of patients on monotherapy may have worsening of metabolic control during the first 5 years of therapy, and concurrent use of two or more medications with different mechanisms of action may be necessary.[9,28]
  - Insulin therapy should be considered for patients presenting in DKA or with very high glucose levels (A1C >10% [>86 mmol/mol]). Insulin therapy can sometimes be stopped after glucose toxicity is corrected but may need to be continued in patients with persistent insulin deficiency.[9,28]
  - Because pancreatic β-cell function is required for the glucose-lowering effects of all noninsulin therapies, many patients will require insulin replacement therapy at some point. Insulin therapy can be initiated with basal insulin or premix insulin or insulin co formulations in addition to other therapies.

TABLE 23-6 Noninsulin Medications for Diabetes

	Renal Dosing Necessary?	Main Adverse Effects
Oral therapies		
Biguanide: Inhibits hepatic glucose output and stimulates glucose uptake by peripheral tissues. Weight neutral. Hold for 48 h after radiographic contrast procedure. Avoid in patients with cardiogenic or septic shock, moderate or severe CHF, severe liver disease, hypoxemia, and tissue hypoperfusion.		
Metformin (available in liquid and long-acting formulations)	Reduce dose to 500 mg 2 × daily if eGFR <45 mL/min/1.73 m^2; stop if eGFR <30 mL/min/1.73 m^2	GI symptoms (20%–30%); lactic acidosis (3/100,000 patient-years)
Sulfonylureas (SFU): Increase insulin secretion by binding specific β-cell receptors. Give 30–60 min before food. **Never** give if fasting. Start with lowest dose and increase over days to weeks to optimal dose (usually half the maximum approved dose).		
Glyburide (glibenclamide)	Avoid if CrCl <50 mL/min	Hypoglycemia, weight gain; avoid with renal insufficiency; caution in elderly
Glipizide	Yes; if CrCl <50 mL/min	Same; fewer problems in kidney disease
Glimepiride	Start lowest dose and titrate slowly	Same; fewer problems in kidney disease
Gliclazide[a]		Same; fewer problems in kidney disease
Meglitinides: Increase insulin secretion; much shorter onset and half-life than SFUs. Dose before each meal. **Never** give if fasting.		
Nateglinide	No	Hypoglycemia, weight gain; not as severe as SFUs
• Give 10 min before meal • Metabolized by cytochrome P450		
Repaglinide	Yes; if CrCl ≤40 mL/min	Same
• Give 30 min before meal		
Mitiglinide[a]		Same

(*Continued*)

TABLE 23-6 Noninsulin Medications for Diabetes (Continued)

α-Glucosidase inhibitors: Block polysaccharide and disaccharide breakdown and decrease postprandial hyperglycemia. Give with food. Start with low dose and increase weekly. Do not use in patients with intestinal disease.		
Acarbose	Avoid if serum Cr >2.0 mg/dL (176.8 μmol/L)	Gas, bloating, diarrhea, abdominal pain (25%–50%); transaminase elevations
Miglitol	Avoid if serum Cr >2.0 mg/dL (176.8 μmol/L)	Gas, bloating, diarrhea, abdominal pain (25%–50%)
Voglibose[a]	No; not renally excreted; not studied in CKD	Same
Thiazolidinediones: Increase insulin sensitivity in muscle, adipose tissue, and liver. Start with low dose and increase after several weeks. Avoid in patients with New York Heart Association class III/IV heart failure. Caution in patients with coronary artery disease, hypertension, long-standing diabetes, left ventricular hypertrophy, preexisting edema or edema on therapy, insulin use, advanced age, renal failure, and aortic or mitral valve disease (Diabetes Care. 2004;27:256).		
Pioglitazone • Alters levels of medicines metabolized by CYP3A4	No	Edema, heart failure, fractures in women, possible increased risk of bladder cancer, mild pancytopenia
DPP-4 inhibitors: Inhibit enzyme that breaks down endogenous GLP (incretin secreted from intestinal L cells). Increased GLP reduces blood glucose by inhibiting glucagon release and stimulating insulin secretion. Avoid in patients with a history of pancreatitis.		
Alogliptin	Yes; if eGFR <60 mL/min	Anaphylaxis, angioedema, skin reactions, liver injury, URI
Linagliptin	No	Anaphylaxis, angioedema, exfoliative skin reactions, URI
Saxagliptin	Yes; if eGFR ≤50 mL/min/1.73 m^2	Urticaria, facial edema, URI
Sitagliptin	Yes; if eGFR <50 mL/min/1.73 m^2	AKI, ESRD, anaphylaxis, angioedema, exfoliative skin reactions, URI

(*Continued*)

TABLE 23-6 Noninsulin Medications for Diabetes (Continued)

	Renal Dosing Necessary?	Main Adverse Effects
Vildagliptin[a] (not indicated in severe hepatic impairment, LFT >3 × upper limit of normal)	Yes; if eGFR <50 mL/min/1.73 m^2; not indicated in severe renal impairment	Blistering skin lesions in animals, increased LFTs
SGLT-2 inhibitors: Inhibit sodium glucose cotransporter 2 in the proximal renal tubule, decreasing glucose reabsorption by the kidney.		
Canagliflozin	Yes; if eGFR 45–<60 mL/min/1.73 m^2 use the lower dose, stop if eGFR <45 mL/min/1.73 m^2	Female genital mycotic infections, urinary tract infections, polyuria; hypotension, volume depletion, renal failure; increased LDL-C
Dapagliflozin	Not indicated for eGFR <60 mL/min/1.73 m^2	Same; possible increased risk for bladder cancer
Empagliflozin	Not indicated for eGFR <45 mL/min/1.73 m^2	Same
Bile acid sequestrants		
Colesevelam hydrochloride (contraindicated in bowel obstruction or GI motility disorders; pregnancy class B; can be used in renal and hepatic disease; take on an empty stomach)	No	Constipation, reduced absorption of some medications; raises triglycerides
Dopamine agonists		
Bromocriptine mesylate (do not use with other dopamine agonists or antagonists)	No	Nausea, asthenia, dizziness, headache, constipation, diarrhea
GLP-1 analogs		
Semaglutide (dosed once daily)	NO; monitor for GI side effects	Nausea, GI distress, vomiting

(Continued)

TABLE 23-6 Noninsulin Medications for Diabetes (Continued)

SC injectable therapies		
GLP-1 analogs: Structurally similar to endogenous GLP-1 but resist breakdown by DPP-4. They have a longer half-life and reach higher levels in blood and tissues. They are given by injection and can improve satiety and result in weight loss. Avoid in patients with history of pancreatitis. Avoid in patients with history of medullary thyroid cancer or MEN2 given increased C-cell tumors in rodents (all except immediate-release exenatide).		
Albiglutide (dosed weekly)	No; monitor for GI side effects in patients with renal impairment	URI, diarrhea, nausea, injection site reaction
Dulaglutide (dosed weekly)	No; monitor for GI side effects in patients with renal impairment	Diarrhea, nausea, vomiting, abdominal pain, decreased appetite
Exenatide (dosed twice daily)	Do not use in severe renal impairment or ESRD; caution with moderate renal impairment or history of renal transplant	Nausea, vomiting, GI distress, reported cases of pancreatitis
Exenatide extended release (dosed weekly)	Do not use in severe renal impairment or ESRD; caution with moderate renal impairment or history of renal transplant	Nausea, vomiting, injection site reaction, headache, diarrhea, dyspepsia
Liraglutide (dosed once daily)	Caution when initiating or escalating dose in patients with renal impairment	Headache, nausea, diarrhea, urticaria
Amylin analogs: Blunt postprandial blood glucose response		
Pramlintide acetate (given as a separate injection with meals; insulin dose reduction is required when starting)	Not defined with CrCl <20 mL/min	Nausea, vomiting, diarrhea, headache, hypoglycemia

(*Continued*)

TABLE 23-6 Noninsulin Medications for Diabetes (Continued)

	Renal Dosing Necessary?	Main Adverse Effects
Recent advances		

Several research groups worldwide are working on the novel approaches to control and eventually eliminate diabetes and its manifold complications. Some of these are mentioned below:

(a) Hydroxychloroquine (HCQ) has a novel mechanism of action, that is, postreceptor inhibition of insulin degradation for reducing blood glucose levels. Considering the antihyperglycemic potential, anti-inflammatory activity, and pleiotropic effects such as lipid-lowering action, antiplatelet action, antithrombotic action, and nephroprotective action, HCQ is emerging as a cost-effective therapeutic option for uncontrolled diabetes patients

(b) Immunomodulators: Otelixizumab and teplizumab; humanized anti-CD3/TCR complex and block T-cell activation which in turn may lead to a reduced autoimmune attack on beta islet cells. In various clinical trials (e.g., AbATE trial), these drugs have shown promising results in the treatment of type 1 DM

(c) Recombinant human GAD vaccine has shown slowdown of autoimmune destruction in LADA; long-term studies are needed to establish its efficacy

(d) Bionic pancreas: Composed of algorithmically controlled insulin–glucagon pump linked to continuous glucose monitoring. These closed-loop systems automatically dose and deliver insulin, and in some cases glucagon, in response to interstitial glucose measurements derived from continuous glucose monitoring and require less patient interaction

(e) Glimins—new class of oral antidiabetic drug—imeglimin; it targets mitochondrial bioenergetics and improves mitochondrial function, thus protecting beta cells from oxidative stress-induced damage. It also seems to improve insulin secretion and action

Please refer to country-specific prescribing information before using any of the antidiabetes therapies.

[a]Not available in the United States.

AKI, acute kidney injury; CKD, chronic kidney disease; CHF, congestive heart failure; Cr, creatinine; CrCl, creatinine clearance; DPP-4, dipeptidyl peptidase-4; eGFR, estimated glomerular filtration rate; ESRD, end-stage renal disease; GAD, glutamic acid decarboxylase; GI, gastrointestinal; GLP, glucagon-like peptide; LADA, latent autoimmune diabetes in adults; LDL-C, low-density lipoprotein cholesterol; LFT, liver function test; MEN2, multiple endocrine neoplasia type 2; URI, upper respiratory infection.

- The toxicity profile of some oral and injectable antidiabetic agents may preclude their use in patients with preexisting illnesses.
- Doses of noninsulin antidiabetes therapies may need to be reduced for declining kidney function. (Table 23-6)
- Cardiovascular outcome trials (CVOTs) with antidiabetes medications have shown that none increase the risk of CVD. Studies with DPP-4 inhibitors have shown CVD safety but no benefit.[29]
- The SGLT-2 inhibitor, empagliflozin, showed reduction in the composite major adverse cardiovascular endpoint (MACE) comprising death, MI, and stroke, with significant reduction in all-cause and cardiovascular mortality.[30] Similar benefit was noted with canagliflozin; however, an increase in amputations was noted.[31] Both empagliflozin and canagliflozin have been shown to slow down the progression of kidney disease in persons with diabetes.[31,32]
- Two of the GLP-1 receptor agonists (liraglutide and semaglutide) reduced the three-point MACE, while two others had neutral effects (lixisenatide, exenatide) when compared with placebo.[33–36] Liraglutide has also shown reduction in renal disease progression.[37]

• **Insulin therapy** in T2DM is indicated in the following:
  - Patients in whom oral or injectable agents have failed to achieve or sustain glycemic control
  - Metabolic decompensation: DKA, HHS
  - Newly diagnosed patients with severe hyperglycemia
  - Patients with chronic kidney disease that precludes use of noninsulin therapies
  - Pregnancy and other situations in which oral agents are contraindicated

• **The success of insulin therapy** depends on both the adequacy of the insulin TDD (0.6 to >1.0 units/kg of body weight per day) and the appropriateness of the insulin regimen for a given patient to achieve target glucose and A1C values.
  - A once-daily injection of intermediate- or long-acting insulin at bedtime or before breakfast (basal insulin) added to oral or injectable agents may achieve the target A1C goal.
  - Premeal insulin may be required if basal insulin plus other agents are not adequate. Short- or rapid-acting insulin administered before meals can be added to basal insulin. Alternatively, a premixed insulin can be given twice daily before breakfast and dinner. In general, the secretagogues are discontinued when premeal insulin is added, but sensitizing and other agents are continued on the basis of the individual patient needs.
  - The TDD of insulin required to achieve glycemic targets varies widely in patients with T2DM and is based on BMI, the continuation of oral agents, and the presence of comorbid conditions. Large doses of insulin (>100 units/d) may be required for optimal glycemic control. Weight gain with insulin use is a concern.
  - Insulin-induced hypoglycemia, the most dangerous side effect, may increase CV event rates and death. Avoidance of hypoglycemia while achieving an A1C as low as 7% can be safely achieved requires close collaboration between physician, patient, and diabetes educators. The frequency of hypoglycemia increases as patients approach normal A1C levels or when deterioration of kidney function occurs.

• **Concentration:** The standard insulin concentration is 100 units/mL (U-100), with vials containing 1000 units in 10 mL. A highly concentrated form of regular insulin containing 500 units/mL (Humulin U-500) is available for the rare patient with severe insulin resistance (usually T2DM). The vial size for U-500 insulin is 20 mL. Pens containing 3 mL are also available for U100 and U500 insulins. Concentrated forms of insulin glargine, a formulation that is 300 units/mL (U-300), and insulin degludec, formulated with 200 units/mL (U-200), are available in pens.

- **Mixed insulin therapy:** Short- and rapid-acting insulins (regular, lispro, aspart, and glulisine) can be mixed with NPH insulin in the same syringe for convenience. The rapid-acting insulin should be drawn first, cross-contamination should be avoided, and the mixed insulin should be injected immediately. Commercial premixed insulin preparations do not allow dose adjustment of individual components but are convenient for patients who are unable or unwilling to do the mixing themselves. Premixed insulins are an option for patients with T2DM who have a regular eating and activity schedule and, in general, should not be used in T1DM.

CHRONIC COMPLICATIONS OF DIABETES MELLITUS

- Prevention of long-term complications is one of the main goals of diabetes management. Appropriate treatment of established complications may delay their progression and improve quality of life.
- **Microvascular complications** include diabetic retinopathy (DR), nephropathy, and neuropathy. These complications are directly related to hyperglycemia. Tight glycemic control has been shown to reduce the development and progression of these complications.

Diabetic Retinopathy

GENERAL PRINCIPLES

Classification

- DR is classified as preproliferative retinopathy (microaneurysms, retinal infarcts, lipid exudates, cotton wool spots, and/or microhemorrhages) with or without macular edema and proliferative retinopathy.
- Other ocular abnormalities associated with diabetes include cataract formation, dyskinetic pupils, glaucoma, optic neuropathy, extraocular muscle paresis, floaters, and fluctuating visual acuity. The latter may be related to changes in BG levels.
- The presence of floaters may be indicative of preretinal or vitreous hemorrhage, and immediate referral for ophthalmologic evaluation is warranted.

Epidemiology

The incidence of DR and vision impairment has dropped significantly with improved management of glycemia, blood pressure, and lipids in patients with both T1DM and T2DM. Early identification and treatment of DR have further reduced vision impairment once it is diagnosed. DR is less frequent in T2DM, but maculopathy may be more severe. DR is still the leading cause of vision loss in adults younger than age 65 years.[38] In the Southeast Asian region, India has the lowest prevalence of DR (9.6%–22.4%) and Singapore has the highest prevalence (up to 35%).[39]

DIAGNOSIS

Annual examination by an ophthalmologist is recommended at the time of diagnosis of all T2DM patients and at the beginning of puberty or 3–5 years after diagnosis for patients with T1DM. Dilated eye examination should be repeated annually by an optometrist or ophthalmologist because progressive DR can be completely asymptomatic until sudden loss of vision occurs. Early detection of DR is critical because therapy is more effective before severe maculopathy or proliferation develops. Any patient with diabetes and visual symptoms should be referred for ophthalmologic evaluation.[40]

TREATMENT

The first line of treatment is glycemic control, which has been shown to reduce the incidence and progression of DR in patients with T1DM or T2DM. Blood pressure control was also shown to be effective in the United Kingdom Prospective Diabetes Study (UKPDS), and treatment with either an ACE inhibitor (ACE-I) or ARB has demonstrated additional utility in preventing DR. Fenofibrate, used with simvastatin, reduced the risk of progression of DR in the ACCORD and FIELD clinical trials.[38] Preproliferative retinopathy is not usually associated with loss of vision unless macular edema is present (25% of cases). The development of macular edema or proliferative retinopathy (particularly new vessels near the optic disk) requires elective laser photocoagulation therapy to preserve vision. Intraocular injections of vascular endothelial growth factor–neutralizing antibodies (**ranibizumab, bevacizumab, brolucizumab, aflibercept**) or glucocorticoids improve vision outcomes in macular edema but have side effects. Vitrectomy is indicated for patients with vitreous hemorrhage or retinal detachment.

Diabetic Nephropathy

GENERAL PRINCIPLES

Epidemiology

Approximately 25%–45% of patients with either type of diabetes develop clinically evident diabetic nephropathy during their lifetime. Diabetic nephropathy is the leading cause of end-stage renal disease (ESRD) in the United States and a major cause of morbidity and mortality in patients with diabetes.[40]

Risk Factors

The newest ADA guidelines no longer distinguish between microalbuminuria and macroalbuminuria, defining albuminuria as urinary albumin-to-creatinine ratio ≥30 mg/g.[40] The mean duration from diagnosis of T1DM to the development of overt proteinuria has increased significantly and is now >25 years. The time from the occurrence of proteinuria (albumin/creatinine >300 mg/g) to ESRD has also increased and is now >5 years. In T2DM, albuminuria can be present at the time of diagnosis. Poor glycemic control is the major risk factor for diabetic nephropathy, but hypertension and smoking are contributors. Obesity may contribute to kidney damage in T2DM. Owing to the widespread use of ACE inhibitor and ARB agents for the treatment of hypertension, impaired kidney function may occur in the absence of albuminuria.[40] Stages of diabetic nephropathy are listed in Table 23-7.

Prevention

Prevention of diabetic nephropathy starts at the time of diagnosis with achievement of glycemic, blood pressure, and lipid targets. Smoking cessation is also important. Annual screening for albuminuria and measurement of serum creatinine identify those with early damage who are at risk of progression. Annual screening should be performed in T1DM patients who have had diabetes for >5 years and all T2DM patients starting at diagnosis.

Associated Conditions

- Patients with proteinuria (albumin/creatinine >300 mg/g) are at higher risk for anemia because of loss of transferrin and poor production of erythropoietin and should be screened at any stage of CKD and treated.
- **Patients with CKD are at higher risk for CVD and mortality**, so management of other CV risk factors is particularly important in this group of patients.

TABLE 23-7 Stages of Diabetic Nephropathy

Stage	Urinary Albumin (mg/g Cr) or Urinary Protein (g/g Cr)	GFR (eGFR) (mL/min/1.73 m^2)
1 (Prenephropathy)	Normoalbuminuria (<30)	≥30
2 (Incipient nephropathy)	Microalbuminuria (30–299)	≥30
3 (Overt nephropathy)	Macroalbuminuria (≥300)	≥30
	Or	
	Persistent proteinuria (≥0.5)	
4 (Kidney failure)	Any albuminuria/proteinuria status	<30
5 (Dialysis therapy)	Any status on continued dialysis therapy	

- Hypovitaminosis D should be corrected, and secondary hyperparathyroidism should be prevented or treated as early as possible.
- Patients with diabetes and CKD may be at risk for hyperkalemia and metabolic acidosis, which should be identified and managed accordingly.

DIAGNOSIS

Diagnostic Testing

- Measurement of the albumin-to-creatinine ratio (normal, <30 mg of albumin/g of creatinine) in a random urine sample is recommended for screening. At least two to three measurements within a 6-month period should be performed to establish the diagnosis of diabetic nephropathy.[30,40]
- Measurement of serum creatinine and serum urea nitrogen should be performed annually, along with calculation of the estimated GFR. Patients with diabetes may have reduced kidney function without manifesting albumin in their urine. Testing and treatment of associated disorders such as anemia, secondary hyperparathyroidism, hyperkalemia, and acid–base disturbances should begin when the estimated GFR is <60 mL/min/1.73 m^2 or during stage 3 CKD (see Chapter 13, Renal Diseases).

TREATMENT

Intensive control of both diabetes and hypertension is important to reduce the rate of progression of CKD due to diabetes. Lower blood pressure targets, less than 130/80 mm Hg, are recommended for persons with diabetes and evidence of kidney damage or dysfunction.[9,15]

Medications

- Antihypertensive treatment with ACE inhibitor or ARB drugs is recommended as first-line therapy for all patients with diabetes and hypertension. These agents have been shown to reduce progression of both retinopathy and nephropathy and may be considered in patients with normal blood pressure or prehypertension.
- Diuretics are considered second line, followed by calcium channel blockers, β-blockers, or centrally acting agents.[9,15,40]

Lifestyle/Risk Modification

- Dietary protein intake of 0.8 g/kg/d (based on ideal body weight) is recommended. Further reduction does not alter glycemic control, CVD risk, or kidney function decline.[40,41]
- Avoidance of renal toxins is important for preservation of kidney function.

Diabetic Neuropathy

GENERAL PRINCIPLES

Classification

Diabetic neuropathy can be classified as (1) subclinical neuropathy, determined by abnormalities in electrodiagnostic and quantitative sensory testing; (2) diffuse symmetrical polyneuropathy with distal symmetric sensorimotor losses ± autonomic syndromes; and (3) focal syndromes.[42]

Epidemiology

Distal symmetric polyneuropathy (DPN) is the most common neuropathy in developed countries and accounts for more hospitalizations than all the other diabetic complications combined. Sensorimotor DPN is a major risk factor for foot trauma, ulceration, and Charcot arthropathy and is responsible for 50%–75% of nontraumatic amputations.[40,42]

Prevention

- Sensation in the lower extremities should be documented at least annually, using a combination of modalities such as a light-touch monofilament, tuning fork (frequency of 128 Hz), pinprick, or temperature.
- Foot examination should be conducted at least annually to evaluate the presence of musculoskeletal deformities, skin changes, and pulses, in addition to the sensory examination.

TREATMENT

- **Painful peripheral neuropathy** responds variably to treatment with tricyclic antidepressants (e.g., amitriptyline 10–150 mg PO at bedtime), topical capsaicin (0.075% cream), or anticonvulsants (e.g., carbamazepine 100–400 mg PO bid, gabapentin 900–3600 mg/d, or pregabalin 150–300 mg/d). Patients should be warned about adverse effects, including sedation and anticholinergic symptoms (tricyclics), burning sensation (capsaicin), and blood dyscrasias (carbamazepine). α-Lipoic acid (600 mg bid) and high-dose thiamine (50–100 mg tid) have been tested in early DPN. Vitamin B_{12} should be checked and replaced if low.
- **Orthostatic hypotension** is a manifestation of autonomic neuropathy, but other etiologies (e.g., dehydration, anemia, medications) should be excluded. Treatment is symptomatic and includes postural maneuvers, use of compressive garments (e.g., Jobst stockings), and intravascular expansion using sodium chloride 1–4 g PO qid and fludrocortisone 0.1–0.3 mg PO daily and other agents such as midodrine, an alpha adrenoceptor agonist, in doses of 2.5–5 mg bid which can be used. Hypokalemia, supine hypertension, and congestive heart failure (CHF) are some adverse effects of fludrocortisone.
- **Intractable nausea and vomiting** may be manifestations of impaired GI motility from autonomic neuropathy. **DKA** should be ruled out when nausea and vomiting are acute. Other causes of nausea and vomiting, including adrenal insufficiency, should be excluded.
    - **Management of diabetic gastroenteropathy** can be challenging. Frequent, small meals (six to eight per day) of soft consistency that are low in fat and fiber provide intermittent relief. Parenteral nutrition may become necessary in refractory cases.

- **Pharmacologic therapy** includes the prokinetic agent metoclopramide, 10–20 mg PO (or as a suppository) before meals and at bedtime, and erythromycin, 125–500 mg PO qid. Extrapyramidal side effects (tremor and tardive dyskinesia) from the antidopaminergic actions of metoclopramide may limit therapy.
- **Cyclical vomiting** that is unrelated to a GI motility disorder or other clear etiology may also occur in patients with diabetes and appears to respond to amitriptyline 25–50 mg PO at bedtime.

- **Diabetic cystopathy,** or bladder dysfunction, results from impaired autonomic control of detrusor muscle and sphincteric function. Manifestations include urgency, dribbling, incomplete emptying, overflow incontinence, and urinary retention. Recurrent urinary tract infections are common in patients with residual urine. Treatment with bethanechol 10 mg tid or intermittent self-catheterization may be required to relieve retention.
- **Chronic, persistent diarrhea** in patients with diabetes is probably multifactorial. Celiac disease and inflammatory bowel diseases should be ruled out, particularly in patients with T1DM. Pancreatic mass is reduced with long-standing diabetes, so the possibility of exocrine pancreatic dysfunction should be considered. Bacterial overgrowth has been considered as an etiology but is difficult to diagnose. Empiric treatment with broad-spectrum antibiotics (e.g., azithromycin, tetracycline, cephalosporins) along with metronidazole may be beneficial. Antifungal agents and probiotic replacement can be tried. If diarrhea persists, loperamide or octreotide 50–75 mg SC bid can be effective in patients with intractable diarrhea.

MACROVASCULAR COMPLICATIONS OF DIABETES MELLITUS

Coronary Heart Disease

GENERAL PRINCIPLES

- Coronary heart disease (CHD), stroke, and peripheral vascular disease (PVD) are responsible for 80% of deaths in persons with diabetes[9,15] (see Chapter 4, Ischemic Heart Disease).
- **Coronary artery disease** (CAD) occurs at a younger age and may have atypical clinical presentations in patients with diabetes.[15] CAD occurs at least a decade earlier in Indians with diabetes, when compared to in their Western counterparts.[39]
  - MI carries a worse prognosis, and angioplasty gives less satisfactory results in patients with diabetes.
  - Persons with diabetes have an increased risk of ischemic and nonischemic heart failure (HF) and sudden death.[43]

Risk Factors

Risk factors for macrovascular disease that are common in persons with diabetes include insulin resistance, hyperglycemia, albuminuria, hypertension, hyperlipidemia, cigarette smoking, and obesity.

Prevention

- CV risk factors should be assessed at least annually and treated aggressively (see treatment goals in the following text). Stress tests, with or without imaging, should be reserved for those with typical or atypical chest pain or those with abnormalities on ECG.[44]
- Screening asymptomatic persons with cardiac stress test has not been shown to reduce mortality or events in asymptomatic patients with T2DM.[44]

- Aspirin 81–325 mg/d has proven beneficial in secondary prevention of MI or stroke in patients with diabetes and may be considered for persons over age 40 years with diabetes.

TREATMENT

- Aggressive risk factor reduction lowers the risk of both microvascular and macrovascular complications in patients with diabetes.
  - Glycemic control should be optimized to A1C <7% (<53 mmol/mol) and as close to normal as possible in the first few years after diagnosis. Patients with long-standing T2DM may have increased risk of mortality with very tight glycemic control (A1C <6.5% [<48 mmol/mol]), particularly if multiple agents are required and the risk of hypoglycemia increases.
  - Hypertension should be controlled to a target blood pressure of <140/90 mm Hg (or <130/80 mm Hg if this can be achieved without adverse effects).
  - Hyperlipidemia should be treated appropriately, with a high-intensity statin in patients with known CVD. High-density lipoprotein cholesterol levels of >50 mg/dL (1.3 mmol/L) and triglyceride levels of <150 mg/dL (1.7 mmol/L) should be achieved.
  - Cigarette smoking should be actively discouraged, and weight loss should be promoted in obese patients.

Heart Failure

GENERAL PRINCIPLES

HF is more common and carries a worse prognosis in persons with diabetes than in persons without diabetes. The hazard ratio for HF among those with prediabetes is 1.2–1.7 in different populations; while in persons with diabetes, the HR is about 2.5. The prognosis for survival is much worse in persons with diabetes and HF compared with those without diabetes.[45]

DIAGNOSIS

Clinical Presentation

HF is suspected after an ischemic event, confirmed by echocardiography or during cardiac catheterization. Diabetes affects both the structure and function of the myocardium, leading to left ventricular concentric remodeling, hypertrophy, and impaired myocardial energetics. Symptoms include reduced exercise tolerance, shortness of breath, and edema.

TREATMENT

Guidelines do not recommend a different approach to the management of HF in persons with diabetes.[46] Treating diabetes in persons with HF requires consideration of available data about the differential impact of antidiabetes agents on admission for HF and mortality. Prior to 2006, metformin was contraindicated for the treatment of diabetes in HF, but when studies showed possible reduced mortality, the FDA eliminated the contraindication. Metformin is considered safe in mild to moderate HF and may be associated with better outcomes.[44,45] Observational trial data and post hoc analyses of randomized clinical trials testing sulfonylureas and insulin have provided conflicting results. Thiazolidinediones are known to cause fluid retention and increase the risk of HF events. The DPP-4 inhibitors have neutral CV effects overall.

Saxagliptin and alogliptin had increased risk of HF in large CVOTs; however, these effects have not been seen in retrospective analyses or observational cohorts. The GLP-1 receptor agonists have had neutral to positive effects on MACE endpoints but have had neutral effects in HF patients. The SGLT-2 inhibitors have had consistently positive effects on HF hospitalization and are currently being studied in populations with HFrEF and HFpEF.[29,30,45–47] The newest consensus statement from the European Association for the Study of Diabetes and the ADA recommends the preferential use of a GLP1-RA (liraglutide or semaglutide) or SGLT-2 inhibitor (empagliflozin or canagliflozin) with proven CV benefit in individuals with atherosclerotic CVD. If HF and CKD are prominent in individuals with or without CVD, then empagliflozin or canagliflozin are the recommended agents.[48]

Peripheral Vascular Disease

GENERAL PRINCIPLES

Diabetes and smoking are the strongest risk factors for PVD. In patients with diabetes, the risk of PVD is increased by age, duration of diabetes, and presence of peripheral neuropathy. PVD is a marker for systemic vascular disease involving coronary, cerebral, and renal vessels. Persons with diabetes and PVD have increased risk for subsequent MI or stroke regardless of the PVD symptoms. In India, the prevalence of PVD appears to be less than in the Western world.[39]

DIAGNOSIS

Clinical Presentation

Symptoms of PVD include intermittent claudication, rest pain, tissue loss, and gangrene, but patients with diabetes may have fewer symptoms because of concomitant neuropathy.

Physical Examination

Physical examination findings include diminished pulses, dependent rubor, pallor on elevation, absence of hair growth, dystrophic toenails, and cool, dry, fissured skin.

Diagnostic Testing

- The ankle-to-brachial index (ABI), defined as the ratio of the systolic blood pressure in the ankle divided by the systolic blood pressure at the arm, is the best initial diagnostic test. An ABI <0.9 by a handheld 5- to 10-MHz Doppler probe has a 95% sensitivity for detecting angiogram-positive PVD.[15]
- ABI should be performed in patients with diabetes with signs or symptoms of PVD.

TREATMENT

- Risk factors should be controlled, with similar goals described for CAD (see the previous text).
- Antiplatelet agents such as clopidogrel (75 mg/d) have additional benefits when compared with aspirin in patients with diabetes and PVD.[15]
- Patients with intermittent claudication could also benefit from exercise rehabilitation and cilostazol (100 mg bid). This medication is contraindicated in patients with CHF.

MISCELLANEOUS COMPLICATIONS

Erectile Dysfunction

GENERAL PRINCIPLES

Epidemiology

It is estimated that 40%–60% of men with diabetes have erectile dysfunction (ED), and the prevalence varies depending on the age of the patient and duration of diabetes. In addition to increasing age, ED is associated with smoking, poor glycemic control, low high-density lipoprotein, neuropathy, and retinopathy.

Etiology

ED in men with diabetes is multifactorial. It can result from nerve damage, impaired blood flow (vascular insufficiency), adverse drug effects, low testosterone, psychological factors, or a combination of these etiologies.

DIAGNOSIS

Evaluation should include a measurement of total or bioavailable testosterone. If the total testosterone is <300 ng/dL (10.4 nmol/L), the test should be repeated in the morning (does not have to be fasting, but a blood draw before 9:00 AM. is appropriate) along with a prolactin, LH, and prostate-specific antigen (PSA).

TREATMENT

- If testosterone is low, and both PSA and prostate examination are normal, then testosterone replacement can be tried with either testosterone enanthate, 200 mg every 2–3 weeks, or a topical gel (AndroGel or Testim).
- A trial of phosphodiesterase type 5 inhibitors (sildenafil, tadalafil, vardenafil) is often warranted in addition to hormonal correction (if indicated). Typical doses include sildenafil 50–100 mg, vardenafil 10 mg, or tadalafil 10 mg 1 hour prior to sexual activity. Tadalafil can also be administered as a daily medication at lower doses (2.5–5 mg/d). Referral to a urology specialist should be considered if the problem persists. CV status should be considered before starting these agents. **This drug class should not be used concurrently with nitrates** to prevent severe and potentially fatal hypotensive reactions. Macular edema should also be ruled out before starting these agents.

Hypoglycemia

GENERAL PRINCIPLES

Classification

Hypoglycemia is uncommon in patients not treated for diabetes. Iatrogenic factors usually account for hypoglycemia in the setting of diabetes, whereas hypoglycemia in the population without diabetes could be classified as fasting or postprandial hypoglycemia. **Iatrogenic hypoglycemia** complicates therapy with insulin or SFUs and is a limiting factor to achieving glycemic control during intensive therapy in patients with diabetes.[49]

Risk Factors

Hypoglycemia resulting from too intensive diabetes management may increase the risk of mortality in older patients with a long duration of diabetes and should be avoided.

- Risk factors for iatrogenic hypoglycemia include skipped or insufficient meals, unaccustomed physical exertion, misguided therapy, alcohol ingestion, and drug overdose.
- Recurrent episodes of hypoglycemia impair recognition of hypoglycemic symptoms, thereby increasing the risk for severe hypoglycemia (hypoglycemia unawareness).
- Hypoglycemia unawareness results from defective glucose counterregulation with blunting of autonomic symptoms and counterregulatory hormone secretion during hypoglycemia. Seizures or coma may develop in such patients without the usual warning symptoms of hypoglycemia.
- Hypoglycemia unrelated to diabetes therapy is an infrequent problem in general medical practice.

DIAGNOSIS

Clinical Presentation

- Hypoglycemia is a clinical syndrome in which low serum (or plasma) glucose levels lead to symptoms of sympathetic–adrenal activation (sweating, anxiety, tremor, nausea, palpitations, and tachycardia) from increased secretion of counterregulatory hormones (e.g., epinephrine).
- Neuroglycopenia occurs as the glucose levels decrease further (fatigue, dizziness, headache, visual disturbances, drowsiness, difficulty speaking, inability to concentrate, abnormal behavior, confusion, and ultimately loss of consciousness or seizures).

Differential Diagnosis

Plasma or capillary BG values should be obtained, whenever feasible, to confirm hypoglycemia.

- Any patient with a serum glucose concentration of <60 mg/dL (3.3 mmol/L) should be suspected of having a hypoglycemic disorder, and further evaluation is required if the value is <50 mg/dL (2.8 mmol/L).
- These levels are usually accompanied by symptoms of hypoglycemia, and absence of symptoms with these levels of glucose suggests the possibility of artifactual hypoglycemia. Detailed evaluation is usually required in a healthy appearing patient, whereas hypoglycemia may be readily recognized as part of the underlying illness in a sick patient.[50] Major categories include fasting and postprandial hypoglycemia.
- **Fasting hypoglycemia** can be caused by inappropriate insulin secretion (e.g., insulinoma), alcohol abuse, severe hepatic or renal insufficiency, hypopituitarism, glucocorticoid deficiency, or surreptitious injection of insulin or ingestion of an SFU.
    - These patients present with neuroglycopenic symptoms, but episodic autonomic symptoms may be present. Occasionally, patients with recurrent seizures, dementia, and bizarre behavior are referred for neuropsychiatric evaluation, which may delay timely diagnosis of hypoglycemia.
    - **Definitive diagnosis** of fasting hypoglycemia requires hourly BG monitoring during a supervised fast lasting up to 72 hours, and measurement of plasma insulin, C-peptide, and SFU metabolites if hypoglycemia (<50 mg/dL [2.8 mmol/L]) is documented. Patients who develop hypoglycemia and have measurable plasma insulin and C-peptide levels without SFU metabolites require further evaluation for an insulinoma.
- **Postprandial hypoglycemia** often is suspected, but seldom proven, in patients with vague symptoms that occur 1 or more hours after meals.
    - **Alimentary hypoglycemia** should be considered in patients with a history of partial gastrectomy or intestinal resection in whom recurrent symptoms develop 1–2 hours

after eating. The mechanism is thought to be related to too rapid glucose absorption, resulting in a robust insulin response. These symptoms should be distinguished from dumping syndrome, which is not associated with hypoglycemia and occurs in the first hour after food intake. Frequent small meals with reduced carbohydrate content may ameliorate symptoms.

- **Functional hypoglycemia:** Symptoms that are possibly suggestive of hypoglycemia, which may or may not be confirmed by plasma glucose measurement, occur in some patients who have not undergone GI surgery. This condition is referred to as "functional hypoglycemia." The symptoms tend to develop 3–5 hours after meals. Current evaluation and management of functional hypoglycemia are imprecise; some patients show evidence of impaired glucose tolerance and may respond to dietary therapy.

TREATMENT

Isolated episodes of mild hypoglycemia may not require specific intervention. Recurrent episodes require a review of lifestyle factors; adjustments may be indicated in the content, timing, and distribution of meals, as well as medication dosage and timing. Severe hypoglycemia is an indication for supervised treatment.

- **Readily absorbable carbohydrates** (e.g., glucose and sugar-containing beverages) can be administered orally to conscious patients for rapid effect. Alternatively, milk, candy bars, fruit, cheese, and crackers may be used in some patients with mild hypoglycemia. Hypoglycemia associated with acarbose or miglitol therapy should preferentially be treated with glucose. Glucose tablets and carbohydrate supplies should be readily available to patients with DM at all times.
- **IV dextrose** is indicated for severe hypoglycemia, in patients with altered consciousness, and during restriction of oral intake. An initial bolus, 20–50 mL of 50% dextrose, should be given immediately, followed by infusion of 5% dextrose in water (D5W) (or D10W) to maintain BG levels above 100 mg/dL (5.6 mmol/L). Prolonged IV dextrose infusion and close observation are warranted in SFU overdose, in the elderly, and in patients with defective counterregulation.
- **Glucagon**, 1 mg IM (or SC), is an effective initial therapy for severe hypoglycemia in patients unable to receive oral intake or in whom an IV access cannot be secured immediately. Vomiting is a frequent side effect, and therefore, care should be taken to prevent the risk of aspiration. A glucagon kit should be available to patients with a history of severe hypoglycemia; family members and roommates should be instructed in its proper use.

PATIENT EDUCATION

- **Education** regarding etiologies of hypoglycemia, preventive measures, and appropriate adjustments to medication, diet, and exercise regimens is an essential task to be addressed during hospitalization for severe hypoglycemia.
- **Hypoglycemia unawareness** can develop in patients who are undergoing intensive diabetes therapy. These patients should be encouraged to monitor their BG levels frequently and take timely measures to correct low values (<60 mg/dL [3.3 mmol/L]). In patients with very tightly controlled diabetes, slight relaxation in glycemic control and scrupulous avoidance of hypoglycemia may restore the lost warning symptoms.

Summary

- In adults with recently diagnosed type 2 DM and no clinically significant cardiovascular disease, glycemic control aimed at the near-normal range should be considered. The goal is to prevent the development of microvascular and macrovascular complications over the lifetime, provided this can be achieved without substantial hypoglycemia.
- In patients with diabetes at higher risk, especially those with multiple ASCVD risk factors or aged 50–70 years, it is reasonable to use high-intensity statin therapy. High-intensity statin therapy will achieve approximately a 50% reduction in LDL-C.
- If glycemic target is not achieved within 3 months after LSM, then glucose-lowering agent should be initiated promptly.
- Instead of metformin monotherapy, early combination therapy could be considered to reduce the risk of failure of glycemic control in some patients with newly diagnosed T2DM.
- The ADA recommends that the early introduction of insulin should be considered if there is evidence of ongoing catabolism (weight loss), if symptoms of hyperglycaemia are present, or when A1C levels (≥10%) or blood glucose levels (≥300 mg/dL) are very high.
- The active use of CGM devices is now recommended from the early stage of diagnosis of diabetes requiring insulin management.
- Distinguishing features of type1 DM include younger age (<35 years), lower BMI (<25 kg/m^2), weight loss, ketoacidosis, and glucose ≥360 mg/dL at diagnosis.

Scan the QR code to access chapter references.

24 Endocrine Disorders

Amy E. Riek, R. MeiZhang, William E. Clutter, and Anudeep Gaddam

Evaluation of Thyroid Function[1]

GENERAL PRINCIPLES

The major hormone secreted by thyroid is **thyroxine** (T_4), which is converted by deiodinases in many tissues to the more potent **triiodothyronine** (T_3). Both are bound reversibly to plasma proteins, primarily **thyroxine-binding globulin**. Only the free (unbound) fraction enters cells and produces biologic effects. T_4 secretion is stimulated by **thyroid-stimulating hormone** (**TSH**) secreted from the pituitary gland. In turn, TSH secretion is inhibited by T_4, forming a negative feedback loop that keeps free T_4 levels within a normal range. Diagnosis of thyroid disease is based on clinical findings, examination of the thyroid, and measurement of plasma TSH and thyroid hormones.

DIAGNOSIS

Clinical Presentation

Thyroid examination determines the size and consistency of the thyroid and the presence of nodules, tenderness, or a thrill.

Diagnostic Testing (Figure 24-1)

- **Plasma TSH is the best initial test in most patients with suspected thyroid disease.** TSH levels are elevated in primary hypothyroidism and are suppressed in hyperthyroidism. Thus, a **normal plasma TSH level excludes nearly all causes of hyperthyroidism,**

Thyroid Function Test Interpretation			
TSH	Free T4	Free T3	Condition
Normal	Normal	Normal	• None
Low	High	High	• **Hyperthyroidism**
Low	Normal	Normal	• Subclinical hyperthyroidism
Low	Normal	High	• T3 toxicosis
Low	High	Normal	• Thyroiditis • T4 ingestion • Hyperthyroidism in the elderly or with comorbid illness
Low	Low	Low	• Euthyroid sick syndrome • Central hypothyroidism
High	Normal	Normal	• Subclinical hypothyroidism • Recovery from euthyroid sick syndrome
High	Low	Low	• **Primary hypothyroidism**
High	High	High	• TSH producing pituitary adenoma

Figure 24-1 Summary of thyroid function test and interpretation.

as well as primary hypothyroidism. Because even slight changes in thyroid hormone levels affect TSH secretion, **abnormal TSH levels are not specific for clinically important thyroid disease.** Changes in plasma TSH lag behind changes in plasma T_4, and TSH levels may be misleading when plasma T_4 levels are changing rapidly, as during treatment of hyperthyroidism.

  - TSH levels may be suppressed in severe nonthyroidal illness, in mild (or subclinical) hyperthyroidism, and during treatment with dopamine or high doses of glucocorticoids. In addition, TSH levels remain suppressed for some time after hyperthyroidism is corrected.
  - Plasma TSH is mildly elevated (up to 10 μU/mL) in some euthyroid patients recovering from nonthyroidal illnesses and in mild (or subclinical) hypothyroidism.
  - TSH levels are usually within the reference range in secondary hypothyroidism and cannot be used to diagnose this rare form of hypothyroidism.

- **Plasma-free T_4** confirms the diagnosis and assesses the severity of hyperthyroidism when plasma TSH is low. It is also used to diagnose secondary hypothyroidism and adjust thyroxine therapy in patients with pituitary disease. Most laboratories measure free T_4 by immunoassay.
- **Free T_4 measured by equilibrium dialysis** is the most reliable measure of unbound T_4, but results are seldom rapidly available. It is needed only in rare cases in which the diagnosis is not clear from measurement of plasma TSH and free T_4 by immunoassay.
- **Effect of nonthyroidal illness on thyroid function tests:** Many illnesses alter thyroid tests without causing true thyroid dysfunction (the nonthyroidal illness or euthyroid sick syndrome). These changes must be recognized to avoid mistaken diagnosis.
  - **Low T_3** occurs in many illnesses, during starvation, and after trauma or surgery. Conversion of T_4 to T_3 is decreased, and plasma T_3 levels are low. Plasma-free T_4 and TSH levels are normal. This may be an adaptive response to illness, and thyroid hormone therapy is not beneficial.
  - **Low T_4** occurs in severe illness. TSH levels decrease early in severe illness, sometimes to <0.1 μU/mL. In prolonged illness, free T_4 may also fall below normal. During recovery, TSH rises, sometimes to levels slightly above the normal range (rarely >20 μU/mL).
  - Some drugs affect thyroid function tests (see Table 24-1). Iodine-containing drugs (**amiodarone** and radiographic contrast media) and immune modulators may cause hyperthyroidism or hypothyroidism in susceptible patients. In general, plasma TSH levels are a reliable guide to whether true hyperthyroidism or hypothyroidism is present.
  - Biotin, commonly taken as an over-the-counter supplement, can interfere with immunoassays for TSH, free T_4, and/or free T_3 at high concentrations. It has a short half-life and should be held for 2 days before laboratory testing.

Hypothyroidism[2–4]

GENERAL PRINCIPLES

- **Primary hypothyroidism** (due to disease of the thyroid itself) accounts for >90% of cases. The prevalence is around 4%–5% in the Western world; in India it is around 11%, with females being most commonly affected. In adults, the most common cause continues to be autoimmune disease, especially in the postiodinization era.[5] Interestingly, studies conducted show that while the incidence of congenital hypothyroidism has dramatically decreased in the post iodinization phase in India, the prevalence of goiter has not come down significantly, indicating the possible role of goitrogens in diet.[6]
- **Chronic lymphocytic thyroiditis (Hashimoto disease)** is the most common cause in developed nations and may be associated with Addison's disease and other endocrine deficits. Its prevalence is greater in women and increases with age.

TABLE 24-1 Effects of Drugs on Thyroid Function Tests

Effect	Drug
Decreased free and total T_4	
True hypothyroidism (TSH elevated)	Iodine (amiodarone, radiographic contrast) Lithium Some tyrosine kinase inhibitors Some immune modulators (e.g., interferon-α, checkpoint inhibitors)
Inhibition of TSH secretion	Glucocorticoids Dopamine
Multiple mechanisms (TSH normal)	Phenytoin
Decreased total T_4 only	
Decreased TBG (TSH normal)	Androgens
Inhibition of T_4 binding to TBG (TSH normal)	Furosemide (high doses) Salicylates
Increased free and total T_4	
True hyperthyroidism (TSH <0.1 μU/mL)	Iodine (amiodarone, radiographic contrast) Some immune modulators (e.g., interferon-α, checkpoint inhibitors)
Inhibited T_4 to T_3 conversion (TSH normal)	Amiodarone
Increased free T_4 only	
Displacement of T_4 from TBG in vitro (TSH normal)	Heparin, low-molecular-weight heparin
Increased total T_4 only	
Increased TBG (TSH normal)	Estrogens, tamoxifen, raloxifene
Variable effect	
Interferes with immunoassays causing lab artifact (no effect on actual thyroid levels)	Biotin

T_3, triiodothyronine; T_4, thyroxine; TBG, thyroxine-binding globulin; TSH, thyroid-stimulating hormone.

- **Iatrogenic hypothyroidism** due to thyroidectomy or radioactive iodine (RAI; iodine-131) therapy is also common.
- Transient hypothyroidism occurs in postpartum thyroiditis and subacute thyroiditis, usually after a period of hyperthyroidism.
- Infiltrative disorders: sarcoidosis, hemochromatosis.
- Irradiation of neck.
- **Drugs that may cause hypothyroidism** include iodine-containing drugs, lithium, interferon (IFN)-α, IFN-β, interleukin-2, thalidomide, bexarotene, sunitinib, amiodarone, and checkpoint inhibitors.
- **Congenital hypothyroidism** (agenesis/dyshormonogenesis).

- Secondary hypothyroidism due to TSH deficiency is uncommon but may occur in any disorder of the pituitary or hypothalamus. It can occur secondary to parasellar neoplasia, vascular injury, and Sheehan syndrome. However, it rarely occurs without other evidence of pituitary disease.

DIAGNOSIS

Clinical Presentation

History

Most symptoms of hypothyroidism are nonspecific and develop gradually. They include cold intolerance, fatigue, somnolence, poor memory, constipation, menorrhagia, myalgias, and hoarseness. Hypothyroidism is readily treatable and should be suspected in any patient with compatible symptoms.

Physical Examination

Signs include slow tendon reflex relaxation, bradycardia, facial and periorbital edema, dry skin, and nonpitting edema (myxoedema). Mild weight gain may occur, but hypothyroidism does not cause marked obesity. Rare manifestations include hypoventilation, pericardial or pleural effusions, deafness, and carpal tunnel syndrome.

Myxoedema coma is a life-threatening condition due to untreated severe hypothyroidism. It manifests with severe hypothermia, bradycardia, hypotension, hypoventilation, hypoglycemia, hyponatremia, and coma.

Diagnostic Testing

- Laboratory findings may include hyponatremia and elevated plasma levels of cholesterol, triglycerides, and creatine kinase.
- In suspected primary hypothyroidism, plasma TSH is the best initial test.
  - A normal value excludes primary hypothyroidism, and an elevated value (>10 μU/mL) confirms the diagnosis.
  - Mild elevation of plasma TSH (<10 μU/mL) may be because of recovery from nonthyroidal illness, but it usually indicates mild (or subclinical) primary hypothyroidism, in which thyroid function is impaired but increased secretion of TSH maintains normal plasma-free T_4 levels. These patients may have nonspecific symptoms that are compatible with hypothyroidism and a mild increase in serum cholesterol and low-density lipoprotein cholesterol. They develop clinical hypothyroidism at a rate of 2.5% per year.
- Antibodies against thyroid peroxidase and thyroglobulin (Tg) are very common and should prompt evaluation for hypothyroidism. However, they do not change the management of hypothyroidism and therefore need not be typically measured.
- If secondary hypothyroidism is suspected because of evidence of pituitary disease, plasma- free T_4 should be measured. Plasma TSH levels are usually within the reference range in secondary hypothyroidism and cannot be used alone to make this diagnosis. Patients with secondary hypothyroidism should be evaluated for other pituitary hormone deficits and for disorders of the pituitary or hypothalamus (see Disorders of Anterior Pituitary Function section).
- **In severe nonthyroidal illness,** the diagnosis of hypothyroidism may be difficult. Plasma-free T_4 measured by routine assays may be low.
  - **Plasma TSH is the best initial diagnostic test.** A normal TSH value is strong evidence that the patient is euthyroid, except when there is evidence of pituitary or hypothalamic disease or in patients treated with dopamine or high doses of glucocorticoids. Marked elevation of plasma TSH (>10 μU/mL) establishes the diagnosis of primary hypothyroidism.

- Moderate elevations of plasma TSH (<10 µU/mL) may occur in euthyroid patients recovering from nonthyroidal illness and are not specific for hypothyroidism. Plasma-free T_4 should be measured if TSH is moderately elevated or if secondary hypothyroidism is suspected, and patients should be treated for hypothyroidism if plasma-free T_4 is low. Thyroid function in these patients should be reevaluated after recovery from illness.

- Ultrasound of neck, ECG, and echocardiography can be done.

TREATMENT

- **Thyroxine** is the drug of choice. The average replacement dose is 1.6–2.3 µg/kg PO daily, and most patients require doses between 75 and 150 µg/d. In elderly patients, the average replacement dose is lower. The need for lifelong treatment should be emphasized. Thyroxine should be taken 1 hour before a meal, because some foods interfere with its absorption, and should not be taken with other medications (mainly antacids).
- **Initiation of therapy:** Young and middle-aged adults should be started on 1.6 µg/kg/d. This regimen gradually corrects hypothyroidism because several weeks are required to reach steady-state plasma levels of T_4. In otherwise healthy elderly patients, the initial dose should be 50 µg/d. Patients with cardiac disease should be started on 25 µg/d and monitored carefully for exacerbation of cardiac symptoms.
- **Dose adjustment and follow-up**
  - **In primary hypothyroidism, the goal of therapy is to maintain plasma TSH within the normal range.** Plasma TSH should be measured 6–8 weeks after initiation of therapy. The dose of thyroxine should then be adjusted in 12- to 25-µg increments at intervals of 6–8 weeks until plasma TSH is normal. Thereafter, annual TSH measurement is adequate to monitor therapy. TSH should also be measured in the first trimester of pregnancy because the thyroxine dose requirement often increases at this time (see Special Considerations section). Overtreatment, indicated by a subnormal TSH, should be avoided because it increases the risk of osteoporosis and atrial fibrillation.
  - **In secondary hypothyroidism, plasma TSH cannot be used to adjust therapy.** The goal of therapy is to maintain the **plasma-free** T_4 in the upper half of the reference range. The dose of thyroxine should be adjusted at 6- to 8-week intervals until this goal is achieved. Thereafter, annual measurement of plasma-free T_4 is adequate to monitor therapy.

SPECIAL CONSIDERATIONS

- **Situations in which thyroxine dose requirements change:** Difficulty in controlling hypothyroidism is most often because of **poor compliance** with therapy. Other causes of increasing thyroxine requirement include the following:
  - Malabsorption because of intestinal disease or drugs that interfere with thyroxine absorption (e.g., calcium carbonate, ferrous sulfate, cholestyramine, sucralfate, aluminum hydroxide)
  - Drug interactions that increase thyroxine clearance (e.g., estrogen, rifampin, carbamazepine, phenytoin) or block conversion of T_4 to T_3 (amiodarone)
  - Gradual failure of remaining endogenous thyroid function after RAI treatment of hyperthyroidism
- **Pregnancy:** Thyroxine dose increases by an average of 40%–50% in the first half of pregnancy. In women with primary hypothyroidism, plasma TSH should be measured as soon as pregnancy is confirmed and monthly thereafter through the second trimester. The thyroxine dose should be increased as needed to maintain plasma TSH <2.5 µU/mL to avoid fetal hypothyroidism.

- **Subclinical hypothyroidism** should be treated if any of the following are present: (1) symptoms compatible with hypothyroidism, (2) hypercholesterolemia that warrants treatment or (3) plasma TSH >10 μU/mL, and (4) pregnancy. Untreated patients should be monitored annually, and thyroxine should be started if symptoms develop or serum TSH increases to >10 μU/mL.
- **Urgent therapy** for hypothyroidism is rarely necessary. Most patients with hypothyroidism and concomitant illness can be treated in the usual manner. However, hypothyroidism may impair survival in critical illness by contributing to hypoventilation, hypotension, hypothermia, bradycardia, or hyponatremia—**myxoedema coma.**
  - Hypoventilation and hypotension should be treated intensively, along with any concomitant diseases. Confirmatory tests (plasma TSH and free T_4) should be obtained before thyroid hormone therapy is started.
  - **Thyroxine, 50–100 μg IV, can be given q6–8h for 24 hours**, followed by 75–100 μg IV daily until oral intake is possible. No clinical trials have determined the optimum method of thyroid hormone replacement, but this method rapidly alleviates hypothyroidism while minimizing the risk of exacerbating underlying coronary disease or heart failure. **Rapid correction is warranted only in extremely ill patients. Vital signs and cardiac rhythm should be monitored carefully to detect early signs of exacerbation of heart disease. Hydrocortisone, 50 mg IV q8h, is recommended during rapid replacement of thyroid hormone because this therapy may precipitate adrenal crisis in patients with adrenal failure.**

Hyperthyroidism[4,7]

GENERAL PRINCIPLES

- **Thyrotoxicosis** is a clinical state that results from any condition leading to high thyroid hormone action in tissues.
- **Hyperthyroidism** is a form of thyrotoxicosis caused by high synthesis and release of thyroid hormone from the thyroid gland.
- **Graves' disease** causes most cases of hyperthyroidism, especially in young patients. Prevalence of 1.6% of subclinical and 1.3% overt hyperthyroidism in India.[5] This **autoimmune** disorder may also cause **proptosis** (exophthalmos) and pretibial myxoedema, neither of which is found in other causes of hyperthyroidism.
- **Toxic multinodular goiter** (MNG) may cause hyperthyroidism, more commonly in older patients.
- Unusual causes include **iodine-induced hyperthyroidism** (precipitated by drugs such as **amiodarone** or radiographic contrast media), thyroid adenomas, subacute thyroiditis (painful tender goiter with transient hyperthyroidism), painless thyroiditis (nontender goiter with transient hyperthyroidism, most often seen in the postpartum period), and surreptitious ingestion of thyroid hormone. TSH-induced hyperthyroidism is extremely rare.

DIAGNOSIS

Clinical Presentation

History

- Symptoms include heat intolerance, weight loss, weakness, palpitations, oligomenorrhea, and anxiety.
- **In the elderly,** hyperthyroidism may present with only atrial fibrillation, heart failure, weakness, or weight loss (apathetic hyperthyroidism), and a high index of suspicion is needed to make the diagnosis.

TABLE 24-2 Differential Diagnosis of Hyperthyroidism

Type of Goiter	Diagnosis
Diffuse, nontender goiter	Graves' disease or painless thyroiditis
Multiple thyroid nodules	Toxic multinodular goiter
Single thyroid nodule	Thyroid adenoma
Tender painful goiter	Subacute thyroiditis
Normal thyroid gland	Graves' disease, painless thyroiditis, or factitious hyperthyroidism

Physical Examination

- Signs include brisk tendon reflexes, fine tremor, proximal weakness, stare, and eyelid lag. Cardiac abnormalities may be prominent, including sinus tachycardia, atrial fibrillation, thyroid acropachy, and exacerbation of coronary artery disease or heart failure.
- Key differentiating physical examination findings (Table 24-2) include the following:
  - The presence of proptosis or pretibial myxoedema, seen only in Graves' disease (although many patients with Graves' disease lack these signs)
  - A diffuse nontender goiter, consistent with Graves' disease or painless thyroiditis
  - Recent pregnancy, neck pain, or recent iodine administration, suggesting causes other than Graves' disease
- **Thyroid storm**—crisis due to sudden release of large amount of thyroid hormone as a result of stress, infection, trauma, or surgery. It usually manifests with atrial fibrillation, hypertension, heart failure, dehydration, and seizures.

Diagnostic Testing

- In rare cases, **24-hour radioactive iodine uptake** (**RAIU**) is needed to distinguish Graves' disease or toxic nodules (in which RAIU is elevated) from postpartum thyroiditis, iodine-induced hyperthyroidism, or factitious hyperthyroidism (in which RAIU is very low).
- In suspected hyperthyroidism, plasma TSH is the best initial diagnostic test.
  - A normal TSH level virtually excludes clinical hyperthyroidism. If plasma TSH is low, **plasma-free T_4** should be measured to determine the severity of hyperthyroidism and as a baseline for therapy. If plasma-free T_4 is elevated, the diagnosis of clinical hyperthyroidism is established.
  - **If plasma TSH is <0.1 μU/mL but free T_4 is normal,** the patient may have clinical hyperthyroidism because of elevation of plasma T_3 alone, and plasma T_3 should be measured in this case.
  - **Mild (or subclinical) hyperthyroidism** may suppress TSH to <0.1 μU/mL, and thus suppression of TSH alone does not confirm that symptoms are due to hyperthyroidism.
  - TSH may also be suppressed by **severe nonthyroidal illness** (see Evaluation of Thyroid Function section).

TREATMENT

- Some forms of hyperthyroidism (subacute or postpartum thyroiditis) are transient and require only **symptomatic therapy**. A **β-adrenergic antagonist** (such as **atenolol** 25–100 mg daily) relieves symptoms of hyperthyroidism, such as palpitations, tremor, and anxiety, until hyperthyroidism is controlled by definitive therapy or until transient forms of hyperthyroidism subside. The dose is adjusted to alleviate symptoms and tachycardia and then reduced gradually as hyperthyroidism is controlled.

- Three methods are available for definitive therapy (none of which controls hyperthyroidism rapidly): RAI, thionamides, and thyroidectomy.
  - During treatment, patients are followed by clinical evaluation and measurement of plasma-free T_4. Plasma TSH is useless in assessing the initial response to therapy because it remains suppressed until after the patient becomes euthyroid.
  - Regardless of the therapy used, all patients with Graves' disease require lifelong follow-up for recurrent hyperthyroidism or development of hypothyroidism.
- **Choice of definitive therapy**
  - **In Graves' disease, RAI therapy is our preferred treatment for almost all patients.** It is simple and highly effective but **cannot be used in pregnancy** (see Hyperthyroidism in Pregnancy section). Thionamides achieve long-term control in fewer than half of patients with Graves' disease, and they carry a small risk of life-threatening side effects (agranulocytosis, liver dysfunction). Thyroidectomy may be used in patients who refuse RAI therapy, have significant Graves' ophthalmopathy, or who relapse or develop side effects with thionamide therapy.
  - **Other causes of hyperthyroidism:** We prefer to treat toxic nodules with RAI (except in pregnancy or during breastfeeding), though thionamides or partial thyroidectomy can also be used. Transient forms of hyperthyroidism because of thyroiditis should be treated symptomatically with atenolol. Iodine-induced hyperthyroidism is treated with thionamides and atenolol until the patient is euthyroid. Although treatment of some patients with amiodarone-induced hyperthyroidism with glucocorticoids has been advocated, **nearly all patients with amiodarone-induced hyperthyroidism respond well to thionamide therapy**.
- **RAI therapy**
  - A single dose permanently controls hyperthyroidism in 90% of patients, and further doses can be given if necessary.
  - A **pregnancy test** is done immediately before therapy in potentially fertile women.
  - A 24-hour RAIU is usually measured and used to calculate the dose.
  - Thionamides interfere with RAI therapy and should be stopped at least 3 days before treatment. If iodine treatment has been given, it should be stopped at least 2 weeks before RAI therapy.
  - **Follow-up:** Usually, several months are needed to restore euthyroidism. Patients are evaluated at 4- to 6-week intervals, with assessment of clinical findings and plasma-free T_4.
    - If thyroid function stabilizes within the normal range, the interval between follow-up visits is gradually increased to annual intervals.
    - If symptomatic hypothyroidism develops, thyroxine therapy is started (see Hypothyroidism section).
    - If symptomatic hyperthyroidism **persists after 6 months, RAI treatment can be repeated.**
  - **Side effects**
    - **Hypothyroidism** occurs in most patients within the first year and thereafter continues to develop at a rate of approximately 3% per year.
    - Because of the release of stored hormone, a slight rise in plasma T_4 may occur in the first 2 weeks after therapy. This development is important only in **patients with severe cardiac disease**, which may worsen as a result. Such patients should be treated with thionamides to restore euthyroidism and to deplete stored hormone before treatment with RAI.
    - There have been mixed results as to whether RAI has a clinically important effect on the course of Graves' eye disease, but early treatment to prevent hypothyroidism after RAI seems to be beneficial, and patients should be counseled to stop smoking, as this is a known contributor to worsening of the eye disease.
    - It does not increase the risk of malignancy or cause congenital abnormalities in the offspring of women who conceive after RAI therapy.

- **Thionamides:** Methimazole and propylthiouracil (PTU) inhibit thyroid hormone synthesis. PTU also inhibits extrathyroidal deiodination of T_4 to T_3. Once thyroid hormone stores are depleted (after several weeks to months), T_4 levels decrease. These drugs have no permanent effect on thyroid function. **In the majority of patients with Graves' disease, hyperthyroidism recurs within 6 months after therapy is stopped.** Spontaneous remission of Graves' disease occurs in approximately one-third of patients during thionamide therapy, and in this minority, no other treatment may be needed. Remission is more likely in mild, recent onset hyperthyroidism and if the goiter is small. Because of a better safety profile, **methimazole should be used instead of PTU** except in specific situations (see the following text).
  - **Initiation of therapy:** Before starting therapy, patients must be warned of side effects and precautions. Usual starting doses are methimazole, 10–40 mg PO daily, or PTU, 100–200 mg PO tid; higher initial doses can be used in severe hyperthyroidism.
  - **Follow-up:** Restoration of euthyroidism takes up to several months.
    - Patients are evaluated at 4-week intervals with assessment of clinical findings and plasma-free T_4. If plasma-free T_4 levels do not fall after 4–8 weeks, the dose should be increased. Doses as high as methimazole, 60 mg PO daily, or PTU, 300 mg PO qid, may be required.
    - Once the plasma-free T_4 level falls to normal, the dose is adjusted to maintain plasma- free T_4 within the normal range.
    - No consensus exists on the optimal duration of therapy, but periods of 6 months to 2 years are usually used. Patients must be monitored carefully for recurrence of hyperthyroidism after the drug is stopped.
  - **Side effects** are most likely to occur within the first few months of therapy.
    - Minor side effects include rash, urticaria, fever, arthralgias, and transient leukopenia.
    - **Agranulocytosis** occurs in 0.3% of patients treated with thionamides. Other life-threatening side effects include **hepatitis**, vasculitis, and drug-induced lupus erythematosus. These complications usually resolve if the drug is stopped promptly.
    - **Patients must be warned to stop the drug immediately if jaundice or symptoms suggestive of agranulocytosis develop (e.g., fever, chills, sore throat)** and to contact their physician promptly for evaluation. Routine monitoring of the white blood cell count is not useful for detecting agranulocytosis, which develops suddenly. Thionamides should not be given again once a patient develops agranulocytosis.
- **Total thyroidectomy:** This procedure provides long-term control of hyperthyroidism in most patients.
  - Surgery may trigger a perioperative exacerbation of hyperthyroidism, and patients should be prepared for surgery by one of two methods.
    - **A thionamide** is given until the patient is nearly euthyroid. **Supersaturated potassium iodide** (**SSKI**), 40–80 mg (one to two drops) PO bid, is then added 1–2 weeks before surgery. Both drugs are stopped postoperatively.
    - **Atenolol** (50–100 mg daily) is started 1–2 weeks before surgery. The dose of atenolol is increased, if necessary, to reduce the resting heart rate below 90 bpm and is continued for 5–7 days postoperatively. SSKI is given as mentioned earlier.
  - **Follow-up:** Clinical findings and plasma-free T_4 and TSH should be assessed 4–6 weeks after surgery.
    - If thyroid function is normal, the patient is seen at 3 and 6 months and then annually.
    - If symptomatic hypothyroidism develops, thyroxine therapy is started.
    - Hyperthyroidism persists or recurs in 3%–7% of patients.
    - **Complications** of thyroidectomy include **hypothyroidism** and **hypoparathyroidism**. Rare complications include permanent vocal cord paralysis, due to recurrent laryngeal nerve injury, and perioperative death. The complication rate appears to depend on the experience of the surgeon.

SPECIAL CONSIDERATIONS

- **Subclinical hyperthyroidism** is present when the plasma TSH is below normal but the patient has no symptoms that are definitely caused by hyperthyroidism, and plasma levels of free T_4 and T_3 are normal.
  - Subclinical hyperthyroidism increases the risk of **atrial fibrillation** in patients older than 65 years and those with heart disease and predisposes to **osteoporosis** in postmenopausal women; it should be treated in these patients. Treatment should also be considered in asymptomatic individuals without risk factors but with TSH persistently <0.1 μU/mL.
  - Asymptomatic young patients with mild Graves' disease can be observed for spontaneous resolution of hyperthyroidism or the development of symptoms or increasing free T_4 levels that warrant treatment.
- **Urgent therapy** is warranted when hyperthyroidism exacerbates heart failure or acute coronary syndromes and in rare patients with severe hyperthyroidism complicated by fever and delirium (thyroid storm). Concomitant diseases should be treated intensively, and confirmatory tests (serum TSH and free T_4) should be obtained before therapy is started.
  - **PTU 300 mg PO q6h or methimazole 60 mg/d PO should be started immediately.**
  - **Iodide** (SSKI, two drops PO q12h) should be started to inhibit thyroid hormone secretion rapidly.
  - **Propranolol,** 40 mg PO q6h (or an equivalent dose IV), should be given to patients with angina or myocardial infarction, and the dose should be adjusted to prevent tachycardia. β-Adrenergic antagonists may benefit some patients with heart failure and marked tachycardia but can further impair left ventricular systolic function. In patients with clinical heart failure, it should be given only with careful monitoring of left ventricular function.
  - Plasma-free T_4 is measured every 4–6 days. When free T_4 approaches the normal range, the doses of methimazole and iodine are gradually decreased. RAI therapy can be scheduled 2–4 weeks after iodine is stopped.
- **Hyperthyroidism in pregnancy:** If hyperthyroidism is suspected, plasma TSH should be measured. Plasma TSH declines in early pregnancy but rarely to <0.1 μU/mL due to the stimulatory effect of hCG on TSH receptors.
  - If TSH is <0.1 μU/mL, the diagnosis should be confirmed by measurement of plasma-free T_4.
  - RAI is contraindicated in pregnancy, and therefore, patients should be treated with **PTU in the first trimester** because of its lower risk of severe congenital defects, whereas **methimazole can be used in later pregnancy**. The dose should be adjusted at 4-week intervals to maintain the plasma-free T_4 near the upper limit of the normal range to avoid fetal hypothyroidism. The dose required often decreases in the later stages of pregnancy.
  - **Atenolol, 25–50 mg PO daily,** can be used to relieve symptoms while awaiting the effects of PTU.
  - The fetus and neonate should be monitored for hyperthyroidism. The **maternal plasma level of thyroid receptor antibodies should be assessed in early pregnancy**, and if elevated or if the patient requires thionamide treatment during pregnancy, it should be repeated at weeks 18–22 and again at weeks 30–34 to assess this risk.
- **Amiodarone-induced thyrotoxicosis** (AIT) develops in 3% of amiodarone-treated patients. AIT is classified as type 1 or type 2. Type 1 AIT occurs in patients with underlying thyroid pathology such as autonomous nodular goiter or Graves' disease. Type 2 AIT is a result of amiodarone causing a subacute thyroiditis with release of preformed thyroid hormones into the circulation. Patients with type 2 AIT benefit by a trial of glucocorticoids, whereas those with type 1 should receive antithyroid therapy with thionamides.

Goiter, Thyroid Nodules, and Thyroid Carcinoma[8,9]

GENERAL PRINCIPLES

- The evaluation of goiter is based on examination of the thyroid and evaluation of thyroid function. If the thyroid is enlarged, the examiner should determine whether the enlargement is **diffuse or nodular**. Both forms of goiter are common, especially in women.
- Thyroid scans and ultrasonography (US) provide no useful additional information about goiters that are diffuse by palpation and should not be performed in these patients. In contrast, all palpable thyroid nodules should be evaluated by US.
- In rare patients, more commonly in those with MNG, the gland compresses the trachea or esophagus, causing dyspnea or dysphagia, and treatment is required. Thyroxine treatment has little, if any, effect on the size of MNGs. Subtotal thyroidectomy is most commonly used to relieve compressive symptoms. RAI therapy will reduce gland size and relieve symptoms in most patients if surgery is not an option, though much higher doses are necessary if the patient is euthyroid.
- **Diffuse goiter**
  - Almost all euthyroid diffuse goiters in the United States are due to **chronic lymphocytic thyroiditis (Hashimoto thyroiditis)**. Because Hashimoto thyroiditis may also cause hypothyroidism, plasma TSH should be measured.
  - Diffuse euthyroid goiters are usually asymptomatic, and therapy is seldom required. Patients should be monitored regularly for the development of hypothyroidism.
  - Diffuse hyperthyroid goiter is most commonly because of Graves' disease, and treatment of the hyperthyroidism usually improves the goiter (see Hyperthyroidism section).
- **Nodular goiter**
  - Between 30% and 50% of people have nonpalpable thyroid nodules that are detectable by ultrasound. These nodules rarely have any clinical importance, but their incidental discovery may lead to unnecessary diagnostic testing and treatment.
  - Nodules are more common in older patients, especially women, and 5%–10% of thyroid nodules are thyroid carcinomas.

DIAGNOSIS

Clinical Presentation

History

Clinical findings that increase the risk of carcinoma include the presence of cervical lymphadenopathy, a history of radiation to the head or neck, and a family history of medullary thyroid carcinoma or multiple endocrine neoplasia syndromes type 2A or 2B.

Physical Examination

A hard, fixed nodule, recent nodule growth, or hoarseness due to vocal cord paralysis suggests malignancy.

Diagnostic Testing

- All patients with one or more palpable thyroid nodules on examination or thyroid nodules identified by other imaging modality should undergo a dedicated **thyroid ultrasound** as this is the most informative imaging for malignancy risk in thyroid nodules.
- **Guidelines from the American Thyroid Association classify malignancy risk and biopsy recommendations based on nodule characteristics and size using thyroid USG (ACR-TIRADS staging).**

- Nodules are characterized into the following risk classes based on their ultrasound appearance: high suspicion (>70%–90% malignancy risk), intermediate suspicion (10%–20% malignancy risk), low suspicion (5%–10% malignancy risk), very low suspicion (<3% malignancy risk), and benign (<1% malignancy risk).
- High and intermediate suspicion nodules warrant evaluation by fine needle aspiration (FNA) when they are >1 cm. Low suspicion nodules should be evaluated at >1.5 cm and very low-risk nodules at 2 cm. Benign nodules require no further follow-up.
- In a few patients, **hyperthyroidism** develops as a result of "toxic" nodules that overproduce thyroid hormone (see Hyperthyroidism section). These nodules can be identified with a radionuclide scan and do not require FNA evaluation as the malignancy risk is only 1%–2%.

TREATMENT

Patients with thyroid carcinoma or suspicion for thyroid carcinoma by FNA cytology typically initially undergo surgical resection with either **hemi- or total thyroidectomy**, sometimes followed by **adjuvant therapy with RAI** and should be managed in consultation with an endocrinologist.

FOLLOW-UP

- **Further follow-up depends on FNA results.** Benign nodules should undergo repeat ultrasound depending on initial ultrasound risk: high risk in 6–12 months and low-intermediate in 12–24 months. The utility of following very low-risk nodules is unclear. Nodules with benign cytology should also be reevaluated periodically by palpation. Thyroxine therapy has little or no effect on the size of thyroid nodules and is not indicated.
- Nodules with **nondiagnostic cytology** because of insufficient sampling should undergo **repeat biopsy**.
- The management of thyroid nodules with **indeterminate cytology** is less clear. Nodules with atypia of undetermined significance or follicular lesion by cytology can be further evaluated with **molecular diagnostic testing** to estimate risk and guide surgical decision-making.

Adrenal Failure[10,11]

GENERAL PRINCIPLES

- Adrenal failure may be due to disease of the adrenal glands (**primary adrenal failure, Addison disease**), with deficiency of both cortisol and aldosterone and elevated plasma adrenocorticotropic hormone (ACTH), or due to ACTH deficiency caused by disorders of the pituitary or hypothalamus (**secondary adrenal failure**), with deficiency of cortisol alone.
- **Primary adrenal failure** is most often due to **autoimmune adrenalitis**, which may be associated with other endocrine deficits (e.g., hypothyroidism).
- Adrenal failure may also develop in patients with infiltrative or infectious diseases of the adrenal glands, such as adrenal lymphoma, metastases, disseminated cytomegalovirus, mycobacterial infection, or fungal infection. Of note, some of the causative infections are more common in immunosuppressed individuals.
- **Hemorrhagic adrenal infarction** (**Waterhouse–Friderichsen syndrome** due to *Neisseria meningitidis*) can occur in the postoperative period, in coagulation disorders and

hypercoagulable states, and in sepsis. Adrenal hemorrhage often causes abdominal or flank pain and fever; CT scan of the abdomen reveals high-density bilateral adrenal masses.

- Less common etiologies include adrenoleukodystrophy that causes adrenal failure in young men and drugs such as ketoconazole and etomidate that inhibit steroid hormone synthesis.
- **Secondary adrenal failure** is most often due to **glucocorticoid therapy**; ACTH suppression may persist for a year after therapy is stopped. Any disorder of the pituitary or hypothalamus can cause ACTH deficiency, but other evidence of these disorders is usually obvious.
- **Checkpoint inhibitors** commonly used for immunotherapy to treat various cancers can cause hypophysitis or, less commonly, adrenalitis, potentially leading to secondary or primary adrenal failure, respectively.

DIAGNOSIS

Clinical Presentation

- Adrenal failure should be suspected in patients with otherwise unexplained hypotension, weight loss, persistent nausea, hyponatremia, hyperkalemia, or hypoglycemia.
- **Clinical findings** in adrenal failure are nonspecific, and without a high index of suspicion, the diagnosis of this potentially lethal but readily treatable disease is easily missed.
  - Symptoms include anorexia, nausea, vomiting, weight loss, weakness, and fatigue. Orthostatic hypotension and hyponatremia are common.
  - Symptoms are usually chronic, but **shock** may develop suddenly and is fatal unless promptly treated. Often, this adrenal crisis is triggered by illness, injury, or surgery. All these symptoms are due to cortisol deficiency and occur in both primary and secondary adrenal failure.
- Hyperpigmentation (because of marked ACTH excess) and hyperkalemia and volume depletion (because of aldosterone deficiency) occur only in primary adrenal failure.

Diagnostic Testing

- The **cosyntropin stimulation test** is used for diagnosis. Cosyntropin, 250 μg, is given IV or IM, and **plasma cortisol is measured 30 and 60 minutes later**. The normal response is a stimulated plasma cortisol >18 μg/dL. This test detects primary and secondary adrenal failure, except within a few weeks of onset of pituitary dysfunction (e.g., shortly after pituitary surgery; see Pituitary Adenomas and Hypopituitarism section).
- The clinical presentation usually helps to distinguish between primary and secondary adrenal failure. Hyperkalemia, hyperpigmentation, or other autoimmune endocrine deficits are more suggestive of primary adrenal failure, whereas deficits of other pituitary hormones, symptoms of a pituitary mass (e.g., headache, visual field loss), or known pituitary or hypothalamic disease are more suggestive secondary adrenal failure.
- If the cause is unclear, the **plasma ACTH** level distinguishes primary adrenal failure (in which it is markedly elevated) from secondary adrenal failure. **High renin and low aldosterone levels** are suggestive of primary adrenal insufficiency.
- Most cases of primary adrenal failure are due to autoimmune adrenalitis, but other causes should be considered. Radiographic evidence of adrenal enlargement or calcification indicates that the cause is infection or hemorrhage.
- Patients with secondary adrenal failure should be tested for other pituitary hormone deficiencies and should be evaluated for a pituitary or hypothalamic tumor (see Pituitary Adenomas and Hypopituitarism section).

TREATMENT

- **Adrenal crisis** with hypotension must be treated immediately. Patients should be evaluated for an underlying illness that precipitated the crisis.
- **If the diagnosis of adrenal failure is known, hydrocortisone, 50 mg IV q6h,** should be given, and **0.9% saline with 5% dextrose** should be infused rapidly until hypotension is corrected. The dose of hydrocortisone is decreased gradually over several days as symptoms and any precipitating illness resolve and then changed to oral maintenance therapy. Mineralocorticoid replacement is not needed until the dose of hydrocortisone is <100 mg/d.
- **If the diagnosis of adrenal failure has not been established,** a single dose of **dexamethasone,** 10 mg IV, should be given, and a rapid infusion of 0.9% saline with 5% dextrose should be started. A **Cosyntropin stimulation test** should be performed, regardless of the time of day. Dexamethasone is used because it does not interfere with measurement of plasma cortisol. After the Cortrosyn stimulation test is complete, hydrocortisone, 100 mg IV q8h, should be given until the test result is known.
- High-dose hydrocortisone provides sufficient mineralocorticoid activity to cover for suspected primary adrenal insufficiency until diagnosis is clarified.
- **Maintenance therapy** in all patients requires cortisol replacement with prednisone. Most patients with primary adrenal failure also require replacement of aldosterone with fludrocortisone.
  - **Prednisone,** 5 mg PO every morning, should be started. The dose is then adjusted with the goal being the lowest dose that relieves the patient's symptoms, to prevent osteoporosis and other signs of Cushing syndrome. Most patients require doses between 4.0 and 7.5 mg PO daily. Concomitant therapy with rifampin, phenytoin, or phenobarbital accelerates glucocorticoid metabolism and increases the dose requirement.
  - **During illness, injury, or the perioperative period, the dose of glucocorticoid must be increased.** For minor illnesses, the patient should double the dose of prednisone for 2–3 days. If the illness resolves, the maintenance dose is resumed.
  - **Vomiting requires immediate medical attention,** with IV glucocorticoid therapy and IV fluid. Patients can be given a 4-mg vial of dexamethasone to be self-administered IM for vomiting or severe illness if medical care is not immediately available.
  - **For severe illness or injury,** hydrocortisone, 50 mg IV q6h, should be given, with the dose tapered as severity of illness wanes. The same regimen is used in **patients undergoing surgery,** with the first dose of hydrocortisone given preoperatively. The dose can be tapered to maintenance therapy by 2–3 days after uncomplicated surgery.
- **In primary adrenal failure, fludrocortisone, 0.1 mg PO daily,** should be given. The dose is adjusted to maintain blood pressure (supine and standing) and serum potassium within the normal range; the usual dosage is 0.05–0.20 mg PO daily.
- **Patients should be educated in management of their disease,** including adjustment of prednisone dose during illness. They should wear a medical identification tag or bracelet.

Cushing Syndrome[12]

General Principles

- Cushing syndrome (CS) is most often **iatrogenic** because of therapy with glucocorticoid drugs—exogenous CS.
- **ACTH-dependant CS: ACTH-secreting pituitary microadenomas (Cushing disease)** account for 80% of cases of endogenous CS, ectopic ACTH-secreting tumors.
- **ACTH-independent CS:** Adrenal tumors, macronodular adrenal hyperplasia, primary pigmented nodular adrenocortical disease (**PPNAD**), account for the remainder.

DIAGNOSIS

Clinical Presentation

- Findings include truncal obesity, rounded face, fat deposits in the supraclavicular fossae and over the posterior neck, hypertension, hirsutism, amenorrhea, and depression. More specific findings include thin skin, easy bruising, reddish striae, proximal muscle weakness, and osteoporosis.
- Hyperpigmentation or severe hypokalemic alkalosis suggests CS due to ectopic ACTH secretion.
- Diabetes mellitus develops in some patients.

Diagnostic Testing (Figure 24-2)

- **Diagnosis** is based on increased cortisol excretion, lack of normal feedback inhibition of ACTH and cortisol secretion, or loss of the normal diurnal rhythm of cortisol secretion. Three initial tests are available:
  - An **overnight dexamethasone suppression test** may be performed (1 mg dexamethasone given PO at 11:00 PM; plasma cortisol measured at 8:00 AM. the next day; normal range: plasma cortisol <1.8 µg/dL); or
  - **Salivary cortisol** may be measured at home during the nadir of normal plasma cortisol at 11:00 PM.
  - 24-Hour urine-free cortisol measurement.
- All these tests are very sensitive, and a normal value virtually excludes the diagnosis. If the overnight dexamethasone suppression test or 11:00 PM. salivary cortisol is abnormal, 24-hour urine cortisol should be measured.
  - If the 24-hour urine cortisol excretion is more than 3–4 times the upper limit of the reference range in a patient with compatible clinical findings, the diagnosis of CS is established.
  - Testing should not be done during severe illness or depression, which may cause false-positive results. Phenytoin therapy also causes a false-positive test by accelerating metabolism of dexamethasone.
- After the diagnosis of CS is made, tests to determine the cause and appropriate treatment are best done in consultation with an endocrinologist.

TREATMENT

Management depends on the etiology of CS and can include surgery, radiotherapy, and medications (Figure 24-3).

Treatment if surgery fails:

- Pituitary irradiation
- Medical therapy - Adrenal enzyme inhibitors (oral ketoconazole, metyrapone, osilodrostat mitotane, intravenous etomidate), glucocorticoid-receptor antagonists (mifepristone (RU-486)
- Medical adrenalectomy with Mitotane.

Incidental Adrenal Nodules[13]

GENERAL PRINCIPLES

- Adrenal nodules are a common incidental finding on abdominal imaging studies.
- Most incidentally discovered nodules are benign adrenocortical tumors that do not secrete excess hormone.

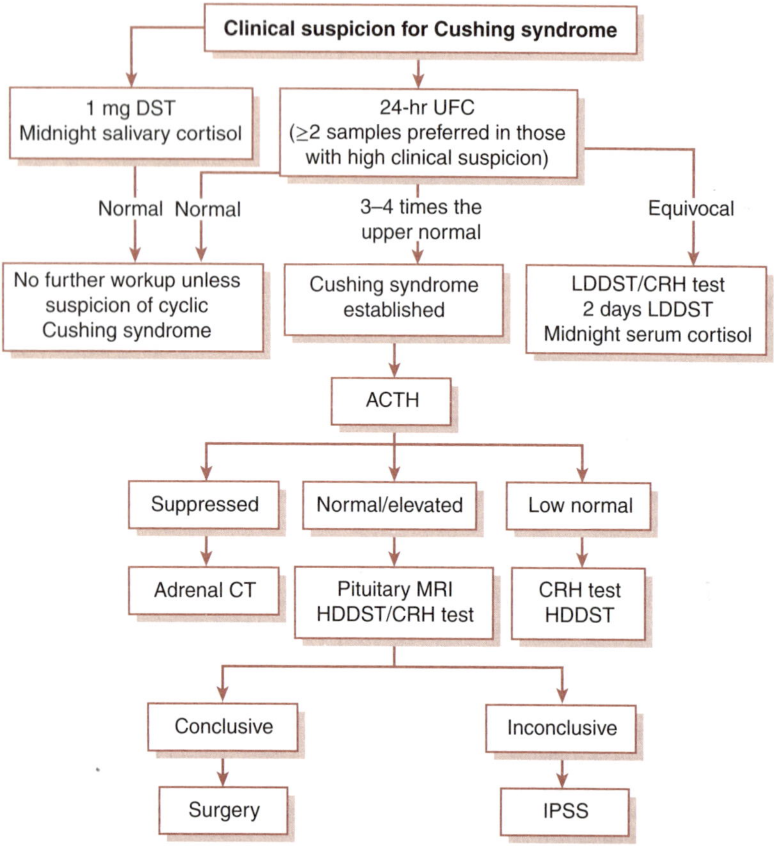

Figure 24-2 Diagnostic algorithm for Cushing syndrome. DST, 1-mg dexamethasone suppression test; UFC, urinary free cortisol; LDDST, 2-day low-dose dexamethasone suppression test; CRH, corticotropin-releasing hormone; HDDST, high-dose DST; IPSS, inferior petrosal sinus sampling.

DIAGNOSIS

Clinical Presentation

Patients should be evaluated for hypertension, symptoms suggestive of pheochromocytoma (episodic headache, palpitations, and sweating), and signs of CS (*see* Cushing Syndrome section).

Differential Diagnosis

- In patients without a known malignancy elsewhere, the diagnostic issues are whether a syndrome of hormone excess or an adrenocortical carcinoma is present.
- The differential diagnosis includes adrenal adenomas causing CS or primary hyperaldosteronism, pheochromocytoma, adrenocortical carcinoma, and metastatic cancer.
- The imaging characteristics of the nodule may suggest a diagnosis but are not specific enough to obviate further evaluation.

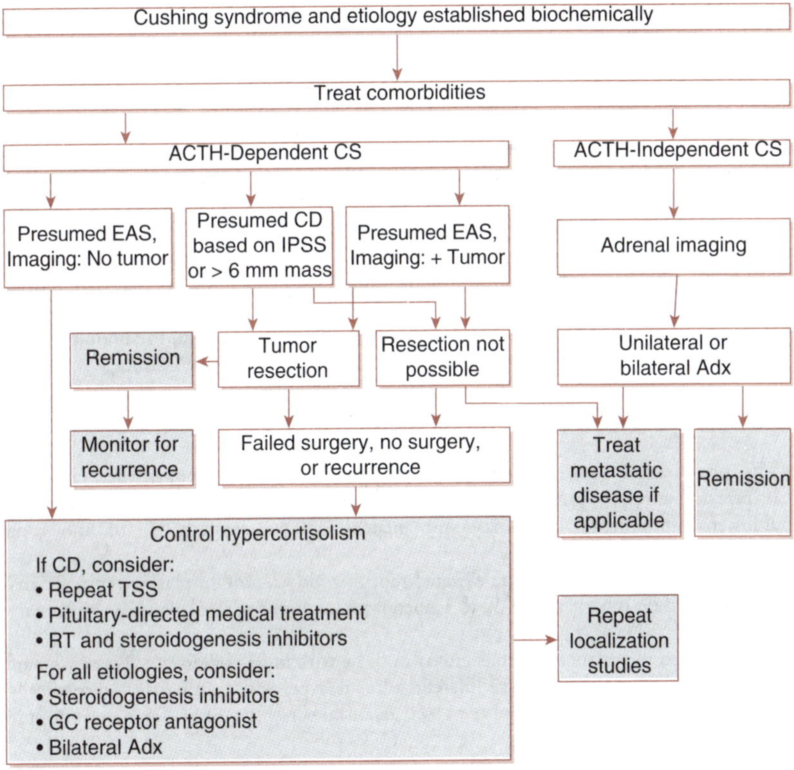

Figure 24-3 An algorithm for treatment of Cushing syndrome. Adx, adrenalectomy; CS, Cushing syndrome; EAS, ectopic ACTH secretion; GC, glucocorticoid; IPSS, inferior petrosal sinus sampling; TSS, transsphenoidal selective adenomectomy. Derived from Nieman LK, Biller BM, Finding, JW, et al. The diagnosis of Cushing's syndrome: an Endocrine Society Clinical Practice Guideline. *J Clin Endocrinol Metab*. 2008;93:1526–1540.

Diagnostic Testing

- **Serum cortisol, plasma sodium, potassium, metanephrines, and dehydroepiandrosterone sulfate** should be measured, and an **overnight dexamethasone suppression** test should be performed.
- **Patients who have potentially resectable cancer elsewhere** and in whom an adrenal metastasis must be excluded may require positron emission tomography.
- Patients with hypertension (especially if they have hypokalemia) should be evaluated for primary hyperaldosteronism by measuring the **ratio of plasma aldosterone (in nanograms per deciliter** [**ng/dL**]**) to plasma renin activity (in ng/mL/h)**. If the ratio is <20, the diagnosis of primary hyperaldosteronism is excluded, whereas a ratio >50 makes the diagnosis very likely. Patients with an intermediate ratio should be further evaluated in consultation with an endocrinologist.
- An abnormal overnight dexamethasone suppression test should be evaluated further (see Cushing Syndrome section).

- Elevation of plasma dehydroepiandrosterone sulfate or a large nodule suggests adrenocortical carcinoma.

TREATMENT

- Most incidental nodules are <4 cm in diameter, do not produce excess hormone, and do not require therapy. One **repeat imaging procedure** 3–6 months later is recommended to ensure that the nodule is not enlarging rapidly (which would suggest an adrenal carcinoma).
- A policy of resecting all nodules >4 cm in diameter appropriately treats the great majority of adrenal carcinomas while minimizing the number of benign nodules that are removed unnecessarily.
- If clinical or biochemical evidence of a pheochromocytoma is found, the nodule should be resected after appropriate α-adrenergic blockade with phenoxybenzamine.

PRIMARY HYPERALDOSTERONISM (CONN SYNDROME)

- The presentation classically described is hypertension and hypokalemia. However, in practice, most patients present without hyperkalemia. The two primary causes are aldosterone-producing adenomas and bilateral adrenal hyperplasia of the zona glomerulosa.
- Diagnosis is confirmed with the elevated morning aldosterone to plasma renin activity ratio. If the ratio is higher than 20 to 1; then it points to the adrenal gland as the primary source.
- The preferred treatment is adrenalectomy in those with unilateral disease. Those who are poor surgical candidates or have bilateral adrenal hyperplasia can be treated medically with mineralocorticoid antagonists as well as antihypertensive drugs for blood pressure control.

Pituitary Adenomas and Hypopituitarism[11,14]

GENERAL PRINCIPLES

- The anterior pituitary gland secretes **prolactin**, **growth hormone**, and four **trophic hormones**, including corticotropin (ACTH), thyrotropin (TSH), and the gonadotropins, luteinizing hormone and follicle-stimulating hormone. Each trophic hormone stimulates a specific target gland.
- Anterior pituitary function is regulated by hypothalamic hormones that reach the pituitary via portal veins in the pituitary stalk. The predominant effect of hypothalamic regulation is to stimulate secretion of pituitary hormones, except for prolactin, which is inhibited by hypothalamic dopamine secretion.
- Secretion of trophic hormones is also regulated by negative feedback by their target gland hormone, and the normal pituitary response to target hormone deficiency is increased secretion of the appropriate trophic hormone.
- **Anterior pituitary dysfunction** can be caused by disorders of either the pituitary or hypothalamus.
- **Pituitary adenomas** are the most common pituitary disorder. They are classified by size and function.
  - **Microadenomas** are <10 mm in diameter and cause clinical manifestations only if they produce excess hormone. They are too small to produce hypopituitarism or mass effects.

  - **Macroadenomas** are >10 mm in diameter and may produce any combination of pituitary hormone excess, hypopituitarism, and mass effects (headache, visual field loss).
  - **Secretory adenomas** produce prolactin, growth hormone, or ACTH.
  - **Nonsecretory macroadenomas** may cause hypopituitarism or mass effects.
  - **Nonsecretory microadenomas** are common incidental radiographic findings, seen in approximately 10% of the normal population, and do not require therapy.
- **Other pituitary or hypothalamic disorders,** such as head trauma, pituitary surgery or radiation, and postpartum pituitary infarction (Sheehan syndrome), may cause hypopituitarism. Other tumors of the pituitary or hypothalamus (e.g., craniopharyngioma, metastases) and inflammatory disorders (e.g., sarcoidosis, Langerhans cell histiocytosis, lymphocytic hypophysitis) may cause hypopituitarism or mass effects. Some immunomodulatory medications, most notably checkpoint inhibitors used for cancer treatment, can cause hypophysitis and hypopituitarism.

DIAGNOSIS

Clinical Presentation

- **Hypopituitarism may be suspected in the presence of clinical signs of target hormone deficiency (e.g., hypothyroidism) or pituitary mass effects.**
- In **hypopituitarism** (deficiency of one or more pituitary hormones), gonadotropin deficiency is most common, causing amenorrhea in women and androgen deficiency in men. Secondary hypothyroidism or adrenal failure rarely occurs alone. Secondary adrenal failure causes deficiency of cortisol but not of aldosterone; hyperkalemia and hyperpigmentation do not occur, although life-threatening adrenal crisis may develop.
- **Hormone excess** most commonly results in **hyperprolactinemia**, which can be due to a secretory adenoma or due to nonsecretory lesions that damage the hypothalamus or pituitary stalk. Growth hormone excess (**acromegaly**) and ACTH and cortisol excess (**Cushing disease**) are caused by secretory adenomas. Hormone excess can be present concurrently with other hormone deficiencies.
- **Mass effects** because of pressure on adjacent structures, such as the optic chiasm, include headaches and loss of visual fields or acuity. Hyperprolactinemia may also be due to mass effect. **Pituitary apoplexy** is sudden enlargement of a pituitary tumor due to hemorrhagic necrosis.
- **Asymptomatic pituitary adenomas are commonly incidentally discovered on imaging.**

Diagnostic Testing

- **Incidental Adenoma**
  - If an incidental microadenoma is found on imaging done for another purpose, the patient should be evaluated for clinical evidence of hyperprolactinemia, Cushing disease, or acromegaly.
  - Plasma **prolactin and insulin-like growth factor 1** (IGF-1) should be measured, and tests for CS should be performed if symptoms or signs of this disorder are evident.
  - If no pituitary hormone excess exists, therapy is not required. Whether such patients need repeat imaging is not established, but the risk of enlargement is clearly small.
  - Incidental discovery of a macroadenoma is unusual. Patients should be evaluated for hormone excess and hypopituitarism. Most macroadenomas should be treated because they are likely to grow further.
  - **Laboratory evaluation** begins with evaluation of **target hormone function**, including **plasma-free T_4** and a **Cosyntropin stimulation test** (see Adrenal Failure section).
  - If recent onset of secondary adrenal failure is suspected (within a few weeks of evaluation), the patient should be treated empirically with glucocorticoids and should be tested 4–8 weeks later because the Cosyntropin stimulation test cannot detect secondary adrenal failure of recent onset.

- In men, plasma testosterone should be measured. The best evaluation of gonadal function in women is the menstrual history.
- **If a target hormone is deficient**, its trophic hormone is measured to determine whether target gland dysfunction is secondary to hypopituitarism. An elevated trophic hormone level indicates primary target gland dysfunction. In hypopituitarism, trophic hormone levels are not elevated and are usually within (not below) the reference range. Thus, **pituitary trophic hormone levels can be interpreted only with knowledge of target hormone levels**, and **measurement of trophic hormone levels alone is useless in the diagnosis of hypopituitarism.** If pituitary disease is obvious, target hormone deficiencies may be assumed to be secondary, and trophic hormones need not be measured.

• **Anatomic evaluation of the pituitary gland and hypothalamus is best done by MRI and should be performed in the setting of any pituitary hormone excess or deficiency.** However, hyperprolactinemia and Cushing disease may be caused by microadenomas too small to be seen. The prevalence of incidental microadenomas should be kept in mind when interpreting MRIs. Visual acuity and **visual fields** should be tested when imaging suggests compression of the optic chiasm.

TREATMENT

- Secondary adrenal failure should be treated immediately, especially if patients are to undergo surgery (see Adrenal Failure section).
- Treatment of secondary hypothyroidism should be monitored by measurement of **plasma-free T_4** (see Hypothyroidism section).
- Infertility because of gonadotropin deficiency may be correctable, and patients who wish to conceive should be referred to an endocrinologist.
- Treatment of hypogonadism in premenopausal women requires replacement of estrogen and progesterone. This can be conveniently done with combination oral contraceptives.
- Treatment of hypogonadism in men requires testosterone replacement, with either topical testosterone gel, 40–50 mg applied daily, or by injection of testosterone enanthate or testosterone cypionate, 100–200 mg IM every 3 weeks.
- Treatment of growth hormone deficiency in adults has been advocated by some, but the long-term benefits, risks, and cost-effectiveness of this therapy are not established.
- Treatment of pituitary macroadenomas generally requires transsphenoidal surgical resection, except for prolactin-secreting tumors.

Hyperprolactinemia[15,16]

GENERAL PRINCIPLES

- In women, the most common causes of pathologic hyperprolactinemia are prolactin-secreting pituitary **microadenomas** and **idiopathic hyperprolactinemia** (Table 24-3).
- In men, the most common cause is a prolactin-secreting **macroadenoma.**
- Hypothalamic or pituitary lesions that cause deficiency of other pituitary hormones often cause hyperprolactinemia.
- **Medications** are an important cause in both men and women.

DIAGNOSIS

Clinical Presentation

- In women, hyperprolactinemia causes amenorrhea or irregular menses and infertility. Only approximately half of these women have galactorrhea. Prolonged estrogen deficiency

TABLE 24-3 Major Causes of Hyperprolactinemia
Pregnancy and Lactation
Prolactin-secreting pituitary adenoma (prolactinoma)
Idiopathic hyperprolactinemia
Drugs (e.g., phenothiazines, atypical antipsychotic medications, metoclopramide, verapamil, domperidone, cimetidine, ranitidine)
Interference with synthesis or transport of hypothalamic dopamine
Hypothalamic lesions
Nonsecretory pituitary macroadenomas
Primary hypothyroidism
Chronic renal failure

increases the risk of osteoporosis. Plasma prolactin should be measured in women with amenorrhea, whether or not galactorrhea is present. Mild elevations should be confirmed by repeat measurements.

- In men, hyperprolactinemia causes androgen deficiency and infertility but not gynecomastia; mass effects and hypopituitarism are common.
- The history should include medications and symptoms of pituitary mass effects or hypothyroidism.

Diagnostic Testing

Pituitary imaging should be performed in most cases because large nonfunctional pituitary or hypothalamic tumors may present with hyperprolactinemia. Testing for hypopituitarism is needed only in patients with a macroadenoma or hypothalamic lesion (see Pituitary Adenomas and Hypopituitarism section).

TREATMENT

- For **microadenomas and idiopathic hyperprolactinemia**, most patients are treated because of infertility or to prevent estrogen deficiency and osteoporosis. Indications for treatment include adenoma >1 cm, bothersome symptomatic galactorrhea, or hypogonadism.
- Some women may be observed without therapy by periodic follow-up of prolactin levels and symptoms. In most patients, hyperprolactinemia does not worsen, and prolactin levels sometimes return to normal. Enlargement of microadenomas is rare.
- **Dopamine agonists bromocriptine** and **cabergoline** suppress plasma prolactin and restore normal menses and fertility in most women.
  - Initial dosages are bromocriptine, 1.25–2.50 mg PO at bedtime with a snack, or cabergoline, 0.25 mg twice a week.
  - Plasma prolactin levels are initially obtained at 2- to 4-week intervals, and doses are adjusted to the lowest dose required to maintain prolactin in the normal range. In general, the maximally effective doses are bromocriptine 2.5 mg tid and cabergoline 1.5 mg twice a week.
  - **Side effects** include nausea and orthostatic hypotension, which can be minimized by increasing the dose gradually and usually resolve with continued therapy. Side effects are less severe with cabergoline.
  - Initially, women should use barrier contraception because fertility may be restored quickly.
  - **Women who want to become pregnant** should be managed in consultation with an endocrinologist.

  - **Women who do not want to become pregnant** should be followed with clinical evaluation and plasma prolactin levels every 6–12 months. Every few years, plasma prolactin may be measured after the dopamine agonist has been withdrawn for several weeks to determine whether the drug is still needed. Follow-up imaging studies are not warranted unless prolactin levels increase substantially.
- **Prolactin-secreting macroadenomas** should be treated with a dopamine agonist, which usually suppresses prolactin levels to normal, reduces tumor size, and improves or corrects abnormal visual fields in 90% of cases.
  - If mass effects are present, the dose should be increased to maximally effective levels over a period of several weeks. Visual field tests, if initially abnormal, should be repeated 4–6 weeks after therapy is started.
  - Pituitary imaging should be repeated 3–6 months after initiation of therapy. If tumor shrinkage and correction of visual abnormalities are satisfactory, therapy can be continued indefinitely, with periodic monitoring of plasma prolactin levels.
  - The full effect on tumor size may take more than 6 months. Further pituitary imaging is probably not warranted unless prolactin levels rise despite therapy.
  - **Transsphenoidal surgery** is indicated to relieve mass effects if the tumor does not shrink or if visual field abnormalities persist during dopamine agonist therapy. However, the likelihood of surgical cure of a prolactin-secreting macroadenoma is low, and most patients require further therapy with a dopamine agonist.
  - **Women with prolactin-secreting macroadenomas should not become pregnant** unless the tumor has been resected surgically or has decreased markedly in size with dopamine agonist therapy because the risk of symptomatic enlargement during pregnancy is 15%–35%. Contraception is essential during dopamine agonist treatment for macroadenoma.

Acromegaly[17]

GENERAL PRINCIPLES

Acromegaly is the syndrome caused by growth hormone excess in adults and is due to a growth hormone–secreting pituitary adenoma in the vast majority of cases.

DIAGNOSIS

Clinical Presentation

Clinical findings include thickened skin and enlargement of hands, feet, jaw, and forehead. Arthritis or carpal tunnel syndrome may develop, and the pituitary adenoma may cause headaches and vision loss. Mortality from cardiovascular disease is increased.

Diagnostic Testing

- **Plasma IGF-1,** which mediates most effects of growth hormone, is the initial screening test. Marked elevations establish the diagnosis.
- If IGF-1 levels are only moderately elevated, the diagnosis can be confirmed by giving 75 mg glucose orally and measuring serum growth hormone every 30 minutes for 2 hours. Failure to suppress growth hormone to <1 ng/mL confirms the diagnosis of acromegaly. Once the diagnosis is made, the pituitary should be imaged.

TREATMENT

- The treatment of choice is transsphenoidal resection of the pituitary adenoma. Most patients have macroadenomas, and complete tumor resection with cure of acromegaly

is often impossible. If IGF-1 levels remain elevated after surgery, radiotherapy is used to prevent regrowth of the tumor and to control acromegaly.
- The somatostatin analog **octreotide** in depot form can be used to suppress growth hormone secretion while awaiting the effect of radiation. A dose of 10–40 mg IM monthly suppresses IGF-1 to normal in about 60% of patients. Side effects include cholelithiasis, diarrhea, and mild abdominal discomfort. Other analogs are lanreotide and pasireotide.
- **Pegvisomant** is a growth hormone antagonist that lowers IGF-1 to normal in almost all patients. The dose is 10–30 mg SC daily. Few side effects have been reported, but patients should be monitored for pituitary adenoma enlargement and transaminase elevation.

Hyperparathyroidism

- Primary hyperparathyroidism is where oversecretion of parathyroid hormone from the parathyroid gland itself is due to adenoma or hyperplasia.
- Secondary hyperparathyroidism is due to compensatory oversecretion of parathyroid hormone (PTH) in response to abnormally low calcium in the blood due to other pathological processes such as renal failure, hyperphosphatemia, gastrointestinal malabsorption, or vitamin D deficiency.
- Tertiary hyperparathyroidism is rare and is characterized by the development of autonomous hypersecretion of PTH causing hypercalcemia.
- Pathological hallmark is hypercalcemia which can cause symptoms of excessive thirst and urination, constipation, bone pain, fatigue, depression, and possibly kidney stones (bones, stones, groans, and moans).
- Parathyroidectomy remains the definitive cure for primary hyperparathyroidism. Medical therapy with calcimimetics like cinacalcet effectively normalize calcium levels but have specific indications for use.

Hypoparathyroidism

- Most commonly occurs when parathyroid gland is removed with elective surgery, or it is damaged during a thyroid resection. It can also be due to autoimmune disorders (polyglandular syndromes).
- Clinical features are due to hypocalcemia, abdominal pains, muscle cramping and numbness, and tingling. Chvostek and Trousseau signs will be positive.
- Treatment is by supplementing calcium and Vitamin D. PTH therapy has been approved for the treatment of patients with hypoparathyroidism that is difficult to control with conventional therapy, such as patients that require large doses of supplements who have had emergency department visits or hospitalizations for hypocalcemia.

Osteomalacia[18,19]

GENERAL PRINCIPLES

- Osteomalacia is characterized by defective mineralization of osteoid. Bone biopsy reveals increased thickness of osteoid seams and decreased mineralization rate, assessed by tetracycline labeling.
- Suboptimal vitamin D nutrition, indicated by plasma 25-hydroxy vitamin D (25[OH]D) levels <30 ng/mL, is very common and contributes to the development of osteoporosis.
- Etiology includes the following:
  - Dietary vitamin D deficiency
  - Malabsorption of vitamin D and calcium because of intestinal, hepatic, or biliary disease
  - Disorders of vitamin D metabolism (e.g., renal disease, vitamin D–dependent rickets)

- Vitamin D resistance
- Chronic hypophosphatemia
- Renal tubular acidosis
- Hypophosphatasia

DIAGNOSIS

Clinical Presentation

- Clinical findings include diffuse skeletal pain, proximal muscle weakness, waddling gait, and propensity to fractures.
- Osteomalacia should be suspected in a patient with osteopenia, elevated serum alkaline phosphatase, and either hypophosphatemia or hypocalcemia.

Diagnostic Testing

- Serum alkaline phosphatase is elevated. Serum phosphorus, calcium, or both may be low.
- **Serum 25(OH)D** levels may be low, establishing the diagnosis of vitamin D deficiency or malabsorption.
- Radiographic findings include osteopenia and radiolucent bands perpendicular to bone surfaces (pseudofractures or Looser zones). Bone density is decreased.

TREATMENT

- **Dietary vitamin D deficiency** can initially be treated with ergocalciferol or cholecalciferol 50,000 international units (IU) PO weekly for 8 weeks to replete body stores, followed by long-term therapy with 2000 IU/d.
- **Malabsorption of vitamin D** may require continued therapy with high doses such as 50,000 IU PO per week. The dose should be adjusted to maintain serum 25(OH)D levels above 30 ng/mL. Calcium supplements, 1 g PO daily, are required. Serum 25(OH) D and serum calcium should be monitored every 6–12 months to avoid hypercalcemia.

Paget Disease[20]

GENERAL PRINCIPLES

Paget disease of bone is a focal skeletal disorder characterized by rapid, disorganized bone remodeling. It usually occurs after the age of 40 years and most often affects the pelvis, femur, spine, and skull.

DIAGNOSIS

Clinical Presentation

- Clinical manifestations include bone pain and deformity, degenerative arthritis, pathologic fractures, neurologic deficits because of nerve root or cranial nerve compression (including deafness), and, rarely, high-output heart failure and osteogenic sarcoma.
- Most patients are asymptomatic, with disease discovered incidentally because of elevated serum alkaline phosphatase or a radiograph taken for other reasons.

Diagnostic Testing

- **Serum alkaline phosphatase** is elevated, reflecting the activity and extent of disease. Serum and urine calcium are usually normal but may increase with immobilization, as after a fracture.

- The **radiographic appearance is usually diagnostic**, including both osteolytic and osteosclerotic lesions, depending on the presentation. A bone scan will reveal areas of skeletal involvement, which can be confirmed by radiography.

TREATMENT

- **Indications for therapy** include (1) bone pain because of Paget disease, (2) nerve compression syndromes, (3) pathologic fracture, (4) elective skeletal surgery, (5) progressive skeletal deformity, (6) immobilization hypercalcemia, and (7) asymptomatic involvement of weight-bearing bones or the skull.
- **Bisphosphonates** inhibit excessive bone resorption, relieve symptoms, and restore serum alkaline phosphatase to normal in most patients. **Zoledronic acid**, 5 mg IV by a single infusion, is the drug of choice. The effectiveness of therapy is monitored by measuring serum alkaline phosphatase annually. Therapy can be repeated if serum alkaline phosphatase rises above normal. Bisphosphonates are not recommended in patients with renal insufficiency.

Summary

- Graves' disease is by far the commonest form of thyrotoxicosis in South Asian population. Periodic paralysis is commonly encountered among thyrotoxic patients due to associated hypokalaemia.
- The common causes of hypothyroidism in adults in our region are post-radioactive iodine therapy and Hashimoto's thyroiditis.
- Consider starting levothyroxine at a dosage of 1.6 μg/kg of body weight per day for adults under the age of 65 years with primary hypothyroidism and no history of cardiovascular disease.
- Acute adrenal crisis manifests with hypotension, hyponatremia, hyperkalemia, and hypoglycemia.
- Cushing disease requires accurate diagnosis, careful treatment selection, and long-term management to optimize patient outcomes.
- Prolactinomas, comprising 30%–50% of all pituitary tumors, frequently occur in females aged 20–50 and cause hypogonadism and infertility.

Scan the QR code to access chapter references.

25 Arthritis and Rheumatologic Diseases

Deepali Prabir Sen and Athulya G. Asokan

Basic Approach to the Rheumatic Diseases

Arthritis is any disease process affecting a joint or joints, causing pain, swelling, and stiffness. Arthritis can be categorized as inflammatory or noninflammatory depending on the pattern of joint involvement and the evidence of inflammatory findings on joint exam. Periarthritis, which mimics arthritis, involves the soft tissues surrounding the joint like tendons and bursal structures. Periarthritis needs to be differentiated from true arthritis. Pain from a true articular process is usually present in all directions of motion and throughout the range of motion of a particular joint, whereas pain from a **periarticular process** is usually evident at a single point or direction in the range of motion. In **periarthritis**, pain often is elicited by palpation over a specific area corresponding to a tendon, ligament, or bursa and it occurs primarily with active movement, while in inflammatory arthritis it can occur with active and passive movements.

DIAGNOSIS

Cardinal features of inflammatory arthritis include the presence of morning stiffness lasting at least 30 minutes, worsening of symptoms with inactivity, and polyarticular involvement. Physical examination may reveal swelling, warmth, or erythema over the joint. Presence of constitutional symptoms such as fatigue, fever, and malaise often suggest underlying systemic inflammation. Associated symptoms such as skin rashes, uveitis, scleritis, mouth ulcers, and serositis among others may give clues to an underlying systemic connective tissue disease. Synovial fluid analysis should be sent for cell count, microscopic examination for crystals, Gram stain, and cultures. Ancillary lab tests and imaging are helpful in supporting a diagnosis if their use is directed by the specific findings on the history and physical examination.

TREATMENT

The etiology of most rheumatologic disorders is unknown. Therapeutic approaches involve either local or systemic administration of analgesic, anti-inflammatory, immunomodulatory, or immunosuppressive drugs.[1]

Medications

- **NSAIDs** exert their effects by inhibiting the constitutive (COX-1) and inducible (COX-2) isoforms of cyclooxygenase, producing a mild to moderate anti-inflammatory and analgesic effect. Individual responses to these agents are variable. If one drug is not effective during a 2- to 3-week trial, another should be tried.
  - **Side effects**
  - **Gastrointestinal (GI) toxicity** manifests clinically as dyspepsia, nausea, vomiting, or GI bleeding. Nausea and dyspepsia often respond to the addition of a histamine-2 (H_2)–blocking agent or proton pump inhibitor or to a change in NSAID. Direct GI irritation can be minimized by administration after food, by the use of enteric-coated

preparations, and by use of the lowest effective dose. All NSAIDs, however, have a systemic effect on the GI mucosa, resulting in increased permeability to gastric acid. Most serious GI bleeds during NSAID use occur without prior GI symptoms. **Risk factors for GI bleed** include a history of duodenal–gastric ulceration, age >60 years, smoking, ethanol use, high dose of NSAIDs, and concomitant use of corticosteroids, anticoagulants (i.e., aspirin, warfarin, clopidogrel), or selective serotonin reuptake inhibitors. The use of proton pump inhibitors such as **omeprazole** 20 mg PO daily decreases the risk of NSAID-induced gastric or duodenal ulceration. **Misoprostol**, a synthetic prostaglandin E analog, is another alternative but may cause diarrhea and is an abortifacient. Consider *Helicobacter pylori* testing prior to beginning NSAIDs, especially in patients with high risk of duodenal–gastric ulceration.

  - **Acute renal failure** due to reversible renal ischemia is the most common form of renal toxicity; however, nephrotic syndrome and acute interstitial nephritis may also occur. **Risk factors** for acute renal failure include preexisting renal dysfunction, congestive heart failure (CHF), cirrhosis with ascites, and a concomitant angiotensin-converting enzyme (ACE) inhibitor or angiotensin receptor blocker (ARB). Periodic monitoring of renal function is recommended, particularly in elderly patients.
  - **Platelet dysfunction** can be caused by all NSAIDs, particularly aspirin, which is a covalent inhibitor of COX. NSAIDs should be used cautiously or avoided in patients with a bleeding diathesis and those taking warfarin. NSAIDs should be discontinued 5–7 days before surgical procedures.
  - **Hypersensitivity reactions** are often seen in patients with a history of asthma, nasal polyps, or atopy. NSAIDs may cause a variety of type I hypersensitivity–like reactions, including urticaria, asthma, and anaphylactoid shock, presumably by increasing leukotriene synthesis. Patients with a hypersensitivity reaction to one NSAID should avoid all NSAIDs and selective COX-2 inhibitors.
  - **Other side effects: Central nervous system** (CNS) toxicity (headaches, dizziness, dysphoria, confusion, aseptic meningitis) is uncommon. Tinnitus and deafness can complicate NSAID use, particularly with high-dose salicylates. **Blood dyscrasias**, including aplastic anemia, have been observed as isolated case reports with ibuprofen, piroxicam, indomethacin, and phenylbutazone. **Dermatologic reactions** and **elevations in transaminases** have also been described. **A metabolic acidosis and respiratory alkalosis** can be seen with high doses of salicylates. Nonacetylated salicylates have been reported to have less toxicity but also may be less effective. The use of NSAIDs in general may be associated with an increased risk for **cardiovascular thrombotic events** and might diminish the cardioprotective effect of aspirin. Among NSAIDs, naproxen has the least risk of cardiovascular events.

- **Selective COX-2 inhibitors** exhibit selective inhibition of COX-2, thereby reducing inflammation while preserving the homeostatic functions of constitutive COX-1–derived prostaglandins. The anti-inflammatory and analgesic efficacy is similar to that of traditional NSAIDs. Celecoxib is the only selective COX-2 inhibitor approved in the United States.
  - Some data demonstrate that **GI symptoms** and **GI ulcerations are reduced** with these agents in comparison with NSAIDs. The potential gastroduodenal sparing effect of selective COX-2 inhibitors may be eliminated by concurrent warfarin therapy or by the use of low-dose aspirin therapy for primary or secondary prevention of cardiovascular or cerebrovascular disease.
  - Acute kidney injury might be precipitated in patients taking selective COX-2 inhibitors, similar to COX-1 inhibitors.
  - **Platelet function** is not impaired, making selective COX-2 inhibitors a good anti-inflammatory option for patients with thrombocytopenia, hemostatic defects, or chronic anticoagulation. In patients who are taking warfarin, however, the international

normalized ratio (INR) should be monitored after the addition of a COX-2 inhibitor (as with any medication change). In addition, there has been controversy as to whether the inhibition of prostacyclin but not thromboxane by these agents may promote clotting.

- Patients with hypersensitivity reactions to NSAIDs should not use a COX-2 inhibitor. Celecoxib should be used with caution in patients with sulfonamide allergy.
- An increase in blood pressure and a dose-related **increase in cardiovascular events** (i.e., CHF exacerbation) have been associated with the use of this medication.

- **Glucocorticoids** exert a pluripotent anti-inflammatory effect via the inhibition of inflammatory mediator gene transcription.
  - **Preparations, dosages, and routes of administration:** The goal of therapy **is to suppress** disease activity with the minimum effective dosage. **Prednisone** (PO) and **methylprednisolone** (IV) are generally the preferred drugs because of cost and half-life considerations. IM absorption is variable and therefore is not advised. The following are **relative anti-inflammatory potencies** of common glucocorticoid preparations: cortisone, 0.8; hydrocortisone, 1; prednisone, 4; methylprednisolone, 5; dexamethasone, 25.
  - **Side effects:** Adverse effects are related to dosage and duration of administration and can be minimized by once daily dosing in the morning, with dose reduction or changing to alternate-day administration once the disease is controlled.
    - **Adrenal suppression:** Glucocorticoids suppress the hypothalamic–pituitary–adrenal axis. Assume functional suppression in patients receiving more than 20 mg of prednisone (or the equivalent) daily for more than 3 weeks, patients receiving an evening dose for more than a few weeks, or patients with Cushingoid appearance. Adrenal suppression is unlikely if the patient has received any dose of steroids for less than 3 weeks or if using alternate-day therapy. Adrenal suppression is minimized by dosing in the morning and using a single daily low dose of a short-acting preparation, such as prednisone, for a short period. In patients who are receiving chronic glucocorticoid therapy, hypoadrenalism (anorexia, weight loss, lethargy, fever, and postural hypotension) may occur at times of severe stress (e.g., infection, major surgery) and should be treated with stress doses of glucocorticoids.
    - **Immunosuppression:** Glucocorticoid therapy reduces resistance to infections. **Bacterial infections** in particular are related to the dosage of glucocorticoids and are a major cause of morbidity and mortality. Minor infections may become systemic, quiescent infections may be activated, and organisms that usually are nonpathogenic may cause disease. Local and systemic signs of infection may be partially masked, although fever associated with infection generally is not suppressed. For patients on prolonged high-dose therapy, consider prophylaxis with trimethoprim/sulfamethoxazole (TMP-SMX) and acyclovir to prevent *Pneumocystis jirovecii* and varicella-zoster viral infections.
    - **Endocrine abnormalities:** Endocrine abnormalities include a **Cushingoid habitus**, hirsutism, and induced or aggravated hyperglycemia, rarely associated with ketoacidosis. Hyperglycemia is not a contraindication to therapy and may require treatment with insulin therapy. Fluid and electrolyte abnormalities include hypokalemia and sodium retention, which may induce or aggravate hypertension.
    - **Osteoporosis** with vertebral compression fractures is common among patients who are receiving long-term glucocorticoid therapy. **Supplemental calcium**, 1–1.5 g/d PO, should be given along with **vitamin D**, 1000 units daily PO, as soon as steroid therapy is begun. Bisphosphonates are most often used for prophylactic prevention of bone loss. Teriparatide (recombinant human parathyroid hormone [1–34]) is indicated in postmenopausal women and in premenopausal women or men who are at high risk for osteoporosis or have failed or been intolerant to bisphosphonates. Determination of baseline bone density and calculation of fracture risk are appropriate

in these patients. A weight-bearing exercise program and avoidance of alcohol and tobacco are recommended.

- **Steroid myopathy** generally involves the hip and shoulder girdle musculature. Muscles are weak but not tender, and in contrast to inflammatory myositis, serum creatine kinase, aldolase, and electromyography are normal. The myopathy usually improves with a reduction in glucocorticoid dosage and resolves slowly with discontinuation.
- **Ischemic bone necrosis** (aseptic necrosis, avascular necrosis) caused by glucocorticoid use often is multifocal, most commonly affecting the femoral head, humeral head, and tibial plateau. Early changes can be demonstrated by bone scan or MRI.
- **Other adverse effects:** Weight gain is one of the commonest side effect and often distressing to the patient. Changes in **mental status** ranging from mild nervousness, euphoria, and insomnia to severe depression or psychosis may occur. **Ocular effects** include increased intraocular pressure (sometimes precipitating glaucoma) and the formation of posterior subcapsular cataracts. **Hyperlipidemia**, **menstrual irregularities**, increased perspiration with **night sweats**, and **pseudotumor cerebri** also may occur.

• **Immunomodulatory and immunosuppressive drugs**, also known as **disease-modifying antirheumatic drugs** (**DMARDs**), include a number of pharmacologically diverse agents that exert anti-inflammatory or immunosuppressive effects. They are characterized by a delayed onset of action and the potential for serious toxicity. Consequently, they should be prescribed with the guidance of a rheumatologist and in cooperative patients who are willing to comply with meticulous follow-up. The specific agents will be discussed in relation to the diseases for which they are indicated. Examples of these agents include methotrexate, azathioprine, hydroxychloroquine (HCQ), sulfasalazine, cyclosporine, rituximab, and etanercept.

Nonpharmacologic Therapies

• **Joint aspiration should be performed in one of three instances: effusion of unclear etiology**, symptomatic relief in a patient with known arthritis diagnosis, and monitoring treatment response in **infectious arthritis**. Intra-articular glucocorticoid therapy can be used to suppress inflammation when only one or a few peripheral joints are inflamed and infection has been excluded. Intra-articular hyaluronic acid derivatives are used for the treatment of knee osteoarthritis (OA). The joint should be aspirated to remove as much fluid as possible before injection. **Glucocorticoid preparations** include methylprednisolone acetate, triamcinolone acetonide, and triamcinolone hexacetonide. The dose used is arbitrary, but the following guidelines based on volume are useful: large joints (knee, ankle, shoulder), 1–2 mL; medium joints (wrists, elbows), 0.5–1 mL; and small joints of the hands and feet, 0.25–0.5 mL. **Lidocaine** (or its equivalent), up to 1 mL of a 1% solution, can be mixed in a single syringe with the glucocorticoid to promote immediate relief but is not generally used in the digits.

• **Contraindications:** Cellulitis overlying the site to be injected is an absolute contraindication. Significant hemostatic defects and bacteremia are relative contraindications to joint aspiration and injection.

• **Complications**
  - **Post-injection synovitis** may develop rarely as a result of phagocytosis of glucocorticoid ester crystals. Reactions usually resolve within 48–72 hours. More persistent symptoms suggest the possibility of iatrogenic infection, which occurs rarely (<0.1% of patients). This reaction is more pronounced with intra-articular hyaluronic acid derivatives.
  - Localized skin depigmentation and atrophy along with accelerated deterioration of bone and cartilage may occur when frequent injections are administered over an extended period. Therefore, any single joint should be injected no more frequently than every 3–6 months.

Infectious Arthritis and Bursitis

GENERAL PRINCIPLES

- **Infectious arthritis** is commonly bacterial, although mycobacterial and fungal arthritis can be seen, especially in immunocompromised host. Bacterial septic arthritis is generally categorized into gonococcal and nongonococcal disease.
- **Nongonococcal infectious arthritis** in adults tends to occur in patients with previous joint damage or compromised host defenses. It is caused most often by *Staphylococcus aureus* (60%) and *Streptococcus* spp. Gram-negative organisms are less common and typically seen with IV drug abuse, neutropenia, concomitant urinary tract infection, or postoperative status. Septic arthritis is common when the underlying joint is affected by rheumatoid arthritis or in the setting of a joint prosthesis.
- **Gonococcal arthritis** causes one-half of all septic arthritis in otherwise healthy, sexually active young adults.

DIAGNOSIS

Clinical Presentation

- **Nongonococcal infectious arthritis** usually presents with fever and acute monoarticular arthritis, although multiple joints may be affected by hematogenous spread of pathogens. Knee joints are the most commonly affected. If a joint in the lower extremity is affected, weight-bearing is typically limited.
- **Gonococcal arthritis** often includes migratory or additive polyarthralgias, followed by tenosynovitis or arthritis of the wrist, ankle, or knee, and vesicopustular skin lesions on the extremities or trunk (disseminated gonococcal infection).

Diagnostic Testing

- **Joint aspiration** should be performed and synovial fluid should be sent for Gram stain, cell count with differential, and cultures. Cultures of blood and other possible extra-articular sites of infection also should be obtained.
- Synovial fluid Gram stain may be positive in 50%–70% of nongonococcal infectious arthritis cases.
- Gram staining of synovial fluid is positive in **less than 25% of cases** of gonococcal arthritis. Cultures of synovial fluid are positive in 20%–50% of cases. Bacteriologic assessment of the throat, cervix, urethra, and rectum may aid in establishing the diagnosis.
- Cell counts show WBC count >50,000 cell/mm^3 with neutrophilic predominance.
- Cultures should include mycobacterial and fungal cultures. Cultures may be negative in gonococcal arthritis and with prior exposure to antibiotics.
- Radiographs may show features of joint destruction especially in untreated disease, indeed rapid joint destruction on radiographs is concerning for underlying septic arthritis.[6]

TREATMENT

- **Empiric antimicrobial therapy** should be started immediately based on the clinical situation.
  - With a positive Gram stain and culture, antibiotic coverage can be tailored accordingly.
  - With a nondiagnostic Gram stain, antibiotics should be chosen to cover *S. aureus, Streptococcus* spp., and *Neisseria gonorrhoeae*. Vancomycin 15 mg/kg IV every 12 hours and ceftriaxone 1 g IV every 24 hours are good initial treatment choices. Cefepime instead of ceftriaxone is preferred if *Pseudomonas* infection is suspected.

  - IV antimicrobials are given for at least 2–4 weeks, followed by 1–2 weeks of oral antimicrobials, with the course of therapy tailored to the patient's response.
  - Treatment of gonococcal arthritis is with an IV antibiotic, generally ceftriaxone, 1–2 g IV daily. After clinical improvement is noted, usually 48 hours after IV antibiotics, therapy is continued with an oral antibiotic to complete 7–14 days of treatment. Cefixime, 400 mg PO bid, or amoxicillin, 500–850 mg PO bid, may be used. **Treatment of coexisting *Chlamydia* infection** with azithromycin or doxycycline should also be considered.
  - Oral and intra-articular antimicrobials are not appropriate as initial therapy.
- **Drainage** of the affected joint is needed to decrease the possibility of permanent joint damage. **Surgical drainage** or arthroscopic lavage and drainage are indicated for (1) a septic hip; (2) joints in which the anatomy, large amounts of tissue debris, or loculation of pus prevent adequate needle drainage; (3) septic arthritis with coexistent osteomyelitis; (4) joints that do not respond in 3–5 days to appropriate therapy; and (5) prosthetic joint infection.
- **General supportive measures** include splinting of the joint, which may help to relieve pain. However, prolonged immobilization can result in joint stiffness. An **NSAID** is useful to reduce pain and increase joint mobility but should not be used until response to antimicrobial therapy has been demonstrated by symptomatic and laboratory improvement.

SPECIAL CONSIDERATIONS

Nonbacterial infectious arthritis is common with many viral infections, especially hepatitis B, rubella, mumps, infectious mononucleosis, parvovirus, enterovirus, chikungunya virus, and adenovirus.

- It is generally self-limiting, lasting for <6 weeks, and responds well to a conservative regimen of rest and NSAIDs.
- Arthralgias (often severe) or reactive arthritis can also be a manifestation of HIV infection.
- Fungi and mycobacterium can cause septic arthritis and should be considered in patients with chronic monoarticular arthritis.
- **Poncet's arthritis** or tubercular rheumatism is a parainfective symmetric nondestructive polyarthritis seen in patients with active tuberculosis in which no mycobacterial involvement can be found and no other causes of polyarthritis detected. The symptoms resolve completely with antituberculous therapy. This differs from tubercular arthritis which is usually monoarticular and is caused by direct tubercular infection of the joint.

Septic Bursitis

GENERAL PRINCIPLES

- Usually involves the olecranon or prepatellar bursa and can be differentiated from septic arthritis by localized, fluctuant superficial swelling and by **relatively painless joint motion** (particularly extension).
- Most patients have a history of previous trauma to the area or an occupational predisposition (e.g., "housemaid's knee," "writer's elbow").
- *S. aureus* is the most common pathogen of septic bursitis.[7]

DIAGNOSIS AND TREATMENT

- Aspiration of the joint is performed, with antibiotic therapy guided by Gram stain and culture of bursa fluid. Aspiration can be repeated if fluid reaccumulates. Surgical drainage is indicated only if adequate needle drainage is not possible.

- Oral antibiotics (guided by Gram stain and culture of bursa fluid) and outpatient management are usually appropriate. Preventive measures (e.g., knee pads) should be used in patients with occupational predispositions to septic bursitis.

Lyme Disease

GENERAL PRINCIPLES

Lyme disease is caused by the tick-borne spirochete *Borrelia burgdorferi*.

DIAGNOSIS

- Typical manifestations begin with an erythematous annular rash (**erythema migrans**) and flu-like symptoms.
- Arthralgias, myalgias, meningitis, neuropathy, and cardiac conduction defects may follow in weeks to a few months. Months later, in untreated patients, an intermittent or chronic oligoarticular arthritis, characteristically including the knee, may develop.
- The diagnosis is based on the clinical picture, exposure in an endemic area, and **supported by serology**. A two-tiered serologic assay with enzyme-linked immunosorbent assay (ELISA) and IgG western blot for *B. burgdorferi* shall be uniformly positive by the time frank arthritis develops. False positives occur, however, and may signify prior infection. *B. burgdorferi* DNA can be detected by polymerase chain reaction in synovial fluid in 85% of cases.[8]

TREATMENT

Antibiotic therapy is required, generally with doxycycline 100 mg PO bid or amoxicillin 500 mg PO tid for 28 days. NSAIDs are a useful adjunct for arthritis.[9]

Crystalline Arthritis

GENERAL PRINCIPLES

Definition

Crystalline arthritis is caused by deposition of microcrystals in joints and periarticular tissues. Common types of crystalline arthritis are **gout**, **pseudogout**, and **apatite disease**.

Classification

- Clinical phases of gout can be divided into asymptomatic hyperuricemia, acute gouty arthritis with intercritical asymptomatic periods, and chronic arthritis.
- **Asymptomatic hyperuricemia** is defined as serum uric acid levels >7 mg/dL without arthritis or evidence of urate nephropathy.
- Men are much more commonly affected by gouty arthritis than women. Most premenopausal women with gout have a family history of the disease.

Etiology

- **Gout** is characterized by hyperuricemia that can be because of underexcretion or overproduction of uric acid. Urate crystals may be deposited in the joints, subcutaneous tissues (tophi), and kidneys. Intrinsic renal disease impairs excretion of uric acid. Several genetic polymorphisms are also associated with changes in uric acid excretion. Medications such as loop diuretics, low-dose aspirin, cyclosporine, and ethanol all interfere with renal excretion of uric acid.

Starvation, lactic acidosis, dehydration, preeclampsia, and diabetic ketoacidosis also can induce hyperuricemia. Overproduction of uric acid occurs in myeloproliferative and lymphoproliferative disorders, hemolytic anemia, and polycythemia. Overproduction may also occur because of intake of purine rich diet.

- **Pseudogout** results when calcium pyrophosphate dihydrate crystals deposited in bone and cartilage are released into synovial fluid and induce acute inflammation. **Risk factors** include older age, advanced OA, neuropathic joint, gout, hyperparathyroidism, hemochromatosis, diabetes mellitus, hypothyroidism, and hypomagnesemia.

DIAGNOSIS

Clinical Presentation

- **Acute gouty arthritis** presents as an excruciating attack of pain, usually in a single joint of the foot or ankle. Inflammation of the first metatarsophalangeal joint called as **podagra** is a classic presenting feature of gout. The talar, subtalar, ankle, and knee can also be involved in some cases. Occasionally, a polyarticular onset can mimic rheumatoid arthritis (RA). Acute gouty arthritis attacks can be precipitated by surgery, dehydration, diuretics, fasting, binge eating, or heavy ingestion of alcohol.
- **Chronic gouty arthritis:** With time, acute gouty attacks occur more frequently, asymptomatic periods are shorter, and chronic joint deformity may appear. Over time, chronic gouty arthritis may cause a symmetric large and small joint involvement known as a pseudorheumatoid arthritis pattern.
- **Pseudogout** may present as an **acute monoarthritis or oligoarthritis**, mimicking gout, or as a **chronic polyarthritis** resembling RA or OA. Usually the knee or wrist is affected, although any synovial joint can be involved.[10]
- **Apatite/basic calcium phosphate crystals** may cause periarthritis, tendonitis, or a destructive arthritis. Shoulders are the most affected joint, either in the form of calcific periarthritis or with true joint arthritis, which is called Milwaukee shoulder.

Diagnostic Testing

- Laboratory
  - A definitive diagnosis of gout or pseudogout is made by finding **intracellular crystals** in synovial fluid examined with a compensated polarized light microscope. **Urate crystals** are needle-shaped and strongly negatively birefringent. **Calcium pyrophosphate dihydrate crystals** are rhomboidal and weakly positively birefringent. Hydroxyapatite complexes and basic calcium phosphate complexes can be identified only by electron microscopy and mass spectroscopy.
  - Serum uric acid level is normal in 30% of patients with acute gout.
  - **Apatite disease** should be suspected when no crystals are present in the **synovial fluid**.
- Imaging
  - Punched out lytic lesion with sclerotic margin and overhanging edge may be seen on imaging with gout (**Martel sign**).
  - Calcium deposition in the cartilage or chondrocalcinosis is a finding that is supportive of (but not diagnostic for) pseudogout. If pseudogout is suspected, films of the wrists, knees, and pubic symphysis may be ordered, as these are the most common sites for chondrocalcinosis.
  - Hydroxyapatite disease may be suspected by finding poorly defined cloud-like calcific deposits in the periarticular area on imaging. Sometimes there is associated OA.

TREATMENT

- **Asymptomatic hyperuricemia** is not routinely treated. However, patients should be monitored closely for the development of complications if the serum uric acid level is at least 12 mg/dL in men or 10 mg/dL in women, and urate-lowering therapy should then be considered. Lifestyle measures such as avoidance of alcohol and limiting intake of sugar and foods rich in purines should be discussed with all patients.
- **Management of gout** includes treatment of acute flares, urate-lowering therapy, and management of risk factors.
- **Acute gout**
  - Although the acute gouty attack will subside spontaneously over several days, prompt treatment can abort the attack within hours.
  - **NSAIDs** are the treatment of choice because of ease of administration and low toxicity. Clinical response may require 12–24 hours, and initial doses should be high, followed by rapid tapering over 2–8 days. One approach is to use indomethacin, 50 mg PO q8h for 2 days, followed by 25 mg PO q8h for 3–7 days. Long-acting NSAIDs are generally not recommended for acute gout.
  - **Glucocorticoids** are useful when NSAIDs are contraindicated. An intra-articular injection of glucocorticoids produces rapid dramatic relief. Alternatively, prednisone, 40–60 mg PO daily, can be given until a response is obtained and then should be tapered rapidly.
  - **Colchicine is most effective if given in the first 12–24 hours** of an acute attack and usually brings relief in 6–12 hours. A dose of 1.2 mg is given at onset of symptoms, and 0.6 mg is taken 1 hour after the initial dose (1.8 mg over 1 hour). This regimen decreases the GI side effects noted with previous higher dose therapies. Colchicine 0.6 mg PO daily or bid, can be used prophylactically for frequent attacks. The dosage needs to be adjusted in patients with renal insufficiency. Colchicine 0.6 mg every other day or every 3 days should be considered in patients with a creatinine clearance between 10 and 34 mL/min. **Maintenance colchicine, 0.6 mg PO daily or bid, should be given for a few days before manipulation of the uric acid level to prevent precipitation of an acute attack.** In patients without tophi, prophylactic colchicine can be discontinued after 6 months once serum urate levels are <6 mg/dL and no acute attacks have been documented by the patient. In patients with tophi, duration of prophylaxis is uncertain but consider discontinuation 6 months after resolution of tophi. Adverse effects of colchicine include gastrointestinal symptoms (nausea and diarrhea), myotoxicity, and myelosuppression.
- **Urate-lowering therapy** can be instituted if there are three or more gout flares. Presence of tophi, joint damage, and urate nephropathy are also indications for urate-lowering therapy.
  - **Allopurinol**, a xanthine oxidase inhibitor, is an effective therapy for hyperuricemia in most patients.
    - **Dosage and administration:** Initial dosage varies and should be adjusted for renal and hepatic dysfunction. Daily doses can be increased by 100 mg every 2–4 weeks to achieve the minimum maintenance dosage that will keep the uric acid level below 6 mg/dL, which is below the limit of solubility of monosodium urate in serum. The concomitant use of a uricosuric agent may hasten the mobilization of tophi. **Allopurinol should be continued during an acute gout flare if already started, and use of NSAIDs, colchicine, or steroids to abort the attack should be considered.**
    - **Side effects: Hypersensitivity reactions** from a minor skin rash to a diffuse exfoliative dermatitis associated with fever, eosinophilia, and a combination of renal and hepatic injury occur in up to 5% of patients. Patients who have mild renal insufficiency and are receiving diuretics are at greatest risk. Severe cases are potentially fatal and usually

require glucocorticoid therapy. Allopurinol may potentiate the effect of oral anticoagulants and blocks metabolism of azathioprine and 6-mercaptopurine, necessitating a 60%–75% reduction in dosage of these cytotoxic drugs.

- **Febuxostat** is a nonpurine selective inhibitor of the xanthine oxidase. It is significantly more expensive than allopurinol. The starting dose is 40 mg/d, with titration to 80 mg/d if needed. Liver function test elevation may be seen and should be monitored.
- **Uricase** catabolizes uric acid to the more soluble compound allantoin. It is available in the United States for the treatment of tumor lysis syndrome in a recombinant form (**rasburicase**). IV **pegloticase** is a recombinant polyethylene glycol–conjugated form of uricase given every 2 weeks that has been shown to provide sustained reductions in plasma uric acid levels, in a substantial proportion of patients with chronic gout who are refractory to, or intolerant of, conventional urate-lowering therapy. Pegloticase will often cause precipitous uric acid reductions almost down to zero. Rapid fall in uric acid levels is often accompanied by gout flares. There is a high risk of anaphylaxis and infusion reactions with this medication, and thus, it is administered in a controlled setting with healthcare professionals who are familiar with the medication. The drug is discontinued if serum uric acid levels fail to reach target or are noted to rise above 4 mg/dL before the next infusion as this may increase risk of anaphylactic reactions.
- **Uricosuric drugs** lower serum uric acid levels by blocking renal tubular reabsorption of uric acid. A 24-hour measurement of creatinine clearance and urine uric acid should be obtained before therapy is started because these drugs are **ineffective with glomerular filtration rates of <50 mL/min**. They are also not recommended for patients who already have high levels of urine uric acid (800 mg/24 h) because of the risk of urate stone formation. Risk of urate stone formation can be minimized by maintaining a high fluid intake and by alkalinizing the urine. If these drugs are being used when an acute gouty attack begins, they should be continued while other drugs are used to treat the acute attack.
- **Probenecid**
  - Initial dosage is 500 mg PO daily, which can be raised in 500-mg increments every week until serum uric acid levels normalize or urine uric acid levels exceed 800 mg/24 h. The maximum dose is 3000 mg/d. Most patients require a total of 1–1.5 g/d in two to three divided doses.
  - Salicylates and probenecid are antagonistic and should not be used together.
  - Probenecid decreases renal excretion of penicillin, indomethacin, and sulfonylureas.
  - Side effects are minimal.
- **Sulfinpyrazone** has uricosuric efficacy similar to that of probenecid; however, it also inhibits platelet function. The initial dosage of 50 mg PO bid can be increased in 100-mg increments weekly until serum uric acid levels normalize to a maximum dose of 800 mg/d. Most patients require 300–400 mg/d in three to four divided doses.
- **Lesinurad** is a new agent that inhibits urate transporter, **URAT1**, causing uricosuric effects. It is used in combination with a xanthine oxidase inhibitor.
- Drugs that block interleukin-1 such as anakinra and canakinumab have been tried, especially during gout flare-ups.

- **Management of risk factors:** Aspirin (uricoretentive), diuretics, high alcohol intake, and foods high in purines (sweetbreads, anchovies, shellfish, sardines, liver, and kidney) should be avoided. Weight loss should be encouraged.
- **Pseudogout**
  - As in gout, the therapy of choice for most patients is a brief high-dose course of an **NSAID. Oral corticosteroids, intra-articular corticosteroids**, and **colchicine** may also relieve symptoms promptly.
  - **Maintenance therapy** with colchicine may diminish the number of recurrent attacks. Allopurinol or uricosuric agents have no role in treating pseudogout.

- Treatment of underlying disease (hyperparathyroidism, hypothyroidism, hemochromatosis) will also help in disease management.
- Treatment of **apatite disease** is similar to that for pseudogout.

Rheumatoid Arthritis

GENERAL PRINCIPLES

RA is a systemic disease of unknown etiology that is characterized by a symmetric inflammatory polyarthritis, extra-articular manifestations (rheumatoid nodules, pulmonary fibrosis, serositis, scleritis, vasculitis), and serum rheumatoid factor (RF) in up to 80% of patients. The course of RA is variable but tends to be chronic and progressive.

DIAGNOSIS

Clinical Presentation

- Most patients describe the insidious onset of pain, swelling, and morning stiffness in the hands and/or wrists or feet.
- Synovitis may be evident on examination of the metacarpophalangeal, proximal interphalangeal, wrist, or other joints. The axial skeleton is usually spared, except for the cervical spine. Rheumatoid nodules may be palpated most commonly on extensor surfaces.
- Suspect the diagnosis in patients presenting with symmetric arthritis in three or more joints especially involving small joints and associated with morning stiffness lasting more than 30 minutes. Features of polymyalgia rheumatic (PMR) may also be present, in addition to the typical features of RA. The episodic pattern of RA with sequential involvement of one to several joints for hours to days is called "palindromic rheumatism."

  The ACR/EULAR has specified criteria defining RA (Table 25-1). These criteria help outline the symptoms at presentation.

  RA may present with extra-articular manifestations as outlined in Table 25-2.[11]

Diagnostic Testing

- Erythrocyte sedimentation rate (ESR) and C-reactive protein (CRP) levels correlate with the severity of disease as well as radiographic changes.
- RF may be positive in 80% of patients. Cyclic citrullinated peptide (CCP) antibodies may be detected in 50%–60% of patients with early RA.
- CCP antibodies are more specific (>90%) for RA than the RF, which can also be elevated in the setting of hepatitis C and other chronic infections.
- Hand and wrist radiographs may show early changes of erosions or periarticular osteopenia.
- Musculoskeletal MRI and ultrasonography are more sensitive than plain radiographs and may be used in equivocal cases to demonstrate clinically inapparent synovitis or erosions.
- Synovial fluid examination reveals an inflammatory effusion, with neutrophilic leukocytosis and a cell count ranging from 1500 to 25,000/cubic mm.
- Composite scales measuring the disease activity—the Disease Activity Score using 28 joints (DAS-28), Simplified Disease Activity Assessment Index (SDAI), and Clinical Disease Assessment Index (CDAI)—are used for disease monitoring and treatment.

TREATMENT

Most patients can benefit from an early aggressive treatment program that combines medical, rehabilitative, and surgical services designed with three distinct goals: (1) early suppression of inflammation in the joints and other tissues, (2) maintenance of joint and muscle function and prevention of deformities, and (3) repair of joint damage to relieve pain or improve function.[2]

TABLE 25-1 American College of Rheumatology (ACR)/European League Against Rheumatism (EULAR) Criteria for the Classification of Acute Rheumatoid Arthritis: 2010

	Classification criteria for RA (Score-based algorithm: add scores of categories A–D. A score ≥6/10 is needed for classification of a patient as having definite RA. A score <6/10 not classifiable as RA, but status needs to be reassessed over time)	
A	**Joint involvement**	
	1 large joint	0 point
	2–10 large joints	1 point
	1–3 small joints (with or without involvement of large joints)	2 points
	4–10 small joints (with or without involvement of large joints)	3 points
	>10 joints (at least 1 small joint)	5 points
B	**Serology (at least one test result is needed for classification)**	
	Negative RF and negative ACPA	0 point
	Low-positive RF or low-positive ACPA (≤3 times ULN)	2 points
	High-positive RF or high-positive ACPA (≥3 times ULN)	3 points
C	**Acute-phase reactants (at least one test result is needed for classification)**	
	Normal CRP and normal ESR	0 point
	Abnormal CRP or abnormal ESR	1 point
D	**Duration of symptoms**	
	<6 weeks	0 point
	≥6 weeks	1 point

ACPA, anticitrullinated protein antibody; CRP, C-reactive protein; ESR, erythrocyte sedimentation rate; RF, rheumatoid factor, ULN, upper limit of normal.

- **DMARDs** appear to alter the natural history of RA by retarding the progression of bony erosions and cartilage loss. Because RA may lead to substantial long-term disability (and is associated with increased mortality), the standard of care is to initiate therapy with such agents early in the course of RA. Once a clinical response has been achieved, the chosen drug usually is continued indefinitely at the lowest effective dosage to prevent relapse.
    - **An established diagnosis of RA along with any evidence of disease activity is an indication to initiate disease-modifying therapy.** Initial monotherapy with NSAIDs or steroids is no longer considered appropriate under usual circumstances.
    - **Methotrexate** typically is the initial choice for moderate to severe RA. **Leflunomide** is also an alternative. **HCQ** or **sulfasalazine** can be used as the initial choice in very mild RA. If response to the initial agent is unsatisfactory after an adequate trial (or if limiting toxicity supervenes), other DMARDs or a biologic agent can be added or substituted.
- **Methotrexate**, a purine inhibitor and folic acid antagonist, is useful in treating synovitis, regardless of the underlying disease process. The drug binds to DHFR and has high affinity for enzymes that require folate cofactors, including **thymidylate synthetase** (TS) **and 5-aminoimidazole-4-carboxamide ribonucleotide** (AICAR) **transformylase.** RA is its most common indication. It is also useful for treatment of Felty syndrome.
    - **Dosage and administration:** Typically, methotrexate is administered as a single PO dose once a week starting with 7.5–10 mg. Clinical response is usually noted in 4–8 weeks. The dosage can be increased by 2.5- to 5-mg increments every 2–4 weeks to a maximum

TABLE 25-2	Extra-articular Manifestations
Pulmonary	Rheumatic lung nodules, pleural effusions, interstitial lung disease, fibrosing alveolitis, and pulmonary vasculitis. Caplan syndrome is the coexistence of seropositive RA and rounded fibrotic peripheral lung nodules with coal worker pneumoconiosis/silicosis
Hematologic manifestations	**Felty syndrome** is the triad of RA, neutropenia, and splenomegaly. Anemia of chronic disease and thrombocytosis are other presentations
Ocular	Severe ocular dryness is the most common ocular manifestation. Scleritis and episcleritis may progress to perforation of the orbit (scleromalacia perforans). Brown syndrome is due to tendinitis of the superior oblique muscles presenting as diplopia
Vasculitis	Rheumatoid vasculitis can affect any blood vessel, but the most common manifestation is distal arteritis ranging from nail fold infarcts to gangrene of the fingertips
Cardiac manifestations	Pericardial effusions, and rarely fibrinous pericarditis and constrictive pericarditis. RA accelerates atherosclerosis and is a risk factor for coronary artery disease
Neurologic manifestations	Peripheral nerve entrapment syndromes such as carpal tunnel syndrome (median nerve at wrist) and tarsal tunnel syndrome (anterior tibial nerve at ankle), myelopathy due to spinal cord (compression by acquired atlantoaxial dislocation), and mononeuritis multiplex

of 25 mg/wk or until improvement is observed. Dosages above 20 mg/wk are generally given by SC injection to promote absorption.

- **Contraindications and side effects:** Methotrexate is **teratogenic** and should not be used during pregnancy. It should also be avoided in patients with significant hepatic or renal impairment. **Folic acid supplementation** at a dosage of 1–2 mg daily may reduce toxicity without attenuating efficacy. Concomitant use of TMP-SMX should be avoided. Serologic testing for hepatitis B and C should be included before initiation of therapy.
  - **Minor side effects** include GI intolerance, stomatitis, rash, headache, and alopecia.
  - **Bone marrow suppression** may occur, particularly at higher doses. Blood and platelet counts should be obtained before initiation, every 4 weeks during the first 3–4 months or if the dose is changed, and every 8 weeks thereafter. **Macrocytosis** may precede serious hematologic toxicity and is an indication for folate supplementation, dose reduction, or both.
  - **Cirrhosis** occurs rarely with long-term use. Aspartate transaminase (AST), alanine transaminase (ALT), and serum albumin should be obtained initially at 4- to 8-week intervals during the first 3–4 months of therapy or if the dose is changed. Patients on a stable dose should be monitored every 8–12 weeks after 3 months of therapy and every 12 weeks after 6 months of therapy. Liver biopsy should be considered if the liver function tests are persistently abnormal or if the liver function tests are abnormal in 6 of 12 monthly determinations (five of nine determinations if measured every 6 weeks). Alcohol consumption increases the risk of methotrexate hepatotoxicity.
  - **Hypersensitivity pneumonitis** may occur but usually is reversible. Distinction from the interstitial lung disease (ILD) associated with RA may be difficult. Patients with preexisting pulmonary parenchymal disease may be at increased risk.

New or worsening symptoms of dyspnea or cough in a patient on methotrexate should prompt evaluation for pneumonitis.
  - **Rheumatoid nodules** may develop or worsen, paradoxically, in some patients on methotrexate.
- **Sulfasalazine** is useful for treating synovitis in the setting of RA and seronegative spondyloarthropathies (SpA).
  - **Dosage:** Initial dosage is 500 mg PO daily, with increases in 500-mg increments weekly until a total daily dose of 2000–3000 mg (given in evenly divided doses) is reached. Clinical response usually occurs in 6–10 weeks.
  - **Contraindications and side effects: Sulfasalazine should be used with extreme caution in patients with glucose-6-phosphate dehydrogenase deficiency. Sulfasalazine should not be used in patients with sulfa allergy.** Nausea is the principal adverse effect and can be minimized by the use of the enteric-coated preparation of the drug. Hematologic toxicity, including a reduction in any cell line and aplastic anemia, rarely occurs. Periodic monitoring of blood and platelet count is recommended.
- **HCQ** is an antimalarial agent that is used to treat dermatitis, alopecia, and synovitis in systemic lupus erythematosus (SLE) and mild synovitis in RA. It decreases the secretion of monocyte-derived proinflammatory cytokines.
  - **Dosage:** HCQ typically is given at a dosage of 4–6 mg/kg PO daily (200–400 mg) after meals to minimize dyspepsia and nausea.
  - **Contraindications and side effects: HCQ should be used with caution in patients with porphyria, glucose-6-phosphate dehydrogenase deficiency, or significant hepatic or renal impairment.** It is safe during pregnancy. The most common side effects are allergic skin eruptions and nausea. Serious ocular toxicity (**corneal deposits and retinopathy**) occurs, but it is rare with currently recommended dosages. Ophthalmologic evaluation should be performed on an annual basis.
- **Leflunomide** is a pyrimidine inhibitor that has been approved for the treatment of RA. It is converted to malononitrilamide, which inhibits the mitochondrial enzyme **dihydroorotate dehydrogenase.**
  - **Dosage and administration:** Treatment is begun with 10 or 20 mg PO daily. Clinical response is generally seen within 4–8 weeks.
  - **Contraindications and side effects:** Leflunomide is **teratogenic** and has a very long half-life. Women who plan to become pregnant must discontinue the drug and complete a course of elimination therapy with cholestyramine, 8 g PO tid for 11 days. Plasma levels should then be verified to be <0.02 mg/L on two separate tests at least 14 days apart before pregnancy is considered. Leflunomide is **contraindicated in patients with significant hepatic dysfunction** or in those who are receiving rifampin. **GI side effects** are the most common. **Diarrhea** occurs in up to 20% of patients and may require discontinuation of the drug. Dosage reduction to 10 mg/d may provide relief while maintaining efficacy and loperamide can be used for symptomatic relief. **Elevations in serum transaminase levels** may occur and should be measured at baseline and then monitored periodically. The dosage should be reduced for confirmed twofold elevations, and greater elevations should be treated with cholestyramine and discontinuation of leflunomide. **Rash** and **alopecia** may occur during therapy.
- **Anticytokine therapies** directed at specific cytokines have been developed. These agents are considered **biologic DMARDs.**
  - **Tumor necrosis factor (TNF) inhibitors** have been approved for treatment of RA. These agents are used in patients with moderate to severe RA who have failed a trial of one or more DMARDs. The effect of these agents on synovitis can be dramatic, with responsive patients sometimes reporting the onset of symptomatic benefits within 1–2 weeks. In addition to their symptomatic benefits, these agents appear to retard joint damage significantly.

- Etanercept is a fusion protein that consists of the ligand-binding portion of the human TNF receptor linked to the Fc portion of human IgG. It binds to TNF, blocking its interaction with cell surface receptors, thus inhibiting the inflammatory and immunoregulatory properties of TNF. It is given in a dosage of 25 mg SC twice a week or 50 mg SC weekly.
- **Infliximab** is a chimeric monoclonal antibody that binds specifically to human TNF-α, blocking its proinflammatory and immunomodulatory effects. It is given by IV infusion in conjunction with methotrexate to reduce production of neutralizing antibodies against infliximab. The recommended treatment regimen includes infliximab infusions of 3 mg/kg at initiation, at 2 and 6 weeks, and every 8 weeks thereafter, along with methotrexate at a dose of at least 7.5 mg/wk.
- **Adalimumab** is a recombinant human IgG-1 monoclonal antibody that is specific to human TNF-α. It is given in a dosage of 40 mg SC every other week.
- **Golimumab** is a human monoclonal antibody that binds to human TNF-α. It can be given as a monthly injection or an infusion every 8 weeks after an initial loading dose.
- **Certolizumab pegol** is a pegylated humanized Fab′ fragment of an anti–TNF-α monoclonal antibody. It is given monthly after an initial loading dose.

- **Contraindications and side effects**
  - **Serious infections and sepsis,** including fatalities, have been reported during the use of TNF-blocking agents. These drugs are contraindicated in patients with acute or chronic infections, and if serious infection or sepsis occurs, the drug should be stopped. Those with a history of recurrent infections and those with underlying conditions that may predispose to infection should be treated with caution and counseled to be vigilant for signs and symptoms of infection. Upper respiratory and sinus infections are most common. Tuberculosis (TB) has also been noted, and **a tuberculin skin test and CXR should be obtained before beginning therapy**. These agents are also contraindicated in patients with CHF (usually with a left ventricular ejection fraction <30%). Patients undergoing elective surgery should discuss with their rheumatologist regarding the optimum duration to hold medications peri-operatively, this may depend upon the half life of the drug and postoperative wound healing.
  - **Local injection site reactions** are common with SC administration, particularly during the first month of therapy. Reactions are generally self-limited and do not require discontinuation of therapy. Serious systemic allergic reactions are rare but may occur with infliximab infusions.
  - **Other adverse effects** may include induction of antinuclear antibodies and, rarely, a lupus-like illness. A demyelinating disorder has been described as well as exacerbations of preexisting multiple sclerosis. The risk of nonmelanoma skin cancer is increased in patients who receive TNF blockers. It is unclear whether the frequency of occurrence of lymphoma is increased in patients who receive these agents. A black box warning, however, has been placed on the package insert of these agents.

- **Interleukin inhibitors**
  - **Anakinra** is a recombinant interleukin (IL)-1 receptor antagonist that is approved for use in RA. It blocks binding of IL-1 to its receptor, thus inhibiting the proinflammatory and immunomodulatory actions of IL-1.
    - It is given in a dosage of 100 mg SC daily. Similar to TNF blockers, it should not be prescribed to patients with ongoing or recurrent infections.
    - **Adverse effects** include an increased frequency of bacterial infections and injection site reactions.
- **B-cell–directed therapy: Rituximab** is a monoclonal antibody directed against CD20, a cell surface receptor found on B cells. CD20-positive B cells in peripheral blood are rapidly depleted after two infusions of 1 g of rituximab 2 weeks apart. Methotrexate is generally used as background therapy. The infusion can be repeated in 6- to 12-month intervals, based on patient symptoms.

- **Contraindications and side effects:** Rituximab has rarely been reported to cause reactivation of JC virus, leading to the clinical syndrome of progressive multifocal leukoencephalopathy (PML), which is uniformly fatal.
- **Infusion reactions** are more common with the first dose and rarely fatal. Antihistamines, IV steroids, and acetaminophen are routinely given prior to infusion.
- **Infectious complications** are a concern, as with all biologics, but appear to be less frequent than in anti-TNF–treated patients.
- With recurrent rituximab infusions, patients may sometimes develop low immunoglobulin levels leading to permanent hypogammaglobulinemia.

- **Tocilizumab** is an antagonist of soluble and membrane-bound IL-6 receptors. It is given as an IV infusion or as an SC injection at a dose of 162 mg either weekly or every other week depending on the patient's weight. Side effects include increased infections, neutropenia, and elevations in cholesterol.
- **Abatacept** is a fusion protein comprising the CTLA-4 molecule and the Fc portion of IgG-1. It blocks selective co-stimulation of T cells. It is given as an IV infusion of 500–1000 mg every 4 weeks. It is also available as an SC formulation that can be given 125 mg SC weekly with or without an initial loading dose. It is approved in patients with an inadequate response to biologic or nonbiologic DMARDs.
  - **Infections** occur slightly more often than in placebo-treated patients. Opportunistic infections have not been observed. **Infusion reactions** are much less common than with rituximab or infliximab.
  - **Chronic obstructive pulmonary disease exacerbations and respiratory infections** are more common in patients with moderate to severe obstructive lung disease when treated with abatacept.
- **Tofacitinib** is an oral agent that inhibits Janus kinases or JAK that are needed for intracellular signaling in immune and hematopoietic cells. Tofacitinib can be used orally as 5 mg bid or an extended release tablet at 11 mg daily. Tofacitinib can be used as monotherapy or in combination with a synthetic DMARD such as methotrexate.
  - Common side effects are cytopenia and hepatic enzyme elevation.
  - There is an increased risk of shingles.
  - LDL cholesterol elevation can be seen and lipid panel should be checked before and after start of therapy.
- **Combinations of DMARDs** can be used if the patient has a partial response to the initial agent.
  - Common combination therapies include methotrexate with HCQ, sulfasalazine, or both. Methotrexate is commonly combined with TNF antagonists because there is evidence for additive efficacy and for a decrease in the formation of human antichimeric antibodies against the TNF blocker. Methotrexate is often used in combination with rituximab or abatacept. Methotrexate and leflunomide may have additive hepatotoxicity, and this combination should be used cautiously.
  - **Combination therapy with two biologic agents is contraindicated because of increased infectious complications.**
- **NSAIDs or selective COX-2 inhibitors** may be used as an adjunct to DMARD therapy.
- **Glucocorticoids are not curative** but may delay the formation of erosions with other DMARDs and are among the most potent anti-inflammatory drugs available.
  - **Indications for glucocorticoids** include (1) symptomatic relief while waiting for a response to a slow-acting immunosuppressive or immunomodulatory agent, (2) persistent synovitis despite adequate trials of DMARDs and NSAIDs, and (3) severe constitutional symptoms (e.g., fever and weight loss) or extra-articular disease (vasculitis, episcleritis, or pleurisy).

- ◦ **Oral administration** of prednisone 5–20 mg daily usually is sufficient for the treatment of synovitis, whereas severe constitutional symptoms or extra-articular disease may require up to 1 mg/kg PO daily. Although alternate-day glucocorticoid therapy reduces the incidence of undesirable side effects, some patients do not tolerate the increase in symptoms that may occur on the off day.
- ◦ **Intra-articular administration** may provide temporary symptomatic relief when only a few joints are inflamed. The beneficial effects of intra-articular steroids may persist for days to months and may delay or negate the need for systemic glucocorticoid therapy.

Nonpharmacologic Therapies[3–5]

- **Acute care** of inflammatory arthritides involves joint protection and pain relief. Proper joint positioning and splints are important elements in joint protection. Heat is a useful analgesic.
- **Subacute disease** therapy should include a gradual increase in passive and active joint movement.
- **Chronic care** encompasses instruction in joint protection, work simplification, and performance of activities of daily living. Adaptive equipment, splints, orthotics, and mobility aids may be useful, and specific exercises designed to promote normal joint mechanics and to strengthen affected muscle groups are useful.

Surgical Management

- **Corrective surgical procedures** including synovectomy, total joint replacement, and joint fusion may be indicated in patients with RA to reduce pain and to improve function.
- **Carpal tunnel syndrome** is common, and surgical repair may be curative if local injection therapy is unsuccessful.
- **Synovectomy** may be helpful if major involvement is limited to one or two joints and if a 6-month trial of medical therapy has failed, but usually it is only of temporary benefit.
- **Surgical fusion of joints** usually results not only in freedom from pain but also in total loss of motion; this is tolerated well in the wrist and thumb.
- **Cervical spine fusion** of C1 and C2 is indicated for significant cervical subluxation (>5 mm) with associated neurologic deficits. Patients with long-standing RA undergoing elective surgical procedures should have a lateral cervical spine radiograph in flexion and extension performed to screen for subluxation.

Immunizations

- Immune response to influenza and pneumococcal vaccinations in patients receiving methotrexate and biologic therapies may be attenuated, although usually adequate. **Influenza** vaccinations should be given to patients prior to starting therapy with all nonbiologic DMARDs, and **pneumococcal** vaccinations should be given to patients started on leflunomide, methotrexate, or sulfasalazine if the patients' vaccinations were not current. In addition, periodic pneumococcal vaccinations and annual influenza vaccinations should be considered for all patients receiving biologic agents, in accordance with the Centers for Disease Control and Prevention (CDC) recommendations for appropriate use and timing of these vaccinations.
- Hepatitis B vaccination is recommended if risk factors for this disease exist and if hepatitis B vaccination has not previously been administered.
- A new recombinant herpes zoster vaccine is available and can be used for immunization for patients on biologic therapy.
- Live vaccines are contraindicated during biologic therapy but should be considered before initiation of biologic therapy or high-dose steroids.

COMPLICATIONS

- **Patients with RA and a single joint inflamed out of proportion to the rest of the joints must be evaluated for coexistent septic arthritis.** This complication occurs with increased frequency in RA and carries 20%–30% mortality.
- **Sjögren syndrome,** characterized by failure of exocrine glands, occurs in a subset of patients with RA, producing sicca symptoms (dry eyes and mouth), parotid gland enlargement, dental caries, and recurrent tracheobronchitis. **Treatment** is symptomatic with artificial tears and saliva or with pilocarpine up to 5 mg PO qid. Cevimeline, 30 mg tid, can also be considered. Assiduous dental and ophthalmologic care is recommended, and drugs that suppress lacrimal–salivary secretion further should be avoided.
- **Felty syndrome:** The triad of RA, splenomegaly, and granulocytopenia also occurs in a small subset of patients, and these patients are at risk for recurrent bacterial infections and nonhealing leg ulcers.
- **Joint deformities:** Approximately 70% of patients show irreversible joint damage on radiography within the first 3 years of disease. Work disability is common, and life span may be shortened.
- Cardiovascular disease is accelerated in rheumatoid arthritis and is the commonest cause of death. RA is considered a coronary artery disease risk factor equivalent to diabetes and aggressive risk factor management should be instituted.

Osteoarthritis

GENERAL PRINCIPLES

OA, or **degenerative joint disease**, is characterized by deterioration of articular cartilage with subsequent formation of reactive new bone at the articular surface. The joints most commonly affected are the distal and proximal interphalangeal joints of the hands, the first carpometacarpal joint and joints of the hips, knees, and cervical and lumbar spine.

Secondary OA occurs with pre-existing joint abnormality which includes trauma or injury, inflammatory arthritis, avascular necrosis, infectious arthritis, Paget disease, metabolic disorders (hemochromatosis, Wilson disease), hemoglobinopathy, Ehlers–Danlos syndrome, or Marfan syndrome.[12]

Epidemiology

The disease is more common in the elderly but may occur at any age, especially as sequelae to joint trauma, chronic inflammatory arthritis, or congenital malformation. OA of the spine may lead to spinal stenosis (neurogenic claudication), with aching or pain in the legs or buttocks on standing or walking.

TREATMENT

- **Acetaminophen** in a dosage of up to 1000 mg qid is the initial pharmacologic treatment.
- **Low-dose NSAIDs or selective COX-2 inhibitors** are the next step, followed by full-dose treatment (see Treatment under the Basic Approach to Rheumatic Diseases section). Because this patient population is often elderly and may have concomitant renal or cardiopulmonary disease, NSAIDs should be used with caution.
- **The data for glucosamine sulfate and chondroitin sulfate** are contradictory. Some studies suggest that it may reduce symptoms as well as the rate of cartilage deterioration, whereas others have shown that these agents have little benefit in patients with OA. Glucosamine

should not be administered to patients who are allergic to **shellfish**. Synthetic and naturally occurring hyaluronic acid derivatives can be administered via intra-articular route and may reduce pain and improve mobility in select patients.

- **Intra-articular glucocorticoid injections** often are beneficial but probably should not be given more than every 3–6 months (see General Principles under Basic Approach to the Rheumatic Diseases section). Systemic steroids should be avoided.[13]
- **Tramadol**, a μ-opioid agonist, may be useful as an alternative analgesic agent. Narcotics may be useful for short-term pain relief and in patients in whom other therapeutic modalities are contraindicated, but in general, they should be avoided for long-term use.
- **Topical NSAIDs, lidocaine, or capsaicin** may provide symptomatic relief with minimal toxicity.
- **Gabapentin** has also been used to help with neural pain modification in patients with severe symptoms of arthritis who are unresponsive to the previously mentioned modalities.
- **Duloxetine** has been approved by the US Food and Drug Administration (FDA) for treatment of OA and chronic lower back pain.

Nonpharmacologic Therapies

- Activities that involve excessive use of the joint should be identified and avoided. Poor body mechanics should be corrected, and misalignments such as pronated feet may be aided by orthotics. An exercise program to prevent or correct muscle atrophy can also provide pain relief. When weight-bearing joints are affected, support in the form of a cane, crutches, or a walker can be helpful. Weight reduction may be of benefit, even for non–weight-bearing joints. Thumb splints may be useful for OA of the first carpometacarpal joint. Consultation with occupational and physical therapists may be helpful.
- **OA of the spine** may cause radicular symptoms from pressure on nerve roots and often produces pain and spasm in the paraspinal soft tissues. Physical supports (cervical collar, lumbar corset), local heat, and exercises to strengthen cervical, paravertebral, and abdominal muscles may provide relief in some patients.
- **Epidural steroid injections** may reduce radicular symptoms.

Surgical Management

- **Surgery** can be considered when patients suffer from disabling pain or deformity. Joint replacement surgery usually relieves pain and increases function in selected patients. Most of the prosthetic joints wear out in 10–15 years and repeat surgery is required.
- **Laminectomy and spinal fusion** should be reserved for patients who have severe disease with intractable pain or neurologic complications.

Spondyloarthropathies (SpA)

The **SpA** are an interrelated group of disorders characterized by one or more of the following features: spondylitis, sacroiliitis, enthesopathy (inflammation at sites of tendon insertion), and asymmetric oligoarthritis. Extra-articular features of this group of disorders may include inflammatory eye disease, urethritis, and mucocutaneous lesions. The SpA aggregate in families, where they are associated with HLA-B27 antigen.[14]

These disorders include ankylosing spondylitis, reactive arthritis, psoriatic arthritis, and arthritis associated with inflammatory bowel disease.

More recently, these disorders have been broadly classified as predominantly axial SpA, affecting the spine, pelvis, and the thoracic cage, or predominantly peripheral SpA, affecting the extremities. The Assessment of Spondyloarthritis International Society (ASAS) has formulated criteria for axial and peripheral spondyloarthritis as given in Tables 25-3(A) and 25-3(B).[15]

TABLE 25-3(A) ASAS Criteria for Classification of Axial Spondyloarthritis (to be Applied for Patients with Back Pain ≥3 mo and Age of Onset <45 Years)[a]

Sacroiliitis on Imaging Plus ≥1 SpA Feature	Or	HLA-B 27 Plus ≥2 Other SpA Features
Sacroiliitis on imaging • Active (acute) inflammation on MRI highly suggestive of SpA-associated sacroiliitis[b] And/or • Definite radiographic sacroiliitis according to modified New York criteria (bilateral grade ≥2 or unilateral grade 3 or 4)		**SpA features** • Inflammatory back pain • Arthritis • Enthesitis (heel) • Anterior uveitis • Dactylitis • Psoriasis • Crohn disease or ulcerative colitis • Good response to NSAIDs • Family history of SpA • HLA-B27 • Elevated CRP

ASAS, Assessment of Spondyloarthritis International Society; CRP, C-reactive protein; SpA, spondyloarthritis.

[a]Sensitivity 83%, specificity 84%.The imaging arm (sacroiliitis) alone has a sensitivity of 66% and a specificity of 97%.

[b]Bone marrow edema and/or osteitis on short tau inversion recovery (STIR) or gadolinium-enhanced T1 image.

TABLE 25-3(B) ASAS Classification Criteria of Peripheral Spondyloarthritis (SpA)

Peripheral arthritis and/or Enthesitis and/or Dactylitis

PLUS

≥1 SpA feature	**OR**	**≥2 other SpA features**
• Uveitis • Psoriasis • Crohn's/colitis • Preceding infection • HLA-B27 • Sacroiliitis on imaging		• Arthritis • Enthesitis • Dactylitis • Inflammatory back pain (ever) • Family history of SpA

Sensitivity 77.8%, specificity 82.2%.

Ankylosing Spondylitis

DIAGNOSIS

- **Ankylosing spondylitis** clinically presents as inflammation and bony ankylosis of the joints and ligaments of the spine and sacroiliac joints.
- Patients are usually young men who classically describe nighttime low back pain and prolonged morning stiffness, which improves with exercise.
- Hips and shoulders are the peripheral joints that are most commonly involved. Progressive fusion of the apophyseal joints of the spine occurs in many patients.
- Bilateral SI joint involvement is considered characteristic of ankylosing spondylitis. In addition, spine radiographs may show evidence of bridging osteophytes or syndesmophytes between vertebral bodies. Radiological signs described are "squaring" of the vertebral bodies, Romanus lesions, or the "shiny corner sign," "dagger sign," and "bamboo spine sign." MRI may detect bone marrow edema (BME) on short tau inversion recovery (STIR) and T2-weighted images with fat suppression, often presenting much earlier in the disease.
- Extra-articular manifestations of ankylosing spondylitis include acute anterior uveitis (25%–35%), restrictive pulmonary disease, aortic insufficiency, inflammatory bowel disease, osteoporosis, cardiac conduction blocks, and cauda equina syndrome.
- Rheumatoid factor by definition is negative, and the ESR is inconsistently elevated.

TREATMENT

Behavioral

- Physical therapy emphasizing extension exercises and posture is recommended to minimize possible late postural defects and respiratory compromise.
- Patients should be instructed to sleep supine on a firm bed without a pillow and to practice postural and deep-breathing exercises regularly.
- Cigarette smoking should be strongly discouraged.

Medications

- **Non-salicylate NSAIDs,** such as indomethacin, are used to provide symptomatic relief, and **selective COX-2 inhibitors** are also effective (see General Principles under Basic Approach to the Rheumatic Diseases section).
- **Methotrexate and sulfasalazine** provide benefit for peripheral disease in some patients (see Treatment under Rheumatoid Arthritis section).
- **TNF blockade** is beneficial in patients with axial symptoms and help with improvement of symptoms as well as range of movement. TNF blockade should be used early if a definitive diagnosis can be made.[16]
- **Secukinumab** is an interleukin-17 monoclonal antibody that has been approved for treatment of ankylosing spondylitis. Doses of 150 mg should be given at weeks 0, 1, 2, 3, 4, and then once every 4 weeks. Infection is the commonest side effect.
- **Pamidronate,** a bisphosphonate, may provide modest clinical benefits. Systemic glucocorticoids are not commonly used and can worsen osteopenia.

Surgical Management

Many patients develop osteoporosis in the fused spondylitic spine and are at risk of spinal fracture. Surgical procedures to correct some spine and hip deformities may result in significant rehabilitation in carefully selected patients.

Arthritis of Inflammatory Bowel Disease

GENERAL PRINCIPLES

Arthritis of inflammatory bowel disease occurs in up to 46% of patients with either Crohn disease or ulcerative colitis. It may also occur in some patients with intestinal bypass and diverticular disease.

DIAGNOSIS

Clinical features include **spondylitis, sacroiliitis,** and **peripheral arthritis,** particularly in the knee and ankle. Peripheral joint and spinal disease may not always correlate with the activity of the colitis.

TREATMENT

- **NSAIDs** relieve joint pain and inflammation in patients with arthritis because of inflammatory bowel disease (IBD). However, GI intolerance because of NSAIDs may be increased among this group of patients, and NSAIDs may exacerbate underlying IBD.
- **Sulfasalazine, methotrexate, azathioprine, and systemic glucocorticoids** may also be effective (see Treatment under Rheumatoid Arthritis section).
- **TNF antagonists, infliximab, adalimumab, golimumab, and certolizumab pegol,** may benefit both the colitis and arthritis.
- **Ustekinumab,** which is an interleukin-23/interleukin-17 inhibitor, has been approved for Crohn disease and may be helpful with Crohn-related arthritis (please see section Psoriatic Arthritis).
- Local **injection of glucocorticoids and physical therapy** are useful adjunctive measures.

Reactive Arthritis

GENERAL PRINCIPLES

- **Reactive arthritis** refers to the inflammatory arthritis that occasionally follows certain GI or genitourinary infections. The triad of arthritis, conjunctivitis, and urethritis was formerly referred to as **Reiter's syndrome.**
- *Chlamydia trachomatis* is the most commonly implicated genitourinary infection. *Shigella flexneri, Salmonella* spp., *Yersinia enterocolitica,* or *Campylobacter jejuni* are the most commonly implicated GI infections. *Clostridium difficile* can also trigger the arthritis.
- Of patients, 50%–80% are HLA-B27 positive. Males and females are equally affected after GI infections, although males more commonly develop the above classic triad after a *Chlamydia* infection.

DIAGNOSIS

Clinical Presentation

The clinical syndrome may include **asymmetric oligoarthritis, urethritis, conjunctivitis,** and characteristic **skin and mucous membrane lesions.** Characteristic scaly rash on the palms and soles of the feet is noted, which is called as **keratoderma blennorrhagica.** The syndrome is usually transient, lasting from one to several months, but chronic arthritis may develop in 4%–19% of patients.[19]

Diagnostic Testing

The triggering infection may have been asymptomatic. Testing for stool pathogens is low yield if the diarrheal illness has resolved, but urine testing for *Chlamydia* may be helpful if the clinical syndrome is consistent with reactive arthritis.

TREATMENT

- Conservative therapy is indicated for control of pain and inflammation in these diseases.
- Spontaneous remissions are common, making evaluation of therapy difficult.
- **NSAIDs** (especially indomethacin) are often useful, and **selective COX-2 inhibitors** also provide relief (see General Principles under Basic Approach to the Rheumatic Diseases section).
- **Sulfasalazine** or **methotrexate** may be of benefit for arthritis that does not resolve after several months (see Treatment under Rheumatoid Arthritis section).
- Trial of an **anti–TNF-α** agent might be considered in patients who do not respond to sulfasalazine or methotrexate.
- In unusually severe cases, **glucocorticoid therapy** may be required to prevent rapid joint destruction (see General Principles under Basic Approach to the Rheumatic Diseases section).
- Treatment for chlamydia infection, if detected, is appropriate. Prolonged empiric antibiotic therapy has not been shown to be beneficial.
- **Conjunctivitis** is usually transient and benign, but ophthalmologic referral and treatment with topical or systemic glucocorticoids are indicated for **iritis**.

Psoriatic Arthritis

GENERAL PRINCIPLES

Classification

Five major patterns of joint disease occur: (1) asymmetric oligoarticular arthritis, (2) distal interphalangeal joint involvement in association with nail disease, (3) symmetric rheumatoid-like polyarthritis, (4) spondylitis and sacroiliitis, and (5) arthritis mutilans.[17]

Epidemiology

Prevalence varies; however, it has been reported that as many as 30% of patients with psoriasis have some form of inflammatory arthritis.

TREATMENT

- **NSAIDs**, particularly indomethacin, are used to treat the arthritic manifestations of psoriasis in conjunction with appropriate measures for the skin disease.
- **Intra-articular glucocorticoids** may be useful in the oligoarticular form of the disease, but injection through a psoriatic plaque should be avoided. Severe skin and joint diseases generally respond well to **methotrexate** (see Treatment under Rheumatoid Arthritis section).
- **Sulfasalazine and leflunomide** may also have disease-modifying effects in polyarthritis.
- **TNF-α blockers** may produce dramatic improvement in both skin and joint disease.
- **Ustekinumab** is a human monoclonal antibody to the shared p40 subunit of IL-12 and IL-23 that interferes with receptor binding to immune cells. It is administered subcutaneously. In patients who weigh less than 100 kg, the dose is 45 mg SC at week 0 and 4. It is then given every 12 weeks. For patients who weigh more than 100 kg, the dose is

90 mg SC given at the same intervals as the lower dose. It may be administered alone or in combination with methotrexate. Patients should be screened for TB prior to initiating this medication and periodically while on it. Monitor for infections and injection site reactions. Monitor all patients for the development of nonmelanoma skin cancer because this has been reported.
- **Apremilast** is an orally administered phosphodiesterase-4 inhibitor. It suppresses multiple proinflammatory cytokines involved in the innate and adaptive immunity. Initial starting dose is 10 mg daily, which is slowly uptitrated to a maximum dose of 30 mg twice daily. GI upset and headaches have commonly been reported.[18]
- **Secukinumab** has been approved for psoriasis as well as psoriatic arthritis in the same doses as ankylosing spondylitis (see above).
- **Abatacept and tofacitinib** have both been approved for use in psoriatic arthritis (see section Rheumatoid Arthritis).

COMPLICATIONS

Colonization of psoriatic skin with *S. aureus* increases the risk of wound infection after reconstructive joint surgery.

Adult-Onset Still Disease

GENERAL PRINCIPLES

Adult-onset Still Disease (AOSD) is a rare inflammatory multisystem disease occurring in adults presenting as fever (quotidian/double quotidian), rash, arthritis, sore throat, hepatosplenomegaly, and serositis. This is the adult form of systemic juvenile rheumatoid arthritis. The rash is classically evanescent, salmon-colored, macular or maculopapular which is usually nonpruritic, and occurs with the fever.

Diagnostic Testing

- AOSD is primarily a diagnosis of exclusion and should be considered only after excluding other differential diagnoses. Infections such as tuberculosis, infective endocarditis, and Lyme disease; granulomatous disease such as sarcoidosis and Crohn disease; malignancies such as leukemia and lymphoma; connective tissue disorders such as systemic lupus erythematosus, mixed connective tissue disease (MCTD), and polyarteritis nodosa, etc., should be ruled out before diagnosis.[20]
- Neutrophilia, thrombocytosis, elevated LDH and liver enzymes, raised ESR, and CRP are the usual lab findings.
- Marked elevation of ferritin (>3000 mg/mL) is found in more than 70% of the patients. Reduced level (<20%) of glycosylated fraction of ferritin is a more useful marker.
- Rheumatoid factor and antinuclear antibody tests are negative.
- The Yamaguchi criteria is used for the diagnosis of AOSD.

TREATMENT

- NSAIDs can be used for pain relief and reducing inflammation.
- Glucocorticoids can be given to reduce systemic inflammation.
- DMARDs such as methotrexate may be used as steroid-sparing agents.
- Trial of biologics such as anti-TNF-α antagonist, IL-1 antagonist (anakinra), and interleukin-6 receptor antibody (Tocilizumab) can be used in patients not responding to the above-mentioned treatment.[21]

- Cyclosporine can be used for patients presenting with macrophage activation syndrome, a rare and fatal complication of AOSD characterized by leukopenia, hypertriglyceridemia, transaminitis, and intravascular coagulation.

Systemic Lupus Erythematosus

GENERAL PRINCIPLES

Definition

SLE is a multisystem disease of unknown etiology that primarily affects women of child-bearing age. The female-to-male ratio is 9:1. It is most common in the second and third decades of life and in African Americans.

Pathophysiology

Pathophysiology is multifactorial and incompletely understood, with interplay of genetic predisposition and environmental factors.

DIAGNOSIS

- Disease manifestations are protean, ranging in severity from fatigue, malaise, weight loss, and fever to potentially life-threatening cytopenias, nephritis, cerebritis, vasculitis, pneumonitis, myositis, and myocarditis.
- The 2019 European Alliance of Associations for Rheumatology (EULAR)/American College of Rheumatology (ACR) classification criteria for systemic lupus erythematosus and the new classification criteria are used for the diagnosis (Figure 25-1).
- Commonly associated other serology includes anti-SSA (Ro) and anti-SSB (La) antibodies in approximately 30% of patients and anti-RNP in 40% of patients.[22]

TREATMENT

Medications

- **NSAIDs** usually control SLE-associated arthritis, arthralgias, fever, and mild serositis but not fatigue, malaise, or major organ system involvement. The response to **selective COX-2 inhibitors** is similar. Hepatic and renal toxicities of NSAIDs appear to be increased in SLE.
- **HCQ** 200 mg bid may be effective in the treatment of rash, photosensitivity, arthralgias, arthritis, alopecia, and malaise associated with SLE and in the treatment of **discoid and subacute cutaneous lupus erythematosus.** The drug is not effective for treating major organ manifestations, but long-term usage reduces both disease progression as well as number of flares. In lupus patients with associated antiphospholipid antibody, HCQ reduces incidence of thrombosis. For the potential ophthalmologic complications, patients need regular eye examination.
- **Glucocorticoid therapy**
    - **Indications** for systemic glucocorticoids include life-threatening manifestations of SLE, such as glomerulonephritis, CNS involvement, thrombocytopenia, hemolytic anemia, and debilitating manifestations of SLE that are unresponsive to conservative therapy.
    - **Dosage:** Patients with severe or potentially life-threatening complications of SLE should be treated with prednisone, 1–2 mg/kg PO daily, which can be given in divided doses. After disease is controlled, prednisone should be tapered slowly, with the dosage being reduced by no more than 10% every 7–10 days. More rapid reduction may result in relapse. **IV pulse therapy** in the form of methylprednisolone, 500–1000 mg IV daily for

Entry criterion

Antinuclear antibodies (ANA) at a titer of ≥1:80 on HEp-2 cells or an equivalent positive test (ever)

↓

If absent, do not classify as SLE

If present, apply additive criteria

↓

Additive criteria

Do not count a criterion if there is a more likely explanation than SLE.
Occurrence of a criterion on at least one occasion is sufficient.
SLE classification requires at least one clinical criterion and ≥10 points.
Criteria need not occur simultaneously.
Within each domain, only the highest weighted criterion is counted toward the total score.

Clinical domains and criteria	Weight
Constitutional	
Fever	2
Hematologic	
Leukopenia	3
Thrombocytopenia	4
Autoimmune hemolysis	4
Neuropsychiatric	
Delirium	2
Phychosis	3
Seizure	5
Mucocutaneous	
Non-scarring alopecia	2
Oral ulcers	2
Subacute cutaneous OR discoid lupus	4
Acute cutaneous lupus	6
Serosal	
Pleural or pericardial effusion	5
Acute pericarditis	6
Musculoskeletal	
Joint involvement	6
Renal	
Proteinuria >0.5 g/24 h	4
Renal biopsy Class II or V lupus nephritis	8
Renal biopsy Class III or IV lupus nephritis	10

Immunology domains and criteria	Weight
Antiphospholipid antibodies	
Anti-cardiolipin antibodies OR Anti-β2GP1 antibodies OR Lupus anticoagulant	2
Complement proteins	
Low C3 OR low C4	3
Low C3 AND low C4	4
SLE-specific antibodies	
Anti-dsDNA antibody OR Anti-Smith antibody	6

Total score:

↓

Classify as Systemic Lupus Erythematosus with a score of 10 or more if entry criterion fulfilled.

Figure 25-1 New classification criteria for systemic lupus erythematosus.

3–5 days, has been used in SLE in such life-threatening situations as rapidly progressive renal failure, active CNS disease, and severe thrombocytopenia. Patients who do not show improvement with this regimen probably are unresponsive to steroids, and other therapeutic alternatives must be considered. A course of oral prednisone should follow completion of pulse therapy.

- **Immunosuppressive therapy**[23]
  - Indications for immunosuppressive therapy in SLE include life-threatening manifestations of SLE such as glomerulonephritis, CNS involvement, thrombocytopenia, hemolytic anemia, and the inability to reduce corticosteroid dosage or severe corticosteroid side effects.
  - Choice of an immunosuppressive therapy is individualized to the clinical situation. **Cyclophosphamide** is used for life-threatening manifestations of SLE. High-dose monthly IV pulse cyclophosphamide (0.5–1 g/m^2) may be less toxic but is also less immunosuppressive than low-dose daily oral cyclophosphamide (1–1.5 mg/kg/d). **Azathioprine** (1–3 mg/kg/d) and **mycophenolate mofetil** (500–1500 mg bid) are also used as steroid-sparing agents for serious lupus manifestations. There is increasing evidence that mycophenolate mofetil may be as effective as cyclophosphamide in certain classes of lupus nephritis with fewer side effects, and it is particularly preferred in the younger population where fertility maintenance is a concern. **Methotrexate** (7.5–20 mg weekly) is often used for musculoskeletal and skin manifestations. **Rituximab** has been shown in uncontrolled observational studies to be effective in cases of severe SLE not responding to conventional treatment; however, placebo-controlled studies have been disappointing. **Belimumab** inhibits B-lymphocytic stimulator (BLyS) signaling, thereby decreasing B cell survival, and differentiation into immunoglobulin-producing plasma cells. It was approved by the FDA in 2012 for the treatment of adult autoantibody-positive lupus patients who are receiving standard therapy after it was shown in trials to reduce SLE disease activity and flares.

Nonpharmacologic Therapies

- **Conservative therapy** alone is warranted if the patient's manifestations are mild.
- **General supportive measures** include adequate sleep and fatigue avoidance.
- All patients, not just those with photosensitive rashes, are advised on use of sunscreens with sun protection factor (SPF) of 30 or greater, protective clothing, and sun avoidance. Isolated skin lesions may respond to **topical steroids.**
- Consider prophylaxis against *Pneumocystis* pneumonia in patients treated with cyclophosphamide. Also consider adding prophylaxis for the prevention of bladder and gonadal toxicity from this agent. Appropriate immunizations should be considered prior to initiation of immunosuppressive therapy, especially against influenza and pneumococcus. Immunization with live vaccines is contraindicated in immunosuppressed patients, but varicella-zoster vaccine may be recommended prior to initiation of therapy.

SPECIAL CONSIDERATIONS

- Patients with lupus have accelerated **coronary and peripheral vascular disease**, especially with high disease activity and chronic steroid use, and cardiovascular risk factors should be managed aggressively.
- **Transplantation and chronic hemodialysis** have been used successfully in SLE patients with renal failure. Clinical and serologic evidence of disease activity often remits when renal failure ensues.
- **Pregnancy in SLE:** An increased incidence of second-trimester spontaneous miscarriages and stillbirths has been reported in women with antibodies to cardiolipin or lupus anticoagulant. SLE patients may experience flares during pregnancy if the lupus is active

at the time of conception. Differentiation between active SLE and preeclampsia is often difficult. Women in whom SLE is well controlled are less likely to have a flare of disease during pregnancy.
- **Neonatal lupus** may occur in offspring of anti-SSA– or anti-SSB–positive mothers, with skin rash and heart block as the most common manifestations.
- **Drug-induced lupus** typically has a sudden onset and is associated with serositis and musculoskeletal manifestations. Renal and CNS manifestations are rare. Serology includes positive ANA and **antihistone antibodies**, negative anti-SM, and anti–double-stranded DNA antibodies, along with normal complement levels. The disease usually resolves with drug discontinuation. Offending drugs include procainamide, hydralazine, minocycline, diltiazem, isoniazid, chlorpromazine, quinidine, methyldopa, and anti-TNF biologics.

Systemic Sclerosis

GENERAL PRINCIPLES

Definition

Systemic sclerosis (scleroderma) is a systemic illness characterized by progressive fibrosis of the skin and visceral organs. The etiology is unknown, but many manifestations of scleroderma are secondary to vasculopathy.

Classification

- Scleroderma can be subdivided based on anatomic skin distribution into **localized scleroderma** (morphea and linear scleroderma) and **systemic sclerosis** (diffuse cutaneous, limited cutaneous, and systemic sclerosis sine scleroderma). The limited cutaneous form involves the extremities distal to the knees and elbows as well as the face. Diffuse cutaneous scleroderma involves the skin of the proximal extremities and the trunk. Systemic sclerosis sine scleroderma affects the internal organs without skin involvement. The **CREST syndrome** is **c**alcinosis, **R**aynaud phenomenon, **e**sophageal dysmotility, **s**clerodactyly, and **t**elangiectasias.
- **Nephrogenic systemic fibrosis** is a potential complication of MRI with gadolinium contrast in patients with renal failure. It is associated with skin thickening and internal organ fibrosis resembling scleroderma, without Raynaud phenomenon or ANA positivity.

DIAGNOSIS

Clinical Presentation

- Nearly all patients with systemic sclerosis have **Raynaud phenomenon**. It is typically the presenting feature. Nail fold capillary changes are also common.
- **Diffuse scleroderma** is associated with scleroderma "renal crisis," and multiple internal organs are affected. Long-term survival is poor.
  - **GI involvement:** Decreased gut motility can occur, leading to bacterial overgrowth, malabsorption, diarrhea, and weight loss. Occasionally, severe constipation and intestinal pseudo-obstruction occur. Classic endoscopic findings include colonic wide-mouth diverticula, patulous esophagus, esophageal strictures, and gastric antral vascular ectasia (GAVE), also known as watermelon stomach.
  - **Renal involvement:** The appearance of sudden hypertension and renal insufficiency indicates potential scleroderma renal crisis. It is associated with a microangiopathic hemolytic anemia and carries a poor prognosis.[24]
  - **Cardiopulmonary involvement:** Patchy myocardial fibrosis can result in heart failure or arrhythmias. Pulmonary involvement includes pleural effusions and inflammatory alveolitis leading to interstitial fibrosis and pulmonary hypertension.

- ◦ **Other organ systems: Skin** involvement appears initially with edematous and erythematous "salt and pepper" pigmentation changes before progressing to skin tightening and thickening. **Musculoskeletal** manifestations range from arthralgias to arthritis with joint contractures because of the regional skin involvement.
- **Limited scleroderma** is more often associated with primary pulmonary hypertension in the absence of ILD or biliary cirrhosis.

Diagnostic Testing

More than 95% of scleroderma patients are ANA positive, and 20%–40% are anti–Scl-70 positive (associated with diffuse disease). Up to 40% of patients with limited scleroderma have anticentromere antibody. RNA polymerase III antibody has been found to increase the risk of scleroderma renal crisis and malignancy.

TREATMENT

Therapeutic options for scleroderma are limited. Treatment focuses on organ involvement and symptoms.

- **Skin:** No therapeutic agent is effective for these cutaneous manifestations. **Physical therapy** is important to retard and reduce joint contractures.[25]
- **GI involvement**
  - ◦ Reflux esophagitis generally responds to standard therapy (e.g., H^2-receptor antagonists, proton pump inhibitors, and promotility agents).
  - ◦ Treatment with broad-spectrum antimicrobials in a rotating sequence including **metronidazole** often improves malabsorption. Metoclopramide may reduce bloating and distention.
  - ◦ Occasionally, esophageal strictures require mechanical **esophageal dilation.**
- **Renal involvement:** Aggressive blood pressure control with **ACE inhibitors** is indicated in scleroderma renal crisis. ARBs do not appear to be as effective.
- **Cardiopulmonary involvement:** Coronary artery vasospasm can cause angina pectoris and may respond to calcium channel antagonists. Pulmonary involvement, such as pulmonary hypertension, is treated with standard therapies for these conditions.
- Rapidly progressive skin disease can be treated with mycophenolate mofetil, which can prevent progression.
- Patients with interstitial lung disease may benefit from glucocorticoids, mycophenolate mofetil, and cyclophosphamide.

Raynaud Phenomenon

GENERAL PRINCIPLES

Raynaud phenomenon is a vasospasm of the digital arteries and can result in ischemia of the digits. It manifests as repeated episodes of color changes of the digits after cold exposure or emotional stress. Primary Raynaud disease has no predisposing factors and is milder. Secondary Raynaud disease occurs in individuals with a predisposing factor, usually a collagen vascular disease.

TREATMENT

Medications

- **Calcium channel antagonists** (of the dihydropyridine group) are the preferred initial agents, although they may exacerbate gastroesophageal reflux and constipation.

- Alternative vasodilators such as prazosin are occasionally helpful but can have limiting side effects, including orthostatic hypotension.
- Other agents that might improve vasospasm include **topical nitroglycerin** applied to the dorsum of the hands, phosphodiesterase inhibitor (e.g., **sildenafil**), and endothelin receptor antagonist (e.g., **bosentan**).
- Daily low-dose aspirin therapy is often prescribed for its antiplatelet effects.
- Patients with severe ischemic digits should be hospitalized, and conditions such as macrovascular disease, vasculitis, or a hypercoagulable state should be ruled out. An IV infusion of a prostaglandin or prostaglandin analog may be considered.
- Patients should be instructed to avoid exposure to cold, protect the hands and feet from trauma, limit caffeine intake, and discontinue cigarette smoking.

Surgical Management

- **Sympathetic ganglion blockade** with a long-acting anesthetic agent may be useful when a patient has progressive digital ulceration that fails to improve with medical therapy.
- Surgical digital sympathectomy may be beneficial.

Sjögren Syndrome

GENERAL PRINCIPLES

Sjögren syndrome is a slowly progressive multisystem autoimmune disease characterized by dysfunction of exocrine glands. This disease may manifest as an entity alone or in association with other autoimmune diseases such as SLE, scleroderma, rheumatoid arthritis, mixed connective tissue disorder, inflammatory myopathy, and autoimmune thyroid disorder.

DIAGNOSIS

Clinical Presentation

History

- Sjögren syndrome can present with glandular and extraglandular manifestations.
- History suggestive of sicca symptoms such as dry eyes and dry mouth and parotid enlargement indicates glandular involvement. Women may present with vaginal dryness.
- Raynaud phenomenon, inflammatory arthritis, renal tubular acidosis, and cutaneous vasculitis are some of the major extraglandular manifestations.
- Some patients may rarely have symptoms of pancreatic insufficiency such as diarrhea and malabsorption.
- Eye examination may reveal reduced tear meniscus and reduced light reflex. The tongue and buccal mucosa may appear dry with diminished sublingual salivary pool on oral cavity examination.
- Persistent parotid enlargement, purpura, hepatosplenomegaly, or lymphadenopathy should raise the suspicion for lymphoma, as the incidence risk is high in patients with Sjögren syndrome.
- Most lymphomas are extranodal and glandular mucosa-associated lymphoma is the commonest. Leukopenia, cryoglobulinemia, low serum C4 complement levels, and autoantibodies (anti-Ro/SS-A, anti-La/SS-B) may suggest development of lymphoma.

Diagnostic Testing

- Diagnosis of primary Sjögren syndrome is based on the sicca symptoms and the antibodies in the serum to Ro/SS-A or La/SS-B or both.
- Minor salivary gland biopsy may reveal focal lymphocytic sialadenitis.

TREATMENT

- Artificial tears and bicarbonate-buffered solutions are useful for dryness of eyes and can be self-administered. Optic cyclosporine and oral pilocarpine, 5 mg QID, or cevimeline, 30 mg TID, have been shown to reduce the ocular dryness. For severe dryness, nasolacrimal duct plugs, soft contact lenses, and even corneal transplantation can be attempted.
- Lubrication with water, local stimulation using sugar-free lozenges, systemic stimulation using oral pilocarpine, 5 mg QID, or cevimeline, 30 mg TID, have been shown to be effective in treating dry mouth symptoms.
- HCQ or methotrexate plus steroids are effective in patients with arthritis.
- Bicarbonate replacement (0.5–2 mmol/kg in four divided doses) is useful in patients with renal tubular acidosis.
- Immunosuppressive agents may be needed for major organ involvement including vasculitis.

Mixed Connective Tissue Disease

GENERAL PRINCIPLES

Patients with limited cutaneous scleroderma presenting with features of SLE, polymyositis (PM), and RA may have MCTD.

High titers of autoantibodies to U1-RNP may be seen in these overlap syndromes.

Clinical Presentation

- Raynaud syndrome and myalgia are the usual initial symptoms. Arthralgia and even erosive polyarthritis may be seen in some patients.
- Skin rashes suggestive of SLE and dermatomyositis (DM) can be present. Sclerodactyly, soft tissue calcinosis, and cutaneous telangiectasia can develop over time.
- Pulmonary fibrosis, pericarditis, esophageal dysmotility, and membranous glomerulonephritis are some of the systemic manifestations.

Diagnostic Testing

- Elevated ESR, hypergammaglobulinemia, and high titers of anti-U1RNP antibodies are seen in patients with MCTD. Systemic sclerosis-specific autoantibodies are usually absent.

TREATMENT

- MCTD patients have good response to glucocorticoids. Compared to systemic sclerosis, MCTD has a better long-term prognosis.

Vasculitis

GENERAL PRINCIPLES

- **Vasculitis** is characterized by inflammation of blood vessels, leading to tissue damage and necrosis. This diagnosis includes a broad spectrum of disorders with various causes that involve vessels of different types, sizes, and locations. The immunopathologic process may involve immune complexes.
- Although in most cases the inciting agent has not been identified, some are associated with chronic hepatitis B and C.
- Vasculitis "mimics" should be excluded before considering the diagnosis. These include infections, neoplasms, coagulopathies, drugs, and others as enlisted in Table 25-4.

TABLE 25-4 Conditions That Can Mimic Vasculitis
• **Infectious diseases**: bacterial endocarditis, disseminated gonococcal infection, pulmonary histoplasmosis, coccidioidomycosis, syphilis, HIV infection, Lyme disease, Rocky Mountain spotted fever, Whipple disease
• **Coagulopathies/thrombotic microangiopathies**: antiphospholipid syndrome, thrombotic thrombocytopenic purpura
• **Neoplasms**: atrial myxoma, lymphoma, carcinomatosis
• **Drug toxicity**: cocaine, levamisole, amphetamines, ergot alkaloids, methysergide, arsenic
• **Others**: sarcoidosis, atheroembolic disease, antiglomerular basement membrane disease (Goodpasture syndrome), amyloidosis, migraine, fibromuscular dysplasia, heritable disorders of connective tissue, segmental arterial mediolysis (SAM), reversible cerebral vasoconstrictive syndrome

DIAGNOSIS

Systemic manifestations including fever, weight loss, mononeuropathy, rash, arthritis, abdominal pain, sinusitis, pulmonary hemorrhage and glomerulonephritis are common for vasculitis. Table 25-5 summarizes the clinical features, diagnosis, and treatment of the most common forms of vasculitis.[26]

Diagnostic Testing

- Anemia, elevated ESR, low complement levels, and urinalysis abnormalities (proteinuria, hematuria, and cellular casts) are often seen.
- c-ANCA that represents antibody to proteinase-3 is specific for granulomatosis with polyangiitis.
- Characteristic finding of vasculitis on biopsy from the affected tissues, such as skin, muscle, artery, and nerve, can be important in establishing the diagnosis. Sural nerve and gastrocnemius muscle are common sites for biopsy.
- Renal biopsy findings tend to be nonspecific.

TREATMENT

The response to therapy and long-term prognosis of these disorders are highly variable.

- **Glucocorticoids** are the initial therapy. Although vasculitis that is limited to the skin may respond to lower doses of corticosteroids, the initial dosage for visceral involvement should be high (prednisone, 1–2 mg/kg/d). If life-threatening manifestations are present, a brief course of high-dose pulse therapy with methylprednisolone, 500 mg IV q12h for 3–5 days, should be considered.
- Strong immunosuppressives are used in the induction treatment of necrotizing vasculitis when major organ system involvement is present. **Cyclophosphamide** has historically been the initial choice. **Rituximab** is now an approved alternative for remission induction especially in ANCA-induced vasculitis.
- **Methotrexate, azathioprine**, and **mycophenolate mofetil** can be used for maintenance therapy and as initial therapy in less severe presentations.
- **Plasma exchange** can be considered in patients with severe renal disease or pulmonary hemorrhage.
- **Tocilizumab** has been found effective in the treatment of large-vessel vasculitis.

TABLE 25-5 Clinical Features and Diagnostic and Treatment Approaches to Vasculitis

Vasculitis Syndrome	Clinical Features	Diagnostic Approach	Treatment
Large-Vessel Involvement			
Temporal arteritis	Headache, located temporally in >50% Jaw claudication Commonly associated with PMR	ESR >50 mm/h Temporal artery biopsy	Prednisone, 60–80 mg/d Tocilizumab
Takayasu arteritis (affects the aorta and primary branches)	Women more commonly affected Greatest prevalence in Asians Commonly presents between ages 20–30 Constitutional symptoms Finger ischemia Arm claudication	Aortic arch arteriogram	Prednisone, 60–80 mg/d Infliximab
Medium-Vessel Involvement			
Polyarteritis nodosa	Skin ulcers Nephritis Mononeuritis Mesenteric ischemia	Skin biopsy Renal biopsy Sural nerve biopsy Mesenteric angiogram Hepatitis B, C testing ANCA negative	Prednisone 60–100 mg/d Cyclophosphamide 1–2 mg/kg/d can be added
Kawasaki disease	Seen in children Fever Conjunctivitis Lymphadenopathy Mucocutaneous erythema Coronary aneurysms	Clinical Coronary angiogram	IV immunoglobulin Aspirin Anticoagulation

(Continued)

TABLE 25-5 Clinical Features and Diagnostic and Treatment Approaches to Vasculitis (Continued)

Small-Vessel Involvement			
Granulomatosis with polyangiitis (c-ANCA vasculitis)	Sinusitis Pulmonary infiltrates Nephritis	c-ANCA, sinus biopsy Lung biopsy Renal biopsy	Prednisone 60–100 mg/d *and* cyclophosphamide 1–2 mg/kg/d Rituximab Plasmapheresis
Microscopic polyangiitis	Pulmonary infiltrates Nephritis	p-ANCA Renal biopsy	Prednisone 60–100 mg/d Cyclophosphamide 1–2 mg/kg/d can be added
Eosinophilic granulomatosis with polyangiitis (Churg-Strauss)	Asthma, allergic rhinitis Fleeting pulmonary infiltrates Mononeuritis multiplex	p-ANCA Peripheral eosinophilia Elevated IgE levels Biopsy (sural nerve/skin) with eosinophilic granulomas	Prednisone 60–100 mg/d Cyclophosphamide if renal, GI, CNS, or cardiac involvement
Vasculitis in SLE or RA	Skin ulcers Polyneuropathy	Skin or sural nerve biopsy	Prednisone 60–80 mg/d Cyclophosphamide 1–2 mg/kg/d can be added
Cutaneous leukocytoclastic vasculitis	Palpable purpura	Skin biopsy	NSAIDs, antihistamine, colchicine, dapsone Low-dose prednisone Discontinue inciting drug
Henoch-Schönlein purpura	Palpable purpura Nephritis Mesenteric ischemia	Skin biopsy Renal biopsy IgA immune complex deposition	Supportive treatment Prednisone 20–60 mg/d may be needed

ANCA, antineutrophil cytoplasmic antibodies; c-ANCA, cytoplasmic antineutrophil cytoplasmic antibodies; CNS, central nervous system; ESR, erythrocyte sedimentation rate; GI, gastrointestinal; p-ANCA, perinuclear antineutrophil cytoplasmic antibodies; PMR, polymyalgia rheumatica; RA, rheumatoid arthritis; SLE, systemic lupus erythematosus.

Polymyalgia Rheumatica

DIAGNOSIS

Clinical Presentation

Polymyalgia rheumatica (PMR) presents in elderly patients as proximal limb girdle pain, morning stiffness lasting at least 30 minutes, and constitutional symptoms.[27] It is associated with **temporal arteritis (TA)** in up to 40% of patients (see Table 25-5).

Diagnostic Testing

- There is no established diagnostic criterion. The diagnosis remains clinical.
- The ESR is >50 mm/h.

TREATMENT

- If PMR is present without evidence of TA, **prednisone**, 10–15 mg PO daily, usually produces dramatic clinical improvement within a few days.
- Patients who are suspected of having TA should be treated promptly with high-dose steroids to prevent blindness, and rheumatology should be consulted immediately.
- Tocilizumab has been approved for the treatment of temporal arteritis.
- The ESR should return to normal during initial treatment. Subsequent therapeutic decisions should be based on ESR and clinical status.
- Glucocorticoid therapy can be tapered gradually to a maintenance dosage of 5–10 mg PO daily but should be continued for at least 1 year to minimize the risk of relapse.

Cryoglobulin Syndromes

GENERAL PRINCIPLES

Cryoglobulins are serum immunoglobulins that reversibly precipitate in the cold. Cryoglobulins are categorized as type 1 (monoclonal, no RF activity) or as those with RF activity, the "mixed" types 2 (monoclonal) and 3 (polyclonal).

Etiology

- Patients with **type 1** usually have an underlying hematologic disorder such as myeloma, lymphoma, or Waldenström macroglobulinemia.
- **Types 2 and 3** are associated with small-vessel vasculitis and can be present in patients with chronic inflammatory diseases such as hepatitis B and C virus infection, endocarditis, SLE, and RA. The majority of patients with mixed cryoglobulinemia have hepatitis C, although only 5% of patients with hepatitis C and cryoglobulins develop vasculitis.
- **"Essential"** cryoglobulinemia (cryoglobulinemia without an etiology) has become exceedingly rare since the discovery of hepatitis C.

DIAGNOSIS

- Symptoms in monoclonal cryoglobulinemia are related to hyperviscosity (blurring of vision, digital ischemia, headache, lethargy).
- Clinical manifestations of mixed cryoglobulinemia are mediated by immune complex deposition (arthralgias, palpable purpura, glomerulonephritis, and neuropathy).[29]

TREATMENT

- Secondary cryoglobulinemia responds to **treatment of the underlying disorder**. It may recur when treatment is stopped.
- Patients with progressive renal failure, distal necrosis, advanced neuropathy, or other severe manifestations should be treated aggressively with **prednisone** and immunosuppression.
- **Plasmapheresis** can be used in addition to immunosuppression in severe disease.

Polymyositis and Dermatomyositis (PM & DM)

GENERAL PRINCIPLES

- Polymyositis and dermatomyositis are idiopathic inflammatory myopathies but have many distinctions.
- **PM** presents as weakness and occasionally tenderness of the proximal musculature. Skin manifestations are absent.
- **DM** is associated with proximal muscle weakness and a characteristic skin rash. Gottron papules and a heliotrope rash are hallmark features of DM, but other skin manifestations may be seen. DM may sometimes occur without myositis.
- PM and DM can occur alone or in association with a variety of neoplasms. Patients with rheumatic diseases such as SLE or RA can also have myositis.
- Antisynthetase syndrome is myositis spectrum disease that is associated with several anti-synthetase antibodies including anti-Jo1, anti-PL7, anti-PL12, anti-OJ, anti-EJ, anti-KS, anti-Ha, and anti-Zo. This syndrome often presents acutely with fever, arthritis, characteristic rash on the hands called as mechanics hands, and interstitial lung disease.

DIAGNOSIS

Clinical Presentation

- The cardinal feature of myositis is proximal muscle weakness without pain. Patients may have difficulty in getting out of the car, chair, or bathtub, climbing stairs, or using their arms above their head. Distal muscle strength is usually normal.
- Dysphagia with nasal regurgitation may occur if there is weakness of the striated muscle of upper esophagus.
- Dyspnea due to interstitial lung disease and inflammatory arthritis causing joint pain may occur in antisynthetase syndrome.
- Physical examination may reveal proximal muscle weakness such as difficulty in rising up from a deep squat or raising the head from supine position.

Diagnostic Testing

- Elevated muscle enzyme levels (creatine kinase, aldolase, transaminases, lactate dehydrogenase [LDH]).
- Myositis-specific or associated antibodies such as Jo-1. Anti–Jo-1 antibodies are strongly associated with ILD, Raynaud phenomenon, and arthritis. These antibodies have therapeutic and prognostic implications and should be assessed in all patients.
- Characteristic findings can be seen on electromyogram (EMG); these include insertional activity, but these changes are not specific and can be seen in infectious or metabolic myopathies.
- A muscle biopsy can establish the diagnosis but may not be required if myositis-related antibodies are present in the right clinical setting. MRI is useful for the detection of inflammation and necrosis and can aid in identifying a biopsy location.[30]

- Screening for common neoplasms, such as colon, lung, breast, and prostate cancer, should be considered in these patients as well as individual risk-based assessment. Risk factors for malignancy in the setting of myositis include the presence of DM, cutaneous vasculitis, male sex, and advanced age.

Treatment

- When PM or DM occurs without associated disease, it usually responds well to **prednisone**, 1–2 mg/kg PO daily. Systemic complaints, such as fever and malaise, respond first, followed by muscle enzymes, and finally, muscle strength. Once serum enzyme levels normalize, the prednisone dosage should be reduced slowly to maintenance levels of 10–20 mg PO daily. Appearance of steroid-induced myopathy and hypokalemia may complicate therapeutic assessment.
- Patients who do not respond to glucocorticoids or who need steroid-sparing treatment may respond to **methotrexate, mycophenolate mofetil**, or **azathioprine**.
- IV infusion of **immunoglobulin** may hasten improvement of severe dysphagia.
- Severe cases are typically treated with **rituximab**. Rituximab is effective in patients with antisynthetase syndrome especially those that are Jo-1 positive.
- PM or DM associated with neoplasia tends to be less responsive to glucocorticoid therapy but may improve after removal of the malignant tumor.
- **Physical therapy** is essential in the management of myositis.

Fibromyalgia

GENERAL PRINCIPLES

- Fibromyalgia is a common cause of musculoskeletal pain. It is described as a pain amplification syndrome unified by sleep disturbance, exaggerated pain sensitivity, and multiplicity of symptoms with paucity of findings on clinical examination and lab testing.

DIAGNOSIS

- Symptoms include diffuse nonarticular pain, sleep disturbances, fatigue, headache, irritable bowel syndrome, paresthesias, depression, and vasomotor symptoms in hands and feet.
- Tenderness on palpation is present in at least 11 out of 18 predetermined tender points included in the initial ACR classification criteria for fibromyalgia.
- Laboratory studies are normal.[28]

Treatment

- Treatment aims to improve sleep, relieve pain, and enhance physical conditioning.
- Tricyclic antidepressants (e.g., amitriptyline, 10–50 mg QHS), trazodone (25–100 mg QHS), and cyclobenzaprine (10–20 mg QHS) may be used to aid sleep.
- Antidepressants such as venlafaxine, duloxetine, and milnacipran may be beneficial.
- Pregabalin is FDA approved for the treatment of fibromyalgia. Gabapentin can also be used.
- An aerobic exercise program is essential and can be supplemented by stretching exercises.
- Cognitive-behavioral therapy programs are also effective.

Summary

- Early initiation of conventional synthetic disease modifying antirheumatic drug treatment greatly reduces the risk of future joint damage and disability in patients with rheumatoid arthritis.
- For organ-threatening or life-threatening SLE, treatment usually includes an initial period of high-intensity immunosuppressive therapy to control disease activity, followed by a longer period of less intensive therapy to consolidate response and prevent relapses.
- The discovery of the role of tumour necrosis factor (TNF) and subsequently interleukin-17A (IL-17A) in the pathophysiology of SpA revolutionized the treatment of this condition.
- The IL-1 signaling pathway was identified to play a central role in the pathogenesis of AOSD and IL-1 inhibitors is favorable reflecting a targeted approach as standard of care.
- Genetic factors and obesity are prominent contributors to hyperuricemia and gout, while dietary factors contribute to less variance in serum urate, though can still have some contribution to population attributable risk.
- Comprehensive management comprises establishing the diagnosis of true vasculitis after ruling out vasculitis mimics, finding the etiology if feasible, assessing the caliber of the vessels involved, deciphering the pathological process of vessel damage, investigating for the existence and extent of systemic involvement, and finally planning therapy.

Scan the QR code to access chapter references.

26 Medical Emergencies

Sue Lin Hilbert, Mark D. Levine, Evan S. Schwarz, and Mohammed Shaheen

PRIMARY ASSESSMENT IN MEDICAL EMERGENCIES

Primary Assessment	Mode of Assessment	Interpretation and Action
Airway	• Is the patient speaking to you? • Are there any abnormal sounds from the oral cavity such as snoring, gurgling, or gasping? • Is there any obvious trauma to the face or neck? Any mass or swelling? • Is there any visible foreign body in the airway/oral cavity?	• Airway patency maneuvers such as head tilt, jaw thrust, chin-lift. • Suctioning of secretions and vomitus. • Insertion of oropharyngeal or nasopharyngeal airway. • Insertion of laryngeal mask airway or supraglottic device. • Insertion of endotracheal tube for definitive airway protection.
Breathing	• Is the patient able to speak in full sentences without getting breathless? • Is the trachea central? • Is the chest movement equal on both sides? • Are breath sounds equal on both sides with no obvious signs of reduced air entry? • Any open wounds or obvious chest trauma; paradoxical respiration? • Is the patient's oxygen saturation within permissible levels?	• Oxygen support as required, using simple delivery mechanisms such as simple mask, nasal cannula, or nonrebreather mask. • Needle decompression for a tension pneumothorax, three-way occlusive dressing for an open pneumothorax, chest tube for a large closed pneumothorax causing hemodynamic instability. • Address acute exacerbation of asthma, COPD, pneumonia, and pulmonary edema with relevant medical management.
Circulation	• Are the patient's extremities cold and clammy? • Does the patient look dehydrated or dry? • Is the patient maintaining his blood pressure? • How is the capillary refill time? • How are the patient's pulses? • Are there any major sources of volume loss identifiable?	• Secure IV access. Preferably two large bore IV cannulas; however, in difficult situations, interosseous access needs to be prioritized over cannulation. • Address source of volume loss with necessary intervention, such as packing of open wounds or pressure dressing. • Address volume loss by administering fluids or blood products.

(Continued)

(Continued)

Primary Assessment	Mode of Assessment	Interpretation and Action
		• If it continues to remain hypotensive, consider vasopressor support. • An eFAST examination and a blood gas analysis are important adjuncts to your primary survey.
Disability/ deformity	• Is the patient alert, oriented, and responding? • What is the patient's level of consciousness according to the Glasgow Coma Scale or AVPU-Scale? • Are the patient's pupils responding to light? • Are there any obvious deformities on the limbs or bones that need to be addressed?	• The patient's level of consciousness is both an indicator of their diagnosis as well as their prognosis. • Assess for these parameters dynamically and on the go. • Dropping level of consciousness should be taken as a sign to restart the primary survey from airway onwards. Just because airway has been addressed initially doesn't mean that the situation cannot change as the patient deteriorates.
Exposure	• Does the patient have any signs of toxin exposure or poisoning on his body? • Does the patient's presentation fit into any of the known toxidromes? • Any clues on head-to-toe examination that can lead to the diagnosis?	• Consider exposing the patient while keeping their dignity intact, along with decontamination, if there is suspicion of toxin exposure, thermal injury, environmental illnesses, venomous animal bites, or severe trauma.
Glucose	• Did you obtain a point-of-care random blood glucose level, especially in an unresponsive patient?	• Address hypoglycemia or hyperglycemia as necessary. Do not forget blood glucose as it can be easily missed during primary survey.

AIRWAY EMERGENCIES

Emergent Airway Management

GENERAL PRINCIPLES

Recognition of the need to manage a patient's airway must be made in a timely and rapid fashion. Most prehospital and in-hospital life support algorithms recommend early airway protection, as respiratory failure can occur suddenly and without obvious signs and symptoms. Increasing evidence shows that to prevent poor outcomes, the most experienced provider should perform the intubation.

Etiology

The need to emergently manage an airway typically arises because of

- Loss of airway protective reflexes
- Respiratory failure
- Cardiopulmonary arrest

TREATMENT

- In a situation where an impending airway collapse is anticipated, it is always recommended to establish a definitive airway. A definitive airway is defined as a self-sustaining tube placed in the trachea with an inflatable cuff that is secured below the level of the vocal cords.
- If the provider is not prepared to establish a definitive airway, temporary support of the airway should be performed.
- In emergency medicine practice, rapid sequence intubation (RSI) is the most frequently used and successful means of intubating the trachea.
- Basic maintenance of airway and/or ventilation is performed with
  - High-flow nasal cannula oxygen at 15 L/min (apneic oxygenation increases desaturation time).
  - Nonrebreather (NRB) oxygen mask at 15 L/min.
  - Bag valve mask (BVM).
  - Supraglottic airway devices. Supraglottic airway devices can be inserted blindly and provide up to 1–2 hours of protected airway. This is a very effective airway protection strategy, especially in low-resource prehospital settings.
- While preparing for definitive airway control, the following steps should be performed:
  - Place the patient upright to decrease dependent lung volume before intubation.
  - Place the patient on NRB mask for 3 minutes if possible.
  - If the patient needs ventilator assistance, deliver eight vital capacity breaths via BVM.
  - Place a positive end expiratory pressure valve set to 5–20 cm H_2O on the BVM, which adds positive pressure to both bagging and passive oxygenation.

Difficult Airway

The mnemonic **"LEMON"** is a helpful tool to assess the likelihood of a patient having a difficult airway:

- "L": Look for signs of obesity, micrognathia, evidence of previous head and neck surgery or irradiation, facial hair, poor dentition, dentures, large teeth, a narrow face, a high and arched palate, a short or thick neck, and facial or neck trauma.
- "E": Evaluate the 3-3-2 rule. Normal mouth opening is three of the patient's fingerbreadths. Hyomental distance should be at least three fingerbreadths, whereas the thyrohyoid distance should be at least two fingerbreadths.

- "M": Mallampati classification, which is performed with the patient seated and neck extended. Open the patient's mouth fully; protrude the patient's tongue, and say "ah."
  - Class I: soft palate, uvula, fauces, and pillars visible—no difficulty
  - Class II: soft palate, uvula, and fauces visible—no difficulty
  - Class III: soft palate and base of uvula visible—moderate difficulty
  - Class IV: only the hard palate is visible—severe difficulty
- "O": Obstruction. Evaluation for foreign bodies, stridor, and other forms of sub- and supraglottic obstruction should be performed prior to laryngoscopy.
- "N": Neck mobility. Patients with cervical spondylosis, degenerative or rheumatoid arthritis, and cervical trauma have to be considered with regard to neck mobility.
- When preparing for intubation in an individual with a difficult airway, the most important task is to call for help from an expert intubator. Alert them early and request their presence, but do not delay airway protection while waiting.

Emergent Airway Adjuncts

- **Gum elastic bougie** is a flexible rubbery stick with a "hockey stick" tip. The bougie can be used blindly but is better suited for direct laryngoscopy where the person intubating cannot visualize the cords. The goal is to obtain the best view possible and for the coude tip of the bougie to be distal and anterior. When the bougie is in the trachea, the tracheal rings are felt as the bougie is slid back and forth. Alternatively, the bougie can be advanced down the oropharynx as deep as possible without losing control of it. If in the esophagus, the bougie will slide all the way down past the stomach with minimal resistance. If in the trachea, the bougie will quickly hit a bronchus and meet resistance. Once in the trachea, one can simply slide an endotracheal tube (ETT) over the bougie and verify placement as usual.
- **Laryngeal mask airway (LMA)** is an easy-to-use rescue device for nearly all airway events. It is an ETT with a balloon at the end that is inflated to cup the trachea while occluding the esophagus. It should not be used in patients with an upper airway obstruction that cannot be cleared or patients with excessive airway pressures such as with chronic obstructive pulmonary disease (COPD), asthma, or pregnancy. There are models of LMAs (which are preferred) that allow an ETT to be passed through them when a definitive airway is desired. Excessive bagging through an LMA can lead to emesis.
- **Supraglottic airway devices** are placed blindly in the oropharynx and inflated with air. An upper balloon obstructs the oropharynx, whereas a lower balloon obstructs the esophagus, allowing ventilation in a similar fashion to an LMA with the same limitations. Intubation is not possible through the supraglottic device as it is with an intubating LMA.
- **Fiber-optic/digital airway devices** are considered by many to be the new standard of care. These devices allow the person intubating to get a view of the vocal cords via a camera or fiber-optic scope without direct oropharyngeal visualization, making intubation much easier. Excessive secretions or blood can obstruct the camera, so the operator needs to be capable of direct laryngoscopy as well as indirect fiber-optic laryngoscopy.
- Operator comfort is the most important determinant of successful airway management. It is important to know what equipment are available to you, which equipment you are most confident using, and what equipment is compatible with the ventilators available in your setting. If you do not feel confident handling the airway, it is best to ask for assistance early on.

Pneumothorax

GENERAL PRINCIPLES

- Pneumothorax may occur spontaneously or as a result of trauma.
- **Primary spontaneous pneumothorax** occurs without obvious underlying lung disease.

- **Secondary spontaneous pneumothorax** results from underlying parenchymal lung disease including COPD and emphysema, interstitial lung disease, necrotizing lung infections, *Pneumocystis jirovecii* pneumonia, TB, and cystic fibrosis.
- **Traumatic pneumothorax** occurs as a result of penetrating or blunt chest trauma.
- **Iatrogenic pneumothorax** occurs after thoracentesis, central line placement, transbronchial biopsy, transthoracic needle biopsy, or barotrauma from mechanical ventilation and resuscitation.
- **Tension pneumothorax** results from continued accumulation of air in the chest that is sufficient to shift mediastinal structures and impede venous return to the heart. This results in abnormal gas exchange, hypotension, and ultimately, cardiovascular collapse.
  - The causes include barotrauma due to mechanical ventilation, a chest wound that allows ingress but not egress of air, or a defect in the visceral pleura that behaves in the same way ("ball valve" effect).
  - Suspect tension pneumothorax when a patient experiences hypotension and respiratory distress on mechanical ventilation or after any procedure in which the thorax is violated.

DIAGNOSIS

Clinical Presentation

History

- Patients commonly complain of ipsilateral chest or shoulder pain, usually of acute onset. A history of recent chest trauma or medical procedure can suggest the diagnosis.
- Dyspnea is usually present.

Physical Examination

- Although examination of the patient with a small pneumothorax may be normal, classic findings include decreased breath sounds and more resonance to percussion on the ipsilateral side.
- With a larger pneumothorax or with underlying lung disease, tachypnea and respiratory distress may be present. The affected hemithorax may be noticeably larger (due to decreased elastic recoil of the collapsed lung) and relatively immobile during respiration.
- If the pneumothorax is very large, and particularly if it is under tension, the patient may exhibit severe distress, diaphoresis, cyanosis, and hypotension. In addition, the patient's trachea may be shifted to the contralateral side.
- If the pneumothorax is the result of penetrating trauma or pneumomediastinum, subcutaneous emphysema may be felt.
- Clinical features alone do not predict the relative size of a pneumothorax, and in a stable patient, further diagnostic studies must be used to guide treatment strategy. However, tension pneumothorax remains a clinical diagnosis, and if suspected in the appropriate clinical scenario, immediate intervention should be undertaken before further evaluation.

Diagnostic Testing

Electrocardiography

An **ECG** may reveal diminished anterior QRS amplitude and an anterior axis shift. In extreme cases, tension pneumothorax may cause electromechanical dissociation.

Imaging

- A **CXR** will reveal a separation of the pleural shadow from the chest wall. If the posteroanterior radiograph is normal and pneumothorax is suspected, a lateral or decubitus film may aid in diagnosis.[1] Air travels to the highest point in a body cavity; thus, a pneumothorax in a supine patient may be detected as an unusually deep costophrenic sulcus and excessive lucency over the upper abdomen caused by the anterior thoracic air. This observation is particularly important in the critical care unit, where radiographs of the mechanically ventilated patient are often obtained with the patient in supine position.

- Although tension pneumothorax is a clinical diagnosis, radiographic correlates include mediastinal and tracheal shift toward contralateral side and depression of the ipsilateral diaphragm.
- **Ultrasonography** is a useful tool for bedside diagnosis of pneumothorax, especially on patients who must remain supine or who are too unstable to undergo CT scanning. Placement of the probe in the intercostal spaces provides information regarding the pleura and underlying lung parenchyma. During normal inspiration, the visceral and parietal pleura move along one another and produce a "sliding sign" phenomenon. In addition, the air-filled lung parenchyma below the pleura produces a raylike opacity known as "comet tails." Presence of the sliding sign and comet tails on ultrasound during inspiration rule out a pneumothorax with high reliability at the point of probe placement. Conversely, absence of these signs is a highly reliable predictor for the presence of pneumothorax. Several places on the chest should be evaluated, including places that air is most likely to accumulate such as the anterior and lateral chest.[2] Studies have shown that in the hands of an experienced clinician with ultrasound training, chest ultrasound is more sensitive than CXR.[3]
- Chest CT is the gold standard for diagnosis and determining the size of pneumothorax. Although not always necessary, it may be particularly useful for differentiating pneumothorax from bullous disease in patients with underlying lung conditions.[4]

TREATMENT

Treatment depends on cause, size, and degree of physiologic derangement.

- **Primary pneumothorax**
  - A small, primary, spontaneous pneumothorax without a continued pleural air leak may resolve spontaneously. Air is resorbed from the pleural space at roughly 1.5% daily, and therefore, a small (approximately 15%) pneumothorax is expected to resolve without intervention in approximately 10 days.
  - If the pneumothorax has not increased in size (6 hour repeat CXR) and symptoms have not changed, the patient may be discharged if they are asymptomatic (apart from mild pleurisy). Obtain follow-up radiographs to confirm resolution of the pneumothorax in 7–10 days. Air travel is discouraged during the follow-up period because a decrease in ambient barometric pressure may cause a larger pneumothorax.
  - If the pneumothorax is **small but the patient is mildly symptomatic**, far from home, or unlikely to cooperate with follow-up, admit the patient and administer high-flow oxygen; the resulting nitrogen gradient will speed resorption.
  - If the patient is **more than mildly symptomatic or has a larger pneumothorax**, simple aspiration is a reasonable initial management strategy. However, aspiration may not be successful for very large pneumothoraces. In patients in whom aspiration fails, proceed with thoracostomy tube insertion.[1]
  - **Pleural sclerosis** to prevent recurrence is recommended by some experts but, in most cases, is not used after a first episode unless a persistent air leak is present.
- **Secondary pneumothorax**
  - Individuals with a secondary spontaneous pneumothorax are usually symptomatic and require lung re-expansion.
  - Often, a bronchopleural fistula persists and a larger thoracostomy tube and suction are required.
  - **Consult a pulmonologist** about pleural sclerosis for persistent air leak and to prevent recurrence.
  - **Surgery** may be required for persistent air leak and should be considered for high-risk patients for prevention of recurrence.

- **Iatrogenic pneumothorax**
  - Iatrogenic pneumothorax is generally caused either by introducing air into the pleural space through the parietal pleura (e.g., thoracentesis, central line placement) or by allowing intrapulmonary air to escape through breach of the visceral pleura (e.g., transbronchial biopsy). Often, no further air leak occurs after the initial event.
  - If the pneumothorax is small and the patient is minimally symptomatic, he or she can be managed conservatively. If the procedure that caused the pneumothorax required sedation, admit the patient, administer oxygen, and repeat the CXR in 6 hours to ensure the patient's stability. If the patient is completely alert and the CXR shows no change, the patient can be discharged.
  - If the patient is symptomatic or if the pneumothorax is too large for expectant care, a pneumothorax catheter with aspiration or a one-way valve is usually adequate and can often be removed the following day.
  - Iatrogenic pneumothorax due to barotrauma from mechanical ventilation almost always has a persistent air leak and should be managed with a chest tube and suction.
- **Tension pneumothorax**
  - When the clinical situation and physical examination strongly suggest this diagnosis, decompress the affected hemithorax immediately with a 14–gauge needle. Place the needle in the second intercostal space, midclavicular line, just superior to the rib. Release of air with clinical improvement confirms the diagnosis.
  - Recognize that an obese patient or a patient with a large amount of breast tissue may not have resolution of tension with a standard angiocatheter because of the inability to reach the chest wall or weight of the tissue kinking off the catheter. These patients may require a longer needle than a standard angiocatheter to reach the intrathoracic space for decompression or require insertion of a larger gauge reinforced catheter to stent open the pathway for air release.
  - The latest Trauma Life Support guidelines recommend the fifth intercostal space, midaxillary line as the recommended location for needle decompression in adults due to less subcutaneous fat or breast tissue in the area. In pediatric patients, the second intercostal approach is considered the best.
  - If long-needle decompression or reinforced catheter insertion is unsuccessful, and the diagnosis is highly probable in an unstable patient, surgical decompression can be performed by incision of the pleura in the fourth to fifth anterior axillary line above the rib in the same space in which thoracostomy tubes are inserted. This technique has been shown to be effective; however, safety and complication rates are not able to be determined because of lack of studies.[5] The full technique for this procedure is beyond the scope of this book.
  - Seal any chest wound with an occlusive dressing and arrange for placement of a thoracostomy tube.

HEAT-INDUCED INJURY

Exertion, environmental exposure, or a combination of both can lead to an elevation of core temperature and the subsequent continuum of pathologies that comprise heat-induced injuries. There are no strict diagnostic criteria for heat-induced injuries, except the general assertion that heat stroke should include a core temperature >40°C and central nervous system (CNS) dysfunction. Diagnosis and treatment are based primarily on exposure history, potential predisposing factors, and clinical presentation.

Heat Exhaustion

GENERAL PRINCIPLES

Heat exhaustion often results from a combination of water and sodium depletion. Water depletion is the result of either overwhelming losses, such as profuse sweating or vomiting, or inadequate replacement. Persons at risk include the elderly, patients taking diuretics, and those working in hot environments with limited water replacement. Salt depletion occurs in unacclimatized individuals who replace fluid losses with large amounts of hypotonic solution.

DIAGNOSIS

- The patient presents with headache, nausea, vomiting, dizziness, weakness, irritability, and/or cramps.
- The patient may have postural hypotension, diaphoresis, and normal or minimally increased core temperature.

TREATMENT

- Treatment consists of removing excess or restrictive clothing, resting the patient in a cool environment, accelerating heat loss by fan evaporation, and using salt-containing solutions for fluid repletion.
- If the patient is not vomiting and has stable blood pressure, an oral, commercial, balanced salt solution is adequate.
- If the patient is vomiting or hemodynamically unstable, check electrolytes and give 1–2 L of 0.9% saline IV.
- The patient should avoid exertion in a hot environment for 2–3 additional days.

Heat Syncope

GENERAL PRINCIPLES

- Heat syncope is a variant of postural hypotension.
- Exertion in a hot environment results in peripheral vasodilation and pooling of blood, with subsequent loss of consciousness. The affected individual has normal body temperature and regains consciousness promptly when supine, which separates this syndrome from heat stroke.

TREATMENT

Treatment is the same as for heat exhaustion.

Heat Stroke

GENERAL PRINCIPLES

- Heat stroke occurs in two varieties: classic and exertional. Both are present with high core temperatures that result in direct thermal tissue injury. Secondary effects include acute renal failure from rhabdomyolysis. Even with rapid therapy, mortality rates can be very high for body temperatures above 41.1°C (106°F). The distinction between classic and exertional heat stroke is not important because the therapeutic goals are similar in both and a delay in cooling increases mortality rate.

- The cardinal features of heat stroke are **hyperthermia (>40°C [104°F]) and altered mental status.** Although patients presenting with classic heat stroke may have anhidrosis, this is not considered a diagnostic criterion because 50% of patients are still diaphoretic at presentation.
- The CNS is very vulnerable to heat stroke with the cerebellum being highly sensitive. Ataxia may be an early sign. Seizures are common. Extent of neurological injury depends on magnitude temperature and duration of exposure.[6]

DIAGNOSIS

Diagnosis is based on the history of exposure or exercise, a core temperature usually of 40.6°C (105°F) or higher, and changes in mental status ranging from confusion to delirium and coma.

Differential Diagnosis

- Drug associated
  - Toxicity
    - Anticholinergic
    - Stimulant toxicity
    - Salicylate toxicity
  - Neuroleptic malignant syndrome (NMS) is associated with antipsychotic drugs. It is worth noting that NMS and malignant hyperthermia are both accompanied by severe muscle rigidity.
  - Serotonin syndrome
  - Malignant hyperthermia
  - Drug withdrawal syndrome (ethanol withdrawal)
  - Drug fever
- Infections
  - Generalized infections (sepsis, malaria, etc.)
  - CNS infections (meningitis, encephalitis, brain abscess)
- Endocrine
  - Thyroid storm
  - Pheochromocytoma
- Hypothalamic dysfunction due to stroke or hemorrhage
  - Status epilepticus
  - Cerebral hemorrhage[7]

Diagnostic Testing

Laboratories

- Laboratory studies should be directed toward identifying potential end organ damage or other underlying etiology and may include complete blood count (CBC); partial thromboplastin time; prothrombin time; electrolytes; blood urea nitrogen (BUN); creatinine, glucose, calcium, and creatine kinase levels; liver function tests (LFTs); and urinalysis.
- If an infectious etiology is suspected, obtain appropriate cultures.
- If there is a concern for cardiac ischemia, obtain an ECG and troponin.

Imaging

If a CNS etiology is considered likely, CT/MR imaging followed by spinal fluid examination is appropriate.

TREATMENT

- If patient is obtunded or hemodynamically unstable, acute life support measures should be initiated, such as intubation or central venous access.
- **Immediate cooling** should be started as early as possible preferably within 30 minutes of illness recognition.[7]
    - For most young, athletic, or otherwise healthy patients, cold water immersion therapy is considered the most efficient cooling method in both the field and hospital settings.[8] Ideally, this consists of immersing the patient up to the neck in a slurry of ice and water but may be impractical in many settings and can interfere in other resuscitative efforts.
    - Evaporative measures are also very effective and often more feasible. In this case, remove the patient's clothing to achieve maximum body surface exposure. Mist the patient continuously with tepid water (20–25°C [68–77°F]) and cool the patient with a large electric fan.
    - Ice packs should be placed at points of major heat transfer, such as the groin, axillae, and chest, to further speed cooling, but there is no evidence to suggest they be used as a primary cooling method.
    - Neither antipyretics nor **Dantrolene sodium** is indicated.[8]
- Monitor core temperatures continuously by rectal probe or Foley catheter. Oral and tympanic membrane temperatures may be inaccurate.
- Discontinue cooling measures when the core temperature reaches 39°C (102.2°F), which should ideally be achieved within 30 minutes. A temperature rebound may occur in 3–6 hours and should be retreated.
- **For hypotension, administer crystalloids:** If refractory, treat with vasopressors and monitor hemodynamics. Avoid pure α-adrenergic agents because they cause vasoconstriction and impair cooling. Administer crystalloids cautiously to normotensive patients.

Complications

- **Rhabdomyolysis** may occur. Treat as described in Chapter 13, Renal Diseases.
- **Hypoxemia and acute respiratory distress syndrome** may occur. Treat as described in Chapter 8, Critical Care.
- Treat seizures with benzodiazepines and antiepileptics, such as phenytoin or levetiracetam.

Monitoring/Follow-Up

Patients should be placed on telemetry.

COLD-INDUCED ILLNESS

Exposure to the cold may result in several different forms of injury. A risk factor is accelerated heat loss, which is promoted by exposure to high wind or by immersion. Extended cold exposure may result from alcohol or drug abuse, injury or immobilization, and mental impairment.

Chilblains

GENERAL PRINCIPLES

- Chilblains are among the mildest form of cold injury and result from exposure of bare skin to a cold, windy environment (0.6–15.6°C [33–60°F]).
- The ears, fingers, and tip of the nose typically are injured, with itchy, painful erythema on rewarming.

TREATMENT

Treatment involves rapid rewarming (see Frostnip section), moisturizing lotions, analgesics, and instructing the patient to avoid re-exposure.

Immersion Injury (Trench Foot)

GENERAL PRINCIPLES

Immersion injury is caused by prolonged immersion (longer than 10–12 hours) at a temperature <10°C (<50°F).

TREATMENT

Treat by rewarming followed by dry dressings. Treat secondary infections with antibiotics.

Frostnip (Superficial Frostbite)

GENERAL PRINCIPLES

Superficial frostbite involves the skin and subcutaneous tissues.

DIAGNOSIS

Areas with first-degree involvement are white, waxy, and anesthetic; have poor capillary refill; and are painful on thawing. Second-degree involvement is manifested by clear or milky bullae.

TREATMENT

The **treatment of choice** is rapid rewarming. Immerse the affected body part for 15–30 minutes; hexachlorophene or povidone iodine can be added to the water bath. Narcotic analgesics may be necessary for rewarming pain. Typically, no deep injury ensues and healing occurs in 3–4 weeks.

Deep Frostbite

GENERAL PRINCIPLES

- Deep frostbite involves death of skin, subcutaneous tissue, and muscle (third degree) or deep tendons and bones (fourth degree).
- Diabetes mellitus, peripheral vascular disease, an outdoor lifestyle, and high altitude are additional **risk factors**.

DIAGNOSIS

- The tissue appears frozen and hard.
- On rewarming, there is no capillary filling.
- Hemorrhagic blisters form, followed by eschars. Healing is very slow, and demarcation of tissue with autoamputation may occur.
- The majority of deep frostbite occurs at temperatures <6.7°C (44°F) with exposures longer than 7–10 hours.

TREATMENT

- The treatment is rapid rewarming as described earlier. **Rewarming should not be started until there is no chance of refreezing.**
- Administer analgesics (IV opioids) as needed.
- Early surgical intervention is not indicated.
- **Elevate** the affected extremity, prevent weight-bearing, separate the affected digits with cotton wool, prevent tissue maceration by using a blanket cradle, and prohibit smoking.
- Update tetanus immunization.
- Intra-arterial vasodilators, heparin, dextran, prostaglandin inhibitors, thrombolytics, and sympathectomy are not routinely justified.
- Role of antibiotics is unclear.[9]
- Amputation is undertaken only after full demarcation has occurred.

Hypothermia

GENERAL PRINCIPLES

Definition

Hypothermia is defined as a core temperature of <35°C (95°F).

Classification

Classification of severity by temperature is not universal. Hypothermia is classified as mild at 32–35°C (90–95°F), moderate at 28–32°C (82–90°F), and severe at <28°C (82°F).

Etiology

- The most common cause of hypothermia in the United States is cold exposure due to alcohol intoxication.
- Another common cause is cold water immersion. Hypothyroidism, drugs (general anesthetics, β-blockers, meperidine, clonidine, neuroleptics), autonomic dysfunction, and carbon monoxide poisoning can all cause hypothermia.

DIAGNOSIS

Clinical Presentation

Presentation varies with the temperature of the patient on arrival. All organ systems can be involved.

- **CNS effects**
  - At temperatures **below 32°C (89.6°F)**, mental processes are slowed and the affect is flattened.
  - At **32.2°C (90°F)**, the ability to shiver is lost, and deep tendon reflexes are diminished.
  - At **28°C (82.4°F)**, coma often supervenes.
  - **Below 18°C (64.4°F)**, the electroencephalogram is flat. On rewarming from severe hypothermia, central pontine myelinolysis may develop.
- **Cardiovascular effects**
  - After an initial increased release of catecholamines, there is a decrease in cardiac output and heart rate with relatively preserved mean arterial pressure. ECG changes manifest initially as sinus bradycardia with T-wave inversion and QT interval prolongation and may manifest as atrial fibrillation at temperatures of <32°C (<89.6°F).
  - **Osborn waves** (J-point elevation) may be visible, particularly in leads II and V_6.

 - An increased susceptibility to ventricular arrhythmias occurs at temperatures **below 32°C (89.6°F)**.
 - At temperatures of **30°C (86°F)**, the susceptibility to ventricular fibrillation is increased significantly, and unnecessary manipulation or jostling of the patient should be avoided.
 - A decrease in mean arterial pressure may also occur, and at temperatures of **28°C (82.4°F)**, progressive bradycardia supervenes.
- **Respiratory effects**
 - After an initial increase in minute ventilation, respiratory rate and tidal volume decrease progressively with decreasing temperature.
 - Arterial blood gases (ABGs) measured with the machine set at 37°C (98.6°F) should serve as the basis for therapy without correction of pH and carbon dioxide tension (PCO_2).[10]
- **Renal manifestations:** Cold-induced diuresis and tubular concentrating defects may be seen.
- Shivering typically ceases between 30°C and 32°C and paradoxical undressing may be observed.

Differential Diagnosis

- Cerebrovascular accident
- Drug overdose
- Diabetic ketoacidosis
- Hypoglycemia
- Uremia
- Adrenal insufficiency
- Myxedema

Diagnostic Testing

Laboratories

- Basic laboratory studies should include CBC, coagulation studies, LFTs, BUN, electrolytes, creatinine, glucose, creatine kinase, calcium, magnesium, amylase levels, urinalysis, ABGs, and ECG.
- Obtain toxicology screen if mental status alteration is more profound than expected for temperature decrease.
- Serum potassium is often increased.
- Elevated serum amylase may reflect underlying pancreatitis.
- Hyperglycemia may be noted but should not be treated because rebound hypoglycemia may occur with rewarming.
- Disseminated intravascular coagulation may also occur.

Imaging

Obtain chest, abdominal and cervical spine radiographs to evaluate all patients with a history of trauma or immersion injury.

TREATMENT

Medications

- Administer supplemental oxygen.
- Give **thiamine** to most patients with cold exposure because exposure due to alcohol intoxication is common.
- Administration of **antibiotics** is a controversial issue. Although some authorities recommend antibiotic administration for 72 hours, pending cultures, antibiotics should be reserved for when the physician suspects an infection. In general, the patients with

hypothermia due to exposure and alcohol intoxication are less likely to have a serious underlying infection than those who are elderly or who have an underlying medical illness.

Other Nonpharmacologic Therapies

- **Rewarming:** The patient should be rewarmed with the goal of increasing the temperature by 0.5–2.0°C/h (32.9–35.6°F/h), although the rate of rewarming has not been shown to be related to the outcome.
- **Passive external rewarming**
  - This method depends on the patient's ability to shiver.
  - It is effective only at core temperatures of **32°C (89.6°F) or higher**. Patients cannot shiver below 32°C.
  - Remove wet clothing, cover the patient with blankets in a warm environment, and monitor.
- **Active external rewarming**
  - It is indicated for patients with hypothermia and stable circulation.[11]
- **Active core rewarming is preferred for treatment of severe hypothermia**, although there is minimal data on outcomes.[12]
  - **Heated oxygen** is the initial therapy of choice for the patient whose cardiovascular status is stable. This therapeutic maneuver can be expected to raise core temperatures by 0.5–1.2°C/h (32.9–34.2°F/h).[13] Administration through an ETT results in more rapid rewarming than delivery via face mask. Administer heated oxygen through a cascade humidifier at a temperature of 45°C (113°F) or lower.
  - **IV fluids** can be heated in a microwave oven or delivered through a blood warmer.
  - **Intravascular heat exchange via catheter** is a recent addition to the options on this list. Less invasive and more familiar to most physicians than the more extreme options, this option can increase body temperature up to 3°C/h. This is simply a central venous catheter placed by the familiar modified Seldinger technique. After placement, warm fluids are run through the catheter (not into the venous system) allowing for cool blood to rewarm as it passes.
  - **Heated nasogastric or bladder lavage** is of limited efficacy because of low-exposed surface area and is reserved for the patient with cardiovascular instability.
  - **Heated peritoneal lavage** with fluid warmed to 40–45°C (104–113°F) is more effective than heated aerosol inhalation, but it should be reserved for patients with cardiovascular instability. Only those who are experienced in its use should perform heated peritoneal lavage, in combination with other modes of rewarming.
  - **Closed thoracic lavage** with heated fluid by thoracostomy tube has been recommended but is unproved.[14] It can be considered in patients where extracorporeal circulation is not an option.
  - **Hemodialysis** can be used for the severely hypothermic, particularly when due to an overdose that is amenable to treatment in this way.
  - **Extracorporeal circulation** (cardiac bypass and extracorporeal membrane oxygenation [ECMO]) is used only in hypothermic individuals who are in cardiac arrest; in these cases, it may be dramatically effective.[15] Extracorporeal circulation may raise the temperature as rapidly as 10–25°C/h (50–77°F/h). Although bypass must be preformed in an operating room, ECMO can be initiated in the emergency department. In patients treated with extracorporeal methods, survival without neurologic impairment is reported to range from 47%–63%.[11]

Resuscitation

- Maintain the airway and administer oxygen. Patients < 32°C (89.6°F) should be moved gently owing to the risk of triggering ventricular fibrillation.

- If intubation is required, the most experienced operator should perform it (see Airway Management and Tracheal Intubation section in Chapter 8, Critical Care).
- Conduct **cardiopulmonary resuscitation** (**CPR**). Perform simultaneous vigorous core rewarming; as long as the core temperature is severely decreased, it should not be assumed that the patient cannot be resuscitated. Although reliable defibrillation requires a core temperature of 32°C (89.6°F) or higher, patients with temperatures below 32°C (89.6°F) can be defibrillated. Administration of vasopressors is controversial. Standard teaching was to withhold vasopressors in patients with temperatures <30°C (86°F) but some research indicates an increased rate of return of spontaneous circulation with vasopressors.[16] However, patients may be resistant to most treatment modalities until their core temperature is >32°C (89.6°F). Prolonged efforts (to a core temperature >32°C [89.6°F]) may be justified because of the neuroprotective effects of hypothermia.
- Do not perform Swan-Ganz catheterization because it may precipitate ventricular fibrillation.
- If ventricular fibrillation occurs, begin CPR as per the advanced cardiac life support protocol (Appendix C). Amiodarone may be administered as per the protocol, although there is no evidence to support its use or guide dosage; some experts suggest reducing the maximum cumulative dose by half. Rewarming is key.
- Monitor ECG rhythm, urine output, and if possible central venous pressure in all patients with an intact circulation.

Disposition

- Admit patients with an underlying disease, physiologic derangement, or core temperature <32°C (<89.6°F), preferably to an ICU.
- Consider discharge for individuals with mild hypothermia (32–35°C [89.6–95°F]) and no predisposing medical conditions or complications when they are normothermic, and an adequate home environment can be ensured.

Monitoring/Follow-Up

- Monitor core temperature.
- A standard oral thermometer registers only to a lower limit of 35°C (95°F). Monitor the patient continuously with a Foley catheter thermometer with a full range of 20–40°C (68–104°F)

OTHER EMERGENCIES

The other emergencies are discussed in the respective chapters (please refer):

Emergencies in cardiology (acute coronary syndrome, acute pulmonary edema, hypertensive emergencies, acute pericarditis, infective endocarditis, arrhythmias)	Chapters 4, 5, 6, 7
Emergencies in pulmonology (acute severe asthma, pulmonary embolism, acute exacerbation of COPD)	Chapters 9, 10
Emergencies in endocrinology (diabetic ketoacidosis, hyperosmolar nonketotic state, hypoglycemia, hyperthyroid crisis, myxedema coma, acute adrenal insufficiency)	Chapters 23, 24
Emergencies in nephrology (pyelonephritis, obstructive uropathy, acute renal failure, hyponatremia, hyperkalemia)	Chapters 12, 13
Emergencies in gastroenterology/hepatology (GI bleed, fulminant hepatic failure, acute pancreatitis)	Chapters 18, 19

(Continued)

(Continued)

Hematologic/oncologic emergencies (neutropenic sepsis, disseminated intravascular coagulation, thrombocytopenia, superior vena cava obstruction, tumor lysis syndrome, SIRS and sepsis, blood transfusion reaction	Chapters 8, 20, 21, 22
Neurologic emergencies (stroke, subarachnoid hemorrhage, meningitis encephalitis, status epilepticus)	Chapter 27
Allergy, anaphylaxis	Chapter 11
Poisoning/overdoses	Chapter 28

Summary

- Optimal treatment in heatstroke patients relies on early recognition and expedition of rapid cooling.
- Hypothermia arises from inadequate heat retention or massive heat loss due to various causes. Symptoms range from mild to severe. Severe hypothermia may result in death if not treated promptly.
- For patients with associated symptoms and showing signs of instability, needle decompression is the treatment of a pneumothorax.

Scan the QR code to access chapter references.

27 Neurologic Disorders

James A. Giles, Robert C. Bucelli, and Abu Thajudeen

Alterations in Consciousness

GENERAL PRINCIPLES

Definition

- **Coma** is a state of complete behavioral unresponsiveness to external stimulation. Evaluation and treatment should be performed concurrently and expeditiously because multiple etiologies can lead to irreversible brain damage. The need for neurosurgical intervention must be determined promptly.
- **Delirium** is an acute state of confusion that can result from diffuse or multifocal cerebral dysfunction and is characterized by relatively rapid reduction in the ability to focus, sustain, or shift attention. Changes in cognition, fluctuations in consciousness, disorientation, and even hallucinations are common.

Epidemiology

- About 30% of patients over 60 years and 80% of ICU patients experience delirium during hospitalization.
- Delirious patients often have prolonged stays and are at greater risk for subsequent cognitive decline.

Etiology

- Coma results from diffuse or multifocal dysfunction that involves both cerebral hemispheres and the reticular activating system in the brainstem.
- Etiologies of altered mental status are listed in Table 27-1.
- Mild systemic illness (e.g., urinary tract infections), introduction of new medications, fever, and/or sleep deprivation are common causes of delirium in the elderly and patients with chronic central nervous system (CNS) dysfunction of any etiology.

DIAGNOSIS

- Initial assessment should focus on recognizing the development and progression of altered consciousness. The examiner should query for history of trauma, seizures, stroke, medication changes, and alcohol or drug use as possible etiologies. A collateral source can be extremely helpful and is often necessary.
- The AWOL tool is a useful, quick bedside measure that can be used to assess patients' risk of delirium at the time of admission.[1] The AWOL score is derived from assigning one point for each of the following variables (age ≥80, inability to spell the word "world" backward, disorientation to location, and nurse-rated illness severity [with a point given for patients considered to be at least moderately ill]). In the pilot study describing this tool, 2% of patients with a score of 0 went on to develop delirium, whereas 64% of patients with a score of 4 went on to develop delirium.
- If trauma has or may have occurred, **immobilize the spine immediately** and then proceed with imaging to identify or exclude fracture or instability. Consultation with additional services (e.g., neurosurgery) may be needed.

TABLE 27-1 Causes of Altered Mental Status

Metabolic derangements/diffuse etiologies • Hypernatremia/hyponatremia • Hypercalcemia • Hyperglycemia/hypoglycemia • Hyperthyroidism/hypothyroidism • Acute intermittent porphyria • Hypertensive encephalopathy/reversible posterior leukoencephalopathy • Hypoxia/hypercapnia • Global cerebral ischemia from hypotension
Infections • Meningitis/encephalitis • Sepsis • Systemic infections with spread to CNS
Drugs/toxins/poisons • Prescription medications and side effects of medications • Drugs of abuse • Withdrawal situations • Medication side effects • Inhaled toxins
Inborn errors of metabolism
Nutritional deficiency (i.e., thiamine)
Seizures • Subclinical seizures • Postictal state
Head trauma
Vascular • Ischemic stroke (only certain stroke locations cause altered mental status) • Hemorrhage
Structural • Hydrocephalus • Tumor
Systemic organ failure • Hepatic failure • Renal failure
Psychiatric
Autoimmune/inflammatory • Vasculitis (primary CNS or systemic) • Encephalitis • Autoantibody-mediated encephalopathies (e.g., anti–voltage-gated potassium channel complex antibodies such as anti-Lgi-1 and anti-Caspr-2)

CNS, central nervous system.

Clinical Presentation

- Search for signs of systemic illness associated with coma (e.g., cirrhosis, hemodialysis fistula/graft, rash of meningococcemia) or signs of head trauma (e.g., lacerations, periorbital or mastoid ecchymosis, hemotympanum). The physical and neurologic examination may reveal systemic illness (e.g., pneumonia or elevated temperature) or neurologic signs (meningismus or paralysis) that can help narrow the differential diagnosis.

- **Herniation** occurs when mass lesions or edema cause shifts in brain tissue. The diagnosis of brain herniation **requires immediate recognition and treatment.** If a risk of herniation is present, the patient should be monitored in a neurosurgical/neurologic critical care unit, and frequent "neuro checks" should be performed to evaluate for signs of impending herniation.
  - **Nonspecific signs and symptoms of increased intracranial pressure** include headache, nausea, vomiting, hypertension, bradycardia, papilledema, sixth nerve palsy, transient visual obscurations, and alterations in consciousness.
  - **Uncal herniation** is caused by unilateral supratentorial lesions. The earliest sign is a dilated pupil ipsilateral to the mass, diminished consciousness, and hemiparesis, first contralateral to the mass and later ipsilateral to the mass (Kernohan notch syndrome).
  - **Central herniation** is caused by medial or bilateral supratentorial lesions. Signs include progressive alteration of consciousness, Cheyne–Stokes or normal respirations followed by central hyperventilation, mid position and unreactive pupils, loss of upward gaze, and posturing of the extremities.
  - **Tonsillar herniation** occurs when pressure in the posterior fossa forces the cerebellar tonsils through the foramen magnum, compressing the medulla. Signs include altered level of consciousness and respiratory irregularity or apnea.
- In general, the neurologic assessment should ascertain the patient's ability to focus, sustain, and shift attention appropriately. Because of fluctuations, repeated examinations are often necessary.
  - **Level of consciousness** can be semiquantitatively assessed and followed by using the Glasgow Coma Scale (GCS) (Table 27-2). Scores range from 3 (unresponsive) to 15 (normal). **The Pupil Reactivity Score gives information about loss of pupil reactivity to light. GCS-P has been shown to be superior to GCS score in predicting**

TABLE 27-2 GCS-P Score

Glasgow Coma Scale		
Eyes	**Verbal**	**Motor**
Spontaneous 4	Orientated 5	Obey commands 6
To sound 3	Confused 4	Localizing 5
To pressure 2	Words 3	Normal flexion 4
None 1	Sounds 2	Abnormal flexion 3
	None 1	Extension 2
		None 1

The Pupil Reactivity Score summarizes information about loss of pupil reactivity to light and is calculated as follows.

Pupils Unreactive to Light	Pupil Reactivity Score
Both pupils	2
One pupil	1
Neither pupil	0

The GCS-P is calculated by subtracting the Pupil Reactivity Score (PRS) from the Glasgow Coma Scale (GCS) total score:

GCS-P = GCS – PRS

outcomes of the patient. The GCS-P is calculated by subtracting the Pupil Reactivity Score (PRS) from the Glasgow Coma Scale (GCS) total score:

- **GCS-P = GCS - PRS***

- **Respiratory rate and pattern (Figure 27-1)**
  - Cheyne–Stokes respirations (rhythmic crescendo–decrescendo hyperpnea alternating with periods of apnea) occur in metabolic coma and supratentorial lesions, as well as in chronic pulmonary disease and congestive heart failure (CHF).
  - Hyperventilation is commonly seen in the setting of metabolic acidosis, hypoxemia, pneumonia, or other pulmonary diseases but can also occur with an upper brainstem injury.
  - Apneustic breathing (long pauses after inspiration), cluster breathing (breathing in short bursts), and ataxic breathing (irregular breaths without pattern) are signs of brainstem injury and are commonly associated with impending respiratory arrest.
- **Pupil size and light reactivity (Figure 27-2)**
  - Anisocoria (asymmetric pupils) in a patient with altered mental status requires immediate diagnosis (i.e., stat head CT) or exclusion and treatment of possible herniation.
  - Anisocoria may be physiologic or produced by mydriatics (e.g., scopolamine, atropine) and therefore requires well-documented serial examinations.
  - Small but reactive pupils are seen in narcotic overdose, metabolic encephalopathy, and pontine lesions.
  - Fixed mid position pupils imply midbrain lesions or transtentorial herniation.
  - Bilaterally fixed and dilated pupils occur with severe anoxic encephalopathy or drug intoxication (scopolamine, atropine, glutethimide, or methanol).
- **Eye movements**
  - To test the oculocephalic reflex ("doll's eyes" maneuver, assuming no cervical injury is present), the examiner quickly turns the head laterally or vertically (head impulse test). Intact brainstem oculomotor function, in the setting of coma, will result in conjugate eye movements opposite to the direction of head movement.
  - Another means of testing the vestibulo-ocular reflex is via cold caloric testing. This can be used if cervical trauma is suspected or if eye movements are absent with the head impulse test described above. Brainstem oculomotor function is intact if there are conjugate eye movements toward the ear lavaged with ice cold water. Vertical gaze can be assessed with simultaneous lavage of both ears (cold water → eyes depress, warm water → eyes elevate).
  - In the absence of a history to suggest a drug-induced cause (e.g., barbiturates, phenytoin, paralytics) or a preexisting disorder such as progressive external ophthalmoplegia, absence of all eye movements indicates a bilateral pontine lesion.

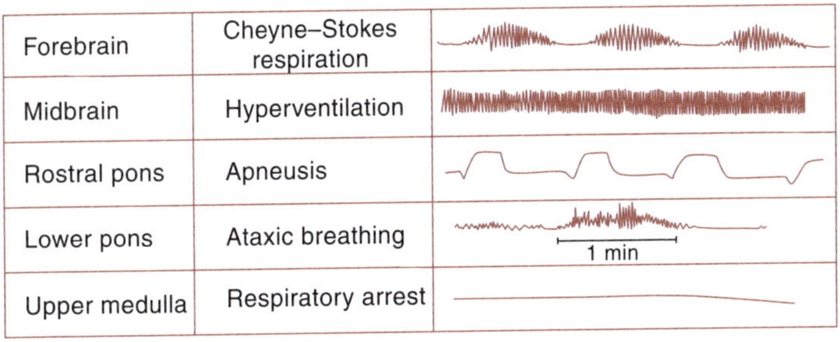

Figure 27-1 Respiratory patterns.

---

* https://www.glasgowcomascale.org/what-is-gcs-p/.

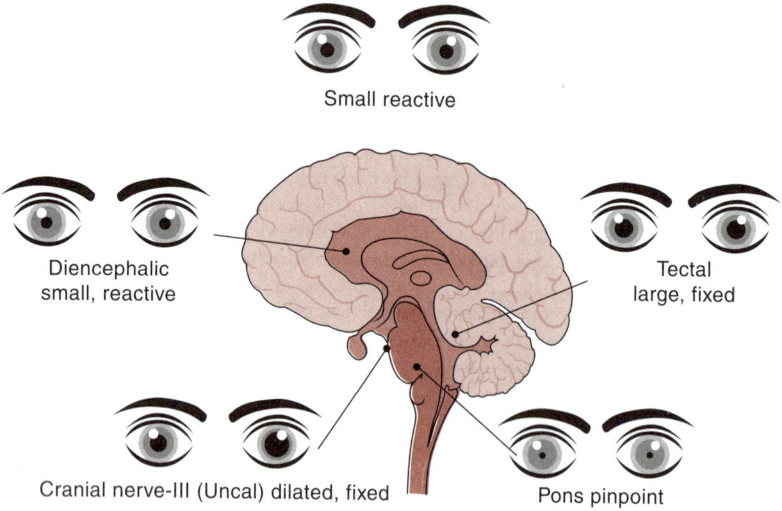

Figure 27-2 Pupillary changes and their localization.

- ◦ Dysconjugate gaze suggests a brainstem lesion.
- ◦ A conjugate gaze preference to one side suggests a unilateral pontine or frontal lobe lesion. Oculocephalic and oculovestibular tests can help localize the lesion in the setting of a concurrent hemiparesis. In pontine lesions, gaze preference is toward the paretic side, and eyes may move toward but do not cross midline. In frontal lobe lesions, gaze preference is away from the paresis, and eye movements are conjugate and move to both sides of midline.
- ◦ Impaired vertical eye movement occurs in midbrain lesions and central herniation. Conjugate depression and impaired elevation suggest a tectal lesion (e.g., pinealoma) or hydrocephalus.
- **Motor responses** also help with localization. Asymmetric motor responses (spontaneous or stimulus induced, including noxious stimuli if necessary) also have localizing value (Figure 27-3).

Diagnostic Testing

Laboratory Studies

Serum electrolytes, creatinine, glucose, calcium, complete blood count (CBC), and urinalysis should be obtained. Drug levels should be ordered if appropriate. An accurate medication list and any history to suggest intoxication are critical features of the evaluation. Toxicology screen of blood and urine should be considered.

Imaging

A head CT should be obtained to evaluate for structural abnormalities. Brain magnetic resonance imaging (MRI) can be useful if head CT is nondiagnostic and there is suspicion for an ischemic or parenchymal lesion (especially of the posterior fossa).

Diagnostic Procedures

- Lumbar puncture (LP) should be considered in patients with fever and/or new headache or those with high risk of infection. A funduscopic examination and/or head imaging should be performed prior to performing the LP to assess risk of herniation. Basic cerebrospinal

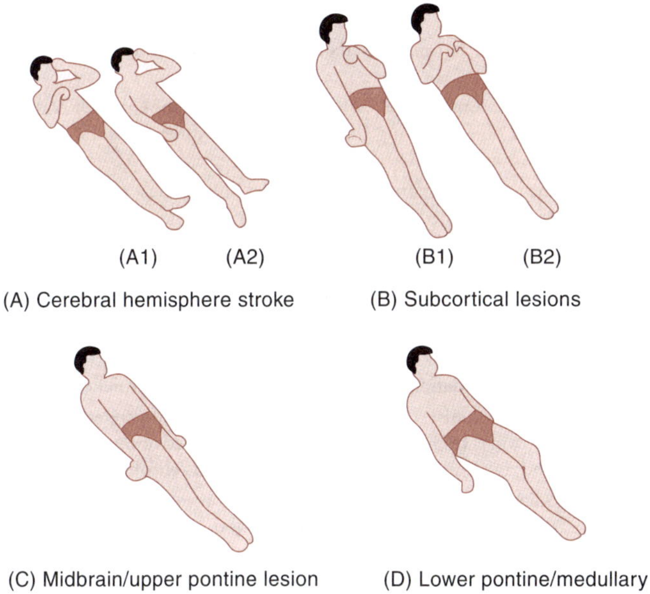

Figure 27-3 Motor responses and localization. Motor response to pain: the symmetry or asymmetry of the motor response can assist localization. (A) Left hemisphere lesion: the two figures illustrate localization of pain with the left hand and flexion (A1) or extension (A2) on the right. (B) Subcortical: unilateral left-sided lesion exerting a variable contralateral effect. The figures illustrate flexion to pain with the left hand with either extension (B1) or flexion (B2) with the right and hyperextension in both lower limbs. (C) Midbrain upper pontine: a bilateral upper and lower limb extension response. (D) Lower pontine/medullary: a bilateral extensor upper limb posture with either flaccidity or minimal diminished flexor response in lower limbs.

fluid (CSF) studies (e.g., protein, glucose, cell count, Gram stain, and aerobic culture) should be obtained with additional studies depending on the possible etiology.

- Electroencephalography (EEG) can be considered to rule out seizures. Nonconvulsive status epilepticus (NCSE) is a common cause of unexplained encephalopathy in the critically ill population. Inter-ictal abnormalities can be suggestive of specific etiologies (e.g., periodic lateralized epileptiform discharges in herpes simplex virus [HSV] encephalitis, triphasic waves in hepatic or uremic encephalopathy, and β activity or voltage suppression in barbiturate or other sedative intoxications).

TREATMENT

Coma

- Ensure adequate airway and ventilation, administer oxygen as needed, and maintain normal body temperature.
- Establish secure IV access and adequate circulation.
- Neurosurgical consult may need to be obtained for intracranial pressure monitoring and treatment, if applicable.

Delirium

- Repeated attempts should be made to reorient the patient and possibly have a sitter present if necessary.
- A quiet room with close observation is necessary. Patients should have a well-lit environment with familiar objects during the day and dark, quiet (minimize stimulation if possible) environments at night.
- Physical and pharmacologic restraints should be used only as a last resort and with appropriate documentation in the medical record. If restraints are needed, they should be carefully adjusted and checked periodically to prevent excessive constriction.

Medications

- IV thiamine (100–500 mg), followed by dextrose (50 mL of 50% dextrose in water = 25 g dextrose), should be administered. Thiamine is administered first because dextrose administration in thiamine-deficient patients may precipitate Wernicke encephalopathy.
- IV naloxone (opiate antagonist), 0.01 mg/kg, should be administered if opiate intoxication is suspected (coma, respiratory depression, small reactive pupils). Naloxone may provoke opiate withdrawal syndrome in patients on opioids chronically.
- Flumazenil (benzodiazepine antagonist), 0.2 mg IV, may reverse benzodiazepine intoxication, but its duration of action is short, and additional doses may be needed. Flumazenil should be used with caution in certain patient populations (e.g., epileptics) because it reduces the seizure threshold.
- In delirious patients, sedatives should be avoided if possible. If necessary, low doses of quetiapine (12.5–25 mg), lorazepam (1 mg), or chlordiazepoxide (25 mg) can be used. Remember to always consider comorbidities before administering these medications.

Other Nonpharmacologic Therapies

If herniation is identified or suspected, treatment consists of measures to lower intracranial pressure while surgically treatable etiologies are identified or excluded. All of the listed measures are only **temporizing methods**. Consultation with neurosurgery should be performed concurrently.

- Elevate the head of the bed to at least 30 degrees.
- Endotracheal intubation is usually performed to enable hyperventilation to a partial pressure of carbon dioxide (PCO_2) of 25–30 mm Hg. This reduces intracranial pressure within minutes by cerebral vasoconstriction. Bag-mask ventilation can be performed if manipulation of the neck is precluded by possible or established spinal instability. Reduction of PCO_2 below 25 mm Hg is not recommended because it may reduce cerebral blood flow.
- Administration of IV mannitol (1–2 g/kg over 10–20 minutes) osmotically reduces free water in the brain via elimination by the kidneys and does not require a central line for administration. This effect peaks at 90 minutes. Remember that, given its potent diuretic effect, mannitol can precipitate renal failure if volume is not adequately replaced. Hypertonic saline (5% or 23.4% saline) is not only an alternative option but also has side effects and requires central venous access.
- Dexamethasone, 10 mg IV, followed by 4 mg IV q6h, reduces the edema surrounding a tumor or an abscess but is not indicated for diffuse cerebral edema or the mass effect associated with malignant cerebral infarcts.
- Coagulopathy should be corrected if intracranial hemorrhage is diagnosed and before surgical treatment or invasive procedures (e.g., LP) are performed. Each patient's circumstances should be carefully assessed before therapeutic anticoagulation is reversed.

Surgical Management

Surgical evacuation of epidural, subdural, or intraparenchymal (e.g., cerebellar) hemorrhage and shunting for acute hydrocephalus should be considered in the appropriate clinical circumstances. However, some structural lesions are not amenable to surgical treatment.

SPECIAL CONSIDERATIONS

- **Brain death** occurs from irreversible brain injury sufficient to permanently eliminate all cortical and brainstem functions. Because the vital centers in the brainstem sustain cardiovascular and respiratory functions, brain death is incompatible with survival despite mechanical ventilation and cardiovascular and nutritional supportive measures. Brain death is distinguished from persistent vegetative state (PVS) in which the absence of higher cortical function is accompanied by intact brainstem function. Patients in a PVS are unable to think, speak, understand, or meaningfully respond to visual, verbal, or auditory stimuli, yet with nutritional and supportive care, their cardiovascular and respiratory functions can sustain viability for many years. Research using functional MRI (fMRI) has broadened our understanding of the marked variability in function present across PVS patients and even demonstrated instances of misdiagnosis. However, the role of fMRI in the assessment of comatose patients remains to be determined.
    - Brain death criteria vary by institution. Refer to your institution's policy for details.
- **Alcohol withdrawal** typically occurs when illness or hospitalization interrupts continued alcohol intake. **In South Asian regions, cases of methanol co-ingestion with ethanol have been reported and it can further cause diagnostic challenges and toxicity.***
    - Tremulousness, irritability, anorexia, and nausea characterize minor alcohol withdrawal. Symptoms usually appear within a few hours after reduction or cessation of alcohol consumption and resolve within 48 hours. Treatment includes a well-lit room, reassurance, and the presence of family or friends. **Thiamine**, 100–500 mg IM/IV, followed by 100 mg PO daily; multivitamins containing **folic acid**; and a balanced diet as tolerated should be administered. Serial evaluation for signs of major alcohol withdrawal is essential.
    - Alcohol withdrawal seizures, typically one or a few brief generalized convulsions, occur 12–48 hours after cessation of ethanol intake. **Anti-epileptic drugs (AEDs) are not indicated for typical alcohol withdrawal seizures.** Other causes for seizures (see Seizures section) must be excluded. If hypoglycemia is present, thiamine should be administered before glucose.
    - Severe withdrawal or **delirium tremens** consists of tremulousness, hallucinations, agitation, confusion, disorientation, and autonomic hyperactivity (fever, tachycardia, diaphoresis), typically occurring 72–96 hours after cessation of drinking. Symptoms generally resolve within 3–5 days. Delirium tremens complicates 5%–10% of cases of alcohol withdrawal, with mortality up to 15%. Other causes of delirium must be considered in the differential diagnosis (see Table 27-1).
    - Mild withdrawal symptoms can be managed with chlordiazepoxide PO 25–50 mg q6–8h (maximum total daily dose 300 mg) with a subsequent dose taper or, preferably, with a symptom-triggered treatment protocol, e.g., CIWA-Ar.[2] In patients with severe hepatic failure, oxazepam (15–30 mg PO, q6–8h as needed), which is excreted by the kidney, is preferred. For patients with severe withdrawal symptoms, seizures, and/or delirium tremens, diazepam or lorazepam IV are effective agents. Diazepam 10 mg IV every 5–20 minutes or lorazepam IV 2–4 mg every 15–20 minutes should be given until symptom control is achieved. Treatment can then be transitioned to a symptom-triggered or scheduled regimen.

---

* Barceloux DG, Randall Bond G, Krenzelok EP, et al. Methanol guidelines—AACT/EAPCCT American Academy of Clinical Toxicology practice guidelines on the treatment of methanol poisoning. *J Toxicol Clin Toxicol.* 2002(4): 415–446.

- Maintenance of fluid and electrolyte balance is important. Alcoholic patients are susceptible to hypomagnesemia, hypokalemia, hypoglycemia, and fluid losses, which may be considerable because of fever, diaphoresis, and vomiting.

Alzheimer Disease

GENERAL PRINCIPLES

Alzheimer disease (AD) is the most common neurodegenerative disorder in older individuals (>60 years old), typically characterized by memory problems and inability to independently perform activities of daily living.

Epidemiology

South East Asia region population is rapidly aging. The proportion of people aged 60 or above was 9.8% in 2017. Mental health, including dementia, is a very important disease to be addressed.*

- Inherited forms of AD manifest typically before age 65 years and are associated with mutations in amyloid precursor protein (*APP*) gene on chromosome 21, presenilin-1 gene on chromosome 14, and presenilin-2 gene on chromosome 1.
- The greatest risk factor for late-onset/sporadic AD is the presence of the apolipoprotein ε4 variant.
- Lifetime risk doubles if a sibling or parent is diagnosed with AD.
- It is common for AD patients to present at late stages of the disease after an unrelated medical illness unmasks signs and symptoms of the disease that had previously gone unrecognized by the family.
- Pseudodementia (cognitive impairment related to comorbid depression) should be considered in the appropriate clinical context.

Pathophysiology

Pathologic diagnosis requires presence of both neurofibrillary tangles because of tau and neuritic plaques composed of amyloid.

DIAGNOSIS

Clinical Presentation

- Memory impairment is required for diagnosis of AD.
- Episodic memory for newly acquired information is impaired, whereas memory for more remote events is not affected.
- Declarative memory for facts and events is affected, whereas procedural memory and motor learning are spared at earlier stages of the disease.
- With progression of disease, language, visuospatial skills, abstract reasoning, and executive function deteriorate. Some patients will also develop apraxia, alexia, and delusions.

Differential Diagnosis

See Table 27-3.

Diagnostic Testing

Progression of disease can be assessed by the Mini–Mental State Examination, the Montreal Cognitive Assessment (MoCA), and the Clinical Dementia Rating Scale.

Laboratory Studies

- Definitive diagnosis of AD requires histopathologic confirmation (i.e., autopsy).
- Reversible causes of dementia such as B12 deficiency, neurosyphilis, and thyroid abnormalities should be ruled out.

---

* https://www.who.int/southeastasia/health-topics/ageing

TABLE 27-3 Differential Diagnosis of Alzheimer Dementia
Frontotemporal dementia Changes in personality, behavior, and executive functioning
Vascular dementia Stepwise course because of repeated strokes or stroke-like events
Dementia with Lewy bodies Visual hallucinations, dream enactment behavior (i.e., REM behavior disorder), cognitive fluctuations, parkinsonism, sensitivity to neuroleptics
Normal pressure hydrocephalus Triad of dementia, urinary incontinence, and gait instability ("wacky, wet, and wobbly")
Vitamin B12 deficiency
Neurosyphilis
Thyroid dysfunction
HIV
Creutzfeldt–Jakob disease
Autoimmune encephalopathies (including paraneoplastic syndromes)

REM, rapid eye movement.

Imaging

- Brain MRI can suggest potential alternative diagnoses.
- MRI may show diffuse atrophy with hippocampal atrophy that is seen with AD.
- [^{18}F] Fluorodeoxyglucose (FDG) positron emission tomography (PET) or perfusion single-photon emission computed tomography may demonstrate hypometabolism and hypoperfusion, respectively, within the parietotemporal cortex.
- Amyloid PET tracers (florbetapir) can measure amyloid deposition in the brain and are approved for clinical use but are quite expensive. New PET tracers for tau are being actively developed.

Diagnostic Procedures

- Neuropsychological testing can establish a baseline cognitive status. This testing can sometimes differentiate dementia from depression (i.e., pseudodementia).
- Both structural MRI and PET imaging may assist in early diagnosis.
- CSF measures of reduced $A\beta_{42}$ and increased tau can be obtained and may assist in the diagnosis.

TREATMENT

- Cholinesterase inhibitors including donepezil, rivastigmine, and galantamine can be considered for early AD.
- Memantine, a noncompetitive *N*-methyl-D-aspartate receptor antagonist, can be considered for moderate to severe dementia.
- A combination of the above medications is sometimes used in more advanced AD patients. Additional therapies (including anti-amyloid agents) are being investigated.

Seizures

GENERAL PRINCIPLES

Definition

- Seizure: Stereotyped spells caused by abnormal electrical brain activity. A more complex definition is uncontrolled excessive electrical discharges in the brain that may produce a sudden change in brain function causing physical convulsion, minor physical signs, thought disturbances, or a combination of symptoms.
- **Epilepsy** is defined as having two or more unprovoked seizures.

- Status epilepticus is defined by >30 minutes of continuous seizure activity or recurrent seizures without full recovery between episodes. However, in practice, a seizure lasting >5 minutes in adults (>10 minutes in children) should be treated as status epilepticus. Generalized convulsive status epilepticus (GCSE) is a medical emergency.
- Nonconvulsive status epilepticus (NCSE) is defined by electrographic seizures with clinically absent or subtle motor activity and impairment or loss of consciousness. NCSE should be treated promptly to avoid irreversible cerebral injury.
- An aura is a simple partial seizure manifesting as sensory, autonomic, or psychic symptoms.
- A prodrome is a sensation or feeling that a seizure will soon occur. Distinguishing a prodrome from an aura can be clinically challenging.

Classification

- Focal seizures begin at a single locus in the brain.
  - **Focal seizure *without* impairment of consciousness (simple partial):** Consciousness is not impaired. The symptoms can be motor (hand jerking), sensory (focal tingling, visual, auditory), autonomic (sensation of epigastric rising), or psychic (déjà vu).
  - **Focal seizure *with* impairment of consciousness or "dyscognitive" focal seizures (complex partial):** Consciousness is impaired. The symptoms vary based on whether they involve the temporal (automatisms such as lip smacking or picking at clothes, staring, behavior arrest), frontal (hypermotor behaviors, bicycling, pelvic thrusting, and automatisms), or occipital lobes (unformed images, visual hallucinations). Frontal seizures are often misdiagnosed as nonepileptic seizures (i.e., pseudoseizures) because of their often complex, sometimes bizarre, semiology and the frequent absence of electrographic seizure activity on standard EEG.
- Generalized seizures originate from the bilateral hemispheres and, by definition, consciousness is lost.
  - May begin as a generalized seizure or a focal seizure with secondary generalization.
  - Include tonic, clonic, tonic-clonic, atonic, myoclonic, and absence.

  The International League Against Epilepsy (ILAE) classification (2017) is discussed in Figure 27-4

  Seizures are now divided into groups depending on:
    - where they start in the brain (onset)
    - whether or not a person's awareness is affected
    - whether or not seizures involve other symptoms, such as movement
    - Depending on where they start, seizures are described as being focal onset, generalised onset or unknown onset.

Epidemiology

- Nearly 80% of people with epilepsy live in low- and middle-income countries.
  In low- and middle-income countries, epilepsy occurs in 139 per 100,000 population (https://www.who.int/news-room/fact-sheets/detail/epilepsy).

Etiology

Etiologies for seizures include those listed in Table 27-4. For patients with a known seizure disorder presenting with an increase in seizure frequency, the most common causes are AED noncompliance, subtherapeutic anticonvulsant levels, or infection.

DIAGNOSIS

Clinical Presentation

History

- Query for family history of epilepsy, developmental delay, trauma, medical historical information including preexisting medical conditions, current and recently discontinued medications, drug allergies, recreational drug use, and possible precipitating events.

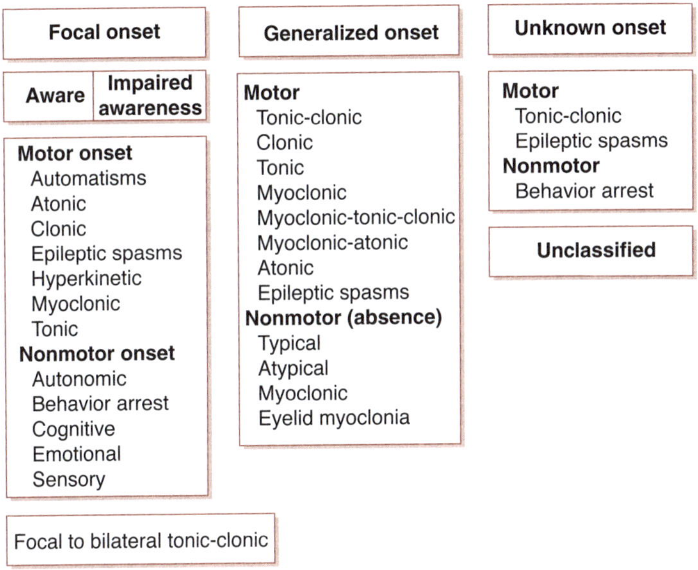

Figure 27-4 The International League Against Epilepsy (ILAE) classification of seizures.

TABLE 27-4 Etiologies of Seizures

- CNS infections
- Fever
- Hypoxic brain injury
- Stroke (ischemic or hemorrhagic)
- Cerebral venous thrombosis
- Vascular malformations
- Tumors/carcinomatous meningitis
- Head injury
- Eclampsia
- Hypertensive encephalopathy/reversible posterior leukoencephalopathy
- Hyperthyroidism
- Congenital brain malformations
- Hereditary (Sturge-Weber, tuberous sclerosis, Dravet syndrome, and other channelopathies)
- Toxic metabolic (porphyria, uremia, liver failure)
- Drug withdrawal (alcohol, barbiturates, benzodiazepine, AEDs)
- Drug intoxication (TCAs, bupropion, clozapine, tramadol, cocaine, amphetamine)
- Electrolyte abnormalities/metabolic
  - Hyponatremia or hypernatremia
  - Hypocalcemia
  - Hypomagnesemia
  - Hypophosphatemia
  - Hypoglycemia/hyperglycemia

AEDs, anti-epileptic drugs; CNS, central nervous system; TCAs, tricyclic antidepressants.

- Ask the patient about any prodrome/aura. An eyewitness account of the event is critical, and a video of the event can be extremely helpful. Inquire about the temporal features (i.e., seizures are typically acute onset with a rapid crescendo), **incontinence**, **tongue biting**, and how the patient behaved after the event ended (e.g., confusion, somnolence) and for how long these persisted.

Physical Examination

- Vital signs and blood sugar should be obtained immediately on all patients. As discussed previously, empiric thiamine should be given when treating hypoglycemia. Ictal and/or postictal fever can occur.
- Look for nuchal rigidity, rash, asterixis, or signs of trauma.
- Convulsive seizures are usually easily identified.
- Features of the seizure can aid in identifying the ictal focus (e.g., complex automatisms in frontal lobe seizures, lip smacking and postictal nose wiping in temporal lobe seizures, ictal laughter in hypothalamic seizures).
- Carefully observe for subtle signs of nonconvulsive seizures, such as automatisms, facial or extremity twitching, eye deviation, and periods of relatively preserved mental status alternating with periods of impaired consciousness.
- Patients may present during the postictal period, defined as the time between the end of the seizure and the return to baseline mental status. During this time, patients may act confused, obtunded, and have amnesia for events since the seizure. This period can typically last from minutes to hours or, rarely, days in the elderly and those with prior CNS injury.
- Postictal paresis (also called Todd paralysis) is a transient neurologic deficit that lasts for hours or, rarely, days after an epileptic seizure.

Differential Diagnosis

Alternate diagnoses that may mimic seizures include the following:

- Syncope, especially convulsive syncope in which seizure-like motor activity is observed. The Calgary Seizure Syncope score is a useful and reliable clinical tool in distinguishing these two entities.[4]
- Nonepileptic seizures ("pseudoseizures") (see the following text).
- Transient ischemic attack (TIA).
- Complicated migraine.
- Toxic metabolic encephalopathy.
- Tremors, dyskinesias (episodic movement disorders).
- Nonepileptic myoclonus following a hypoxic event.
- Sleep disorders.
- Rigors.

Diagnostic Testing

Laboratory Studies

Initial laboratory studies should include blood glucose, electrolytes (sodium, calcium, magnesium, and phosphorus), CBC, urinalysis, urine drug screen, and AED levels if indicated.

Imaging

Neuroimaging is usually indicated to identify structural etiologies.

- Start with a head CT in the acute setting. The administration of contrast can assist in diagnosis of possible tumors.

- Brain MRI with and without contrast, protocolled to evaluate for an ictal focus, is almost always indicated in the evaluation of new-onset seizures and is certainly indicated in patients with recurrent unprovoked seizures.

Diagnostic Procedures

- LP should be done if there is concern for CNS infection. Send for routine CSF studies as well as herpes simplex virus polymerase chain reaction (HSV-PCR). Save extra CSF for any additional testing.
- CSF testing for acid fast bacilli, adenosine deaminase, and cartridge-based nucleic acid amplification test needs to be performed to rule out CNS tuberculosis.
- EEG is not required for initial diagnosis and management of GCSE. If mental status is not improving as expected after convulsive seizures stop, EEG may be necessary to exclude conversion to NCSE. Unless the patient is known to typically have an extraordinarily prolonged postictal period, NCSE should be considered in any patient who fails to return to baseline within an hour of a seizure. Approximately 50% of patients who present with GCSE will go on to develop NCSE within 24 hours of cessation of clinical seizure activity.
- Routine EEG is indicated for all new-onset seizures.[5]
- Video EEG is the gold standard test for the evaluation of suspected nonepileptic seizures. A notable (30%–50% in some studies) number of patients with nonepileptic seizures ("pseudoseizures") will also have epileptic seizures.

TREATMENT

- **Initiation of AED therapy is usually not indicated after a single unprovoked seizure** because about two-thirds of patients who had a single seizure will not have seizure recurrence.[6] However, patients with a single unprovoked seizure and either an abnormal EEG or evidence of an ictal focus on head CT or brain MRI warrant initiation of AED therapy given a much higher likelihood of seizure recurrence.
- In general, AEDs should not be started in patients with provoked seizures.
- A diagnosis of epilepsy is made after two or more unprovoked seizures. AED treatment is generally started after the second seizure because the patient has a substantially increased risk (approximately 75%) for repeated seizures after two events.
- Treatment of status epilepticus must be prompt because efficacy of treatment decreases with increased seizure duration and GCSE carries an all-cause mortality of 30% (see Figure 27-5 for treatment of status epilepticus).[7] Within 5–30 minutes of GCSE onset, the body's homeostatic mechanisms begin to fail and patients' risk of permanent brain injury increases, as does risk of systemic complications including hyperthermia, pulmonary embolism, cardiovascular and respiratory insufficiency, and other life-threatening complications. Prolonged NCSE will also result in brain injury but on a timescale of days as opposed to minutes (see Figure 27-6).
- Long duration of seizure is a predictor of lack of response to first-line drugs.*

Medications

- The selection of a specific AED for a patient must be individualized according to the drug effectiveness for seizure type(s), potential adverse effects of the drug, interactions with other possible medications, cost, and mechanism of drug action (Table 27-5).[8]
- About half of all patients with a new diagnosis of epilepsy will be seizure free with the first AED prescribed.[9]

---

*Murthy JM, Jayalaxmi SS, Kanikannan MA. Convulsive status epilepticus: clinical profile in a developing country. *Epilepsia.* 48;2008:2217–2223.

Step 1
5-10 minutes

Give oxygen, get vital signs, obtain IV access, begin ECG and pulse oximetry monitoring, draw blood, ABG, fingerstick glucose

- Lorazepam 2 mg IV over 1 minute
- Repeat after 1 minute until max dose 0.1 mg/kg

If no IV access:
Diazepam 20 mg PR
Midazolam 10 mg IM

↓

Step 2
10-30 minutes

Choose from the following antiepileptics:

Valproic acid 40 mg/kg IV
Levetiracetam 20 mg/kg IV
Fosphenytoin 20 mg/kg (consider further 10 mg/kg dose)*
Lacosamide 400 mg IV
or
Proceed directly to Step 3

↓

Step 3
30-60 minutes

Intubate, start continuous EEG monitoring

- Midazolam 0.2 mg/kg bolus, followed by IV infusion 0.1 mg/kg/h
- Propofol 1-2 mg/kg bolus followed by IV infusion 2 mg/kg/h†
- Pentobarbital 5 mg/kg (at 50mg/min) followed by IV infusion 1 mg/kg/h

Rebolus and titrate infusions to seizure suppression or EEG background (burst) suppression

*Check phenytoin level 2 hours after load. Level should be 20–25 μg/mL
†Using propofol at high doses for >2 days may result in potentially lethal propofol toxicity

Figure 27-5 Treatment of status epilepticus. ABG, arterial blood gas; EEG, electroencephalogram; PR, per rectum.

- Treatment should be started with a single drug that can be titrated until adequate control or until side effects are experienced.
- **Combination therapy (polytherapy) should be attempted only after at least two adequate sequential trials of single agents have failed.** Failure to control epilepsy with adequate trials of two drugs meets criteria for treatment-resistant epilepsy, and a referral for presurgical evaluation should be considered.[10]
- **Patients who are on antitubercular and antiretroviral drugs must be carefully monitored for AED toxicities and AED failure due to drug interactions.**

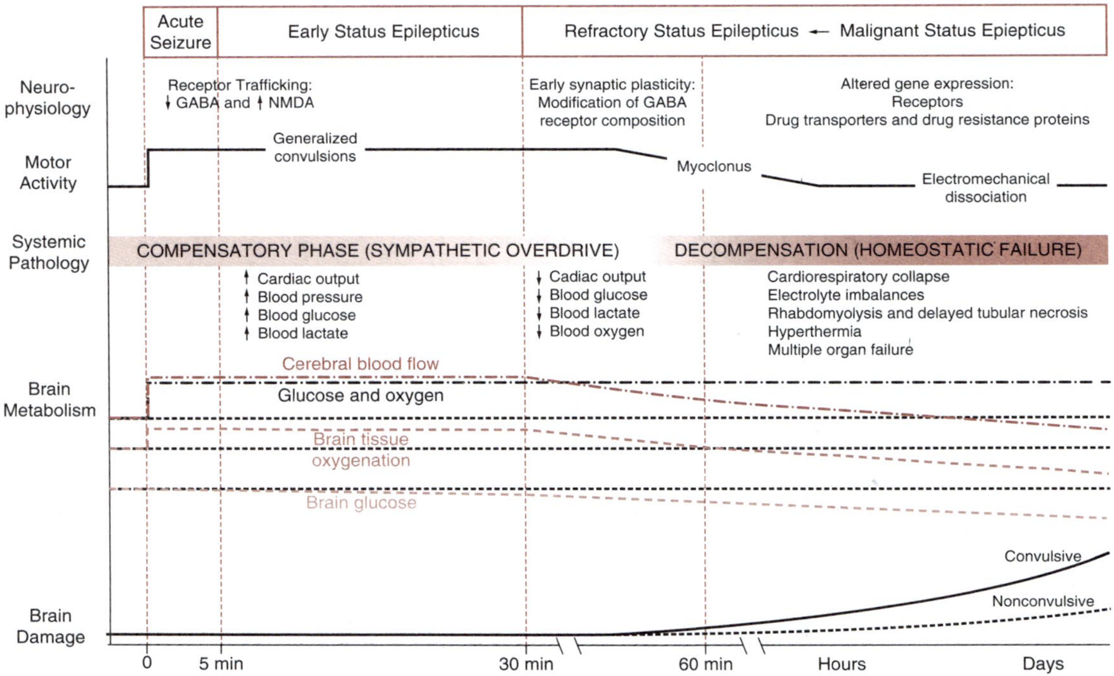

Figure 27-6 Brain and systemic pathology in prolonged convulsive and nonconvulsive status epilepticus. From Hirsch LJ, Gaspard N. Status epilepticus. *Continuum.* 2013;19:767.

TABLE 27-5 Antiepileptic Drugs and their Dosages, Common Drug Reactions, and Contraindications

AED	Initial dosage	Maximal maintenance dosage (per day)	Adverse drug reaction	Contraindication
Carbamazepine	100–200 mg bid	1200 mg	Neurological: somnolence, lethargy, dizziness, diplopia, ataxia General: hyponatremia, GI problems, leukocytopenia, LFT elevation, rash, osteoporosis	SJS, DRESS, bone-marrow suppression, AVB, MAOI medication
Ethosuximide	250 mg bid	1000 mg	Neurological: somnolence, dizziness, ataxia, anorexia, psychosis General: GI problems, weight loss, leukocytopenia, anemia	SJS, DRESS, pancytopenia, lupus, porphyria
Gabapentin	100 mg tid	2400 mg	Neurological: somnolence, lethargy, dizziness, diplopia, ataxia, tremor General: GI problems, weight gain	Pancreatitis, absence seizure
Lacosamide	50 mg bid	400 mg	Neurological: somnolence, lethargy, dizziness, diplopia, ataxia, headache General: cardiac arrhythmia	
Lamotrigine	25 mg qd	400 mg	Neurological: ataxia, dizziness, diplopia, aseptic meningitis General: rash, osteoporosis	SJS, DRESS
Levetiracetam	250 mg bid	3000 mg	Neurological: somnolence, lethargy, dizziness, diplopia, ataxia, falling, hostility, psychosis, mood disorder	Suicidal or homicidal ideation
Oxcarbazepine	150–300 mg bid	2400 mg	Neurological: somnolence, lethargy, dizziness, ataxia, headache General: hyponatremia, GI problems	SJS, AVB, bone-marrow suppression, MAOI medication

(Continued)

TABLE 27-5 Antiepileptic Drugs and their Dosages, Common Drug Reactions, and Contraindications (Continued)

Perampanel	2 mg hs	12 mg	Neurological: somnolence, lethargy, dizziness, diplopia, ataxia, falling, hostility, psychosis, mood disorder	Suicidal or homicidal ideation
Phenobarbital	60 mg per day	240 mg	Neurological: somnolence, lethargy, dizziness, diplopia, ataxia, headache, rash, psychosis, mood disorder, cognitive slowing General: osteoporosis, anemia	SJS, DRESS
Phenytoin	100 mg or 150 mg bid	600 mg	Neurological: somnolence, lethargy, dizziness, diplopia, ataxia, nystagmus, cerebellar atrophy General: gingival hypertrophy, osteoporosis, pancytopenia, lymphadenopathy	SJS, bone-marrow suppression, recent myocardial infarction, second- or third-degree AVB
Pregabalin	≤75 mg bid	600 mg	Neurological: somnolence, lethargy, dizziness, ataxia General: dry mouth, weight gain, edema	Angioedema
Topiramate	25 mg qd or bid	500 mg for monotherapy, 800 mg for combination therapy	Neurological: cognitive slowing, dizziness, anorexia General: weight loss, GI problems	Glaucoma, hyperammonemia, hypohidrosis with hyperthermia, urolithiasis

(Continued)

TABLE 27-5 Antiepileptic Drugs and their Dosages, Common Drug Reactions, and Contraindications (Continued)

AED	Initial dosage	Maximal maintenance dosage (per day)	Adverse drug reaction	Contraindication
Valproic acid	10–15 mg/kg/day (divalproex) 20–30 mg/kg/day (sodium valproate)	60 mg/kg/day	Neurological: dizziness, diplopia, ataxia, tremor General: hyperammonemia, thrombocytopenia, alopecia, GI problems, weight gain	Urea-cycle disorder, unfulfilled PPP, significant hepatic or pancreatic dysfunction, porphyria, coadministration with carbapenems or mefloquine
Vigabatrin	500 mg bid	3000 mg	Neurological: somnolence, lethargy, diplopia, ataxia, nystagmus, cognitive slowing General: anemia, weight gain, arthralgia	Permanent bilateral visual field constriction, blurred vision
Zonisamide	100 mg qd	600 mg	Neurological: somnolence, lethargy, dizziness, ataxia, mood disorders, anorexia, cognitive slowing General: weight loss	SJS, DRESS, urolithiasis, hypohidrosis with hyperthermia

AED, antiepileptic drug; AVB, atrioventricular block; DRESS, drug reaction with eosinophilia and systemic symptoms; GI, gastrointestinal; LFT, liver function test; MAOI, monoamine oxidase inhibitor; PPP, pregnancy prevention program; SJS: Stevens-Johnson syndrome.

Lifestyle Modifications

- Patients should not start other medications (e.g., over-the-counter medications or herbal remedies) without contacting their physician because drug interactions may occur.
- Patients should keep a seizure calendar to identify possible seizure triggers. Screen patients for poor sleep hygiene. Women may have catamenial (perimenstrual) seizures.
- Women should ideally inform their physicians well in advance of any plans for pregnancy or at the very least immediately on finding out they are pregnant given the teratogenicity associated with certain AEDs, the increased risk of teratogenicity with polytherapy versus monotherapy, and the potential need for medication adjustment during pregnancy.
- Patients should reduce alcohol intake because heavy consumption (three or more drinks per day) is associated with an increased risk of seizures.

REFERRAL

Neurologic consultation may be helpful for managing status epilepticus and for evaluation and management of new-onset seizures.

PATIENT EDUCATION

Patients with epilepsy, especially those left untreated, have a small risk of sudden death in epilepsy.[11] Patients with epilepsy should not swim unsupervised, bathe in a bathtub of standing water, use motorized tools, or be in position to fall from heights during a seizure (i.e., patients should avoid situations in which they could harm themselves or others if they were to have a seizure). Driver licensing requirements for patients with epilepsy vary from state to state. A complete listing of state laws can be found at https://www.epilepsy.com/driving-laws.

MONITORING/FOLLOW-UP

- Regular follow-up visits should be scheduled to check drug concentrations, blood counts, and hepatic and renal function. Side effects after initiating AED should be monitored.
- Again, correctable causes for seizures (e.g., hyponatremia, drug toxicity, alcohol withdrawal) do not require long-term anticonvulsant therapy.

Multiple Sclerosis

GENERAL PRINCIPLES

Definition

- Multiple sclerosis (MS) is a chronic, progressive, immune-mediated disorder of the CNS, initially characterized by inflammatory demyelination followed later in its course by neurodegeneration.
- Although the disorder is presumed to be autoimmune in nature, the antigen(s) driving the immune response remains unknown.

Classification

- Forms of MS include the most common form, relapsing-remitting MS (RRMS), associated with episodic neurologic dysfunction followed by a complete or partial recovery in between episodes. The majority of patients are initially diagnosed with RRMS.

- A less common variant is primary progressive MS (PPMS), a form of the disease characterized by progressive neurologic dysfunction from onset without relapses or remissions.
- Secondary progressive MS (SPMS) is also characterized by a course of progressive neurologic dysfunction but follows an initial relapsing-remitting course.
- The least common form is one of a progressive relapsing course in which patients have a steady, progressive decline from the time of onset with superimposed exacerbations (i.e., worsening).
- Classification is important in that progressive forms of the disease, in general, do not respond to many of the first-line disease-modifying therapies (DMTs) effective in RRMS (e.g., interferon-β) but do respond to other therapies (e.g., ocrelizumab in PPMS).

Epidemiology

- Approximate prevalence rate of MS in India is 0.17–1.33/10,000 population which is lesser compared to the Western population. However due to advances in imaging, more cases are being diagnosed nowadays.*
- The worldwide prevalence is estimated at over 2.3 million and growing.

Etiology

The exact etiology of MS remains unknown. The pathophysiologic pattern of MS is characterized by inflammatory cell infiltration, demyelination, axonal damage, and gliosis culminating in neurodegeneration.

DIAGNOSIS

Clinical Presentation

- At disease onset, symptoms are variable and can include visual dysfunction (i.e., optic neuritis), sensory abnormalities, motor dysfunction, ataxia, fatigue, and bowel/bladder dysfunction.
- For the majority of patients, remission occurs after the initial episode, but repeated flares lead to RRMS.
- Eventually, patients can progress to SPMS (see above).

Differential Diagnosis

- The differential diagnosis of MS is too extensive to be covered here but is reviewed in great detail by Sand and Lublin.[12]
- Important differential diagnoses to consider include neuromyelitis optica (NMO), another immune-mediated demyelinating disorder of the CNS. NMO, in the majority of cases, is associated with antibodies against the aquaporin-4 antigen. NMO and MS can be differentiated on some clinico-laboratory parameters (Table 27-6).
- Another autoantibody-mediated demyelinating disorder of the CNS that shares clinical features with MS and NMO is anti–myelin oligodendrocyte glycoprotein (MOG) disease.

Diagnostic Testing

- A cornerstone of diagnostic testing and monitoring/follow-up is MRI of the brain and spinal cord (in many cases). It is worth noting that "MRI-negative" MS does not exist. Lesions on MRI are part of the diagnostic criteria (McDonald criteria) for the disease. However, in patients unable to undergo MRI scans, additional laboratory studies (CSF analysis) can be used, in the appropriate clinical context to support a diagnosis of MS.

---

*Pandit L, Kundapur R. Prevalence and patterns of demyelinating central nervous system disorders in urban Mangalore, South India. Mult Scler. 2014;20:1651–3

TABLE 27-6 Differences Between NMO and MS

Features	Neuromyelitis Optica	Multiple Sclerosis
Optic neuritis	Bilateral usually	Unilateral
Vision	Severely affected	Less affected
MRI white matter abnormalities	Uncommon	Common
Transverse myelitis	More than three segments involved	Usually involves a single segment
Oligoclonal bands	Rare	Common
CSF protein	Elevated	Elevated but to a lesser extent compared to NMO
Response to disease modifying agents	Poor	good

(Hedieh Hoorbakht. Farid Bagherkashi. Optic Neuritis, its Differential Diagnosis and Management. The Open Ophthalmology Journal, 2012, 6, 65–72)

- CSF analysis is second to MRI in its value as a diagnostic marker of MS. Ninety-five percent of patients with MS will have oligoclonal bands specific to the CSF (on comparison to serum).

Diagnostic Criteria (Table 27-7)

TABLE 27-7 Criteria for Diagnosis of Multiple Sclerosis in Patients with an Attack at Onset

≥2 attacks; objective clinical evidence of ≥2 lesions or objective clinical evidence of 1 lesion with reasonable historical evidence of a prior attack
≥2 attacks; objective clinical evidence of 1 lesion *Dissemination in space, demonstrated by:* • ≥1 T2 lesion on MRI in at least 2 out of 4 MS-typical regions of the CNS (periventricular, juxtacortical, infratentorial, or spinal cord) OR • Await a further clinical attack implicating a different CNS site
1 attack; objective clinical evidence of ≥2 lesions *Dissemination in time, demonstrated by:* • Simultaneous presence of asymptomatic gadolinium-enhancing and non-enhancing lesions at any time OR • A new T2 and/or gadolinium-enhancing lesion(s) on follow-up MRI, irrespective of itstiming with reference to a baseline scan OR • Await a second clinical attack

(Continued)

TABLE 27-7 Criteria for Diagnosis of Multiple Sclerosis in Patients with an Attack at Onset (Continued)
1 attack; objective clinical evidence of 1 lesion (clinically isolated syndrome) *Dissemination in space and time, demonstrated by:* *For dissemination in space* • ≥1T2 lesion in at least 2 out of 4 MS-typical regions of the CNS (periventricular, juxtacortical, infratentorial, or spinal cord) OR • Await a second clinical attack implicating a different CNS site AND *For dissemination in time* • Simultaneous presence of asymptomatic gadolinium-enhancing and non-enhancing lesions at any time OR • A new T2 and/or gadolinium-enhancing lesion(s) on follow-up MRI, irrespective of itstiming with reference to a baseline scan OR • Await a second clinical attack
Criteria for diagnosis of multiple sclerosis in patients with a disease course characterized by progression from onset (primary progressive multiple sclerosis) Insidious neurologic progression suggestive of primary progressive multiple sclerosis *1 year of disease progression (retrospectively or prospectively determined)* *AND* *2 out of the 3 following criteria:* • Evidence for dissemination in space in the brain based on ≥1 T2+ lesions in the MS-characteristic periventricular, juxtacortical, or infratentorial regions • Evidence for dissemination in space in the spinal cord based on ≥2 T2+ lesions in thecord • Positive cerebrospinal fluid (isoelectric focusing evidence of oligoclonal bands and/or elevated IgG index)

Adapted from Fowler VG, Durack DT, Selton-Suty C, Athan E, Bayer AS, Chamis AL, Dahl A, DiBernardo L, Durante-Mangoni E, Duval X, Fortes CQ, Fosbøl E, Hannan MM, Hasse B, Hoen B, Karchmer AW, Mestres CA, Petti CA, Pizzi MN, Preston SD, Roque A, Vandenesch F, van der Meer JTM, van der Vaart TW, Miro JM. The 2023 Duke-International Society for Cardiovascular Infectious Diseases Criteria for Infective Endocarditis: Updating the Modified Duke Criteria. Clin Infect Dis. 2023 Aug 22;77(4):518–526.

TREATMENT

- Acute relapses are often treated with corticosteroids.
- There is no cure for MS. Disease-modifying therapies (DMTs) remain the cornerstone of treatment.
- Approved injectable DMTs for the treatment of RRMS include interferon-β (IFN-β) preparations (Betaseron, Extavia, Avonex, and Rebif), glatiramer acetate (Copaxone), and mitoxantrone (Ralenova).
- Currently approved oral agents include fingolimod (Gilenya), teriflunomide (Aubagio), and dimethyl fumarate (Tecfidera).
- IV infusions of monoclonal antibodies, natalizumab (Tysabri), ocrelizumab (Ocrevus), rituximab (Rituxan), alemtuzumab (Lemtrada), have been shown to be effective.
- There has been a substantial growth in the number of DMTs available to treat MS in recent years. See Table 27-8 for more details.

TABLE 27-8 Disease-Modifying Therapies Approved for Use in Relapsing-Remitting Multiple Sclerosis

Drug	Mechanism of Action	Efficacy	Side Effects
Injectables			
Interferon-β preparations—IM or SC (Betaseron, Extavia, Avonex, Rebif, and Plegridy)	Modulates B- and T cell function Reverses blood–brain barrier disruption Modulation of cytokine expression	30% reduction in relapses Reduction in disability Reduction in MRI lesions	Flu-like symptoms Injection site reactions Transaminitis (monitor HFP)
Glatiramer acetate (Copaxone, Glatopa)—SC	Stimulates regulatory T cells Neuroprotection and repair(?)	30% reduction in relapses Reduction in disability Reduction in MRI lesions	Injection site reactions
Orals			
Fingolimod (Gilenya)	Sphingosine-1-phosphate receptor modulator Inhibits egress of lymphocytes from lymph nodes toward CNS	Reduces annual number of relapses and MRI lesions Reduces the risk of disability progression	First-dose bradycardia Skin malignancies Herpes infection Cardiac arrhythmia Macular edema Lymphopenia Hypertension
Teriflunomide (Aubagio)	Dihydroorotate dehydrogenase inhibitor Downregulation of T- and B cell proliferation via de novo synthesis of pyrimidines (drug derived directly from leflunomide)	Reduces annual number of relapses and MRI lesions Reduces the risk of disability progression	Lymphopenia UTIs Elevated liver enzymes Teratogenicity (washout necessary)
Dimethyl fumarate and diroximel Fumarate	Nuclear factor (erythroid-derived 2)- like 2 pathway inhibitor Shifts dendritic cell differentiation Suppresses inflammatory cytokine production	Reduces annual number of relapses and MRI lesions Reduces the risk of disability progression	Lymphopenia Abdominal pain Diarrhea Flushing

(Continued)

TABLE 27-8 Disease-Modifying Therapies Approved for Use in Relapsing-Remitting Multiple Sclerosis (Continued)

Drug	Mechanism of Action	Efficacy	Side Effects
Infusions			
Natalizumab (Tysabri)—IV	Humanized monoclonal antibody that blocks the interaction of α4β1-integrin on leukocytes with vascular cell adhesion molecules to prevent migration of leukocytes from the blood to the CNS	68% reduction in relapses Reduction in disability Reduction in MRI lesions by 92% relative to placebo	Infusion reactions including anaphylaxis Progressive multifocal leukoencephalopathy (need to monitor JCV antibodies/titers)
Alemtuzumab (Lemtrada)—IV	Humanized monoclonal antibody against CD52 Depletes circulating lymphocytes and monocytes	50% reduction in relapses relative to interferon-β Reduction in MRI lesions relative to interferon-β	Infusion reactions Infections (URI, UTI, oral herpes) Secondary autoimmune disorders
Ocrelizumab (Ocrevus) - IV	Humanized monoclonal antibody against CD20 (B cell depletion)	Approximately 50% reduction in relapses relative to interferon-β Reduction in MRI lesions relative to interferon-β First drug to slow down disease progression in PPMS	Infusion-related reaction, nasopharyngitis, upper respiratory tract infection, headache, and urinary tract infection Avoid live vaccines Follow CD19 counts Baseline hepatitis serologies
Mitoxantrone	DNA intercalator	Relative reduction in relapses compared with placebo: 61%	Dose-related cardiomyopathy, promyelocytic leukemia
Ofatumumab- SC	Anti-CD20 mAb	Relative reduction in ARR compared with teriflunomide: 54%	Injection-related reaction, nasopharyngitis, headache, upper respiratory tract infection, and urinary tract infection

ARR, annualized relapse rate; CNS, central nervous system; MRI, magnetic resonance imaging; URI, upper respiratory tract infection; UTI, urinary tract infection.

REFERRAL

In general, all patients with suspected MS or MS should be referred to a neurologist for formal diagnostic testing and initiation of DMT if indicated.

Cerebrovascular Disease

GENERAL PRINCIPLES

- Stroke is a medical emergency that requires rapid diagnosis and treatment. Remember that "Time Is Brain."
- The hallmark of stroke is the abrupt interruption of cerebral blood flow to a specific brain region, resulting in a **sudden-onset focal neurologic deficit.**
- Fluctuation of functional deficits after stroke onset or a brief deficit known as TIA suggests tissue at risk for infarction that may be rescued by reestablishing perfusion.
- **Stroke occurring in less than 45-year-olds is considered as young stroke.**

Epidemiology

More than 795,000 strokes occur per year in the United States (one stroke every 40 seconds in the US population), and it is the fourth leading cause of death in the United States (one death every 4 minutes).

Etiology

- **Ischemic stroke** can be subclassified into atherothrombotic, embolic, hypoperfusion, or hypercoagulable state (the latter being relatively rare).
  - **Atherothrombosis** results from reduced flow within an artery or embolism of thrombus into the distal segment of an artery.
    - Atherosclerosis is the most common etiology of thrombus formation in large vessels.
    - Less common etiologies include dissection, fibromuscular dysplasia, moyamoya, and giant cell arteritis.
    - Lipohyalinosis, usually because of hypertension, is the most common etiology of small-vessel disease.
  - **Cardioembolic** strokes account for about 20% of all ischemic strokes. High-risk cardiac sources include atrial fibrillation, sustained atrial flutter, rheumatic valve disease, atrial or ventricular thrombus, dilated cardiomyopathy, prosthetic valve, bacterial endocarditis, nonbacterial endocarditis (antiphospholipid antibody syndrome, marantic endocarditis, Libman–Sacks endocarditis), sick sinus syndrome, and coronary artery bypass graft surgery.
  - **Hypoperfusion** occurs because of general circulatory problems and often results in bilateral symptoms. Infarction commonly occurs in border zones between large vessels, resulting in watershed infarcts.
  - **Hypercoagulable states** may predispose to arterial thrombosis. These include sickle cell disease, polycythemia vera, essential thrombocythemia, thrombotic thrombocytopenic purpura, antiphospholipid antibody syndrome, hyperhomocysteinemia, etc. Factor V Leiden, protein C and S deficiency, and antithrombin (AT)-III deficiency typically result in venous, not arterial, infarcts.
- **Hemorrhagic stroke** occurs in about 20% of all cases.
  - The location of an **intraparenchymal hemorrhage** (IPH) may suggest its etiology.
    - Hemorrhage in the basal ganglia, thalamus, or pons is often because of chronic systemic hypertension.
    - Amyloid angiopathy typically causes lobar hemorrhages and is a common etiology in the elderly.

- Head trauma, anticoagulants, drugs (cocaine or amphetamines), arteriovenous malformation (AVM), tumor, blood dyscrasia, hemorrhagic conversion of an ischemic stroke, and vasculitis are other possible hemorrhagic stroke etiologies.
  - **Aneurysmal subarachnoid hemorrhage** (for this section, SAH will refer to aneurysmal subarachnoid hemorrhage unless designated otherwise) is caused by the rupture of an arterial aneurysm resulting in bleeding into the subarachnoid space (which contains CSF). Hypertension, cigarette smoking, genetic factors, and septic emboli (resulting in mycotic aneurysms) can all contribute to aneurysm formation.
- **Cerebral venous sinus thrombosis** (CVST) is the occlusion of a venous sinus(es) by a thrombus. It occurs in hypercoagulable states such as late pregnancy or postpartum, cancer, and thrombophilias, as well as with trauma and adjacent inflammation/infection. It may manifest with ischemic infarcts and/or hemorrhage.
- **The prevalence of stroke in young adults, defined as age < 50 years, is estimated to be about 10–14% of all strokes. It has various etiologies which are summarized in Table 27-9.**

Risk Factors

Major significant risk factors for ischemic stroke include hypertension, prior TIA/stroke, carotid stenosis, diabetes mellitus, dyslipidemia, heart failure, cigarette smoking, alcohol consumption, oral contraceptive use, obesity, genetics, and age.

TIA is a focal or global neurological deficit lasting less than 24 hours with no imaging abnormality. Based on vascular territory it is classified into the anterior circulation TIA (amaurausis fugax, transient hemiplegias, transient aphasias, transient UMN facial palsy,

TABLE 27-9 Etiologies of Ischemic Stroke in Young
• Carotid and vertebral dissection
• Fibromuscular dysplasia
• Homocystinuria
• Illicit drug usage: Cocaine, Heroin
• Moyamoya disease
• Takayasu's arteritis
Cardioembolism • Rheumatic valvular heart disease • Dilated cardiomyopathy • Patent foramen ovale
• Protein C and S deficiency, factor V Leiden, antithrombin III deficiency, and prothrombin mutation
• Myeloproliferative disorder
• Antiphospholipid syndromes
• Sickle cell disease
• Vasculitis
• Oral contraceptives and hormone supplements
• Genetic (MELAS/CADASIL)
• Cerebral venous thrombosis
• Migraine

MELAS, mitochondrial encephalopathy, lactic acidosis, and stroke-like episodes; CADASIL, cerebral autosomal dominant arteriopathy with subcortical infarcts and leukoencephalopathy

and transient sensory deficit in the limbs) or posterior circulation TIA (transient ataxias, giddiness, nystagmus, dysphagias, and cerebellar abnormalities). Based on etiology it can be classified into **low flow TIA** (few episodes in a day) and **embolic TIA** (multiple episodes in a day). If a patient develops both anterior and posterior circulation TIAs, the source of emboli is probably cardiac. If he develops TIA in the same vascular territory it may be artery to artery embolism. TIA has high risk (up to 30%) of predisposing to a full-fledged CVA within the next 1 week.*

DIAGNOSIS

Clinical Presentation

History

- Time of onset is critical if thrombolytic therapy is to be administered. Time of onset is when the patient was last known well and **not** when the patient was found with their deficit.
- Onset of symptoms is typically sudden. Ask about progression or fluctuation of symptoms and when the patient was **last normal**.
- Prior TIA symptoms (e.g., transient monocular loss of vision, aphasia, dysarthria, paresis, or sensory disturbance) suggest atherosclerotic vascular disease, the most common cause for stroke.
- Inquire about cardiac arrhythmias and atherosclerotic risk factors.
- A history of neck trauma or recent chiropractic maneuvers warrants evaluation for arterial dissection.
- SAH commonly presents with sudden onset of a severe headache (i.e., the "worst headache of my life"). Lethargy or coma, fever, vomiting, seizures, and low back pain may also be present.
- IPH presents with neurologic deficits accompanied by headache, vomiting, and possibly lethargy.
- CVST often presents with signs and symptoms of elevated intracranial pressure, such as a positional headache with diurnal variability (waking from sleep, worse in the morning), bilateral sixth nerve palsies, blurred vision (typically peripheral with sparing of central vision initially), and papilledema.

Physical Examination

- A careful neurologic examination can reliably establish the anatomic location of a stroke in most cases.
- In general, carotid artery distribution (anterior circulation) strokes produce combinations of functional deficits (hemiparesis, hemianopsia, cortical sensory loss, often with aphasias or agnosias) contralateral to the affected hemisphere.
- Vertebrobasilar strokes (posterior circulation) produce unilateral or bilateral motor/sensory deficits, usually accompanied by cranial nerve and brainstem signs (vertigo, diplopia, ataxia).
- Horner syndrome (ptosis, miosis, anhidrosis) contralateral to an acute hemiparesis suggests carotid dissection. A Horner syndrome with nystagmus and ipsilateral loss of facial pain and temperature sensation with contralateral loss of body pain and temperature sensation is diagnostic of a lateral medullary stroke because of a posterior inferior cerebellar artery infarct (i.e., Wallenberg syndrome).
- General physical examination should be focused on possible etiologic factors. Examine for abnormal pulses, arrhythmias, murmurs, carotid bruits, and embolic phenomena.

---

*Easton JD, Saver JL, Albers GW, et al. Definition and evaluation of transient ischemic attack. *Stroke*. 2009;4040: 2276–2293.

Differential Diagnosis

Mimics of stroke include postseizure paralysis (Todd paresis), migraine with neurologic deficit (i.e., complicated migraine), and hypo- or hyperglycemia.

Diagnostic Testing

Laboratory Studies

- In the acute setting (e.g., acute evaluation for thrombolytic therapy), these should include blood glucose and may include CBC and coagulation studies (INR, PTT, anti-factor Xa level, thrombin time).
- The following are indicated but not emergent: Basic metabolic panel, troponin, lipid profile, and hemoglobin A1C. Tests such as erythrocyte sedimentation rate (ESR), C-reactive protein (CRP) and blood cultures (if endocarditis suspected), rapid plasma reagin, antinuclear antibody, antiphospholipid antibodies, drug toxicology screen, and HIV are not part of a "standard screen" but may be indicated in certain clinical contexts.

Electrocardiography

ECG should be done to look for atrial fibrillation or ischemic changes.

Imaging

- **Noncontrast head CT** scan should be obtained acutely to rapidly differentiate hemorrhagic from ischemic strokes. It can identify acute hemorrhages in most cases. It is insensitive for acute ischemic strokes. It is often the rate-limiting step in making decisions on thrombolytic therapy. Head CT scan is diagnostic of SAH in 90% of SAH patients in the first 24 hours.
- **Emergent vascular imaging** (typically **CT angiography** with or without CT perfusion scanning) is now performed in all patients presenting with suspected large-vessel occlusion (carotid, proximal MCA, or basilar artery) to screen for lesions amenable to endovascular thrombectomy.
- **MRI** scan is the most sensitive imaging study for stroke diagnosis. Diffusion-weighted images detect stroke the earliest. If a diagnosis of stroke is clear from clinical examination, MRI is not always necessary because it is unlikely to affect management in a great majority of cases.
- *Magnetic resonance angiography (MRA)* and *venograms* are useful noninvasive tests to evaluate large arteries and veins, respectively. MRA of the neck with contrast can serve as a screen for carotid stenosis.
- **Carotid Doppler** studies enable noninvasive estimation of carotid stenosis and should be done for anterior circulation strokes unless some form of angiography has already been performed for another indication.
- **Two-dimensional transthoracic echocardiography** is helpful to demonstrate intracardiac thrombi, valve vegetations, valvular stenosis or insufficiency, and right-to-left shunt (bubble study). In some patients, transesophageal echocardiography may be necessary to evaluate the left atrium for thrombi.

Diagnostic Procedures

- **Cerebral angiography** is the definitive study for vascular malformations but may miss small aneurysms. Some surgeons prefer having this procedure performed before proceeding with carotid endarterectomy (CEA).
- If suspicion for SAH is high and head CT is negative, an **LP** should be performed.
    - Tubes 1 and 4 should be sent for cell count. If the number of red blood cells (RBCs) decreases dramatically from tube 1 to tube 4, a traumatic LP is more likely than SAH.
    - Bloody CSF should be centrifuged and examined for xanthochromia (yellow color). Xanthochromia results from RBC lysis and takes several hours to develop, indicating SAH rather than a traumatic LP.

TREATMENT

- Vital signs, including oximetry and continuous telemetry, should be monitored.
- Hypertension management after ischemic stroke:
  - Perfusion pressure in areas of the brain distal to the arterial occlusion may be low. Cerebral perfusion depends in part on mean systemic arterial pressure. Thus, a degree of hypertension may be necessary to maintain adequate perfusion pressure to injured areas.
  - Aggressive lowering of blood pressure (BP) has been associated with neurologic deterioration, although there exists an ongoing debate in the field on this topic (see the following text).[13]
  - Patients with acute stroke often present hypertensive. BP tends to fall on its own over several days following a stroke.
  - Although management of hypertension in the setting of acute stroke remains controversial, BP should not be lowered acutely unless necessary for treatment of acute coronary syndrome, CHF, hypertensive crisis with end-organ involvement, or SBP >220 mm Hg or DBP >120 mm Hg.[14] BP lowering should proceed cautiously, with 15% during the first 24 hours being a reasonable goal.
- Treatment of intracranial hemorrhage consists of supportive care, gradual reduction in BP, and elevation of head of bed by 15 degrees.
- Treatment of SAH depends on etiology (surgical clipping vs. intravascular coiling).
  - Supportive measures include bed rest, sedation, analgesia, and laxatives to prevent sudden increases in intracranial pressure.
  - Patients with SAH tend toward volume contraction, and although there is insufficient evidence to support a benefit for volume expansion, guidelines do emphasize the importance of maintaining euvolemia to avoid delayed cerebral ischemia (DCI).
  - Induced hypertension (unless contraindicated by cardiac comorbidities or in patients with baseline elevated BP) is still recommended in patients with vasospasm/DCI because it has been shown to improve cerebral blood flow in these patients.
  - Endovascular angioplasty is recommended in patients with symptomatic vasospasm of proximal cerebral arteries that fail to respond to induced hypertension. In many instances, endovascular therapies are combined with intra-arterial vasodilator therapies (e.g., calcium channel blockers).
  - Other nonpharmacologic (hemodilution) and pharmacologic (statins, endothelin receptor antagonists, magnesium) therapies have failed to demonstrate a definitive benefit in patients with SAH.
  - Future therapies for preventing and treating cerebral vasospasm hinge on gaining a better understanding of the mechanisms underlying cerebral vasospasm and DCI.

Medications

- Recombinant tissue plasminogen activator (t-PA), including alteplase and tenecteplase, remains the only US Food and Drug Administration (FDA)–approved pharmacologic therapy for acute ischemic stroke. The recommended dose is 0.9 mg/kg (maximum 90 mg total dose), 10% of the total dose is administered as an initial IV bolus over one minute, and the remaining dose is infused over 60 minutes.
  - Administration of t-PA must commence within 4.5 hours of stroke onset but should be started as close to onset as possible (i.e., do not delay to see if the patient "gets better" if they present early in the window).[15]
  - Hyperacute MRI may be used to estimate the time of onset for patients with strokes of unknown onset time to make decisions regarding thrombolysis.[16]
  - t-PA treatment increases risk for symptomatic brain hemorrhage, compared with placebo, but without any significant impact on 3- and 12-month mortality rates.

  - Exclusion criteria differ by stroke center protocol (Table 27-10). The acute stroke team should be contacted emergently to evaluate **all** acute strokes because some patients ineligible for IV t-PA may be candidates for other interventions, such as thrombectomy.
  - Advanced radiology can assist with selection of patients with large-vessel occlusions who would benefit from endovascular thrombectomy (Table 27-11).
  - Aspirin and anticoagulants should be held for the first 24 hours after t-PA.
- Aspirin reduces atherosclerotic stroke morbidity and mortality and is typically given at an initial dose of 325 mg within 24–48 hours of stroke onset. The dose may be reduced to 81 mg in the post–acute stroke period.
- Other antiplatelet-aggregating drugs (clopidogrel, aspirin/dipyridamole) are available and may be of benefit for certain patients. Both of these drugs have a significant advantage over aspirin in secondary stroke prevention. Dual antiplatelet therapy for secondary prevention may benefit select patients, though is also associated with increased risk of hemorrhage.
- Heparin, low molecular weight heparin (LMWH), and warfarin anticoagulation are **not** recommended routinely for acute ischemic stroke.
- Anticoagulation with a DOAC or warfarin is indicated to prevent recurrent embolic strokes because of atrial fibrillation. Target INR for warfarin therapy is 2–3.[14]
- Nimodipine, a calcium channel blocker, improves outcome in SAH patients and may reduce the incidence of associated cerebral infarction with few side effects. However, the mechanism by which nimodipine offers neuroprotection remains unclear (i.e., no evidence that it prevents vasospasm).
- Anticoagulation with heparin/LMWH followed by warfarin is indicated for venous sinus thrombosis both with and without hemorrhagic infarcts. Trials of NOACs for this indication are ongoing. Boluses of heparin to correct the aPTT should be avoided in the setting of hemorrhage. aPTTs should be closely monitored and maintained between 60 and 80 seconds.

Other Nonpharmacologic Therapies

- Recently published trials have demonstrated a clear benefit to endovascular thrombectomy in select patients with acute ischemic stroke. This may be combined with IV t-PA.
- CT angiography and CT perfusion scans may be used to select patients who will benefit from thrombectomy up to 24 hours after the time they were last known well.[17,18]
- These studies represent the first major breakthrough in acute ischemic stroke therapy since the introduction of IV t-PA in 1996.
- Physical, occupational, and speech therapy are extremely important in stroke rehabilitation and have a clear beneficial impact on poststroke outcomes.
- Stroke patients with obvious dysphagia, dysarthria, or a facial droop should be kept nothing by mouth until an experienced individual can assess their swallowing abilities.

Surgical Management

- CEA decreases the risk of stroke and death in patients with recent TIAs or nondisabling strokes and ipsilateral high-grade (70%–99%) carotid stenosis.[19]
  - The CREST (Carotid Revascularization Endarterectomy vs. Stenting) trial provides evidence to suggest that carotid stenting is of equal efficacy to CEA, but carries a higher periprocedural stroke risk.[20]
  - Neurology and surgery recommendations should be sought before deciding between the two approaches.
- CEA for asymptomatic high-grade carotid stenosis (≥60%) reduces the 5-year risk of ipsilateral stroke in men, provided that the operator's surgical/angiography complication rate is <3%.[21,22]
- See the earlier section on nonpharmacologic therapies for information on endovascular therapies in acute ischemic stroke.

TABLE 27-10 Inclusion and Exclusion Criteria for tPA for Acute Ischemic Stroke (Washington University Stroke Center Protocol)

tPA Inclusion Criteria

1. Age ≥18 yr
2. Clinical diagnosis of ischemic stroke causing disabling neurologic deficit
3. Onset of stroke symptoms well established to be less than 4h30 before treatment would begin

tPA Exclusion Criteria

1. Intracranial hemorrhage on noncontrast head CT
2. Serious head trauma within 3 mo
3. Active bleeding or suspected underlying coagulopathy including thrombocytopenia (<100); INR>1.7, therapeutic anticoagulation (verify with coagulation testing).[a]
4. Sustained SBP >185 or DBP >110 at the time of treatment
5. Nondisabling or rapidly improving symptoms
6. Symptoms suggest subarachnoid hemorrhage despite negative CT scan
7. Infective endocarditis suspected as cause of stroke
8. For 3–4h30 window, severe stroke (NIHSS >25)

Relative Exclusion Criteria

Balance potential benefit of tPA in reducing long-term disability with risk of hemorrhagic complications. Consultation with a stroke team and other subspecialists is advised.

1. Major surgery or serious trauma within 30 d
2. Intracranial or spinal surgery within 3 mo
3. Serum glucose <50 mg/dL or >400 mg/dL (reassess after treatment for blood sugar)
4. Stroke within past 3 mo
5. History of intracranial hemorrhage
6. GI/GU hemorrhage within 21 d or known structural GI malignancy at risk of bleeding
7. Primary or metastatic intracranial, intra-axial neoplasm
8. Seizure at onset (with deficits thought related to postictal paresis)
9. Recent arterial puncture at a noncompressible site
10. Large (>10 mm) unsecured intracranial aneurysm
11. Intracranial arteriovenous malformation
12. Extensive regions of clear hypoattenuation on CT (large subacute stroke)

Based on the current American Heart Association/American Stroke Association Guidelines: Powers WJ, Rabinstein AA, Ackerson T, et al. 2018 Guidelines for the early management of patients with acute ischemic stroke: a guideline for healthcare professionals from the American Heart Association/American Stroke Association. Stroke. 2018;49:e46–e110. doi:10.1161/STR.0000000000000158.

[a]Because time is critical, thrombolytic therapy should not be delayed while waiting for the results of the PT, PTT, or platelet count unless a bleeding abnormality or thrombocytopenia is suspected; the patient has been taking warfarin, heparin, dabigatran, rivaroxaban, or apixaban; anticoagulation use is uncertain.

CT, computed tomography; DBP, diastolic blood pressure; GI, gastrointestinal; GU, genitourinary; INR, international normalized ratio; NIHSS, National Institutes of Health Stroke Scale; SBP, systolic blood pressure; tPA, tissue plasminogen activator.

TABLE 27-11 Inclusion and Exclusion Criteria for Endovascular Thrombectomy (Washington University Stroke Center Protocol)

Endovascular Thrombectomy Inclusion Criteria

1. Age ≥18 yr
2. Clinical diagnosis of ischemic stroke causing disabling neurologic deficit
   a. NIHSS ≥6 if <16 h from time last seen well
   b. NIHSS ≥10 if 16–24 h from time last seen well
3. Ability to initiate thrombectomy in appropriate time window (24 h based on current trials)
4. For posterior circulation strokes (e.g. basilar thrombus), time window is at the discretion of the stroke and neurointerventional attending physicians

Imaging Inclusion Criteria

1. Noncontrast head CT: absence of intracranial hemorrhage/mass/mass effect
2. Noncontrast head CT/MRI: absence of evidence of large, completed infarct
3. CT/MR angiography: large-vessel occlusion, e.g. ICA, MCA (M1/M2), vertebral or basilar artery
4. CT perfusion within 6–16 h[a]: core infarct volume ≤70 mL, core-penumbra mismatch volume ≥15 mL, core-penumbra mismatch ratio ≥1.8
5. CT perfusion within 16–24 h[b]: core infarct volume ≤30 mL (if age <80), core infarct volume ≤20 mL (if age ≥80)

Endovascular Thrombectomy Exclusion Criteria

1. Premorbid disability (mRS≥2) or comorbidities that affect recovery potential
2. Intracranial hemorrhage, mass, or mass effect as cause of stroke symptoms
3. Current severe uncontrolled hypertension, SBP >185 or DBP >110, despite reasonable treatment
4. Active bleeding or suspected underlying coagulopathy including thrombocytopenia (<30), INR>3, therapeutic anticoagulation (verify with coagulation testing)

[a]Based on the results of the DEFUSE 3 trial.[17]
[b]Based on the result of the DAWN trial.[18]
CT, computed tomography; DBP, diastolic blood pressure; INR, international normalized ratio; MRI, magnetic resonance imaging; mRS, modified Rankin Scale; NIHSS, National Institutes of Health; SBP, systolic blood pressure.

- Hemicraniectomy increases survival and can improve functional outcomes in select patients with large hemispheric infarcts and severe edema (e.g., "malignant" middle cerebral artery infarcts). Neurosurgical consultation should be obtained early in these cases.
- Cerebellar infarction or hematomas may result in brainstem compression or obstructive hydrocephalus and may also warrant urgent neurosurgical intervention.

Lifestyle/Risk Modification

Modifiable risk factors (Table 27-12) include the following.

- BP reduction even in normotensive stroke patients is beneficial.[23]
- Diabetes control is important with care taken to avoid hypoglycemia and hyperglycemia.
- Smoking cessation.
- Patients under age 75 with no concerns for safety of statin therapy should be placed on "high-intensity" statin therapy (e.g., atorvastatin 40–80 mg or rosuvastatin 20–40 mg), whereas patients over 75 or patients for whom there is concern for safety of statin therapy should be placed on "moderate-intensity" statin therapy (e.g., atorvastatin 10–20 mg, rosuvastatin 5–10 mg, simvastatin 20–40 mg, pravastatin 40–80 mg).[24]

TABLE 27-12 Secondary Stroke Prevention ("BLASTED")

- **B**lood pressure
- **L**DL
- **A**SA (**a**ntiplatelet), **A**1C
- **S**troke management and rehabilitation team (varies from facility to facility)
  - PT, OT, ST, stroke educator, smoking cessation counseling
- **T**elemetry: cardiac rhythm monitoring
- **E**chocardiography
- **D**oppler for carotid stenosis, **d**iabetes (A1C, diabetes educator, etc.)

ASA, acetylsalicylic acid; LDL, low-density lipoprotein; OT, occupational therapy; PT, physical therapy; ST, speech therapy.

- Identify and treat obstructive sleep apnea.
- Oral contraceptives or hormonal therapies may need to be discontinued in women with stroke.

COMPLICATIONS

- Cerebral edema following ischemic stroke peaks at 48–96 hours after stroke, and patients need to be watched closely during this time.
- Hemorrhagic conversion of an ischemic stroke is more likely in patients who are receiving anticoagulation or in patients with large strokes, particularly those with embolic ischemic infarcts.

Headache

GENERAL PRINCIPLES

Classification

- **Primary headache syndromes** include migraines with (classic) or without (common) aura, the hemicranias and indomethacin-responsive headaches, tension headaches, chronic daily headaches, and cluster headaches.
- **Secondary headaches** have specific etiologies, and symptomatic features vary depending on the underlying pathology (i.e., SAH, tumor, hypertension, posterior reversible encephalopathy syndrome or reversible posterior leukoencephalopathy, reversible cerebral vasoconstriction syndrome [RCVS], analgesic overuse, iatrogenic).
- **Migraine without aura (common):** At least five attacks that last 4–72 hours. Symptoms should include at least two of the following: unilateral location, pulsating or throbbing, moderate to severe in intensity, aggravated by activity, and at least one of these associated features: nausea/vomiting, photophobia, and/or phonophobia.
- **Migraine with aura (classic):** Same as above, except at least two attacks with an associated aura that lasts from 4 minutes to 1 hour (longer than 60 minutes is a red flag). The aura should have a gradual onset, should be fully reversible, and can occur before, with, or after headache onset.
- **Cluster headache:** Unilateral orbital or temporal pain with lacrimation, conjunctival injection, nasal congestion, rhinorrhea, facial swelling, miosis, ptosis, and eyelid edema.
- **Rebound headache** (analgesic overuse headache) occurs in the setting of chronic use of analgesics or narcotics.
- **Trigeminal neuralgia** presents as episodic sharp stabbing pain that is unilateral. Rule out MS or an alternative etiology with MRI.

- **Temporal arteritis** presents as a dull unilateral headache with a thick tortuous artery over temporal region. The disease is almost exclusively limited to individuals over 60 years of age with jaw claudication, low-grade fever, and an elevated ESR and CRP.
- **Tension type headaches** are bilateral pressing or tightening headaches which last from few minutes to weeks which are not associated with emesis. This may be due to dysfunction of pain perception in pathways involving pericranial myofascial tissues.*

Etiology

Secondary headache etiologies include the following:

- Subdural hematoma (SDH), intracerebral hemorrhage, SAH, AVM, brain abscess, meningitis, encephalitis, vasculitis, obstructive hydrocephalus, and cerebral ischemia or infarction.
- Idiopathic intracranial hypertension (commonly known as pseudotumor cerebri) presents with headache, papilledema, diplopia, and elevated CSF pressure (at least >20 cm H_2O in relaxed lateral decubitus position). CVST should be ruled out in all patients presenting with suspected idiopathic intracranial hypertension.
- Extracranial causes include giant cell arteritis, sinusitis, glaucoma, optic neuritis, dental disease (including temporomandibular joint syndrome), and disorders of the cervical spine ("cervicogenic" headache).
- Systemic causes include fever, viremia, hypoxia, carbon monoxide poisoning, hypercapnia, systemic hypertension, allergy, anemia, caffeine withdrawal, and vasoactive or toxic chemicals (nitrites).
- Depression is a common cause of long-standing, treatment-resistant headaches. Specific inquiry about vegetative signs of depression and exclusion of other causes help support this diagnosis.

DIAGNOSIS

Clinical Presentation

History

- The sudden onset of severe headache ("**the worst headache of my life,**" also known as a "thunderclap headache") or a severe persistent headache that reaches maximal intensity within a few seconds/minutes warrants immediate investigation for possible SAH.
- Other headache syndromes that can present with a thunderclap headache include RCVS, posterior cerebral artery infarcts, CVST, arterial dissections, CNS vasculitis, pituitary apoplexy, intracerebral hemorrhage, and some of the indomethacin-responsive headache syndromes.
- History should focus on the following:
  - Age at onset
  - Frequency, intensity, and duration of attacks
  - Triggers, associations (menstrual cycle), associated symptoms (e.g., photophobia, phonophobia, nausea, vomiting), and alleviating factors
  - Location and quality of pain (e.g., sharp, dull)
  - Number of headaches per month, including number of disabling headaches
  - Family history of migraines
  - Sleep and diet hygiene (caffeine intake)
  - Use of pain medications, including over-the-counter medications
- Certain "**red flag**" symptoms must be identified to diagnose the following life-threatening causes of headaches:
  - Sudden onset: suspect CVST, SAH, and meningitis.

---

*Chowdhury D. Tension type headache. *Ann Indian Acad Neurol.* 2012;15(1):S83–S88.

- Focal neurological deficits: CVST and space occupying lesions.
- Systemic symptoms like fever, neck stiffness, loss of weight, meningitis, and tumors.
- Associated projectile vomiting: raised ICT due to infection, neoplasm, and vascular.
- Onset >60 years: temporal arteritis.

Physical Examination

- On general examination, check BP and pulse, listen for possible bruits, palpate head and neck muscles, and check temporal arteries.
- If neck stiffness and meningismus (resistance to passive neck flexion) are present on examination, then consider meningitis.
- If papilledema is observed on examination, then consider an intracranial mass, meningitis, CVST, or idiopathic intracranial hypertension.

Diagnostic Testing

Imaging

Neuroimaging is generally not indicated for known primary headache syndromes but may be required to exclude secondary etiologies (listed earlier) in cases that have not been previously diagnosed or in patients presenting with new headaches, especially those who present with atypical features or abnormal examination findings.

Diagnostic Procedures

LP is indicated in a patient with severe headache with suspicion of SAH even if the head CT scan is negative. However, head CT is over 99% sensitive for detecting SAH if obtained within 6 hours of headache onset.

TREATMENT

- **Acute treatment of migraine,** the most common primary headache syndrome, is directed at aborting the headache. This is easier at onset and often very difficult when the attack is well established. Accordingly, the threshold for treating at the first sign of a headache should be low. Patients have often used nonprescription analgesics (acetylsalicylic acid [ASA], acetaminophen, NSAIDs) and oral prescription medications (butalbital with aspirin or acetaminophen), which are the first-line treatments and are most effective early in the course of an attack. Emergent treatments include serotonin agonists and other parenteral medications.
- Scheduled IV NSAID (e.g., ketorolac) in combination with antiemetics (typically prochlorperazine) and IV fluids is an effective first-line regimen in many cases.
- Antidopaminergic therapies including haloperidol and droperidol are also effective first-line therapies. A baseline ECG should be obtained to evaluate for a prolonged QT_c.
- **Triptans** (serotonin receptor $5HT_{1B}$ and $5HT_{1D}$ agonists) are effective abortive medications available in multiple formulations and may be effective even in a protracted attack. Triptans should not be used in patients with coronary artery disease, cerebrovascular disease, uncontrolled hypertension, hemiplegic migraine, or vertebrobasilar migraine.
- **Dihydroergotamine** is a potent venoconstrictor with minimal peripheral arterial constriction. Cardiac precautions and a baseline ECG are indicated in all patients. This medication is contraindicated when there is a history of angina, myocardial infarction, or peripheral vascular disease. Alternative therapies should also be considered in elderly patients.
- **Ergotamine** is a vasoconstrictive agent effective for aborting migraine headaches, particularly if administered during the prodromal phase. Ergotamine should be taken at symptom onset in the maximum dose tolerated by the patient; nausea often limits the dose. Rectal preparations are better absorbed than oral agents. This medication is also

contraindicated in patients with a history of angina, myocardial infarction, or peripheral vascular disease.

- Additional abortive therapies with less evidence supporting their use include IV valproic acid, IV/PO methylprednisolone, IM ziprasidone, and IV magnesium.
- Chronic daily headaches should not be treated with narcotic analgesics so as to prevent addiction, rebound headaches, and tachyphylaxis.
- Treatment of secondary headaches is directed at the primary etiology, such as surgical treatment of cerebral aneurysm causing SAH, evacuation of SDH, calcium channel blockers in RCVS, or shunting in obstructive hydrocephalus.
- **Prophylactic medications** should be considered if a patient has at least three disabling migraines per month.
  - It is important to review a patient's use of all medications and comorbidities because they may influence choice of medication and offer additional factors contributing to the headache syndrome.
  - Possible prophylactic medications include propranolol, topiramate, tricyclic antidepressants (TCAs) (amitriptyline, nortriptyline), and now less commonly, valproic acid. Second-line agents include verapamil, selective serotonin reuptake inhibitors (SSRIs), and serotonin-norepinephrine reuptake inhibitors (SNRIs). Weaker evidence exists for other AEDs and for calcium channel blockers.
  - Alternative (nonprescription) therapies for migraine prophylaxis include butterbur, riboflavin, magnesium, and acupuncture.
  - Botulinum toxin (onabotulinumtoxin A) is FDA approved for migraine prophylaxis in adult patients with chronic migraine (defined as ≥15 headache days per month).

Lifestyle Modifications

- Patients should keep a headache calendar to identify possible triggers.
- Patients should reduce alcohol, caffeine, and other triggers that may increase risk of migraines.

REFERRAL

Neurosurgical consultation is indicated for managing SAH, SDH, vascular malformations, tumors, and other space-occupying lesions resulting in mass effect. Neurologic consultation is indicated if a patient is not well controlled on a first-line prophylactic agent with appropriate use of an abortive therapy.

Head Trauma

GENERAL PRINCIPLES

Definition

- **Traumatic brain injury (TBI)** can occur with head injury because of contact and/or acceleration/deceleration forces.
- **Concussion:** Trauma-induced alteration in mental status with normal radiographic studies that may or may not involve loss of consciousness.
- **Contusion:** Trauma-induced lesion consisting of punctate hemorrhages and surrounding edema.

Classification

- Closed head injuries may produce axonal injury.

- Contusion or hemorrhage can occur at site of initial impact, "coup injury," or opposite to the side of impact, "countercoup injury."
- Penetrating injuries (including depressed skull fracture) or foreign objects cause brain injury directly.
- Secondary increases in intracranial pressure may compromise cerebral perfusion.

Epidemiology

- Head injury is the most common cause of neurologic illness in young people. Developing economies record higher rates of road traffic injuries, with 93% of fatalities coming from low- and middle-income countries.*
- Two-thirds of TBIs are considered "mild," whereas 20% are severe and 10% are fatal. Note that although designated as "mild," mild TBI can still translate into significant disability (permanent in 15%).
- Rates of TBI are highest in the very young, adolescents, and the elderly.

DIAGNOSIS

Clinical Presentation

- Patients will often present with confusion and amnesia, including loss of memory for the traumatic event as well as inability to recall events both immediately before and after trauma.
- Patients may complain of nonspecific signs including headache, vertigo, nausea, vomiting, and personality changes.
- Intracerebral hematomas may be present initially or develop after a contusion.
- Epidural hematoma is usually associated with skull fractures across a meningeal artery and may cause precipitous deterioration after a **lucid interval**.
- SDH is most common in aged, debilitated alcoholics, and/or in anticoagulated patients. Antecedent trauma may be minimal or absent.

Physical Examination

- Careful examination for penetrating wounds and other injuries.
- Hemotympanum, mastoid ecchymosis (Battle sign), periorbital ecchymosis ("raccoon eyes"), and CSF otorrhea/rhinorrhea are indicative of a basilar skull fracture.
- Neurologic examination should focus on the level of consciousness, focal deficits, and signs of herniation. The GCS should be used for an assessment. Serial examinations must be performed and documented to identify neurologic deterioration.
- Degree of impairment because of trauma can be classified using injury severity scores, with GCS being the most common.
- Treatment and diagnostic assessment of patients with severe head injury at admission are done according to the Advanced Trauma Life Support (ATLS) protocol.
- The Standardized Assessment of Concussion is a standardized tool for the sideline evaluation of athletes who suffer a head injury.

Diagnostic Testing

- Head CT should be considered for patients with GCS <15 2 hours after trauma, suspected skull fracture, repeated episodes of vomiting after trauma, age >65 years, dangerous mechanism (e.g., pedestrian struck by motor vehicle, occupant ejected from motor vehicle, fall from ≥3 feet or ≥five stairs), drug or alcohol intoxication, or persistent anterograde amnesia.

---

* https://www.who.int/health-topics/road-safety#tab=tab_1.

- Noncontrast head CT scan in the emergency room can rapidly identify intracranial hemorrhage and contusion.
  - A lenticular-shaped extra-axial hematoma is characteristic of epidural hematoma.
  - Bone window views may help to locate fractures, if present.
- Cervical radiographs ± CT of the neck must be performed to exclude fracture or dislocation.
- MRI can assist in evaluation of TBI patients with persistent sequelae because it is more sensitive for demonstrating small areas of contusion or petechial hemorrhage, axonal injury, and small extra-axial hematomas.

TREATMENT

- Hospital admission is recommended for patients at risk for immediate complications from head injury. These include patients with GCS <15, abnormal CT scan, intracranial bleeding, cerebral edema, seizures, or abnormal bleeding parameters.
- When admitted, continuously monitor vital signs and oximetry. ECG should be performed. Arterial pressure monitoring in conjunction with intracranial monitoring may be indicated.
- Immobilize the neck in a hard cervical collar to avoid spinal cord injury from manipulating an unstable or fractured cervical spine.
- **Avoid hypotonic fluids** to limit cerebral edema.
- Steroids are not indicated for head injury.
- Avoid hypoventilation and systemic hypotension because they may reduce cerebral perfusion.
- Anticipate and conservatively treat increased intracranial pressure:
  - Head midline and elevated 30 degrees.
  - In the mechanically ventilated patient, modest hyperventilation (PCO_2 approximately 35 mm Hg) reduces intracranial pressure by cerebral vasoconstriction; excessive hyperventilation may reduce cerebral perfusion. Remember that these are merely temporizing measures and neurosurgical consultation is always warranted if there is concern for increased intracranial pressure because of head injury.
- Neurologic deterioration after head injury of any severity requires an immediate repeat head CT scan to differentiate an expanding hematoma that necessitates surgery from diffuse cerebral edema that requires monitoring and reduction of intracranial pressure.
- The use of AEDs in the acute management of TBI can reduce the incidence of early seizures but does not prevent development of epilepsy at a later time. Furthermore, certain AEDs can have adverse effects on cognition, and so these agents should only be used when clinically indicated, with careful consideration of the specific agent chosen. There is no evidence to support AED use for seizure prophylaxis.
- Because a second injury, referred to as the "second impact syndrome," may lead to severe complications including death, guidelines have been proposed for when individuals can return to play.[25]

Surgical Management

- Neurosurgical consultation is indicated for patients with contusion, intracranial hematoma, cervical fracture, skull fractures, penetrating injuries, or focal neurologic deficits.
- In cases of closed head injury complicated by increased intracranial pressure, intracranial pressure monitoring assists medical management.
- Evacuation of chronic SDH is determined by the symptoms and degree of mass effect.

Acute Spinal Cord Dysfunction

GENERAL PRINCIPLES

- Spinal cord dysfunction is demonstrated by a level below which motor, sensory, and autonomic functions are interrupted.
- **Traumatic spinal cord injury** (TSCI) may be obvious from history or examination but should also be considered in unconscious, confused, or inebriated patients with trauma.
- **Spinal cord concussion** refers to posttraumatic spinal cord symptoms and signs that resolve rapidly (hours to days).

Etiology

See Table 27-13.

DIAGNOSIS

Clinical Presentation

- **Spinal cord compression** often presents with back pain at the level of compression, progressive walking difficulties, sensory impairment, urinary retention with overflow incontinence, and diminished rectal tone. Rapid deterioration may occur.
- **Transverse myelitis or myelopathy** can present with symptoms and signs similar to cord compression.
- **Spinal shock** with hypotonia and areflexia may be present soon after traumatic event.
- Acute presentations suggest traumatic or vascular insults, whereas a subacute course suggests an enlarging mass lesion or infectious process. Autoimmune/inflammatory disorders can present in both ways.
- **Radicular signs** (lancinating pain, paresthesias, and numbness in the dermatomal distribution of a nerve root, with weakness and decreased tone and reflexes in muscles supplied by the root) suggest concurrent inflammation or compression of the corresponding nerve root. Tenderness to spinal percussion over the lesion may be present.
- **Spinal cord syndromes (Figure 27-7).**
    - **Complete cord syndrome:** Bilateral flaccid paralysis (quadriplegia or paraplegia) and loss of all sensation (anesthesia) below a dermatomal level, initially with areflexia and sphincter dysfunction (urinary retention/loss of rectal tone). With time, patients develop spasticity and hyperreflexia caudal to the lesion with possible lower motor neuron signs (areflexia and flaccid paralysis) at the level of the lesion and extensor plantar responses (Babinski signs).
    - **Brown-Séquard syndrome:** Unilateral cord lesion resulting in contralateral pain and temperature loss, with ipsilateral weakness and proprioceptive loss.
    - **Anterior cord syndrome** often results from anterior spinal artery lesion and produces bilateral pain and temperature loss and weakness below the site of the lesion with preserved proprioception and vibratory sensation.
    - **Cauda equina syndrome** from compression of the lower lumbar and sacral roots produces sensory loss in a saddle distribution, asymmetric flaccid leg weakness, decreased reflexes, and urinary/bowel incontinence due to an areflexic bladder and loss of rectal tone.
    - **Conus medullaris syndrome** has similar features to cauda equina syndrome with one important difference being the presence of mixed upper and lower motor neuron signs because of involvement of the caudal spinal cord.
    - **Central cord syndrome** is often characterized by motor impairment in upper extremities more than lower extremities, bladder dysfunction, and variable degree of sensory loss at the site of the lesion. Trauma is a common cause.

TABLE 27-13 Causes of Acute Spinal Cord Dysfunction

Structural • Tumor (primary or metastatic) • Herniated disk • Epidural abscess or hematoma • Osteomyelitis • Trauma ± fracture of bony elements • Atlantoaxial instability (e.g., rheumatoid arthritis) • Fibrocartilaginous
Ischemia/infarction (particularly after aortic surgery) • Aortic dissection or surgery • Embolic (cardiogenic, gaseous embolus) • Prolonged hypotension with underlying vascular disease • Intravascular lymphoma
Toxic • Nitrous oxide (typically in the setting of vitamin B_{12} deficiency) • Heroin
Vascular malformations (e.g., AVM) **Inflammatory/infectious (transverse myelitis)** • Multiple sclerosis • Neuromyelitis optica (classically longitudinally extensive, >3 spinal segments) • Anti–myelin oligodendrocyte protein (anti-MOG) disease • Acute disseminated encephalomyelitis • Parainfectious processes (e.g., after *Mycoplasma pneumoniae*) • Sarcoidosis • Paraneoplastic (amphiphysin and CRMP-5) • Systemic lupus erythematosus • Sjögren syndrome • Behçet disease • Viruses (e.g., enterovirus, HSV, HIV, VZV, CMV, WNV) • Fungal (extremely rare) • Lyme disease • TB • Syphilis

AVM, arteriovenous malformation; CMV, cytomegalovirus; CRMP-5, collapsing response mediator protein 5; HSV, herpes simplex virus; TB, tuberculosis; VZV, varicella-zoster virus; WNV, West Nile virus.

Diagnostic Testing

Imaging

- The presence and extent of spinal cord injuries should be confirmed with neuroimaging.
- Plain radiographs of the spine may reveal metastatic disease, osteomyelitis, discitis, fractures, or dislocation.
- Emergent MRI scan of the entire cord can confirm the exact level and extent of the lesion(s). CT myelography may be necessary in individuals unable to undergo MRI.
- CT of the spine with and without contrast can also be used to evaluate for epidural abscess, osteomyelitis, and/or discitis in patients unable to undergo MRI.

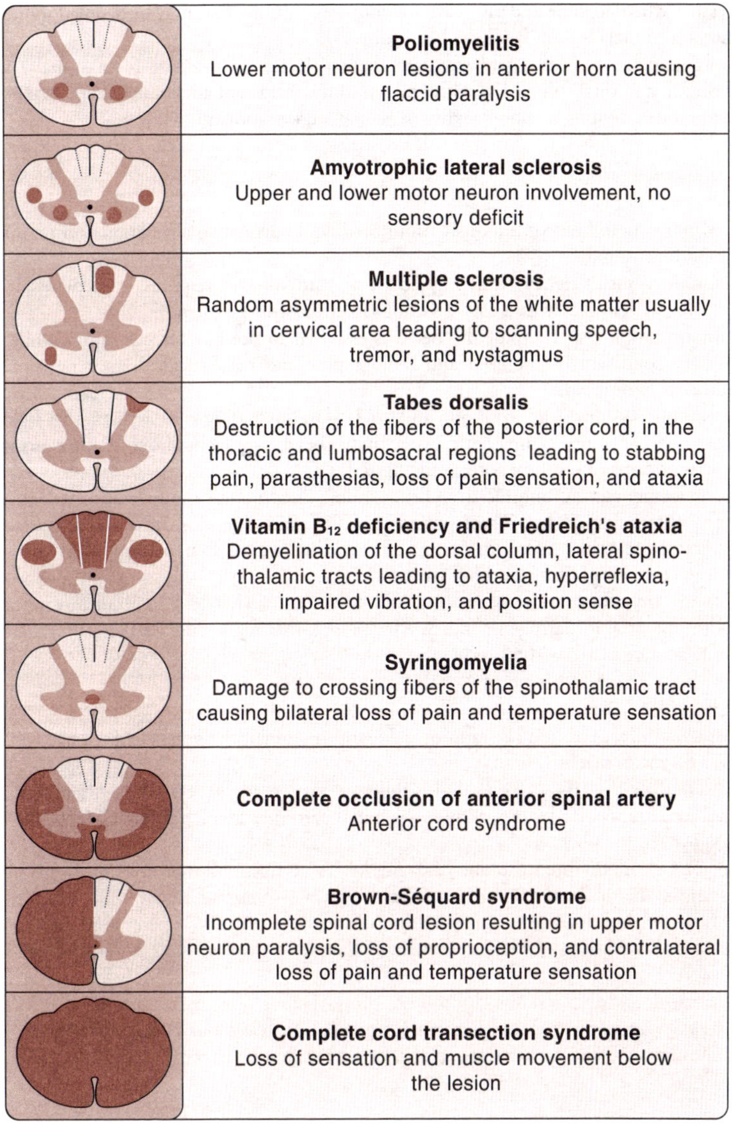

Figure 27-7 Spinal cord syndromes.

Diagnostic Procedures

- LP: Inflammatory and infectious etiologies often require CSF analysis for pleocytosis, malignant cells, abnormal protein/glucose, oligoclonal bands, and IgG index; if indicated, tests for specific pathogens and cytology/flow cytometry can be considered. If possible, imaging should be performed prior to performing an LP to rule out abscess, tumor, or other structural contraindication to LP. Remember to always check an opening pressure when possible and save CSF for additional studies that may be deemed indicated once additional clinical data have been gathered.

- Spinal angiogram is the gold standard diagnostic test to evaluate for a spinal AVM. However, a normal spine MRI with and without contrast, of adequate quality, makes the likelihood of finding an abnormality on spinal angiography quite low.

TREATMENT

- Vital signs should be continuously monitored, and adequate oxygenation and perfusion should be ensured.
- Respiratory insufficiency from high cervical cord injuries requires immediate airway control and ventilatory assistance, without manipulation of the neck.
- Immobilization, especially of the neck, is essential to prevent further injury while the patient's condition is stabilized and radiographic and neurosurgical assessment of the injuries is performed.
- Autonomic dysfunction is common and can lead to fluctuating vital signs and BP. Bladder distension can cause sympathetic overactivity (headache, tachycardia, diaphoresis, and hypertension) as a result of autonomic dysreflexia.
  - Management of autonomic dysreflexia should incorporate the help of a spinal cord rehabilitation specialist. These patients require strict attention to bowel and bladder functions (e.g., manual disimpaction, promotility agents, straight catheterization) as a means to prevent an autonomic crisis.
  - Do not treat fluctuations in vital signs blindly because changes can occur precipitously with potential for iatrogenic injury. Always look first for a cause and treat fluctuations in heart rate or BP with caution.

Medications

- Treatable infections require appropriate antimicrobial therapies (e.g., acyclovir for varicella-zoster myelitis).
- **Dexamethasone,** 10–20 mg IV bolus followed by 2–4 mg IV q6–8h, is often administered for compressive lesions, tumors, or spinal cord infarction, although benefit has not been proven for all etiologies.
- For TSCI, **methylprednisolone**, 30 mg/kg IV bolus, followed by an infusion of 5.4 mg/kg/h for 24 hours when initiated within 3 hours of injury, and infusion for 48 hours when initiated within 3–8 hours of injury, may improve neurologic recovery.
- The first-line therapy for the treatment of transverse myelitis is high-dose intravenous glucocorticoids.
- Pharmacologic deep venous thrombosis prophylaxis is extremely important. LMWH is superior to unfractionated heparin for prevention of venous thromboembolism and pulmonary embolism. Inferior vena cava filters should be considered in bedbound patients.

Surgical Management

Neurosurgical consultation should be obtained because in many cases, spinal cord compression can be decompressed and stabilized. Penetrating injury, foreign bodies, comminuted fractures, misalignment, and hematoma may require surgical treatment.

SPECIAL CONSIDERATIONS

Emergent radiation therapy combined with high-dose steroids is usually indicated for cord compression because of malignancy and generally requires a histologic diagnosis.

MONITORING/FOLLOW-UP

Long-term supportive care is important for patients with spinal cord dysfunction. Pulmonary and urinary infections, skin breakdown, joint contractures, spasticity, and irregular bowel and bladder elimination are common long-term problems.

Parkinson Disease

GENERAL PRINCIPLES

- Parkinson disease (PD) is a chronic, progressive neurodegenerative disease characterized by at least two of three cardinal features: resting tremor, bradykinesia, and rigidity. Often, postural instability is seen later in the disease.
- The neurologic examination remains the gold standard diagnostic test for PD.
- Cognitive dysfunction and dementia are common in PD (one-third of patients in most studies; six times higher than age-matched controls). Considerable overlap can occur between AD and PD.
  - One-third of PD patients are depressed.
  - Olfactory dysfunction, autonomic dysfunction, and sleep disorders are also common in PD and have a significant impact on quality of life.

Epidemiology

Parkinson's disease caused 2,11, 296 deaths globally and 3.2 million DALYs.

Increasing life expectancy is contributing to higher prevalence.*

DIAGNOSIS

Clinical Presentation

- The parkinsonian tremor is a resting pill rolling tremor (3–7 Hz) that is often asymmetric.[26]
- Bradykinesia is characterized by generalized slowness of movement, especially in finger movement dexterity and gait (often shuffling).
- Cogwheel rigidity is often observed with a ratchety pattern of resistance and relaxation as examiner moves limbs ("cog wheeling" is because of the rigidity with a superimposed tremor).
- Postural instability can be assessed by the "pull" test, where the examiner pulls the patient by the shoulders while standing behind the patient.
- Other signs that are often associated but not required for diagnosis include masked-like facies, decreased eye blink, increased salivation, hypokinetic dysarthria, micrographia, constipation, anosmia, and sleep disorders, particularly rapid eye movement sleep behavior disorder.
- Dementia seen with PD is typically subcortical with psychomotor retardation, memory difficulty, and altered personality. Accordingly, a brief cognitive assessment (e.g., MoCA) could be considered as a screening test for cognitive dysfunction.
- Disorders which mimic idiopathic Parkinson disease but have symmetrical onset, atypical or absent tremor, autonomic dysfunction which is prominent and early, profound postural disturbances, gaze abnormalities, corticospinal, and cerebellar involvement with early dementia are called Parkinson plus syndromes. They respond poorly to levodopa. They are progressive supranuclear palsy, multiple system atrophy, corticobasal degeneration, and dementia lewy body (Table 27-14).†

* Wanneveich M, Moisan F, Jacqmin-Gadda H, et al. Projections of prevalence, lifetime risk and life expectancy of Parkinson disease (2010–2030) in France. *Mov Disord.* 2018;33(9):1449–1455.

† Mitra K, Gangopadhaya PK, Das SK. Parkinsonism plus syndrome—a review. *Neurol India.* 2003;51(2):183–188.

TABLE 27-14	Parkinson Plus Syndromes
Multiple systems atrophy	• Autonomic failure—Shy–Drager syndrome • Cerebellar involvement • Pyramidal tract degeneration • Postural hypotension • Sphincter disturbance (impotence/urinary incontinence) • Cerebellar signs
Progressive supra-nuclear palsy	• Supranuclear paralysis of eye movements – frequent falls • Pyramidal signs • Cognitive impairment • Axial rigidity • Failure of vertical gaze
Corticobasal Degeneration	• Extreme rigidity • Focal myoclonus, dystonia • Alien limb phenomenon • Apraxia
Lewy body dementia	• Early progressive dementia • Nocturnal wanderings ± confusion • Hallucinations
Drug-induced parkinsonism	• Symmetrical disease • Younger patient • Seen in persons taking dopamine antagonists/lithium
Vascular parkinsonism	• Sudden onset • Stuttering progression • Minimal tremor • Lower limbs affected >upper limbs

Differential Diagnosis

See Table 27-15.

Diagnostic Testing

MRI of the brain (or head CT with contrast in patients unable to undergo MRI) should be performed to exclude specific structural abnormalities.

TABLE 27-15	Differential Diagnosis of Parkinson Disease

• Essential tremor
  ◦ Action tremor
• Dementia with Lewy bodies
  ◦ Visual hallucinations, fluctuating cognition, sensitivity to neuroleptics
• Parkinson plus diseases: corticobasal degeneration, multiple system atrophy, progressive supranuclear palsy
• Alzheimer disease
• Frontotemporal dementia
  ◦ Changes in personality
• Huntington disease
• Wilson disease and other neurodegenerative disorders with metal accumulation
• Toxic/iatrogenic
  ◦ Carbon monoxide, manganese, neuroleptics, other dopamine receptor antagonists	

TREATMENT

Medications

- **PD patients should not be given neuroleptics or any dopamine-blocking medications under any circumstances** (prochlorperazine, metoclopramide) because this can have devastating consequences ranging from worsening PD symptoms to death.[27] If a neuroleptic is absolutely necessary, quetiapine and clozapine are the safest, but the risk/benefit profile needs to be considered. Pimavanserin has also been approved specifically for PD psychosis.
- Treatment of PD can be divided into neuroprotective and symptomatic therapy.
- Initiation of symptomatic treatment for a PD patient is determined by the degree to which the patient is functionally impaired.

First Line

- Carbidopa–levodopa (CL) is the most effective symptomatic therapy for PD and is often considered when both the patient and the physician decide that quality of life of the patient is being affected by PD. It requires frequent dosing and is associated with the highest risk of dopaminergic motor complications. Levodopa is more likely to cause dyskinesia than other options within the first five years, and thus the minimum effective dose should be used and patients should be counseled regarding this risk
- MAO-B inhibitors such as selegiline, rasagiline, and safinamide can also be used in combination with levodopa-based preparations to allow for a reduction in the levodopa dose.
- Dopamine agonists (pramipexole, ropinirole) can be used as monotherapy or in combination with other PD medications. They are ineffective in patients who show no response to levodopa. They are often used in patients who develop significant dyskinesias or motor fluctuations on CL, but these drugs are less efficacious and have more adverse effects.
- Many patients can be managed with CL alone without need for agonist therapy.

Second Line

- Amantadine and catechol-*O*-methyl transferase inhibitors (entacapone, tolcapone, and opicapone) can help supplement the effects of dopamine replacement therapy and are beneficial with regard to the dyskinesias and fluctuations, respectively, commonly experienced by patients.
- Anticholinergic drugs (benztropine, orphenadrine, procyclidine, and trihexyphenidyl [Benzhexol]) are used only in younger patients in whom tremor is the predominant symptom.

Third Line

Deep brain stimulation and Duodopa (intestinal infusion of carbidopa/levodopa gel) have benefit in PD patients who progress to develop motor fluctuations and dyskinesias unresponsive to oral medications. It is important to note that advanced therapies are not a cure for PD and patients will continue to progress.

COMPLICATIONS

- Patients can develop neuroleptic malignant syndrome (NMS) after sudden withdrawal of levodopa or dopamine agonists and following exposure to neuroleptics or other antidopaminergic drugs.
- Serotonin syndrome can occur when monoamine oxidase inhibitors (MAOIs) are combined with TCAs or SSRIs.

Ataxias

Ataxias are disorders which cause abnormalities in rate, range, force, and direction of movement. Ataxias can be broadly classified into sensory ataxia, cerebellar ataxia, or vestibular ataxia (Table 27-16). A positive Romberg's sign strongly favors a sensory ataxia. If the ataxia is symmetric toxins, infections, postinfectious syndrome, paraneoplastic, vitamin B12 deficiency, and endocrine causes like hypothyroidism must be suspected. If the ataxia is asymmetrical demyelination, tumors, and vascular causes are to be suspected. Genetic ataxias are spinocerebellar ataxia, Friedreich ataxia, ataxia telangiectasia, episodic ataxias, and dentatorubropallidoluysian atrophy. The primary aim of the treatment is to identify reversible causes like thyroid disorders, vitamin deficiencies, surgically resectable tumors, and address them.

TABLE 27-16 Differences Between Vestibular, Sensory, and Cerebellar Ataxia

	Vestibular	Sensory	Cerebellar
Nystagmus	Present	Absent	Often present
Vertigo	Present	Absent	May be present
Dysarthria	Absent	Absent	May be present
Stance	May be able to stand with feet together, typically worse with eyes closed	Often able to stand with feet together and eyes open but not with eyes closed (Romberg sign)	Unable to stand with feet together, eyes either open or closed
Limb ataxia	Absent	Present (legs)	Usually present (all limbs, only legs unilateral or one limb)
Ankle reflexes	Normal	Impaired	Normal
Vibration and position sense	Normal	Depressed or absent	Normal

NEUROMUSCULAR DISEASE

Guillain-Barré Syndrome

GENERAL PRINCIPLES

Definition

Guillain-Barré syndrome (GBS) is an acute polyradiculoneuropathy syndrome and a common cause of acute flaccid paralysis. There are many GBS subtypes with marked geographic variability in their prevalence. The clinical syndrome is classically characterized by ascending weakness, distal paresthesias, and areflexia. Classically, GBS follows a viral infection, vaccination, or surgery, but in many instances, no prodrome is identified.

Acute immune/inflammatory demyelinating polyneuropathy **(AIDP) is the commonest type of GBS in the world but studies have shown that** acute motor axonal neuropathy **(AMAN) variant is more common in Asian countries.***

Classification

- AIDP variant is the most common GBS variant in North America. It is an acute immune-mediated polyneuropathy/radiculopathy with presumed autoantibodies (as yet unidentified) directed against myelin antigens.
- Axonal variants of GBS include AMAN, acute motor and sensory axonal neuropathy (AMSAN), acute motor conduction block neuropathy (AMCBN), Miller Fisher syndrome (MFS), and pharyngeal-cervical-brachial (PCB) weakness. Many of these syndromes are associated with antiganglioside antibodies directed against gangliosides located in the axolemma near the nodes of Ranvier. These axonal variants are much more common in Japan, China, and third-world countries than they are in the United States. Antibody associations include the following:
    - IgG anti-GM1 antibodies in AMAN and AMCBN
    - IgG anti-GQ1b and less commonly IgG anti-GT1a in MFS, a syndrome consisting of ophthalmoparesis, ataxia, and areflexia
    - IgG anti-GT1a and less commonly IgG anti-GQ1b in PCB weakness syndrome

Pathophysiology

- GBS results from an attack of peripheral myelin or axons mediated by autoantibodies originally generated in response to an infection that typically precedes the onset of neuropathy symptoms by days to weeks. These antibodies cross-react with the myelin or nodal axolemma antigens via molecular mimicry.
- This concept is well established in the axonal variants where there is definitive evidence of molecular mimicry between *Campylobacter jejuni* lipo-oligosaccharides and the ganglioside antigens listed above. In fact, GBS was the first disease to illustrate the concept of molecular mimicry and fulfills all four criteria ("Witebsky postulates") for designation as an autoimmune disease.
- This concept is less well established in AIDP, given the absence of a known autoantibody/myelin antigen. Prodromal infections commonly associated with AIDP include cytomegalovirus and Epstein–Barr virus.

DIAGNOSIS

Clinical Presentation

- AIDP typically presents with progressive, symmetric ascending paralysis.
- Mild asymmetries are common, but major asymmetries are a red flag suggestive of an alternative diagnosis.
- Reflexes are almost always hypoactive or absent. Exceptions exist, especially with the axonal variants (in particular with Fisher–Bickerstaff syndrome, which has elements of MFS along with hypersomnolence in the setting of concurrent brainstem encephalitis).
- Sensory symptoms, such as paresthesias in the hands and feet, are often present, but objective sensory loss is uncommon.
- Facial and/or oropharyngeal weakness occurs in about 70% of AIDP patients.
- Respiratory failure, necessitating intubation, occurs in 25%–30% of patients.[28]
- Pain in the back, hips, and thighs is common. Pain is one of the most common presenting symptoms of GBS in the pediatric population.

---

* Bae JS, Yuki N, Kuwabara S, et al. *Guillain–Barre syndrome in Asia. J Neurol Neurosurg Psychiatry.* 2013;85(8):907–913.

- Autonomic instability is common (approximately 60%) and potentially life threatening. Common manifestations include tachycardia/bradycardia, hypotension alternating with hypertension, and ileus.

Differential Diagnosis

See Table 27-17.

Diagnostic Testing

Imaging

MRI of the spine is indicated in atypical cases or in those with concern for one of the differentials listed earlier that could result in myeloradiculopathy. Nerve root contrast enhancement and/or thickening can be seen with GBS.

Diagnostic Procedures

- **LP should be performed to narrow the differential and evaluate for albuminocytologic dissociation.**
- CSF protein is usually elevated about 1 week after symptom onset. It may be normal if checked earlier (e.g., 85% of patients with normal CSF within first 2 days).
- CSF leukocytosis is uncommon, and if present (especially >25 cells/μL), an alternative diagnosis should be considered. (Note CSF pleocytosis may be present if associated with HIV)

TABLE 27-17 Differential Diagnosis of Acute Immune Demyelinating Polyneuropathy

- Acute/initial presentation of chronic inflammatory demyelinating polyneuropathy
- Paraproteinemic/paraneoplastic polyradiculopathy/polyneuropathy
- Diabetic/nondiabetic lumbosacral radiculoplexopathies
- Sarcoidosis
- Mononeuritis multiplex (confluent)
- West Nile and polioviruses (usually has fever, CSF pleocytosis, and often asymmetric paralysis)
- HIV
- Lyme disease (if in endemic area)
- Postdiphtheric paralysis
- Tick paralysis and other neurotoxins
- Myasthenia gravis (MFS variant)
- Critical illness myopathy
- Prolonged neuromuscular junction blockade
- Periodic paralysis
- Thiamine deficiency (MFS variant in particular)
- Botulism
- Arsenic
- Lead
- Chemotherapy
- Acute intermittent porphyria
- Carcinomatous or lymphomatous meningitis with root involvement
- Functional weakness/conversion disorder

See http://neuromuscular.wustl.edu/time/nmacute.htm for further information.
CSF, cerebral spinal fluid; MFS, Miller Fisher syndrome variant of Guillain-Barré Syndrome (associated with ataxia, areflexia, and ophthalmoparesis).

- Nerve conduction studies (NCS) and electromyography (EMG) are a very important part of the evaluation but should not delay initiation of treatment, particularly in severe cases. NCS should include evaluation of the proximal nerve segments via "late" responses (F-waves and H-reflexes). EMG-NCS performed early in the disease course may have very few abnormalities and can even be normal but serves an important role in the diagnostic evaluation, even when normal. A repeat study after a few weeks can be extremely useful for classification and prognostication, particularly when there is a baseline study available for comparison.

TREATMENT

- Follow **respiratory function closely**, including oximetry and frequent bedside measurements of vital capacity (VC) and negative inspiratory force (NIF).
- We use the "20/30" rule in identifying patients who will likely require ventilatory support: <20 mL/kg of forced VC (FVC) (approximately 1.5 L for an average-size adult) and an NIF >–30 cm H_2O. These parameters provide a more sensitive measure for impending respiratory failure than do the presence of hypoxia, dyspnea, and acidosis. The threshold for elective intubation should be low.
- If NIF/FVC testing is not available at the bedside, a quick and indirect measure is to ask the patient to count to as high a number as possible on one breath. Each number equals 100 mL of VC (e.g., a count to 10 = 1 L).
- Paroxysmal hypertension should not be treated with antihypertensive medications unless absolutely necessary (e.g., signs of end-organ injury or comorbid coronary artery disease). If necessary, extremely low doses of titratable short-acting agents are preferred.
- Hypotension is usually caused by decreased venous return and peripheral vasodilation. Mechanically ventilated patients are particularly prone to hypotension. Treatment consists of intravascular volume expansion; occasionally, vasopressors may be required (see Chapter 8, Critical Care).
- Continuous telemetry monitoring is necessary to monitor for cardiac arrhythmias.
- Prevention of exposure keratitis of the eye, venous thrombosis, and vigilance for hyponatremia, including syndrome of inappropriate diuretic hormone, should be priorities.

Medications

- **Plasma exchange (PLEX) and IV immunoglobulin (IVIG)** are comparably effective in improving outcomes and shortening duration of disease when administered early to patients who cannot walk or have respiratory failure.[29] The decision between the two depends on the individual patient's comorbidities and medical history.
- Corticosteroids are not indicated and may actually delay recovery.
- Neuropathic pain medications may be needed.

Other Nonpharmacologic Therapies

Physical therapy to prevent contractures and to improve strength and function should be started early.

COMPLICATIONS

Complications from prolonged hospitalization and ventilation may occur. These include aspiration pneumonia, sepsis, pressure ulcers, and pulmonary embolism.

PROGNOSIS

- The disease typically progresses over 2–4 weeks, with all patients, by definition, reaching their nadir by 4 weeks.
- This is followed by a plateau of several weeks in duration.
- Recovery takes place over months.
  - Overall, about 80% of patients recover completely or have only minor deficits.[30]
  - A total of 5%–10% of patients (usually elderly patients and those with more severe disease) have significant permanent residual disability, and 3% remain wheelchair bound.
- Of course, there are many exceptions, and many patients have a shorter course and/or a quicker recovery.
- About 5% of the patients die because of respiratory or autonomic complications despite optimal medical therapy.
- By definition, GBS is a monophasic disease, and a recurrence of symptoms should lead you to revisit the original diagnosis (e.g., consider chronic inflammatory demyelinating polyneuropathy). Repeat electrodiagnostic studies are critical in determining the etiology of an apparent "recurrent GBS" and emphasize the importance of obtaining a baseline study soon after presentation.

CHRONIC INFLAMMATORY DEMYELINATING POLYNEUROPATHY

It is a chronic acquired immune mediated polyneuropathy with onset like GBS but lasting for >8 weeks. It presents with a stepwise progressive/relapsing weakness more common in 50–60 years of age. Pathologically nerve biopsy shows evidence of repeated demyelination and remyelination. Prednisolone remains the cornerstone of treatment with acute episodes managed by ivig/plasma exchange. Differential diagnosis includes distal acquired demyelinating symmetrical (DADS) neuropathy, multifocal acquired demyelinating sensory and motor (MADSAM) neuropathy, and multifocal motor neuropathy (MMN).*

Myasthenia Gravis

GENERAL PRINCIPLES

Definition

Myasthenia gravis (MG) is an autoimmune disorder that involves antibody-mediated postsynaptic dysfunction of the neuromuscular junction of skeletal muscle resulting in fatigable weakness.

Classification

- Generalized disease is most common and affects a variable combination of ocular, bulbar, respiratory, and appendicular muscles.
- Ocular MG is confined to eyelid and oculomotor function. It accounts for 10%–40% of all MG cases. The longer a patient with ocular MG goes without evidence of generalization, the less likely he or she is to develop generalized MG (<5% will advance to generalized MG if there are no symptoms of generalization by 2 years).

---

*Dimachkie MM, Barohn RJ. Chronic inflammatory demyelinating polyneuropathy. *Curr Treat Options Neurol.* 2013;15(3):350–366.

Epidemiology

Bimodal distribution with peak incidence in women in the second and third decades and in men in the sixth and seventh decades. **In the Western world the disease is more common in females whereas a large study from India shows male predominance in this part of the world.***

Pathophysiology

MG is an acquired autoimmune disorder resulting from the production of autoantibodies against the postsynaptic acetylcholine receptor (AChR) or, less commonly, against receptor-associated proteins, including muscle-specific receptor tyrosine kinase (MuSK) or low-density lipoprotein receptor-related protein 4 (LRP4). However, despite the identification of these additional antigens, "seronegative" forms still account for up to 10% of MG patients. One must consider hereditary/congenital forms of MG and avoid mistakenly lumping these patients or the anti-LRP4 or anti-MuSK patients into this group.

Associated Conditions

- MG is often associated with thymus hyperplasia; 10% may have a malignant thymoma. Hyperplasia is more common in those under 40 years of age. Thymoma is more common in MG patients over 30 years of age. There are data to support thymectomy in all patients with generalized MG under the age of 65, regardless of the presence of thymic hyperplasia or thymoma.[31] Thymectomy for non–thymoma-associated generalized MG in patients over the age of 65 years is generally reserved for treatment refractory cases and can be considered on a case-by-case basis.
- Autoimmune thyroiditis (hyper- more common than hypo-) is present in approximately 15% of patients with MG. MG patients also have an increased risk of other autoimmune diseases including lupus, rheumatoid arthritis, polymyositis, and pernicious anemia.

DIAGNOSIS

Clinical Presentation

History

- The cardinal feature of MG is fluctuating weakness that is worse after exercise or prolonged activity and improves with rest.
- More than 50% of patients present with ptosis that may be asymmetric.
- Other common complaints include blurred vision or diplopia, trouble smiling, and difficulties with chewing, swallowing, and speaking (e.g., winded at end of sentences, "staccato" [interrupted] speech, nasal speech, or weak voice).
- Weakness of neck flexors and extensors and proximal arm weakness are common. MG is one of the few neuromuscular disorders to cause prominent neck extensor weakness, creating a "head drop."
- **Myasthenic crisis** consists of respiratory failure or the need for airway protection and occurs in approximately 15%–20% of MG patients.[32] Patients with bulbar and respiratory muscle weakness are particularly prone to respiratory failure, which may develop rapidly and unexpectedly. They require as much vigilance and monitoring as do patients with GBS.
- Respiratory infection, surgery (e.g., thymectomy), medications (e.g., aminoglycosides, quinine, quinolones, β-blockers, lithium, magnesium sulfate), pregnancy, and thyroid dysfunction can precipitate crisis or exacerbate symptoms. However, it is important to note that none of these medications should be withheld if required to treat a concurrent illness.

---

*Singhal BS, Bhatia NS, Umesh T, Menon S. Myasthenia gravis: a study from India. *Neurol India.* 2008;56:352–355.

Anticholinergic medications are a notable exception to this rule for obvious reasons, and in the absence of a life-threatening indication, their use should be avoided.

Physical Examination

- Presenting signs include ptosis, diplopia, dysarthria, dysphagia, extremity weakness, and respiratory difficulty.
- Fatigability on examination is a useful diagnostic feature.
- Ptosis may worsen after prolonged upward gaze (usually by 60 seconds). Patients may also begin to develop diplopia after sustained gaze in one direction.
- Carefully evaluate the airway, handling of secretions, ventilation, and the work of breathing.
- NIF and FVC are useful at the bedside to assess for respiratory muscle weakness. The breath count test described earlier in the GBS section is also useful in this population. The same general rules for ventilatory support (inability to protect airway or ventilate adequately) apply.

Differential Diagnosis

- Lambert-Eaton myasthenic syndrome (LEMS) is an autoimmune disease affecting the presynaptic voltage-gated calcium channels of the neuromuscular junction. It is frequently associated with malignancy (small cell lung cancer). LEMS also presents with fluctuating weakness, but the weakness improves for a brief period after exercise. Weakness in LEMS is classically more prominent in the legs relative to the arms, and unlike MG, oculobulbar deficits are uncommon. A quick bedside examination finding that may be present is to evaluate for facilitation of reflexes that are absent or diminished at rest but present or increased after 10 seconds of isometric exercise.
- Amyotrophic lateral sclerosis (ALS) may present with bulbar weakness and a "head drop." However, ALS can be differentiated from MG by presence of upper motor neuron signs in the former. Electrodiagnostic studies are also very useful in distinguishing the two.
- The differential also includes botulism (covered in more detail below), congenital forms of myasthenia, mitochondrial disorders (e.g., chronic progressive external ophthalmoplegia), and acquired and hereditary myopathies or other motor neuronopathies (other than ALS).

Diagnostic Testing

A good rule of thumb is to have two lines of diagnostic evidence (usually serologic and electrodiagnostic) in the appropriate clinical context to make a diagnosis of autoimmune MG.

Laboratory Studies

- Serum **AChR binding antibodies** are detected in 85%–90% of adult generalized MG patients and in 50%–70% of ocular MG patients.
- **MuSK antibodies** are detected in about 30%–70% of AChR antibody–negative MG patients.
- Thyroid function should be checked to evaluate for autoimmune thyroiditis.

Imaging

Chest CT is indicated to screen for a **thymoma.**

Diagnostic Procedures

Electrodiagnostic studies are an important step in diagnosing MG.

- Repetitive nerve stimulation (RNS) at 2–5 Hz typically shows >10% decrement in the amplitude of the compound muscle action potential (CMAP) in MG. If the patient is taking pyridostigmine, it should be held (if possible) because it could mask a decrement.

RNS has a higher yield when it is performed on **weak** proximal muscles. Accordingly, it is only positive in 50% of patients with ocular MG.

- It should be noted that a decrement on slow RNS is not 100% specific for MG and can also be seen in LEMS, botulism, motor neuronopathies/neuropathies, and myopathies.
- In LEMS, the response is incremental with fast RNS (20–50 Hz). Because fast RNS is extremely painful, an adequate supplement is to look for an increment in CMAP amplitude after 10 seconds of tetanic isometric exercise (pre- and postexercise CMAPs).
- Single-fiber EMG has a sensitivity of >95% for both generalized and ocular MG when performed on facial muscles. However, the specificity is much lower (abnormalities also seen in LEMS, botulism, motor neuronopathies/neuropathies, and myopathies). It is usually reserved for those with suspected disease (based on clinical symptoms) but negative antibody and RNS testing.
- Edrophonium testing is no longer routinely used.
- Myasthenic weakness is often improved by cold. Although the history obtained from the patient may suggest this phenomenon, the "**ice pack test**" is an easy and safe, objective "bedside" measure of this phenomenon and is often helpful in the evaluation of ocular MG. For 2–5 minutes an ice pack is applied to upper eyelid. If ptosis improves by >2 mm or more, the test is considered positive.

TREATMENT

- Treatment of MG is individualized and depends on the severity of the disease, age, comorbidities, and response to therapy.
- **Myasthenic crisis** requires prompt recognition and aggressive support.
    - Consider intensive care unit (ICU) level care and elective intubation for FVC <20 mL/kg or NIF >–30 cm H_2O (similar parameters to the "20/30" rule used for GBS).
    - Given the potential for fairly rapid improvement with acute immunomodulatory therapies (see below), noninvasive ventilation (e.g., bilevel positive airway pressure) can also be considered, in patients with adequate airway protection, as a means to avoid invasive ventilation.
    - Treat superimposed infections and metabolic derangements.
    - **Plasmapheresis** and IVIG are both used to treat MG crises/exacerbations and have equal efficacy with a similar rate of adverse effects.[33] However, expert guidelines support the use of plasmapheresis over IVIG in myasthenic crisis, given its greater short term efficacy and quicker onset of action, unless there are comorbidities or elements of the individual's medical history that make IVIG the better option.[34] As for GBS, the decision ultimately depends on the individual patient's comorbidities and medical history.
    - Because the effects of PLEX or IVIG are relatively rapid in onset but short lived, corticosteroids are typically started soon after initiating PLEX, usually at a dose of 10–20 mg/d and slowly titrated (e.g., by 5 mg every 3 days) to a dose of 50 mg/d.
    - Anticholinesterases should be temporarily withdrawn from patients who are receiving ventilation support to avoid cholinergic stimulation of pulmonary secretions.
    - Neuromuscular blocking agents should be avoided.

Medications

First Line

Anticholinesterase drugs can produce symptomatic improvement in most forms of MG (anti-MuSK MG is frequently an exception).

Pyridostigmine should be started at 30–60 mg PO tid–qid and titrated for symptom relief.

Second Line

- Immunosuppressive drugs are typically used when additional benefit is needed beyond cholinesterase inhibitors.
- High doses of **prednisone** can be used to achieve rapid improvement. **However, up to 50% of patients experience a transient worsening of weakness on initiation of prednisone therapy.** Hence, it is important to start low and increase slow (see above), especially if the patient has not been or is not being treated with PLEX or IVIG.
- Azathioprine, mycophenolate mofetil, cyclosporine A, tacrolimus, and cyclophosphamide are steroid-sparing immunomodulatory agents that have all been used to treat MG with varying degrees of evidence to support their efficacy.
- There is strong evidence that rituximab (anti-CD20 chimeric monoclonal antibody) has great efficacy in treating anti-MuSK MG. Its utility in medically refractory anti-AChR MG disease is currently under investigation.
- Eculizumab (Soliris), a humanized monoclonal antibody that binds with high affinity to human terminal complement protein C5, is approved for use in treatment refractory anti-AChR MG.

Surgical Management

- Thymectomy is indicated in all patients with thymoma, regardless of age, and in patients with generalized MG that are 65 years of age or younger.[30]
- Thymectomy in ocular MG patients and generalized MG patients over the age of 65 is considered on a case-by-case basis.

Other Neuromuscular Disorders

GENERAL PRINCIPLES

- **Myopathies:** Rapidly progressive proximal muscle weakness can be caused by many drugs including but not limited to ethanol, steroids, colchicine, cyclosporine, and cholesterol-lowering drugs (particularly in combination). Other common causes include HIV or HIV therapies, particularly zidovudine, and hypothyroidism.
  - **Critical illness myopathy** is increasingly recognized in patients with critical illness. **Myosin loss myopathy** accounts for a percentage of patients with critical illness myopathy and is commonly associated with clinical features of respiratory failure (e.g., difficulties weaning from the ventilator), severe weakness, and classic risk factors include exposure to high-dose corticosteroids and/or neuromuscular-blocking agents. The diagnosis of myosin loss myopathy requires pathologic confirmation (i.e., a muscle biopsy must be performed).
  - **Polymyositis (PM) and dermatomyositis (DM)** fall into a class of diseases now referred to as the idiopathic immune and inflammatory myopathies (IIMs). Most forms respond well to immunomodulatory therapy with a notable exception being the inclusion body myopathies. DM and PM can also be a component of a syndrome affecting multiple different organ systems. Perhaps the best examples are antisynthetase syndromes, such as Jo-1 myositis, which involves skin, joint, lung, and muscle. Patients suspected of having DM or PM should have myositis-specific and myositis-associated autoantibodies checked and should be screened for interstitial lung disease, which has a high degree of morbidity if left untreated (see Chapter 25, Arthritis and Rheumatologic Diseases).
- **Rhabdomyolysis** may produce rapid muscle weakness, leading to hyperkalemia, myoglobinuria (by definition true rhabdomyolysis causes myoglobinuria), and renal failure (for management, see Chapter 12, Fluid and Electrolyte Management, and Chapter 13, Renal Diseases). The potential etiologies include metabolic (deficits of lipid or carbohydrate metabolism), excessive exercise/exertion (including seizures/dystonia), drugs (abuse and

prescribed), ischemic, compression/crush (trauma), infection/inflammatory, noxious (toxins), and electrolyte abnormalities (diabetic ketoacidosis, hyperosmolar hyperglycemic nonketotic syndrome, hypokalemia). Statin drugs causing rhabdomyolysis are increasingly evident nowadays and being of Asian origin increases incidence of rhabdomyolysis with the use of statins.*

- **Botulism** is a disorder of the **neuromuscular junction** caused by ingestion of an exotoxin produced by *Clostridium botulinum*, acquired through a wound or via an iatrogenic route.
  - The exotoxin interferes with release of acetylcholine from presynaptic terminals at the neuromuscular junction.
  - In infants, it is commonly attributed to gastrointestinal (GI) colonization in the first 6 months of life when normal gut flora is not yet present. Classically, it is associated with ingestion of raw honey, but inhalation/ingestion of soil-based spores and wound botulism from "skin popping" (i.e., injection of drugs of abuse underneath the skin) are likely more common means of absorption.
  - Symptoms begin within 12–36 hours of ingestion in food-borne botulism and within 10 days in wound botulism.
  - Symptoms include **autonomic dysfunction** (xerostomia, blurred vision, urinary retention, and constipation), followed by **cranial nerve palsies**, **descending weakness**, and **possibly respiratory distress.**
  - **Serum assays for botulinum toxin** may aid diagnosis in adults.
  - Management includes removing nonabsorbed toxin with **cathartics**, **supportive care**, and neutralizing absorbed toxin with **equine trivalent** (A, B, E) **antitoxin** (more immunogenic because it contains both the Fab and Fc portions) or **heptavalent** (A, B, C, D, E, F, G) **antitoxin** (less immunogenic as Fc portion is cleaved off and has $F(ab)_2$ portions). Penicillin G is often administered, but no formal clinical trials have been performed. There is some evidence that botulism immune globulin can shorten hospital stay by approximately 2 weeks.[35]
  - Recovery is slow and occurs spontaneously, but with appropriate ventilatory and supportive care, most make a full recovery.

Disorders with Rigidity

GENERAL PRINCIPLES

- **NMS** is associated with the use of neuroleptic drugs, certain antiemetic drugs (e.g., metoclopramide, promethazine), and sudden withdrawal of dopamine agonists (L-dopa in PD) and can even occur as an "off" phenomenon in PD patients experiencing severe "on–off" fluctuations.
  - Features include hyperthermia, altered mental status, muscular rigidity, and dysautonomia.
  - Laboratory abnormalities include a leukocytosis and a markedly elevated creatine kinase with myoglobinuria.
  - Treatment includes discontinuing precipitating drug(s), restarting medications that were stopped (in the case of a PD patient), cooling and paralytics (if necessary), monitoring and supporting vital functions (arrhythmias, shock, hyperkalemia, acidosis, renal failure, and management of rhabdomyolysis), and administering dantrolene and/or bromocriptine. Treatment is essentially identical to that used for malignant hyperthermia (see the following text).

*Antons KA, Williams CD, Bake SK, et al. Clinical perspectives of statin-induced rhabdomyolysis. *Am J Med.* 2006;119(5):400–409.

- **Serotonin syndrome** results from excessive serotonergic activity, especially following recent dosage changes of SSRIs, MAOIs, and TCAs.
  - It presents as a **triad of mental status change, autonomic overactivity**, and **neuromuscular abnormalities.** Distinguishing features of serotonin syndrome from NMS include the degree of mental status change, seizures, and the marked hyperreflexia. However, in certain circumstances, the two can be difficult to distinguish from one another.
  - Hyperthermia, tremor, nausea, vomiting, and clonus are common signs.
  - Treatment includes removal of offending drugs, aggressive supportive care, cyproheptadine, and benzodiazepines.[36]
- **Malignant hyperthermia** is the acute development of high fever, obtundation, and muscular rigidity following triggering factors (e.g., halothane anesthesia, succinylcholine).
  - The most common etiology is an autosomal dominant mutation in the ryanodine receptor (*RYR1*), making a screen of the family history a critical part of the preoperative evaluation. Abnormalities in this calcium channel predispose patients to an elevation in intracytoplasmic calcium triggered by certain anesthetics. Other ion channels have also been identified, and children with dystrophinopathies and other forms of muscular dystrophy are also at an increased risk.
  - **Serum creatine kinase is markedly elevated.** Renal failure from myoglobinuria and cardiac arrhythmias from electrolyte imbalance can be life threatening.
  - Successful management requires prompt recognition of early indicators of the syndrome (increased end-tidal carbon dioxide, tachycardia, acidosis, and/or muscle rigidity; note, hyperthermia comes later if at all); discontinuation of the offending anesthetic agent; aggressive supportive care that focuses on oxygenation/ventilation, circulation, correction of acid–base and electrolyte derangements; and administration of **dantrolene sodium**, 1–10 mg/kg/d, for at least 48–96 hours to reduce muscular rigidity.
- **Tetanus** typically presents with generalized muscle spasm (especially trismus) caused by the exotoxin (tetanospasmin) from *Clostridium tetani*, a Gram-positive bacillus commonly found in intestinal flora and soil.
  - The organism usually enters the body through wounds. Onset typically occurs within 7–21 days of an injury.[37]
  - Patients who are **unvaccinated or have reduced immunity** are at risk, underscoring the importance of prevention by tetanus toxoid boosters following wounds. Tetanus may occur in **drug abusers who inject SC.**
  - Management consists of supportive care, particularly airway control (laryngospasm) and treatment of muscle spasms (benzodiazepines, barbiturates, analgesics, and sometimes neuromuscular blockade). Cardiac arrhythmias and fluctuations in BP can occur. Recovery takes months. Shorter incubation periods (≤7 days) portend more severe courses and a worse prognosis.
  - The patient should be kept in quiet isolation, sedated but arousable.
  - Specific measures include wound debridement, **penicillin G or metronidazole**, and **human tetanus immunoglobulin** (3000–6000 units IM).
  - **Active immunization** is needed after recovery (total of three doses of tetanus and diphtheria toxoid spaced at least 2 weeks apart).

NEUROLATHYRISM

It is a toxin-induced myelopathy caused by consumption of a plant, Lathyrus sativus (Kesari dhal), which contains the toxic compound beta-N-Oxalylamino-L-alanine. It results in progressive neuroparalysis and crippling. This is primarily due to toxin-mediated damage to pyramidal tract resulting in a UMN type of paralysis. Avoidance of the crop, steeping, and boiling may reduce the incidence of the disease.

Summary

- In the evaluation of coma, thorough clinical examination and laboratory investigations including imaging is vital.
- Alzheimer disease is the most common type of dementia. Although dementia mostly affects older adults, it is not a part of normal aging.
- Status epilepticus is a medical emergency where the seizures are prolonged and require urgent medical intervention, resulting in long-lasting consequences and fatalities if left untreated or unattended.
- Multiple sclerosis is a complex autoimmune neurologic disorder that results in both neurologic and non-neurologic symptoms, disability, and mortality.
- TIAs have a 30% risk of full-fledged stroke in the next 1 week.

Scan the QR code to access chapter references.

28 Toxicology

S. Eliza Dunn, Evan S. Schwarz, Michael E. Mullins, and Suraj B. Utmani

TOXIDROMES

GENERAL PRINCIPLES

- According to the 2021 Annual Report of the National Poison Data System (NPDS), there were over 2.8 million cases of known or suspected human toxic exposures managed by the United States poison control centres.[1] Of these 4497 resulted in death of the patient. Overdoses are common in the emergency department, and although they are rarely fatal, it is important to follow some general guidelines while caring for the poisoned patient.
- Patients who present to the hospital with an overdose or toxic exposure can be challenging for the clinician. This section will begin with a review of the general approach to the poisoned patient, followed by a discussion of specific ingestions.
- When managing the poisoned patient, as with all patients, it is vital to make sure the patient has a patent airway, intact breathing, and palpable pulses. Beyond the basics of general emergency management, it is important to remember physiologic principles when approaching the poisoned patient. Quite often, patients can be categorized into one of six common toxidromes based on simple clinical examination findings. However, there are more than five unique toxidromes.

Definition

A **toxidrome**, or toxic syndrome, is a constellation of clinical examination findings that assists in the diagnosis and treatment of the patient who presents following an exposure to an unknown agent. The set of clinical manifestations, biological tests, and/or ECG suggestive of a poisoning defines a toxidrome or toxic syndrome. The toxicologic physical examination should include documentation of **vital signs, pupillary diameter, and skin findings** (dry, flushed, or diaphoretic), as well as the presence or absence of **bowel sounds and urinary retention.**

Classification

There are six **general toxidromes** that encompass a variety of xenobiotic exposures (Table 28-1). They include the following:

- **Sympathomimetic:** This toxidrome is characterized by widespread activation of the sympathetic nervous system (SNS). The vital sign abnormalities include **hypertension** due to α-adrenergic stimulation and **tachycardia** due to increased β-adrenergic tone. Patients may also present with pyrexia. Physical examination will reveal **pupillary dilatation, diaphoresis,** and occasionally, altered mental status. Drugs that can cause this type of toxidrome include cocaine, amphetamines, and the newer synthetic analogues (both the cannabinoids and cathinones). Likewise, vasopressors and β-adrenergic agonists can cause a partial syndrome depending on which agent is being used.
- **Cholinergic:** This toxidrome is characterized by the widespread activation of the parasympathetic nervous system. Classically, the vital signs associated with a cholinergic toxidrome include **bradycardia** due to increased vagal tone, **respiratory depression** due to

TABLE 28-1 Classification of Toxidromes

Syndromes	Vital Signs	Mental Status	Pupil	Skin	Peristalsis	Others
Sympathomimetics	Increased	Agitated	Dilated	Increased sweating	No change/ increased	Tremors, seizures
Cholinergic	Decreased	Depressed	Constricted	Increased sweating	Increased	Salivation, lacrimation, urination, fasciculation, bronchorrhea, paralysis
Anticholinergic	Increased	Delirium	Dilated	No sweating	Decreased	Dry mucous membrane, urinary retention
Opioids	Decreased	Depressed	Constricted	-	Decreased	Hyporeflexia
Sedative hypnotic	Decreased	Depressed	-	-	Decreased	Hyporeflexia, ataxia

paralysis, and **decreased oxygen saturations** on pulse oximetry, due to **bronchoconstriction and bronchorrhea.** Excess acetylcholine (ACh) affects muscarinic receptors leading to the development of pinpoint pupils and the SLUDGE syndrome of **salivation, lacrimation, urination, defecation, gastrointestinal (GI) distress, and emesis.** Excess ACh at the neuromuscular junction results in a depolarizing blockade of the muscles, leading to **fasciculations** and **paralysis.** In the central nervous system (CNS), cholinergic overload is associated with the development of **seizures** and **coma.** Agents linked with the development of this toxidrome all block the function of acetylcholinesterase (AChE), resulting in the accumulation of ACh in the synapse. These agents include organophosphate insecticides and nerve gases, as well as carbamate pesticides. Carbamates are also used therapeutically in anesthesia, myasthenia gravis, and the treatment of anticholinergic toxidromes. Certain types of mushrooms can also cause cholinergic symptoms.

- **Anticholinergic:** This toxidrome should perhaps be more appropriately described as an antimuscarinic syndrome. Its features include **tachycardia** due to vagal blockade and **hyperthermia** (which may be mild to severe). CNS effects include **agitation, delirium,** and in severe cases, seizures. Other peripheral effects include **mydriasis; dry,** flushed skin; **urinary retention;** and **decreased intestinal motility.** The mnemonic "red as a beet, dry as a bone, blind as a bat, mad as a hatter, hot as a hare, full as a flask" can be used to remember the classical symptoms and signs of this poisoning. These patients classically demonstrate a "picking or plucking" motions (woolgathering). For reasons that are not fully understood, some patients will only present with a **central anticholinergic toxidrome** (i.e., the delirium without the peripheral findings). Anticholinergic toxicity can be confused with sympathomimetic toxicity; however, the absence of sweating indicates anticholinergic toxicity. Therapeutic agents that cause this toxidrome include atropine, scopolamine, and antihistamines such as diphenhydramine.
- **Opioids:** The opioids produce a classic vital sign combination of **respiratory depression** and oxygen desaturations in conjunction with **miosis, decreased GI motility,** and **coma.** Opioids produce this toxidrome by binding to one of the four G protein receptors on the cell membrane, leading to analgesia. However, respiratory depression, miosis, and physical dependence are secondary, undesirable effects. Other agents that produce a similar toxidrome include the imidazolines, including clonidine, dexmedetomidine, tetrahydrozoline, and oxymetazoline.
- **Sedative hypnotic/myorelaxation syndrome:** The benzodiazepines bind to γ-aminobutyric acid (GABA) receptors in the brain and cause a clinical picture of **sedation or coma** in the setting of **normal** vital signs. A common misconception is that ingested benzodiazepines cause respiratory depression. Although this may be true in the setting of IV administered benzodiazepines or when benzodiazepines are taken in combination with other sedative agents, patients with a **benzodiazepine ingestion generally do not develop respiratory compromise.** Other sedatives can cause similar sedation or coma with respiratory depression.
- **Serotonin syndrome: It is** seen with substances such as the SRIs, monoamine oxidase inhibitors, lithium, tricyclic antidepressants, ecstasy, and L-tryptophan. The clinical picture includes the following:
  - Neurological symptoms including agitation, confusion, hallucinations, myoclonus, tremor, seizure, and coma
  - Autonomic features such as mydriasis, sweating, tachycardia, tachypnea, hyperthermia, chills, hypotension, diarrhea, or even respiratory arrest
  - Metabolic changes such as hyperglycemia, leukocytosis, hypokalemia, hypocalcemia, disseminated intravascular coagulation, lactic acidosis, and rhabdomyolysis

DIAGNOSIS

Diagnostic Testing

If patients do not fall into any of the aforementioned categories, suspect a mixed or undifferentiated exposure, and several diagnostic tests should be ordered.

Laboratories

- **Finger stick blood glucose (FSBG):** This test should be considered one of the vital signs in the patient with altered mental status.
- **Chemistry:** A basic metabolic profile should be ordered on any patient with a toxic exposure. The two important pieces of information gleaned from the basic metabolic panel (BMP) include the presence or absence of a low bicarbonate and the creatinine. If the patient has a low bicarbonate, a metabolic acidosis is present and the clinician should calculate the **anion gap.** Beware of patients with a falsely elevated chloride and therefore either a falsely low or negative anion gap. Patients who present with an elevated anion gap acidosis are often subjected to a battery of unnecessary studies because the differential diagnosis is enormous. To tailor the diagnosis, the clinician should focus on a mechanistic approach and check serum **ketones** and **lactate.** If these are negative and the **creatinine** is normal, then one should suspect the presence of a toxic alcohol and send the appropriate studies.
- **Blood gas:** In most cases of intoxication, pH rather than oxygenation is of great relevance. Therefore, it is reasonable to send **venous blood gases (VBGs)** rather than arterial blood gases (ABGs) in routine cases of poisoning. However, if adequate oxygenation is a concern (e.g., cyanide, carbon monoxide poisoning, methemoglobinemia), then an ABG should be sent. Co-oximetry can be sent from either arterial or venous samples. High anion gap metabolic acidosis is seen in poisoning with methanol, salicylates, paraldehyde, ethylene glycol, and paracetamol.
  - Measurement of osmolar gap (difference between osmolarity measured with delta cryoscopic method and calculated osmolarity: $2 \times Na + 1.15 \times [GLU/18 + BUN/2.8]$). Normal (10–15 mOsmol/kg) indicates the presence of low-molecular-weight and high-concentration particles. An osmolar gap $\geq$25 mOsmol/kg in a patient with metabolic acidosis is suggestive of alcohol or glycol poisoning.
- **Serum drug screen:** In general, the studies included on this panel include acetaminophen, salicylate, and ethanol concentrations. Rarely, laboratories may include a tricyclic antidepressant (TCA) screen.
  - In practice, the piece of information that is critical on this panel is the serum **acetaminophen** (*N*-acetyl-para-aminophenol [APAP]) because patients with this ingestion are often asymptomatic on presentation, and approximately 1 in 500 overdoses have been found to have an unsuspected and treatable APAP concentration.[2]
  - Acute **salicylate** ingestions, although very serious, produce a clinical syndrome that is readily identifiable at the bedside. Chronic salicylate toxicity should be suspected in elderly patients taking aspirin who present with altered mental status and tachypnea or patients with an unexplained anion gap metabolic acidosis.
  - **Ethanol** concentrations are ***not*** predictive of intoxication, despite the forensic definition of 80 mg/dL as the legal limit for driving. Intoxication is a clinical diagnosis. One of the pitfalls of routinely obtaining ethanol levels is that serious medical conditions may coexist in these often fragile patients. These conditions are frequently missed when the patient is thought to be drunk. The test is useful to exclude ethanol as the cause of altered mental status.
  - **TCA** screens are notoriously unreliable and cross-react with many therapeutic agents. In the absence of the characteristic ECG findings and vital sign abnormalities, a positive result is meaningless and is the source of confusion, leading to unnecessary treatment.

- **Urine drug screen:** This rarely contributes to the management of the patient. These serve as possible proof of an exposure but do not confirm intoxication. Many of the assays produce false-positive or false-negative results and may, in fact, cause harm by leading the clinician to attribute a patient's condition to intoxication rather than a medical emergency. Additionally, these tests are expensive to conduct and therefore are of limited value in the management of the poisoned patient. The urine drug screen tends to vary between hospitals but often tests for the following substances:
  - **Amphetamines:** The assay for amphetamines commonly cross-reacts with over-the-counter cold medications. Many designer amphetamines will not be detected.
  - **Opioids:** This assay frequently misses the presence of the synthetic opioids such as fentanyl, fentanyl analogues, methadone, and meperidine; therefore, it is important to rely on the toxidrome for the diagnosis.
  - **Cocaine:** This assay is not directed at the parent compound; rather, it detects the metabolite benzoylecgonine. Because the parent compound is very short lived, this test is very reliable for the identification of recent use but in no way confirms intoxication.
  - **Cannabinoids:** Like cocaine, detection of the tetrahydrocannabinolic acid metabolite is a reliable indicator of use; however, its presence does not have any bearing on the diagnosis of intoxication. In general, synthetic cannabinoids will ***not*** cause a positive test result.
  - **Benzodiazepines:** The detection of benzodiazepines most commonly relies on the detection of oxazepam; therefore, some commonly used benzodiazepines (such as lorazepam, clonazepam, alprazolam) are often missed during this screening.[3] Given that benzodiazepine overdoses tend to be benign, the utility of this component is questionable at best.
  - **Phencyclidine (PCP):** Screening assays may cross-react with dextromethorphan, ketamine, and diphenhydramine to produce a false-positive result. Once again, the clinical picture is more important in the diagnosis of PCP intoxication, and the presence of PCP on a drug screen does not alter the management of a patient.
- Specific laboratory testing will be further addressed in the following text.

Electrocardiography

- The ECG is a critical part of the toxicologic evaluation, and certain overdoses produce characteristic ECG changes that guide diagnosis and treatment plans.
- In general, the important cardiac toxins tend to prolong the PR interval (reflecting nodal blockade), the QRS (reflecting sodium channel blockade), or the QT interval (potassium channel blockade).
- ECG changes specific to certain toxins will be further discussed in the following text.

Imaging

- In general, there is a limited role of diagnostic imaging in toxicology. However, there are a few cases when imaging may be helpful in the diagnosis and management of the poisoned patient. The most useful imaging study in overdose is the abdominal radiograph, which may reveal radiodense material in the stomach or gut in the following ingestions[4]:
  - Chloral hydrate
  - Heavy metals
  - Iron
  - Phenothiazines
  - Enteric-coated preparations
  - Sustained-release preparations
- Occasionally, subtle abnormalities on the abdominal film will detect the presence of "rosettes" or elongated packets in the GI tract of body packers (patients who swallow

hundreds of packets of drugs in an attempt to smuggle them). The abdominal film is of limited utility in body stuffers.[5] CT scans are also unreliable in these patients.

TREATMENT

As with any patient, it is crucial to maintain the airway, check for adequacy of breathing and circulation, and check an FSBG in the patient with altered mental status or coma.

- **Prevention of absorption:** Traditionally, gastric emptying by either inducing **emesis** or **lavage** has been a mainstay in the treatment of the acutely overdosed patient. However, the literature regarding these methods of decontamination suggests that they are of little benefit.[6] Furthermore, numerous studies have suggested that patients present approximately 3–4 hours after ingestion on average, which tends to make it less likely that there will be a large recovery of pills.[7] Therefore, the routine administration of **ipecac** to children and "stomach pumping" have fallen by the wayside except in very specific circumstances. Contraindications to gastric lavage include ingestion of corrosives and most hydrocarbons, patients with depressed gag reflexes who are not intubated, and clinically insignificant ingestions. Complications include aspiration and perforation of the esophagus or bronchus.
  - **Activated charcoal (AC)** has largely replaced both of these methods of gastric emptying.[8] However, the clinical utility of this method of decontamination is limited if the ingestion occurred more than 1 hour before presentation.[9] As such, fewer toxicologists routinely recommend the administration of AC.[10] Contraindications to activated charcoal use include mechanical bowel obstruction and ileus. In addition, patients at risk for decreased mental status or seizures should not be given AC owing to concerns for aspiration. Certain ingestions benefit from multidose AC because they either bind to concretions in the stomach (aspirin) or they decrease enterohepatic or enteroenteric reabsorption (phenobarbital, phenytoin, theophylline). The usual dosage is 1–2 g/kg for children and adults, usually given as a single dose combined with a cathartic.
  - **Whole-bowel irrigation** is appropriate in patients who have ingested sustained-release medications, body packing, or metals that do not bind to AC. The optimal dose of polyethylene glycol is 1–2 L/h until the rectal effluent is clear. This dose is a large amount of fluid to ingest, so it is often necessary to place a nasogastric tube to achieve this rate of emptying. Contraindications to whole bowel irrigation include mechanical obstruction, ileus, perforation, and GI bleeding.
  - In cases **of life-threatening** ingestions such as colchicine or nondihydropyridine calcium channel blockers (CCBs), it is appropriate to consider **lavage** as well as **AC**.
  - **Cathartics** have no role in the management of overdose. They are often present in the premixed AC solutions. If this is the case, only one dose should be administered.
- **Enhanced elimination**
  - **Forced diuresis** with normal saline (NS) and Ringer's lactate was thought to enhance the elimination of low-molecular weight agents such as lithium in dehydrated individuals. In general, this strategy should be avoided.
  - **Urinary alkalinization** with IV sodium bicarbonate enhances the elimination of weak acids and is useful in the setting of salicylate overdose. Typical doses are 1–2 mEq/kg, with a goal of maintaining the urinary pH at approximately 7–8. Specific recommendations will be further discussed in the following text.
  - There is no role for **urinary acidification** in the management of overdoses.
  - **Hemodialysis and hemoperfusion** are reserved for life-threatening ingestions of substances that have a low volume of distribution, have a molecular weight of <500 Da, have a low endogenous clearance, are water soluble, and have little protein binding. This treatment modality will be further discussed under specific substances.

- **Antidotes** (Table 28-2) will be discussed under specific toxicities. Antidotes are typically given once the patient has been stabilized, usually within a few hours of the ingestion. The regional poison center or a medical toxicologist should be contacted for specific treatment guidelines.
- **Disposition**
  - Patients who have taken an overdose as a suicidal gesture should all receive a psychiatric evaluation before discharge.
  - Most cases of unintentional overdose do not result in significant morbidity, and in cases where the patient is stable and asymptomatic, a brief period of observation may be all that is necessary.
  - In cases where potentially toxic agents have been ingested, most patients should be monitored for 4–6 hours before discharge.

TABLE 28-2 Common Poisons and Their Antidotes

Poison	Antidote
Acetaminophen	*N*-Acetylcysteine (Acetadote®, Mucomyst®)
Anticholinergics	Physostigmine
Anticoagulants	Vitamin K
Calcium channel blockers	Calcium chloride Calcium gluconate Glucagon Insulin/glucose
Carbon monoxide	Oxygen
Cholinergics	Atropine Pralidoxime (2-PAM)
Cyanide	Cyanide antidote kit (Lilly Kit) Amyl nitrite Sodium nitrite Sodium thiosulfite Hydroxycobalamin (Cyanokit) Sodium thiosulfate alone
Digoxin	Digoxin FAB (Digibind)
Heparin	Protamine
Heavy metals Arsenic Copper Lead Mercury	 Dimercaprol EDTA Penicillamine Succimer (DMSA)
Iron	Deferoxamine
Isoniazid	Pyridoxine
Methanol	Ethanol
Ethylene glycol	Fomepizole (Antizol)
Opioids	Naloxone

ANALGESICS, ANTIPYRETICS, AND ANTI-INFLAMMATORY DRUG

Acetaminophen

GENERAL PRINCIPLES

APAP is available worldwide as an over-the-counter analgesic and antipyretic and has become the most common pharmacologic agent involved in toxicologic fatalities.[11] The recommended maximum dose for adults is 4 g/d.

Classification

- An analgesic. Within the United States, APAP is sold under the trade name Tylenol. The most common trade name for APAP outside the United States is Paracetamol.
- Because of its use as an analgesic and antipyretic, APAP has become a common ingredient in various cold and flu remedies. It is also used in the treatment of fevers, headaches, and acute and chronic pain.
- APAP is often sold in combination preparations together with NSAIDs, opioid analgesics, or sedatives (e.g., Tylenol #3, Percocet, Vicodin, NyQuil, Tylenol PM).

Epidemiology

APAP is the leading cause of toxicologic fatalities per year in the United States, and APAP-induced hepatotoxicity is the most frequent cause of acute liver failure.[12] Notably, APAP is a classic cause of drug-induced hepatotoxicity in a dose-dependent manner. **Paracetamol**-induced hepatotoxicity rate in a multiethnic Asian population is low at 7.3%. Mortality and morbidity were nonexistent despite high doses of **paracetamol** ingestion and delayed presentations to hospital.

Etiology

- APAP is available as tablets, capsules, liquids, and suppositories. In addition to the more common immediate-release form, there is also an extended-release preparation (e.g., Tylenol Arthritis Pain).
- Unintentional overdosing is more common than intentional ingestion in suicide attempts, especially in elderly patients on chronic pain regimens including several APAP-containing painkillers.[13]
- All patients with presumed APAP overdose should be adequately assessed, evaluated, and treated. However, only the minority of poisoned patients require inpatient care.[14]

Pathophysiology

- **Absorption:** APAP serum levels peak 30–60 minutes after oral ingestion; the extended-release preparations peak after 1–2 hours. Absorption is often delayed in overdose, and peak levels are usually reached after 2–4 hours. The overdose kinetics of extended-release APAP are not yet well established.
- **Overdose:** The hepatic conjugation pathways become saturated in overdose. A cascade of biochemical changes occurs in the liver, and centrilobular cell necrosis results.[15]
  - Acetaminophen is metabolized predominantly via glucuronidation (47%–62%) and sulfation (25%–36%) by phase II metabolism in liver as nontoxic conjugate products. However, a small percentage is metabolized via oxidation (5%–8%) by the cytochrome P450 (2E1) pathway to a toxic metabolite, *N*-acetyl-*p*-benzoquinone imine (NAPQI). NAPQI is conjugated by glutathione to nontoxic cysteine and mercapturic acid conjugates.

- In cases of acetaminophen toxicity, the phase II conjugation enzymes are saturated, and a higher fraction of acetaminophen is conjugated via oxidation to NAPQI. The conjugation of NAPQI by glutathione occurs until glutathione is depleted from hepatic reserves, after which the toxic NAPQI and other free radicals accumulate and cause damage to the hepatocytes.

Risk Factors

- Decreased glutathione stores (fasting, malnutrition, anorexia nervosa, chronic alcoholism, febrile illness, chronic disease)
- P450 enzyme inducers (ethanol, isoniazid [INH], phenytoin and other anticonvulsants, barbiturates, smoking)

DIAGNOSIS

Clinical Presentation

- **First 24 hours**—Asymptomatic stage (stage 1):
  - Early symptoms are very nonspecific and primarily related to the GI tract (nausea, vomiting, anorexia).
  - High-dose APAP can cause pallor or lethargy in some patients. Rarely, very high doses can inhibit aerobic metabolism.
  - This initial phase has few symptoms and patients appear pretty unremarkable. Therefore, always think of other coingestants if a patient exhibits extreme vital sign abnormalities or other significant symptoms during the first 24 hours.
- **24–48 hours**—Hepatotoxic stage (stage 2):
  - Right upper quadrant tenderness is the most common symptom.
  - Transaminitis, bilirubinemia, and elevated prothrombin time (PT)/international normalized ratio (INR) are also common findings during the second phase.
- **2–4 days**—Fulminant hepatic failure stage (stage 3): Significant hepatic dysfunction develops (i.e., a peak in hepatic enzyme elevation along with jaundice, coagulopathy with high risk of spontaneous bleeding, hypoglycemia, anuria, and cerebral edema with coma or even death). In 25% of patients, acute tubular necrosis and renal failure are seen.
- **4–14 days**—Recovery stage (stage 4): If stage 3 is survived, the hepatic dysfunction usually resolves over the following days/weeks.

History

- To predict the risk of hepatotoxicity after acute overdose, a reliable time of ingestion must be obtained from the patient or family/friends.
- Also obtain information about the amount of APAP that has been ingested, in what form (e.g., combination preparations, extended-release form), and over what period of time.
- Inquire about other coingestants (alcohol, other medications, other drugs).

Physical Examination

Assess airway, breathing, and circulation (ABCs) and mental status. The assessment of mental status is crucial, especially in patients who are nauseated or vomiting, to intervene with airway protection in time.

Diagnostic Criteria

- In general, a dose of 150 mg APAP per kilogram is the potentially toxic limit that requires therapeutic intervention. This limit includes an added 25% safety margin that was added by the US Food and Drug Administration (FDA) to adjust for patients with multiple risk factors for increased liver toxicity.[16]

- If the total amount of ingested APAP is >150 mg/kg or cannot be obtained from the patient history, it is crucial to predict the risk of toxicity.
- Obtain an APAP serum level at 4 hours or later after ingestion.
- Plot the APAP concentration on the **Rumack-Matthew nomogram** (APAP serum concentration vs. time after ingestion) to assess the possibility of hepatic toxicity. NOTE: The nomogram should only be used for acute ingestions and cannot be used until 4 hours after the ingestion.
- During treatment of APAP overdose, it is important to assess the risk of progressive liver failure. The King's College Hospital (KCH) criteria provide prognostic markers that help to predict the probability of developing severe liver damage[17]:
  - pH <7.3, 2 days after ingestion
  - All of the following: PT >100 (INR >6), serum creatinine >3.3 mmol/L, severe hepatic encephalopathy (grade III or IV)
- Elevated serum phosphate levels >1.2 mmol/L (>3.72 mg/dL) on days 2–4 (additional criterion, not originally part of KCH criteria).[18]
- Arterial serum lactate >3.0 mmol/L (>27 mg/dL) after fluid resuscitation (additional criterion, not originally part of KCH criteria).[19]

Diagnostic Testing

- **APAP serum level at 4 hours** after ingestion or later (see earlier discussion).
- **Liver function tests (LFTs)**—Aspartate aminotransferase (AST) is a relatively sensitive nonprognostic marker for hepatic injury.
- **PT/INR, serum bicarbonate, blood pH, serum lactate, renal function panel, and serum phosphate** level are the prognostic markers for hepatic injury.
- APAP may interfere with some blood sugar test kits causing measurements higher or lower than actual; always recheck FSBG over the course of hospitalization.[20]

TREATMENT

Gastric lavage is not useful in APAP overdose; however, it may be indicated in presence of certain other coingestants.

Medications

- **AC:** Only potentially indicated in patients with isolated APAP exposure (with no other evidence of mentally altering substances) who present less than 4 hours after ingestion. Give **1 g/kg PO**.
- ***N*-Acetylcysteine (NAC):** NAC is the specific antidote to prevent APAP-related hepatotoxicity.[21] NAC replenishes depleted glutathione stores. It should be administered early (i.e., within 8 hours after ingestion) to prevent any liver damage. NAC is a nonspecific antioxidant and will still provide some liver protection if given beyond this time window.[22]
  - **Oral dosing:** Loading dose of 140 mg/kg PO, then 70 mg/kg PO every 4 hours for a total of 17 doses (i.e., 1330 mg/kg over 72 hours).[23]
  - **IV dosing:** Prepare the infusion by adding 30 g of a 20% NAC solution (150 mL) to 1 L dextrose 5% in water (D5W). This will result in a final concentration of 30 mg/mL. Load with a dose of 150 mg/kg NAC IV over 1 hour. Thereafter, continue to give 12.5 mg/kg/h IV for 20 hours (i.e., 400 mg/kg over 21 hours) (according to IV NAC treatment protocol used by Toxicology Service at Barnes-Jewish Hospital).[24] This is a different dosing strategy than what is recommended in the package insert. Multiple hospitals have modified their dosing strategy to decrease administration errors.
  - **NAC administration** can be safely stopped before the completion of the total regimen as soon as the APAP level returns to 0, INR <2.0, and AST normalizes (or reaches

less than half of the peak level during acute intoxication), and the patient is clinically improving.

- **NAC indications:** NAC treatment should be started in the following:
  - Any patient after acute poisoning with a toxic APAP level according to the nomogram.
  - Patients who present beyond 8 hours after acute ingestion. Start NAC therapy while awaiting the initial APAP serum level. Continue treatment if the serum concentration is in the toxic range per nomogram.
  - Patients who present more than 24 hours after acute ingestion and still have a detectable serum APAP level or elevated AST.
  - Patients with chronic APAP exposure (i.e., >4 g/d in adults, >120 mg/kg/d in children) who present with elevated transaminases.
  - Patients with signs of fulminant hepatic failure. NAC treatment should be started immediately, and transfer to a transplant center should be arranged without fail. NAC has been shown to improve survival of patients in fulminant hepatic failure.[25–27]
- **Oral versus IV NAC:**
  - IV administration of NAC is the preferred route because it is used in all of the studies of patients with fulminant hepatic failure.
  - Oral administration may be slightly safer compared to the IV form; however, NAC has a rather bad odor and taste. Rash, flushing, urticaria, nausea/vomiting, angioedema, bronchospasm, tachycardia, and hypotension have been reported as adverse reactions to IV administration.[28]
  - If oral NAC is given, dilute the NAC with juice, provide a drinking straw and place a lid on the glass, and give IV antiemetics (e.g., metoclopramide, ondansetron).
  - Consider oral over IV NAC in patients who are prone to anaphylactoid reactions (e.g., severe asthmatics) and in patient whom IV access is difficult to obtain (IVDU).
  - NAC is effective either way when given within 8 hours after ingestion.[23]
  - AC adsorbs oral NAC. Both PO and IV NAC regimens provide enough excess of the drug to ensure adequate therapeutic effects. Nevertheless, it is advised to administer AC 2 hours apart from NAC when given PO but do not delay administration of NAC to do this.
- **Criteria to be present for discontinuation of IV NAC:**
  - Undetectable acetaminophen concentration.
  - Improving hepatic aminotransferases <100 IU/mL.
  - Improving prognostic markers (e.g., creatinine, lactate, pH, prothrombin time/INR, phosphate).
  - A minimum of 12 hours of NAC has been given.

COMPLICATIONS

- Overdose with extended-relief APAP:[29]
  - Get APAP serum level 4 hours after ingestion.
  - If toxic per nomogram, treat with full NAC course.
  - If below toxic level per nomogram, repeat the APAP level at 8 hours after ingestion, although this is controversial. Many do not repeat the APAP level if the initial is below the nomogram.
  - If now toxic, treat with full course. If remains below toxic level, no therapy is necessary.
- Patients with progressing liver failure need to be admitted to an intensive care unit (ICU) bed with close monitoring for hyperglycemia, electrolyte imbalances, GI bleeding, acid–base disturbances, cerebral edema, infections, and renal failure.

REFERRAL

- Involve a clinical toxicologist in all cases where toxic APAP levels are documented. Discuss the initiation of NAC treatment with the toxicology service where possible.
- Inform your regional poison control center (1-800-222-1222).
- Involve the liver or transplant service early in patients presenting with poor prognostic factors for hepatic failure.
- Patients with toxic liver failure should be transferred to a transplant center as early as possible.[30,31]

Colchicine

GENERAL PRINCIPLES

Definition

Colchicine is the active alkaloid extracted from two plants of the Liliaceae family: *Colchicum autumnale* (autumn crocus) and *Gloriosa superba* (glory lily). It has been used in the therapy of gout for centuries.

Etiology

Colchicine has a very narrow therapeutic index. Severe poisoning and death can result from the ingestion of as little as 0.8 mg/kg of body weight.[32]

Pathophysiology

Colchicine is an effective inhibitor of intracellular microtubule formation, leading to impaired leukocyte chemotaxis, and phagocytosis, resulting in a decrease in the inflammatory cascade.[33] In overdose, colchicine causes mitotic arrest, leading to cellular dysfunction and death.[34]

Prevention

Patients who are started on colchicine for gout symptoms should be explicitly directed to stop taking the medication as soon as symptoms of diarrhea occur. They should also be told that increasing the dose in an acute flare can result in significant toxicity; therefore, if they are unable to control the symptoms at home, they should seek expert care early.

DIAGNOSIS

Clinical Presentation

Patients who present with a colchicine overdose tend to develop a syndrome that progresses through three phases. The initial phase usually begins several hours after the overdose and is characterized by nausea, vomiting, and diarrhea. Over the next 1–7 days, patients may develop multiorgan failure requiring intensive support or sudden cardiac death; death is common at this stage. In the final phase, patients develop alopecia and myoneuropathies.

History

Patients with inadvertent overdoses will present with a recent history of an acute gouty flare, followed by the development of nausea, vomiting, and diarrhea within a few hours after the overdose. Colchicine poisoning presents (1) 10–24 hours after ingestion—GI phase mimicking gastroenteritis; and (2) 24 hours to 7 days after ingestion—multiorgan dysfunction and sepsis. Recovery typically occurs within a few weeks of ingestion.

Physical Examination

The examination tends to be somewhat unremarkable in these patients. They may exhibit signs of dehydration with tachycardia and dry mucous membranes. They may also have decreased urine output. As the toxicity progresses, patients may develop signs of worsening distress and confusion requiring aggressive resuscitation measures. As the disease evolves, fatal cardiac arrhythmias and refractory cardiovascular collapse may occur, usually within a week of overdose.[35] Reversible alopecia has been reported in survivors.[34]

Differential Diagnosis

As with any ingestion, the differential diagnosis is large. However, GI symptoms are common in patients with overdoses of methylxanthines, podophyllin, digoxin and other cardioactive steroids, chemotherapeutic agents, heavy metals, and salicylates.

Diagnostic Testing

There is a very interesting sequence of laboratory findings that should lead one to consider colchicine poisoning in patients.

Laboratories

- **Complete blood cell count** (**CBC**)**:** In the initial phase of poisoning that lasts for approximately 12–24 hours, patients develop a leukocytosis. In the next 48–72 hours, signs of bone marrow suppression evolve, starting with a profound decline in the leukocyte count and subsequent pancytopenia.
- **BMP:** Colchicine poisoning has also been associated with renal failure and adrenal hemorrhage;[36] therefore, electrolytes should be monitored.
- **LFTs:** Colchicine overdoses have been reported to cause hepatotoxicity; therefore, LFTs should be monitored.
- **Coagulation studies:** Disseminated intravascular coagulation (DIC) occasionally occurs; therefore, a full panel, including fibrinogen and fibrin split products, should be obtained.
- **Colchicine concentrations:** Colchicine has a narrow therapeutic index, and plasma concentrations >3 ng/mL may produce significant toxicity. However, this laboratory test is not readily available, and toxicity should be suspected if clinical symptoms and laboratory studies are supportive. This test should be thought of as a confirmatory study.
- **Other studies:** Creatine kinase (CK; or creatine phosphokinase), troponin, lipase, and other electrolytes should be obtained depending on the clinical scenario.

Electrocardiography

An ECG should be obtained at presentation, given the patient's predilection for developing cardiac arrhythmias, and the patient should be admitted with continuous cardiac monitoring.

Imaging

Colchicine toxicity has been associated with the development of acute respiratory distress syndrome (ARDS). Therefore, a CXR should be obtained.

TREATMENT

Colchicine overdoses are often fatal and require aggressive supportive measures. As always, airway protection is of paramount importance followed by adequacy of breathing and support of circulation.

Medications

In cases of severe neutropenia, consider **granulocyte colony-stimulating factor** (G-CSF) administration.

Other Nonpharmacologic Therapies

- If the patient is **not** vomiting, consider **gastric lavage** and **AC**. If the patient is altered and vomiting, consider early **endotracheal intubation**. **Fluids** and direct-acting **vasopressors** should be used in cases of hypotension. **Hemodialysis** is not useful for clearing colchicine, given its large volume of distribution; however, it should be used in the setting of colchicine-induced renal failure.
- All symptomatic patients should be admitted to the ICU. Patients without symptoms should be monitored for 8–12 hours before discharge.

SPECIAL CONSIDERATIONS

Given its narrow therapeutic window and pharmacokinetics, colchicine should be used cautiously in patients with underlying renal or liver dysfunction. Likewise, colchicine is a P450 drug and is subject to many drug–drug interactions.[37] A thorough review of the patient's medication list should be conducted before starting this agent as toxic concentrations can accumulate rapidly. In this setting, consider using alternative therapies for the management of acute gouty flares.

Nonsteroidal Anti-inflammatory Drugs

GENERAL PRINCIPLES

- NSAIDs are widely prescribed as analgesics for the management of inflammatory diseases. There are many different classes available; however, the discussion in the following text relates to over-the-counter preparations available in the United States and includes ibuprofen, ketoprofen, and naproxen as well as the selective cyclooxygenase (COX)-2 inhibitors.
- NSAIDs exert their therapeutic effects by inhibiting COX and thereby preventing the formation of prostaglandins. This mechanism accounts for both their therapeutic and toxic side effects, which include ulceration of the GI mucosa and renal dysfunction. In the vast majority of cases, overdose is benign.

DIAGNOSIS

Clinical Presentation

Overdose histories are often unreliable. Consider NSAID overdose in patients who present with **GI distress**. **Massive overdose** with ibuprofen occasionally presents with **coma, a metabolic acidosis, and seizures**.

Diagnostic Testing

Obtain a **BMP** to evaluate renal function and hydration status. An **APAP** concentration should be obtained because many patients confuse over-the-counter analgesics.

TREATMENT

Usually supportive care is all that is necessary for the management of this overdose. IV fluids (IVF) are beneficial for maintaining hydration in vomiting patients.

Medications

- **Antiemetics and antacids** are beneficial in patients with significant distress.
- **Benzodiazepines** should be used for the management of seizures associated with massive ibuprofen overdose.

Opioids

DIAGNOSIS

Clinical Presentation

The sine qua non of opioid intoxication is respiratory depression, a depressed level of consciousness, and **miosis.** However, the pupils may be dilated with acidosis or hypoxia or after overdoses with meperidine or diphenoxylate plus atropine. Overdose with fentanyl or derivatives such as α-methyl fentanyl ("China white") or other synthetic opioids may result in negative urine toxicology screens.

Illicit opioid use continues to be a growing problem with more than 40,000 deaths due to opioid overdoses in 2016 in the United States.[38] Newer synthetic opioids such as U-47700, the W series (e.g., W18), and fentanyl analogues are adulterating large amounts of the heroin supply. Additionally, prescription opioid medications bought illicitly may actually contain large amounts of synthetic opioids. This has led to multiple deaths.

Diagnostic Testing

Laboratories

Drug concentrations and other standard laboratory tests are of little use. Pulse oximetry and **ABGs** are useful for monitoring respiratory status. Capnography measuring end-tidal CO_2 is more sensitive in detecting impending respiratory arrest as hypercapnia precedes hypoxemia.

Electrocardiography

- **Methadone** has been reported to cause a **prolonged QT_c**. Obtain an ECG in suspected overdose.
- **Propoxyphene** exhibits type IA antidysrhythmic effects due to sodium channel blockade and may present with a **wide complex QRS** on ECG.[39]

Imaging

A CXR should be obtained if pulmonary symptoms are present.

TREATMENT

- Treatment includes airway maintenance, ventilatory support, and judicious use of opioid antagonist.
- Avoid gastric lavage.
- Limit use of whole-bowel irrigation to body packers. Body packers rarely require surgery, except in cases of intestinal obstruction.
- Endoscopic removal should generally not be attempted owing to the danger of rupture.

Medications

- **Naloxone hydrochloride** specifically reverses opioid-induced respiratory and CNS depression and hypotension.
  - The lowest effective dose should be used. The goal of treatment is adequate.
  - Spontaneous respiration and not alertness. The initial dose is 0.04–2 mg IV, although the lowest effective dose should be used to prevent withdrawal.
  - Larger doses (up to 10 mg IV) may be required to reverse the effects of propoxyphene, diphenoxylate, buprenorphine, or pentazocine. Larger doses may also be necessary to reverse some of the newer synthetic opioids, although this has not been firmly established. Interestingly, large doses of naloxone following buprenorphine overdose can result in paradoxical respiratory depression.

- In the absence of an IV line, naloxone can be administered sublingually,[40] via endotracheal tube, IM, or intranasally.[41] Isolated opioid overdose is unlikely if there is no response to a total of 10 mg naloxone. Repetitive doses may be required (duration of action is 45 minutes), and this should prompt hospitalization and initiation of a continuous infusion despite the patient's return to an alert status.
- Methadone overdose may require therapy for 24–48 hours, whereas levo-α-acetylmethadol may require therapy for 72 hours. A continuous IV drip that provides two-thirds of the initial dose of naloxone hourly, diluted in D5W, may be necessary to maintain an alert state.[42,43]
- Ventilatory support should be provided for the patient who is unresponsive to naloxone and for pulmonary edema.
- Naloxone can be prescribed for any patient who is at risk of an overdose. Information regarding prescribing laws, Good Samaritan laws, and pharmacy distribution of naloxone can be found at Prescribetoprevent.org.

- **Disposition**
  - If the patient is alert and asymptomatic for 1–6 hours after a single dose of naloxone or for 1–4 hours after a single treatment for an IV overdose, he or she can be discharged safely.[44]
  - Methadone and buprenorphine overdoses need to be admitted.
  - Body packers should be admitted to an ICU for close monitoring of the respiratory rate and level of consciousness and remain so until all packets have passed, as documented by CT.

SPECIAL CONSIDERATIONS

- Heroin may be adulterated with scopolamine, cocaine, clenbuterol, or caffeine, complicating the clinical picture. Less common complications include hypotension, bradycardia, and pulmonary edema.
- Be aware of body packers who smuggle heroin in their intestinal tracts. Deterioration of latex or plastic containers may result in drug release and death.[45]

Salicylates

GENERAL PRINCIPLES

- Salicylates, such as aspirin, salicylic acid, and oil of wintergreen, are compounds which are easily available over the counter (OTC). Salicylate toxicity may result from **acute or chronic** ingestion of acetylsalicylic acid. Toxicity is usually mild after acute ingestions of <150 mg/kg, moderate after ingestions of 150–300 mg/kg, and generally severe with overdoses of 300–500 mg/kg.
- Toxicity from chronic ingestion is typically due to intake of >100 mg/kg/d over a period of several days and usually occurs in elderly patients with chronic underlying illness. Diagnosis is often delayed in this group of patients, and mortality is approximately 25%. Significant toxicity due to chronic ingestion may occur with blood concentrations lower than those associated with acute ingestions.
- Topical preparations containing methyl salicylate or oil of wintergreen can cause toxicity with excessive topical use or if ingested.

DIAGNOSIS

Clinical Presentation

- Nausea, vomiting, tinnitus (or hearing changes), tachypnea, hyperpnea, and malaise is common. Hyperthermia results from uncoupled mitochondrial oxidative phosphorylation and suggests a poor prognosis.
- Severe intoxications may include lethargy, acidosis, convulsions, hypoglycemia, and coma, which may result from cerebral edema and energy depletion in the CNS.
- Noncardiogenic pulmonary edema may occur and is more common with chronic ingestion, cigarette smoking, neurologic symptoms, and older age.
- Severe overdoses of >300 mg/kg may present with tachypnea, dehydration, pulmonary edema, altered mental status, seizures, or coma.

Diagnostic Testing

Laboratories

- Obtain electrolytes, blood urea nitrogen (BUN), creatinine, glucose, and salicylate concentration.
- Obtain either ABGs or VBGs.
- ABGs may reveal an early respiratory alkalosis, followed by metabolic acidosis.
    - Approximately 20% of patients exhibit either respiratory alkalosis or metabolic acidosis alone.[46]
    - Most adults with pure salicylate overdose have a primary metabolic acidosis and a primary respiratory alkalosis.
    - After mixed overdoses, respiratory acidosis may become prominent.[46]
- Serum salicylate concentrations drawn after acute ingestion of salicylates assist in prediction of severity of intoxication and patient disposition. However, **do not rely on the Done nomogram.**
    - Salicylate concentrations >70 mg/dL at any time represent moderate to severe intoxication.
    - Salicylate concentrations >100 mg/dL are very serious and often fatal. This information is useful only for acute overdoses of non–enteric-coated aspirin.
    - Enteric-coated aspirin may have delayed absorption and delayed peak concentration.
    - Chronic ingestion can cause toxicity with lower salicylate concentrations.
    - Bicarbonate concentrations and pH are more useful than salicylate concentrations as prognostic indicators in chronic intoxication.
    - **Be aware of units.** The majority of hospitals report salicylate concentrations in mg/dL. However, some hospitals still report concentrations in mg/L, which has caused multiple interpretation errors.

Imaging

- Repeated blood salicylate concentrations that fail to adequately decline could indicate the formation of a bezoar or concretion and may require imaging. Salicylate concretions may require endoscopy, multiple-dose AC, or bicarbonate lavage.
- Consider whole-bowel irrigation with polyethylene glycol.

TREATMENT

Medications

- Administer 50–100 g of **AC** if presentation is within 1 hour of ingestion.
- **Multidose charcoal** may be useful in severe overdose[47] or in cases in which salicylate concentrations fail to decline (due to possible gastric bezoar formation or pyloric contraction).

- In an acute overdose, most patients will be volume depleted and benefit from receiving 1–2 L of saline. Caution should be used in patients with renal failure or congestive heart failure (CHF).
- **Alkaline diuresis** is indicated for symptomatic patients with salicylate blood concentrations >30–40 mg/dL.
  - Administer 150 mEq (three ampules) sodium bicarbonate in 1000 mL D5W at a rate of 10–15 mL/kg/h if the patient is clinically volume depleted until urine flow is achieved.
  - Maintain alkalinization using the same solution at 2–3 mL/kg/h, and monitor urine output, urine pH (target pH, 7–8), and serum potassium. Successful alkaline diuresis requires the simultaneous administration of potassium chloride. Hypokalemia will prevent adequate alkalinization.
  - Give **40 mEq potassium chloride** IV piggyback (IVPB) over 4–5 hours. Give additional potassium chloride either orally or IV as needed to maintain serum potassium concentration above 4 mEq/L.
  - **Use caution with alkaline diuresis in older patients**, who may have cardiac, renal, or pulmonary comorbidity, because pulmonary edema is more likely to occur in this population.
  - Sodium acetate may be substituted for sodium bicarbonate during a drug shortage. Sodium acetate cannot be administered as a rapid IV bolus. To administer an infusion, 150 mEq (three ampules) is placed in 1000 mL D5W.[48,49]
- **Do not use acetazolamide** (carbonic anhydrase inhibitor). Although acetazolamide alkalinizes the urine, it increases salicylate toxicity because it also alkalinizes the CNS (trapping more salicylate in the brain) and worsens acidemia.
- **Hyperventilate any patient requiring endotracheal intubation.** In salicylate-poisoned patients with tachypnea and hyperpnea, the respiratory alkalosis partially compensates for the metabolic acidosis. Mechanical ventilation with neuromuscular paralysis, sedation, and "normal" ventilator rates will remove the respiratory alkalosis, worsen acidosis, and cause rapid deterioration or death. Administering one to two ampules of sodium bicarbonate (50–100 mEq) immediately before the intubation should be considered. Patients requiring intubation will most likely also require hemodialysis.
- **Treat altered mental status with IV dextrose**, despite normal blood glucose.
- Treat cerebral edema with hyperventilation and osmotic diuresis.
- Treat **seizures** with a **benzodiazepine** (diazepam, 5–10 mg IV q15 min up to 50 mg) followed by **phenobarbital**, 15 mg/kg IV. Give **dextrose** 25 g IV immediately following seizure control.

Other Nonpharmacologic Therapies

- **Hemodialysis** is indicated for blood concentrations >100 mg/dL after acute intoxication. However, patients with rising levels despite therapy, acidosis, pulmonary or cerebral edema, and patients who cannot receive a large amount of fluid may also require hemodialysis even with concentrations <100 mg/dL. Hemodialysis rapidly removes salicylate and corrects acidosis. Hemodialysis may be useful with chronic toxicity when salicylate concentrations are as low as 40 mg/dL in patients with any of the following: persistent acidosis, severe CNS symptoms, progressive clinical deterioration, pulmonary edema, or renal failure.
- Treatment of pulmonary edema may also require mechanical ventilation with a high fraction of inspired oxygen concentration and positive end-expiratory pressure (in addition to high respiratory rate).

SPECIAL CONSIDERATIONS

- Admit moderately symptomatic patients for at least 24 hours. Repeat serum salicylate concentration, electrolytes, BUN, creatinine, and glucose at least every 6 hours to confirm declining salicylate concentration, improving bicarbonate concentration, and stable potassium concentration. Measure urine pH at least every 6 hours (if patient has urinary bladder catheter) or with each spontaneous void to confirm urinary alkalinization.

- Admit patients with severe overdoses to an ICU. Even in patients with hemodynamic stability, the nursing requirements may be too intensive to be managed on the floor. Monitor laboratory studies as with moderately ill patients. Closely monitor ABGs or VBGs. Arrange for immediate hemodialysis. Use great caution with mechanical ventilation, and hyperventilate any patient who requires mechanical ventilation.

ANTICONVULSANTS

Phenytoin and Fosphenytoin

GENERAL PRINCIPLES

Classification

There are five major mechanisms by which anticonvulsants exert therapeutic activity. In overdose, these features are enhanced:

- **Inhibition of sodium channels:** carbamazepine, lacosamide, lamotrigine, oxcarbazepine, phenytoin, valproic acid, topiramate, and zonisamide
- **Inhibition of calcium conductance:** ethosuximide, zonisamide, valproic acid, pregabalin, and gabapentin
- **Inhibition of excitatory neurotransmitters (NMDA):** perampanel, felbamate, lamotrigine, and topiramate
- **Stimulation of inhibitory neurotransmitter (GABA):** benzodiazepines, phenobarbital, tiagabine, and vigabatrin
- **Interaction with SV2A proteins:** levetiracetam

Pathophysiology

- Phenytoin has been a first-line treatment for seizures since its introduction. Fosphenytoin was developed as a response to some of the toxicity associated with IV phenytoin administration. Fosphenytoin is a prodrug that is converted to phenytoin after IV or IM injection and therefore will be referred to as phenytoin in the following text.
- **Neither of these drugs is indicated for the treatment of toxin-induced seizures,**[50] **including ethanol withdrawal seizures.**[51]
- Phenytoin exerts therapeutic activity by binding to sodium channels and inhibiting reactivation.[52] Phenytoin exhibits saturable kinetics, and at plasma levels >20 µg/mL, toxic effects become rapidly apparent.
- Acute toxicity is associated with the development of a **neurologic syndrome** that appears to be cerebellar in origin. **Cardiotoxicity** is **not** associated with phenytoin **ingestion;**[53] however, it has been **reported with IV administration** of phenytoin. Rapid IV administration slows cardiac conduction and decreases systemic vascular resistance and myocardial contractility. The cardiac toxicity associated with IV phenytoin administration is due in part to the presence of propylene glycol and ethanol in the diluent, which are known myocardial depressants and vasodilators.[54] The introduction of fosphenytoin has decreased the incidence of cardiac complications as it does not contain propylene glycol as a diluent.

Risk Factors

Other than overdose, risk factors for developing phenytoin toxicity are associated with the coadministration of drugs that affect the **cytochrome P450** system like metronidazole, fluconazole, cimetidine and amiodarone. Inducers such as alcohol, rifampicin, barbiturates can decrease the levels of phenytoin. Valproic acid and sulfonylureas can precipitate toxicity by displacing it from the protein binding site.

DIAGNOSIS

There are several classic clinical findings that point to the diagnosis of phenytoin toxicity.

Clinical Presentation

History

Antiepileptic toxicity commonly presents with a triad of symptoms: CNS depression, ataxia, and nystagmus. There is usually a history of seizure disorder, and the medication list will include phenytoin. In intentional overdoses, the patient may be lethargic with slurred speech and an extrapyramidal movement disorder.[55]

Physical Examination

- At plasma concentrations of >15 μg/mL, patients will exhibit **nystagmus. Ataxia** develops at levels of 30 μg/mL. **Confusion** and **frank movement disorders** occur at levels of 50 μg/mL or greater. Levels >100 μg/mL are lethal. Chronic phenytoin ingestion is also associated with **gingival hyperplasia**, which is a very useful clinical finding when uncertain of the diagnosis. **Ingestions** are **not** associated with **cardiotoxicity** or vital sign abnormalities.[56] Rapid **IV** administration of phenytoin results in **hypotension** and **bradycardia.** Death has been reported.[55] Drug reaction with eosinophilia and systemic symptoms (DRESS) is a potentially life-threatening condition presenting 2 months after initiating treatment. There are also case reports of TEN and SJS.
- **Extravasation** injury is a serious complication of IV phenytoin administration and can result in blister pain and peripheral edema described as **the purple glove syndrome**. This injury will occasionally require surgical debridement.[57] This syndrome can also occur in the absence of extravasation. Mechanism is not fully understood and thought to occur due to irritation of the tissues because of added propylene glycol and sodium hydroxide.
- **Given the potential for these complications**, unless a patient is unable to tolerate PO administration, it is preferable to administer phenytoin by the PO route.

Differential Diagnosis

Phenytoin toxicity is similar in presentation to carbamazepine poisoning; however, carbamazepine tends to exhibit cardiotoxicity. Other considerations include a convulsive status epilepticus, meningitis, encephalitis, or other intracerebral lesion.

Diagnostic Testing

Laboratories

- **Serial phenytoin concentrations** (corrected for albumin, because phenytoin is highly protein bound) should be obtained on any patient with a potential history of exposure. Adjusted phenytoin concentration = measured total concentration / [(0.2 × albumin)] + 0.1 : Sheiner Tozer Formula
- CBC: Phenytoin has been reported to occasionally cause agranulocytosis.
- LFTs: Phenytoin is associated with the occasional development of hepatotoxicity.

Electrocardiography

ECGs and telemetry are generally needed in oral overdoses.[56] However, in IV infusions, it is necessary to have the patient in a monitored setting like continuous monitoring of the heart rhythm or serial ECGs.

TREATMENT

- Admission is warranted for patients with ataxia, and serial levels should be obtained while in the hospital.
- Supportive care is the mainstay of treatment for acute or chronic phenytoin toxicity. **Multidose AC** (MDAC) is useful in decreasing the serum half-life; however, given the pharmacokinetic profile of this drug, it is possible to rapidly lower the serum concentration below therapeutic levels and precipitate a seizure. For wide QRS complex more than 100 ms, sodium bicarbonate 2 mmol/kg IV repeated every 2 minute is indicated till rhythm is restored. Consider IV ligocaine 1.5 mg/kg if pH >7.5 and patient is having dysrhythmia.
- **Benzodiazepines** are the mainstay of treatment for seizures.
- Hypotension and bradycardia in the setting of IV administration are usually self-limiting and will resolve with supportive care. In refractory bradycardia or hypotension, advanced cardiac life support principles apply.
- Cases of agranulocytosis are responsive to **G-CSF** administration.
- Hepatotoxicity usually resolves with the discontinuation of the drug.

Surgical Management

In cases of extravasation, it is important to have a surgical evaluation to determine the need for operative debridement.

SPECIAL CONSIDERATIONS

- Because the mainstay of treatment of acute seizures is benzodiazepine administration and IV phenytoin is associated with significant toxicity, it is better to orally load patients whenever possible.
- Phenytoin can also cause **anticonvulsant hypersensitivity syndrome** (AHS), which can be confused for Stevens-Johnson syndrome.[58] AHS can also be seen with carbamazepine and lamotrigine.

OUTCOME/PROGNOSIS

Phenytoin overdoses tend to be benign and self-limiting with supportive care. Deaths are exceedingly unusual even in the setting of massive overdose.

Carbamazepine/Oxcarbazepine

GENERAL PRINCIPLES

Definition

Carbamazepine and oxcarbazepine are structurally related to TCAs. Like fosphenytoin, oxcarbazepine is a prodrug that is metabolized to an active metabolite. Carbamazepine and oxcarbazepine are anticonvulsants.

Pathophysiology

- The therapeutic efficacy of carbamazepine and oxcarbazepine is due to **sodium channel blockade**, which prevents the propagation of an abnormal focus. The therapeutic serum concentration of carbamazepine is 8–12 mg/L. There is no routine laboratory testing for oxcarbazepine; however, the carbamazepine assay will detect the presence of oxcarbazepine.

- The toxicity associated with carbamazepine is likely due to its chemical structure. TCA-like effects include sodium channel blockade, QT prolongation, and anticholinergic features.
- In overdose, carbamazepine is erratically absorbed and may form concretions in the GI tract causing prolonged toxicity.
- Persistently high levels of carbamazepine have been reported to increase antidiuretic hormone secretion leading to syndrome of inappropriate antidiuretic hormone release (SIADH).[59]

Risk Factors

Carbamazepine toxicity may be enhanced by concomitant use of drugs that are metabolized by the cytochrome P450 system.

DIAGNOSIS

There are several key features of carbamazepine toxicity.

Clinical Presentation

History

Toxicity should be suspected in individuals who present with a history of a seizure disorder and altered mental status. **Delayed toxicity** has been reported after an acute overdose given the variability in GI absorption.[60] Patients may exhibit a relapsing syndrome of coma and altered consciousness due to bezoar formation and enterohepatic recirculation.

Physical Examination

- The predominant clinical findings in carbamazepine toxicity are neurologic, cardiovascular and anticholinergic effects. In mild to moderate toxicity, patients may present with ataxia, nystagmus, and mydriasis. In serious overdose, patients may develop **coma** and **seizures**, including status epilepticus. Vital sign abnormalities include **tachycardia**, hyperthermia, urinary retention, absent bowl sounds, due to the anticholinergic effects of the drug, as well as **hypotension, bradycardia**, due to direct myocardial depressant effects.
- The combination of cerebellar findings on examination, in conjunction with an anticholinergic toxidrome, should prompt the clinician to consider carbamazepine as a potential toxicant. Chronic cases may present with leukopenia, agranulocytosis, and aplastic anemia. One of the important causes of drug-induced hyponatremia is chronic CBZ use. DRESS, TEN, and SJS have also been reported.

Differential Diagnosis

Mild-to-moderate carbamazepine toxicity resembles phenytoin toxicity. Other considerations include a convulsive status epilepticus, meningitis, encephalitis, or other intracerebral lesion.

Diagnostic Testing

- Serum carbamazepine concentrations should be obtained on any patient who presents with a history of ingestion. The therapeutic range is from 8 to 12 mg/L. Serial levels should be obtained every 4–6 hours to evaluate for delayed toxicity or prolonged absorption. Disorientation and ataxia if levels <11 mg/L, hallucinations at levels 15 to 25 mg/L, and coma and convulsions >25 mg/L. Concentrations of >40 mg/L are associated with the development of cardiotoxicity.[61]

- Patients with carbamazepine overdoses will often develop signs of cardiac toxicity. ECG findings include QRS and QT_c prolongation and atrioventricular (AV) conduction delays. Cardiotoxicity will occasionally be delayed, so all patients should be admitted with telemetry.

TREATMENT

Medications

Maintain airway protection always and treat seizures with **benzodiazepines**. Gastric decontamination with AC is recommended several hours after ingestion, as CBZ exhibits delayed absorption. Although there is a paucity of data regarding the efficacy of **sodium bicarbonate** in this setting, its use should be considered if the QRS duration is >100 ms, given the structural similarity to TCAs. Hemodialysis or hemoperfusion is indicated only to improve elimination in case of persistent seizures, coma, respiratory depression. Intravenous lipid emulsion therapy has been reported to be successful in few case reports.

Other Nonpharmacologic Therapies

Like phenytoin, carbamazepine's half-life is reduced by the administration of **MDAC** by decreasing enterohepatic recirculation of the drug.[62]

Use caution with administration of MDAC in the setting of this overdose because patients may develop seizures and coma, which pose a significant aspiration risk.

Lamotrigine

GENERAL PRINCIPLES

Definition

Lamotrigine, an anticonvulsant, is widely prescribed as a mood stabilizer as well as for the treatment of partial complex seizures.

Pathophysiology

Lamotrigine exerts its therapeutic effects by blocking presynaptic and postsynaptic sodium channels. In overdose, excess sodium channel blockade may result in widening of the QRS on the ECG and conduction blocks. Idiopathic cases of dermatologic pathology including AHS, Steven–Johnson syndrome, and toxic epidermal necrolysis have been reported with the therapeutic administration of lamotrigine.

DIAGNOSIS

Clinical Presentation

History

Suspect lamotrigine toxicity in patients with a seizure disorder and altered mental status.

Physical Examination

Patients with lamotrigine toxicity present with lethargy, oculogyric crisis, dystonia, ataxia, and nystagmus. Overdose may present with seizures as well.

Differential Diagnosis

Lamotrigine toxicity is similar to other sodium channel–blocking anticonvulsant agents.

Diagnostic Testing

Laboratories

Therapeutic concentrations range from 3 to 14 mg/L; concentrations >15 mg/L are associated with the development of toxicity.

Electrocardiography

Lamotrigine overdose has been associated with the development of conduction delays and QRS widening. Patients should be admitted on telemetry.

TREATMENT

AC should be administered to alert patients with an intact airway. Seizures should be treated with **benzodiazepines**. There are theoretical benefits of administering **sodium bicarbonate**, 150 mEq in 1 L of 5% dextrose, in patients with a QRS >100 ms; however, there is a paucity of experimental data to support this practice. In the setting of bicarbonate administration, close monitoring of **serum potassium** levels is required to avoid life-threatening hypokalemia.

Levetiracetam

GENERAL PRINCIPLES

- Levetiracetam, an anticonvulsant, is becoming increasingly used in the management of several of the different subtypes of epilepsy.
- The mechanism by which levetiracetam exerts its therapeutic effect is not well described; however, it does block N-type calcium channels on the presynaptic terminals of neurons.

DIAGNOSIS

Clinical Presentation

Very little data exist on levetiracetam overdoses. Lethargy and respiratory depression have been reported in the setting of overdose.

Differential Diagnosis

In patients with a seizure disorder and lethargy, intoxication, infectious, and metabolic disorders should be considered.

Diagnostic Testing

Although a test is available for measuring serum levels, this assay is not routinely available.

TREATMENT

Generally, **supportive care** is required. In cases where respiratory depression is evident, the patient should be intubated and ventilated. Avoid AC in patients with an altered mental status and an unprotected airway.

Valproic Acid

GENERAL PRINCIPLES

Valproic acid (VPA), an anticonvulsant, is widely used for the management of seizures and mood disorders like bipolar disorder and exerts its effects by inhibiting the function of voltage-gated sodium and calcium channels as well as enhancing the function of GABA.

Pathophysiology

VPA is metabolized by the hepatocytes through a complicated biochemical process that involves β-oxidation in the mitochondria. This drug may result in fatty infiltrates in the liver and accumulation of ammonia.

Risk Factors

Hepatic dysfunction can occur even at therapeutic levels and therefore should be monitored. The therapeutic range is 50–100 mg/L. In overdose, the risk of hepatic dysfunction and hyperammonemia increases.

DIAGNOSIS

Clinical Presentation

Patients with valproate overdoses may present with drowsiness, confusion, tremor, ataxia, cerebral edema, and coma. Occasionally, patients will present with abdominal pain.

Diagnostic Testing

- Therapeutic concentrations range from 50 to 100 mg/L. VPA levels should be done every 2 to 4 hours till peak is achieved and levels start to fall. CT is not routinely indicated, but if there is focal neurological deficit, it should be done. Patients who present with overdoses should have a **BMP** drawn to evaluate for hypernatremia, hypocalcemia, hyperosmolality, and high anion gap metabolic acidosis.
- In cases of massive overdose, a **CBC** should be sent because cases of pancytopenia have been reported in the literature.[63] Hematopoietic disturbances may occur up to 5 days after overdose.
- Chronic VPA therapy has been associated with the development of hepatotoxicity and may result in a fatal hepatitis. In cases of chronic toxicity, **LFTs** should be sent to evaluate for transaminitis. Likewise, any patient with VPA toxicity should have an **ammonia** level sent. Idiopathic fulminant hepatic failure can also occur.
- There have been occasional reports of pancreatitis;[64] therefore, in massive overdose, consider sending **lipase** as well.
- Hyperammonemia can occur with therapeutic dosing so ammonia levels should be sent in patients on VPA presenting with altered mental status.

TREATMENT

- Most cases of toxicity resolve with supportive care. In patients who are awake with adequate airway protection, **AC** is warranted. Naloxone is reported to reverse CNS depression.
- In patients with hyperammonemia >35 mmol/L (>80 μg/dL) **L-carnitine** therapy should be instituted. In awake patients, oral carnitine is the preferred route at 50–100 mg/kg/d divided every 6 hours up to 3 g/d. In cases where patients are not able to tolerate PO, IV L-carnitine may be administered at 100 mg/kg, up to 6 g, as a loading dose, and then

15 mg/kg every 4 hours. Therapy may be discontinued when the patient's ammonia level declines to <35 mmol/L.

ANTIDEPRESSANTS

Monoamine Oxidase Inhibitors

GENERAL PRINCIPLES

Although several different classes of monoamine oxidase inhibitors (MAOIs) exist, the drugs most frequently implicated in toxicity are the first-generation antidepressant drugs: **phenelzine**, **isocarboxazid**, and **tranylcypromine**. **Clorgiline**, a later-generation drug, is also associated with a similar toxic profile. The third-generation drugs, including **moclobemide**, have a better safety profile.

Pathophysiology

Monoamine oxidase is an enzyme responsible for the inactivation of biogenic amines such as **epinephrine**, **norepinephrine**, **tyramine**, **dopamine**, and **serotonin**. Inhibition of this enzyme results in an increase of synaptic concentrations of biogenic amines. An increase in norepinephrine and serotonin, in particular, is thought to be responsible for mood elevation. MAOIs are structurally similar to amphetamine. In overdose, a significant amount of neurotransmitter is released, resulting in a **sympathomimetic** toxidrome. Phenelzine and isocarboxazid are also hydrazine derivatives and, in overdose, have been associated with the development of **seizure** activity. As neurotransmitters become depleted, patients develop cardiovascular collapse, which is often refractory to therapy. Given the fact that MAOIs affect an enzymatic pathway, there is often a **significant delay** in the development of toxicity after overdose, with most cases occurring in a **24-hour** period after ingestion, although there are cases of toxicity occurring **up to 32-hours** after overdose.[65] This effect may occur with seemingly small overdoses of five or six pills.[66]

Risk Factors

The classic risk factors for developing toxicity include increasing a prescribed dose or eating foods rich in **tyramine**, such as aged cheddar cheese or red wine. Drug–drug interactions occur when a new antidepressant (often a selective serotonin reuptake inhibitor [SSRI]) is introduced without an adequate **washout period** of several weeks after discontinuing the MAOI.

Prevention

Patients should be well educated on the risk associated with these drugs. The **duration of action of these drugs significantly outlasts their half-lives**; therefore, physicians should always use a reference guide or consult a pharmacist before prescribing a new drug in addition to or as a replacement for the MAOI.

Associated Conditions

- MAOIs have been associated with severe **hypertensive crises** in the setting of coingestions of **tyramine**-containing foods such as **aged cheddar and red wine.** Likewise, coingestion of **indirect-acting sympathomimetics**, which cause presynaptic release of norepinephrine, may precipitate a hypertensive crisis. Agents included in this category are **amphetamine-based drugs, dopamine, and pseudoephedrine.**
- **Serotonin syndrome** is also associated with the coingestion of **SSRIs, St. John's wort, meperidine**, and **dextromethorphan**.

DIAGNOSIS

Clinical Presentation

MAOI overdose is associated with a considerable risk of mortality and morbidity.

History

- In overdose, there may be a **significant delay** in the development of symptoms. Anyone who presents with normal vital signs and history of MAOI overdose must be **admitted and monitored** for at least 24 hours.
- Overdose should be suspected in patients who are taking MAOIs and present in extremis with a florid **sympathomimetic** toxidrome.

Physical Examination

Patients may initially present with minimal signs of toxicity. Subsequently, they will develop **agitation, diaphoresis, tachycardia, severe hypertension, dilated pupils**, and **headache**. As their illness progresses, they may develop **hyperthermia, rigidity, and seizures**. Ultimately, there is depletion of neurotransmitter stores, and the patient develops refractory cardiovascular collapse.

Differential Diagnosis

MAOI overdose produces a clinical picture that is similar to severe serotonin syndrome and severe sympathomimetic toxicity. Serotonin syndrome has a relatively faster onset of action and occurs within minutes to hours of ingestion.

Diagnostic Testing

Laboratories

These include routine laboratory tests such as a **BMP**, looking for metabolic acidosis, hyperkalemia, and renal failure; **CK** to look for rhabdomyolysis; and **troponins** to evaluate for myocardial infarction in severe cases. **Coagulation studies** are important because these patients may develop DIC.

Electrocardiography

ECG analysis may reveal a range of disorders from a simple sinus tachycardia to a wide complex dysrhythmia.

Imaging

A **head CT** should be obtained on altered patients and patients complaining of a headache to evaluate for intracranial hemorrhage.

TREATMENT

- The management of first-generation MAOI overdose can be very difficult because the patient may have dramatically variable vital signs. Patients with MAOI overdose should be aggressively managed with **orogastric lavage**, even if they are asymptomatic on arrival to the hospital.
- In hyperthermic patients, **rapid cooling measures** should be instituted.

Medications

First Line

- **AC** (1 g/kg) should be administered to the patient after the airway is secured. Many patients will be awake and alert and may not need immediate intubation; however, these patients should receive AC as well.

- Given the propensity for wildly fluctuating blood pressure (BP), titratable and short-acting agents are the mainstay of treatment in these patients. Hypertension should be managed with **nitroglycerin, nitroprusside, or phentolamine.** If the patient develops hypotension, a direct-acting α-agonist such as **norepinephrine** should be used. **Avoid dopamine** in the setting of MAOI overdose because it often fails to improve BP due to catecholamine depletion.
- **Benzodiazepines** should be used for seizures and agitation. Rigidity that does not respond to benzodiazepine administration may be managed with **nondepolarizing** paralytics. There are case reports describing the resolution of rigidity after the administration of **cyproheptadine.**[67]

Second Line

In patients with refractory seizures, early administration of **pyridoxine** is warranted because MAOIs may deplete pyridoxine concentrations. Doses of 70 mg/kg, not to exceed 5 g, should be administered early as an IV infusion of 0.5 g/min.

SPECIAL CONSIDERATIONS

- Patients with MAOI overdoses require admission with monitoring for at least 24 hours, given the propensity for delayed toxicity. Aggressive decontamination measures should be taken, even if the patient seems to be asymptomatic because decompensation is rapid and frequently fatal.
- The **exception** to this is an overdose of **moclobemide**, which has a much better safety profile and tends to have a benign course because of its short duration of MAO inhibition.

PATIENT EDUCATION

- Patients who are placed on MAOIs should be educated about food and drug interactions and warned about the risk of interactions with herbal supplements, including St. John's wort.
- A washout period of at least 2 weeks after discontinuation of an MAOI should be observed before starting another antidepressant.

Tricyclic Antidepressants

GENERAL PRINCIPLES

- Multiple TCAs are on the market, including amitriptyline, clomipramine, doxepin, imipramine, trimipramine, desipramine, nortriptyline, and amoxapine.
- TCAs interact with a wide variety of receptors with many consequent effects in the setting of an overdose. The primary antidepressant effect is due to the inhibition of serotonin and norepinephrine reuptake. Additionally, TCAs modulate the function of central sympathetic and serotonergic receptors, which is thought to contribute to their antidepressant effects.
- TCAs have antimuscarinic effects, resulting in tachycardia, dry mucous membranes and skin, urinary retention, and decreased GI motility. Patients will also have dilated pupils.[68] Sedation is likely due to antihistamine effects. Furthermore, these agents are potent α_1-antagonists, leading to the development of hypotension and a reflex tachycardia. Cardiac toxicity is due to sodium channel blockade, resulting in a wide complex rhythm on the ECG.[69] TCAs also exhibit a complex interaction with the GABA receptor, which in overdose likely contributes to seizure activity.[70]

DIAGNOSIS

TCA overdose exhibits its own toxidrome. Patients with an acute overdose may present to the emergency department with a normal mental status and vital signs but then rapidly decompensate.

Clinical Presentation

History

As with any overdose, a history is often unreliable. The clinical picture in serious toxicity is fairly stereotypical, and a careful physical examination can help establish the diagnosis.

Physical Examination

- Often present with a rapid onset of **CNS depression**
- **Tachycardia** and **hypotension** due to vasodilatation
- **Dilated pupils, dry mucous membranes,** and **urinary retention** due to the antimuscarinic effects
- May present with **seizure** activity, if significant overdose present

Diagnostic Criteria

The TCA toxidrome is a fairly consistent constellation of signs including hypotension, tachycardia, coma, and seizures.

Diagnostic Testing

Laboratories

- **Serum TCA concentrations** have a **limited role** in the management of acute TCA toxicity because they are **not predictive of severity of illness.**[71] Qualitative measurements of TCA concentrations in the urine are unreliable because there are many common drugs that cross-react on the assay, including diphenhydramine and cyclobenzaprine.
- Serial **VBGs** should be measured in patients undergoing alkalinization. Because bicarbonate treatment can cause profound hypokalemia, serial K^+ should be followed and repleted.
- **Dextrose** should be checked in any patient with altered mental status.

Electrocardiography

The ECG has proved to be a valuable tool in predicting the degree of morbidity in TCA overdose. In one classic study, one-third of patients with a **QRS of ≥100 ms** developed **seizures.** Fifty percent of patients with a QRS of ≥160 ms developed **ventricular dysrhythmias.**[71] A terminal 40-ms axis of >120 degrees is found in patients who are taking TCAs and may help narrow the diagnosis in patients with an altered mental status of unknown etiology. Simply put, the ECG will show an **R′ in aVR** and an S wave in leads I and aVL. An R′ in aVR of >3 mm has been demonstrated to be predictive of neurologic and cardiac complications in TCA-poisoned patients.[72]

TREATMENT

- Patients with TCA overdose require early aggressive intervention.
- In patients with altered mental status, early **intubation, resuscitation, and GI decontamination** are warranted.
- Orogastric lavage may be beneficial in patients who are intubated with large ingestions because of decreased GI motility. Avoid this in small children because they only typically take one to two pills.

- **Hyperventilation** to achieve rapid serum alkalinization may be used as a bridge until bicarbonate therapy is started.

Medications

First Line

- **After the patient's airway is protected**, an AC dose of 1 g/kg is warranted even in delayed presentations.
- **Sodium bicarbonate** has been demonstrated to narrow the QRS, decrease the incidence of ventricular arrhythmias, and improve hypotension.[73] A bolus of 1–2 mEq/kg every 3–5 minutes should be given with continuous ECG monitoring until the QRS narrows or the BP improves. Serial VBGs should be obtained with a goal of maintaining the blood pH at 7.50–7.55.
  - A bicarbonate drip should be titrated to the QRS narrowing and resolution of hypotension. The patient should be monitored in an ICU with serial pH and serum potassium measurements as well as monitoring for fluid overload.
  - Alkalinization should continue for 12–24 hours until the clinical picture and the ECG improve.
- **Temporary pacemakers** have been used to treat refractory symptomatic bradycardias not responsive to sodium bicarbonate.
- **Norepinephrine** is the pressor of choice in hypotensive patients who do not respond to alkalinization because of its direct effects on the vasculature.
- **Lidocaine** may be considered in the presence of ventricular dysrhythmias precipitated by TCA toxicity. However, class **Ia and Ic antidysrhythmics are contraindicated in the management of TCA-poisoned patients.**
- **Benzodiazepines** are the mainstay of treatment for seizures. **Phenytoin should be avoided.**

Second Line

Propofol and **barbiturates** may be beneficial in refractory seizures.

Other Nonpharmacologic Therapies

Cardiopulmonary bypass and **extracorporeal membrane oxygenation** (ECMO) have been used in critically ill patients with refractory hypotension.[74,75]

Selective Serotonin Reuptake Inhibitors

GENERAL PRINCIPLES

Classification

This class of drugs includes **fluoxetine, fluvoxamine, paroxetine, sertraline, citalopram,** and **escitalopram.** These drugs have a much better safety profile than the earlier drugs marketed for the management of depressive disorders and, as such, have largely supplanted MAOIs and TCAs in the treatment of depression.

Pathophysiology

These drugs enhance serotonergic activity by preventing its reuptake into the presynaptic terminal of the neuron, which may partially explain their antidepressant effects. Unlike other antidepressants, SSRIs have limited effects on other receptors and therefore tend to be less toxic in overdose.

DIAGNOSIS

Clinical Presentation

The vast majority of these overdoses have a benign clinical course. However, patients may present with signs of serotonin excess. Patients who have ingested **citalopram** or **escitalopram** may develop delayed toxicity.

History

Overdose histories are unreliable. Many patients who claim to have taken an overdose yet who look well actually took SSRIs.

Physical Examination

Signs of toxicity are usually absent unless the patient has taken a massive overdose. In these cases, patients may present with nausea, vomiting, and tachycardia. Patients with **citalopram** or **escitalopram** ingestions may present with **seizures.**

Diagnostic Testing

Laboratories

- Obtain **BMP** because SSRIs have been implicated in the development of **SIADH.**
- **FSBG** should be checked in patients with an altered mental status or seizures.
- Check CK, lactate, and coagulation profile in patients with serotonin syndrome.

Electrocardiography

Patients will occasionally present with a sinus tachycardia. Patients with citalopram or escitalopram ingestions may develop QT_c prolongation as late as 24 hours after an overdose.[76]

TREATMENT

- The vast majority of overdoses require only 6 hours of observation and supportive care. Patients with intentional **citalopram** and **escitalopram** overdoses should be admitted to the floor with 24 hours of telemetry to monitor for QT_c prolongation.
- In patients who are awake and alert, 1 g/kg of **AC** may be administered.
- Treat seizures or neuromuscular hyperactivity with **benzodiazepines.**
- Treat torsades de pointes (TdP) with **magnesium**, correction of electrolytes, **lidocaine**, and **overdrive pacing.**

Serotonin Syndrome

GENERAL PRINCIPLES

Definition

Serotonin syndrome is a disorder that can be precipitated by the introduction of a serotonergic agent and has been reported to occur even after ingestion of a single pill.[77]

Pathophysiology

Serotonin syndrome is thought to occur secondary to excess stimulation of $5HT_{2A}$ receptors.[78] This syndrome can result from the coadministration of two or more serotonergic agents including SSRIs, MAOIs, meperidine, amphetamines, cocaine, TCAs, and various other drugs. This syndrome consists of a combination of mental status changes, neuromuscular hyperactivity, and autonomic hyperactivity.

DIAGNOSIS

Clinical Presentation

History

Suspect serotonin syndrome in any patient who presents with a rapid onset of tremor and clonus after administration of a serotonergic agent. It is important to avoid the addition of other serotonergic agents in the management of these patients.

Physical Examination

- Patients will present with signs of excess serotonergic activity including restlessness, shivering, diaphoresis, and diarrhea.
- Patients may develop tremors, akathisias, myoclonus, ocular clonus, and muscle rigidity later.
- Vital sign abnormalities include tachycardia, hypertension, and hyperpyrexia.

Diagnostic Criteria

- Serotonin syndrome is diagnosed by the presence of four of the following major criteria: alteration of consciousness, coma, or mood elevation; shivering, myoclonus, rigidity, or hyperreflexia; pyrexia; or diaphoresis or autonomic instability.
- Additional minor criteria include restlessness or insomnia; mydriasis or akathisia; tachycardia; diarrhea; and respiratory or BP abnormalities.[79]

Differential Diagnosis

Patients who present with altered mental status, rigidity, and hyperpyrexia may be misdiagnosed with neuroleptic malignant syndrome (NMS). NMS tends to develop over days to weeks, whereas serotonin syndrome has a faster onset, usually manifesting over a 24-hour period.

Diagnostic Testing

Serotonin syndrome is diagnosed by a constellation of symptoms and signs rather than any specific laboratory findings; however, as the disease evolves, laboratory abnormalities develop.

Laboratories

- As with any critical illness, patients may succumb to multiorgan failure, and therefore, laboratory studies should be obtained on the basis of the presentation.
- Patients may have no laboratory abnormalities if they present early with mild form.
- On the other hand, more severe presentations may develop complications from psychomotor agitation and muscle rigidity including elevated **CK**, **metabolic acidosis**, and an **elevated lactate.**
- Check **BMP** because **renal failure** may occur in the presence of rhabdomyolysis.
- Check **coagulation studies** because patients with hyperthermia may develop **coagulopathy**.

Electrocardiography

The typical ECG will show a sinus tachycardia; however, there are no specific diagnostic ECG criteria associated with serotonin syndrome.

TREATMENT

- The treatment of serotonin syndrome is largely supportive and requires the removal of the offending agent. Aggressive cooling and hydration measures should be taken in the hyperthermic patient. Antipyretics are not useful for the treatment of hyperthermia in serotonin syndrome.

- **Benzodiazepines (diazepam)** should be used liberally to treat psychomotor agitation and myoclonus. In severe cases, **nondepolarizing paralytics** should be used to limit the degree of rhabdomyolysis.
- Severe hypertension and tachycardia can be treated with short-acting esmolol or nitroprusside.
- In patients with mild to moderate symptoms, **cyproheptadine**, an antihistamine with $5HT_{1A}$ and $5HT_{2A}$ antagonism, should be considered. A **4- to 8-mg** initial dose should be given orally, which often results in a rapid reversal of symptoms. If there is no response, the dose may be repeated in 2 hours. Subsequent dosing is 2–4 mg orally every 6 hours until the patient improves or a maximum dose of 32 mg/d is reached.

Lithium

GENERAL PRINCIPLES

Classification

Toxicity may be classified as **acute, chronic, or acute on chronic**. Lithium, an antidepressant, has a narrow therapeutic index, and therefore, risk of toxicity is high in patients on chronic therapy. The therapeutic range is approximately 0.6–1.2 mmol/L (or mEq/L).

Pathophysiology

- The mechanism by which lithium exerts its antimanic properties is not well understood. There is some evidence that lithium enhances serotonin function, which may contribute to its mood-stabilizing properties.[80]
- Acute toxicity is associated with the development of a GI illness because lithium is a metal.
- Chronic toxicity is primarily associated with neurologic dysfunction.
- Although serum levels are helpful in the management of these patients, the clinical picture should be the basis for therapy.
  - Generally, in **chronically** exposed patients, levels of less than 2.5 mEq/L are associated with tremulousness, ataxia, and nystagmus.
  - Levels greater than 2.5 mEq/L are associated with a deteriorating neurologic syndrome and are an indication for aggressive intervention including dialysis.
  - A serum concentration of 4.0 mEq/L in an **acute** overdose is also an indication for dialysis.[81]

Risk Factors

Lithium has peripheral effects, which may enhance its toxicity, including the development of nephrogenic diabetes insipidus. This phenomenon is thought to occur through the reduction in the binding of aquaporins in the collecting duct of the kidney.[82] This development enhances toxicity by causing dehydration, which leads to an increase in proximal tubular reabsorption of lithium.[83] Other dehydration states may enhance toxicity as well.

Prevention

Patients on chronic lithium therapy should have serum levels monitored and regular follow-up with their psychiatrist, which should include evaluation for the clinical signs of toxicity.

Associated Conditions

Lithium therapy has been associated with the development of chronic tubulointerstitial nephropathy,[84] thyroid dysfunction,[85] serotonin syndrome,[86] and other endocrine effects.

DIAGNOSIS

Clinical Presentation

History

Although the history is often unreliable in overdose patients, acutely intoxicated patients may present complaining of nausea and abdominal discomfort. In chronic toxicity, patients may present with worsening confusion.

Physical Examination

- **Acute overdose** presents with a predominately GI syndrome of nausea, vomiting, diarrhea, and abdominal pain. As the illness progresses, patients may develop signs of volume depletion with tachycardia and hypotension. Severe toxicity is associated with neurologic dysfunction including altered mental status, nystagmus, ataxia, or coma.
- **Chronic toxicity** is associated with tremor, nystagmus, and ataxia. Confusion, dysarthria, fasciculations, and myoclonus are frequent physical findings. Seizures are reported in the literature.[87]

Diagnostic Testing

Laboratories

- Obtain serial lithium levels in patients who present with evidence of toxicity.
  - A high initial level may be due to the timing of the last dose; therefore, the clinical picture should guide therapy.
  - **Obtain the serum sample in a lithium-free tube.**
- Other laboratories should include a **BMP** to evaluate electrolyte levels, renal function, and hydration status.
- Lithium induces an elevation in the **white blood cell (WBC) count.**

Electrocardiography

The ECG may show nonspecific T-wave flattening or QT_c prolongation; however, cardiac dysfunction is unusual in this overdose.

TREATMENT

- AC does not bind to lithium and therefore has no role in the management of these overdoses.
- Whole-bowel irrigation with **polyethylene glycol** at a rate of 2 L/h is indicated for overdoses of sustained-release preparations.[88]
- The mainstay of therapy is the infusion of **0.9% saline solution** at twice the maintenance rate. Closely monitor fluid status in these patients to avoid overload.

Other Nonpharmacologic Therapies

Consider **dialysis** for patients who present with signs of severe toxicity, with altered mental status, or with other neurologic dysfunction but are unable to tolerate the required fluid load for enhanced elimination. In patients with acute overdose and a serum lithium concentration >4.0 mEq/L or chronic overdose and a serum level >2.5 mEq/L, dialysis should be considered.

Bupropion

GENERAL PRINCIPLES

Bupropion is an atypical antidepressant of the monocyclic aminoketone class and is structurally related to amphetamines. It acts by selectively inhibiting dopamine and norepinephrine reuptake.

DIAGNOSIS

Bupropion has been associated with more severe symptoms than the other atypical agents. Common features of toxicity include tachycardia, drowsiness, hallucinations, and convulsions. **Seizures** have been reported at therapeutic doses.[89] **QRS prolongation** has also been described in overdose. Symptoms may be **delayed for up to 10 hours** after ingestion of sustained-release pills.

TREATMENT

Treatment of bupropion overdose includes airway protection. **Whole-bowel irrigation** and MDAC should be considered in patients who present early with a normal mental status and ingestion of a sustained-release preparation. This modality is **contraindicated** in seizing patients. Seizures should be treated with **benzodiazepines**. Barbiturates and propofol should be considered in patients with status epilepticus.

ANTIPSYCHOTICS

GENERAL PRINCIPLES

Epidemiology

According to the AAPCC's 2007 report, antipsychotic/sedative hypnotic agents were the fourth leading cause of fatal overdoses in the United States.[90]

Pathophysiology

Antipsychotic agents exert their therapeutic effect largely by binding to dopamine receptors in the CNS, which tends to mitigate the positive symptoms of schizophrenia. Dopamine receptor blockade is also associated with the development of movement disorders, and the newer neuroleptic agents attempt to address this by modulating serotonergic tone. Most antipsychotics affect multiple receptors in the nervous, endocrine, and cardiovascular systems, which accounts for a wide range of toxic symptoms. In general, the older "typical" agents in the phenothiazine class tend to have more cardiac toxicity, with varying degrees of sodium channel blockade (wide QRS) and potassium channel blockade (QT_c prolongation). Furthermore, these agents tend to have more significant extrapyramidal effects. The newer or "atypical" antipsychotics tend to exhibit less cardiac toxicity, but they often have pronounced α_1-antagonism, causing hypotension. The atypicals are also associated with the idiosyncratic development of other medical problems. For example, olanzapine has been associated with the development of fatal diabetic ketoacidosis (DKA),[91] and clozapine was briefly withdrawn from the market because a small percentage of patients developed agranulocytosis.[92]

Phenothiazines

GENERAL PRINCIPLES

These are the prototypic antipsychotic drugs and include chlorpromazine, thioridazine, prochlorperazine, perphenazine, trifluoperazine, fluphenazine, mesoridazine, haloperidol (a butyrophenone), and thiothixene.

DIAGNOSIS

Clinical Presentation

History

The history is often difficult to obtain in these patients.

Physical Examination

- Overdoses are characterized by agitation or delirium, which may progress rapidly to coma. Pupils may be mydriatic, and deep tendon reflexes are depressed. Seizures may occur.
- Vital sign abnormalities may include hyperthermia, hypotension (due to strong α-adrenergic antagonism), tachycardia, arrhythmias (including TdP), and depressed cardiac conduction.

Diagnostic Testing

Laboratories

- Serum concentrations are generally not available or useful.
- FSBG and a BMP should be checked on all patients with altered mentation.

Imaging

Abdominal radiographs may reveal pill concretions.

TREATMENT

- Assess airway and breathing, place an IV, and institute cardiac monitoring.
- Hypotensive patients should receive a 20 mL/kg bolus of NS.
- Consider whole-bowel irrigation for ingestion of sustained-release formulations.
- Treat ventricular arrhythmias with lidocaine. Class Ia agents (e.g., procainamide, quinidine, disopyramide) are contraindicated; avoid sotalol.
- Treat hypotension with IVF administration and α-adrenergic vasopressors (norepinephrine or phenylephrine). **Avoid epinephrine** because vasodilation may occur because of unopposed β-adrenergic response in the setting of strong α-adrenergic antagonism.
- TdP may require magnesium, isoproterenol, or overdrive pacing (see Chapter 7, Cardiac Arrhythmias).
- Treat seizures with benzodiazepines.
- Treat dystonic reactions with benztropine, 1–4 mg, or diphenhydramine, 25–50 mg, IM or IV.
- Treat hyperthermia with cooling.

SPECIAL CONSIDERATIONS

- NMS, which may complicate use of these agents, is characterized by rigidity, hyperthermia, altered mental status, and elevated CK. NMS should be treated with aggressive cooling measures, benzodiazepines (lorazepam), and **bromocriptine** (2.5–10 mg IV tid

until the patient improves, then taper the dose over several days to avoid recrudescence of symptoms). Dantrolene is used in severe cases of NMS.
- Admit patients who have ingested a significant overdose for cardiac monitoring for at least 48 hours.

Clozapine

GENERAL PRINCIPLES

Definition

An atypical neuroleptic.

DIAGNOSIS

Clinical Presentation

- Overdose is characterized by altered mental status, ranging from somnolence to coma.
- Anticholinergic effects occur, including blurred vision, dry mouth (although **hypersalivation** may occur in overdose), lethargy, delirium, and constipation. Seizures occur in a minority of overdoses. Coma may occur.
- Vital sign abnormalities include hypotension, tachycardia, fasciculations, tremor, and myoclonus.

Diagnostic Testing

- Obtain CBC and LFTs; follow the WBC counts weekly for 4 weeks.
- Clozapine levels are not useful.

TREATMENT

- As always, support ABCs. Place an IV and institute cardiac monitoring.
- Consider AC 1 g/kg if the patient presents within an hour of ingestion.
- Treat hypotension with 20 mL/kg of IVF; if resistant, treat with norepinephrine or dopamine.
- Treat seizures with benzodiazepines.
- Consider filgrastim for agranulocytosis.
- Forced diuresis, hemodialysis, and hemoperfusion are not beneficial.
- Admit and monitor patients with severely symptomatic overdoses for 24 hours or more.

Olanzapine

GENERAL PRINCIPLES

Definition

An atypical neuroleptic.

DIAGNOSIS

Clinical Presentation

- Overdose is characterized by somnolence, slurred speech, ataxia, vertigo, nausea, and vomiting.[93]
- Anticholinergic effects occur, including blurred vision, dry mouth, and tachycardia.

- Seizures are uncommon. Coma may occur.
- Vital sign abnormalities include hypotension and tachycardia. Serious dysrhythmias rarely occur.
- **Pinpoint pupils are unresponsive to naloxone.**

TREATMENT

- Pay attention to ABCs, place an IV, and institute cardiac monitoring.
- Give AC if presentation is within 1 hour of ingestion.
- Treat hypotension with fluids and, if ineffective, norepinephrine.
- Give benzodiazepines for seizures.
- Treat DKA aggressively, if present.

Risperidone, Ziprasidone, Quetiapine

GENERAL PRINCIPLES

These are newer neuroleptic agents and reports of overdoses have increased significantly. Quetiapine overdose is associated with more adverse outcomes than other neuroleptic agents[94] and requires aggressive therapy.

DIAGNOSIS

Clinical Presentation

- Clinical effects include CNS depression, tachycardia, hypotension, and electrolyte abnormalities.
- Clinically significant ventricular dysrhythmias are uncommon.
- Quetiapine overdose is associated with respiratory depression[94] and seizures.[95]
- Miosis is a common finding.

Diagnostic Testing

QRS and QT_c prolongation have been reported.[96]

TREATMENT

- Scrupulous attention should be paid to ventilatory and circulatory support.
- Treat hypotension with 20 mL/kg fluid boluses and, if severe and persistent, consider a direct-acting pressor such as norepinephrine.
- Replete electrolytes as needed.
- Diuresis, hemodialysis, and hemoperfusion do not appear to be useful.

ANTIHYPERTENSIVES

β-Adrenergic Antagonists

GENERAL PRINCIPLES

Definition

Of all of the agents available, propranolol tends to exhibit the most toxicity because it is lipophilic, is widely distributed throughout the body, and possesses significant membrane-stabilizing activity. Sotalol, which is classically thought of as a class III antiarrhythmic, also has some β-adrenergic antagonist activity and, in toxic doses, can result in a prolonged QT_c and TdP.

Classification

Cardiovascular agents are a frequent cause of serious poisonings and, according to the 2017 annual report of the National Poison Data System, were the eighth leading cause of fatal drug exposures.[1] Patients with these overdoses require aggressive intervention and close monitoring.

Pathophysiology

The toxicity associated with an overdose of β-blockers is largely due to the effects of antagonism at catecholamine receptors. In general, selectivity is lost in overdose, so bronchospasm may occur in the setting of β_1-selective antagonists.

DIAGNOSIS

Clinical Presentation

- Patients with a significant ingestion of an immediate-release product will exhibit signs of toxicity within 6 hours. The exception to this rule is sotalol, which in overdose can have delayed toxicity and prolonged effects, with one report of QT_c prolongation persisting up to 100 hours after ingestion.[97]
- With the exception of propranolol and sotalol, β-blocker overdose in healthy people tends to be benign, with a significant number of patients remaining asymptomatic after ingestion,[98] although severe intoxication can occur.

History

Suspect β-antagonist overdose in patients with altered mental status, bradycardia, and hypotension.

Physical Examination

Patients with significant ingestions present with bradycardia and CHF. Patients with propranolol ingestions may develop coma, seizures, and hypotension. Propranolol overdoses have a high mortality.[99]

Differential Diagnosis

In patients with symptomatic bradycardia, also consider overdose of CCB, clonidine, or digoxin.

Diagnostic Testing

Laboratories

Patients with β-antagonist overdoses occasionally become hypoglycemic; therefore, a **FSBG** should be obtained. Likewise, any patient with an altered mental status should have a **BMP** sent. Consider obtaining a **lactate** because patients with profound hypotension may develop mesenteric ischemia.

Electrocardiography

The ECG may reveal sinus bradycardia or AV block. In propranolol ingestions, a wide QRS manifesting sodium channel blockade may be present. With sotalol, QT_c prolongation may appear as a delayed presentation and TdP may develop.

TREATMENT

The treatment of β-blocker overdose is largely supportive in mild to moderate cases. The patient should have an IV placed, and continuous cardiac monitoring should be instituted. **Hypoglycemia** should be treated with 50 mL of 50% **dextrose** (D_{50}). Consider **AC** if patients present within 1 hour of ingestion. Intubation and ventilation should be instituted in patients with altered mental status. Likewise, consider **orogastric lavage** in patients with potential for severe toxicity such as propranolol overdoses.

Medications

- Patients with significant toxicity from propranolol or sotalol ingestions should be treated more aggressively.
- **Atropine** 1 mg IV may be given up to 3 mg for symptomatic bradycardia; however, this is usually ineffective because the bradycardia is not vagally mediated.
- **A fluid bolus** of 20 mL/kg should be given and may be repeated; monitor for the development of fluid overload.
- **Glucagon** 2–4 mg IV may be given over 1–2 minutes. Then start infusion of 2–5 mg/h, not to exceed 10 mg/h. One of the significant side effects of glucagon administration is nausea and vomiting; monitor for vagally mediated bradycardia.
- **Calcium gluconate** 3–9 g IV may be given through a peripheral line in patients with hypotension. Alternatively, consider **calcium chloride** 1–3 g through a central line slow IV push over 10 minutes. Calcium chloride is sclerosing and can cause severe extravasation injury.
- Any patient with hypotension is a candidate for **high-dose insulin euglycemia therapy.** Although the mechanism for improvement is unclear, this is routinely used in the management of severe CCB overdose.[100] Animal studies of severe propranolol overdose have shown a survival benefit.[101] This involves a bolus of **1 unit/kg of regular insulin, followed by an infusion of 0.5–1.0 unit/kg/h of regular insulin.** This should be accompanied by a dose of **50 mL of D_{50} and a dextrose drip at 1 g/kg/h of dextrose**, which calculates to 10 mL/kg/h of D_{10} or 2 mL/kg/h of D_{50}.[4] FSBG should be obtained every 30 minutes, and potassium levels should be followed every 2 hours with repletion because **profound hypokalemia** may complicate this treatment modality. The BP response tends to be delayed by 15–30 minutes.
- **Lipid therapy** is emerging as a promising treatment modality in these often fatal poisonings. Theoretically, lipid administration causes lipophilic drugs to partition into the plasma and away from the heart. The current protocol, which can be found at http://www.lipidrescue.org, starts with **1.5 mL/kg of 20% intralipid administration over 1 minute, followed by an infusion rate of 0.25 mL/kg/min.** If there is no response, the patient may have repeat boluses every 3–5 minutes until a **3 mL/kg** total dose, and the infusion rate may be increased to **0.5 mL/kg/min. The maximum total dose recommended is 8 mL/kg.**[102]
- **Catecholamines** should be approached with caution in these patients because α-stimulation in conjunction with β-blockade may precipitate acute heart failure. Therefore, **hemodynamic monitoring** should be instituted with careful titration of **epinephrine at 0.02 μg/kg/min or norepinephrine at 0.10 μg/kg/min. Isoproterenol at 0.10 μg/kg/min** may be useful as well; however, monitor closely for the development of hypotension. It is important to note that high doses of these agents may be required.

Other Nonpharmacologic Therapies

- In cases of refractory hypotension and bradycardia, it is reasonable to consider an intra-aortic balloon pump (IABP)[103] and **ECMO.**[104]

- Transvenous pacing may be attempted, but it is generally difficult to achieve capture, given the degree of myocardial depression.
- Some β-adrenergic antagonists are water soluble and can be eliminated with hemodialysis.[105]

Calcium Channel Blockers

GENERAL PRINCIPLES

Definition

CCBs are widely used for the management of tachyarrhythmias and hypertension. Generally speaking, the overdoses of dihydropyridines (block L type calcium channels in peripheral vasculature) such as amlodipine, nimodipine, nicardipine, and nifedipine, tend to be more benign; although in massive overdose, selectivity may be lost and may result in significant symptoms. Nondihydropyridines (block L type calcium channels in myocardium) verapamil and diltiazem, can produce severe toxicity, even in the setting of a small overdose.

Pathophysiology

CCBs exert their effects by blocking L-type calcium channels on the smooth muscle of the vasculature and the myocardium. This decreases inotropy and chronotropy and results in a decrement of BP and heart rate. In overdose, these effects are accentuated. L-type calcium channels are also involved in the release of insulin from the β-islet cells of the pancreas. In CCB overdose, patients will often present with elevated blood sugars.

DIAGNOSIS

Clinical Presentation

Patients with diltiazem or verapamil overdoses should be considered critically ill and require aggressive intervention.

History

Patients will often present with an unintentional ingestion where they missed a dose and attempted to "catch up" by doubling their next dose. Focused history should include the agent – immediate/sustained release, timing, preexisting cardiac disorder.

Physical Examination

Patients with verapamil or diltiazem overdoses will present with profound **hypotension and bradycardia and generally have a normal mental status until they arrest**. It is thought that CCBs have somewhat of a neuroprotective effect that may explain the preservation of mentation. In the setting of dihydropyridine CCB overdoses, patients usually present with hypotension and a reflex tachycardia. However, specificity can be lost causing these patients to become bradycardic. In severe cases of shock, the mental status can be altered and led to seizure, delirium, and coma.

Differential Diagnosis

CCB toxicity may resemble β-antagonist or clonidine overdoses.

Diagnostic Testing

This is a clinical diagnosis; serum concentrations are not useful in the management of CCB overdose.

Laboratories

- **Fasting blood sugar** should be checked and is elevated in the setting of CCB toxicity. This is part of the toxidrome associated with this particular overdose.
- A **BMP** should be obtained as well to follow serum calcium levels. In patients on a calcium drip, ionized calcium should be followed. Serum lactate > 3 mmol/L – poor prognosis.

Electrocardiography

The ECG may show sinus bradycardia, conduction delays, or even complete heart block. With dihydropyridine overdose, a sinus tachycardia may be present.

TREATMENT

The treatment of dihydropyridine CCB overdose is largely supportive in mild to moderate cases. The patient should have an IV placed, and continuous cardiac monitoring should be instituted. Consider **activated charcoal** if patients present within 1 hour of ingestion. Intubation and ventilation should be instituted in unstable patients. Likewise, consider **orogastric lavage** in patients with potential for severe toxicity. **Whole-bowel irrigation** with polyethylene glycol should be instituted for sustained-release preparations.

Medications

Patients with significant toxicity, such as verapamil or diltiazem ingestions, should be treated more aggressively.

- **Atropine** 1 mg IV may be given up to 3 mg for symptomatic bradycardia; however, this is usually ineffective because the bradycardia is not vagally mediated.
- **A fluid bolus** of 20 mL/kg should be given and may be repeated; monitor for the development of fluid overload.
- **Calcium gluconate** or **calcium chloride** may be given as described in the treatment section of β-blocker overdose. In addition, a calcium gluconate drip may be started and run up to 2 g/h. Close monitoring of calcium is required.
- Any patient with hypotension is a candidate for **high-dose insulin euglycemia therapy**. See discussion of this topic under treatment of β-blocker overdose.
- **Lipid therapy**, as described in the treatment section of β-blocker overdose, should be initiated early.
- **Catecholamines** should be approached with caution in these patients because α stimulation may precipitate acute heart failure. Therefore, **hemodynamic monitoring** should be instituted with careful titration of **epinephrine starting at 0.02 μg/kg/min or norepinephrine at 0.10 μg/kg/min.**
- **It is important to note that calcium is generally ineffective at treating this overdose because the L-type calcium channel is blocked, preventing calcium entry into the cell. Therefore, lipid or insulin should be considered first-line therapy in the management of these patients.[106] However, some still consider vasopressors as first-line therapy.[107]**

Other Nonpharmacologic Therapies

- In cases of refractory hypotension and bradycardia, it is reasonable to consider IABP,[108] cardiopulmonary bypass,[109] and **ECMO**.[110]
- Transvenous pacing may be attempted, but it is generally difficult to achieve capture, given the degree of myocardial depression.

SPECIAL CONSIDERATIONS

Patients with ingestions of a sustained-release preparation should be monitored in an intensive care setting. Immediate-release preparations should be monitored for 6–8 hours before discharge or psychiatric evaluation.

Clonidine

GENERAL PRINCIPLES

- Clonidine is an orally administered agent used in the management of hypertension.
- Clonidine is an imidazoline drug with centrally acting antihypertensive effects related to α_2-agonism, which decreases sympathetic outflow from the CNS.[111] Other drugs in this family include oxymetazoline and tetrahydrozoline, nasal decongestants that exhibit similar toxicity when orally administered. In overdose, peripheral effects include an initial release of norepinephrine with a **transient increase** in BP, followed by hypotension.[112]

DIAGNOSIS

Clinical Presentation

Although the clinical presentation of these overdoses can be quite concerning, most patients recover with supportive care. Patients tend to develop symptoms within 30 minutes to an hour after their overdose.

History

The history is unreliable in these patients because they are often somnolent or comatose on arrival to the hospital.

Physical Examination

Suspect clonidine overdose in patients with hypotension, bradycardia, and CNS depression. Occasionally, patients may develop hypoventilation, which is usually responsive to vocal or tactile stimulation.[113] Pupillary examination reveals miosis, and this finding in the setting of hypotension and bradycardia is highly suggestive of clonidine overdose.

Differential Diagnosis

β-Antagonists, digoxin, and CCB overdose should be included in the differential.

Diagnostic Testing

Laboratories

Serum clonidine concentrations are not routinely used in the management of these patients. An **FSBG** and **BMP** should be obtained on any patient with altered mental status.

Electrocardiography

The ECG generally shows a sinus bradycardia.

TREATMENT

- Patients generally respond with supportive care. In severely poisoned patients, consider intubation and ventilation; however, this is rarely needed.
- **Avoid GI decontamination and AC in these patients because they tend to develop altered mental status quickly.**

- **Atropine** 1 mg IV may be given up to 3 mg for symptomatic bradycardia; however, this is usually not necessary because the bradycardia tends to resolve on its own.
- **A fluid bolus** of 20 mL/kg should be given and may be repeated; monitor for the development of fluid overload.
- An initial dose of 0.4 mg of **naloxone** may be useful in reversing the hypotension and bradycardia associated with clonidine overdose.[114] However, high doses (i.e., 10 mg) may be required, with redosing every 2–3 hours because naloxone has a shorter duration of action than clonidine.[115]

SPECIAL CONSIDERATIONS

Withdrawal syndromes have been reported in patients who have stopped taking clonidine. It is usually manifested as **rebound severe hypertension**, agitation, and palpitations. Treatment is to administer clonidine and taper the dose gradually. Benzodiazepines are also useful in this situation.

Other Antihypertensives

- These agents include **diuretics, α_1-antagonists, angiotensin-converting enzyme** (ACE) **inhibitors, and angiotensin II receptor blockers** (ARBs).
- **Diuretics** tend to be benign in overdose. Occasionally, they cause dehydration and electrolyte imbalances. Laboratory studies should include a BMP. Management usually only requires gentle fluid hydration.
- **α_1-Antagonists** cause peripheral vasodilation, which usually responds to hydration. Occasionally, they cause enough hypotension to require vasopressors. In these cases, norepinephrine should be administered.
- **ACE inhibitors** rarely cause significant toxicity, although there are case reports of fatal overdoses. Treatment is supportive. In patients with hypotension, naloxone may be useful.[116]
- **ARBs** may cause hypotension in overdose. Treatment is supportive.

PARASYMPATHETIC AGENTS

ACh is a neurotransmitter of the peripheral nervous system and CNS, acting on nicotinic and muscarinic receptors.

Anticholinergics

GENERAL PRINCIPLES

Anticholinergic effects are primarily due to blockade of muscarinic receptors (i.e., antimuscarinic effects) and, therefore, mainly affect parasympathetic functions.

Epidemiology

Anticholinergic poisoning occurs either from intentional ingestion of certain plants or over-the-counter medications (e.g., Jimson weed, diphenhydramine)[117] or from accidental overdosing (e.g., medical noncompliance, polypharmaceutical regimens).[118]

Etiology

Drugs and medications with anticholinergic effects include the following:

- **Anticholinergics:** Atropine, scopolamine, benztropine, glycopyrrolate, ipratropium
- **Antihistamines:** Diphenhydramine, promethazine, doxylamine

- **Antipsychotics:** Chlorpromazine, clozapine, olanzapine, quetiapine
- **Antidepressants:** Amitriptyline, nortriptyline, imipramine, desipramine
- **Antiparkinson drugs:** Benztropine, trihexyphenidyl
- **Mydriatics:** Cyclopentolate, homatropine, tropicamide
- **Muscle relaxants:** Cyclobenzaprine
- **Plants:** Belladonna, Jimson weed, *Amanita* mushrooms

Pathophysiology

- Blockade of muscarinic receptors (i.e., parasympathetic autonomic nervous system [ANS], except for the sympathetically innervated sweat glands) leads to the so-called **anticholinergic toxidrome.**
- **Tachycardia** is one of the main symptoms in anticholinergic poisoning. Vagal blockade of cardiac muscarinic receptors leads to unopposed sympathetic stimulation of the myocardium.
- Some anticholinergic drugs can also cross the blood–brain barrier and interact with muscarinic receptors in the cortex and subcortical regions of the brain causing anticholinergic CNS **manifestations.**

Associated Conditions

- Antihistamines and cyclic antidepressants also block sodium channels and cause additional cardiac symptoms such as dysrhythmias and QRS prolongations.
- Potassium channel blockade may result in QT_c prolongation and TdP.

DIAGNOSIS

Clinical Presentation

Anticholinergic Toxidrome

- **Central effects:** Confusion, agitation, euphoria/dysphoria, hallucinations, incoherent thoughts and speech, lethargy, ataxia, choreoathetoid movements, and rarely, seizures or coma.
- **Peripheral effects:** Tachycardia, mouth dryness, decreased perspiration with flushed skin and hyperthermia, dilated pupils with photophobia and blurred vision, decreased bowel sounds, and urinary retention.
- A helpful mnemonic for antimuscarinic effects is "RED as a beet, DRY as a bone, BLIND as a bat, MAD as a hatter, and HOT as a hare."

TREATMENT

- All patients presenting with an anticholinergic toxidrome need **cardiovascular monitoring.** Serial evaluation of vital signs and serial physical examinations are essential to address sudden worsening of the patient's condition (dysrhythmia, seizure).
- GI decontamination is only indicated if the patient is fully awake and cooperative because of the high risk of aspiration or loss of airway control in unconscious or combative patients. **Gastric lavage** for GI decontamination may be appropriate, given decreased stomach emptying and slowed GI motility from the anticholinergic effect; although, it is rarely used.
- Patients with hyperthermia may benefit from cooling measures.

Medications

- **Physostigmine** is a reversible **anticholinesterase** that leads to increased ACh in synapses to overcome receptor blockade. It is useful in the management of severe anticholinergic poisoning with delirium, hallucinations, and seizures.[119,120]
  - In the emergency department setting, the use of physostigmine as a diagnostic tool in patients with high suspicion of anticholinergic agitation or delirium has been found to be relatively safe.[121,122]
  - **Contraindications:** Underlying cardiovascular disease, wide QRS complex or AV block on ECG, asthma, bowel or bladder obstruction, peripheral vascular disease, or gangrene. Its use is also relatively contraindicated in the setting of cyclic antidepressant overdose.
  - **Adult dosing:** 0.5 mg IV over 5 minutes and every 5 minutes up to 2 mg total or until improved level of consciousness.
  - Physostigmine has a short duration of action (20–60 minutes), and redosing might be necessary if agitation recurs.
  - NOTE: Always have **atropine** at bedside for reversal if needed, that is, in case of severe bradycardia or asystole from unopposed cholinergic stimulation or other dysrhythmias from sodium channel blockade (e.g., in TCA overdose).[123]
- **Benzodiazepines** should be used as adjuncts to treat anticholinergic agitation or delirium. There is no benefit of benzodiazepine monotherapy in anticholinergic central symptoms.[122]

Insecticides

GENERAL PRINCIPLES

Insecticides are critical tools for combating insect-borne illness. In the United States, *Aedes* spp. of mosquitoes have migrated as far up as New York State and are the vectors of dengue, Zika, West Nile, and yellow fever. Cases of dengue and Zika have been reported in Florida and the public health impact of these diseases warrants serious prevention measures. Per the World Health Organization, vector-borne illnesses cause over 700,000 preventable deaths per year.[124] Organophosphorus pesticide (Table 28-3) self-poisoning is a major clinical and public -health problem across much of rural Asia. Of the estimated 500,000 deaths from self-harm each year, about 60% are due to pesticide poisoning.

TABLE 28-3 Classification of Insecticide Poisons

Organophosphorus • Diethyl organophosphorus: quinalphos, Chlorpyrifos, diazinon, triazophos, phorate, dimethoate, parathion-ethyl • Dimethyl organophosphorus: monocrotophos, dichlorvos, acephate, malathion, fenthion, mathamidophos, and phosphamidon
Carbamates: methomyl, carbaryl, carbofuran, bendiocarb, aldicarb, propoxur
Organochlorine: endosulfan, endrin
Pyrethroids: cypermethrin, alpha-cypermethrin, deltamethrin, cyhalothrin
Neonicotinoid: imidacloprid, acetamiprid

Cholinesterase Inhibitors

- Cholinesterase inhibitors are chemical compounds that inhibit the enzyme cholinesterase. Blockade of **AChE** function leads to excess ACh in synapses of the ANS and SNS.
- Cholinesterase inhibitors are divided into two classes:
  - Organophosphates (OPs)
  - Carbamates

Organophosphates

GENERAL PRINCIPLES

Epidemiology

- OPs are commonly used as pesticides and insecticides. Some also have medical indications (e.g., malathion in lice shampoo).
- In the developing countries like India, OP and other pesticide poisonings represent the most common cause of overdose deaths.[125]
- OPs are also potent chemical terrorism and warfare agents ("nerve gas" agents) (e.g., sarin in the Tokyo subway attack or in Syria, tabun in the Iraq–Iran War).[126]
- Although self-inflicted OP poisoning with suicidal intent occurs, exposure is primarily occupational or accidental.[127] Because absorption occurs through skin and airways, the handling of OPs requires appropriate protective gear.
- With improvement in understanding of the disease and better healthcare systems, mortality is on decreasing trend.

Pathophysiology

- Inhibition of AChE leads to accumulation of ACh at nicotinic and muscarinic receptors, resulting in **excessive cholinergic stimulation.**
- The severity of symptoms varies depending on the route of exposure (dermal, inhalation, oral, parenteral), dose, lipid solubility of OP, type of OP, and enzyme affinity.[128]
- Initially, most OPs bind AChE reversibly. Some OPs, however, become permanently bound over time, a phenomenon known as "**aging.**" If aging occurs, the only way to overcome the inhibitory effect is for the body to synthesize new enzyme.
- OPs are hepatically metabolized. Some OPs become active toxins after liver metabolism and thus can have delayed effects (e.g., parathion).[129]

DIAGNOSIS

Clinical Presentation

The cholinergic toxidrome is a result of overstimulation of nicotinic and muscarinic receptors.[128,129] Although patients classically present with muscarinic features, because both receptors are being stimulated, patients can present with a mixture of muscarinic and nicotinic effects.

- **Muscarinic effects**
  - **SLUDGE syndrome:** Salivation, Lacrimation, Urination, Diarrhea, GI cramping, Emesis.
  - **Bradycardia, bronchorrhea, bronchoconstriction** (NOTE: Asphyxia and cardiovascular collapse are lethal features of OP poisoning.)
  - **Other effects:** Miosis, diaphoresis.
- **Nicotinic effects**
  - **Ganglionic:** Tachycardia, hypertension, diaphoresis, mydriasis

- ◦ **Neuromuscular:** Neuromuscular depolarization, fasciculations, motor weakness, paralysis with respiratory failure (analogous to succinylcholine, which is related to ACh)
- ◦ **Central:** Confusion, agitation, lethargy, seizures, coma

Diagnostic Testing

- **Cholinesterase concentrations:** There are two different cholinesterases that are routinely measured in red blood cells and plasma,[129] that is, butyrylcholinesterase activity in plasma and acetylcholinesterase in whole blood.
- Both assays are relatively useless in assessing the severity of exposure in acute intoxications because of their wide ranges of normal values. However, the results of such assays are rarely available in time to affect clinical decision making. Generally, a value <25% is taken as supportive evidence of significant exposure to OP or carbamate compound.
- They are mostly used as sensitivity markers to compare changes from baseline enzyme activity (e.g., in chronic occupational exposure or after OP elimination).[128]

TREATMENT

- **Protection:** OP-intoxicated patients pose a significant risk for further contamination of others through direct contact. Health-care personnel should use special **personal protective equipment** (PPE) (gowns, gloves, masks) until the patient is properly decontaminated.[128] If the OP was ingested, PPE may be required until any emesis is discarded because off-gassing from the emesis can result in bystander illness. PPE should not consist of latex or vinyl because OPs are lipophilic and may penetrate such materials.
- **Decontamination**
  - ◦ Remove patient from potential source of poisoning.[130] All clothing, especially leather, should be removed from the patient and discarded in a ventilated area.[130] Skin and hair decontamination requires thorough irrigation with water and might be enhanced through use of alcohol-based soaps.[130] Eyes should be irrigated with only water.[130]
  - ◦ Gastric lavage might be indicated in stable patients who ingested contaminated fluids.[131] Gastric lavage with KMnO4 or Na2SO46
  - ◦ NOTE: All lavaged/aspirated fluids need to be safely discarded.
- **Stabilization**
  - ◦ ABCs: Have a low threshold for early intubation to obtain airway protection. NOTE: Intubation alone may not improve hypoxia due to the large amount of pulmonary edema and bronchospasm. Succinylcholine is generally avoided since clearance of OP compound maybe delayed.
  - ◦ **Avoid** mouth-to-mouth resuscitation because of contamination risk.
  - ◦ Start IVF as an initial bolus of 20 mL/kg.[132]
- **Atropine** is an antimuscarinic agent that competes with ACh for receptor binding.
  - ◦ **Goal: Atropinization** (i.e., drying of bronchial secretions with normalized oxygen saturation [which may require 10–100 times the usual atropine dose]), heart rate >80 bpm, and systolic BP >90 mm Hg.[128]
  - ◦ The initial **adult dose** is 1.8–3 mg IV bolus. Then titrate according to persistence of bronchorrhea by doubling the previously used dose every 2–5 minutes until atropinization is achieved.[128]
  - ◦ The initial **pediatric dose** is 0.02 mg/kg IV. Titrate as in adults.[133]
  - ◦ Once the patient is stabilized, an infusion of atropine should be started with 10%–20% of the initial atropinization dose per hour and should be held once anticholinergic effects occur (e.g., absent bowel sounds, urinary retention, agitation).[128] If the patient develops atropine-induced psychosis, the infusion should be stopped for 1 hour and restarted at 80% the previous infusion rate.

  - If atropine supplies are exhausted, other antimuscarinic agents can be considered (e.g., diphenhydramine, glycopyrrolate).[134]
- **Pralidoxime** (2-PAM): Oximes are nucleophilic agents, for example, pralidoxime forms a complex with OPs that are bound to AChE. The pralidoxime–OP complex is then released from the enzyme and thus regenerates AChE function. Its use is controversial, but the best available evidence suggests that oximes should be administered. Its use has been limited to patients who present early (<2 hours) with diethyl OP compound.
  - Once the AChE-bound OPs start aging, pralidoxime is rendered ineffective. Therefore, if it is used, it is crucial to start pralidoxime therapy early.
  - Pralidoxime also binds to some degree to free OPs and thus prevents further AChE binding.
  - **Adult dosing:** New evidence favors an infusion regimen: 1–2 g of pralidoxime in 100 mL NS IV over 20 minutes, then infusion of 500 mg/h.[128] One trial indicated that a high-dose regimen (2-g loading dose followed by 1 g/h infusion for 48 hours) improved mortality.[135]
  - NOTE: Pralidoxime use longer than 24 hours might be indicated if unaged OPs are redistributed from fat tissue. In such cases, infusions should be continued until the patient remains symptom free for at least 12 hours without additional atropine doses or until the patient is extubated.[128]
  - Cardiac and respiratory failures have been reported after administration of pralidoxime.[136]
- **Benzodiazepines (diazepam)** are the first-line agents for OP-induced seizures.[125] These are also helpful in treating agitation and delirium due to atropine.
- Another antidote that is being investigated as bioscavenger treatment. It includes enzymes like purified human butyryl cholinesterase, which will sequester the highly toxic OP compound.

COMPLICATIONS

- **Intermediate syndrome**
  - This syndrome is a postacute exposure paralysis from persistent ACh excess after the acute cholinergic phase has been controlled and is not related to the severity of the acute phase. Some believe incomplete or insufficient oxime therapy explains this syndrome (*J Toxicol Clin Toxicol.* 1992;30:347).
  - It is characterized by weakness of proximal extremity muscles and the muscles supplied by cranial nerves that occurs hours to days (1–4 days) after acute OP poisoning and can lead to respiratory failure if unnoticed (*PLoS Med.* 2008;5(7):e147).
- It is recommended to assess flexor neck strength regularly in conscious patients. Any sign of weakness is a sign that the patient is at risk of developing peripheral respiratory failure (intermediate syndrome). Also tidal volume should be checked every 4 hours in such patients. Values less than 5 mL/kg suggest a need for intubation and ventilation. This syndrome of weakness is self-limiting and lasts for 1 to 2 weeks with complete resolution usually.
- **OP-induced delayed neurotoxicity (OPIDN)**
  - Besides AChE, some OPs also inhibit other neurotoxic esterases, resulting in polyneuropathy or spinal cord damage due to demyelination of the long nerve fibers.
  - OPIDN usually occurs several days to weeks after acute OP poisoning, leading to temporary, chronic, or recurrent motor or sensory dysfunction (*Annu Rev Pharmacol Toxicol.* 1990;30:405).
- **Cardiovascular complications:** Electrocardiographic findings suggest that QTc prolongation, ST-T segment changes, and T-wave abnormalities are common. Other manifestations include sinus bradycardia or tachycardia, hypotension or hypertension, supraventricular and ventricular arrhythmias, and noncardiogenic pulmonary edema.

Extrapyramidal manifestations like dystonia, rigidity, and tremors (usually resolves within 1 to 2 weeks) can be managed by using trihexyphenidyl, amantadine, and bromocriptine.

- Organophosphate coma: Coma can occur in the acute phase. Patient may either develop an encephalopathy like picture or progress to coma. This clinical clue may mimic brain death except here there will be pinpoint pupils unlike in brain death where it will be fixed and dilated. It can last for 3 to 5 days and resolves spontaneously. An EEG can be used to confirm the clinical suspicion.

MONITORING/FOLLOW-UP

- All patients with severe or moderate poisoning should be admitted to an ICU after initial stabilization for further monitoring and treatment (*Crit Care*. 2004;8(6):R391).
- Asymptomatic patients presenting with a history of unintentional poisoning or patients with only mild symptoms do not always require hospital admission but should be observed for 6–12 hours (*BMJ*. 2007;334:629).

Carbamates

GENERAL PRINCIPLES

Epidemiology

Carbamates are chemical esters of N-methylcarbamic acid and are reversible AChE inhibitors that also lead to ACh excess in the synaptic junction. These are relatively less toxic to humans compared to organophosphates and organochlorides because they act reversibly and for a shorter duration. They are occasionally found in pesticides. In India, pesticides containing aluminum phosphide is one of the leading causes of self-ingested poison.[137] The incidence is 18/100,000 in developed countries and this number is 10 times higher in developing countries.[138] Examples include Propoxur, Carbaryl, Carbofuran, and Carbosulfan.

- **Physostigmine** is a naturally occurring methyl carbamate found in the Calabar bean. Other common carbamates are pyridostigmine and neostigmine.
- **Pyridostigmine** has been used in the treatment of myasthenia gravis.

Pathophysiology

- Inhibition of ACh breakdown through blockage of AChE leads to accumulation of ACh at nicotinic and muscarinic receptors with **excess cholinergic stimulation**.
- Carbamates are reversible enzyme inhibitors; they release AChE spontaneously. There is no "aging" phenomenon with carbamates.

DIAGNOSIS

Clinical Presentation

The clinical picture of the carbamate-induced cholinergic toxidrome is analogous to the one seen in OP poisoning because nicotinic and muscarinic receptors of the ANS and SNS are stimulated.

- Look for **SLUDGE** syndrome, **bradycardia, bronchorrhea,** and **bronchoconstriction** as well as neuromuscular depolarization and be aware of the risk of cardiovascular or respiratory failure. Muscarinic features include – bronchospasm, brochorrhea, miosis, lacrimation, urination, diarrhea, hypotension, bradycardia, vomiting, salivation. Nicotinic features include tachycardia, mydriasis, hypertension, sweating. Neurologic features include confusion, agitation, and coma. Neuromuscular features are muscle weakness, paralysis, and fasciculations.

- Symptoms from carbamate poisoning are generally milder compared to OP poisoning and of shorter duration.

Diagnostic Testing

Diagnosis is based on clinical findings and history of exposure. **Cholinesterase concentrations** are used to compare changes from baseline enzyme activity in exposures but are not useful in acute toxicity.[139] In case there is doubt, an atropine challenge can be tried, where 0.6 to 1.2 mg can be given intravenously, a resultant increase in heart rate by 20 to 25 beats/min usually rules out poisoning or may be indicative of mild toxicity.[140]

TREATMENT

- The same measures of **protection and decontamination** as with OP poisoning apply to carbamates.
- **Stabilization**
  - ABCs: Have a low threshold for early intubation to obtain airway protection.
  - Avoid mouth-to-mouth resuscitation because of contamination risk. Universal precautions of wearing cap, gloves, gown, and goggles should be followed.

Medications

First Line

Atropine is an antimuscarinic agent that competes with ACh for receptor binding. **Goal: Atropinization.** See Treatment under Organophosphates section for dosing guidelines.

Second Line

- Pralidoxime can be considered if there is no clear evidence for isolated carbamate poisoning because additional OP exposure should always be suspected.
- **Benzodiazepines** are the first-line agents for carbamate-induced seizures.

Pyrethroids

GENERAL PRINCIPLES

The chemical substances used to reduce, stop, kill or repel any pest including insects, rodents and weeds to microorganisms are known as pesticide. The insecticidal properties of certain species of Chrysanthemum have been known for centuries. The flower secrets a compound called **pyrethrum** that targets **sodium channels** on the exoskeleton of insects.[141] **Permethrin** is a synthetic derivative of pyrethrum that is the first-line treatment for scabies and lice as well as an insect repellent on bed nets and military uniforms. Mechanism of action - Pyrethroids are about 2250 times more toxic to insects than mammals, the reason being they have a more sensitive sodium channel, small body size, and lower body temperature.[142] Nerve and muscle are the principal targets of the pyrethroid toxicity. It delays closure of voltage sensitive sodium channels, resulting in prolonged sodium influx "tail current" and lastly conduction block.

Epidemiology

According to the AAPCC, pyrethroid exposures increased between 2000 and 2005, which corresponded with the phase out of organophosphate insecticides for residential use. Given the low toxicity of these agents, most outcomes resulted in no or minor symptoms.[143]

Clinical Presentation

History

It is rare that patients with permethrin exposures will present with acute symptoms as permethrin ingestions result in rapid hydrolysis. Additionally minimal toxicities arise when used dermally as prescribed. Occasionally, patients with complain of mild itching, tingling, erythema, paresthesia, or dermatitis.[144] Inhalational exposure results in cough, dyspnea, sneezing, and increased secretions. Oral intake can lead to nausea, vomiting, oral ulceration, dysphagia, and abdominal pain. Convulsions and coma are the dreaded complications and can result in death. Pyrethroid insecticides do not bioaccumulate and have virtually no chronic toxicity despite occasional news reports to the contrary. The NHANES study found no association between pyrethroid exposure and ADHD or learning disability in children.[145]

Physical Examination

Patients may have a mild case of dermatitis on examination. It is important to look for oral ulcerations and do thorough examination.

Differential Diagnosis

Allergic dermatitis

Diagnostic Testing

None

TREATMENT

Systemic toxicity is less common. Generally supportive. Antihistamines, vitamin E, and corticosteroids as needed for dermatitis. Gastric lavage is better avoided.

HERBICIDES

GENERAL PRINCIPLES

Before World War II, there were no herbicides available to farmers. A substantial size of the population was required to farm to maintain an adequate food supply largely because manual weeding required every available hand in agriculture. The development of herbicides revolutionized farming and food security.

Glyphosate

GENERAL PRINCIPLES

Glyphosate is one of the most widely used herbicide in the world because of its broad-spectrum activity and its favorable safety profile. Glyphosate exerts its herbicidal activity by targeting a plant enzyme called 5-enolpyruvyl-shikimate-3-phosphate synthase (EPSPS).[146]

Epidemiology

According to the AAPCC there were 3181 acute glyphosate exposures in 2016, with 3 deaths reported.[1] Additionally, the National Cancer Institute published its updated research in the Agricultural Health Study demonstrating that chronic exposures to glyphosate are not associated with the development of cancer.[147]

DIAGNOSIS

Diagnosis is usually made by history alone.

Clinical Presentation

History

It is unusual for people with accidental ingestions to present with significant symptoms. Large symptomatic ingestions are usually suicide attempts and may result in caustic injury to the upper GI tract due to surfactants in the formulated product. Patients may complain of oropharyngeal, chest and abdominal discomfort, as well as nausea and vomiting. Aspiration can result in respiratory distress.[148]

Physical Examination

Acute ingestions of large volumes of the formulated product may result in caustic injuries to the upper GI tract, with **esophageal** and **stomach ulceration** and **perforation**, or caustic injury to the **larynx** and **airways** leading to **respiratory distress**. This is due to the surfactant in the formulated product. Surfactants are like detergents and after ingestion patients may be vomiting, drooling, stridorous, or wheezing depending on the degree of injury. Critically ill patients may develop cardiovascular collapse.

Diagnostic Testing

Laboratory Testing

Testing for glyphosate does not impact management and is therefore not indicated. Routine **CBC, BMP** may be warranted in critically ill patients.

Imaging

In cases of caustic injury, **CXR** or **CT** to evaluate for perforation may be warranted.

Diagnostic Procedures

In cases of caustic injury consider **GI evaluation** and **endoscopy**. Consider **laryngoscopy** in patients with respiratory distress.

TREATMENT

Supportive care is usually sufficient in mild ingestions. In cases of caustic injury consider **GI evaluation** and **endoscopy**. Hypotension should be treated with **IV fluids** and **vasopressors**.

Paraquat and Diquat

GENERAL PRINCIPLES

Paraquat is a restricted use herbicide that is safe when used per the manufacturer's label but exhibits marked toxicity when ingested. Ingestions of paraquat usually result in **death** from fulminant **respiratory failure**. Paraquat is bis-quaternary ammonium compound that is colorless, water soluble solid. Diquat is structurally related to paraquat.

Epidemiology

Although paraquat poisoning is rare in the United States, it is a leading cause of poisoning mortality in Asia-Pacific and Latin America.[125] Diquat poisoning is much less common.[149] The very high case fatality of paraquat is due to both its inherent toxicity and the lack of any effective treatment.

Pathophysiology

Paraquat undergoes redox recycling by many enzyme systems and generates reactive oxygen species. It causes lipid peroxidation, mitochondrial toxicity, oxidation of NADPH, and apoptosis. The paraquat molecule is actively transported into the lung by a polyamine transporter and cause oxidative injury to the Type I and Type II alveolar cells resulting in acute alveolitis, diffuse alveolar collapse, attachment of neutrophils and activated platelets to vascular endothelium and rapid fibrosis of the alveoli.[150] There are overlapping phases, in the acute "destructive phase" pneumocytes develop swelling and disruption of endoplasmic reticulum and mitochondria. Next is proliferative phase wherein profibroblasts and mature into fibroblasts in 1 week. At last, lung fibrosis develops. Although diquat has a similar toxicity profile, pulmonary injury is less frequent because of the structure of the molecule. Diquat does cause tubular necrosis of the kidney and renal failure is the prominent feature of diquat ingestions.[149]

DIAGNOSIS

Clinical Presentation

Small ingestions of paraquat (10–20 mL of a 20% solution) lead to toxicity in the two key target organs (kidneys and lungs) developing over the next 2–6 days.

History

Suspect paraquat ingestion in agricultural workers who present with **corrosive injury** to the upper GI tract. They will often complain of severe **chest pain** due to esophageal perforation and mediastinitis. **Dyspnea** signifies impending respiratory failure. Symptoms develop rapidly and progress to death within 1–5 days.

Clinical Features

Excessive inhalation of aerosolized paraquat may cause stomatitis, epistaxis, sore throat, and headache. Erythema, eruptions, boil, and ulceration of the skin can occur. GI toxicity is seen in all patients. Mucosal lesions of the mouth and the tongue ("paraquat tongue") begin to appear within the first few days and may become ulcerated with bleeding. Esophageal perforation and mediastinitis can occur. Corrosive injury to the oropharynx can result in "**pseudodiptheria**" or membrane formation over the pharyngeal structures.[151] Patients will present with **drooling, ulceration, nausea, and vomiting**. Liver can get affected and lead to icterus, hepatomegaly. Pancreatic involvement results in pain abdomen and pancreatitis. Pulmonary manifestations include cough, hemoptysis, dyspnea. Rapid decompensation of respiratory function can lead to ARDS. Respiratory failure is **not as prominent** in diquat ingestions. Renal failure can be oliguric or nonoliguric and is secondary to acute tubular necrosis. Neurological features include cerebral edema which manifests as ataxia, seizures, and coma. In the heart, there can be ventricular tachycardia, intraventricular conduction delay, hypotension, and cardiac arrest.

Depending on the quantity ingested patients can be classified into three categories:[219]

Mild poisoning – 20 mg ion/kg body weight. Maybe asymptomatic or may have mild GI symptoms. Usually fully recover.

Moderate to severe poisoning – 20 to 40 mg ion/kg body weight. Severe ulcerations in the GI tract, pulmonary fibrosis, acute renal failure. Death occurs in 2 to 3 weeks from respiratory failure.

Fulminant poisoning – >40 mg ion/kg . They present with severe hypoxia and metabolic acidosis. Multiorgan failure leading to death occurs in a few hours.

Diagnostic Testing

Laboratory Testing

Plasma and urine should be obtained for both qualitative and quantitative testing. Specimens should be sent in plastic containers as paraquat binds to glass. Urine samples with >2 μg/mL paraquat will turn **blue or black** in alkaline sodium dithionite solution, whereas diquat will turn **yellow or green**.[152]

A **CBC** may show leukocytosis and anemia, **BMP** will show progressive elevation of creatinine due to **renal tubular necrosis**—this is the prominent pathologic feature of **diquat** ingestions. **LFTs** and **CK** may show liver and skeletal muscle injury. **Lipase** is useful for diagnosis pancreatic injury and **ABG** is to measure oxygenation.

Imaging

CXR or CT can help identify pneumothorax, pneumomediastinum, and pulmonary fibrosis.

Diagnostic Procedures

In cases of caustic injury consider **GI evaluation** and **endoscopy**. Consider **laryngoscopy** in patients with respiratory distress. The presence of esophageal or gastric ulceration portends a grave prognosis as ulceration enhances absorption.[153]

TREATMENT

Timely intervention is critical for these patients. Contaminated clothing should be immediately removed, and any exposed skin should be gently rinsed with soap and water. Ophthalmic exposures should be copiously irrigated and ophthalmology consult should be obtained. Orogastric decontamination with 1–2 g/kg of **Fuller's earth, bentonite** or even **dirt** should be instituted within minutes of ingestion to adsorb paraquat. Most paraquat formulations contain an emetic to promote prompt GI decontamination. Once at the hospital, consider readminstration of 1–2 g/kg AC.

Other Nonpharmacologic Therapies

Intensive supportive care and **hemodialysis/hemoperfusion** for renal failure are indicated for these patients. Although hemodialysis and hemoperfusion can increase the clearance of paraquat or diquat, they do not tend to affect clinical outcomes.[154]

SPECIAL CONSIDERATIONS

Avoid oxygen: supplemental oxygen exacerbates pulmonary injury by accelerating free radical generation and redox cycling and should be withheld until the patient develops respiratory distress or until hypoxia develops.

Immunosuppressants (cyclophosphamide, MESNA, methylprednisolone, and dexamethasone) and antioxidants (Vitamin E, Vitamin C, NAC, deferoxamine, salicylic acid) have been tried with no major mortality benefits. Mortality rates varies according to the amount ingested: > 60 mL about 100 mL; 40 to 50 mL more than 90%, 20 to 40 mL, 50–60%; 10 to 20 mL, 10–20%; less than 10 mL less than 1% mortality.[220]

Yellow Phosphorous

GENERAL PRINCIPLES

Yellow phosphorous (YP) used in the production of fireworks, firecrackers, ammunition, rodenticides, and fertilizers causes direct hepatotoxicity typically resulting in periportal injury. It can be absorbed through the skin, mucous membranes, respiratory, and gastrointestinal system.

Etiology

The estimated dose of YP that is lethal to the liver is 1 mg/kg, and the ingestion of that amount results in death due to acute liver failure and cardiovascular collapse.

Pathophysiology

The mechanism of toxicity of yellow phosphorus is by means of an exothermic reaction producing phosphoric acid that causes direct tissue damage due to the production of free radicals against organic molecules. The increased predilection for liver damage is not fully understood.

DIAGNOSIS

Clinical Presentation

Clinical presentation has been divided into the following three stages:

- The initial GI stage is characterized by oral burns, vomiting, nausea, diarrhea (smoky stool), abdominal pain and gastrointestinal bleed, which occurs within the first 24 hours after ingestion.
- The second stage (1–4 days), which may last for several days, is essentially a symptom-free period, but liver enzyme levels become elevated, and toxic hepatitis begins to spread.
- The third stage can end in acute liver failure and acute renal failure with metabolic derangements, encephalopathy, coagulopathy, arrhythmia, cardiogenic shock, and abnormal liver tests between 4 and 7 days.

Diagnostic Testing

Laboratory evaluation reveals deranged liver function tests with elevated liver enzymes, aspartate transaminase (AST), and alanine transaminase (ALT) and coagulopathy. Prothrombin time (PT) and internationalized normalized ratio should be reassessed every 6 hours. Other tests needed are ABG, renal function tests, and ECG.

TREATMENT

Gastric decontamination can be employed within 6 hours in cases of rodenticide poisoning. The only definitive treatment for acute liver failure due to the ingestion of YP is liver transplantation because no antidote or medical treatment is available to reverse the toxic effects on the liver.

Studies have shown no clear benefit from *N*-acetylcysteine, corticosteroids, or exchange transfusion; however, NAC (20-hour regimen as for paracetamol toxicity) has been followed in many centers.

Supportive therapy with IV vitamin K, IV fluids, IV antibiotics, and fresh frozen plasma is practiced.

COMPLICATIONS

Serious intoxication resulting from this substance follows a course that is accompanied by multisystem organ failures and has a mortality rate between 20% and 50%.

Aluminum Phosphide

Aluminum phosphide is a solid fumigant pesticide, insecticide, and rodenticide used as a grain preservative. Zinc phosphide also has similar presentation. Aluminum phosphide is available as greenish gray tablet of 3 g. This contains 56% aluminum phosphide and 44% of aluminum carbonate. Other formulations are pellets and granules.

GENERAL PRINCIPLES

The tablet liberates 1 g of phosphine gas when it becomes exposed to moisture or gastric acid. Pure phosphine gas is colorless and odorless; however, garlicky odor is attributed to the impurities. Fatal dose by ingestion route is 0.5 g and inhalation of phosphine is 400–600 ppm. Majority die within 24 hours.

Etiology

Pathophysiology

Aluminum phosphide inhibits respiratory chain enzymes, electron transport, and cytochrome oxidase.

Aluminum phosphide releases phosphine gas in the presence of HCl in the stomach, which gets rapidly absorbed throughout the GI tract, resulting in systemic toxic effects within 30 minutes such as serious cardiac arrhythmias, intractable shock, acidosis, and pulmonary edema.

DIAGNOSIS

Clinical Presentation

- **Inhalation exposure:** Patients commonly have airway irritation and breathlessness followed by chest tightness, headache, diplopia, vomiting, diarrhea, ataxia, numbness, paresthesia, tremor, muscle weakness, diplopia, and jaundice.
- In severe forms (ARDS), cardiac failure, cardiac arrhythmias, convulsion, coma, hepatotoxicity, and nephrotoxicity are seen. Cardiac arrhythmias are pathognomic and all types of rhythm abnormalities can occur.
- **Ingestion exposure**: Nausea, repeated vomiting, diarrhea, headache, and abdominal discomfort may occur in mild cases while in moderate to severe ingestional poisoning, features of hepatic and renal failure, and disseminated intravascular coagulation may also occur.

Diagnostic Testing

Diagnostic testing depends on the clinical suspicion or history. The classic triad of hypotension, severe metabolic acidosis, and cardiac arrhythmia should raise a strong suspicion. Gas chromatography with a nitrogen–phosphorous detector is the most specific and sensitive test.

TREATMENT

Early decontamination with potassium permanganate (1:10000) can help to oxidize the phosphine and can be done within 1 hour of ingestion and supportive care form the mainstay of treatment. Ventilation for respiratory distress, management of electrolyte disturbances among other measures should be emphasized.

Antioxidants, magnesium, and steroids have been tried in small trials. Steroids have limited role. Magnesium acts like an antioxidant and prevents arrhythmias. Glucose-insulin and potassium (GIK) infusion administered to produce hyperinsulinemic euglycemia has shown promising results. In case of failing hemodynamics, ECMO and intra-aortic balloon pump has shown some benefit.

Mortality associated with this poison is very high (30%–100%) in various Asian studies. Indicators of poor prognosis include low pH <7.2, low systolic blood pressure <90 mm Hg, and altered mental status.

SEDATIVES AND HYPNOTICS

Barbiturates

GENERAL PRINCIPLES

These include phenobarbitone, thiopentone, and methohexitone. They act on the GABA BZD receptor chloride channel complex to potentiate the GABAergic inhibition by increasing the duration of the channel opening. The use of barbiturates has largely fallen by the wayside because safer drugs are now available. Barbiturates are still used as induction agents for anesthesia as well as second-line agents for seizure control.

Diagnosis

Suspect barbiturate overdose in patients who present with CNS and respiratory depression.

Clinical Presentation

History

It is often difficult to elicit a history because these patients are generally sedated or comatose on arrival.

Physical Examination

Typical examination findings include **respiratory depression** and **coma**. Other vital sign abnormalities may include hypothermia. Patients may develop cutaneous bullae known as "**barb blisters.**"[155] The blisters may be from being on the ground for a prolonged time and not a direct effect of the barbiturates. **Miosis** may be present.

Differential Diagnosis

The differential diagnosis includes benzodiazepine overdose, opioid overdose, hypoglycemia, ethanol intoxication, other sedatives (e.g., zolpidem, γ-hydroxybutyric acid [GHB]), CNS depressants, and other metabolic causes of coma.

Diagnostic Testing

Laboratories

This should include routine testing for any presentation of coma: **blood glucose, BMP, LFTs, and thyroid function tests.**

Electroencephalography

In barbiturate overdose, electroencephalography recordings may show no electrical activity. This is true for a number of xenobiotics (e.g., baclofen). As such, care must be taken before declaring these patients brain dead.[156]

Imaging

- A **CXR** should be obtained on all of these patients to evaluate for aspiration.
- **Head CT** may help evaluate for the presence of CNS lesions contributing to coma.

Diagnostic Procedures

Consider **lumbar puncture (LP)** in patients with undifferentiated coma to evaluate for meningitis or subarachnoid hemorrhage.

TREATMENT

The most important management strategy in barbiturate overdose is airway and breathing protection. Patients with respiratory depression should be intubated.

Medications

First Line

- Consider **MDAC** in patients with a protected airway and bowel sounds.
- Hypotension should be treated with IVF. If this fails, consider a direct-acting vasopressor such as norepinephrine.

Second Line

Urine alkalinization with sodium bicarbonate is reserved for phenobarbital overdoses refractory to MDAC that do not improve with supportive care. The optimum urinary pH to be achieved is >7.5 and urine output should be more than 2 mL/kg/min. It is inferior to MDAC.[157]

Other Nonpharmacologic Therapies

Consider **hemoperfusion** in the setting of life-threatening phenobarbital overdose that is refractory to conventional management.[158] **Hemodialysis** has been reported to be useful as well.[159] However, renal replacement therapies are generally not necessary because most patients do well with general supportive care.

Benzodiazepines

GENERAL PRINCIPLES

These include diazepam, midazolam, alprazolam, lorazepam, chlordiazepoxide, and oxazepam. The site of action is the GABAa receptor chloride channel complex in the ascending reticular formation and limbic system and increases the pre and post synaptic inhibition. In general, benzodiazepines have a wide safety margin. Deaths are usually related to the presence of a coingestant or ethanol.

DIAGNOSIS

Clinical Presentation

History

This is often difficult to elicit because patients are frequently sedated or comatose.

Physical Examination

The typical presentation of a pure oral benzodiazepine overdose is a sleepy patient, slurring of speech, loss of recent memory, impaired motor function leading to ataxia and hypotonia. In severe cases, coma occurs with normal vital signs. With flurazepam overdose, paradoxical symptoms such as delirium, anxiety, hallucinations, and aggression can occur. Respiratory depression is exceedingly unusual in an oral overdose of benzodiazepines.

Differential Diagnosis

The differential diagnosis includes barbiturate overdose, hypoglycemia, ethanol intoxication, CNS depressants, other sedatives (e.g., zolpidem, GHB), and other metabolic causes of coma.

Diagnostic Testing

Laboratories

- This should include routine testing for any presentation of coma: **blood glucose, BMP, LFTs, and thyroid function tests.** Consider **LP** in patients with undifferentiated coma to evaluate for meningitis or subarachnoid hemorrhage.
- **Urine drug screens** are unreliable in the setting of benzodiazepine overdose because the target metabolite, oxazepam or desmethyldiazepam, is not produced by the metabolism of many of the benzodiazepines. Classically, clonazepam, alprazolam, and lorazepam are not detected. Therefore, routine screening is not recommended.[3]

Imaging

- A **CXR** should be obtained on all of these patients to evaluate for aspiration.
- A **head CT** may help evaluate for the presence of CNS lesions contributing to coma.

TREATMENT

Supportive care with observation is the mainstay of therapy. In patients with coingestions and respiratory depression, intubation and ventilation may be required. Hypotension is managed by aggressive IV fluids. Bradycardia is treated by atropine. Because this is a benign overdose, **gastric lavage and AC are not necessary**. These interventions may cause aspiration in an otherwise stable patient.

Medications

- Traditional recommendations include the use of **flumazenil**; however, given the propensity to precipitate seizures and acute benzodiazepine withdrawal in patients on long-term benzodiazepine therapy, this therapy is generally **avoided. Contraindications** include long duration of BZD therapy, a seizure history, coingestion of a cardiotoxic or epileptogenic drug, or ECG evidence of cyclic antidepressant ingestion.
- In **special cases** such as reversal of iatrogenically induced respiratory depression, reversal of sedation, or pediatric benzodiazepine ingestion, flumazenil may be given as a 0.1 mg/min dose IV over 30 seconds and may be repeated after 1–2 min till the dose of 1–2 mg. Repeat injections may be given, because resedation occasionally occurs. If the patient develops respiratory failure, flumazenil can also be considered.

SYMPATHOMIMETICS

GENERAL PRINCIPLES

Definition

Patients who overdose on sympathomimetic agents exhibit a syndrome of excess adrenergic tone due to direct stimulation of adrenergic receptors or the effects of norepinephrine and epinephrine. Many of the agents in this category are drugs of abuse, although several therapeutic agents can produce a similar toxidrome.

Classification

Agents that fall into this category include amphetamines, cocaine, vasopressors, methylxanthines, synthetic cannabinoids and cathinones, and β-agonists.

Epidemiology

Stimulants and street drugs were the ninth most common human exposure in adults but were the third leading cause of fatal exposures according to the AAPCC in 2021.[1]

Pathophysiology

- Agents that stimulate the SNS generally do so by either causing the release or preventing the reuptake of **endogenous catecholamines** or **directly stimulating** α- and/or **β-receptors.**
- **Methylxanthines** (theophylline, caffeine) and **β-agonists** (albuterol, dobutamine, isoproterenol) enhance chronotropy and inotropy by **facilitating calcium entry into the myocardium.** They also enhance the function of β_2-receptors leading to **bronchodilatation.** Stimulation of the β_2-rich vascular beds to skeletal muscle results in **vasodilatation** as well. Therefore, in a pure β-agonist overdose, **hypotension and tachycardia** predominate.
- **Epinephrine, norepinephrine, cocaine, and amphetamines** have both α and β effects, resulting in **hypertension and tachycardia.**
- Other α-receptors are found on the **iris**, which, when stimulated, results in **pupillary dilatation.**
- Sympathetic stimulation of **sweat glands** is a **cholinergic** effect.
- **Synthetic cannabinoids** act on the cannabinoid receptors but may result in sympathomimetic effects.[160]

Amphetamines

GENERAL PRINCIPLES

Drugs of abuse in this class include **amphetamine, methamphetamine, 3,4-methylenedioxymethamphetamine (MDMA), and the synthetic cathinones (bath salts).** MDMA is a potent inducer and/or reuptake inhibitor of presynaptic serotonin, dopamine, and norepinephrine.

Amphetamine is a CNS stimulant. It was initially used as a nasal decongestant and weight loss drug but became a drug of abuse mainly for its euphoric effects. Amphetamine is a lipophilic drug and has large volume of distribution, crossing the blood brain barrier. Its chemical structure resembles that of sympathomimetics, and consequently, its manifestations are similar to theirs.

DIAGNOSIS

Clinical Presentation

- Suspect amphetamines in any patient presenting with a sympathomimetic toxidrome of **hypertension, tachycardia, dilated pupils,** and **diaphoresis.** Focal neurological deficits, seizures, and delirium can occur in acute intoxication. Anxiety and suicidal ideation have been reported in chronic cases.
  - Meth mouth: Typical finding in chronic abusers in which there is tooth decay, poor dental hygiene, repeated grinding of teeth, and decreased salivation.
  - Tachypnea and dyspnea are common respiratory complaints. Complications include acute pulmonary edema, pulmonary hypertension, pneumonia, pneumothorax, pulmonary hemorrhage, and ARDS.

- Severely intoxicated patients may develop **hyperthermia, seizures, stroke, coma,** and **cardiovascular collapse**. Acute coronary syndrome occurs rarely. Valvular dysfunction can also occur secondary to serotoninergic effects.

History
Drug abusers will often deny illicit use; therefore, the history is often unreliable.

Physical Examination
Patients may have **agitation and altered mental status** depending on the degree of intoxication. **Synthetic cannabinoids** and **methamphetamines** can cause prolonged psychosis. Track marks maybe visible in chronic intravenous abusers.

Differential Diagnosis

The differential includes anything that may result in a sympathomimetic toxidrome including cocaine, ephedrine, pseudoephedrine, and various amphetamine-derived designer drugs.

Diagnostic Testing

Laboratories
Patients with a sympathomimetic toxidrome should be evaluated for end-organ dysfunction.
- A **BMP** is useful to assess the degree of hydration and renal function. MDMA is also associated with the development of hyponatremia due to either SIADH or ingestion of large quantities of water.
- A **CK** should be checked to evaluate for rhabdomyolysis in agitated patients.
- Patients complaining of chest pain should have a **troponin** drawn.
- **Urine drug screens** are often associated with false-negative and false-positive results, are expensive, and **do not contribute to the management of this syndrome.**

Electrocardiography
An ECG should be obtained to evaluate for ischemia and electrolyte disturbances.

Imaging
In select cases, imaging may be useful.
- Obtain a **head CT** in patients complaining of a headache or altered mental status to evaluate for an intracranial hemorrhage.
- Obtain a **CXR** and 2D Echo in patients complaining of chest pain.
- In patients with severe chest pain that radiates to the back or is associated with marked agitation, consider obtaining a **chest CT** to evaluate for aortic dissection.

TREATMENT

Mild to moderate cases usually respond to supportive care, including IV hydration and benzodiazepines. In hyperthermic cases, aggressive cooling measures should be taken, which may include intubation and paralysis. As always, priority should be given to airway protection, breathing, and circulation.

Medications

First Line
- Treat agitation and seizures with **benzodiazepines**. In refractory seizures, consider **barbiturates and propofol.**
- Hypertension and tachycardia may be managed with **CCBs**. ***Avoid*** **β-antagonists because they may be associated with the development of a hypertensive crisis.**

- **Nitroglycerin, nitroprusside, nicardipine,** and **phentolamine** may be used in the setting of severe hypertension.
- Ventricular arrhythmias should be treated with **lidocaine** or **amiodarone.**

Second Line

- Although benzodiazepines remain the treatment of choice, some data suggest that antipsychotics are useful in the management of agitated delirium in these patients.[161] Consider administration of **haloperidol 5.0 mg IV or droperidol 2.5 mg IV** in patients with hallucinations.[162] In particular, antipsychotics may be useful in patients with delirium from bath salts. However, they can lower the seizure threshold in these patients.
- **Ketamine** can be considered in patients with agitated delirium. Its onset of action is faster than benzodiazepines or antipsychotics. Dosing is at 3–5 mg/kg IM or 1–2 mg/kg IV. It should be used with caution as more patients may require intubation compared to sedation with other agents.[163]
- In hyperthermic-agitated patients, consider **paralysis** with a nondepolarizing agent to prevent rhabdomyolysis.

Other Nonpharmacologic Therapies

Patients with renal failure and rhabdomyolysis may require **hemodialysis.**

SPECIAL CONSIDERATIONS

MDMA may cause hyponatremia and serotonin syndrome (see earlier discussion).

REFERRAL

Obtain a chemical dependency consult in patients hospitalized as a result of drug abuse.

Cocaine

GENERAL PRINCIPLES

- Cocaine is derived from the leaves of the coca plant (*Erythroxylum coca*). Cocaine abuse is seen predominantly in the younger age group (15–35 years). It is used to increase vitality, alertness, social disinhibition, euphoria, and decrease fatigue. Cocaine exerts its effects by inhibiting the reuptake of norepinephrine, serotonin, epinephrine, and dopamine via sodium channel blockade. Excess adrenergic tone in the setting of toxicity is reflected by the development of hypertension and tachycardia. Drug-seeking behavior is likely modulated by dopaminergic effects in the ventral tegmental area of the brain.
- It is metabolized to various metabolites, most important being benzoylecgonine. This can be detected in urine for many days after administration. Cocaine has also been implicated in the development of early cardiovascular disease,[164] likely due to a combination of vasospastic,[165] prothrombotic,[166] and atherogenic effects.[167]

DIAGNOSIS

Clinical Presentation

- It can be consumed by various routes like oral, insufflation, intravenous, inhalational, rectal, and vaginal. The most common route is nasal insufflation by snorting or sniffing. Patients with cocaine intoxication often present with complaints of ischemic chest pain secondary to coronary vasoconstriction, increased platelet aggregation and accelerated atherosclerosis besides having a positive chronotropic and inotropic effect.

- Suspect cocaine in any patient presenting with a sympathomimetic toxidrome of **hypertension, tachycardia, dilated pupils,** and **diaphoresis**. Inhaling cocaine can lead to pneumothorax and bronchospasm.
- Cocaine is a stimulant that increases arousal, alertness, vigilance, and provides a sense of euphoria. Severely intoxicated patients may develop headache, **hyperthermia, seizures, coma,** and **cardiovascular collapse**. It also causes pupillary dilatation, loss of vision, and precipitate angle closure glaucoma.
- Cocaine increases hydrochloric acid formation leading to peptic ulcer disease. It can also cause intestinal perforation and ischemic colitis.

History

Drug abusers will often deny illicit use; therefore, the history is often unreliable.

Physical Examination

Patients may have **agitation** and **altered mental status** depending on the degree of intoxication.

Differential Diagnosis

The differential includes anything that may result in a sympathomimetic toxidrome, including amphetamines, ephedrine, pseudoephedrine, and various amphetamine-derived designer drugs.

Diagnostic Testing

Laboratories

Patients with a sympathomimetic toxidrome should be evaluated for end-organ dysfunction.

- A **BMP** is useful to assess the degree of hydration and renal function.
- A **CK** should be checked to evaluate for rhabdomyolysis in agitated patients.
- Patients complaining of chest pain should have a **troponin** drawn.
- **Urine drug screens**, although reliable in determining recent use, should not modify the acute management of these patients.

Electrocardiography

- An ECG should be obtained to evaluate for ischemia and electrolyte disturbances.
- Cocaine is a known sodium channel blocker, which may be reflected as a wide complex rhythm[168] or **Brugada pattern**[169] VT, SVT, and VF on the ECG.
- Cocaine has been reported to increase the QT_c.[170]

Imaging

In select cases, imaging may be useful.

- Obtain a **head CT** in patients complaining of a headache or altered mental status.
- Obtain a **CXR** and 2D Echo in patients complaining of chest pain.
- In patients with severe chest pain that radiates to the back or is associated with marked agitation, consider obtaining a **chest CT** to evaluate for aortic dissection.

TREATMENT

Mild to moderate cases usually respond to supportive care, including IV hydration. In hyperthermic cases, aggressive cooling measures should be taken. As always, priority should be given to airway protection, breathing, and circulation.

Medications

First Line

- Treat agitation and seizures with **benzodiazepines**. In refractory seizures, consider **barbiturates and propofol**. Avoid succinylcholine during intubation.
- Hypertension and tachycardia may be managed with **CCBs**, benzodiazepines, and vasodilators (e.g., nitroglycerin, nitroprusside, phentolamine).
- *Avoid* **β-antagonists because they may be associated with the development of a hypertensive crisis and vasospasm.**
- Sodium channel blockade should be treated with **sodium bicarbonate.**[171] Give **1–2 mEq/kg** as an IV bolus; this may be repeated. Monitor for QRS narrowing. **Sodium acetate** can be substituted for sodium bicarbonate during drug shortages; it can only be administered as a slow infusion.
- Ventricular arrhythmias should be treated with **lidocaine.**

Second Line

In hyperthermic-agitated patients, consider **paralysis** with a nondepolarizing agent to prevent rhabdomyolysis.

Other Nonpharmacologic Therapies

Patients with renal failure and rhabdomyolysis may require **hemodialysis.**

SPECIAL CONSIDERATIONS

- **Body packers** (patients smuggling large amounts of drugs by swallowing multiple packets of drugs) with suspected cocaine toxicity or obstructive symptoms should have emergent surgical intervention. A patient who is running from the police and swallows drugs (**body stuffer**) is unlikely to need surgical intervention and can be managed medically. Consider whole-bowel irrigation in patients who present without signs of toxicity.
- Increasingly, cocaine has been found to be adulterated with **levamisole.** This veterinary dewormer has been demonstrated to cause agranulocytosis and vasculitis, which reverse with cessation of cocaine use. Any patient who presents with an unexpected decrease in their WBC or necrotic skin rash should be counseled to stop using cocaine. G-CSF may be used to treat serious neutropenia.[172]

Theophylline

GENERAL PRINCIPLES

Definition

Theophylline is a methylxanthine obtained from plants used in the treatment of obstructive pulmonary diseases such as asthma and emphysema. Its use has largely fallen by the wayside as alternative, less toxic medications have been developed. However, patients with refractory pulmonary disease may still be prescribed this drug. It is available in both oral and intravenous preparations.

Classification

Toxicity is classified as **acute** or **chronic.** The management strategy is different depending on whether the drug is an **immediate-** or **sustained-release** preparation.

Pathophysiology

Theophylline exerts its therapeutic effects by promoting catecholamine release, which results in enhanced β-agonism.[173] Additionally, at high doses, theophylline is a phosphodiesterase inhibitor, which prolongs the effects of β-agonism by preventing the breakdown of cyclic adenosine monophosphate. Theophylline is also an adenosine antagonist, which in therapeutic doses enhances bronchodilatation. Its therapeutic range is 5–15 mg/L and toxicity develops if the dose exceeds 25 mg/L. In toxic doses, adenosine antagonism is associated with the development of tachydysrhythmias and seizures.

DIAGNOSIS

Clinical Presentation

- **Acute toxicity:** Patients with serum concentrations >**20 μg/mL** will present complaining of **nausea** and multiple episodes of **vomiting, which may be very difficult to control.** On examination, the patient will be **tremulous** and **tachycardic. Hyperventilation** is often present. In more severe cases, **hypotension** and **seizures** occur. **Refractory status epilepticus** is due to adenosine antagonism in the CNS.[174] These effects are most often present at serum concentrations >**90 μg/mL** in the acutely intoxicated patient.
- **Chronic toxicity** usually occurs in patients with a large body burden of theophylline who develop a concurrent illness or are administered a drug that delays the P450 metabolism and theophylline clearance. Subtle symptoms such as nausea and anorexia may occur; tachycardia is usually present. Severe toxicity may occur at serum levels of **40–60 μg/mL.** Patients with these serum concentrations may present with seizures.

Diagnostic Testing

Laboratories

- Therapeutic concentrations are 5–15 μg/mL.
- **Acute toxicity** is associated with the development of **hypokalemia** and **hyperglycemia.** In severe cases, expect a **metabolic acidosis.** Obtain a **BMP and blood glucose.**
- **Serial theophylline** concentrations should be obtained every 1–2 hours until a downward trend is present; remember, with sustained-release preparations, a peak may not be evident for 16 hours or later after ingestion.
- **Calcium, magnesium, and CK** should be checked as well.
- **Chronic toxicity** can occur with lower concentrations than in acute toxicity. Many laboratories (e.g., potassium, glucose) may be unremarkable, unless seizures are present but should still be obtained. **Serial theophylline** concentrations are also warranted in these patients.

Electrocardiography

Adenosine antagonism and increased catecholamines may result in a sinus tachycardia or supraventricular tachycardia (SVT) on the ECG. In overdose, premature ventricular contractions (PVCs) may be apparent.

TREATMENT

Patients with theophylline toxicity do not require gastric lavage because they tend to vomit. Sustained-release preparations occasionally form bezoars. Severely intoxicated patients require intubation and ventilation. Sustained-release formulations should be treated with **whole-bowel irrigation.** Replete potassium and electrolytes as needed.

Medications

- Administer **AC 1 g/kg.** Consider **MDAC** because theophylline clearance is increased by this modality.[175] Ensure patients have adequate airway protection because vomiting and aspiration may occur.
- **Vomiting** should be managed with **ondansetron** or **metoclopramide. Phenothiazines are contraindicated** because they lower the seizure threshold.
- **Seizures** are often refractory and should initially be treated with **benzodiazepines.** If this modality fails, consider moving to **phenobarbital** as a 10 mg/kg loading dose at a rate of 50 mg/min, followed by up to a total of 30 mg/kg at a rate of 50 mg/min, followed by 1–5 mg/kg/d to maintain therapeutic plasma levels. **Propofol** is a reasonable alternative if these fail. Monitor for hypotension.
- **Hypotension** should be treated with 20 mL/kg bolus of IVF, which may be repeated. Direct pressors such as **phenylephrine** and **norepinephrine** may be added if fluid boluses are not sufficient. Because much of the hypotension is mediated by β_2-agonism, **avoid epinephrine.** Consider using short-acting β-antagonists such as **esmolol**, which, although counterintuitive, may reverse β_2-mediated vasodilatation. Monitor for bronchospasm.
- **Arrhythmias** should be treated with β-antagonists. Use short-acting agents such as **esmolol** and monitor for bronchospasm. Because theophylline is an adenosine antagonist, **adenosine may fail to treat SVT.**

Other Nonpharmacologic Therapies

Extracorporeal toxin removal techniques like hemoperfusion (charcoal or resin) or **hemodialysis** is indicated for the following:

- Intractable seizures or life-threatening cardiovascular complications, regardless of drug level
- A theophylline level of >100 mg/mL after an **acute** overdose
- A theophylline level >60 mg/mL in acute intoxication, with worsening symptoms, or inability to tolerate oral charcoal administration
- A theophylline level >60 mg/mL in **chronic** intoxication without life-threatening symptoms
- A theophylline level >40 mg/mL in a patient with chronic intoxication and CHF, respiratory insufficiency, hepatic failure, or age >60 years.[176] The cessation of ECTR can be considered if there is clinical improvement or if serum theophylline levels are less than 15 mg/L.

TOXIC ALCOHOL

GENERAL PRINCIPLES

- High alcohol concentrations increase the measured plasma osmolality and subsequently widen the osmolar gap. A normal gap is <10 mmol/dL and varies from −14 to +10 mmol/dL.[177]
- In presence of a widened gap, the actual serum alcohol level can be estimated if done early after ingestion.[178]
- As the alcohol is metabolized, the osmolar gap falls, and the anion gap rises.[179] Therefore, the osmolar gap should only be used to support the diagnosis of toxic alcohol poisoning and not to draw conclusions about the actual amount of ingested toxin.
- Causes of elevate osmolar gap include ethanol, methanol, ethylene glycol, isopropanol. Nontoxicological causes include DKA, AKA, renal failure. Although a normal osmolar gap does not rule out toxic alcohol poisoning.[(218)]
- Unlike methanol and ethylene glycol, isopropanol (rubbing alcohol) does not form a toxic metabolite.

TREATMENT

The general approach to toxic alcohol ingestions is to:[180]

- Prevent the formation of toxic metabolites by inhibiting alcohol dehydrogenase (ADH) (in methanol and ethylene glycol poisoning only).
- Eliminate the toxic alcohol and toxic metabolites from the blood.
- Correct acid–base imbalance.
- Replenish cofactors.

Methanol

GENERAL PRINCIPLES

Definition

Methanol is used in gasoline, antifreeze, deicers, windshield washer fluid, paint and varnish removers, fuel, photocopy fluid, and embalming fluids. It can be found in "moonshine" liquor and is used as a denaturant for ethanol. It is also known as wood alcohol.

Etiology

Ingestions are mostly intentional, occurring as suicide attempts.

Pathophysiology

Methanol is rapidly absorbed following ingestion and reaches peak concentration in 30 to 60 minutes. It is metabolized by hepatic ADH to formaldehyde which is further converted to extremely toxic formic acid, which is responsible for the anion gap metabolic acidosis in methanol poisoning.[181] Formic acid inhibits mitochondrial cytochrome oxidase thus impairing oxidative metabolism and formation of lactic acid. Toxic dose can be as low as 30 mL. Ingestion of 10 mL can lead to blindness.

DIAGNOSIS

Clinical Presentation

- **Early stage**
  - Early after ingestion, mild CNS depression or headache evolves, but profound obtundation or inebriation can occur as well.
  - These early symptoms are directly caused by methanol before being metabolized.
- **Late stage**
  - After a latent period, a severe anion gap metabolic acidosis without significant lactate or ketone formation develops.
  - Formate accumulation within the retina and optic nerve fibers causes "snow field vision," blurred vision, visual field defects, and blindness.[182]
  - Other CNS symptoms during the late phase are lethargy, convulsion, delirium, and coma. Basal ganglia hemorrhage with dyskinesia or hypokinesia has been observed.[183]
  - Abdominal complaints include nausea, vomiting, pain, and acute pancreatitis.[184]

History

Obtain history of what, when, how, and how much of the toxic substance was ingested.

Physical Examination

- Assess mental status and respiratory and cardiovascular stability.
- Kussmaul respirations may indicate underlying metabolic acidosis.

- Visual field testing may reveal central scotoma or other visual field defects. A thorough funduscopic examination may show hyperemia, disk edema, or atrophy.[185]

Diagnostic Testing

- Address possible causes of an anion gap acidosis:
  - BMP: Acidosis, anion gap, renal function
  - Urinalysis (UA): Ketones
  - Serum lactate
- Blood glucose measurement
- Obtain serum osmolality if toxic alcohol ingestion is suspected.
- ABG or VBG: To assess acid–base status and treatment success.
- Ethanol concentration: If >100 mg/dL, toxic methanol manifestations may be delayed; if elevated in presence of acidosis, the acidosis is unlikely to be related to a toxic alcohol ingestion because ethanol blocks the metabolism of the parent compound (unless the toxic alcohol ingestion occurred hours before the ethanol ingestion).
- Serum methanol concentration: Usually not readily available; therefore, it may not be useful clinically. If you are concerned enough to check a level, you should consider pre-emptively treating it before returning.

TREATMENT

- ABCs and general supportive care.
- GI decontamination: Nasogastric lavage is only indicated in patients who present <30 minutes after ingestion or who ingested large amounts of methanol while maintaining a normal mental status.
- **Do not use AC** because the GI tract rapidly absorbs methanol. AC bears a high risk of aspiration in acutely intoxicated patients.
- Sodium bicarbonate: Give 50 mg IV every 4 hours for arterial pH <7.30.[186]
  - Serum alkalinization limits the amount of undissociated formic acid, which prevents CNS toxicity.
  - Urine alkalinization enhances clearance of formate. CAVEAT: Watch for fluid overload and hypokalemia if giving large amounts of bicarbonate.
- Ethanol (EtOH) therapy: EtOH serum levels of 100 mg/dL block ADH sufficiently to inhibit formation of toxic metabolites.
  - Loading dose of **7.6 mL/kg of 10% ethanol** solution IV (correlates with an EtOH serum level of 100–200 mg/dL)
  - Maintenance dose of **0.8 mL/kg/h (nondrinker), 2.0 mL/kg/h (drinker), or 2.0–3.3 mL/kg/h (on hemodialysis)** of 10% ethanol solution IV[179]
- **Fomepizole** therapy: 4-Methylpyrazole (Antizol) is an FDA-approved competitive inhibitor of ADH for the treatment of methanol poisoning.[187]
  - Loading dose of **15 mg/kg IV** loading dose, maintenance dose of **10 mg/kg IV** every 12 hours for 48 hours, and then 15 mg/kg IV every 12 hours until methanol level <20 mg/dL. It is preferred over ethanol due to ease of administration and safety profile.
  - Dose adjustment may be needed for patients on hemodialysis.[186] If on intermittent hemodialysis, redose can be done after hemodialysis is completed and other dose adjustments are not needed.
  - Continue treatment until methanol levels <20 mg/dL and acidosis resolves.[188]
- Indication: Ethanol or fomepizole therapy should be started if:
  - Strong evidence of methanol ingestion
  - Methanol serum concentration >20 mg/dL
  - Osmolar gap >10 mmol/dL
  - Arterial pH <7.3

  - Serum CO_2 <20 mmol/L
  - Unexplained anion gap metabolic acidosis is present with suspicion for toxic alcohol exposure[186]

Other Nonpharmacologic Therapies

- **Hemodialysis** should be used in addition to the aforementioned therapies to prevent end-organ toxicity.
- **Hemodialysis** corrects metabolic abnormalities and eliminates nonmetabolized methanol. Indications for hemodialysis are a methanol level >50 mg/dL, severe acidemia (bicarbonate <15 mmol/L, pH <7.30), and/or optic injury from toxicity.[189] If the methanol concentration is very elevated, hemodialysis should also be considered even if the patient is not acidotic given the long half-life of methanol and expense of fomepizole.
- Folic acid 1 mg/kg (up to 50 mg) IV every 4–6 hours and folinic acid (leucovorin) 1 mg/kg (up to 50 mg) IV every 4–6 hours enhance formate metabolism and should be given until metabolic acidosis resolves.[190]

SPECIAL CONSIDERATIONS

- Ethanol therapy has significant disadvantages (e.g., complex dosing regimen, hard to titrate therapeutic levels, intensive care requirements, and severe side effect profile). Although very expensive ($500/dose), fomepizole has become the preferred agent in the treatment of methanol intoxication.[191]
- Admit all patients on ethanol infusions to the ICU (risk of hypotension, tachycardia, hypoglycemia, and CNS and respiratory depression).
- Stable patients on fomepizole infusion can be safely admitted to the floor. Adverse effects of fomepizole are usually mild and include headache, nausea, and dizziness but not sedation.[192,193]
- Report all cases of methanol intoxication to the lccal poison control center (1-800-222-1222).
- Get a clinical toxicologist involved early.
- Consult ophthalmology or neurology service if signs of opt.c injury or other neurologic deficits are present.

Ethylene Glycol

GENERAL PRINCIPLES

Etiology

It is an odorless, sweet tasting compound found in coolants, antifreeze compounds, hydraulic brake fluids, glycerin substitutes, paints, and cosmetics. Ingestions are mostly due to intentional suicide attempts.

Pathophysiology

- Ethylene glycol undergoes rapid absorption from the GI tract and is oxidized to glycolic acid and oxalic acid.
- Glycolate accumulation is responsible for the anion gap metabolic acidosis in ethylene glycol poisoning.
- Oxalate accumulation is responsible for the development of calcium oxalate crystals which precipitate in proximal tubules and lead to acute tubular necrosis and renal failure in ethylene glycol poisoning.[194]

DIAGNOSIS

Clinical Presentation

- Neurologic stage (Stage 1) First 12 hours
  - CNS depression with altered mental status, hallucinations, ataxia, slurred speech, and cranial nerve palsies are directly caused by ethylene glycol before metabolization.
  - Seizures, myoclonic jerks, coma, and respiratory depression can occur in severe intoxications.
- Cardiovascular stage (Stage 2) 12 to 24 hours: Glycolate affects the cardiopulmonary system and causes tachycardia, hypotension, heart failure, pulmonary edema, and ARDS. Death can occur during this stage.
- Renal stage (Stage 3) 2 to 3 days
  - Glycolic acid is further metabolized to oxalic acid. Oxalate is a calcium chelator, and accumulation of oxalate leads to **hypocalcemia**.
  - Calcium oxalate can precipitate in the renal tubules, which subsequently causes acute tubular necrosis with flank pain and acute renal failure.[195]
- Within 4–6 hours after ingestion, development of an anion gap metabolic acidosis from glycolic acid formation in the absence of significant lactate or ketone concentrations occurs.
- Abdominal complaints (nausea, vomiting, pain) are also common. Poor prognostic factors include severe acidosis, renal failure, seizures, coma, hyperkalemia, and delay in initiation of treatment.

History

Obtain history of what, when, how, and how much of the toxic substance was ingested.

Physical Examination

- Assess mental status and respiratory and cardiovascular stability.
- Kussmaul respiration may indicate severe metabolic acidosis.

Diagnostic Testing

- Address causes of a high anion gap metabolic acidosis:
  - BMP: Acidosis, anion gap, renal function.
  - UA: Ketones, oxalate crystals (usually a late sign during intoxication).
  - Serum lactate.
  - **Glycolic acid may also be misinterpreted as a high lactic acid on a point-of-care blood gas analyzer.** Serum levels should be obtained in these cases.
- Obtain serum osmolality if toxic alcohol ingestion is suspected.
- ABG or VBG to assess acid–base status and treatment success.
- Ethanol level: If elevated, toxic ethylene glycol manifestations may be delayed; if elevated in presence of acidosis, unlikely to be toxic alcohol ingestion (unless toxic alcohol ingestion occurred hours before ethanol ingestion).
- Obtain serum ethylene glycol concentration: Usually not readily available; therefore, clinically often not useful.
- Serum calcium concentration: Low if increased formation of calcium oxalate.
- Repeated renal function testing: Increased risk of acute kidney injury.
- Urine microscopy: Calcium oxalate might be visible as envelope-shaped crystals.[196]
- Wood lamp examination of urine to detect fluorescence after assumed antifreeze ingestion is not a reliable screening tool.[197]

TREATMENT

- ABCs and supportive care; monitor urine output.
- GI decontamination: Nasogastric lavage is only indicated in patients who present <30 minutes after ingestion or who ingested large amounts of ethylene glycol while maintaining a normal mental status.
- **Do not use AC** because the GI tract rapidly absorbs ethylene glycol. AC bears a high risk of aspiration in acutely intoxicated patients.
- **Thiamine** (vitamin B_1) 100 mg IV every 4–6 hours and **pyridoxine** (vitamin B_6) 50 mg IV every 6–12 hours enhance glycolate metabolism and should be given until metabolic acidosis resolves.[198]
- Sodium bicarbonate: Give 50 mg IV every 4 hours for arterial pH <7.30.[186]
  - Serum alkalinization limits the amount of undissociated glycolic acid, which prevents CNS toxicity.
  - Urine alkalinization enhances clearance of glycolate. CAVEAT: Watch for fluid overload and hypokalemia if giving large amounts of bicarbonate.
- Ethanol therapy: EtOH serum concentrations of 100 mg/dL block ADH sufficiently to inhibit formation of toxic metabolites. See discussion of methanol overdose treatment for dosing.
- **Fomepizole** therapy: 15 mg/kg loading dose followed by 10 mg/kg every 12 hours for a total of 48 hours.
- **Indications:** Ethanol or fomepizole therapy should be started if:
  - Strong evidence of ethylene glycol ingestion
  - Ethylene glycol serum concentration >20 mg/dL
  - Osmolar gap >10 mmol/dL
  - Arterial pH <7.3
  - Serum CO_2 <20 mmol/L
  - Unexplained anion gap metabolic acidosis is present.[186]
- Monitor serum calcium levels and if the patient develops clinical signs of hypocalcemia, start 10% calcium gluconate. Do not give calcium gluconate only for hypocalcemia alone as it will encourage the formation of calcium oxalate crystals.

Other Nonpharmacologic Therapies

- **Hemodialysis** should be used in addition to the aforementioned therapies to prevent end-organ toxicity.
- **Hemodialysis** corrects metabolic abnormalities and eliminates nonmetabolized ethylene glycol. Indications for hemodialysis are an ethylene glycol concentration >50 mg/dL, severe acidemia (bicarbonate <15 mmol/L, pH <7.30), hyperviscosity from very elevated concentrations, and/or optic injury from toxicity.[189] Recent literature demonstrates that in otherwise well patients, hemodialysis may not be required even with markedly elevated ethylene glycol concentrations.[199]

Ethanol

PROBLEM STATEMENT

- Ethanol is the most used recreational substance worldwide. Alcohol abuse causes a great deal of financial burden to the healthcare system besides affecting the individual, family, and society at large. At risk drinking is defined as an average of 15 or more standard drinks per week or 5 or more on an occasion for men and 8 or more drinks weekly or 4 or more on occasion for women as well as individuals above 65 years of age.

In parts of India, adolescent drinking has dramatically increased over the last two decades, with estimates being as high as 74% for those born between 1981 and 1985.
  - Elimination rate: 20–25 mg/dL/h (zero-order kinetics, faster in chronic alcoholics).
- Ethanol is present in all alcoholic beverages, some food extracts, mouthwash, and cold syrups, but it is also industrially used as a solvent in its denatured form.

Pathophysiology and Pharmacokinetics

Ethanol undergoes hepatic metabolism via 2 pathways: Alcohol dehydrogenase (ADH) and microsomal ethanol oxidizing system (MEOS). ADH is the rate limiting step and major pathway. Ethanol is converted to acetaldehyde which is further converted to acetic acid ultimately forming water and carbon dioxide. Acetaldehyde is highly reactive and toxic byproduct. With larger quantities, the cytochrome P450 2E1 is activated and increases the NADPH-NADP ratio.

DIAGNOSIS

Clinical Presentation

- Ethanol is a selective central nervous system depressant at low concentration and a general depressant at high concentration. Initially, ethanol produces euphoria and loss of inhibition which progresses to ataxia, drowsiness, and confusion at blood concentrations >100 mg/dL. Respiratory depression can occur at higher concentrations.[200] The intoxicated patient may demonstrate facial flushing, dilated pupils, diaphoresis, GI distress, hypothermia, and hypotension.
- Chronic alcohol abuse induces tolerance, and patients appear asymptomatic even with high blood concentrations.[201]
- Hypoglycemia is due to an altered NADH/NAD+ ratio with the development of a reduced state. Pyruvate is then shunted from the gluconeogenesis pathway, and lactate production is favored because of increased NADH. Severe hypoglycemia is common in chronic alcoholics and in children.
- Chronic intoxication causes further gluconeogenesis disturbances, an increase in ketogenesis (β-hydroxybutyrate) and eventually the development of alcoholic ketoacidosis (AKA).[202]

Diagnostic Testing

- Obtain glucose concentrations, hepatic function tests, and BMP (especially in chronic alcoholics).
- Serum ethanol concentrations are only relevant to rule out poisoning from other alcohols or in the evaluation of patients presenting with a coma or altered mental status.
- Serum osmolality (if coingestion with other alcohols is suspected).
- May also have mild lactic acidosis if dehydrated or has hepatic dysfunction.

TREATMENT

Treatment is mainly supportive; gastric decontamination is not indicated in ethanol poisoning because it is rapidly absorbed from the stomach, however, hemodialysis may be indicated in severe poisoning (e.g., cardiovascular collapse from ethanol). Administer 100 mg **thiamine** IV followed by 50 mL of D_{50} in water IV to any **comatose alcoholic patient** with hypoglycemia. Thiamine should be administered in all alcoholic patients. Patients may require intubation for respiratory depression or for airway protection.

SPECIAL CONSIDERATIONS

- Increased morbidity and mortality result from chronic toxicity (liver and GI injuries) and AKA.
- Traumatic injuries and severe hypothermia are frequent findings due to risky behavior or decreased judgment capability during acute intoxication.
- Ethanol withdrawal can lead to life-threatening conditions and requires special attention.
- Patients should be observed until signs of clinical intoxication resolve.
- In patients with concern for Wernicke's encephalopathy, would recommend high-dose thiamine (500 mg IV).

CYANIDE

GENERAL PRINCIPLES

Cyanide is one of the most rapidly acting and lethal poisons in existence. Cyanide has an odor of bitter almonds; however, only 50% of the population can detect it.[203]

Etiology

- Inhalation of smoke from industrial or residential fires is the most common source of cyanide exposure in the Western and South Asian countries.
- Other etiologies include artificial nail remover, older rodenticides, electroplating solutions, photographic developer solutions, laboratory reagents, laetrile, plants (e.g., pits from the *Prunus* species if chewed), food such as cassava, and prolonged infusion of sodium nitroprusside.
- Lethal dose: Orally administered HCN 50 to 100 mg and of KCN is 150 to 250 mg.

Pathophysiology

- Cyanide is a chemical asphyxiant. It induces cellular hypoxia by inhibiting complex IV (also known as cytochrome c oxidase or cytochrome oxidase aa_3) in the electron transport chain and thus preventing the formation of adenosine triphosphate. Cyanide toxicity affects the most ATP-dependent organs first like heart and brain. Neurotoxicity is caused by stimulation of NMDA receptors and release of glutamate, eventually causing intracellular calcium release and cell death.
- Hyperlactemia occurs from inhibition of aerobic metabolism.

DIAGNOSIS

Clinical Presentation

- The dose, duration of exposure, route of exposure, and etiology of the exposure all contribute to the severity of the illness. Signs and symptoms can be nonspecific, so physicians must have a high degree of clinical suspicion to avoid missing the diagnosis.[204]
- Transient increases in heart rate, BP, and respiratory rate can be followed by cardiovascular collapse and respiratory failure. Initially, patients can present with bradycardia and hypertension; this is followed by tachycardia and hypotension, before they experience cardiovascular collapse.
- The heart and CNS have high demands for oxygen and are commonly affected. Signs and symptoms include headache, anxiety, lethargy, seizures, coma, respiratory failure, and cardiovascular collapse. Cyanogen chloride exposure causes skin and mucous membrane irritation, lacrimation, rhinorrhea, bronchorrhea, cough, chest tightness, and pulmonary edema. Cyanide does not cause cyanosis.

Symptoms	Duration After Exposure
Hyperpnea and hypertension	15 seconds
Loss of consciousness	30 seconds
Convulsions	30–45 seconds
Respiratory arrest	3–5 minutes
Bradycardia, hypotension, and cardiac arrest	5–8 minutes

- The cherry-red skin that is classically associated with cyanide toxicity is an uncommon finding. If it occurs, it occurs very late in the clinical course. Retinal veins may be bright red.

Laboratories

- Blood and serum concentrations are not available in a timely fashion so are not clinically useful. Smokers may have a slightly elevated baseline concentration compared to nonsmokers.
- Because of inhibition of aerobic metabolism, patients can have elevated lactate concentrations. In smoke inhalation victims, a lactate greater than 10 mmol/L was suggestive of cyanide toxicity.[205] High lactates and high anion gap metabolic acidosis are the two most common and universal findings in these patients.
- Patients may have an "arterialization" of their venous blood because the venous oxygen saturation may be very elevated due to inhibition of aerobic metabolism. The partial pressure of oxygen in venous and arterial samples can be nearly identical. As such, venous samples may appear bright red, similar to arterial samples. This can be seen when comparing ABGs and VBGs that are drawn simultaneously.
- Other more specific tests include measurement of thiocyanate in urine and whole blood cyanide concentration assay. Postmortem measurement of tissue cyanide levels in the liver and heart may be more accurate than blood cyanide levels.

TREATMENT

Two antidotes are available for patients with cyanide toxicity.

- The cyanide antidote kit contains **amyl nitrite pearls** and **sodium nitrite.** The pearls (1 ampoule 0.3 mL) can be broken over handkerchief and placed over the patient's mouth for 15 seconds while IV access is obtained. Sodium nitrite (300 mg) is administered as a 3% solution given over 2–4 minutes IV in adults. Nitrites are given to induce a methemoglobinemia, which cyanide will preferentially bind to instead of the electron transport chain. However, in patients with smoke inhalation, this can be dangerous because they may already have elevated levels of carboxyhemoglobin, and the combination can cause a very severe functional anemia. Nitrites can also cause or exacerbate hypotension. The dose should be modified in patients with underlying anemia. The second part of the antidote is **sodium thiosulfate**, administered as 12.5 g in 50 mL of NS IV over 30 minutes in adults. Its time of onset is slower than the nitrites; at times, it is given prophylactically to patients on nitroprusside infusions.[206]
- **Hydroxocobalamin** (5 g IV) is another antidote. It combines with cyanide to form cyanocobalamin (vitamin B_{12}). It has few side effects. It turns the urine red and causes skin discoloration, which negatively interferes with co-oximetry. It will also interfere with certain laboratory tests such as bilirubin, creatinine, and serum glucose.[207] Although more expensive, it is generally the preferred antidote. Other drugs that can be used are 4 dimethylamino phenol and dicobalt edetate.

- The rest of care is supportive, including adequate volume resuscitation, airway support, and vasopressor and inotropic support as needed.[204]

CARBON MONOXIDE

GENERAL PRINCIPLES

Carbon monoxide (CO) is a colorless, odorless, and tasteless gas that is produced during incomplete combustion of carbon-containing fuels. It is the leading cause of poisoning morbidity and mortality in the United States.[208]

Etiology

Common sources of exposure include smoke inhalation in house fires, inhaling solvents, paint removers, and electric generators, automobile exhaust, smoking, forklifts, and chemicals such as methylene chloride.[209] Incomplete combustion in gas geysers installed in bathrooms have emerged as another important cause.

Pathophysiology

- CO has 250 times more affinity for Hb than oxygen. CO binds with hemoglobin to form carboxyhemoglobin, which causes a functional anemia and shifts the oxyhemoglobin dissociation curve to the left.
- CO inhibits cellular respiration by binding to mitochondrial cytochrome oxidase and disrupting the electron transport chain.[210]
- Nitric oxide levels, which cause vasodilation, are also increased (likely secondary to activation of nitric oxide synthase).[209] It activates inflammatory processes resulting in neurological damage.

DIAGNOSIS

The diagnosis of CO poisoning is challenging because of its many vague signs and symptoms that can wax and wane depending on the patient's source of exposure.

Clinical Presentation

- Patients may present with flu- or viral-like symptoms, which include headache, myalgias, fatigue, lethargy, nausea, vomiting, and dizziness. If these patients remove themselves from the exposure, such as when they leave their house to seek medical attention, the symptoms may improve before they are evaluated by a physician. Cherry red discoloration of the skin is rare and found in severe CO poisoning, it heralds poor outcome.
- The heart and CNS have higher oxygen demands, and thus, patients can present with chest pain, myocardial infarctions, cardiac dysrhythmias, syncope, stroke-like symptoms, seizures, coma, and other psychoneurologic symptoms. On fundus examination, there can be bright red retinal veins, flame- shaped hemorrhages, and papilledema.
- Patients may present with persistent neurologic sequelae (PNS), which occur at the time of exposure, or delayed neurologic sequelae (DNS), which can occur anywhere between 2 and 40 days after the exposure.[211]

Diagnostic Testing

- Carboxyhemoglobin (CO-Hgb) levels are readily available. They can be obtained on either arterial or venous specimens.[212] Levels greater than 5% in nonsmokers and greater than 5%–10% in smokers generally confirm an exogenous exposure. Recent literature suggests that levels may only be slightly elevated in smokers. Either way, levels do not correlate well with a patient's symptoms or prognosis.

- New handheld pulse co-oximeters can be used to noninvasively measure CO-Hgb. Standard pulse oximeters may be falsely reassuring because they cannot detect a difference between oxyhemoglobin and CO-Hgb. This results in a "gap" between the measured pulse oximetry using a finger probe and the true value found by using co-oximetry.
- Levels need to be interpreted in the context of how long it has been since the exposure and when oxygen therapy was initiated. Both will cause the level to be "falsely low." A normal PaO_2 in venous blood in presence of hypoxia will suggest the diagnosis.
- Head CTs may show bilateral lesions in the globus pallidus.
- A lactic acidosis may be present owing to the disruption of aerobic respiration.

TREATMENT

- Treatment involves administering oxygen (normobaric oxygen, NBO). One hundred percent oxygen administered through a nonrebreather will decrease the half-life of CO to 60–90 minutes. Hyperbaric oxygen (HBO) will decrease it to 20–30 minutes. Most patients will need to be transported to tertiary centers to receive HBO; hence, improving PNS or preventing DNS and not just decreasing the half-life of CO is the rationale for the use of HBO.
  - Randomized studies have both supported HBO for CO poisoning[211,213] and concluded that it was ineffective.[214,215] The studies differed in their inclusion criteria, exclusion criteria, treatment protocols, and outcome assessment.
  - Indications for and the benefits of HBO are controversial, and more research is needed.[216] Suggested indications include syncope, coma, neurologic deficits, PNS, cardiac ischemia, severe metabolic acidosis, pregnancy, and CO >25%. Given the controversy, a treatment approach using shared decision-making is recommended.
- Additional care includes airway and ventilator support, vasopressors for hypotension, and treating any additional concurrent injury, such as if the patient has a burn, trauma, or cyanide toxicity from a house fire.

COMPLICATIONS

- If the patient survives the exposure, DNS and PNS are the most feared long-term complications after CO poisoning.
- The signs and symptoms of DNS are variable, and a standard definition does not exist. They can include malaise, fatigue, headache, memory problems, paralysis, dementia, neuropathy, psychosis, and cortical blindness.[211] The methods used to test for DNS and the definition of DNS varied between the different randomized trials cited earlier.

ORAL ANTICOAGULANTS

GENERAL PRINCIPLES

Historically, the vitamin k antagonist warfarin was the oral anticoagulant of choice. However, this required bridging with heparin to avoid rare complications and laboratory monitoring. Additionally, both medications and foods led to significant medication interactions. These concerns led to the development of novel oral anticoagulants (NOACs): direct thrombin inhibitors (dabigatran) and factor Xa antagonists (rivaroxaban, apixaban).

Pathophysiology

- Warfarin and other vitamin k antagonists inhibits vitamin k epoxide reductase leading to a deficiency of factors II, VII, IX, X, C, and S
- NOACs either inhibit factor II or Xa

DIAGNOSIS

- For warfarin, the INR can be followed.
- For the NOACs, PT/INR/PTT does not reliably confirm exposure, or if abnormal, it indicates the degree of excess anticoagulation. Thrombin time, the Ecarin Clotting Time, and antifactor Xa levels can be used to monitor NOACs. However, these may be send out tests or may not be readily available, which likely limits their utility.

Clinical Presentation

In overdose, all can lead to bleeding and complications from bleeding. Brodifacoums are long-acting vitamin k antagonists found in rodenticides. They can lead to significant anticoagulation that can last from weeks to months depending on the exposure. A review of poison center data demonstrated a small, but significant, risk of bleeding following overdose of a NOAC.[217] Tissue necrosis, purple toe syndrome, and hyperkalemia are uncommon adverse events associated with warfarin.

TREATMENT

- Prothrombin complex concentrate (PCC) and/or vitamin k are used to treat supratherapeutic INR levels and bleeding following ingestions of warfarin. Mild ingestions may not require reversal. The CHEST guidelines are used to determine if reversal is needed in patients with supratherapeutic warfarin ingestions. Weeks to months of high dose vitamin k may be needed in patients with brodaficoum exposures.
- Idarucizumab is a monoclonal antibody that binds dabigatran. It is indicated for clinically significant bleeding in patients on dabigatran. It is administered as two 2.5 g doses.[218] Vitamin K and PCC should not be coadministered. Hemodialysis is not particularly effective in removing dabigatran because of delays in initiation as well as limited data regarding its efficacy.

  Andaxanet alpha was approved for the reversal of Xa inhibitors in May 2018.[219]

PLANT POISONS

Common plant poisons and their manifestation and treatment have been discussed in Table 28-4.

SNAKE BITE

GENERAL PRINCIPLES

Five million snakebites occur globally each year, causing between 81,000 and 138,000 deaths and nearly 400,000 amputations and other permanent disabilities.* South Asia has

* World Health Organization. Prevalence of Snakebite Envenoming. Available at www.who.int/snakebites/epidemiology/en

TABLE 28-4 Plant Poisons

	Active Principle	Signs and Symptoms	Treatment
Abrus precatorius	Abrin, glycyrrhizin, and *N*-methyltryptophan	GIT irritation, nausea, vomiting, abdominal pain, diarrhea, vertigo, arrhythmia, convulsions, death	Symptomatic
Ricinus communis	Ricin	Colicky pain in abdomen, diarrhea, dehydration, oliguria, uremia, collapse, and death	Symptomatic
Semecarpus anacardium	Semecarpol, bhilwanol	Black vesicles on skin and itching, blisters in throat, GI irritation, areflexia, delirium, coma, cyanosis, death	Symptomatic
Aconite	Aconitine	Tingling and numbness, GI irritation, increased sweating, giddiness, and impaired speech and vision. Pupils show alternate constriction and dilatation (hippus), multiple ectopic, ventricular fibrillation, and bundle branch blocks	Stomach wash, injection strychnine, digitalis, and atropine
Oleander	Nerin and oleandrin	GI irritation, contact dermatitis, dilated pupils, cardiac failure, hypotension, bradycardia Muscle fasciculations	Stomach wash, morphine, and symptomatic treatment
Datura	Hyoscine, hyoscyamine, and atropine	Dryness of secretions, dilated pupils, increased temperature, delirium, coma	Stomach wash Pilocarpine 15 mg or prostigmin 1 mg SC or repeated doses of 0.5–1 mg IM or IV physostigmine Barbiturates

the highest incidence of venomous snakebites in the world.* Within the region, Bangladesh, India, Nepal, Pakistan, and Sri Lanka together constitute nearly 70% of the global snakebite mortality.† About 50,000 people die of snake bite every year in India.

*Kasturiratne A, Wickremasinghe AR, de Silva N, et al. The global burden of snakebite: a literature analysis and modelling based on regional estimates of envenoming and deaths. *PLoS Med.* 2008;5:e218.

† Simpson ID, Norris RL. The global snakebite crisis—a public health issue misunderstood, not neglected. *Wilderness Environ Med.* 2009;20:43–56.

Etiology

Of 300 different snake species in South Asia, an estimated 70 are venomous.

The "big four" include the common krait (*Bungarus caeruleus*), binocellate cobra (*Naja naja*), Russell's viper (*Daboia russelii*), and saw-scaled viper (*Echis carinatus*). These are distributed across the subcontinent and are largely responsible for deaths and long-term complications from snakebite. Around 90% of snakebite deaths in India are from one of these.*

Pathophysiology

Snake venom is not a single component but is a highly complex mixture of variety of components enzymatic, nonenzymatic proteins, and toxins which work together. Elapidae such as the cobra and krait venoms are neurotoxic and cardiotoxic. Local effects are seen in the former but not in the latter. Viper venom is vasculotoxic and has severe necrotizing local effects. The neurotoxins of elapids and sea snakes are absorbed rapidly into the bloodstream (therefore causing rapid systemic effects), whereas the much larger molecules of viper venom are taken up more slowly through the lymphatics (therefore causing severe local effects).

DIAGNOSIS

Clinical Presentation

The clinical features of snake venom poisoning depend on many factors such as type of snake, age and health of the patient, and site of the snake bite. In some proportion of cases, bites by venomous snakes do not result in envenomation called dry bites.

Local Reaction

The local reactions are most profound with viper bite characterized by local swelling, pain, necrosis, compartment syndrome, and gangrene. In cases of bite from cobra or krait, the immediate local actions are burning or tingling pain, irritation, swelling, and inflammation.

Systemic Features

- **Clotting defects and hemolysis:** These are characteristic of envenomation by Viperidae. Persistent bleeding from fang puncture wounds, venepuncture, or injection sites; epistaxis; hematemesis; cutaneous ecchymoses; hemoptysis; subconjunctival, retroperitoneal, and intracranial hemorrhages have been reported.
- **Neurotoxicity:** Elapid and sea snake venoms have significant neurotoxicity. manifests with ptosis and external ophthalmoplegia; later the face, palate, jaws, tongue, vocal cords, neck muscles, and muscles of deglutition become paralyzed. Airway obstruction or paralysis of the intercostal muscles and diaphragm causes respiratory failure.
- **Myotoxicity:** Sea snakes cause myalgias, myopathy, and rhabdomyolysis.
- **Cardiotoxicity:** Viper and elapid venom can cause arrhythmias, bradycardia, tachycardia, or hypotension.
- **Nephrotoxicity:** Renal failure is secondary to ischemia in viper bites.
- **Shock:** Secondary to fright, hypovolemia (due to extravasation of fluids and blood loss), myocardial depression, and hemorrhage into the adrenals and pituitary.

Diagnostic Testing

- The species responsible can be inferred from the clinical syndrome of symptoms and signs.

*Alirol E, Sharma SK, Bawaskar HS, Kuch U, Chappuis F. Snake bite in South Asia: a review. *PLoS Negl Trop Dis.* 2010;4:e603.

- **Twenty-minute whole blood clotting time:** The test should be carried out every 30 minutes from admission for 3 hours and then hourly after that. If incoagulable blood is discovered, the 6-hourly cycle should then be adopted to test for the requirement for repeated doses of ASV. If the tube is not made of ordinary glass or if it has been used before and cleaned with detergent, its wall might stimulate clotting and test should be considered invalid.
- **Blood:** leukocytosis, thrombocytopenia, hemolysis, prolonged clotting and prothrombin time, and hypofibrinogenemia.
- **Metabolic:** acidosis, hyperkalemia.
- **Urine:** presence of Hb, albumin, blood, and azotemia.
- **ECG:** presence of arrhythmias.

TREATMENT

First Aid

Do it R.I.G.H.T. Following points should be taken into account for first aid:

- **Reassure** the patient: It is very important, as many people die just because of the neurogenic shock resulting from fear of death. Majority of the snakes are nonpoisonous. It may be assured to the patient that it may be possible that he or she may have been bitten by a nonpoisonous snake, if the snake is not traceable. Even in poisonous snake bite, reassure the patient that he or she may not die and everything is being done.
- **Immobilize** same way as a fractured limb. Use bandages or cloth to hold the splints. Do not compress by tight ligatures.
- **Get to Hospital immediately.**
- **Tell the physician** about systemic symptoms such as dropping eyelids, double vision, dribbling, and taste of blood in the victim's mouth, that develop on the way to hospital.

Indications of ASV

- Systemic envenomation
  1. Hemostatic abnormalities – Spontaneous systemic bleeding, coagulopathy (WBCT >20 min) or thrombocytopenia.
  2. Neurotoxic signs – Ptosis, external ophthalmoplegia, paralysis
  3. Cardiovascular abnormalities – Hypotension, shock, cardiac arrhythmia
  4. Acute renal failure – Oliguria/anuria, rising BUN/creatinine, hemoglobinuria/myoglobinuria
- Local envenomation: Local swelling involving more than half of the bitten limb, swelling of digits after bite, rapid extension of swelling and development of an enlarged tender lymph node draining the bitten limb.

Dosage of ASV

There is no absolute contraindication to ASV.

Intravenous: Starting with 10 vials of reconstituted, freeze dried ASV diluted in 200–300 mL of isotonic saline over 1 hour ensures that there is sufficient neutralizing power to neutralize the average amount of venom injected → further doses based on 20-minute WBCT/clinical need.

- Watch for symptoms and signs of anaphylaxis. Skin/conjunctival hypersensitivity testing does not reliably predict antivenom reactions and is not recommended. If anaphylaxis develops then stop ASV. Give 0.5 mg of 1:1000 adrenaline IM, repeat after 10–15 minutes if no improvement. ASV can then be restarted slowly for 10–15 minutes.

Supportive Therapy

- Tetanus prophylaxis.
- Antibiotics as indicated.

- Surgical debridement/fasciotomy for compartment syndromes.
- Management of respiratory paralysis. Ventilatory support must be considered and instituted early. Neostigmine methyl sulfate (50–100 μg/kg body weight) for neurotoxic cases.
- Hemostatic disturbances: fresh frozen plasma, cryoprecipitates, and platelet concentrates if required.
- Hemodialysis: if renal failure, severe acidosis.

SCORPION BITE

GENERAL PRINCIPLES

Scorpion stings are acute life-threatening medical emergency which are common in rural areas of many tropical and subtropical regions of the world. Of the 1500 total scorpion species in the world, around 30 are found to be lethal to humans.

Etiology

Among the neurotoxic ones, *Centruroides* and *Parabuthus* predominate while *Buthus*, *Mesobuthus*, and *Androctonus* cause lethal cardiotoxicity. In India, 86 species of scorpions have been identified; Mesobuthus tamulus and Palamneus gravimanus are medically important.

Pathophysiology

Most of the scorpion stings are minor, despite more than a million stings occurring annually. The venom is deposited deep into the subcutaneous tissue and is completely absorbed within few hours. The toxin in the venom that have the greatest significance is α-toxin, this causes massive endogenous release of catecholamines as well as other vasoactive peptide hormones leading to an "autonomic storm." The venom leads to prolonged depolarization by causing incomplete inactivation of sodium channels resulting in a slow influx of sodium. This results in membrane hyperexcitability and unregulated axon firing.

DIAGNOSIS

Clinical Presentation

- Local inflammatory reaction (swelling, redness, rise in temperature) and severe pain, local necrosis.
- Positive tap test: Tapping leads to an increase in paresthesia in some patients.
- Systemic manifestations may develop early or can be delayed up to 24 hours. Hypertension can develop commonly and is due to sympathetic overactivity. Similarly, there can be restlessness, piloerection, marked tachycardia, mydriasis, toxic myocarditis, cardiac failure, pulmonary edema, and cardiogenic shock.[216]
- Seizure-like activity, pharyngeal muscles and uncontrolled diaphragmatic, and intercostal neuromuscular activity may result in respiratory distress.
- Priapism may occur secondary to cholinergic stimulation.
- Clinical grading:
  - Grade I- Local pain and paresthesia without systemic manifestation.
  - Grade II- Pain and paresthesia distant from site of sting with or without tachycardia and without cardiorespiratory signs
  - Grade III- Peripheral circulatory failure, cardiovascular, and respiratory manifestations
  - Grade IV- Central nervous system manifestation and multisystem involvement

Diagnostic Testing

Basic laboratory studies, including a complete blood count, a comprehensive metabolic panel, PT/INR, PTT, lipase, and ECG, are recommended.

TREATMENT

- Mild pain can be relieved by application of ice packs and oral analgesics. Severe excruciating pain may require ring block with lignocaine and bupivacaine.
- Prazosin is the antidote to scorpion sting and reverses the hormonal and metabolic effects of alpha receptor stimulation. Dose is 1 mg as tablet, repeating the dose after 3 hours may be necessary depending on the clinical response and subsequently after 6 hours (maximum dose 5 mg per day).[217]
- Atropine is contraindicated.
- Antivenom is reserved for patients displaying skeletal muscle or cranial nerve dysfunction who are stung by *Centruroides* scorpions. It is available in the United States, under the name Anascorp, which is an intravenous scorpion-specific F(ab')2 equine antivenom (dose is 5–25 mL, diluted in two or three volumes of isotonic saline over an hour).
- Mechanical ventilation and inotropes (dobutamine) may be needed for patients with complications.

COMPLICATIONS

- Include neurotoxicity, skeletal muscle dysfunction, hyperthermia, rhabdomyolysis, pulmonary edema, and multiple organ failures.

Summary

- Common toxidromes include anticholinergic toxidrome, cholinergic toxidrome, sympathomimetic toxidrome, opioid toxidrome, and sedative-hypnotic toxidrome.
- Decontamination and administration of specific antidotes are key to the management.
- Insecticides, herbicides, and rodenticides are common poisons encountered in medical practice.
- Opioids, benzodiazepines, antidepressants, paracetamol, and NSAIDs can cause toxicity if taken in excessive doses.
- Snake bite envenomation include hemotoxicity, neurotoxicity, and local reaction. Prompt identification and administration of antivenom is of prime importance.

Scan the QR code to access chapter references.

29 Medical Disorders in Pregnancy

Mohammed Shaheen, Murali Mohan Rama Krishna Reddy, and Archith Boloor

Physiologic Changes in Pregnancy

See Table 29-1.

TABLE 29-1 Physiologic Changes in Pregnancy

Organ System	Changes Occurring in Pregnancy
General hemodynamics	Plasma volume and red cell mass increases in pregnancy. Expansion of plasma volume is greater than increase in red blood cell mass; hence, there is a fall in hematocrit. There is no change in MCV or MCHC. Platelet count reduces in pregnancy, but remains within normal limits. Concentration of clotting factors, especially factors VIII, IX, and X, increases. Fibrinogen levels increase by around 50%, whereas concentration of endogenous anticoagulants decreases.
Cardiac system	By 8 weeks of pregnancy, cardiac output increases by 20% which goes up to 40% by the end of pregnancy. This is achieved by an increase in stroke volume, and rarely by increase in heart rate. Systemic vascular resistance is reduced by 20%–35% due to peripheral vasodilation. Blood pressure decreases in the first and second trimesters and returns to prepregnancy value in the third trimester. Over 90% of pregnant women have a bounding pulse and may have an ejection systolic murmur.
Renal system	Due to renal vasodilation, renal blood flow and GFR increase by about 50%. Concentration of serum urea and creatinine reduces. Due to increased renal blood flow, the size of the kidneys increases by about 1–1.5 cm, reaching maximum size by the second trimester. Due to increase in capillary permeability and GFR, more glucose and protein are excreted in urine than in a nonpregnant individual.
Respiratory system	Due to an increase in metabolic rate and oxygen consumption, there is a 40%–50% increase in minute ventilation due to an increase in the tidal volume. This compensates for the increased oxygen demand. As a result of this hyperventilation, arterial pO_2 increases and $PaCO_2$ falls, leading to a mild, fully compensated respiratory alkalosis which is normal in pregnancy.

(*Continued*)

TABLE 29-1 Physiologic Changes in Pregnancy (Continued)

Organ System	Changes Occurring in Pregnancy
Gastrointestinal tract	The gravid uterus displaces the stomach upwards, leading to an increased intragastric pressure. Hormones secreted in pregnancy also cause a decrease in the tone of esophageal sphincter. This may contribute toward reflux, nausea, or vomiting.
Endocrine changes	Increased production of thyroxine-binding globulin by the liver causes a rise in the level of total T3 and total T4. Serum concentration of TSH is decreased due to the thyrotropic effect of hCG. Increased serum levels of ACTH, cortisol-binding globulin, and free cortisol make pregnancy a state of physiologic hypercortisolism. This manifests as abdominal striae, facial plethora, or impaired glucose intolerance. The pituitary gland enlarges in pregnancy due to proliferation of prolactin-producing cells in the anterior lobe. Levels of FSH and LH are almost undetectable in pregnancy due to the feedback by estrogen and progesterone. Serum growth hormone levels are increased due to the production of growth hormone by the placenta. The posterior pituitary produces oxytocin which increases during pregnancy to peak at term.
Carbohydrate metabolism	Pregnancy is a diabetogenic state and involves relocating glucose stores to promote the development of the fetus. Insulin sensitivity is increased in early pregnancy, but in the near-term it progresses towards insulin resistance. This begins in the second trimester due to the increase in diabetogenic hormones from the placenta, such as human placental lactogen, growth hormone, cortisol, and progesterone. Fasting glucose levels are usually decreased in pregnancy due to increased peripheral use of glucose. Postpartum, there is a sudden reduction in insulin resistance due to absence of placental hormones.
Protein metabolism	Pregnant women require an increased intake of proteins due to active shunting of amino acids to support the growing fetus. Protein catabolism is reduced in pregnancy due to the usage of lipids as an energy source.
Lipid metabolism	Total serum cholesterol and triglyceride levels in pregnancy are increased. This is due to increased production by the liver and decreased activity of lipoprotein lipase. LDL levels increase by up to 50% and HDL increases in the first half of pregnancy, but falls by the third trimester to about 15% more than the prepregnancy value.
Calcium metabolism	Maternal levels of serum calcium are maintained and fetal demand is met through increased dietary absorption, which doubles from around 12 weeks of gestation. Increased calcium absorption is also associated with an increase in calcium excretion. Pregnancy is also a risk factor for kidney stones due to this physiologic hypercalciuria.

Soma-Pillay P, Nelson-Piercy C, Tolppanen H, Mebazaa A. Physiological changes in pregnancy. *Cardiovasc J Afr.* 2016;27(2):89–94.

Asthma in Pregnancy

GENERAL PRINCIPLES

Asthma is one of the most common chronic diseases complicating pregnancy. It is characterized by recurring episodes of airway obstruction due to hyepersensitivity or bronchial hyperresponsiveness to allergens. It affects roughly 9% of gestating mothers worldwide. Acute exacerbations of asthma in pregnancy are an important and overlooked cause of fetomaternal morbidity. Of the roughly 33% of pregnant women with asthma experience worsening, one-third will find it improved and another third will observe no change.

The increase in the metabolic rate of pregnant women results in an increase in oxygen consumption by about 20%. This, in turn, increases the rate of ventilation by around 30%–40%. This hyperventilated state is mediated in the respiratory center by progesterone. Estrogen also contributes to mucosal and laryngeal edema in about 20%–30% of pregnant women.

Anatomically, the increased size of the uterus pushes upwards on the diaphragm leading to a decrease in the functional residual capacity. The maternal immune response shows a shift from Th1 to Th2 type for the fetus to survive. This upregulation of Th2 may also be a contributing factor.

Excessive first-trimester weight gain, obesity, maternal smoking, and maternal anxiety are known to increase the risk of exacerbation.

DIAGNOSIS

The distribution of exacerbation, however, is nonuniform throughout pregnancy. This is an important diagnostic challenge. In most women in whom the symptoms decrease, the improvement is gradual as the pregnancy progress. In patients whose symptoms worsen, there are two spikes: one at the 14–24-week mark and the subsequent one at the 28- and 32-week period of gestation. Asthma during the last month of pregnancy is relatively less severe.

The symptoms are often worse at night and in the early morning, being triggered by viral infections, pollen and allergen exposure, and other irritants. The most frequent sign is wheezing on auscultation. In severe cases, a silent chest is observed on auscultation due to severe reduction in airflow.

MANAGEMENT

The treatment approach to asthma in pregnancy is the same as that of adult and adolescent asthmatics given under the Global Initiative for Asthma strategy.

The short-acting beta-agonist of choice is salbutamol. This should be given as a reliever drug to patients with mild to moderate asthma. For patients who experience moderate to severe asthma during pregnancy, inclusion of inhaled glucocorticoids reduces the risk of exacerbation. Similarly, withdrawal from the existing usage of inhaled glucocorticoids was shown to increase the risk of exacerbations. Due to availability of more clinical research data, budesonide is the preferred inhaled glucocorticoid for the treatment of asthma during pregnancy. Salmeterol is the recommended long-acting beta-agonist (LABA), once again due to availability of more data. Addition of long-acting muscarinic antagonist (ipratropium) may be considered if LABA-inhaled corticosteroid (ICS) combination is not effective. Leukotriene modifiers can be considered in patients who showed response to it prior to pregnancy. Methylxanthines, cromoglycate drugs, biologics, and immunotherapy are avoided due to lack of safety evidence.

The main concern with asthmatics who become pregnant is their compliance with therapy. Patient education and adequate counseling is necessary. It is important for the patient to recognize the early signs and symptoms of an exacerbation, practice correct use of medications, avoid environmental triggers, and formulate a treatment plan for an acute episode.

Treatment of Acute Exacerbations

Acute exacerbation of asthma during pregnancy is known to increase the risk of preeclampsia, gestational diabetes, abruptio placentae, and placenta previa. Pharmacotherapy does not differ from the generic management of acute asthma; however, it is imperative to closely monitor both the mother and the fetus during such episodes.

Supportive measures advised are to keep the mother in a sitting, propped-up, or lateral position. This reduces the compression on the abdominal aorta by the gravid uterus. Supplemental oxygen is administered at the rate of 3–4 L/min by nasal cannula until the oxygen saturation by pulse oximetry is >95%.

Intravenous magnesium sulfate is known to have some benefit in acute asthma in conjunction with inhaled beta-agonists and intravenous glucocorticoids. It is especially helpful to prevent preeclamptic seizures and to reduce the frequency of uterine contractions.

Peripartum usage of prostaglandin F2-alpha (carboprost) for termination of pregnancy, ripening of cervix, or control of postpartum hemorrhage is contraindicated in asthmatics as it may cause sudden bronchoconstriction. Oxytocin, dinoprostone, and misoprostol are recommended alternatives. Similarly, morphine is not advised for pain control as it can cause histamine release which may inadvertently exacerbate the symptoms.

Anemia in Pregnancy

GENERAL PRINCIPLES

Anemia is one of the most common medical complications related to pregnancy. Normal physiologic changes that occur in pregnancy usually lead to a relative reduction in the Hb concentration. Due to this, the parameters defining pregnancy in anemia are different than those seen in nonpregnant individuals (Table 29-2).

TABLE 29-2 Criteria for Diagnosis of Anemia in Pregnancy

Criteria Given by	Mild	Moderate	Severe	Very Severe
ICMR (in g/dL)	10–10.9	7–9.9	4–6.9	<4
WHO (in g/dL)	8–11	5–7	<5	—
	First Trimester	**Second Trimester**	**Third Trimester**	
CDC *(defined by trimester; no criteria for mild, moderate, or severe) (in g/dL)*	<11	<10.5	<11	

CDC, Centers for Disease Control and Prevention; ICMR, Indian Council of Medical Research; WHO, World Health Organization.

ETIOLOGY

Iron-deficiency anemia is the most common etiologic form of anemia in pregnancy. It must be observed that the increased physiologic demands during pregnancy paired with the poor dietary intake, especially in developing countries such as India, contribute to a very high prevalence of anemia in pregnancy.

DIAGNOSIS

Clinical Presentation

Laboratory assessment in the booking visit is routinely done and may be helpful to diagnose anemia. However, second trimester (24–28 weeks) and third trimester (36 weeks) laboratory evaluations are more sensitive. However, symptoms of anemia such as fatigue, breathlessness, alopecia, and pica and signs such as pallor and koilonychia must be looked for in a brief clinical examination.

Diagnostic Evaluation

Both hemoglobin estimation and peripheral smear are practical and cost-efficient methods of diagnosis. Serum ferritin level below 12 ng/mL is also a good indicator for iron-deficiency anemia as it does not get affected by recent iron intake and reflects iron stores. A value below 30 ng/mL reflects depleted maternal iron stores. Peripheral smear is indicated to know the morphology of anemia.

MANAGEMENT

Oral Iron Therapy

The recommended dose for the treatment of iron-deficiency anemia in pregnancy is 120 mg/d according to the WHO guidelines and between 100 and 200 mg/d as per the British guidelines. Doses higher than this do not improve efficacy but can lead to increased gastrointestinal side effects. All pregnant women should be advised to take an oral iron supplement on an empty stomach or 1 hour after a meal, preferably with a vitamin C–rich product such as orange juice or lemonade. Ferric salts are known to have better tolerance than ferrous salts; however, they have lesser absorption.

Parenteral Iron Therapy

Intravenous preparations have faster absorption, better bioavailability, and fewer side effects. However, they are expensive and pose a risk of oxidant damage. Preparations such as iron-isomaltoside and iron-carboxymaltose allow for larger quantities of elemental iron to be infused over a shorter time. The formula used to calculate the dosage is given by Ganzoni's equation:

$$\text{Dose of iron required (mg)} = (2.4 \times [\text{target Hb} - \text{current Hb}] \times \text{prepregnancy weight [in kg]}) + 1000 \text{ mg for replenishment of stores}$$

Blood Transfusion

Blood transfusion poses the risk of RBC alloimmunization in pregnancy. Another potential complication that may happen in pregnancy is volume overload. However, the most recent RCOG guidelines state that hemoglobin below 7 g/dL may be considered as threshold for transfusion. Routine usage of transfusion is not recommended and must be individualized based on the availability of oral and parenteral iron preparations.

Folic Acid Deficiency

The recommended intake of 1 mg/d of folic acid preconceptionally and throughout the first trimester is usually enough to prevent the development of megaloblastic anemia due to folic acid deficiency. However, it must be noted that in individuals with seizure disorders who are on antiepileptics such as valproate, a high-dose prophylaxis of 4 mg is advised. A matter of concern is that in women with megaloblastic anemia, it is important to rule out vitamin B_{12} deficiency as folate therapy can mask and delay the diagnosis of vitamin B_{12} deficiency.

Prevention

Prophylaxis in nonpregnant women through increased dietary consumption of iron-rich foods and deworming during the second/third trimester using oral antihelminthics such as a single tablet of albendazole 400 mg along with iron supplementation during pregnancy is shown to have great results.

Cardiac Disease in Pregnancy

GENERAL PRINCIPLES

Due to improved medical and maternal care, more women with congenital and acquired heart conditions can bear children safely. However, due to the tremendous physiologic load of pregnancy on the cardiovascular system, cardiac disease in pregnancy continues to be associated with significant risk.

Less than 1% of pregnancies are complicated by cardiac disease; however, it remains the leading indirect cause of maternal death worldwide. Epidemiologic factors vary largely based on ethnicity, geographic location, and lifestyle. Death in these patients, though very rare, is usually due to myocardial infarction, aortic dissection, or cardiomyopathy.

Cardiovascular diseases are categorized based on the risk they carry during pregnancy (Table 29-3).

TABLE 29-3 Risk Assessment of Cardiac Diseases During Pregnancy

WHO Criteria for Risk Assessment of Cardiac Disease in Pregnancy	Common Disorders
WHO I: Risk no higher than the general population	Uncomplicated mild pulmonary stenosis Mitral valve prolapse Successfully repaired atrial or ventricular septal defects Isolated atrial or ventricular ectopias
WHO II: Small risk of increased maternal mortality or morbidity	Unrepaired atrial or ventricular septal defects Repaired tetralogy of Fallot Most arrhythmias
WHO II–III	LV dysfunction with ejection fraction >30% Hypertrophic cardiomyopathy Marfan without dilation of aorta Repaired coarctation of aorta Aortic dilatation less than 45 mm in bicuspid aortic valve disease

(*Continued*)

TABLE 29-3 Risk Assessment of Cardiac Diseases During Pregnancy (Continued)

WHO III: Significantly increased risk; expert cardiac and obstetric care required at all stages	Mechanical valve Unrepaired cyanotic heart disease Fontan circulation Complex congenital heart disease Aortic dilatation of 40–45 mm in Marfan Aortic dilatation of 45–50 mm in bicuspid aortic valve disease
WHO IV: Pregnancy is contraindicated	Pulmonary arterial hypertension Severe aortic or mitral stenosis Severe heart failure with ejection fraction less than 30% Previous peripartum cardiomyopathy with residual LV damage Aortic dilatation of more than 45 mm in Marfan Aortic dilatation of more than 50 mm in bicuspid aortic valve disease

LV, left ventricular; WHO, World Health Organization.

CLINICAL PRESENTATION AND DIAGNOSIS

Several of the symptoms seen in cardiac disease are mimicked by pregnancy in itself. Hence, a clear and elaborate history is essential to diagnose the various cardiac disorders in pregnancy. Breathlessness, palpitations, pedal edema, and syncope are the commonly seen symptoms. Signs include a bounding pulse, systolic murmur, raised JVP, S3 and/or S4 heart sounds, among others.

Evaluation of cardiac disease in pregnancy requires advanced workup. Routine blood work and an electrocardiogram can function as the starting point for diagnosis. It is important to note that normal pregnancy can cause ECG changes that may mimic a cardiac disorder. Due to a rotation of the heart from the right to the left, a mild left-axis deviation may be seen. Dilation of all the chambers of the heart due to the volume overload can manifest as dysrhythmias on an ECG. The most commonly seen dysrhythmias in pregnancy are atrial/ventricular premature beats and even supraventricular tachycardia. Nonspecific ST-segment changes can be seen in up to 15% of normal pregnancies.

Peripartum Cardiomyopathy

The diagnostic criteria for peripartum cardiomyopathy is discussed in Table 29-4.

TREATMENT AND MANAGEMENT

Most cardiac disorders in pregnancy are treated based on the disease progression and require a multidisciplinary approach. Prior treatment regimens may be continued by replacing known teratogenic drugs.

TABLE 29-4 Diagnostic Criteria for Peripartum Cardiomyopathy

Demakis Criteria	ECG Criteria
Features suggestive of heart failure within the last month of pregnancy up to 5 months postpartum	Left ventricular ejection fraction <45%
Absence of determinable cause for the heart failure	Left ventricular fractional shortening <30%
Absence of heart failure before the last month of pregnancy	Left ventricular end-diastolic dimension >2.7 cm/m^2 of body surface area

In patients with ventricular dysfunction or prior cardiac failure, the second trimester of pregnancy may exacerbate the symptoms drastically. ACE inhibitors and ARBs which are usually used in the treatment of heart failure are contraindicated due to their teratogenicity, causing renal failure, oligohydramnios, and intrauterine growth restriction (Potter sequence). Hydralazine, nitrates, and cardioselective beta-blockers may be used to achieve the desired effect. Patients with peripartum cardiomyopathy are treated in the same way during pregnancy, but ACE inhibitors and ARBs may be resumed after delivery.

Beta-blockers are the drug of choice in pregnant women with mitral stenosis. Due to the high rates of mortality and morbidity in these patients, hospital admission is advised in the third trimester of the pregnancy and the patient must be monitored well. Aortic stenosis is more difficult to treat; however, it is much rarer in pregnancy.

Treatment of an acute myocardial infarction should proceed as it does with nonpregnant individuals: emergency angioplasty with bare metal stents is recommended due to the availability of good clinical research data. Clopidogrel may be used as an antiplatelet for a short course following the stenting. It is contraindicated to perform thrombolysis since coronary artery dissection is a very common cause of acute myocardial infarction in pregnancy.

Studies have shown that caesarean sections are much more common in women with cardiac disease. This may be due to the perceived safety of an elective cesarean section over a failed trial of labor. However, cesarean sections are associated with more blood loss, sudden hemodynamic changes, and increased risk of infection, and affect the mode of delivery in subsequent pregnancies. Therefore, in a resource-rich setting with a specialist team, vaginal delivery is recommended. Adequate use of combined spinal–epidural and operative delivery using a forceps or vacuum can allow for a "pain-free, push-free" delivery.

Postpartum follow-up involves assessment for deterioration following pregnancy. This is also an important time to discuss contraceptive options with the family and further counsel them regarding the cardiac status of the mother. Reintroduction of drugs that were withheld during pregnancy may be done within 2–4 weeks of pregnancy.

Pregnancy-Induced Hypertension

GENERAL PRINCIPLES

Hypertensive disorders of pregnancy is an all-encompassing term that includes both pregnancy-induced hypertension and preexisting hypertension. It complicates up to 6%–10% of pregnancies and poses significant risk of mortality and morbidity to both the mother and the child. The ACOG defines gestational hypertension as blood pressure greater than or equal to 140 mm Hg systolic or 90 mm Hg diastolic taken on two separate occasions 4 hours apart after 20 weeks of pregnancy, provided that the previous readings were normal.

Gestational hypertension also includes preeclampsia and eclampsia which are life-threatening hypertensive emergencies seen in pregnant individuals.

The main risk factor in the development of hypertensive disease in pregnancy is uteroplacental insufficiency. Therefore, conditions that can contribute to this are considered predecessors to pregnancy-induced-hypertension. These include renal disease, diabetes, thrombophilias, and autoimmune diseases. Additionally, women who are younger than 20 years or older than 40 years, are first-time mothers, or have a mother or sister who has had gestational hypertension have been shown to be at higher risk for developing gestational hypertension and pose more risk to transition into preeclampsia.

CLINICAL PRESENTATION AND DIAGNOSIS

Hypertensive disorders are classified based on the time and context at which they are identified. This classification varies worldwide, but the following are accepted across international guidelines:

- **Gestational hypertension:** Hypertension that appears de novo after 20 weeks of gestation and normalizes within 12 weeks postpartum.
- **Chronic hypertension:** Hypertension that antedates pregnancy before 20 weeks of gestation or persisting after 12 weeks postpartum. Hypertension due to gestational trophoblastic disease has to be ruled out.
- **Preeclampsia:** Gestational hypertension in association with proteinuria greater than 300 mg in 24 hours. It is considered severe preeclampsia if the proteinuria is greater than 5 g in 24 hours.
- **Eclampsia:** Gestational hypertension in association with proteinuria and seizures that cannot be attributed to any neurological disease.

The classical definition of two blood pressure readings above 140 or 90 mm Hg 4 hours apart is not routinely used in clinical practice. A single reading above 160 mm Hg systolic and/or 110 mm Hg diastolic is considered to be a feature of severe hypertension and must be managed aggressively.

TREATMENT

The target blood pressure to be achieved at any point is below 160/110 mm Hg. However, achieving control below this level remains debatable. Also, how quickly the blood pressure may be controlled is also not well defined due to a paucity of clinical data. It is recommended that the diastolic blood pressure is never reduced below 80–90 mm Hg to maintain adequate uteroplacental blood flow.

Common drugs used in the treatment of hypertension, as given by the American College of Obstetrics and Gynecology Guidelines of 2019, are as listed in Table 29-5.

Development of preeclampsia however poses a challenge to the management of the patient. Preeclampsia with features of severe disease is an indication for delivery if it is after 34 weeks of gestation. Attempting to prolong the delivery through expectant management in severe cases of preeclampsia is debatable due to the high risk of fetomaternal complications.

In the absence of severe disease, it is still recommended to deliver the baby at 37–38 weeks of gestation.

Treatment of Eclampsia

The main aim of therapy here is to prevent maternal hypoxia and trauma, treat severe hypertension, prevent recurrence of seizures, and prompt delivery. Magnesium sulfate is

TABLE 29-5 Antihypertensive Drug Usage in Pregnancy

Pharmacological Agent	Routine Control of Blood Pressure	Emergency Control of Blood Pressure
Methyldopa	500–3000 mg/d given orally in two to four divided doses	Not commonly used as first line
Hydralazine	Not commonly used as first line	5 mg given intravenously, and then 5–10 mg given every 20–40 minutes up to 20 mg/d Alternatively, an infusion at 0.5/10 mg/h
Nifedipine	Extended-release tablet of 30–120 mg/d given orally	10–20 mg given orally every 4–6 hour up to 180 mg/d
Labetalol	200–2400 mg/d given orally in two to three divided doses	10–20 mg given intravenously, and then 20–80 mg given every 20–30 minutes up to 300 mg/d Alternatively, an infusion at 1–2 mg/h

TABLE 29-6 Treatment of Eclampsia

Route of Administration of Magnesium Sulfate	Loading Dose	Maintenance Dose
Intravenous	4–6 g over 15–20 minutes	1–3 g/h continuous IV infusion
Intramuscular	5 g administered on each buttock for a total of 10 g	5 g administered intramuscularly every 4 hours

the recommended anticonvulsive agent as it reduces the rate of recurrence of seizures by two-thirds.

The usage of magnesium sulfate must be accompanied by continuous monitoring regimen described in Table 29-6. The maintenance dose must be skipped or withdrawn if the maternal patellar reflex becomes absent, respiratory rate drops below 12, or the urine output is less than 100 mL in 4 hours.

The definitive treatment for eclampsia is immediate delivery. Postpartum, antihypertensive medication is continued with the same target blood pressure to reduce the risk of stroke. All routinely used antihypertensives are safe while breast-feeding.

Thromboembolism

GENERAL PRINCIPLES

Pregnancy and postpregnancy puerperium are known to be in a prothrombotic state. The effects of the physiologic changes in pregnancy pertaining to procoagulant state manifest in the late first trimester and persist till a few weeks following delivery. The main clinical challenge is that most often, symptoms of pregnancy overlap with the symptoms of an acute thromboembolic event and hence diagnosis and treatment get delayed.

The risk of developing venous thromboembolism is 4–50 times higher in pregnant women than in their nonpregnant counterparts. Among pregnant women, the risk of VTE is two to five times more in the postpartum period than in the antepartum. The geographic distribution of cases tends to show a higher risk of DVT in African women. Also, pregnant women are more likely to develop DVT on the left lower extremities.

All three components of the Virchow's triad play their role in increasing the risk of venous thromboembolism in pregnancy. Increased venous capacitance due to pregnancy-associated changes and compression of the lower abdominal veins by the gravid uterus contribute to stasis. Labor and the physiologic stress caused by it are implicated in vascular endothelial injury. This is aggravated severely in assisted methods of vaginal delivery such as application of forceps or vacuum. Progressive increase in coagulation factors and a decrease in levels of protein S, along with suppression of fibrinolysis, contribute to a hypercoagulable state.

CLINICAL PRESENTATION AND DIAGNOSIS

The clinical presentation is the same as that in nonpregnant individuals, however with a predilection toward the left side of the lower body. This is due to the compression of the left common iliac vein by both the right ovarian artery and the right common iliac artery. Symptoms include a swollen, tender leg in venous thromboembolism and breathlessness, sharp-stabbing chest pain, and syncope in pulmonary embolism.

The fetomaternal effects as direct sequelae of a thromboembolic event are not significant. However, in an untreated maternal pulmonary embolism, there is a 30% risk of death. This can be brought down through appropriate medical management.

Diagnosis is also done in the same way as done in nonpregnant individuals. Radiographic studies, specifically a Doppler ultrasonogram or magnetic resonance imaging, of the suspected veins in the case of DVT and/or CT pulmonary angiogram for pulmonary embolism are done. The main challenge here is to weigh the risk of radiation exposure to the fetus versus the importance of establishing the diagnosis in the mother.

A point to note is that D-dimer measurements do not have any significant benefit in diagnosis as in pregnancy, the physiologic changes to the coagulation system can show a high D-dimer value. Conversely, it can be argued that it may be used to negate a diagnosis: a low value of D-dimer can be used to rule out a thromboembolic episode.

TREATMENT AND MANAGEMENT

Depending on their risk category, women with low-to-moderate risk are recommended postnatal prophylaxis, usually in the form of low-molecular-weight heparin. Women with high antenatal risk for a thromboembolic event are advised low-molecular-weight heparin, good mobilization, and elastic compression stockings.

In the suspicion of an acute venous thromboembolism, prompt therapy is the mainstay of management. Clinicians are advised to start on empiric therapy using low-molecular-weight heparin. Warfarin is contraindicated during pregnancy.

Nausea and Vomiting of Pregnancy

GENERAL PRINCIPLES

Up to 90% of women are affected by nausea during their pregnancy, more so in the first trimester of pregnancy. This is combined with vomiting in about 50%–55% of the population. When this pernicious vomiting of pregnancy becomes intractable leading to weight loss and/or volume depletion, it is known as hyperemesis gravidarum. Incidences of hyperemesis gravidarum are however much rarer, ranging from 1% to 3% depending on the target population.

hCG levels peak during the first trimester, which corresponds with the onset of nausea and vomiting. Also, pregnancies with larger placental area such as molar pregnancies and twin gestations have increased nausea and vomiting, possibly due to higher levels of hCG. Estrogen is also implicated as the levels of blood estradiol mirror the onset and fall of nausea and vomiting of pregnancy.

CLINICAL PRESENTATION AND DIAGNOSIS

Due to the lack of an accepted definition or criterion for hyperemesis gravidarum, it is diagnosed clinically. The most common symptom for diagnosis is vomiting leading to significant dehydration as evidenced by ketonuria or electrolyte abnormalities. Weight loss of more than 5% of the prepregnancy weight without an underlying pathologic cause should also prompt the clinician to establish a diagnosis.

The patient is evaluated through urinalysis to check for ketones. Elevated hemoglobin or hematocrit can be a manifestation of hemoconcentration due to dehydration. Significant dehydration can result in increased creatinine due to acute kidney injury. Electrolyte abnormalities set in due to reduced oral intake of fluids.

Radiographic studies, mainly ultrasounds, can be used to diagnose a gestational trophoblastic disease, an ectopic pregnancy, or a multiple gestation.

TREATMENT/MANAGEMENT

The nausea and vomiting in pregnancy guidelines of the American College of Obstetrics and Gynecology state that initial treatment is using nonpharmacological interventions. This includes supplementation of ginger in the diet, 250 mg of extract powder four times a day or changing the patient's prenatal vitamins to folic acid only.

In the event of continuing symptoms, first-line pharmacological therapy is using a combination of pyridoxine and doxylamine. Second-line drugs are antihistaminics and dopamine antagonists such as dimenhydrinate, diphenhydramine, prochlorperazine, or promethazine (Table 29-7). Ondansetron is avoided until 12 weeks.

In case of dehydration setting in, intravenous fluid boluses or continuous infusion of normal saline must be given along with intravenous metoclopramide, ondansetron, or promethazine. Electrolytes must be replaced as required.

Complications

Increased incidences of low birth weight and premature infancy are seen in the setting of nausea and vomiting in pregnancy. In severe cases of hyperemesis, Wernicke encephalopathy in the mother due to vitamin B_1 deficiency is seen. Hypokalemia can also cause

TABLE 29-7 Treatment of Vomiting in Pregnancy

Drug	Regimen
Vitamin B_6 and doxylamine	10 mg four times a day or 20 mg BD each, oral
Dimenhydrinate	25–50 mg six hourly, oral
Diphenhydramine	25–50 mg six hourly, oral
Prochlorperazine	25 mg 12 hourly, rectal
Promethazine	12.5–25 mg six hourly, oral, or rectal

significant morbidity in the mother. Higher rates of depression and anxiety are experienced by mothers with hyperemesis during pregnancy.

Hepatic Disorders of Pregnancy

Hepatic disorders of pregnancy can be divided into three: those that are induced by pregnancy (such as acute fatty liver of pregnancy [AFLP] or intrahepatic cholestasis), those that develop during pregnancy but are unrelated to it, and preexisting hepatobiliary disorders that complicate pregnancy.

Table 29-8 summarizes the common hepatic disorders in pregnancy.

INTRAHEPATIC CHOLESTASIS OF PREGNANCY (ICP)

ICP is the most common pregnancy-specific liver disorder. The pathophysiology and reasons for epidemiologic distribution are poorly understood, with prevalence ranging from 1% to 25%. Advanced maternal age, multiple gestation, ethnic distribution, and similar history in the past or in family members as well as chronic hepatitis C infections are all risk factors for the development.

A second-trimester onset of mild to intractable itching is usually the primary symptom in ICP. It has a predilection toward the soles and palms. Other symptoms include steatorrhea, nausea, poor appetite, right upper quadrant pain, and insomnia. The symptoms rarely progress toward hepatic failure, and if signs of hepatic failure are seen, then it is usually advised to evaluate for other causes. Increase in total serum bile acid concentration is often noted. Elevated liver enzymes may help to differentiate from viral hepatitis; however, they are not helpful in the diagnosis of ICP.

The principle of management of ICP is to control the symptoms and to prevent maternal or fetal complications. Ursodeoxycholic acid is the preferred drug in ICP and is given in doses of 15 mg/kg/day until the onset of labor. The drug is well tolerated by patients and in most cases symptomatic improvement is seen within 1 week. The dose can be increased up to 21 mg/kg/d. Additional drugs that have satisfactory results are cholestyramine, rifampicin, hydroxyzine, and chlorpheniramine.

An early vaginal delivery is recommended to avoid fetal demise. The ideal time of delivery should be decided by weighing the risks of prematurity against the risk of complications to the mother. The ACOG recommends delivery at 36–37 weeks, and an earlier delivery if indicated based on the clinical circumstances.

Postpartum, the pruritus usually resolves within 3–4 days and the biochemical profile comes to normal within 1–2 weeks. Breast-feeding is not contraindicated, and follow-up of liver enzymes should be done 6–8 weeks prior to delivery. ICP has a very high recurrence rate in subsequent pregnancies.

ACUTE FATTY LIVER OF PREGNANCY (AFLP)

AFLP is a rare, but serious obstetric emergency that is characterized by maternal hepatic dysfunction which may or may not lead to hepatic failure, risking severe fetomaternal complications and even death.

Epidemiologic studies to establish the ethnic or geographic distribution of AFLP are lacking. However, the prevalence is rare, ranging from 0.005% to 0.015%. Multiple gestation, first pregnancy, obesity, preeclampsia, and low BMI are risk factors for the development of AFLP. Fetal long-chain 3-hydroxyacyl-CoA dehydrogenase (LCHAD) deficiency is seen in 20% of patients who develop AFLP.

TABLE 29-8 Common Hepatic Disorders in Pregnancy

Disease	Hyperemesis Gravidarum	Liver Failure due to Pre-eclampsia	Intrahepatic Cholestasis	AFLP	HELLP Syndrome
Trimester	1st	>20 weeks	2nd–3rd	2nd–3rd	3rd to Postpartum
Frequency	0.3%–2%	<10%	0.1%–5%	0.01%	0.2%–0.6%
Clinical features	Nausea, vomiting, dehydration, weight loss, features of ketosis	Hypertension, proteinuria, headache, epigastric pain, blurring of vision, edema of extremities	Jaundice rarely, pruritus	Abdominal pain, proteinuria, encephalopathy	Abdominal pain, vomiting, proteinuria, headache, edema of extremities
Ascites	Nil	Nil	Nil	May be present	Nil
Platelet count	Normal	Decreased	Normal	Decreased	Decreased
Hemolysis	Nil	++	Nil	Nil	+++
Bilirubin and bile acids	Bilirubin remains low. No change in bile acids.	Bilirubin remains low. No change in bile acids.	Conjugated hyperbilirubinemia. Bile acids may be increased 50–100 times.	Mildly increased bilirubin. No change in bile acids	Bilirubin remains low. No change in bile acids
AST/ALT	1–2 times normal	1–100 times normal	1–5 times normal	5–10 times normal	1–100 times normal
LDH	Normal	Mildly increased	Normal	Mildly increased	Usually above 600 IU/L
ALP	No change	Mildly increased	Increased	Increased	Increased
Uric acid	No change	Increased	No change	Highly increased	Increased
Treatment	Supportive therapy, anti-emetics, vitamin (B_1, B_6, B_{12}) replacement, admission if dehydration is severe.	Good control of blood pressures, careful monitoring for progression into eclampsia	Ursodeoxycholic acid may be administered. Delivery preferably at 36–37 weeks	Delivery to be done early. Preferably at 34–36 weeks	Delivery to be done early. May need to go as early as 24–34 weeks as long as antenatal corticosteroids are given
Complications	Resolves spontaneously by 18 weeks	Maternal and perinatal mortality	Late IUFD	Liver rupture, necrosis, maternal and perinatal mortality	Maternal and perinatal mortality
Recurrence	+++	++	+++	Rare	++

AFLP, acute fatty liver of pregnancy; ALP, alkaline phosphatase; AST/ALT, aspartate aminotransferase/alanine aminotransferase; HELLP, HEELP, hemolysis, elevated liver enzymes, and a low platelet count; IUFD, Intrauterine fetal demise; LDH, lactate dehydrogenase.

Patients usually present with symptoms around the third trimester. AFLP begins with nonspecific symptoms such as nausea, vomiting, headaches, and loss of appetite, and rapidly progresses to signs and symptoms of acute hepatic failure such as jaundice, ascites, and encephalopathy. Most patients are hypertensive, 20%–40% of patients are diagnosed with preeclampsia, and some patients even develop renal failure.

Women with AFLP have liver enzymes that are around 8–10 times the upper limit. This, with the clinical picture, should be used to make a prompt diagnosis. Radiologic studies provide no diagnostic value with fatty infiltration of the liver seen on ultrasound.

Management of AFLP is the delivery of the fetus, as prompt delivery ensures resolution of the disease. Due to the overlapping of symptoms of HELLP, preeclampsia, and AFLP, it must be stressed that the initial management and supportive measures for the mother must not be delayed while waiting to establish the diagnosis.

A diagnosis of AFLP necessitates a multidisciplinary approach. Patients often require intensive monitoring with close attention to their fluid status because aggressive fluid replacement can lead to pulmonary edema. Physical examination, pulse oximetry, fluid balance, urinary output, and mental status assessment are important parameters to monitor the patient.

Once the patient is stable, vaginal delivery is considered if the patient is expected to deliver within 24 hours of induction. If that is not the case, a cesarean section is advised.

Postpartum, AFLP resolves completely within 1–2 days, normal liver function returning within 1 week. Parents have to be counseled about the possibility of recurrence in future pregnancies.

Thyroid Disorders in Pregnancy

GENERAL PRINCIPLES

Thyroid hormone dysfunction is the second most common endocrine disorder seen in pregnant women, preceded only by diabetes. Maternal hypothyroidism is an easily treatable condition that is associated with significant risk to the fetus: low birth weight, fetal distress, and impaired neuropsychological development.

Hyperthyroidism in pregnancy is very rare and presents itself in less than 0.5% of women globally. Hypothyroidism, however, has a higher incidence. Almost 2%–3% of pregnant women present with subclinical hypothyroidism, with the numbers increasing in places of endemic iodine deficiency. Overt hypothyroidism is seen in around 0.8%–1% of pregnant women.

Etiology

In normal physiology of pregnancy, the thyroid gland undergoes hyperplasia with increased vascularity. In the first trimester, there is an increased level of beta-hCG. Beta-hCG is structurally similar to TSH and can stimulate the TSH receptors directly. This leads to an increased amount of free T3 and T4, suppressing TSH secretion. The normal physiologic levels of TSH by trimester as defined by the American Thyroid Association are given in Table 29-9.

TABLE 29-9 Thyroid-Stimulation Hormone (TSH) Reference Ranges in Pregnancy

Trimester	TSH Reference Value (mIU/L)
First trimester	0.1–4.0
Second trimester	0.5–5.0
Third trimester	0.5–5.0

CLINICAL PRESENTATION AND DIAGNOSIS

The most common presentation is that of a woman with subclinical or clinical hypothyroidism preconceptionally or immediately after conceiving. The presence of a high TSH value with low-normal levels of free thyroid hormones in the first trimester should prompt further investigation. The presence of thyroid antibody even in euthyroid cases is implicated in postpartum thyroid dysfunction and, in rare cases, miscarriages and perinatal death.

Hyperthyroidism usually leads to difficulty in conception and is secondary to Graves' disease. Typically, this presents with hyperemesis gravidarum requiring intravenous fluids, poor fetal growth, and pregnancy-induced hypertension.

Another endocrinal disorder seen in pregnant women is postpartum thyroiditis. It is defined as the development of hypothyroidism, thyrotoxicosis, or both in the year following delivery, in women without history or previous evidence of thyroid disorders. Surprisingly, it occurs in 7%–10% of postpartum women, although this varies depending on iodine intake and genetic factors.

TREATMENT

Treatment for hypothyroidism is initiated as soon as possible. For newly diagnosed cases, a replacement dose of 2–2.4 μg/kg/day of levothyroxine is recommended. For women who were previously on levothyroxine, the requirement in pregnancy is 30%–50% more than that of the preconception dosage. Patients must be followed up 4–6 weeks after initiation of treatment, with the goal of therapy to titrate serum TSH levels below 2.5 mIU/L while maintaining free T4 levels in the high-normal range.

Medical therapy for hyperthyroidism is restricted to overt hyperthyroidism due to Graves' disease, toxic multinodular goiter, or thyroid adenoma. Propylthiouracil is recommended as the first-line antithyroid drug in the first trimester and methimazole in the second and third trimesters of pregnancy. Carbimazole is associated with congenital abnormalities and hence is avoided until late second trimester. Maternal agranulocytosis, fetal hypothyroidism, and fetal goiter are risks that must be expected. Tachycardia and tremors can be managed symptomatically.

Gestational Diabetes

GENERAL PRINCIPLES

The most common medical and endocrine complication of pregnancy, gestational diabetes mellitus (GDM) affects 14%–20% of all pregnancies worldwide. Its trends are increasing only parallel to the global concerns of obesity and other lifestyle illnesses. The lack of uniform strategies for GDM screening and the risk of morbidity and mortality for both the mother and child are matters of medical importance.

Epidemiology and Etiology

The physiologic changes in pregnancy are all aimed at mobilizing stored glucose toward the fetus. Hence, pregnancy is inherently a diabetogenic state. The production of placental hormones which act as insulin antagonists (such as estrogen, progesterone, cortisol, and human placental lactogen) especially in the second half of pregnancy pushes the maternal body toward a state of insulin resistance. The maternal pancreas is unable to keep up with the increased demand and manifests as hyperglycemia. GDM is thus defined as variable degree of glucose intolerance with its onset and/or first recognition during pregnancy.

Overt diabetes or pre-GDM is another entity wherein the patient has glucose intolerance antedating the pregnancy.

The prevalence rates are higher for Asian, Hispanic, African, Indian, and Middle Eastern women. Women with first-degree relatives who have diabetes, ethnicities that are more prone to diabetes, polycystic ovary syndrome, BMI more than 30 kg/m^2, and a previous GDM diagnosis are all at higher risk for developing GDM in the current pregnancy.

CLINICAL PRESENTATION AND DIAGNOSIS

Gestational diabetics usually present with symphysiofundal height not corresponding to the period of gestation, exhibiting a larger uterine size. This may be due to increased amniotic fluid or a macrosomic baby. However, in practice, it is far more common to have asymptomatic cases. Hence, it is inevitable to have an effective screening strategy in place. An oral glucose tolerance test (OGTT) at 24–28 weeks is recommended. An earlier OGTT can be followed in very high-risk individuals. The risk factors are most recently defined by the NICE guidelines (National Institute of Health and Clinical Excellence, 2015):

- Previous macrosomic infant (4.5 kg or above)
- Previous gestational diabetes
- First-degree relative with diabetes
- Obesity (BMI more than 30 kg/m^2)
- Specific ethnic family origin with a high prevalence of diabetes: South Asian *(specifically women whose country of family origin is India, Pakistan, or Bangladesh)*, Black Caribbean, and Middle Eastern *(specifically women whose country of family origin is Saudi Arabia, United Arab Emirates, Iraq, Jordan, Syria, Oman, Qatar, Kuwait, Lebanon, or Egypt)*
- Macrosomia in current pregnancy *(variably defined in different studies, e.g., fetal abdominal circumference measured with ultrasound >90th centile, or fetal weight estimated using formulae based on ultrasound measurements)*
- Glycosuria ≥1+ on more than one occasion or ≥2+ on one occasion
- Previous unexpected and unexplained perinatal death
- Polycystic ovary syndrome
- Polyhydramnios
- Fasting blood glucose (FBG) more than 105 mg/dL or random blood glucose more than 125 mg/dL

GDM is diagnosed by the values determined by the deranged values in an OGTT using 100 g of glucose as given in Table 29-10.

TABLE 29-10 Diagnostic Criteria for Gestational Diabetes Mellitus

Timing of Test	Carpenter and Coustan (mg/dL)	NDDG (mg/dL)	WHO, 1999 (Uses 75 g of Glucose) (mg/dL)	IADPSG (Uses 75 g of Glucose) (mg/dL)	ADA (Uses 100 g GTT Following a 1-hour 50 g GCT) (mg/dL)
Fasting	95	105	125	95	>95
First hour	180	190	—	—	>180
Second hour	155	165	140	155	>155
Third hour	140	145	—	—	>140

ADA, American Diabetes Association; IADPSG, International Association of Diabetes and Pregnancy Study Group; NDDG, National Diabetes Data Group; WHO, World Health Organization.

MANAGEMENT AND TREATMENT

The main tenet of management is achieving good glycemic control. In gestational diabetes, this is usually done using lifestyle modification and pharmacotherapy. Lifestyle modification involves nutritional control, physical activity, and weight control. Large fluctuations in blood glucose levels must be strictly avoided by administering a carbohydrate-controlled diet: more consumption of low-glycemic-index carbohydrates and a high-fiber, high-protein diet is recommended.

Insulin is the best treatment recommended. Tight glycemic control, with fasting levels ≤95 mg/dL, 1-hour postprandial levels ≤140 mg/dL, and 2-hour postprandial levels ≤120 mg/dL, improves outcomes. The drugs recommended in pregnancy are metformin and glyburide/glibenclamide, which are reasonable alternatives for women who decline to take or are unable to comply with insulin therapy. The long-term effects of transplacental passage of oral antihyperglycemic agents are not known.

Vaginal delivery at term is recommended at 37–38 weeks. It is advisable to not prolong the pregnancy once term gestation is achieved as the risk for sudden perinatal mortality is high.

Postpartum, the mother is screened and continuously monitored for blood glucose. In majority of the patients, the values will be normal. However, it is advisable to screen 12 weeks postpartum and at least every 3 years thereafter.

Sheehan Syndrome (Postpartum Pituitary Necrosis)

Sheehan syndrome is characterized by anterior pituitary insufficiency secondary to pituitary ischemia and necrosis following massive obstetric hemorrhage and shock. It is a primary cause of anterior pituitary insufficiency in adult females, commonly presenting with a failure to lactate. Other symptoms, such as fatigue, cold intolerance, hypotension, menstrual abnormalities, and genital atrophy are noted. ACTH stimulation is the best initial test, and an MRI of the pituitary gland and hypothalamus is the investigation of choice. Hormone replacement therapy is the mainstay of treatment.

Epilepsy and Seizure Disorders in Pregnancy

Women with epileptic disorders were earlier counseled to avoid pregnancy. However, with modern obstetrics and medical management, epilepsy is no longer considered a contraindication to pregnancy and about 90% of pregnant women with seizure disorder will have good outcomes. Prepregnancy consultation and adherence to therapy can drastically reduce the range of perinatal complications that may arise.

PRECONCEPTIONAL MANAGEMENT

Women with epilepsy who are of childbearing potential must be counseled regarding pregnancy and childbirth. This includes the importance of birth control, adherence to antiepileptic drugs, risk of antiepileptic drugs on pregnancy outcomes, and folic acid supplementation. Ideally, all women with epilepsy should have a planned pregnancy. Most antiepileptic drugs have enzyme-inducing activity and are known to cause faster metabolism of hormonal contraceptives. Hence, newer antiepileptic drugs such as levetiracetam and intrauterine device (copper or levonorgestrel) or intramuscular depot (DMPA) are recommended. Folic acid is supplemented for all women with epilepsy at a higher dose of 1 mg daily, initiated preconceptionally and continued throughout pregnancy.

MANAGEMENT DURING PREGNANCY

Lamotrigine and levetiracetam are preferred as first-line therapy for pregnant women with seizure disorders. Studies show that these drugs have the most consistent results with least neurodevelopmental teratogenic effects. However, doses may need to be increased by around 20%–40% in pregnancy as these drugs are metabolized faster in the pregnant mother. Valproate must be avoided completely. It may be used only when all other antiepileptic drugs have not provided adequate seizure control and must be started at the lowest possible dose. There is abundant data showing the teratogenic effects of sodium valproate with usage leading to major congenital malformations, autism spectrum disorders, and neurodevelopmental abnormality. Folic acid dosage may be increased to 4 mg daily if the patient is started on sodium valproate. Screening frequency for aneuploidy is not altered and depends on maternal age.

MANAGEMENT AT DELIVERY

The mode of delivery should be governed by obstetric situations and not by epilepsy. All women with epilepsy can be delivered vaginally unless there are contraindications for the same. However, there is an increased risk of seizures during the 3 peripartum days, that is, 1 day prior to delivery, day of delivery, and 1-day postdelivery. It is essential to have adequate pain management and the dose of the antiepileptic should not be skipped. Fetal monitoring must be done continuously as maternal seizures are associated with increased risk for placental abruption.

MANAGEMENT POSTPARTUM

The main concern postpartum is the worsening of seizures due to sleep deprivation and safety of the newborn. Hence, couples are counseled and advised to allow adequate time for the mother to rest while taking care of the newborn. The husband should play an active role so that the mother can obtain uninterrupted sleep. For women who have had myoclonic seizures in the past, a baby harness is advised. Furthermore, the mother and the child must not be left alone. Breast-feeding should be advised as there are no contraindications while using antiepileptic drugs. Even though all the antiepileptic drugs are present in measurable quantities in breast milk, there is little evidence to prove that this causes clinical effects in the newborn. Hence, the advantage of breast-feeding outweighs the possible demerits.

Posterior Reversible Encephalopathy Syndrome

GENERAL PRINCIPLES

Posterior reversible encephalopathy syndrome (PRES) is a recently described neuroradiologic entity characterized by headache, altered mentation, seizures, and visual loss. It has various associations with hypertensive encephalopathy, renal failure, autoimmune disorders, and treatment with cytotoxic drugs. A high level of suspicion is required in any pregnant woman presenting with seizures and blindness to diagnose PRES.

CLINICAL PRESENTATION AND DIAGNOSIS

PRES is characterized by its association with elevated blood pressure. The development of neurologic symptoms may be acute or subacute, ranging from few hours to sometimes 1–2 weeks. Signs of encephalopathy such as loss of cognition, stupor, or somnolence are usually present initially. Both focal and generalized seizures are seen in about 60%–70% of the patients. These seizures may also result in status epilepticus in about 5% of the patients, which poses a severe risk to the life of the mother.

Due to the involvement of the occipital lobes, visual acuity disturbances, hemianopia, hallucinations, and sometimes cortical blindness can be a presenting symptom. Less specific neurologic symptoms such as nausea, headache, and projectile vomiting may be associated with raised intracranial tension.

There is no universally recognized diagnostic criterion for PRES. However, every clinician must have a certain degree of suspicion when a pregnant woman presents with acute-onset neurologic symptoms with antecedent hypertension. Radiologic evidence of vasogenic edema seen in an MRI with reversibility of the clinicoradiologic findings after treatment is required for complete diagnosis.

TREATMENT AND MANAGEMENT

Due to the nonavailability of a therapeutic protocol, treatment of PRES is mainly management of the symptoms and management of the underlying pathology leading to the development of PRES. Control of hypertension is an essential component of treating PRES. The antihypertensive agent is selected based on general recommendations for the treatment of hypertension in pregnancy. The aim of therapy is to reduce the blood pressure by 25% every 24–48 hours. Anticonvulsive drugs are frequently required to reduce the risk of status epilepticus. Usually, these can be tapered off once the individual is asymptomatic and the radioimaging has normalized. Due to studies showing that hypomagnesemia adversely affects the outcome in patients with PRES, serum levels should be monitored and maintained at the high-normal range. This provides added benefit due to its anticonvulsive and vasodilatory effects. Management of labor is done in the same way as in pregnancy-induced hypertension. Neurologic and radiologic abnormalities of PRES resolve within days to weeks, if treated appropriately.

Systemic Lupus Erythematosus

Systemic lupus erythematosus (SLE) is an autoimmune multisystem disorder characterized by intermittent relapses and remissions. It predominantly affects women of childbearing age; however, it is not known to directly affect fertility. Pregnancy in women with SLE is shown to have a higher risk of feto-maternal complications, and adequate planning of pregnancy and a multidisciplinary approach are necessary to treat such patients.

Pregnancy is known to cause increased frequency of relapses in patients with SLE. A major clinical challenge with respect to SLE is differentiating the symptoms from the normal changes in pregnancy. Postnatally, most SLE patients end up having a flare of the disease. Due to the effects of SLE on the renal system, some patients may end up having irreversible chronic kidney disease as an aftereffect of pregnancy. Patients with SLE are at an increased risk of developing preeclampsia and may have early miscarriages, missed abortions, preterm births, and fetal growth restriction. Fetuses may show congenital heart blocks, due to the transplacental crossing of anti-Ro/SSA or anti-La/SSB autoantibodies to fetal cardiac tissue, or they may have neonatal lupus.

Management begins with preconceptional counseling. Women with SLE who wish to bear children are advised to conceive only after the disease and flares have been quiescent for at least 6 months prior. The presence of active SLE at the time of conception has a very poor prognosis and must be avoided.

Several studies have shown that continuation of hydroxychloroquine in pregnancy is associated with positive outcome. Hydroxychloroquine should therefore not be discontinued, unless contraindicated. Even though it both crosses the placenta and excretes into breast milk, safety concerns are minimal as both levels are well within the range of safety for the infant. Low-dose aspirin may also be administered to the mother, starting at 12–14 weeks of gestation to prevent the development of preeclampsia. Care should be taken to differentiate lupus nephritis from preeclampsia with severe features, especially renal involvement.

Drugs that are contraindicated in pregnancy with SLE are methotrexate, leflunomide, mycophenolate mofetil, and cyclophosphamide. Vaginal delivery is recommended, and labor is induced at 37–38 weeks. Patients should be monitored closely by a rheumatologist postpartum as most women develop an exacerbation within 1–2 weeks of delivery.

Infectious Diseases in Pregnancy

VIRAL HEPATITIS

The prevalence of hepatitis in pregnancy is less than 5%, usually either hepatitis B or C. However, hepatitis does not alter the course of pregnancy, neither does pregnancy usually alter the natural course of an acute hepatitis infection. There is an evidence of hepatitis B carriers undergoing a reactivation into active state as a result of the physiologic stress of pregnancy; similarly, some hepatitis C patients may undergo faster disease progression.

In women with severe acute viral hepatitis, the risk of spontaneous preterm labor is very high. Early diagnosis and admission help to thwart the risks posed to the fetus. Moreover, the main concern is the vertical transmission to the fetus. Hence, the management of acute viral hepatitis is mainly governed by identifying the disease early and ensuring prevention of mother-to-child transmission. A routine screening for hepatitis B with serum HBsAg and the practice of immunization against hepatitis B during pregnancy, if not previously immunized, is recommended.

During labor, it is advised to not use any investigations that may increase chances of blood contact to the fetus, such as scalp blood sampling. There is no consensus on the benefits of a cesarean section; hence, a vaginal delivery is recommended at term. Babies of mothers who have hepatitis B positive are treated with hepatitis B immunoglobulins and early hepatitis B immunization.

MALARIA

Most South Asian countries are endemic for malaria. In these countries, malaria is a common infectious disease that complicates pregnancy. It is interesting to note that pregnancy has a propensity to increase the chances of infection by malaria, the severity of the disease being affected by the parasite, immune status of the individual, and severity of anemia caused by it.

The main concern with malaria is that the parasite can grow floridly in the placenta due to the availability of high-capacitance vessels with good blood flow. Placental malaria occurs in about 20%–60% of pregnant patients with malaria.

Patients present similar to their nonpregnant counterparts: fever with chills and rigor, malaise, nausea and vomiting, and easy fatigability. Patients may also manifest with severe anemic symptoms.

The aim of control of malaria in pregnancy should begin with prevention. Mothers living in endemic areas are advised to sleep with medicated mosquito nets, maintain adequate hygiene of the surrounding areas, and use insecticides as necessary. Those who are traveling to endemic areas should preferably delay the travel until the pregnancy is completed or may take prophylaxis.

Chloroquine 300 mg given weekly, starting 1 week before travel and continuing to 4 weeks after return, is considered the best option for traveler prophylaxis

TABLE 29-11 Treatment of Malaria

Malaria	First Trimester	Second Trimester	Third Trimester
Uncomplicated *falciparum* malaria	**Chloroquine resistant**: Artemether (20 mg) lumefantrine (120 mg) for 3 days Alternatively, ACT or quinine plus clindamycin for 7 days **Chloroquine sensitive**: Chloroquine or hydroxychloroquine	**Chloroquine resistant**: Three-day course of artemisinin combination therapy: Artemether-lumefantrine, artesunate-amodiaquine, artesunate-mefloquine, dihydroartemisinin-piperaquine Alternatively, quinine + clindamycin for 7 d **Chloroquine sensitive**: Chloroquine or hydroxychloroquine	
Severe *falciparum* malaria	Parenteral artesunate as given to nonpregnant individuals in all trimesters Alternatively, quinine or artemether may be used; quinine is associated with recurrent hypoglycemia		
Chloroquine-resistant non-*falciparum* malaria	Artemether-lumefantrine or ACT or quinine	ACT or quinine sulfate	
Chloroquine-sensitive non-*falciparum* malaria	Chloroquine or hydroxychloroquine or ACT	Chloroquine or hydroxychloroquine; may use ACT if not resolving	

in pregnant women. It is safe in pregnancy and also safe while breast-feeding. Mefloquine at a weekly dose of 250 mg may also be given; however, it is recommended to avoid mefloquine during the first trimester. Patients should be treated with chloroquine prophylaxis for the duration of the pregnancy to prevent relapse following treatment of *Plasmodium vivax or Plasmodium ovale* infection. Treatment is summarized in Table 29-11.

URINARY TRACT INFECTIONS AND ACUTE PYELONEPHRITIS

Urinary tract infections are very common in pregnant women. Asymptomatic bacteriuria occurs in 2%–7% of sexually active women; this is compounded in pregnant women due to the structural and physiologic changes to the renal tract during pregnancy. This leads to an increased risk of development of acute pyelonephritis. Without adequate treatment, about 30%–40% of women with asymptomatic bacteriuria will develop a cystitis and pyelonephritis during pregnancy. It is important to treat it as bacteriuria may potentially cause preterm birth, low birth weight, and, in rare cases, perinatal mortality as well.

As in nonpregnant women, the most common organism that causes UTI is *E. coli* (70%–90%). Other organisms include *Klebsiella* species, *Enterobacter* species, and GBS. As with all community-acquired infections, the increasing antibiotic resistance poses a concern in the treatment against uropathogens. Diagnosis is made by isolating the same bacterial strain in two separate midstream clean-catch voided urine specimens in quantities of greater than or equal to 10^5 cfu/mL. However, in clinical practice, it may be diagnosed with a single urine specimen.

Treatment is aggressive use of antibiotics according to the sensitivity pattern of the isolated organism. Most of the time, standard doses of amoxicillin, third-generation cephalosporins, nitrofurantoin, and fosfomycin are effective. Fluoroquinolones are contraindicated in pregnancy. Additional measures such as adequate hydration, symptomatic management for systemic symptoms, and bed rest may be advised. A repeat urine culture is performed 1 week following treatment to ensure a cure. Pyelonephritis requires admission to the hospital for fluid, IV third-generation cephalosporins, and a follow-up culture to determine cure. Suppressive antibiotics based on culture sensitivity are advised for the rest of the pregnancy in patients with pyelonephritis. GBS prophylaxis with IV penicillin at the time of labor is recommended where urine cultures show growth of it.

HIV

Pregnancy does not alter the progression of HIV. HIV also does not have any effect on the course of pregnancy. The management of pregnant women with HIV infection mainly revolves around the prevention of mother-to-child transmission. The risk of transmission has reduced drastically due to better patient compliance, the availability of more effective drugs, universal testing in pregnant women, and appropriate breast-feeding.

The risk of vertical transmission is highest in treatment-naïve patients and in advanced disease with high viral loads. Vertical transmission usually occurs transplacentally during the pregnancy, at the time of delivery due to intermixing of blood, and postpartum while breast-feeding. Withholding breast-feeding reduces the transmission rates by 20%–25%. Women with viral loads higher than 400 copies/mL are recommended to undergo a cesarean section.

Routine screening of pregnant women for HIV is mandatory during the initial visit. Repeat testing for HIV during the third trimester and/or during delivery for high-risk pregnant women with prior negative test should be done. The use of anti-HIV medication during pregnancy is known to reduce the risk of vertical transmission. If a woman is already on HAART, the regimen must be altered to avoid teratogenic ART medication such as zidovudine and delavirdine. For treatment-naïve individuals, HAART is started at the time of diagnosis, regardless of CD4 count and viral load, and continued lifelong. Invasive procedures such as internal fetal monitoring (using fetal scalp electrodes), amniocentesis, and fetal blood sampling must be avoided during pregnancy.

The National AIDS Control Organization (NACO) in India proposed the initiation of a fixed-dose combination of tenofovir (TDF 300 mg) + lamivudine (3TC 300 mg) + dolutegravir (DTG 50 mg) for all pregnant women irrespective of gestational age. It is recommended due to its low pill burden, good tolerance, and low monitoring requirements. In resource-limited settings, the mode of delivery is not affected by the HIV infection status of the pregnant woman. Although cesarean sections are associated with reduced rates of perinatal transmission in women with viral loads >1000 copies/mL, this practice cannot be extended to resource-limited settings.

Neonatal screening for HIV is initiated at birth and continues till 3 months of age. Postexposure prophylaxis for the child is recommended and women are advised to not breast-feed. However, in resource-deficient settings where breast-feeding is essential to provide nutrition for the growing child, this is a gray zone. The NACO in India proposes that the mother continues to breast-feed exclusively for 6 months, while the low-risk child is given syrup nevirapine daily for 4–6 weeks as prophylaxis.

Resistance to any ART drug during pregnancy requires a drug switch based on its safety profile. Regular follow-up with CD4 counts and viral loads in HIV positive mothers on lifelong ART is advised. Infants determined to be infected with HIV should receive prompt pediatric referral for HIV care and immediate initiation of ART.

In developing countries, tuberculosis remains a global health issue, infecting almost 5–6 million new people every year. HIV is the biggest trigger for reactivation of tuberculosis, and almost one-quarter of the patients with HIV die due to symptomatic manifestations of TB. With respect to pregnancy and HIV, this is a point that must be kept in mind by every clinician. However, *Mycobacterium* does not transmit vertically to the child. As such, the risks to a pregnant woman with tuberculosis do not vary significantly from those of their nonpregnant counterparts. On confirmation of diagnosis, the individual must be started on antitubercular treatment with the exception of streptomycin.

MASTITIS

Cellulitis of periglandular tissue is caused by trauma from breast feeding and the introduction of bacteria into ducts, with Staphylococcus aureus being the most commonly implicated bacteria. Symptoms appear 2–4 weeks postpartum with unilateral breast pain and tenderness, along with other signs of inflammation and possible discharge. Fever, chills, and rigor can also be seen. The mainstay of treatment involves the continuation of breast feeding to prevent the accumulation of infected material and the administration of oral antibiotics such as amoxiclav, dicloxacillin, azithromycin, clindamycin, or cephalexin. Supportive measures like antipyretics or NSAIDs can be used. Patients who do not show improvement in 2–3 days will require evaluation with ultrasonography to assess for an abscess, which requires incision and drainage.

Summary

- Anemia in pregnancy is common and, if left untreated, can result in unfavorable maternal and fetal outcomes.
- Hypertension in pregnancy must be diagnosed early and managed carefully. If left uncontrolled, it can lead to eclampsia, HELLP syndrome, and adverse outcomes for both the mother and the baby.
- Gestational diabetes can result in preterm births, macrosomia, and various congenital anomalies.
- Thrombophilia, such as Factor V Leiden mutation and antiphospholipid syndrome, may lead to complications such as deep vein thrombosis, pulmonary embolism, or placental insufficiency.
- Intrahepatic cholestasis of pregnancy must be differentiated from acute fatty liver of pregnancy and HELLP syndrome.
- Thyroid diseases and connective tissue disorders also account for poor fetal outcomes; hence, they need to be treated appropriately.
- Guillain-Barré syndrome and its variants are post-infectious immune-mediated polyradiculoneuropathies commonly associated with acute ascending areflexic motor weakness.
- Myasthenia gravis (MG), an autoimmune neuromuscular disorder, is characterized by fluctuating weakness involving ocular, bulbar, limb, and/or respiratory muscles.

Scan the QR code to access chapter references.

30 Geriatrics

Sheetal Raj M.

The world geriatric population is expected to increase to 16% by the year 2050[1] and the fastest increase among this is expected to be in Asia, Northern Africa, and Latin America. The life expectancy beyond 65 years is expected to increase by 19 years from the current 17 years by 2050. By 2030, 1 in 6 people in the world will be aged 60 years or over. Increasing population aging will result in proportionate increase in financial and social burdens on the society. While public transfer systems and benefit schemes offer relief in Europe and the Americas, personal assets remain the only source of financial support in South and South East Asian region, thus placing huge financial and social burdens on older adults and their families.

With the change in demographics across the world and the projected increase in the older adult population, we can say with reasonable certainty that most of the knowledge from chapters in the rest of this book will invariably be used in the care of older adults.

A knowledge of the fundamentals of geriatric medicine will aid the physician to avoid the common pitfalls in the care of older adults.

KEY CONCEPTS IN PRACTICE OF GERIATRIC MEDICINE

Interpreting disease presentation among older adults is extremely challenging to a physician. Knowing certain key common principles[2,3] regarding the physiology and disease presentation greatly simplifies the approach to their treatment.

- **Atypical disease presentation**
  - Unlike younger patients, older adults present with symptoms not referable to the affected organ. For example, urinary tract infection and pneumonia may present as confusion and fall with hip fracture. Typical symptoms of pyrexia and cough with expectoration are uncommon.
- **"Weakest link" theory**
  - Systems previously afflicted by a disease will have weakened reserves and older adults with acute ailments will present with symptoms attributable to the weakened system rather than the current locus of the acute illness. For example, a case of recent stroke may present with worsening weakness of the limbs, which on evaluation might reveal underlying pneumonia and sepsis.
- **Missing symptoms**
  - A case of myocardial infarction in an 80-year-old with severe osteoarthritis may present with dyspnea caused by pulmonary edema, rather than with chest pain. In such a patient typical symptoms of angina (chest pain brought on by exertion) may be missing as they probably avoid walking due to the severe osteoarthritis.
- **Masking of symptoms**
  - A patient admitted with a history of fall and fracture neck of femur may mask an underlying hemiparetic limb in a confused older adult who is living alone.
- **Differing healthcare goals in older adults**
  - Unlike younger patients with severe illness, older patients may give preference to maintenance of independence and achievement of symptom relief over cure or life-prolonging treatments.

- **Red flag sign for suspected elder abuse**
  - Presence of clinical signs discordant with the reported mechanism of injury should alert the physician to suspected abuse.
- **Multimorbidity**
  - The law of parsimony or the Occam's razor, which is the well-accepted diagnostic model in internal medicine, loses its value in the diagnosis of disease in older adults. In geriatric medicine, do not try to make one unifying diagnosis to explain all the symptoms. Among older adults, multiple symptoms often imply multiple diagnoses and one presentation such as syncope may have multiple contributing causes, each of which needs to be identified and addressed.
  - Most older adults have two more coexisting comorbid illnesses, which interact to create implications which alter the experience of human suffering. Most evidence-based guidelines are disease specific and fail to address the complexities arising out of multimorbidity.
- **Adverse drug reactions more common among older adults**
  - A dose of NSAID prescribed for osteoarthritis may precipitate cardiac failure in an otherwise stable case of coronary artery disease.
- **Tolerance of acute illness very poor in older adults with reduced physiologic reserves**
  - For example, older adults with pneumonia often develop an acute cardiac event such as a myocardial infarction or concurrent cardiac failure during hospitalization for the acute illness.
- **Prevention several times more efficient and lifesaving than treatment in older adults**
  - Preventive measures such as vaccination for pneumonia and use of antiplatelets are more effective than treatment of subsequent stroke or pneumonia among older adults.
- **Remarkable change in symptoms and quality of life among older adults by small interventions**
  - For example, maintenance of a bladder diary and movement of the bed closer to the bathroom may resolve completely the problem of incontinence in a patient with severe osteoarthritis.

CLINICAL ASSESSMENT IN OLDER ADULTS

Assessment in older adults focuses on aspects and outcomes that are different from the usual medical evaluation. Comprehensive geriatric assessment (CGA)[3,4] is a multidimensional diagnostic process to identify deficits in physical, functional, and psychosocial domains with a coordinated integrated plan for treatment and follow-up. Although described as a diagnostic process, geriatric assessment includes evaluation, goal setting, and management of the deficits. It also focuses on holistic evaluation and has the following major components: physical evaluation, assessment of functional status, psychological and cognitive assessment, and assessment of socioenvironmental factors (Figure 30-1).

CGA can be performed by the trained geriatrician individually or by an interdisciplinary team consisting of at least a physician, a nurse, and a social worker. Additional team members such as pharmacist, dietician, physical therapist and occupational therapist may be added depending on the availability of resources. CGA is known to help in better identification of older adult problems, improved quality of life, and greater independence in activities of daily living.

Assessment of older adults places a significant focus on functional status both as an assessment parameter and as an outcome to be achieved and maintained.

FUNCTION IN OLDER ADULTS[2]

Function refers to a set of behaviors which enable an older adult to live independently. Functional capacity is a potent predictor of outcomes in older hospitalized patients.

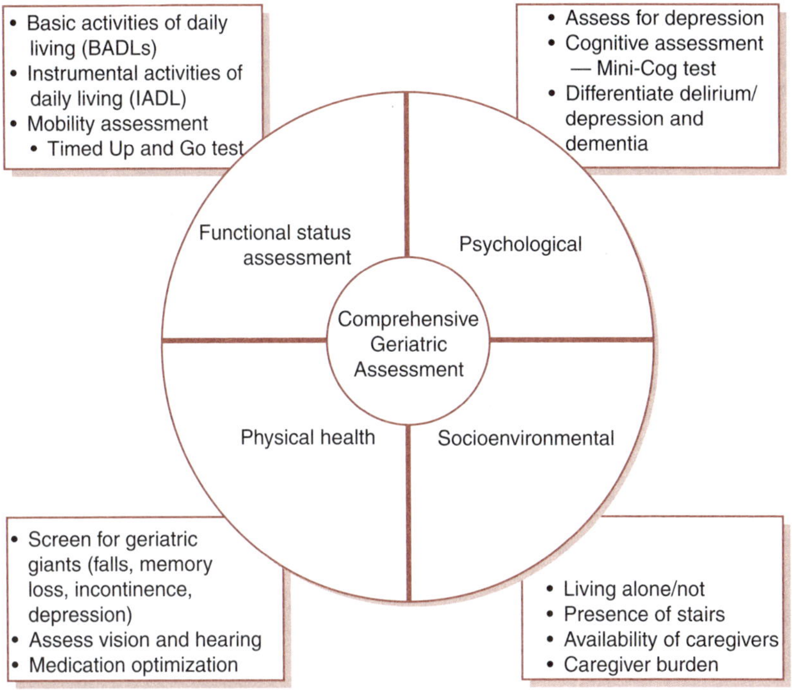

Figure 30-1 Components of comprehensive geriatric assessment.

Poor functional status results in prolonged hospital stay, poor clinical outcome after acute illness, and high caregiver burden.

Assessment of functional status commonly involves the following three major components:

- **Basic Activities of Daily Living** (**BADLs**) include the ability to independently bathe, dress, toilet, feed, transfer, and be continent.
- The **Instrumental Activities of Daily Living** (**IADLs**) are complex tasks performed by the older adults to enable them to live independently and safely in their environment in conformity to their culture. They include: shopping, using a telephone, doing finances, house-keeping, preparing food, etc.
- **Mobility** is the ability of an individual to ambulate safely in his or her own environment.

Functional status can be assessed using various validated scales such as the Katz Index for BADLs or the Lawton's Scale for the assessment of IADLs. Mobility can be assessed using a Timed Up and Go test which can easily be performed at the bedside. IADLs are lost first, followed by ADLs. Loss of ADLs indicates severe decline and high caregiver burden.

GERIATRIC SYNDROMES OR GERIATRIC GIANTS[2–4]

First coined by Sir Bernard Isaacs, the term geriatric giants refers to syndromes which cross organ systems and disease boundaries to manifest as clinical problems which are commonly faced in the older adult population. This description of geriatric syndromes points to the patient-centric approach that defines geriatric medicine as opposed to the disease-centric approach that is commonly taught and also to the enormity of the burden faced by older adults. Common geriatric giants are: falls, incontinence, memory loss, and depression. Additional giants[5] such as frailty, sarcopenia and anorexia of aging have been newly described. Validated bedside tools are available for the screening of common geriatric syndromes. Some geriatric syndromes will be discussed here.

Memory Loss/Forgetfulness/Confusion

Older adults presenting with a history of memory loss are evaluated for the evidence of major or minor neurocognitive disorder according to the DSM-5 criteria. With the introduction of the DSM-5 the term dementia was replaced with the term neurocognitive disorder. However due to its familiarity with most physicians the term dementia will be used interchangeably with the term major neurcognitive disorder in this chapter. Patients are also evaluated for depression using the 15- to 30-point Geriatric Depression Scale. Hypoactive and hyperactive delirium are assessed and monitored using various validated scales. Dementia can be a risk factor for delirium. **Delirium** should be suspected in an inattentive patient with an acute onset of mental status changes with a fluctuating course with altered consciousness or with evidence of disorganized thoughts.

During clinical evaluation, confirm the diagnosis of dementia using validated tools. Chronic psychiatric disorders and lifelong personality disorders may confound the diagnosis. Depression, schizophrenia, post-traumatic stress disorders, and CNS neoplasms are other common differential diagnoses in dementia patients with behavioral and psychological symptoms of dementia (BPSD).

Evaluation of patients presenting with complaints, suggesting cognitive impairment, should proceed as given in the subsequent text (Figure 30-2).

Stages and Course of Dementia

- Early stage (first or second year of disease): It is often overlooked as part of aging. It is characterized by language difficulties, getting lost in familiar places, mood changes, depression, loss of interest in hobbies, etc.
- Middle stage (second to fifth year of disease): The patient demonstrates pronounced limitations, becomes restricted in activities and begins to lose ADLs, and becomes dependent for ADLs.
- Last stage (fifth year onwards): The patient becomes totally dependent for all activities and becomes bed ridden/chair bound. Death may occur due to complications such as pneumonia/UTI/decubitus ulcers/malnutrition.

Management of Major Neurocognitive Disorder (Dementia)

- Early diagnosis
- Optimization of physical health, cognition, activity, and well-being
- Detection and treatment of BPSD[3]
- Educating the caregiver and providing long-term support to him or her

Behavioral and Psychological Symptoms of Dementia

Agitation (defined as purposeless verbal and motor behaviors that put the patient or others at risk of harm) is the most common problem, and is seen in up to 75% of the patients with dementia. Other problem behaviors include: wandering, depression, repeated stories and statements, psychosis, hoarding and rummaging, aggression, violence, and hypersexuality. Behavioral and psychological symptoms lead to caregiver stress, burnout, or depression, and may be a trigger for frequent elder abuse. They are disruptive and can lead to social isolation, accelerate the need for placement in long-term care homes, and lead to increased use of restraints (and their associated problems) and increased contact with healthcare systems, leading to drug overuse and adverse effects.

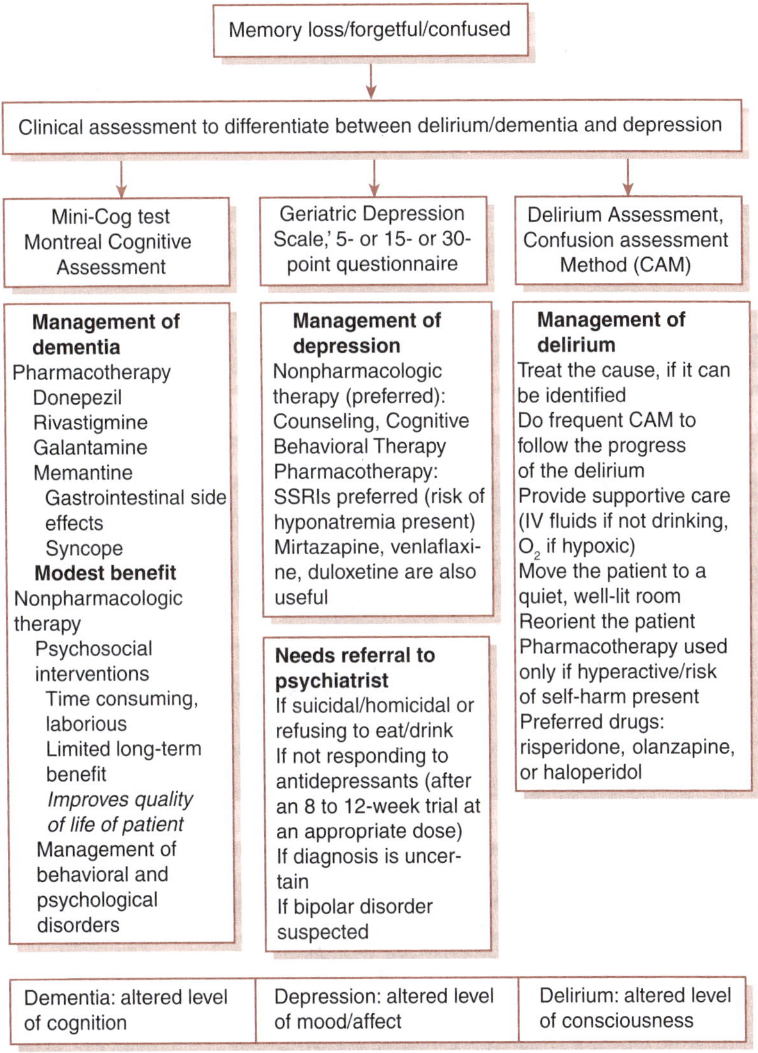

Figure 30-2 Evaluation of patients with cognitive impairment.

Before initiating any interventions for BPSD, **rule out discomfort** (untreated pain, bladder distension), and rule out **unmet needs** such as hunger, constipation, and noisy/warm/cold environment.

Nonpharmacologic Management of BPSD

Diagnose and treat any underlying depression or delirium. A wide range of **psychosocial interventions** have been proposed for the patient and caregivers:

- Cognitive interventions: memory retraining, use of mnemonics, and memory aids (early disease).

- Functional performance interventions: stimulus control, verbal and physical prompting, and physical guidance.
- Environmental interventions: noise management (white noise, nature sound recordings, classical music), lighting management (dimmed lighting at mealtime, contrasting food colors), way-finding cues, and identification and elimination of stress-inducing triggers.
- Pleasure-inducing interventions: pet therapy, recreational therapy, art therapy, music therapy, and reminiscence therapy.
- Patient and family responses to interventions: ongoing individualization to meet changing needs.
- Family interventions: combinations of traditional psychotherapy and educative/supportive interventions, respite services, and training to manage the patient.

Caregiver training: Educating the carer is the primary management strategy in major neurocognitive disorders. It improves coping mechanisms, but has no effect on ADLs. Caregivers are taught that most behavioral disturbances are responses to discomfort or unmet needs, or are attempts to communicate.

Pharmacotherapy for BPSD

- Early identification and empirical treatment of known or potential pain. Use of paracetamol, low-dose morphine, and adjuvant analgesics is advised. Tramadol is associated with multiple adverse effects and high risk of falls and fracture and should be avoided in older adults.
- Levetiracetam can be used in case of seizures.
- Selective serotonin reuptake inhibitors (SSRIs) have been preferred to antipsychotics in the treatment of aggression and agitation in BPSD (escitalopram and sertraline).
  - Common adverse effects: hyponatremia and QT prolongation.
- Antipsychotics for BPSD: risperidone, olanzapine, quetiapine, and aripiprazole have been used for the management of aggression and agitation in dementia patients, with modest benefits and high incidence of adverse effects.
- Psychotropics for BPSD work only if there is psychosis and/or aggression, depression, anxiety, or sleep disturbance.
- Repetition and wandering do not respond to administration of psychotropics.

The US FDA has issued a black box warning indicating a high risk of death in patients who are treated with antipsychotics for BPSD. Use of drugs for the management of BPSD should be considered only when nonpharmacologic methods fail and when all causes for discomfort have been resolved and symptoms are severe enough for them to cause self-harm or harm to the caregivers.

At present there are no US FDA-approved drugs for use in behavioral and psychological disorders in dementia.

Advance Care Planning in Neurocognitive Disorder

A patient who has been diagnosed with a minor neurocognitive disorder or major neurocognitive disorder in early stages may appropriately receive all medical interventions (e.g., mammograms, pneumococcal vaccination, and antibiotics) that a patient without dementia might receive. Conversely, similar care for a patient who is immobile, mute, and unable to eat in the advanced stages of dementia may be inappropriate. These discussions are under the purview of palliative care and decisions should be based on the wishes of the patient/family after appropriate counseling regarding futility.

Geriatric depression is extremely common and presents with hopelessness, excessive guilt, inertia, suicidality or somatization. It can mimic dementia and is known as **pseudodementia** (Figure 30-2). Treatment of depression may lead to resolution of cognitive impairments.

Electroconvulsive therapy (ECT) is safe in older adults and can be used as per clinical indication. There are no absolute contraindications to ECT in older adults; however, there are situations which may cause increased complications. Caution should be exercised in patients with brain tumors, recent stroke (within the past 3 months), and recent myocardial infarction (within the past 3 months).

Frailty

Frailty[6] is the loss of an individual's ability to withstand stress, occurring due to loss of physiologic reserve in various organs due to a disease. It is a combination of unintentional weight loss, self-reported exhaustion, and reduced gait speed, strength, and activity. Although weight loss and sarcopenia are primary components that define frailty, some patients who are obese can also be frail and are at an equal risk of healthcare burdens arising out of frailty.

Frailty is an independent risk factor for functional decline leading to disability, hospitalization, institutionalization, and death.

Prevention and treatment of frailty: Individualized physical activity training which includes multicomponent exercises (including resistance training) along with high-quality protein intake can have a positive impact on the prevention and progression of frailty.

Depression

Depression is characterized by a combination of depressed mood, loss of interest or pleasure, changes in weight and sleep, psychomotor agitation or retardation, fatigue, feelings of worthlessness or guilt, difficulty concentrating, and recurrent thoughts of suicide or death. The prevalence of depressive disorders in older adults with cancer ranges from 1.8% to 10.0%, whereas up to 28% have clinically notable depressive symptoms.

Sarcopenia

Sarcopenia is age-related loss of muscle mass.[5] It increases the risk for falls, fractures, dependency, use of hospital services, institutionalization, and mortality. It can be treated and prevented using a high-protein diet and resistance training.

Anorexia of Aging

It is a multifactorial decrease in appetite and food intake that occurs in older adults, resulting in malnutrition if not detected and treated.[5] It is characterized by wasting (cachexia and sarcopenia), decreased endurance, physical performance, gait speed, and impaired mobility. It adversely impacts survival independent of age, gender, and presence of multiple comorbidities.

Strategies to combat anorexia of aging are the following:

- Addressing reversible contributing factors/comorbidities
- Prescription review
- Improving food texture and palatability
- Protein supplementation: 1–1.2 g/kg body weight

Polypharmacy

This term refers to the use of "too many drugs" and has been identified as a common risk factor for medication errors and adverse drug events in older adults. It was defined as the use of ≥5 drugs in a single prescription or use of any combination of drugs that results in an adverse drug interaction. However, the term polypharmacy has become obsolete, as it is not always possible to reduce the number of prescribed drugs due to the increase in chronic progressive illnesses among older adults and ever-increasing therapeutic options for their management.

Medication optimization[3,4,7–9] is the new term which refers to medication review to ensure that older adults are on the optimum dose and number of drugs.

Older adults are the major consumers of medications including prescribed and over-the-counter (or borrowed) drugs. Changing physiology due to aging and the presence of comorbidities make it common for older adults to have an increased number of adverse drug reactions. Ten percent to 30% of unplanned hospitalizations in older adults occur due to adverse drug events, 30%–50% of which are preventable.[8] Medications errors and adverse drug event form the key issues that affect prescribing in older adults.

Medication use process consists of the steps given in Figure 30-3.

Errors of monitoring are responsible for most of the adverse drug events in older adults, especially more so in those who are living in long-term care homes. Adverse drug events caused by lapses in any of the steps of medication use are preventable.

Adverse drug event commonly seen in older adults are of three types:

- Adverse drug reactions: An unintended and noxious response to a drug that occurs when the drug is prescribed at the normal dose for the specified indication.
- Adverse drug withdrawal effect: This refers to clinical symptoms and signs that result from discontinuation of the drug.
- Treatment failure: This is a failure to achieve the goals of therapy due to inadequate dose of drug administered (due to poor compliance, inadequate dose, or drug).

Understanding the Pharmacology of the Aging Adult

The common **pharmacokinetic** changes seen with aging in older adults are given in Table 30-1.

Drug half-life: The half-life of a drug depends on the volume of distribution and drug clearance. The following is the formula for $t_{1/2}$:

$$t_{1/2} = \frac{0.693 \times V_d}{CL}$$

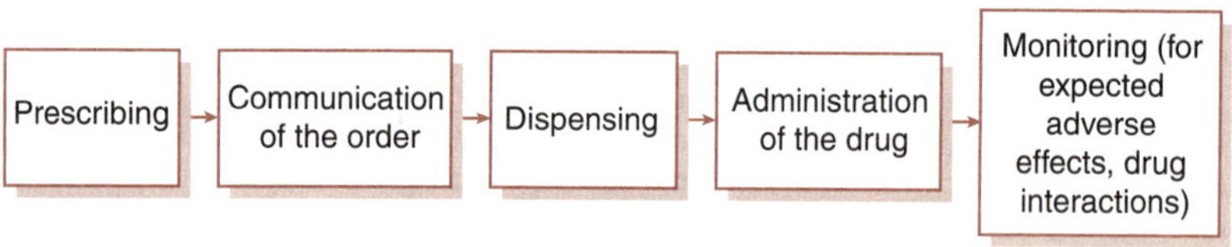

Figure 30-3 Steps in the medication use process.

TABLE 30-1 Drug Pharmacokinetics in Older Adult

Phase of Pharmacokinetics	Changes due to Aging
Gastrointestinal absorption	Unchanged passive diffusion and no change in bioavailability for most drugs
Distribution	Increased volume of distribution and increased $t_{1/2}$ for fat-soluble drugs Decreased volume of distribution and increased plasma concentration for water-soluble drugs
Hepatic clearance	Decreased clearance and increased $t_{1/2}$ for some oxidatively metabolized drugs and for drugs with high hepatic extraction ratio
Renal clearance	Decreased clearance and increased $t_{1/2}$ for renally excreted drugs

A decrease in clearance which is seen with aging results in an increase in half-life. Also, aging causes an increase in volume of distribution of lipid-soluble drugs thereby causing an increase in half-life. The half-life of a drug determines the accumulation and elimination kinetics of a drug and also its dosing interval. When a drug is initiated, it takes approximately four half-lives for the drug to reach steady-state concentration of >90%. Also, when a drug that was at steady state is stopped, plasma concentration of the drug drops to <10% of the steady state after approximately four half-lives.

It is also observed that the effect of aging on the increase in volume of distribution is less than its effect on clearance, thus resulting in an overall increase in half-life of most drugs when compared to in younger subjects. *Hence, older adults have longer half-lives for most drugs; thus, they require a longer duration to achieve steady state after drug initiation, take longer to eliminate a drug after the drug is stopped, and also need increased dosing intervals.*

Thus, the dictum in prescribing for older adults is "**to start low and go slow**" in order to minimize adverse drug events.

Renal clearance: In normal aging, the glomerular filtration rate (GFR) reduces by 5%–40%. Serum creatinine is not a useful measure of renal function in older adults due to the sarcopenia (muscle loss that gets replaced by fat) that is commonly seen with advancing age. Calculation of renal clearance is necessary to determine maintenance doses of renally excreted drugs. The Cockcroft and Gault equation (Refer chapter 13) is the preferred formula to calculate renal clearance in older adults. The MDRD formula is not validated for extremes of age and it often overestimates the creatinine clearance. In patients with a body mass index >30 mg/m^2; the Cockcroft and Gault equation is used after adjusting for body weight. The Cockcroft and Gault equation underestimates the creatinine clearance in older adults who are frail.[7] Alternative methods such as measurement of Cystatin C has been explored as a non-creatinine based method to calculate GFR more effectively in older adults. While the Cockcroft and Gault equation is useful to calculate maintenance doses for most renally excreted drugs, for drugs with a narrow therapeutic index, it is better to rely on therapeutic drug monitoring and clinical response.

Pharmacodynamic studies in older adults have revealed **increased sensitivity** of older adults to the following drugs: benzodiazepines, warfarin, opioids, metoclopramide, levodopa, and antipsychotics.

Decreased efficiency of homeostatic mechanisms causing gait instability, orthostatic hypotension, cognitive deficits, and bowel and bladder disturbances puts older adults at an increased risk of geriatric syndromes such as falls, delirium, and incontinence.

Various **drug–disease/herb interactions** are listed in Tables 30-2 and 30-3.

Strategies to Optimize Pharmacotherapy in Older Adults

Following are some of the principles to combat the medication errors and adverse drug events in older adults:

- Consider whether medication therapy is necessary.
- Conduct a brown bag review (review all prescription, nonprescription drugs, and supplements which are taken by the patients).
- Start low and go slow.
- Prescribe the least expensive drugs.
- Use tools such as the Beer's criteria and START or STOP criteria to periodically identify inappropriate medications.
- Incorporate changes in the design of health systems.
  - Introduce electronic prescription writing.
  - Make available to physicians comprehensive data regarding medication safety and prescribing.

TABLE 30-2	Drug–Disease Interaction
Diseases or Geriatric Syndrome	**Drugs or Drug Classes which Interact Commonly**
Heart failure	NSAIDs, COX-2 inhibitors; pioglitazone, cilostazol; dronedarone and nondihydropyridine CCBs (avoid only for systolic heart failure)
Syncope	AChEIs; peripheral α-blockers (e.g., doxazosin, prazosin, terazosin); tertiary TCAs (e.g., amitriptyline, clomipramine, doxepin, imipramine, trimipramine); chlorpromazine; thioridazine; olanzapine
Delirium	Anticholinergics; benzodiazepines; chlorpromazine; corticosteroids; H2 receptor antagonists; sedative–hypnotics; antipsychotics
Dementia	Anticholinergics; benzodiazepines; H2 receptor antagonists; nonbenzodiazepine hypnotics (eszopiclone, zolpidem, zaleplon); antipsychotics
History of falls/ fracture	Anticonvulsants; antipsychotics; benzodiazepines; nonbenzodiazepine hypnotics (eszopiclone, zaleplon, zolpidem); TCAs; SSRIs; opioids
Insomnia	Oral decongestants (e.g., pseudoephedrine and phenylephrine); stimulants (e.g., amphetamine, methylphenidate, modafinil); theophylline and caffeine
Parkinson disease	All antipsychotics (except for aripiprazole, quetiapine, and clozapine); antiemetics (metoclopramide, prochlorperazine, promethazine)
History of gastric or duodenal ulcers	Aspirin (>325 mg/d); non–COX-2 selective NSAIDs

TABLE 30-3	Lists Some Commonly Seen Drug–Herb Interactions	
Drug or Drug Class	**Herb**	**Clinical Effect Seen**
Warfarin	Ginseng	Decreases INR
	Garlic, danshen, gingko, devil's claw, dong quai, papaya, glucosamine	Increases INR
Aspirin, NSAIDs, dipyridamole, clopidogrel–ticlopidine	Gingko	Increases bleeding time
Aspirin	Tamarind	Increases drug concentration
Levodopa	Gingko	Increases off-periods in Parkinson disease
Heparin	Fenugreek	Increases bleeding risk

- Improve health services.
  - Use clinical pharmacy consultation to reduce errors.
  - Use geriatric medicine services to optimize prescriptions.
- Conduct patient and caregiver education and training.
  - Use of printed booklets helps to improve adherence and also aids in withdrawal of drugs to which patients are addicted.
  - Counseling by a clinical pharmacist helps to reduce adverse drug events.

Summary

- Comprehensive geriatric assessment involves evaluating multiple domains of health, including physical, cognitive, functional, social, and psychological aspects that helps to identify medical conditions, functional limitations, and social support systems that may impact the health and well-being of older adults.
- The geriatric giants include immobility, instability, incontinence, and intellectual impairment.
- Frailty, sarcopenia, depression, and anorexia of aging are other major problems of concern.
- Multimorbidity and polypharmacy also need to be addressed in the elderly.
- Comprehensive geriatric assessment, interdisciplinary management, and targeted interventions are crucial for addressing geriatric syndromes and improving outcomes in older adults.

Scan the QR code to access chapter references.

31 Pain Management

Sheetal Raj M.

He jests at scars that never felt a wound.

—*Shakespeare*

Pain

An unpleasant sensory and emotional experience associated with, or resembling with actual or potential tissue damage.[1]

Effective pain management necessitates an understanding of the concept of **total pain**.

Total pain (Figure 31-1) is the suffering that encompasses the physical, emotional, social, and spiritual components of a person's distress.[2] Inability to address the nonphysical components of pain will result in persistence of distress and use of unnecessary medications resulting in drugs' side effects and delirium.

Pain can be classified in various ways according to duration, pathologic mechanism, temporal factors, etc. (Tables 31-1 to 31-4).[2,5–7]

A third pain type, called nociplastic pain, is defined by the IASP as "pain that arises from altered nociception despite no clear evidence of actual or threatened tissue damage causing the activation of peripheral nociceptors or evidence for disease or lesion of the somatosensory system causing the pain."

It can be considered a form of primary pain, which is defined as pain in one or more anatomical regions that (1) "persists or recurs for longer than 3 months", (2) "is associated with significant emotional distress," and (3) has symptoms that "are not better accounted for by another diagnosis."[8]

Patients with serious illnesses are more often suffering from chronic pain that is undertreated. The rest of the discussion on pain in this chapter focusses primarily on chronic pain.

Pain assessment should include a detailed investigation into each of the above-mentioned subtypes of pain and should institute treatment specific to the cause.[3]

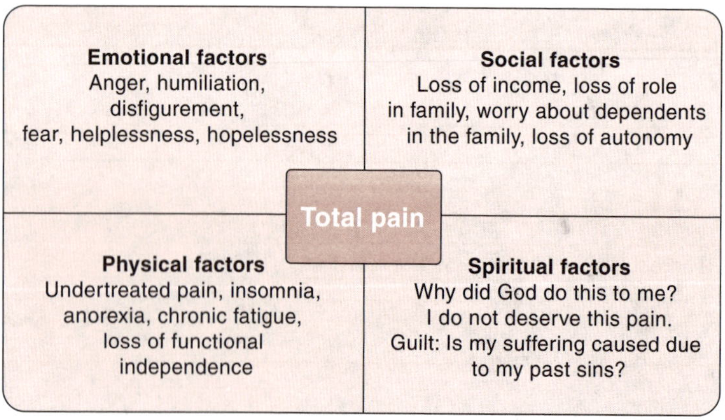

Figure 31-1 Total pain.

TABLE 31-1 Differentiating Acute and Chronic Pain

Acute Pain	Chronic Pain
• Sudden onset, short duration, and is clearly associated with a cause • Protective for the patient as it draws attention to the site of injury • Patient often self-reports pain • Often accompanied by physical signs of distress such as tachycardia, sweating, tachypnea, rise in blood pressure, pupillary dilatation	• Pain that lasts/persists or recurs for longer than 3 months • May have negative impact on the patient • Physical signs of distress may be absent despite the patient being in severe pain • Patient may not self-report pain unless asked • Causes change in personality, depression, loss of libido, anorexia, insomnia

TABLE 31-2 Features of Nociceptive and Neuropathic Pain

	Nociceptive	Neuropathic
	Caused due to stimulation of free nerve endings in somatic or visceral tissues	Type of pain that arises as a direct consequence of a lesion or disease affecting the somatosensory system Occurs due to compression or injury to nerves
Subtypes	• Somatic • Visceral	• Nerve compression • Nerve injury • Sympathetically mediated pain
Description	Gnawing, colicky (visceral) Sharp, aching, throbbing (somatic)	Lancinating, heat, burning, shooting, pricking
Localization	Diffuse (visceral), localized (somatic)	Neurodermatomal, glove and stocking distribution
Abnormal sensations	None	Allodynia, hyperalgesia, numbness
Preferred analgesic	Somatic pain: Nonopioids, NSAIDs Visceral pain: Nonopioids, NSAIDs, antispasmodics, corticosteroids (if there is tumor edema) Opioids are effective in both if pain is severe	Adjuvant analgesics Opioids Nerve blocks, spinal analgesia TENS

TABLE 31-3 Differentiating Somatic and Visceral Pain

Somatic Pain	Visceral Pain
Caused by injury to skin, soft tissue, muscles, and bone	Caused by inflammation or distention in the visceral organs such as bowels, liver, uterus (includes referred pain)
Well localized Described as sharp, aching, gnawing	Poorly localized Described as colicky, bloating, cramping, waxing, and waning Associated with autonomic symptoms such as sweating, nausea, and vomiting

TABLE 31-4	Types of Pain Based on Temporal Relation
Persistent pain/ baseline pain	Present throughout in the background and is of constant intensity
Breakthrough pain[3]	Pain flares occurring in a patient with controlled baseline pain. It is transient (lasts less than 30 min) It can be triggered by voluntary or involuntary movements (e.g., brought on by change of dressing, personal cares)
Incident pain[4]	Transitory increase in pain often brought on by movement. It can be predictable and is absent at rest. It is a subtype of breakthrough pain
End-of-dose pain[3]	Pain occurring at end of the dose interval of analgesics

Pain Assessment

Assessment of pain should involve an enquiry into the site, quality, character, temporal features, and aggravating and relieving factors of pain.[9] PQRST is a commonly used mnemonic to ascertain the detailed characteristics of pain[5] (Table 31-5).

Assessment of the physical characteristics of pain should be followed by an assessment and enquiry into the functional implications of the physical pain and also an immediate assessment and acknowledgment of the emotional, social, and spiritual components of the pain. Patients in chronic pain are more likely to have unresolved nonphysical symptoms.

TOOLS FOR ASSESSMENT OF PAIN

Some easy-to-use bedside tools are the Numerical Pain Rating Scale (NRS) and the Wong-Baker FACES Pain Rating Scale. In the NRS,[10] the patients are asked to indicate their current, best, and worst pain scores on a scale between 0 and 10, with 0 suggestive of no pain at all and 10 suggestive of worst imaginable pain.

The Wong–Baker FACES scale is used to rate the severity of pain in children, elderly, and patients who have language barriers.[7]

The Brief Pain Inventory,[11] formulated by the WHO group on evaluation of pain, measures pain severity as well as the functional implications of pain to the patient.

The Critical Care Pain Observation Tool (CPOT) was devised to allow pain assessment in the critically ill patients who are unable to self-report pain.[11,12] Critically ill patients exhibit behaviors in response to noxious stimuli and these responses are used to rate pain severity in the CPOT.[12]

The Pain Assessment in Advanced Dementia Scale[11] (PAINAID) measures pain in patients with dementia who are unable to communicate. It measures breathing pattern, vocalization, consolability, body language, and facial expression to assess the pain.

TABLE 31-5	Assessment of Characteristics of Pain Using "PQRST"
P–provocative/palliative factors	What worsens the pain? What activities cause pain relief?
Q–quality	How does it feel?
R–radiation	Does it spread to any other part of the body?
S–severity	How intense is the pain (measured using various pain rating scales)? How does it affect your everyday activities?
T–temporal factors	When is it present? Does it vary during the day and night?

WHO ANALGESIC LADDER[13]

The three-step WHO ladder serves as a simple but relevant tool in management of pain relief due to cancer pain. Following assessment of the quality and intensity of pain, the WHO ladder serves as a general guide for decision making for most types of pain (Figure 31-2).

GENERAL PRINCIPLES FOR ANALGESIC ADMINISTRATION

The WHO guidelines for pain relief in cancer set forth the guiding principles given in Figure 31-3 for administration of analgesics.[6]

The goals for pain relief are set based on the level of pain reduction needed to provide an *acceptable quality of life to the patient*. The benefit of pain relief must be balanced against the risk of adverse drug reactions such as respiratory depression.[6]

An NRS score ≤3 is considered satisfactory on serial pain assessment. Whenever the patient reports a persistently higher score, the assessor should move up to the next step of the WHO analgesic ladder. The WHO ladder should serve as a general guide in deciding the choice of pain medication based on pain severity, and does not represent a strict protocol for pain relief. For example, in cases with severe pain, it may be wise to start at Step 3 rather than let the patient suffer.

Global Pain Assessment

As pain is defined as "an emotional and sensory experience"; the evaluation of pain must take into account the cultural values, religious beliefs, age, and knowledge and beliefs of the patient regarding the pain and social support systems, and a comprehensive care plan should be prepared, based on individual patient factors and sound clinical judgment.

Pain evaluation must take into account **the meaning of pain** for the patient.[2] Psychosocial and spiritual factors color the experience of human suffering. Inability to acknowledge and address these factors may result in intractable pain.[6] Psychosocial and spiritual assessment and counseling may be needed to address these factors. Depression, fear, and anxiety are

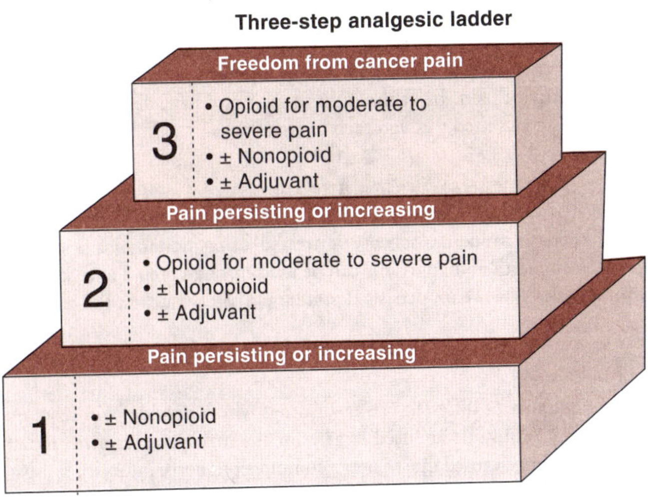

Figure 31-2 Picture of WHO ladder.

By the Clock	By Mouth	For the Individual	With Attention to Detail
• Analgesics should be scheduled according to duration of action of the drug and not on PRN basis.	• Oral route of administration is preferred as it is pain free.	• Although the WHO analgesic ladder provides general guidance, individual factors should be considered while prescribing analgesics. Careful assessment of pain and evaluation of drug's side effects should be done before deciding prescription.	• Patient's waking and bedtime should be considered while prescribing first dose and last dose of the day. Patients should be educated about reasons for drug use, anticipated adverse reactions, and remedies for the same.

Figure 31-3 WHO guiding principles for analgesia.

commonly encountered in patients with severe chronic pain. Some patients may need specialist consultation and pharmacologic management for the treatment of psychological distress.[14]

Use of Analgesics

There are three main classes of analgesics:

1. Nonopioids
2. Adjuvants
3. Opioids (weak and strong)

Use of the WHO analgesic ladder provides us a broad-spectrum view of analgesic use based on the severity of pain. In Tables 31-6 to 31-8, we have discussed each step of the ladder and the analgesics used through each of these steps.

STEP 1 OF THE WHO ANALGESIC LADDER

Here pain of mild to moderate severity is treated using nonopioids ± adjuvant drugs (Table 31-6). Nonopioids and adjuvants can be used through Step 2 and Step 3 in combination with opioids. When pain persists despite use of Step 1 drugs, the patient is moved to Step 2.

Adjuvant Analgesics

These are a unique mix of different classes of drugs which provide pain relief under specific circumstances. Adjuvants are used largely for the management of neuropathic pain. Neuropathic pain can be caused due to nerve compression, nerve injury, or sympathetically mediated processes. It occurs due to neuronal hyperexcitability and spontaneous activity at the site of injury.

TABLE 31-6 Step 1 of the WHO Analgesic Ladder

Drug Class	Drug Names and Typical Regimen	Remarks
Nonopioids		
Paracetamol[5,6,14]	Tablet: 100–500 mg Starting dose: 500–1000 mg, PO every 6 h. Maximum dose: 4 g daily Oral liquid: 125 mg/5 mL Suppository: 100, 125, 250 mg Injection (for IV infusion): 10 mg/mL	Does not have anti-inflammatory action, gastric safe In renal failure (creatinine clearance ≤30 mL/min), dosing interval must be ≥q6h USE with CAUTION in hepatic impairment (not to exceed 2 g in chronic alcoholics) Not to exceed 3 g/day if given unmonitored

NSAIDs	• Acetylsalicylic acid
	  • *Suppository:* 50–150 mg
	  • *Tablet:* 100–500 mg
	  • Starting dose 325–650 mg PO q4h
	  • Maximum dose: not to exceed 4 g/d
	Note: Use should not exceed 10 d, due to risk of adverse effects
		Precautions: Salicylate poisoning may cause respiratory stimulation, hyperventilation, and eventual respiratory failure

	• Ibuprofen
	  • 400–800 mg PO every 8 h
	  • Usual maximum dose: 2.4 g daily (3.2 g in inflammatory disease)
	  • Usual maintenance dose: 0.6–1.2 g/daily
	• Diclofenac
	  • Tablet: 50 mg
	  • IV: 37.5 mg/mL
	  • Starting dose: 50 mg, PO every 8–12 h
	  • Maximum dose: 150 mg
	• Naproxen
	  • Starting dose: 250–500 mg PO, BD
	  • Maximum dose: 1.25 g
	  • Has long elimination half-life
		Has excellent anti-inflammatory action (useful for soft tissue infiltration and bone metastasis), often in combination with opioids
		Use with proton pump inhibitors to reduce gastrointestinal side effects
		Adverse effects: gastrointestinal disturbances; hypersensitivity reactions including rash, angioedema, and bronchospasm; fluid retention (rarely precipitating congestive heart failure in older persons); raised blood pressure, renal failure; rarely hepatic damage, erythema multiforme (Stevens–Johnson syndrome), toxic dermal necrolysis (Lyell syndrome), colitis, and aseptic meningitis

(Continued)

TABLE 31-6 Step 1 of the WHO Analgesic Ladder (Continued)

Drug Class	Drug Names and Typical Regimen	Remarks
	• Piroxicam • Starting dose: 20–40 mg • Has long elimination half-life	
COX-2 selective NSAIDs	• Etoricoxib • Starting dose: 60–90 mg, PO once a day • Indications: 60 mg (60 mg) for osteoarthrosis, 90 mg (90 mg) for rheumatoid arthritis, 120 mg (120 mg for acute gouty arthritis)	Is gastric safe Adverse effects: causes fluid retention, increased blood pressure, increased risk of thrombosis (can precipitate MI or stroke) May precipitate hypoglycemia in diabetics Contraindicated in cardiac disease, HTN, diabetes
Adjuvants[5,6,*]:		
Corticosteroids	Dexamethasone: 8–16 mg, PO every morning Prednisolone: 15–30 mg, PO every morning *Note: Optimum dosing has not been defined. Prescribe for as short a period as possible due to risk of adverse effects*[6]	Indication: metastatic bone pain, visceral pain, neuropathic pain (nerve compression, spinal cord compression) Monitor for adverse effects: hyperglycemia, steroid psychosis, myopathy
Antidepressants	Amitriptyline, Imipramine } Starting dose: 12.5–25 mg every night (increase by 12.5–25 mg every 3–5 d, up to 100 mg/d)	Indication: neuropathic pain Adverse effects: antimuscarinic effects such as dry mouth, orthostatic hypotension, sedation, confusion, tachycardia, constipation (exercise caution in older adults—increases fall risk)
	Duloxetine: 30–60 mg/d every night	Indication: neuropathic pain
Antiepileptics	• Sodium valproate • Starting dose: 200 mg every night • Titrate up by 200 mg every 3–5 d up to a maximum of 1000 mg/d	Indication: neuropathic pain Adverse effect: drowsiness
	• Carbamazepine • Starting dose: 50–100 mg t.d.s. • Titrate up by 200 mg every 2 weeks up to a maximum dose of 1200 mg/d	Indication: neuropathic pain Adverse reactions: ataxia, dizziness, drowsiness, aplastic anemia, high risk of hypersensitivity

(Continued)

TABLE 31-6 Step 1 of the WHO Analgesic Ladder (Continued)

	• Gabapentin: 300–600 mg, PO q8h (not to exceed 1800 mg/d)	Needs dose modification in renal failure. Do not administer if CrCl ≤30 mL/min on hemodialysis
	• Pregabalin: 50–100 mg, PO, q8h (not to exceed 300 mg/d)	Indication: neuropathic pain needs dose modification in renal failure Adverse effects: drowsiness, ataxia, dizziness
	Note: The WHO guidelines for the management of cancer pain in adults and adolescents do not provide recommendations for OR against the use of antidepressants and anticonvulsants for the treatment of neuropathic pain.	
Bisphosphonates	Pamidronate 90 mg iv every 4 weeks Zoledronic acid 4 mg iv every 4–8 weeks	Used to prevent and treat bone pain[6] Adverse effects: pyrexia, flu-like malaise for 1–2 days
NMDA receptor channel blockers	• Methadone • Injection: 10 mg/mL in various vial sizes (as hydrochloride) • Tablet: 5, 10, 40 mg (as hydrochloride) • Oral liquid: 1, 2 mg/mL, 5 mg/mL (as hydrochloride) • Oral concentrate: 10 mg/mL (as hydrochloride) • Starting dose in opioid-naïve patients: 2.5 mg (1–2 mg in older persons) PO q8h regularly and q6h p.r.n. If necessary, titrate the regular dose upwards once a week, guided by PRN use • <u>Features unique to the pharmacology and use of methadone</u> • Long elimination half-life of up to 190 h which does not match the observed analgesic duration of 6–12 h once it reaches steady state	Indications • Neuropathic pain that is poorly responsive to antidepressants, antiepileptics, and NSAIDs. • Pain unresponsive to morphine, compounded by increasing adverse effects to morphine. • Intolerable undesirable effect of morphine at any dose. • Preferred in renal failure Adverse effects: nausea, vomiting, constipation, dry mouth, biliary spasm, respiratory depression, drowsiness, muscle rigidity, hypotension, bradycardia, tachycardia, palpitation, edema, postural hypotension, hallucinations, vertigo, euphoria, dysphoria, dependence, confusion, urinary retention, ureteric spasm

(Continued)

TABLE 31-6 Step 1 of the WHO Analgesic Ladder (Continued)

Drug Class	Drug Names and Typical Regimen	Remarks
	• Varying potency of methadone with patient's current exposure to opioids • High incidence of drug interaction with a large number of drugs ***CAUTION:*** *Due to the complex nature and wide interindividual variation in the pharmacokinetics of methadone, it should be initiated and titrated only by practitioners experienced with its use*	
	• Ketamine[15]: low-dose ketamine (at subanesthetic doses) can be used PO, subcutaneously, or intravenously for pain refractory to opioids and as an adjuvant analgesic *Note: There are no large studies or trials and no recommendations supporting use of ketamine in Palliative care*	Indications: opioid-resistant pain, neuropathic pain, allodynia, and hyperalgesia Adverse effects: hypersalivation, hypertension, tachycardia, bad dreams, dysphoria, alteration in body image/mood
Muscle relaxants	Diazepam: 5–10 mg ,every night Baclofen: 10 mg PO TDS	Adverse effects: drowsiness, ataxia
Antispasmodics	Hyoscine butylbromide: 60–160 mg/24 h SC Glycopyrronium: 600–1200 μg/24 h SC	Adverse effects: peripheral antimuscarinic effects

*They are a miscellaneous group of drugs used to relieve pain under specific circumstances. They include drugs used to control adverse effects of analgesics and concurrently used psychotropic medications. They are useful in controlling neuropathic pain. They are generally used as add-on drugs along with NSAIDs or opioids.

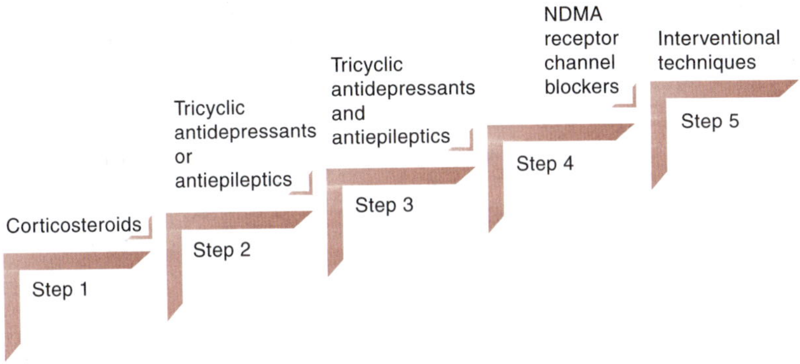

Figure 31-4 Scheme for selection of adjuvant analgesics for neuropathic pain.[5]

Figure 31-4 provides a scheme for drug selection for neuropathic pain. One or two drugs from each category may be selected to provide acceptable pain relief.

More than 50% of the patients with neuropathic cancer pain show good response to a combination of NSAIDs and a strong opioid. On addition of an adjuvant analgesic, >90% of patients show a good response.

STEP 2 OF THE WHO ANALGESIC LADDER

Here, weak opioids are used in combination with nonopioids or adjuvants as per the clinical indication (Table 31-7). Recent studies have suggested that the use of weak opioids often results in poor pain control and increasing side effects. Weak opioids have a ceiling effect on analgesia. Hence, newer recommendations suggest skipping Step 2 of the WHO ladder and prescribing Step 3, that is, low-dose morphine for moderate pain.

Note:

- Weak opioids should be added to a nonopioid prescription and not substituted for it.
- When a weak opioid does not provide acceptable pain relief, step up to a strong opioid such as morphine.

The Case Against Tramadol

Mechanism of Action

Tramadol[16] has a dual mechanism of action as a central opiate agonist and as central nervous system (CNS) reuptake inhibitor of norepinephrine and serotonin.

a. Tramadol exists as two enantiomers: (+)-tramadol and its metabolite *O*-desmethyltramadol, also known as M1. M1 metabolite binds to the mu receptor with 300 times more activity compared to the parent compound.
b. The (+)-tramadol inhibits reuptake of serotonin and norepinephrine, thereby enhancing the inhibitory descending pathways associated with pain transmission in the CNS.

The metabolism of the M1 metabolite occurs in the liver via the enzyme CYP2D6 and subsequent excretion of the metabolites occurs via the kidneys (>90%).

Adverse Events Caused by Tramadol

The common adverse effects noted with tramadol are nausea, vomiting, constipation, headache, dizziness, dry mouth, and insomnia. Serious adverse event such as seizure, hypoglycemia, hyponatremia, and serotonin syndrome have also been reported.

TABLE 31-7 Step 2 of the WHO Analgesic Ladder

Drug Class	Drugs and Typical Regimen	Remarks
Weak opioids	• Tramadol • Tablets: 50–100 mg, PO, BID/TDS • Maximum dose: 400 mg/d	Has less opioid side effects than morphine and codeine Causes nausea, vomiting, and constipation
	• Codeine • Tablet: 15, 30, 60 mg • Starting dose: 30–60 mg every 4 h when necessary • Maximum dose: 240 mg daily • Oral solution: 25 mg/5 mL • Injection: 60 mg/mL	Causes severe constipation
	Note: Codeine depends on the CYP2D6 enzyme for its metabolism. Due to the high interindividual variability in the action of CYP2D6, the benefits and risks of its action are highly unpredictable. Hence, its use is not preferred	
	• Tapentadol • 50–150 mg, PO, every 6–8 h • Maximum dose: 400 mg/d	Can precipitate serotonin syndrome and cause physical/psychological dependence
	• Buprenorphine: 0.2–0.4 mg sublingual or 0.15 mg IV applied every 6–8 h for acute pain, 5–20 μg/h transdermal patch, changed every 7 d	Used as substitution therapy for substance abuse disorder: 4–32 mg/daily Do not use for patients with high and varying analgesic requirements

Serious Adverse Events

Polymorphisms in the enzyme CYP2D6 leading to significant interindividual variability in the expression of this enzyme among the population cause unpredictability in the analgesic action of tramadol. Poor metabolizers of CYP2D6 show low levels of M1 and inadequate pain control and increased serotonin reuptake inhibition is caused by the (+)- tramadol enantiomer. Rapid metabolizers develop respiratory depression due to very high levels of M1.

Serotonin Syndrome

The serotonin syndrome characterized by altered mental status, neuromuscular abnormalities, and autonomic hyperactivity has been reported most commonly with SSRIs and with overdosage of tramadol. However, there are increasing reports of serotonin syndrome occurring with therapeutic dose of tramadol when it has been used in combination with one or more drugs known to cause serotonin syndrome (SSRIS, SNRIs, TCAs, and triptans).

Seizure Risk

There is an increased seizure risk reported from the use of tramadol at recommended dose ranges. The risk further increases with concomitant use of SSRIs, TCAs, baclofen, and other opioids.[17]

Hypoglycemia

Tramadol has been reported to cause increased risk of hypoglycemia in both diabetic and nondiabetic populations in various studies.[18]

TABLE 31-8 Step 3 of the WHO Analgesic Ladder

Drug Class	Drugs and Typical Regimen	Remarks
Opioids	• Morphine ◦ *Injection:* 10 mg (morphine hydrochloride or morphine sulfate) in 1 mL ampoule ◦ *Oral liquid:* 10 mg (morphine hydrochloride or morphine sulfate)/5 mL ◦ *Tablet:* 10 mg (morphine sulfate) ◦ *Tablet (prolonged-release):* 10, 30, 60 mg (morphine sulfate) ◦ Starting dose: 5 mg, PO every 4 h, 2 mg IV/SC every 4 h ***No maximum dose***	Reduce the dose or decrease the frequency of administration in renal failure Coprescribe laxatives (stimulant laxatives preferred)
	• Fentanyl ◦ *Transmucosal lozenge:* 200, 400, 600, 800, 1200, 1600 g (as citrate) ◦ *Transdermal patch (extended-release):* 12, 25, 50, 75, 100 μg/h (as base) (every 72 h) ◦ *Injection:* 50 μg/mL in various vial sizes (as citrate)	Unsuitable for patients with unstable pain Do not use in patients with severe cachexia, fevers, or frequent sweating No maximum dose
	• Methadone: In addition to opioid agonist activity, methadone has NMDA receptor channel blocker activity and is a presynaptic blocker of serotonin reuptake	Details are given under Step 1 (refer Table 31-6)

Used when step 2 medications do not relieve pain or when pain is severe at onset

Hyponatremia

Tramadol increases the risk of hyponatremia and SIADH in older adults.[19]

Age, Hepatic and Renal Failure

Due to the variable metabolism and incidence of adverse drug interactions with multiple drugs, tramadol should be used with caution in older adults, and in those with hepatic and renal failure.

> Due to the variable analgesic potency, risk of serious adverse events and increased risk for abuse tramadol has been increasingly described as ***tramadon't***. Suggestions are afoot to skip the Step 2 of the WHO ladder and replace tramadol with low-dose morphine for better efficacy and lesser side effects.[20]

STEP 3 OF THE WHO ANALGESIC LADDER

Patients with moderate to severe pain or pain persisting after usage of Step 2 drugs can be moved up to Step 3. Oral morphine remains the mainstay of Step 3 of the WHO analgesic ladder. Patients who have severe pain while on morphine or those who are unable to use morphine in view of intolerable side effects can be prescribed alternative strong opioids such as fentanyl or methadone. Methadone is indicated in patients who have severe pain while on morphine or have intolerable neuropathic pain.

Initiation of Morphine

Oral morphine is the mainstay of analgesia in Step 3. Starting dose is 5–10 mg every 4 hours, with a double dose given at night to allow for a good night's sleep without awakening due to pain.

For example, tab. morphine 5 mg 1-1-1-1-2 + 5 mg PRN for breakthrough pain. Rescue dose for breakthrough pain must be one-sixth of the regular dose.

- Dose titration is done as follows: Goal is improved functional status of the patient.
- Review the pain score and functional status of the patient every 2–3 days and add the scheduled doses + PRN doses to obtain the new total morphine dose for the next couple of days. The new dosing schedule is followed until next review and until goals are met.
- In older adults and in those with renal failure, dosing frequency should be increased to q8h or q12h and uptitrated slowly based on tolerability and close monitoring for adverse effects.

Side Effects of Morphine

Most of the side effects of opioids are self-limiting and wear off within the first week of morphine initiation. Patient education and prophylactic medications for nausea and vomiting can be given during first few days of morphine therapy. Constipation often persists for longer and may require coprescription of stimulant laxatives in most cases for the duration of opioid treatment (Table 31-9).

Signs of Opioid Overdose

Opioid overdose is not as common as it is feared with oral morphine. Common features include undue drowsiness, vomiting, delirium, myoclonus, and pinpoint pupils on examination.

Respiratory depression is NOT common with regular analgesic doses of morphine unless there is overdose (accidental/intentional).

Delirium, myoclonus, and persistent drowsiness can be managed by reduction of opioid dose. Intractable side effects despite dose reduction necessitate switch to an alternate opioid.

Respiratory Depression

- Signs: respiratory rate <8–10 breaths/min; SpO_2 <85% with pinpoint pupils.
- Management: Skip the next dose of morphine. Start a titrated dose of IV naloxone. (Note: Naloxone is rarely needed in palliative care.)
- Dosage: 0.08–0.12 mg IV every 2–3 minutes until the patient is breathing adequately.

  After initial response, the intravenous dose may need to be repeated every 20–60 minutes because of the short duration of action. For continuous intravenous infusion, dilute to a concentration of 4 µg/mL with glucose 5% or sodium chloride 0.9%.

TABLE 31-9 Common Side Effects of Oral Morphine

Common Side Effects	Management
Constipation	Stimulant laxatives, bisacodyl 10 mg HS or senna 15 mg Bulk-forming laxatives do not have a role in opioid-induced constipation
Nausea and vomiting	Self-limiting (1 wk) Tab haloperidol 1–3 mg every night or metoclopramide 10 mg TDS
Sedation	Reduce the dose of morphine if persistent sedation for more than 3 d. In rare cases, use methylphenidate 10 mg, PO OD to BD
Itching	It is a central phenomenon and does not respond to H1 blockers. Use ondansetron 8 mg IV stat, and 8 mg PO BD for 3–5 d

- Precautions: opioid-tolerant patients may develop severe withdrawal symptoms during naloxone infusion such as tachycardia, sweating and accelerated hypertension, and loss of analgesia resulting in severe pain.

Commonly misinterpreted facts about oral morphine

- Oral morphine which is slowly uptitrated according to pain scores RARELY causes respiratory depression. Pain is a physiologic antagonist of the central depressive action of opioids.
- The chances of addiction with oral morphine preparations are low.
- Step 3 drugs are not reserved for terminal stages of the disease. Choosing the drug should be based on severity of pain and not on the stage of the disease.
- The ratio between therapeutic effect and lethal dose of morphine (therapeutic ratio) is greater than is widely assumed, which allows for gradual and safe uptitration of oral morphine dose until optimum pain relief is achieved.

Addiction

Addiction is a psychological phenomenon characterized by impaired control over drug use, compulsive use, and continued use despite harm and craving.

Physical Dependence

This is a state of adaptation to a specific drug class, often brought on by abrupt cessation or dose reduction of the drug or administration of an antagonist.

Equianalgesic Doses of Different Opioids

See Table 31-10.

Cessation of Opioid Therapy

Definite guidelines for cessation of opioid therapy do not exist. Tapering of opioids should be individualized based on clinical evaluation of the patient. A rough guide for the same is presented in Table 31-11.

TABLE 31-10 Equianalgesic Doses of Different Routes of Administration of Opioids

Drug	Route	Dose	Conversion Factor
Morphine	Oral	30	1
	IV, IM, SC	10	0.3
	Epidural	3	0.1
	Intrathecal	0.3	0.01
Oxycodone	Oral	20	1.5
Hydromorphone	Oral	8	3.75
Methadone	Oral	10	0.3
Tramadol	Oral	150	0.2
	IV	100	0.1
Meperidine	IV	75	0.13
Fentanyl	IV	0.1	100
Sufentanil	IV	0.01	1000
Buprenorphine	SL	0.3	100

TABLE 31-11 Cessation of Opioid Therapy

Clinical Scenario	Opioid Tapering and Cessation Strategy	Remarks
Short-term use (<2 wks)	Opioids need to be tapered only if patient has residual pain, or else they can be stopped abruptly	Physical dependence unlikely
Long-term use (>4 wks)	Taper by 10% every week to as minimum a dose as is feasible. Once the minimum dose is reached, start increasing dosing interval until the dose is 24 h apart without signs or symptoms of withdrawal and then stop. If withdrawal symptoms appear, increase the previous highest dose and slow the taper to 10% every 2 wks	Some degree of physical dependence likely Signs and symptoms of withdrawal: drug craving, anxiety, insomnia, abdominal pain, vomiting, diarrhea, diaphoresis, mydriasis, tremor, tachycardia, or piloerection
Use between 2 and 4 wks	Taper by 10–50% every week If withdrawal symptoms appear, return to previous highest dose and reduce the percentage of the taper	Physical dependence uncertain
Long-term use/in patients with history of substance use disorder	Consult a specialist in opioid use disorder	

INTERVENTIONAL PAIN MANAGEMENT

Various interventional pain management techniques may be tried in certain cases where clinically appropriate. Some of these measures are listed as follows:

1. Palliative surgery: Palliative surgery such as a diverting colostomy can be considered to relieve abdominal pain caused by malignant bowel obstruction.
2. Nerve blocks/neuroablation: This implies regional anesthetic procedures that can include blocks of spinal nerves, peripheral nerves, and sympathetic ganglia.
3. Kyphoplasty or vertebroplasty: Injection of cement into the focal metastatic areas of the spine will help in spine stabilization as well as in pain relief.
4. Epidural medications of steroids or local anesthetic is used to provide pain relief.
5. Intrathecal pain pumps: Intrathecal injections of opioids are given using pumps, in very small doses, to provide good analgesia with minimal side effects.

NONPHARMACOLOGIC MANAGEMENT OF PAIN[16]

Nonpharmacologic methods are multimodal and are often used together with medications and other pain-relieving methods. Some commonly used modalities are as given in the subsequent text.

1. Physical Therapy

Specific exercise training helps to address fear avoidance and the severe deconditioning which is seen commonly in patients with chronic pain. Therapeutic exercise and stretching also serves to overcome long-established fear avoidance behaviors.

2. Psychological Therapy

2a. Cognitive Behavior Therapy

Cognitive behavior therapy (CBT) is the best and most recommended of the psychological therapies for chronic pain management. It targets maladaptive behavioral responses to the pain, and social and environmental factors. Through a goal-directed concise series of 15–20 sessions, CBT causes significant reduction in stress and severity of pain, more realistic expectations, and more control over symptoms.

2b. Mind–Body Techniques

Several mindfulness techniques, structured exercise programs, deep relaxation techniques, yoga, and tai chi have been recommended for pain severity. The evidence for these therapies is modest but shows improved function and moderate reduction in pain medication.

3. Acupuncture

Acupuncture has been used since several centuries for the treatment of chronic pain and continues to be used. It has been recommended for use in chronic low backache and chronic migraine.

4. Transcutaneous Electrical Nerve Stimulation (TENS)

This is a surface-applied neuromodulation system which is delivered by a trained physical therapist. It has been used in the treatment of chronic pain despite lack of robust evidence of benefit.

Summary

- Effective pain management begins with a thorough assessment of the patient's pain, including its intensity, location, duration, and characteristics.
- It is important to differentiate the types of pain as it has an important bearing on the management.
- Pain management includes pharmacological therapies such as analgesic medications (e.g., nonsteroidal anti-inflammatory drugs, opioids), adjuvant medications (e.g., antidepressants, anticonvulsants), and nonpharmacological therapies such as physical therapy, cognitive-behavioral therapy, acupuncture, massage, and relaxation techniques.
- The WHO Pain Ladder emphasizes a progressive approach to pain management, starting with the least potent medications and escalating to stronger options as needed based on the severity of pain.

Scan the QR code to access chapter references.

32 Palliative Care

Sheetal Raj M.

From inability to let well alone,
From too much zeal for the new and contempt for what is old,
From putting knowledge before wisdom, science before art and cleverness before common sense,
From treating patients as cases and
From making the cure of the disease more grievous than the endurance of the same,
good Lord deliver us.

Sir Robert Hutchison

This quote[1] from Sir Robert Hutchison is never more apt than it is in the context of palliative care. The word palliation is derived from the Latin word "palliare," meaning "to cloak" or to cover up or mitigate.[2] Palliative care includes early prevention comprehensive assessment and management of physical symptoms (including pain), and psychological, social, and spiritual needs.[3]

Palliative Care

Palliative care[3] is defined as the active holistic care of individuals across all ages *with serious health-related suffering* due to *severe illness* and especially of those near the end of life. It also aims to improve the quality of life of patients, their families, and their caregivers.

Suffering is health-related when it is associated with illness or injury of any kind. **Health-related suffering is serious**[3,4] when it cannot be relieved without medical intervention and when it compromises physical, social, spiritual, and/or emotional functioning.

Severe Illness

Severe illness[3,5] is a condition that carries a high risk of mortality, negatively impacts quality of life and daily function, and/or is burdensome in symptoms, treatments, or caregiver stress. It can be used interchangeably with the term *serious illness.*

This new definition[3] of palliative care by the WHO underscores the shift in approach to palliative care from a disease-centered conceptualization to one with emphasis on human suffering.

The estimated global burden of suffering, suggests that, by the year 2060, 47% of all the deaths globally will be due to *serious health-related suffering.* More than 80% of these deaths will occur in Low and Middle-Income Countries (LMIC). By the year 2060, the fastest increase in serious health-related suffering will be seen among, older adults (≥70 years) and people with dementia. These alarming projections underscore the ethical and economic imperative to integrate palliative care into health systems.[5]

In traditional medical education, the curing of physical symptoms was considered to be of foremost importance, with little value given for emotional distress, quality of life, and suffering.

With the increasing burden of chronic progressive illnesses and life-limiting conditions, we face the reality that the prospect of *cure* is largely nonexistent in most cases. This necessitates a shift in focus toward improving quality of life and reducing distress among these patients with serious health-related suffering. ***Palliative care teaches us that diagnosis of a terminal illness does not mean that "nothing else can be done."***[5] With structured knowledge and training, physicians can offer their patients various healthcare options which offer comfort, dignity, and symptom relief. Thus, palliative care emphasizes a shift in focus from cure-based care to comfort-based care.[1]

THE INTERDISCIPLINARY TEAM[2]

The hallmark of quality palliative care is a well-trained interdisciplinary team, which offers round-the-clock, comprehensive care with respect to the multiple domains of needs of the patient/family/caregiver, namely, physical, psychological, social, and spiritual, and availability of resources. Although the composition of interdisciplinary teams varies depending on the availability of trained resources, the *core team is usually made up of physician, nurse and social worker*, and may also include other providers such as physical therapist, chaplain, occupational therapist, volunteers, bereavement counselors, music therapists, dietician, and speech–language therapists. The interdisciplinary team is characterized by a *patient-centric approach*, with care coordination between patients and providers and between providers themselves with a *task-dependent leadership* focused on integration, sharing, and a horizontal hierarchy. The patient is at the center of care and takes active part in the consultative and decision-making process with quality of life and relief of suffering being the primary focus of care.

ETHICS IN PALLIATIVE CARE[2]

The principles and practice of palliative care are governed by the four cardinal principles of medical ethics:

1. Autonomy (respect for the patient as a person, informed consent)
2. Beneficence (do good if you can)
3. Nonmaleficence (minimize harm)
4. Justice (fair use of available resources)

   The four cardinal principles should be balanced against *three dichotomies* (Figure 32-1):

   a. In an attempt to preserve life, if the burdens of life-sustaining treatments outweigh the benefits, then withdrawal of such treatments and providing comfort and relief of suffering should be foremost. Physicians should recognize medical futility.

   b. The principle of double effect states that, "A single act having two possible foreseen effects, one good and one harmful, is not always morally prohibited if the harm effect is not intended".* Clinical decision making is fraught with ambivalence, especially in the care of terminally ill patients, and hence every treatment has an inherent risk. According to the principle of double effect, the focus is on the intention of the physician to provide comfort to the patient and to relieve suffering and thus any side effect/harm arising unintentionally from such a treatment is permissible.

   c. Individual needs should be balanced against those of the society, especially when resources are limited.

The four cardinal principles of ethics should be balanced against the three dichotomies and applied in a background of respect for life and the acceptance of death as an inevitable event.

Scope of Palliative Care[2,3,6–9]

One of the greatest challenges is determining when in the course of illness one should begin palliative care, whether it should follow after cessation of curative therapy, and whether palliative care is the domain of palliative care specialists or of general physicians. Determining prognosis in noncancer illness is difficult and uncertain. Even in cancer, scales such as

*Twycross R. Introducing Palliative Care., 4th edition, sixth economy reprint 2013. Publisher: Institute of Palliative Medicine, Pain and Palliative Care Society, Medical College P.O., Calicut, Kerala, India-673008.

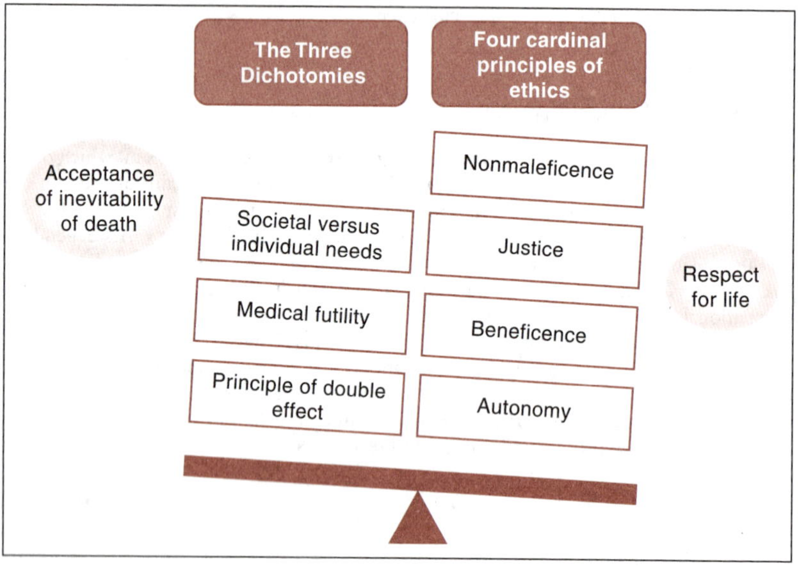

Figure 32-1 The four cardinal principles and the three dichotomies of ethics.

the Palliative Performance Scale and the Eastern Cooperative Oncology Group (ECOG) scale which are used commonly often overestimate prognosis and make it difficult for the oncologist to determine when to stop curative intent therapy.

Illness Trajectories

Illness trajectories[6,8,10] have been described to explain prognosis in chronic progressive diseases (Figure 32-2). These graphs help patients and doctors in understanding and communicating disease prognosis.

Cancer

Here, there is a relatively stable period of high physical function followed by rapid decline over the last few months of life. The period of decline may vary from 1 to 5 months and may be more predictable in solid tumors than in others, thus helping patients and doctors to better anticipate decline. These patients more often receive palliative care than the ones with other disease trajectories. Physical function and spiritual distress may have peaks of worsening at the time of diagnosis and recurrence, and during the terminal phase of illness.

Organ Failure

There occurs steady decline interspersed with multiple periods of acute deterioration followed by recovery, and eventual sudden worsening followed by a seemingly unexpected death. Following each acute deterioration, the patient will be at risk of death, but may recover with a decline in functional status. Prognosis is most uncertain with this pattern. Common examples include: advanced COPD, cardiac failure, and liver failure.

Frailty/Dementia/Old Age

There is a steady, slow decline in functional status and gradual loss of speech and cognition over several years. This is often not recognized as a terminal illness and carries the maximum burden for caregiving.

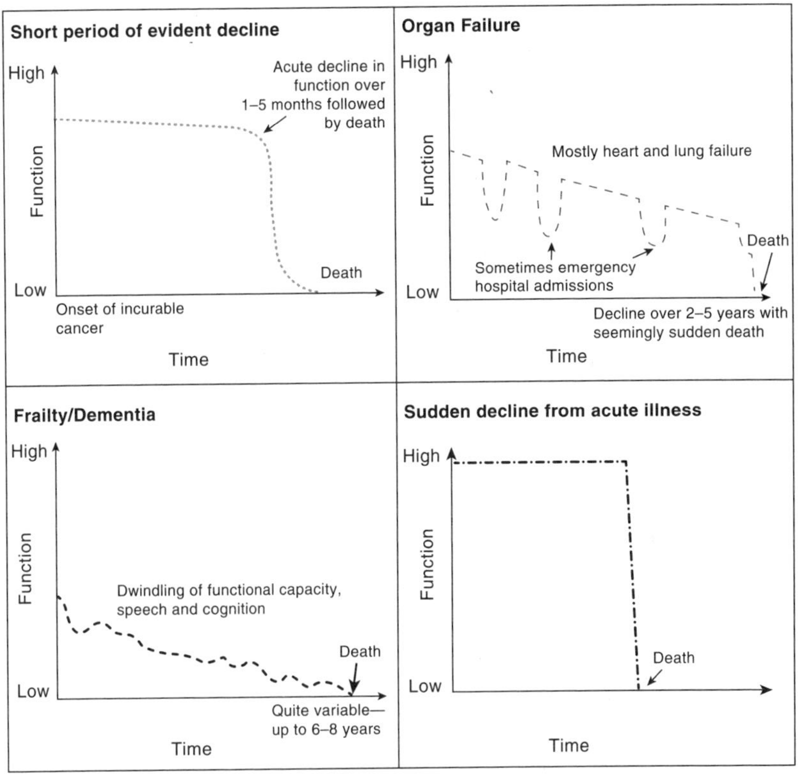

Figure 32-2 Illness trajectories in chronic illnesses—cancer, organ failure, dementia, and sudden death.

Sudden Death

Here, there is a sudden decline from high physical function to very low function/death. Common causes are trauma and acute cardiopulmonary/neurological events. The caregivers may express anger and may be at risk of complicated grief due to the sudden and severe change to a new reality.

The vast majority of deaths worldwide occur due to chronic illnesses with a prolonged period of decline characterized by severe health-related suffering. Present consensus suggests that early initiation of palliative care at the time of diagnosis of serious illness helps to improve quality of life and provide maximum relief of suffering.[2,6] Palliative care should continue to provide support to the patient and family to come to terms with the diagnosis, through treatment and cure/continued treatment, and death and should end with bereavement support to the family for up to 13 months after the death of the patient[2,3,9] (Figure 32-3).

The term serious health-related suffering identifies 20 conditions which commonly cause death or suffering necessitating palliative care intervention. They are: atherosclerosis; cerebrovascular disease; chronic ischemic heart diseases; congenital malformations; degeneration of the CNS; dementia; diseases of the liver; hemorrhagic fevers; HIV disease; inflammatory disease of the CNS; injury, poisoning, and external causes; leukemia; lung diseases; malignant neoplasms (cancers); musculoskeletal disorders; nonischemic heart

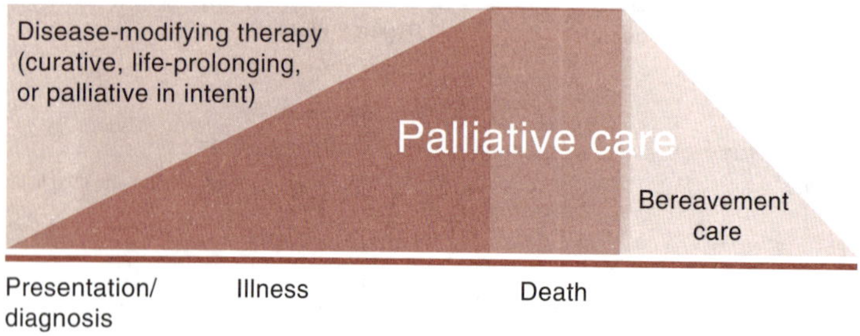

Figure 32-3 Integrated model of curative and palliative care for chronic progressive illness.

diseases; premature birth and birth trauma; protein–energy malnutrition; renal failure; and tuberculosis.[4]

Key Principles of Palliative Care[6]

Palliative care espouses the following key principles which are the determinants of good clinical practice:

- Symptom control
- Effective communication
- Rehabilitation
- Continuity of care
- Terminal care
- Support in bereavement
- Education
- Research

SYMPTOM MANAGEMENT IN PALLIATIVE CARE

Cough

Causes

Causes include tumors of the lung, pleura, mediastinum, chronic respiratory diseases, cardiac failure, acid reflux, drug-induced causes, and chest infection.

Management

Intractable cough can cause sleep disturbance, hamper communication, and cause social embarrassment.

1. Key to management in early stages is to identify the cause of the cough and treat the cough.
2. Identify whether cough is dry or productive.
3. Nonpharmacologic methods
    a. Humidified air, nebulized saline, and chest physiotherapy as an addition to pharmacotherapy
    b. Identification and acknowledgment of the psychological and social impact of the cough
4. Pharmacologic methods
    a. Dry cough or if the patient is too weak to cough effectively
        i. *Dextromethorphan*: Centrally acting opioid derivative; does not produce sedation and other gastrointestinal side effects of opioids

ii. *Morphine*
- Five milligrams q4h, PO to be increased till symptom relief (in opioid-naïve patients). Reduce the starting dose and frequency in older adults and in renal failure.
- Increase opioid dose by 20%–25% in those who are already on a fixed opioid regime for pain relief.

iii. *Codeine*: 30–60 mL QDS

iv. *Intractable cases*: Nebulized lidocaine (5 mL of 0.2% TDS) or bupivacaine (5 mL of 0.25% TDS)

b. Productive cough in which the patient is able to cough effectively
   i. Nebulized saline
   ii. Nebulized mucolytic (*N*-acetylcysteine)
   iii. Steam inhalations (tincture benzoin, carbol, menthol, eucalyptus)
   iv. Chest physiotherapy and postural drainage
   v. Antibiotics (if there are overt signs of bacterial infection such as fever, raised leucocyte counts or purulent sputum)

Breathlessness

Breathlessness is a common symptom in the last few weeks preceding death in most patients with cancer. It is often associated with a feeling of exhaustion and is brought on by minimal exertion, talking, or physical activity.

It can lead to anxiety, panic, and fear of impending death.

Causes of Breathlessness

- **Cancer causing hypoxia:** Lung replacement by tumor mass, obstruction of airway by mass, lymphangitis carcinomatosa, pleural effusion, and massive ascites causing hypoxia
- **Primary cardiorespiratory disease:** Advanced COPD, asthma, cardiac failure, pneumonia, and empyema
- **Concurrent comorbidities:** Acidosis, fever, panic disorder, anxiety, and depression
- **Debility:** Anemia, atelectasis, respiratory muscle weakness, and cachexia–anorexia

Management

1. **Correct the correctable** (Table 32-1): Identify and correct the treatable causes.
2. **Nonpharmacologic methods**
   a. *Counseling of patient and family:* Allay anxiety and fear of death. Help the patient to cope with the loss of functional independence caused by the worsening breathlessness. Assure the patient and family of your presence until the patient feels better.

TABLE 32-1 Treatment of Common Causes of Dyspnea

Causes	Treatment
COPD/bronchial asthma/pneumonia	Bronchodilators, antibiotics, steroids, oxygen
Cardiac failure	Diuretics, nitrates, ACEIs, assist devices
Lymphangitis carcinomatosa	Corticosteroids, diuretics, bronchodilators
Pericardial effusion	Paracentesis, corticosteroids
Pleural effusion	Thoracocentesis, pleurodesis
Ascites	Paracentesis, diuretics
Pulmonary embolism	Anticoagulants
Anemia	Blood transfusion, iron, erythropoietin

b. *General measures:* Avoid hot environments, wear loose clothing, position the patient propped up and near a window with a cool draught or place a table fan adjacent to the patient's bed, implement activity pacing (to achieve a balance between activity and rest by pacing it according to the patient's capacity), music. Hand held fans have shown benefit and can be advocated for the relief of chronic breathlessness as part of self management.*

c. *Physiotherapy*

i. Pursed lip breathing, relaxation therapy, and encourage exertion to the point of breathlessness to improve activity tolerance and to maintain fitness.

3. **Pharmacologic methods:** These methods should be used only when all nonpharmacologic measures fail to provide adequate relief.

a. *Morphine*

i. Mechanism: The mechanism of action of morphine in alleviating dyspnea is poorly understood and often mired in controversy regarding safety concerns (respiratory depression). However it is known to act centrally, peripherally and also by allaying anxiety. It is known to reduce the ventilatory response to carbon dioxide, hypoxia, inspiratory flow resistive loading and to exercise. It also reduces the oxygen consumption both at rest and during exercise among healthy individuals.†

ii. Dose

- Opioid-naïve patients: Starting dose is 2.5 mg q4h to q6h, PO. Optimum dose is obtained by titrating as needed until relief of dyspnea.
- If the patient is already on a fixed dose of morphine for pain: Increase the dose by 25%–50%.

b. *Benzodiazepines:* Anecdotal reports suggest a role for benzodiazepines in relieving breathlessness in those patients who have persistent anxiety or are in panic.

i. Dose: Diazepam, 5–10 mg stat and every night (reduce dose to 2–5 mg in older adults); lorazepam, 0.5–1 mg sublingually, BD or PRN; or midazolam, 1–2 mg SC (for respite sedation in severe breathlessness). Haloperidol can be added if the patient appears fearful.

c. *Oxygen therapy*: It improves oxygenation and reduces work of breathing. However, *oxygen should be given only if there is clear benefit and relief of dyspnea.* The benefit from oxygen may not be much more than that of a fan/draught through an open window. Oxygen should preferably be delivered through nasal prongs to allow social interaction and feeding (avoid face mask). The advantages of continued oxygen therapy should be weighed against the burdens of cost, loss of mobility, psychological impact, and relief of suffocation.

In patients with breathlessness on exertion, trial of oxygen before activity might be of benefit.

d. *Corticosteroids*

i. Mechanism: Reduces tissue edema and increases sense of well being.

ii. Dose: Dexamethasone, 4 or 8 mg, PO, s/c, or IV can be given. Dose should be titrated according to known side effects.

Nausea and Vomiting

Key to management of nausea and vomiting in palliative care lies in providing receptor-guided and individualized therapy which incorporates the multifactorial nature of this much ignored symptom complex.

The emetic pathway is given in Figure 32-4.

---

*Tim Luckett, Jane Phillips, Miriam J. Johnson, Morag Farquhar, Flavia Swan, Teresa Assen, Priyanka Bhattarai, Sara Booth European Respiratory Journal 2017 50: 1700262; DOI: 10.1183/13993003.00262-2017.

†Uronis HE, Currow DC, Abernethy AP. Palliative management of refractory dyspnea in COPD. Int J Chron Obstruct Pulmon Dis. 2006;1(3):289–304. doi:10.2147/copd.2006.1.3.289.

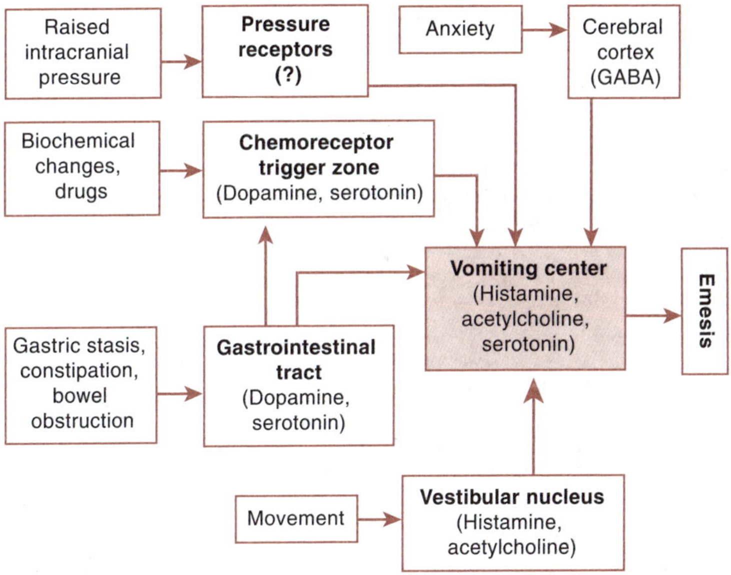

Figure 32-4 The pathogenesis of emesis.

Key Principles of Management of Nausea, Vomiting, and Retching

1. Identify by thorough history and holistic evaluation a possible etiology for the cause of vomiting.
2. Identify the mechanism causing vomiting and the receptors which are most likely to be involved. In most cases, the clinical mechanism and receptor targets causing vomiting fall under one of the following categories: stasis, obstruction, toxin induced, drugs, or emotional factors.
3. Choose an antiemetic regime based on the above-mentioned factors to match the patient's clinical profile, incorporating multifactorial nature of the symptoms.
4. Antiemetics should always be prescribed as a scheduled drug and not on PRN basis. Additional PRN dosing should be prescribed to allow for self-titration by the patient.
5. Correct the correctable once etiology for nausea and vomiting has been identified.
6. Nonpharmacologic measures to address nausea and vomiting* are the following:
   a. Modify the patient's diet to avoid triggers. Fatty, spicy, and salty foods may commonly trigger nausea.
   b. Provide a calm and reassuring environment.
   c. Avoid sights, sounds, or smells which trigger nausea in that patient.
   d. Control malodor from fungating wounds, colostomy, or pressure sores.
   e. Small, frequent meals are preferred to large meals given infrequently.
   f. Address anxiety, fear, and other emotional factors. Specialist consultation may be required if severe. Behavioral approaches such as relaxation and distraction have been found to be useful.
7. Pharmacologic therapies for nausea and vomiting: Table 32-2 lists the common palliative care strategies used for the treatment of nausea and vomiting.

---

* Rajagopal MR, Nandini V, Mathews L, Rajashree KC, Watson M. An Indian primer of palliative care—for medical students and doctors. Kerela: Trivandrum Institute of Palliative Science Publication; 2015.

TABLE 32-2 Antiemetic Choices Based on Etiology and Mechanism of Emesis

Clinical Clue	Mechanism/ Receptor/Site of Action	Drug Class	Dose
Chemical/ metabolic causes (opioids, hypercalcemia, uremia, chemotherapy)	Chemoreceptor trigger zone (CTZ)	Antidopamine Antiserotonin	Haloperidol 1.5–5.0 mg, PO BD or TDS, and PRN *or* 0.5–2 mg IV q8h Metoclopramide 10 mg QDS; 40 mg s/c over 24 h or domperidone 10 mg QDS OR Ondansetron 4–8 mg TDS Metoclopramide needs dose adjustment in renal failure and in older adults
Movement related	Vestibular dysfunction	Antihistaminic Anticholinergic	Promethazine 12–25 mg PO, q4–6h Cyclizine 25–50 mg, TDS, hyoscine hydrobromide 300 μg PO or SC, or 1000 μg/24 h transdermally *or* Cinnarizine
Bowel distension	Cholinergic, vomiting center	Anticholinergic	Scopolamine up to 3 patches q3 days
Gastric stasis	Dopamine, serotonin		Metoclopramide 10 mg TDS
Raised intracranial tension (ICT)	Cerebral cortex, CTZ Vestibular stimulation	Corticosteroids	Dexamethasone 4–8 mg/d for nausea and vomiting, up to 16 mg/d for raised ICT Cyclizine 50 mg PO stat, and BD or TDS
Anxiety, emotional/social factors, fear	Cerebral cortex, GABA	Benzodiazepine	Lorazepam 0.5–1 mg PO or IV q6h as needed

Prokinetics such as metoclopramide should never be combined with antimuscarinic agents (hyoscine butylbromide) as they are competitively blocked by the latter.
Bowel obstruction will be discussed in detail under the section Obstruction.

Refractory Nausea and Vomiting[11]

- **Levomepromazine:** Dose 6.25–25 mg twice a day, or 25–50 mg/d via continuous subcutaneous infusion
- **Olanzapine:** Dose 5–10 mg/d, PO (2.5–5 mg/d PO for older adults)
- **Ondansetron:** Dose 4–8 mg/d PO or IV as third-line agent for refractory nausea and vomiting

The evidence base for the effectiveness of the palliative care approach to management of nausea and vomiting is meager.[11] However, these strategies continue to be used by palliative care physicians worldwide for the past several decades.

Constipation[2,6]

In palliative care, constipation is commonly seen in cancer patients, among older adults with chronic serious illnesses, and as an adverse effect of opioid therapy.

Management

Goals of management of constipation in palliative care are as follows:

1. To reestablish comfortable bowel habits and to relieve pain and discomfort
2. To ensure well-being of the patient and to promote independence
3. To avoid other gastrointestinal symptoms such as nausea, vomiting, abdominal distension, and pain

Assessment

- Perform clinical history and examination to identify severity and cause of constipation.
- Rule out bowel obstruction. Ensure that the patient is passing flatus.
- Rule out impacted feces.
- Assess the state of hydration and nutrition.

Nonpharmacologic Methods

- Ensure adequate hydration and high-fiber diet.
- Encourage physical activity
- Ensure privacy and access to a toilet.
- Correct the reversible factors causing constipation

Pharmacologic Methods (Table 32-3)

- **First-line methods:** Generally, a combination of a stool softener and a stimulant laxative is effective in the management of constipation in palliative care.
  Bulk laxatives contain indigestible fiber and require high fluid intake by the patient, which may be difficult to implement in the palliative care patient and in older adults. Bulking agents are not effective in opioid-induced constipation.
- **Second-line methods:** Rectal suppositories and/or enema can be tried.
- **Third-line methods:** Manual evacuation of feces can be done. Consider use of a peripherally specific opioid antagonist methylnaltrexone in opioid-induced constipation.

TABLE 32-3 Classification of Laxatives[2,6]

Stimulant laxatives	Bisacodyl Dantron Senna Sodium picosulfate	
Softener laxatives	Osmotic laxatives	Lactulose syrup Liquid paraffin and magnesium hydroxide emulsion Macrogols (polyethylene glycols) Magnesium hydroxide suspension (milk of magnesia) Magnesium sulfate
	Surface wetting agents	Docusate sodium
	Lubricants	Liquid paraffin/mineral oil
Bulk-forming laxatives	Ispaghula husk Methylcellulose	

Opioid-Induced Constipation

- **Mechanism:** Reduced intestinal propulsive activity, increasing nonpropulsive activity, and enhanced absorption of fluids and electrolytes
- **Management**
  - Monitor bowel activity proactively in those who are on opioids.
  - Use of stimulant laxatives facilitate propulsive activity thereby counteracting opioid induced constipation. For example, Senna, bisacodyl, or dantron.
  - If >3 days since last bowel action, "uncork" using suppositories, for example, Bisacodyl 10 mg, Glycerine 4 mg, or a microenema.
  - Bulk-forming laxatives do not relieve opioid-induced constipation and may even worsen it.
  - Methylnaltrexone is a peripherally acting opioid antagonist, which does not fully cross the blood–brain barrier and hence acts to relieve constipation without reversing opioid analgesia. It is usually the last line of management.

Obstruction

Obstruction of the gastrointestinal system (Figure 32-5) can present in various ways depending on the degree, type, and site of obstruction.

Conventionally, the management of obstruction entails nasogastric tube for decompression, hydration, and surgical correction of the obstruction. In palliative care, most of these options would have been exhausted and the goal of therapy is relief of symptoms (nausea, vomiting, pain), comfort care, and feasible nutrition.

Management of Obstruction

1. Encourage ambulation
2. In those with no colic, who are passing flatus, the drug of choice is a prokinetic agent (metoclopramide 10 mg TDS).
3. If severe colic
   a. Prokinetics are contraindicated.
   b. Antisecretory and antispasmodic drugs should be prescribed:
      i. Hyoscine butylbromide 120–200 mg by continuous SC infusion, or Octreotide 250–500 μg/24 h by continuous SC infusion
      ii. Glycopyrronium
   c. Stop bulk-forming and osmotic laxatives.
   d. Enema with stool softener can be tried if constipation is a probable contributory factor.

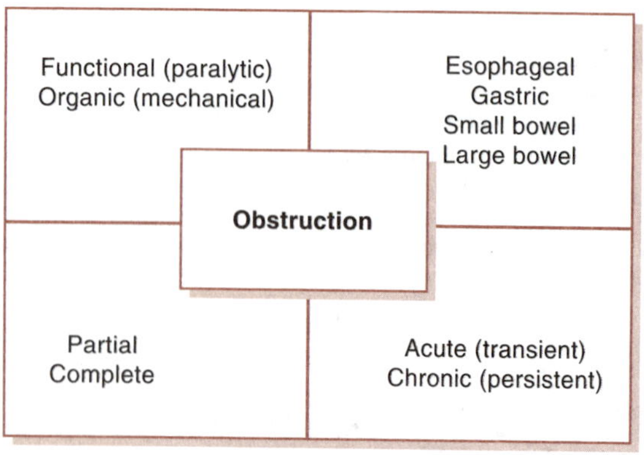

Figure 32-5 Approach to gastrointestinal obstruction.

4. If symptoms do not resolve after 7–10 days of the above-mentioned treatment, a trial of corticosteroids may be tried. A 3-day course of dexamethasone given PO or SC can be tried.
5. Morphine can be given for pain relief, and titrated upwards until relief.
6. Haloperidol 1.5–5 mg PO, SC can be given for nausea.
7. Ice cubes/small-volume fluids of choice can be tried to relieve thirst and dry mouth.

Itch

Pruritus is a common symptom in advanced malignancies. A few common causes are listed in Figure 32-6.

Management

General Measures

Dry skin is a common feature in most palliative care patients; general measures should focus on the management of dryness. Some useful methods are as follows:

- Discontinue the use of soap; use aqueous cream as a soap substitute.
- Avoid hot baths.
- Use emollients after bath.
- Avoid sweating.
- Discourage scratching; keep nails short; allow gentle rubbing.

Pharmacologic Management

1. Topical (for itchy skin rashes and insect bites)
   a. Aqueous cream + 1%–2% menthol
   b. Oily calamine lotion (containing 0.5%–1% phenol)
   c. Antihistamine creams (short-term use only)
2. Topical hydrocortisone cream 1% for contact dermatitis
3. Opioid-induced pruritus
   a. Ondansetron
   b. Opioid antagonists (contraindicated if opioid analgesia is required)
4. HIV: Indomethacin
5. Uremia: Thalidomide, UVB therapy, paroxetine, and mirtazapine
6. Paraneoplastic itch: Paroxetine

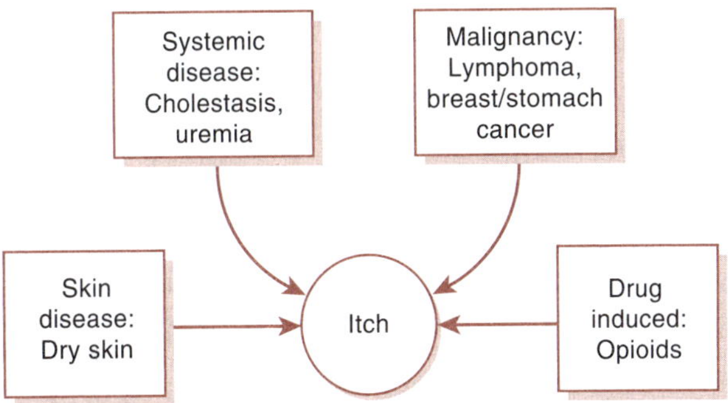

Figure 32-6 Common causes of itch.

Itch in Hodgkin lymphoma	Radiotherapy and/or chemotherapy if applicable	Corticosteroid (Dexamethasone 4–8 mg OD or prednisolone 30–60 mg OD)	H2 receptor antagonists—ranitidine	Mirtazapine 7.5–15 mg, every night
Itch in cholestasis	Stenting of the common bile duct	Naltrexone 12.5–250 mg OD or 17α-alkyl androgen (methyl testosterone 25 mg S/L OD or danazol 200 mg OD to TDS	Rifampicin 75 mg OD to 150 mg BD	Cholestyramine 4 g OD or BD
Paraneoplastic itch	Paroxetine 5–20 mg OD	Substitute mirtazapine 7.5–15 mg every night	Paroxetine + mirtazapine	Substitute thalidomide 100 mg every night

Figure 32-7 Treatment options for itch.

Figure 32-7 shows treatment flowcharts for itch due to cholestasis, Hodgkin lymphoma, and paraneoplastic itch.

Hiccups[12]

- **Persistent hiccups:** Last >48 hours
- **Intractable hiccups:** Last >1 month

Common Causes for Hiccups in Palliative Care

Common causes for hiccups in palliative care are:

- Gastric distension (common)
- Gastroesophageal reflex
- Diaphragmatic irritation
- Uremia

Management of Hiccups

- **Reduce gastric distension:** Metoclopramide 10 mg PO or domperidone 10–20 mg PO, and proton pump inhibitor to treat gastroesophageal reflux
- **Elevation of PCO_2:** Breath holding and rebreathing into a paper bag
- **Muscle relaxant:** Baclofen 5 mg PO, nifedipine 10–20 mg PO/SL, and midazolam 2 mg IV
- **Central suppression of hiccup reflex:** Haloperidol 5–10 mg, PO or IV given TDS, chlorpromazine 10–50 mg PO TDS or QDS or IV, and sodium valproate 200–500 mg PO or IV

Ascites

Management of Ascites in Palliative Care

1. Diuretic therapy
   a. Loop diuretics can be tapered and stopped once clinical response is obtained.
   b. Spironolactone: It is the mainstay of drug therapy in ascites because it counteracts the renin–angiotensin mechanism.
2. Paracentesis: Goal of therapy is to remove as much fluid as is needed to relieve symptoms of distress. Removal of as little as 2 L provides good symptomatic relief. Hypotension due to paracentesis is a rare problem in malignant ascites unlike in ascites due to chronic liver disease.
3. Semipermanent intra-abdominal catheter is useful for patients who are unable to visit the hospital frequently.

Lymphedema

It occurs following obstruction or interruption of lymphatic tissue following surgical resection, radiotherapy, or tumor. It commonly affects the limbs, but can also affect trunk, genitalia, or head.

Effects

- Skin changes: Thickening, fibrosis, oozing, and distortion of limb
- Infections: Blisters and maceration, which can lead to skin infections and cellulitis
- Loss of functional independence
- Psychological impact: Body image disturbance, embarrassment, and depression

Management

Nonpharmacologic management is key to improvement in chronic lymphedema. It involves a combination of the following:

- **Skin care:** The skin should be washed and moisturized daily at bedtime. Avoid trauma to the skin. Antibiotics should be instituted promptly if there is any sign of infection.
- **Massage:** Massage causes manual lymph drainage from the noncontractile lymphatics to the deeper intramuscular collecting lymphatics. This process is done for 60 minutes in each session.
- **Compression bandage:** Soon after massage, compression bandage is applied and maintained for most of the day.
- **Exercise:** Encourage passive or gentle active movements. Support the affected limb while resting.

After a week of intensive massage, compression bandage, and care, the lymphedema will show a significant reduction in most patients. They are then started on a self-managed regime of compression bandaging with as-needed manual lymph drainage.

Communication in Serious Illness[2,6,7,13–15]

Effective communication skills are essential to the delivery of quality palliative care. With the rise in serious health-related suffering all over the world, the number of patients with prolonged disease trajectories is increasing. With the advance in technology over the past few decades, there is an increase in therapeutic options for many chronic medical illnesses. Many of these patients and their families face complex medical decisions and social and financial burdens which lead to a myriad of emotions. Physicians who treat these patients often lack the communication skills training and are unequipped to handle the implications arising from these scenarios, resulting in conflicts, poor compliance to care, and often litigation. Physicians who are not trained in high-quality end-of-life conversations avoid these conversations and instead focus on details of therapeutic interventions rather than on the patient's goals of care, suffering, and the burden of family members.

Every physician involved in treating serious illnesses should have basic training and access to tools required for effective patient communication. In this chapter, we present a few brief concepts and handy tools for communication, for the physician who is involved in the care of seriously ill patients.

Barriers to Effective Communication (Faced by Physicians)

1. Lack of privacy
2. Lack of time
3. Collusion
4. Physician discomfort with discussing end-of-life issues/unpleasant prognosis
5. Not perceiving communication as "*part of their job*"
6. Worry about patient losing hope

7. Lack of familiarity with the patient's language and culture
8. Lack of training and skills needed for effective communication
9. Inability to say "*I do not know*"

Communication Barriers Faced by Patients/Family

1. Fear of hospital/loss of control in unfamiliar surroundings
2. Inability to follow medical jargon
3. Fear and guilt, caused by interpersonal factors
4. Paternalistic healthcare system in which discussion and free questions are discouraged; fear of treatment being denied if questions are raised
5. Language, cultural and social barriers

Behaviors which should be Avoided by Healthcare Professionals as they Lead to Poor Communication

1. Avoid moralizing/lecturing.
2. Avoid threatening/paternalistic culture.
3. Avoid exclamations of surprise, intolerance, or disgust.
4. Avoid being defensive. Do not argue.
5. Avoid distancing behaviors: Distancing behaviors prevent the patients and caregivers from engaging with the doctor on a psychosocial level. They feel discouraged to express negative emotions and fears, which eventually lead to an increase in frustration and resentment often directed toward the healthcare system.
    a. Avoiding labeling a patient (e.g., "She's a breast case" or "He's a troublesome patient")
    b. Paying selective attention to "safe" physical concerns of the patient (e.g., "Doctor, I am worried about my future. I am losing weight and my neck pain has returned." Doctor replies, "Yes, tell me about your neck pain.")
    c. Premature normalizing (e.g., to tell a crying patient, "Don't worry, everyone in your place would feel upset," instead of "I can see you are upset. Can you tell me what is upsetting you?")
    d. Using only closed questions
    e. Jollying along and expecting the patient to keep a brave face ("Come on, it's a bright and sunny day, there's no need to look so sad!")
    f. Inappropriate humor

Differences in education, culture, social factors, and life experiences between patients and healthcare professionals lead to barriers in communication and recognition of these differences is key to mitigation.

It is said that words make up 7% of communication, whereas tone accounts for 38% and nonverbal cues form 55% of the overall communication. Congruence between all three components is essential for effective communication.

Good Communication

Good communication (Figure 32-8) should be unambiguous, delivered with clarity and compassion, and natural. Effective communication skills are best delivered in a background of warmth, genuineness, empathy, acceptance, dignity, and trust.

Given in the subsequent text are some of good communication skills which are useful to the physician treating serious illness.

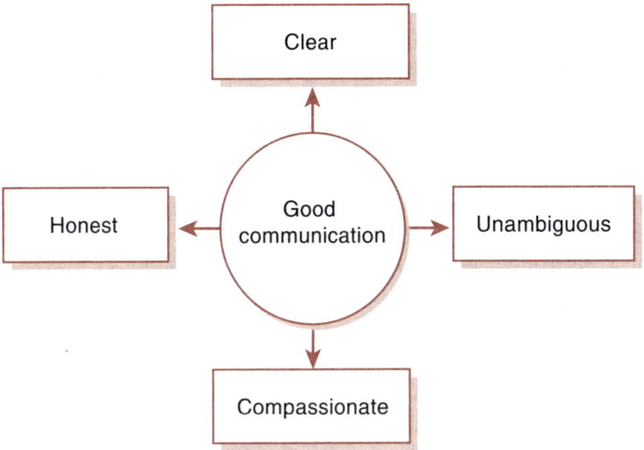

Figure 32-8 Characteristics of good communication.

Active Listening

Nonverbal Techniques	Verbal Cues
Be seated at the eye level.	Stop talking; avoid interruptions.
Make eye contact.	If the patient stops midsentence, encourage him or her to continue by repeating the last three words of the patient. This gives him or her permission to continue.
Nod regularly, to indicate that you are paying attention.	
Posture should reflect attentiveness: Sit erect and lean toward the patient.	Ask about feelings, for example, "How does that make you feel?"
Touch: Place a hand on the patient's hand/shoulder (be culture appropriate).	Validate feelings: "It's natural to feel like that."
Observe the body language of the patient/caregiver.	Summarize to check the accuracy of your understanding of the patient's problems.

Open Questions

Avoid leading and closed questions. Instead, use open questions to elicit the patient's feeling and to encourage communication.

Leading questions elicit the answers that the physician wants to hear. For example, "Are you feeling tired?"
Closed questions These questions produce yes/no answers. For example, "Do you have pain?" "Have you managed well since our last conversation?"
Open questions are *how* and *what* questions. They encourage patients to express their worries and concerns. For example, "How are you feeling today?" "How have you been coping since we last met?"

Silence[6]

Studies have revealed that patient satisfaction scores depend on the physicians' use of silence and reaction time latency between speakers. *Most patients are known to take at least 2 minutes to reply, whereas most physicians interrupt their patients within 18–23 seconds!*[2] Allowing silence during conversation facilitates dialogue between patients and doctors. It allows both the patient and the physician time to gather thoughts and assimilate what has been said so far. Silence may imply intense emotion and an inability to express it in words, and thus it needs to be acknowledged. A prolonged silence can be broken by gentle enquiry, for example, "What are you thinking right now? Why did you pause?" Nonverbal gestures of reassurance will help the patients to wade through their emotions.

Delivering Serious News

Commonly known by the term *breaking bad news*, here we have chosen to use the term *delivering serious news*[16] to reiterate the gentleness and sensitivity with which the news should be conveyed to the patients and/or their families as opposed to the use of the word "breaking" which suggests force! Most physicians have little or no training in end-of-life conversations and report low confidence in doing so effectively. The following text provides an oft-used tool, which is a six-step protocol called SPIKES[17] that has been validated in delivering serious news to cancer patients. Several other toolkits are also useful such as the Serious illness Conversation Guide[18] and the GUIDE[19] tool, which also help to deliver bad news in seriously ill patients. Serious news refers to any news that may be life-threatening, but may also include information regarding failure of treatment, transitions of care, or death of a loved one.

The SPIKES protocol (**Table 32-4**), a six-step protocol, is used as a training tool to teach basic communication skills to medical graduates. Delivering serious news should

TABLE 32-4 The "SPIKES" Protocol

			Remarks
S	Setting	Ensure privacy. Involve significant others. Find a chair. It is better to be seated at eye level during the session. Build a rapport with the patient. Avoid interruptions.	Sitting down relaxes the patient. It also tells the patient that the doctor is not too busy to talk.
P	Perception	Always, before you tell, **ASK**. Check about patient's knowledge about the disease. Correct misconceptions if any. Identify unrealistic expectations.	Use open-ended questions here to elicit information. For example, "What have you been told about your disease so far?"
I	Invitation	Summarize the case. *Obtain permission* to reveal the serious news. **REMEMBER** to allow the *patient to be in control* of the conversation.	Studies across the world have shown that majority of the patients want to know their diagnosis. However, some patients might choose to not know their prognosis as a valid psychological coping mechanism.

(Continued)

TABLE 32-4 The "SPIKES" Protocol (Continued)

			In traditional Eastern societies, the family may prevent the doctor from revealing the diagnosis directly to the patient.
K	Knowledge	Give a warning shot. Provide the serious news in the form of a single-headline sentence. "Chunk and check"—this is a method by which information is given in small chunks, while periodically checking on the patient, for understanding and for emotions. Do not overload a massive volume of information at once. If the patient wishes, stop and reconvene a meeting at a later date to discuss future strategies for care.	Warning shot: For example, "I am sorry to tell you that ...." "I am afraid the test results are not very good ...."
E	Emotion and empathy	***Expect*** emotion and express empathy (use the NURSE mnemonic to express empathy). ***Explore*** for emotions and ***acknowledge*** the patient's feelings.	**Explore:** Can you tell me more about it? Can you tell me what worries you? **Validate** the patient's emotions: "Many other patients have felt the same way you did." "I think anyone would react the same way you did."
S	Strategy and summary	Close the conversation by summarizing to verify patient understanding. Discuss future strategy (tests, referrals, treatment options). **AVOID** saying, "There is nothing more that we can do for you." ***NONABANDONMENT*** is key. Offer a means of contact if further questions arise.	Strategy for the future could be something as simple as the patient scheduling a discussion with a family member.

be done with utmost care and sensitivity keeping in mind the wishes, needs, culture, and resources of the patient.[2]

Empathy and emotions represent the most challenging stage for most physicians during a session on delivering serious news. Empathy[20] has two components: (1) gaining a clear understanding of another person's feelings or situation and (2) communicating that understanding back to the patient in a visible and supportive way. The mnemonic NURSE[21] empowers the physician in responding to emotions and to empathize (Table 32-5).

TABLE 32-5 Responding to Empathy

The "NURSE" Mnemonic		Examples
N	Naming	Name the emotion. Turn down the intensity by a notch when you name it.
U	Understanding	This helps me to understand what you are thinking.
R	Respecting	Praise or offer respect to the patient for his or her efforts in coping. "This must be really difficult to deal with ...."
S	Supporting	Offer your commitment in helping the patient through the suffering.
E	Exploring	Explore and encourage the patient to discuss, for example, "Could you tell me more about how you feel about this?"

Goals-of-Care Discussion[22]

This usually follows the delivery of serious news. Here, the physician should aim to elicit the values, goals, and fears of a patient. This does not refer to discussion about therapeutic interventions and is rather an attempt by the doctor to understand the patient as a fellow human being so that he or she can help the patient to decide on the future course of action in accordance with his or her beliefs.

Values tell us how the patient approaches the world and thereby takes his or her decisions regarding his or her health. *Goals* refer to targets that the patient hopes to reach during the disease progression such as symptom relief, quality of life, being independent, to be mentally alert, and to live long enough to achieve a milestone or attend a long-awaited family event. All goals may not be attainable, but an understanding of the goals and values of a patient will help the healthcare team to align treatment decisions to match the goals. The REMAP tool[23] helps to conduct a goals-of-care discussion (Table 32-6).

TABLE 32-6 The REMAP Tool

Reframe	The physician here reframes the patient's case history to reveal the larger picture, often in the context of a new diagnosis or a change in prognosis. It is important thereby to first elicit the patient's understanding of illness at this point by reframing the context. It could also function as a delivering of serious news in case the patient is completely unaware of the disease prognosis. Use a teach-back technique at the end to ask the patient to repeat his or her understanding of the conversation.
Emotion	Expect emotion after reframe. Respond with empathy. Emotions may be expressed verbally or nonverbally. *It is important to remember that the patient's enquiries about further treatment options may actually be an expression of emotion rather than a medical query.* It is important that the physician recognize and acknowledge the emotion. The NURSE mnemonic can be handy here.
	The physician may have to revisit the emotion several times until it is resolved. If the patient appears overwhelmed, the rest of the interview may have to be cut short and rescheduled.

(Continued)

TABLE 32-6 The REMAP Tool (Continued)

Map	Here, the physician should map out the values of the patient. The discussion should focus on patients' goals for treatment in the context of their values. Ask evocative questions to elicit values. Explore their fears. Patients may express concern about the welfare of dependents such as children, express a wish to die without pain, etc. The values and goals will determine the healthcare choices that they subsequently make. The patient's priorities between life extension and quality of life can be explored here.
Align	The physician verbally reflects back and summarizes the patient's values and goals including ambivalence regarding several core decisions. The patients may further clarify or expand on these values during this phase.
Propose a plan	After the patient signals an affirmation of all the goals and values, the physician can proceed to the planning stage. The physician then proceeds to propose a medical plan which aligns the best possible medical options with the patient's core values. The physician should present a patient-centric plan with the chief aim being achievement of the patient's goals. In cases where the patients or family choose to not get an input from the doctor, they should be allowed to decide their own plans and communicate the same.
	Enquiring whether the plan is acceptable to the patient and allowing questions helps to conclude the conversation.

A goals-of-care discussion helps the doctor to align specific future interventions such as hospitalizations, use of mechanical ventilators, and do not resuscitate orders with the goals, values, and fears of the patient.

Collusion

This occurs when the patient's family conspires with the healthcare provider to conceal the diagnosis/prognosis from the patient. This is usually done to safeguard the patient from worry and sometimes works as a psychological coping mechanism.

Collusion is harmful when it hinders good-quality care, is harmful to the patient, and leads to use of futile medical interventions. A nonconfrontational approach with exploration of the family's reasons for collusion, reassurance, and clarification regarding prognosis may help the physician to break collusion and to align family values with the best interests of the patient.

Elizabeth Kubler Ross described the following four stages of grief:

1. Denial
2. Anger
3. Bargaining
4. Acceptance

Patients facing a difficult prognosis may experience the same. All patients may not experience all stages and may not experience them in sequence.

Denial

This is a common defense mechanism. It occurs when a person attempts to eliminate a threatening reality by ignoring it. This may be associated with underlying anxiety. It needs to be addressed if it interferes with the acceptance of treatment, interpersonal relationships, and planning for the future.

Managing denial:

- Explore whether denial is due to lack of correct information/understanding of medical diagnosis.
- If denial is a sign of underlying fear, explore the patient's feelings; provide emotional support.
- Avoid direct confrontation.
- Assure the patient of constant support from the healthcare team. Reassure regarding nonabandonment.

Anger

- A response to helplessness and fear
- Indicative of poor communication between the healthcare team and the patient
- May result in a withdrawn, uncooperative, depressed patient if suppressed
- May result in litigation
- Often unleashed on a close and nonthreatening person

Managing anger:

- Name and acknowledge the emotion.
- Ensure that both the patient and the physician are seated. Make eye contact.
- Maintain calm and express empathy.
- If there is risk of violence, ensure prompt access to hospital security.

Summary

- Palliative care works on enhancing the quality of life for patients and their families by addressing physical, emotional, social, and spiritual needs.
- The principles of palliative care include autonomy, beneficence, nonmaleficence, and justice.
- Understanding the illness trajectories helps us to plan appropriate treatment.
- Palliative care focuses on providing continuity of care throughout the illness trajectory, from diagnosis through the end of life and into bereavement support for families.
- Individual symptom management, psychosocial support, good and effective communication, and cultural sensitivity form the basis of effective palliative care.
- The "SPIKES" protocol, the REMAP tool can be used for effective communication and goals of care discussion.

Scan the QR code to access chapter references.

33 End-of-Life Care

Sheetal Raj M.

End-of-life care (EoLC)[1–3] is a subset of palliative care and refers to an approach to care whereby the focus is shifted toward comfort care, and away from curative intent therapies. During EoLC, the patients may have less than 12 months to live and death is imminent. The focus of care is on comfort, dignity, good symptom control, quality of life, and ***quality of dying***. EoLC also includes bereavement support to the family for up to 13 months after the death (Figure 33-1).

The acute care model of Western medicine is unsuited for the relief of the suffering seen in chronic progressive medical illnesses. As modern medicine works *to cure always and relieve suffering if one has the time and leaves the comforting to someone else*,[2] we in this chapter on EoLC hope to revisit Hippocrates aphorism, "***to cure sometimes, to relieve often and to comfort always.***"

Advances in technology and rise in chronic progressive medical illnesses have led to prolongation of the process of dying (dialysis, ventilators, intravenous fluids, antibitoics, left ventricular assist devices, etc.) (Figure 32-2). Although death itself is not difficult to diagnose, predicting it is fraught with uncertainty.[2,4] The Gold Standards Framework[1] of the United Kingdom attempted to define criteria for early identification of patients with palliative care needs. They have defined general and specific indicators of clinical decline which aim to help the physician to identify the patients who need EoLC. Identifying the common disease trajectories helps the physician to institute early and appropriate palliative care measures. Accordingly, there are ***three triggers***[1] which help physicians to define patients who need EoLC:

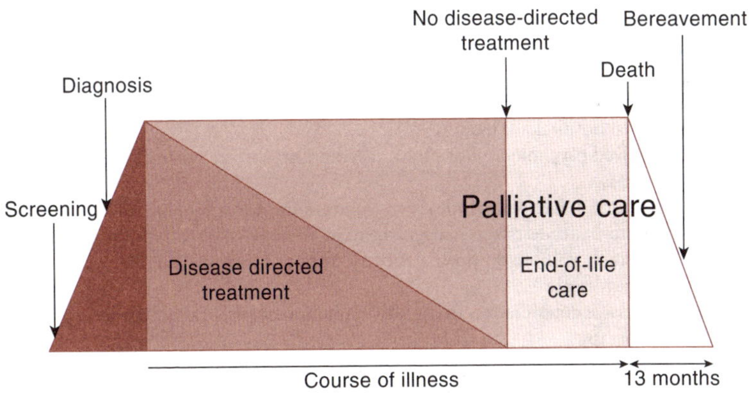

Figure 33-1 Representing the continuum of palliative care and end-of-life care in an illness trajectory.

- **The Surprise Question**
  - Would you be surprised if this patient were to die in the next few months, weeks, or days?

OR

- **General indicators of decline**
  - Functional decline (measured by Barthel Index, Karnofsky Performance Status Score, or the WHO/Eastern Cooperative Oncology Group Performance Status) with increasing dependence or the patient being bed bound or chair bound for >50% of the day
  - Presence of multimorbidity
  - Patient choosing no further active treatment (e.g., no further dialysis)
  - Weight loss of >10% in 6 months
  - Repeated unplanned hospital admissions or crises
  - Serum albumin <2.5 mg/dL
  - A sentinel event such as a major fall or bereavement

OR

- **Disease-specific indicators of decline:** Early identification of disease trajectories helps to anticipate and address the needs of patients in end of life. The following disease-specific criteria are commonly used to identify patients who need EoLC:
  - Cancer (rapid and predictable decline)
    - Presence of metastatic disease along with poor functional status as measured by performance scales (e.g., Palliative Performance Scale with a score ≤50%)
  - Organ failure (erratic decline)
    - Obstructive airway disease (COPD/bronchial asthma)/interstitial lung disease (any two of the following criteria)
      - Stage 4 or 5 MRC grade of dyspnea
      - FeV_1 <30% of predicted
      - Presence of cor pulmonale
      - Patients on long-term oxygen therapy
      - Patients on systemic steroids for the past 6 months
      - Recent ICU admission or infection with drug-resistant organisms
    - Cardiac failure
      - Severe dyspnea, NYHA stage 3 or 4
      - Repeated hospital admissions
      - Unresolved psychological or physical symptoms despite optimal therapy
    - Renal disease
      - Stage 4 or 5 CKD with clinical deterioration in the form of any of the following:
        - Symptomatic despite renal replacement therapy (nausea, vomiting, anorexia, intractable volume overload, pruritus, or poor functional status)
    - Neurologic disease
      1. Progressive deterioration in cognitive function or physical function despite optimal therapy
      2. Dysphagia leading to aspiration pneumonia, respiratory failure, or sepsis
      3. Increasing difficulty with speech and communications

    PLUS
    - Any of the following disease-specific factors:

      A. Stroke
        - Poststroke cognitive impairment

- ▲ Persistent vegetative state or minimally conscious state
- ▲ Lack of improvement within 3 months of onset of stroke

B. Dementia/frailty (gradual decline)
- ▲ Worsening activities of daily living with Barthel score <3 **PLUS**
- ▲ Infections (pressure sores, UTI, etc.)
- ▲ Reduced oral intake

C. Parkinson disease
- ▲ Increasing off periods, dyskinesias, and falls
- ▲ Psychological symptoms such as depression, psychosis, or anxiety
- ▲ Functional decline
- ▲ Drug treatment which is less effective or use of complex treatment regimes

D. Motor neuron disease
- ▲ Vital capacity <70% of predicted
- ▲ Marked rapid decline in physical status
- ▲ Dyskinesias, mobility issues, and falls

The **Palliative Performance Scale**[4] is another useful scale to identify patients with a limited life span who would benefit from EoLC. It uses general criteria such as ambulation, self-care, intake, level of consciousness, and activity levels to identify patients with limited survival and is more patient centered than disease-specific criteria.

A few terms[5] for use in EoLC are as follows:

- **Terminal illness**: An irreversible or incurable disease condition from which death is expected in the foreseeable future.
- **Actively dying**: The hours or days preceding imminent death during which time the patient's physiological functions wane.
- **Life-sustaining treatment**: Life-sustaining treatment comprises any medical treatment that artificially supports or replaces a body function essential to the life of the person. (It includes cardiopulmonary resuscitation [CPR], endotracheal intubation, mechanical ventilation, vasopressor therapy, parenteral or artificial enteral nutrition, dialysis,[4] blood products, antibiotics, and intravenous fluids.)
- **Euthanasia**: Euthanasia is the intentional act of killing a dying patient with terminal illness by the direct intervention of a doctor, for the purpose of good of the patient.

CARE OF THE DYING PATIENT

How to identify that the patient is actively dying

The points given in the subsequent text are clinical aids to help the physician in ***recognizing the dying patient***.[3,4] However, they are not definite clinical criteria and they may merely suggest poor prognosis and may not be indicative of a definite timeline for death. A patient who is sedated or on mechanical ventilation may not show any of these signs or symptoms.

The following clinical signs are usually present *during the last 72 hours of a patient's life*:

- Progressively falling blood pressure
- Tachycardia progressing to bradycardia and asystole
- Peripheral vasoconstriction—cold peripheries
- Altered breathing pattern (Cheyne–Stokes/irregular breathing)
- Change in skin color—duller/grayish blue/mottling, bluish nails
- Patient being increasingly bed bound/no spontaneous movements
- No verbalizing and no response to questions by the patient
- Total detachment from surroundings/nil interest in food/water
- Bedridden patient with diminishing spontaneous movement

- Decreased passage of stools (do not intervene unless there is significant discomfort from distension/impaction)
- Decreased urine output (rule out bladder outlet obstruction)
- Comatose
- Severe cachexia
- Agitation/paranoia/terminal delirium

Clinical features indicative of less than 24-hour survival are as follows:

- Loss of radial pulse
- Onset of jaw jerk with each breath
- Terminal delirium
- Terminal fever
- Pooling of secretions

Psychosocial needs at End of Life

- Need to reconcile, to forgive, to affirm
- Need for closure
- Process of life review for patients and their caregivers

Spiritual needs at End of Life[4]

- To identify the meaning of life and examine their legacy to their loved ones/to society Identify spiritual angst and address it, as it causes the *most severe form of suffering*.

SYMPTOM MANAGEMENT IN EoLC[2,3,6]

Symptom	Principles of Management
Pain	• Route of drug administration may need to be changed • Switch morphine PO to SC or SC infusion (or IV infusion if in hospital setup) • ***Remember*** that unconscious patients may also experience pain
Nausea and vomiting	Use IV metoclopramide. Consider SC or IV haloperidol or cyclizine for refractory cases
Terminal breathlessness	• Reassure the patient and family. Address the fear of suffocating to death • Optimize drug treatment with morphine/benzodiazepine and oxygen • Palliative sedation: It masks the distress caused by the dyspnea. Combine opioid + sedative anxiolytic given by continuous subcutaneous infusion and SC PRN (e.g., morphine + midazolam) • Haloperidol can be added if the patient develops confusion/agitation
Terminal agitation[5]	• Often associated with delirium • Haloperidol 10–30 mg/24 h and/or midazolam 10–60 mg/24 h by continuous subcutaneous infusion • Note that patients with a history of torture/abuse/violence in the past are at higher risk of agitation. Unresolved psychosocial trauma results in greater agitation • Refractory cases: Levomepromazine 25–50 mg stat, followed by 50–200 mg/24 h *or* phenobarbital 100–200 mg SC stat, followed by 800–1600 mg/24 h can be tried
Care of skin and mucosa	• Positioning, care of pressure points • Mouth care: Sponge-tipped swabs can be used to moisten the mouth • Eye care: Methylcellulose eye drops can be used

(*Continued*)

(*Continued*)

Pooling of secretions[5]	Also known as the death rattle , it refers to the rattling noise produced by the pooling of secretions in the hypopharynx oscillating with the respiratory cycles. It occurs in the last few hours of a person's life and is distressing to the relatives and caregivers. It is NOT distressing to the patient
	Management
	• Nonpharmacologic methods
	  • Educate the family/caregivers that the secretions are not distressing to the semiconscious/unconscious patient
	  • AVOID suctioning unless the patient is unconscious, as it causes distress to semiconscious/conscious patients
	  • Semiprone position to encourage postural drainage
	    • Hyoscine hydrobromide 0.4–0.6 mg SC, 1.2–2.4 mg continuous subcutaneous infusion
	• Pharmacologic methods
	  • Antisecretory drugs
	    • Glycopyrronium 0.2–0.4 mg SC stat, followed by 0.6–1.2 mg by continuous subcutaneous infusion
	    • Hyoscine butylbromide 20 mg SC stat, followed by 20–40 mg by continuous subcutaneous infusion
	Note: Bronchial secretions or secretions caused by gastric reflux do not respond to antisecretory agents (pseudo-death rattle)

Terminal hemorrhage[5,7,8]	*Definition*: Massive hemorrhage that is likely to progress rapidly to death due to hypovolemic shock. Most commonly caused due to carotid blowout
	At-risk patients
	• Head and neck cancer patients—postsurgery, postradiation, tumor encasing carotid artery (most common)
	• Hematologic malignancies (with severe thrombocytopenia)
	• Hemoptysis, gastrointestinal bleeding, vaginal bleeding from cervical or uterine cancer
	• Patients with sentinel bleeds are the ones at maximum risk
	Classification: They can be divided based on risk of bleed as follows:
	• Threatened bleed: Imaging that is suggestive of impending rupture *or* presence of an exposed artery
	• Impending bleed: Sentinel bleed caused by a transoral or transcervical bleed typically caused by a carotid pseudoaneurysm, which resolves by pressure or packing. It is a trivial bleed that heralds massive hemorrhage in the next 24–28 h
	• Acute bleed: Massive hemorrhage not controlled by conservative measures
	Management
	• If the patient is ambulant
	  • Early endovascular stenting as prophylaxis
	  • Use pressure with a gloved finger followed by resuscitation with fluids and blood and airway management (impending and acute bleed)

(*Continued*)

(*Continued*)

Symptom	Principles of Management

	• If the patient is bed bound and in the final weeks or days of life, institute EoLC as follows:
	  • Educate the patient and/or family and caregivers regarding the impending bleed. Allay anxiety and reassure them regarding rarity of the event. Ensure adequate preparation without causing panic
	  • Address modifiable risk factors: Stop NSAIDs, aspirin, and anticoagulants
	  • Consider transfusion of platelets, FFP, and vitamin K administration if clinically feasible
	  • Prepare an emergency care plan: Discuss with the patient and/or family and healthcare team whether and where to shift the patient in case of bleed
	  • Prepare a crisis pack containing the following:
	    • Readily available dark-colored towels and linen (to reduce distress caused by bright red blood on white linen)
	    • Universal precautions using goggles/face mask and gloves to shield from arterial spurt
	    • Suctioning device if available and feasible
	    • Warm blankets—as the patient may be cold from hypotension
	    • Predrawn syringes with midazolam/benzodiazepine
	• The A, B, C of managing the event—Assurance, Be there, Comfort and Calm
	  • Continuous company during the event. NEVER leave the patient alone. Position the family so that they can be in close physical contact, but not in direct view of the catastrophic bleed
	  • Provide direct pressure with a gloved finger on the site of bleed
	  • Rapid sedation to palliate fear, dyspnea, and suffocation: Consider a combination of IV or subcutaneous diazepam/midazolam 5–20 mg until the patient is unconscious
	  • Bereavement support: Provide support to family members who witnessed the event. Monitor for complicated grief and post-traumatic stress disorder among family members. Debrief the healthcare team that witnessed the event and offer support where needed

COMMUNICATION IN EoL[2–6]

The key goals of communication during end-of-life discussions are as follows:

- Establishing a consensus about the disease process among the caregivers
  - Prognostic uncertainty in chronic medical illnesses combined with the presence of a multitude of specialists involved in care of these patients makes it difficult to establish a consensus regarding the progress of the patient's suffering. Recognizing the dying patient and identifying medical futility are key challenges to establishing a consensus.
- Honest, accurate, and early disclosure of prognosis to the patient and family
  - Use of the SPIKES model can help in compassionate disclosure of prognosis to the patient/family.
- Discussion of end-of-life decisions with the patient and family
  - After disclosure of poor prognosis, the healthcare team should proceed to explore the Goals of Care preferences of the patient.

- Although, traditionally, a paternalistic culture for medical decision making was followed in the past, (in which the physician takes all decisions unilaterally while the patient plays a passive role), most recent research has suggested a preference for the **shared decision-making model** in all cultures. In shared decision making, both the patient and the physician express their views and share information regarding their preferences, values, and disease progress after which decisions regarding end of life are taken based on a consensus of opinions between the healthcare team and the patient and/or the patient's surrogates, and responsibility for the same is shared by all.
- The standard modalities of **limiting life-prolonging treatment** should be discussed with any patient or surrogate who is considering comfort care only. They are as follows:
  - *Do not intubate/do not resuscitate (DNI/DNR) orders*: This is a decision not to initiate CPR in a terminally ill patient/intubate the patient, when the chances of the patient surviving the procedure are very low. These are bona fide statements signed by the patient when he/she has capacity or by the healthcare surrogate when the patient loses such capacity. It aims to reduce the avoidable physical trauma and possibility of prolongation of suffering in the terminally ill patient.
  - *Withholding of life support/do not escalate order*: This constitutes a decision not to institute new treatment or escalate existing life-prolonging therapies (such as ventilation, intubation, antibiotics, inotropes, dialysis, or intravenous fluids) with the understanding that the patient will probably die from the illness.
  - *Withdrawal of life support*: This is removal of an ongoing life-sustaining treatment with the plan to not substitute an alternative treatment, with the understanding that the patient may die following the change in therapy primarily due to the underlying illness.
- **End-of-life discussions** include the following key topics:
  - *Appointment of a healthcare proxy/surrogate*: This refers to a person or persons other than the healthcare providers who is/are accepted as the representatives of the patient's best interests, who will make decisions on behalf of the patient when the patient loses his/her capacity to make healthcare decisions. In the absence of a designated surrogate chosen by the patient, the next of kin become the surrogate.
  - *Advance directives*: It is a statement made by a person with decision-making capacity stating his/her wishes regarding how to be treated or not at a stage when s/he loses such capacity. This includes living will and healthcare proxies and DNR orders. It also includes the patient's choice of place for EoLC.
  - *Clinically assisted nutrition and hydration (CANH)*: This includes Ryles tube feed, percutaneous gastrostomy, and intravenous fluids. The benefits, burden, and risks of continuing CANH in the end of life are not clear-cut. While it may provide symptom relief and improved quality of life in some patients, it may also prolong the period of suffering in an actively dying patient whose nutritional needs are minimal. A frank discussion should be conducted with the patient/surrogate regarding the risks and benefits of CANH, and also taking into consideration the cultural and religious values of the patient and family. The idea of food as nurture may not be relevant to a dying patient and consensus should be attempted by compassionate discussions with the family. Following a decision to withhold/withdraw CANH, the patient should be periodically monitored and reassessed and the decision revisited if clinically relevant or if requested by the family.
  - *Discussions should also include creation of opportunities for expression of spiritual needs and to address unfinished business.*

Decisions to withhold/withdraw life-prolonging treatment and advance directives are executed based on local law and regulations of each country.

BEREAVEMENT[6]

Bereavement is a period of mourning and grief following death of a loved one. **Mourning** is an overt expression of grief, which is often culturally influenced. **Grief** refers to feeling of sorrow, loss, anger, guilt, or confusion that arises when one experiences a loss. It may also manifest in the form of physical symptoms such as insomnia, nausea, and vomiting; changes in interpersonal relationships; or spiritual distress.

The process of EoLC does not end with the death of the patient, but continues in the form of bereavement support provided by the palliative care team to the family of the deceased for up to 13 months after the death. An interdisciplinary team member is assigned to the family for support and guidance during post-death period for funeral and burial planning.

Uncomplicated grief evolves and allows the family to adjust to the loss over a period of 1–2 years. However, in some cases, grief may be prolonged and may require counseling and psychosocial support. While a visit by a member of the interdisciplinary team or phone calls may be sufficient to help most of the families, some may require specialist support and counseling.

Prolonged grief is commonly seen in the following cases:

- Unexpected/violent death/suicide of a loved one
- Lack of support systems or friendships
- Being unprepared for death
- Close or dependent relationship with the deceased

Bereavement support may be enriched by the help of local support groups or community initiatives, or by enlisting help of the primary physician.

We would like to end this chapter by listing the principles of a "good death."[9] The EoLC physician would do well to remember that control, autonomy, and independence are key themes in ensuring good EoLC.

Principles of a Good Death

- To know when death is coming, and to understand what can be expected
- To be able to retain control of what happens
- To be afforded dignity and privacy
- To have control over pain relief and other symptom control
- To have choice and control over where death occurs (at home or elsewhere)
- To have access to information and expertise of whatever kind is necessary
- To have access to any spiritual or emotional support required
- To have access to hospice care in any location, not only in hospital
- To have control over who is present and who shares the end
- To be able to issue advance directives which ensure that wishes are respected
- To have time to say goodbye, and control over other aspects of timing
- To be able to leave when it is time to go, and not to have life prolonged pointlessly

Summary

- End-of-life care deals with the inevitability of death and focuses on enhancing the quality of life for individuals facing terminal illnesses or advanced age.
- It addresses holistic palliative care, shared decision making, advanced care planning, and bereavement support.
- It is important to identify the signs that a patient is actively dying.
- Symptoms of pain, nausea, vomiting, dyspnoea, agitation should me actively managed.

Scan the QR code to access chapter references.

Appendix A

Immunizations and Postexposure Therapies

Carlos Mejia-Chew and Stephen Y. Liang

Introduction

- **Active immunization** promotes the development of a durable primary immune response (B-cell proliferation, antibody response, T-cell sensitization) directed toward a specific pathogen such that subsequent exposure to that pathogen results in a secondary immune response that protects against infection (Table A-1).
- **Passive immunization** involves the administration of immune globulin resulting in transient protection against infection. It is usually employed in a host with limited capacity to mount a primary immune response, when exposure to a pathogen occurs in a previously unvaccinated host, or to protect against toxin-mediated disease.
- **Postexposure prophylaxis** is therapy given following exposure to a pathogen to prevent the development of disease. This can include active immunization, passive immunization, and/or antimicrobial therapy (Tables A-2 and A-3).
- **Adverse events potentially related to vaccination** should be reported through the Vaccine Adverse Event Reporting System at http://vaers.hhs.gov/ or 1-800-822-7967.
- **More information**, including adult vaccination schedules, recommendations regarding travel, and up-to-date guidelines can be found at the Centers for Disease Control and Prevention (CDC) website, http://www.cdc.gov/. Additional guidance for specific clinical questions can be obtained by contacting the CDC directly at 1-800-232-4636 (1-800-CDC-INFO) or via e-mail at NIPINFO@cdc.gov.

TABLE A-1 Selected Adult Immunization Recommendations in the United States

Vaccine, Dose	Indications & Dosing	Contraindications	Precautions
Haemophilus influenzae type b (Hib) Hib conjugate vaccine: 0.5 mL IM	**Unvaccinated adults with anatomic or functional asplenia (including sickle cell disease) or undergoing elective splenectomy (preferably 14 d before surgery):** Administer 1 dose **Hematopoietic stem cell transplant recipients 6–12 mo after successful transplant:** Administer three doses (4 wk apart)	Severe allergic reaction to any vaccine component or after a previous dose	Moderate or severe acute illness with or without fever
Hepatitis A Single-antigen hepatitis A vaccine (HepA; Havrix, Vaqta): 1 mL IM Combined hepatitis A/hepatitis B vaccine (HepA-Hep B; Twinrix): 1 mL IM	**Any adult seeking protection from hepatitis A virus (HAV)** **Specific indications:** travel to countries with high or intermediate HAV endemicity (including infants 6 mo and older); men who have sex with men (MSM); injection or noninjection drug use; laboratory workers exposed to HAV; clotting factor disorders; chronic liver disease; persons who anticipate close personal contact with an adoptee from a country with high or intermediate HAV endemicity during the first 60 d after arrival in the United States; healthy persons ages 12 mo and older recently exposed to HAV (adults >40 yr may also receive HAV immunoglobulin). **Standard dosing:** Havrix: Administer two doses at 0 and 6–12 mo Vaqta: Administer two doses at 0 and 6–18 mo Twinrix: Administer three doses at 0, 1, and 6 mo	Severe allergic reaction to any vaccine component or after a previous dose	Moderate or severe acute illness with or without fever

(Continued)

TABLE A-1 Selected Adult Immunization Recommendations in the United States (Continued)

Hepatitis B Single-antigen hepatitis B vaccine (HepB; Recombivax HB), standard (10 µg/mL) & high-dose (40 µg/mL) formulations: 1 mL IM Single-antigen hepatitis B vaccine (HepB; Engerix-B) (20 µg/mL): 1 mL IM Combined hepatitis A/hepatitis B vaccine (HepA-Hep B; Twinrix): 1 mL IM	**Any adult seeking protection from hepatitis B virus (HBV)** **Specific indications:** chronic liver disease; HIV infection; percutaneous or mucosal risk of exposure to blood (e.g., household contacts of persons with chronic HBV infection; persons age <60 yr with diabetes mellitus and those ≥60 yr at discretion of treating clinician; adults with ESRD including those receiving dialysis; injection drug users; health care and public safety workers at risk for exposure to blood or body fluids); sexual exposure risk (e.g., sex partners of persons with chronic HBV infection; sexually active persons not in long-term, mutually monogamous relationship; persons seeking evaluation or treatment for a sexually transmitted disease; MSM); persons receiving care in settings where risk of HBV infection is high (e.g., facilities providing STD treatment, HIV testing and treatment, or drug abuse treatment and prevention services; health-care settings targeting services to injection drug users or MSM; correctional facilities; ESRD and hemodialysis programs; institutions for persons with developmental disabilities); travelers to countries with high or intermediate HBV endemicity **Standard dosing:** Administer three doses of standard-dose Recombivax HB, Engerix-B, or Twinrix at 0, 1, and 6 mo **HD patients or other immunocompromised:** Administer three doses of high-dose Recombivax HB at 0, 1, and 6 mo, or eight doses of Engerix-B as four two-dose (2 mL) injections at 0, 1, 2, and 6 mo	Severe allergic reaction to any vaccine component or after a previous dose	Moderate or severe acute illness with or without fever
Human papillomavirus (HPV) 9-valent vaccine (9vHPV; Gardisil 9): 0.5 mL IM	**Females through age 26 yr (including immune compromised) and males through age 21 yr (males aged 22 through 26 yr if MSM or immune compromised):** If age <15 yr, administer two doses at 0 and 6–12 mo If age ≥15 yr, administer three doses at 0, 1–2, and 6 mo	Severe allergic reaction to any vaccine component or after a previous dose	Moderate or severe acute illness with or without fever; **pregnancy**

(Continued)

TABLE A-1 Selected Adult Immunization Recommendations in the United States (Continued)

Vaccine, Dose	Indications & Dosing	Contraindications	Precautions
Influenza Inactivated or recombinant influenza vaccine (IIV or RIV): 0.5 mL IM (5 mL if multidose vial used) Intradermal IIV3 0.5 mL (only aged 18–64 yr) Live attenuated influenza vaccine (LAIV): 0.2 mL intranasal Available in quadrivalent (4) and trivalent (3). Quadrivalent contains the same three influenza viruses (A/A/B) and an additional influenza B vaccine virus	**Annual vaccination is recommended for all persons aged ≥6 mo who do not have contraindications.** **Age 6 mo through 8 yr:** IIV4 (LAIV4 option for age ≥2 yr) **Pregnancy:** IIV4 or RIV4 **Age ≥65 yr:** High-dose IIV3 **All others:** Standard-dose IIV4 or IIV3 **Egg allergy:** RIV4 preferred *Cell culture-based IIV4 or RIV4 should only be administered if age ≥18 yr* **Health-care personnel** who receive LAIV should avoid providing care for severely immune-suppressed persons (i.e., requiring protective environment) until 7 d postvaccination	Severe allergic reaction to any vaccine component or after a previous dose Persons with a history of egg allergy of any severity may receive any licensed, recommended, and age-appropriate influenza vaccine LAIV: **pregnancy, immune suppression** (includes close contacts), children aged 2–4 yr with asthma, children/adolescents on salicylate therapy (aspirin), persons who have taken influenza antiviral medications within previous 48 h	Moderate to severe illness with or without fever; history of Guillain-Barré syndrome (GBS) within 6 wk of previous influenza vaccination LAIV: asthma; chronic medical conditions that may predispose to higher risk of influenza-related complications (e.g., lung disease, cardiovascular disease, diabetes, renal or hepatic disease)

(Continued)

TABLE A-1 Selected Adult Immunization Recommendations in the United States (Continued)

Measles, mumps, rubella Live measles, mumps, and rubella (MMR) vaccine: 0.5 mL SC	**Anyone without evidence of immunity:** Administer one dose **Evidence of immunity:** • Born before 1957 (except for health-care personnel) • Documented vaccination • Laboratory confirmation of immunity or disease **HIV infection with CD4⁺ >200 cells/μL for at least 6 mo without evidence of immunity:** Administer two doses ≥28 d apart **Students in postsecondary educational institutions, international travelers, and household contacts of immune compromised persons:** Administer two doses ≥28 d apart **Women of childbearing age:** Rubella immunity should be determined. If no immunity and nonpregnant, administer 1 dose of MMR; **pregnant women with no rubella immunity**: administer 1 dose on completion or termination of pregnancy and before discharge from the health-care facility **Health-care personnel born in 1957 or later:** If no documentation of vaccination or laboratory confirmation of immunity or disease, administer vaccination (two doses if measles or mumps nonimmune ≥28 d apart; one dose if rubella nonimmune) **Adults who previously received ≤2 doses of MMR identified to be at increased risk for mumps during an outbreak:** Administer one dose	Severe allergic reaction to any vaccine component or after a previous dose; current febrile respiratory or other febrile infection; known **severe immunodeficiency** (e.g., hematologic and solid tumors, receipt of chemotherapy, congenital immunodeficiency, long-term immunosuppressive therapy, HIV infection with $CD4^+$ <200 cells/μL); **pregnancy**	Moderate or severe acute illness with or without fever; recent (≤11 mo) receipt of antibody-containing blood product; history of thrombocytopenia or thrombocytopenic purpura; need for tuberculin skin testing within 4 wk of vaccination (measles component may temporarily suppress reactivity)

(Continued)

TABLE A-1 Selected Adult Immunization Recommendations in the United States (Continued)

Vaccine, Dose	Indications & Dosing	Contraindications	Precautions
Meningococcal (*Neisseria meningitidis*) Quadrivalent meningococcal conjugate vaccine-diphtheria toxoid carrier (MenACWY; Menactra, Menveo): 0.5 mL IM Meningococcal serogroup B vaccine (MenB-4C, Bexsero; MenB-FHbp, Trumenba): 0.5 mL IM	**Adults with anatomical or functional asplenia, HIV infection, persistent complement component deficiency, or eculizumab use:** Administer two doses of MenACWY ≥8 wk apart; revaccinate with 1 dose of MenACWY every 5 yr if risk persists **Adults traveling to living in countries where meningococcal disease is hyperendemic or epidemic, microbiologists routinely exposed to *N. meningitidis*, military recruits, first-year college students living in residence halls if no vaccination at age 16 yr or older:** Administer one dose of MenACWY; revaccinate with one dose of MenACWY every 5 yr if risk persists **Adults with anatomical or function asplenia, persistent complement component deficiency, eculizumab use, microbiologists routinely exposed to *N. meningitidis*, or at risk for meningococcal disease outbreak attributed to serogroup B:** Administer two doses of MenB-4C ≥1 mo apart or three doses of MenB-FHbp at 0, 1–2, and 6 mo	Severe allergic reaction to any vaccine component or after a previous dose	Moderate or severe acute illness with or without fever

(Continued)

TABLE A-1 Selected Adult Immunization Recommendations in the United States (Continued)

Pneumococcal (*Streptococcus pneumoniae*) 13-Valent pneumococcal conjugate vaccine (PCV13): 0.5 mL IM 23-Valent pneumococcal polysaccharide vaccine (PPSV23): 0.5 mL IM or SC	**Immunocompetent adults ≥65 yr:** Administer one dose of PCV13 (if not previously received), followed by one dose of PPSV23 ≥1 yr later. If PPSV23 previously administered but not PCV13, administer PCV13 at least 1 yr after PPSV23 **Adults 19–64 yr AND chronic heart disease (including hypertension), chronic lung disease, chronic liver disease, alcoholism, diabetes mellitus, or tobacco dependence:** Administer one dose of PPSV23. At age ≥65 yr, administer one dose of PCV13 (if not previously received), followed by another dose of PPSV23 ≥1 yr after PCV13 and ≥5 yr after last PPSV23 **Adults 19–64 yr AND immune compromise, HIV infection, anatomic or functional asplenia, chronic kidney disease, or nephrotic syndrome:** Administer one dose of PCV13, followed by one dose PPSV23 at ≥8 wk and second dose at ≥5 yr after 1st PPSV23. If last PPSV23 received before age 65 yr, at age 65 yr, administer another dose of PPSV23 ≥5 yr after last dose **Adults 19–64 yr AND cerebrospinal fluid leak or cochlear implant:** Administer one dose of PCV13, followed by one dose of PPSV23 at ≥8 wk. If PPSV23 received before age 65 yr, at age 65 yr, administer another dose of PPSV23 ≥5 yr after last dose	Severe allergic reaction after a previous dose or to a vaccine component PCV13: severe allergic reaction to any vaccine containing diphtheria toxoid	Moderate or severe acute illness with or without fever

(Continued)

TABLE A-1 Selected Adult Immunization Recommendations in the United States (Continued)

Vaccine, Dose	Indications & Dosing	Contraindications	Precautions
Tetanus, diphtheria, pertussis Tetanus & diphtheria toxoids vaccine (Td): 0.5 mL IM Tetanus, diphtheria & acellular pertussis vaccine (Tdap; Adacel, Boostrix): 0.5 mL IM Other formulations [e.g., diphtheria and tetanus toxoids and acellular pertussis (DTaP)] not recommended for adult use	**Everyone:** Td: Administer every 10 yr Tdap: Administer one dose after age 18 yr as substitute for 1 Td booster **Pregnant women**: Administer one dose every pregnancy (preferably at 27–36 wk gestation) **Adults not previously vaccinated:** Administer three-dose series consisting of Tdap followed by Td 4 wk later and Td 6–12 mo later **Postexposure prophylaxis:** See Table A-2	Severe allergic reaction to any vaccine component or after a previous dose Tdap: encephalopathy (e.g., coma, prolonged seizures) not attributable to other cause within 7 d of administration of previous dose	Moderate or severe acute illness with or without fever; GBS within 6 wk after previous dose of tetanus toxoid-containing vaccine; history of Arthus-type (type III) hypersensitivity reactions after previous dose of diphtheria toxoid–containing vaccine Tdap: progressive or unstable neurologic disorder, uncontrolled seizures, or progressive encephalopathy until treatment regimen established and condition stabilized

(Continued)

TABLE A-1 Selected Adult Immunization Recommendations in the United States (Continued)

Varicella (chickenpox) Live varicella vaccine (VAR, Varivax): 0.5 mL SC	**Anyone without evidence of immunity:** Administer two doses (4–8 wks apart); if one dose given previously, only give second dose **Evidence of immunity:** • Documented vaccination (two doses >4 wk apart) • US born before 1980 **except** if pregnant or health-care personnel • Varicella or zoster infection documented by health-care provider • Laboratory confirmation of immunity or disease	Severe allergic reaction to any vaccine component or after a previous dose; known **severe immunodeficiency** (e.g., hematologic and solid tumors, receipt of chemotherapy, congenital immunodeficiency, long-term immunosuppressive therapy, HIV infection with $CD4^+$ <200 cells/µL); **pregnancy**	Moderate or severe acute illness with or without fever; simultaneous or recent (≤2 wk) receipt of antibody-containing blood product; receipt of specific antivirals (i.e., acyclovir, famciclovir, valacyclovir) 24 h before vaccination; avoid antiviral use for 14 d after vaccination

(Continued)

TABLE A-1 Selected Adult Immunization Recommendations in the United States (Continued)

Vaccine, Dose	Indications & Dosing	Contraindications	Precautions
Herpes zoster (shingles) Recombinant zoster vaccine (RZV; Shingrix): 0.5 mL IM Zoster vaccine live (ZVL; Zostavax): 0.65 mg SC	**Adults ≥50 yr:** Administer two doses of RZV 2–6 mo apart regardless of prior episode of herpes zoster or receipt of ZVL (give RZV at least 2 mo after ZVL) **Adults ≥60 yr:** Administer either two doses of RZV as above (preferred) or single dose of ZVL	Severe allergic reaction to a vaccine component ZVL: known **severe immunodeficiency** (e.g., hematologic and solid tumors, receipt of chemotherapy, congenital immunodeficiency, long-term immunosuppressive therapy, HIV infection with $CD4^+$ <200 cells/μL); **pregnancy**	Moderate or severe acute illness with or without fever ZVL: receipt of specific antivirals (i.e., acyclovir, famciclovir, valacyclovir) 24 h before vaccination; avoid antiviral use for 14 d after vaccination

Adapted from Centers for Disease Control and Prevention. Advisory Committee on Immunization Practices recommended immunization schedule for adults aged 19 years or older—United States, 2018. *MMWR Morb Mortal Wkly Rep.* 2018;67(5):158–160. https://www.cdc.gov/vaccines/schedules/hcp/imz/adult.html.

ESRD, end stage renal disease

TABLE A-2 Selected Adult Postexposure Prophylaxis Recommendations

Disease	Indications and Therapy
Anthrax	Indicated for all contacts. Either ciprofloxacin 500 mg PO q12h (preferred for **pregnant women**), or doxycycline 100 mg PO q12h for 60 days and anthrax vaccine absorbed (AVA) SC series (obtained from the CDC): First dose administered as soon as possible, second and third doses administered at 2 and 4 wk after the first dose. (Alternative antibiotic regimens available; see CDC website.)
Botulinum toxin	Close observation of exposed person; treat with heptavalent botulinum antitoxin (equine immunoglobulin) at first sign of illness (obtained via consultation with state health department).
Diphtheria	Indicated for close (e.g., household) contacts: Benzathine penicillin G 1.2 million units IM once or erythromycin (base) 500 mg PO q12h for 7–10 d and tetanus and diphtheria (Td) booster vaccine (see Table A-1). Diphtheria antitoxin (DAT) 10,000 units IM/IV (after appropriate sensitivity testing) used for prophylaxis only in exceptional circumstances, obtained in consultation with the CDC (770-488-7100).
Hepatitis A	Indicated for unvaccinated household and sexual contacts of infected individual; persons who have shared illicit drugs with the infected individual; coworkers of infected food handlers; all staff and children at day care centers caring for diapered children where ≥1 case has occurred or when cases occur in ≥2 households of center attendees; only classroom contacts in centers not caring for diapered children. **For healthy persons <40 yr**: Administer single-antigen hepatitis A vaccine (see Table A-1). **For persons ≥40 yr, immune compromised, or with chronic liver disease:** Administer single-antigen hepatitis A vaccine (see Table A-1) and immune globulin (IG), 0.1 mL/kg IM, once **within 14 d** of exposure.
Hepatitis B	**Nonoccupational:** If exposure source is known surface antigen positive, unvaccinated or incompletely vaccinated persons should receive vaccine (see Table A-1) and hepatitis B immune globulin (HBIG) 0.06 mL/kg IM once. Vaccinated persons without serologic confirmation of immunity should receive 1 vaccine dose. If exposure source antigen status is unknown, unvaccinated persons should receive the vaccine series, and incompletely vaccinated persons should receive the remaining doses. Vaccinated persons require no further treatment. **Occupational:** See Table A-3.

(Continued)

TABLE A-2 Selected Adult Postexposure Prophylaxis Recommendations (Continued)

Disease	Indications and Therapy
HIV	**Nonoccupational:** Indicated within 72 h of exposure to HIV-infected blood, urogenital secretions, or other body fluids (e.g., condomless sexual intercourse, needle sharing). Administer tenofovir-emtricitabine 300/200 mg (1 tablet) PO daily and raltegravir 400 mg PO q12h for 28 d. Test for HIV at presentation and ensure follow-up for repeat HIV testing at 6 wk. See https://www.cdc.gov/hiv/pdf/programresources/cdc-hiv-npep-guidelines.pdf. If alternative regimens desired, recommend consultation with an HIV specialist. **Occupational:** See Table A-3.
Measles	**Nonoccupational:** If nonimmune (see Table A-1), give measles, mumps, rubella (MMR) vaccine within 72 h of initial exposure. For **pregnant women** (if nonimmune) or severely **immunocompromised** (regardless of prior immunity), give immunoglobulin 400 mg/kg IV (IVIG) once within 6 d of exposure. Monitor for signs/symptoms for at least 1 incubation period. **Occupational:** See Table A-3.
Meningococcus (*Neisseria meningitidis*)	Indicated for close contacts of patients with invasive meningococcal disease, including household contacts, child care center contacts, and persons directly exposed to the patient's oral secretions. Administer ciprofloxacin 500 mg PO once, rifampin 600 mg PO q12h for 2 d, or ceftriaxone 250 mg IM once (preferred in **pregnancy**).
Pertussis (*Bordetella pertussis*, whooping cough)	Indicated for close contacts of symptomatic patients (face-to-face exposure ≤3 ft), persons with direct contact with infected respiratory or oral secretions, persons with high risk of severe illness (e.g., **immunocompromised**, third trimester of **pregnancy**, asthma), or those who will have contact with high-risk persons (including infants age <12 mo). Administer a macrolide antibiotic (azithromycin 500 mg PO day 1, 250 mg PO daily days 2–5; erythromycin 500 mg PO q6h for 14 d; clarithromycin 500 mg PO q12h for 7 d) within 21 d of onset of cough in exposure source.
Plague	Indicated for close contacts of pneumonic plague patients (face-to-face exposure ≤3 ft) that have received ≤48 h of effective antibiotic therapy or persons with direct contact with infected body fluids or tissues (for **pregnant women**, weigh prophylactic benefits with antibiotic risks). Administer doxycycline 100 mg PO q12h or ciprofloxacin 500 mg PO q12h for 7 d.
Rabies	See Rabies Postexposure Prophylaxis section of this Appendix.

(Continued)

TABLE A-2 Selected Adult Postexposure Prophylaxis Recommendations (Continued)

Disease	Indications and Therapy
Tetanus	**For clean, minor wounds:** If vaccination history unknown or <3 doses tetanus toxoid-containing vaccine, give Tdap and complete catch-up vaccination (see Table A-1). If ≥3 doses and >10 yr since last dose, give Tdap (if not yet received) or Td. **For all other wounds:** If vaccination history unknown or <3 doses tetanus toxoid-containing vaccine, give tetanus immune globulin 250 units IM once, as well as Tdap (at separate site) and complete catch-up vaccination. If ≥3 doses and >5 yr since last dose, give Tdap (if not yet received) or Td.
Tularemia	Routine prophylaxis not recommended. If exposure in bioterrorism or mass casualty setting, give doxycycline 100 mg PO q12h or ciprofloxacin 500 mg PO q12h (preferred in **pregnant women**) for 14 d.
Smallpox	Indicated in setting of intentional release of smallpox (variola virus) for exposed persons and persons with contact with infectious materials from smallpox patients, weighing risks and benefits for those with relative contraindications. Administer smallpox (vaccinia) vaccine (ACAM2000; available from the CDC Drug Service at 404-639-3670) ideally within 3 d of exposure; vaccination 4–7 d after exposure may offer some protection.
Varicella	Indicated for exposed persons without evidence of immunity. Vaccinate (see Table A-1) within 3 d of exposure (possibly effective up to 5 d of postexposure). If contraindication to vaccination and at high risk of severe infection (e.g., **pregnant women, immunocompromised, malignancy**), give varicella-zoster immune globulin (VariZIG) 12.5 international units (IU)/kg IM once (minimum, 125 IU; maximum, 625 IU) within 10 d of exposure, which can be obtained from FFF Enterprises (800-843-7477, http://www.fffenterprises.com).

CDC, Centers for Disease Control and Prevention; Tdap, tetanus, diphtheria, pertussis.

TABLE A-3 Selected Postexposure Guidelines for Health Care Personnel[a]

Pathogen	Treatment
HIV	Indicated for exposure to HIV-infected blood, tissue, or body fluids (e.g., semen, vaginal secretions, amniotic fluid)[b] via percutaneous injury, contact with mucous membranes, or contact with nonintact skin. Administer as soon as possible within 72 h after exposure (can consider up to 1 wk in very–high risk cases). Preferred regimen is tenofovir-emtricitabine 300/200 mg (1 tablet) PO daily and raltegravir 400 mg PO bid for 28 d or until exposure source tests negative for HIV (unless acute seroconversion is suspected).[c] Test exposed workers at baseline, 6 wk, 12 wk, and 6 mo for HIV (baseline, 6 wk, and 4 mo if using fourth-generation test). Assistance with choosing a regimen may be obtained by calling the National Clinicians' Post-Exposure Prophylaxis Hotline (PEPline) at 1-888-448-4911 or consulting an HIV expert.
Hepatitis B	For percutaneous injury with blood or blood-contaminated fluids from known surface antigen–positive source: Unvaccinated health-care worker: Administer hepatitis B immunoglobulin (HBIG), 0.06 mL/kg IM, within 96 h of exposure AND start hepatitis B vaccine series (see Table A-1). Vaccinated health-care worker: Known responder: no treatment Nonresponder after one complete series: HBIG × 1 and repeat series Nonresponder after two complete series: HBIG × 2 doses 1 mo apart Antibody response unknown: check anti-HBs titer; if ≥10 IU/mL: no therapy; if <10 IU/mL: HBIG × 1 and vaccine booster.
Hepatitis C	Immunoglobulin and postexposure prophylaxis not effective. Ensure occupational health follow-up for baseline and subsequent follow-up testing.
Measles	If no documented evidence of immunity, give MMR vaccine within 72 h of initial exposure. For **pregnant women** (if nonimmune) or severely **immunocompromised** (regardless of prior immunity), give immunoglobulin 400 mg/kg IV (IVIG) once within 6 d of exposure. Monitor for signs/symptoms for at least one incubation period. Health-care personnel without evidence of immunity should be off duty from day 5 after first exposure to day 21 after last exposure, regardless of whether prophylaxis was given.

[a]All blood and body fluid exposures should be reported to the occupational health department. Source patients should be tested for HIV (with consent), hepatitis B surface antigen (HbsAg), and hepatitis C antibody (anti-HCV).
[b]Body fluids not considered infectious include feces, urine, vomitus, saliva, and tears, unless these are visibly contaminated with blood.
[c]Multiple alternative antiretroviral regimens are available if exposed worker has contraindications to or is otherwise unable to use the preferred regimen, or if the exposure source is known to have resistant virus. See *Infect Control Hosp Epidemiol. 2013;34:875.* Consultation with an HIV specialist is recommended in such cases.

TABLE A-4 Rabies Postexposure Prophylaxis Recommendations

	Therapy	
Vaccination Status	**Vaccine**	**HRIG**
Not previously vaccinated	Yes, on days 0, 3, 7, and 14	Yes, once on day 0
Previously vaccinated	Yes, on days 0 and 3	No

HRIG, human rabies immune globulin.

Rabies Postexposure Prophylaxis

- For all suspected rabies exposures, consultation with local or state health officials is recommended. Contact information can be found at http://www.cdc.gov/rabies/resources/contacts.html.
- Postexposure prophylaxis is generally indicated only for bite wounds from mammals.[1]
  - Bites from bats, skunks, raccoons, foxes, and most other carnivores warrant immediate prophylaxis unless the animal is confirmed to be rabies negative by laboratory testing. Animals should not be held for observation but euthanized as soon as possible.
  - Bites from dogs, cats, and ferrets that are rabid or suspected to be rabid also warrant immediate prophylaxis. If the animal is healthy and can be observed for 10 days, do not begin prophylaxis but observe. If signs or symptoms of rabies develop in the animal, prophylaxis should begin immediately. For bites where the status of the animal is unknown, consult with public health officials.
  - Bites from all other sources (e.g., rodents, hares, livestock) should be considered on an individual basis and prophylaxis initiated only in consultation with public health officials.
- Postexposure prophylaxis consists of wound care, vaccination, and in certain situations, administration of human rabies immune globulin (HRIG) (Table A-4).[2]
  - All wounds should be cleaned thoroughly with soap and water and irrigated with a virucidal solution such as povidone-iodine.
  - Human diploid cell vaccine or purified chick embryo cell vaccine, 1 mL IM, should be administered in the deltoid region, the only acceptable site for vaccination in adults.
  - If HRIG is indicated, give 20 IU/kg IM once. Do not administer in the same syringe as the vaccine. When possible, infiltrate as much of the product around and into the wound(s). The remaining volume can be administered intramuscularly at any site anatomically distant from the site of vaccination. Subsequent vaccine doses at later dates can be given at the same site as previous HRIG.

REFERENCES

1. Manning SE, Rupprecht CE, Fishbein D, et al. Human rabies prevention–United States, 2008: recommendations of the Advisory Committee on Immunization Practices. *MMWR Recomm Rep*. 2008;57(RR-3):1-28.
2. Rupprecht CE, Briggs D, Brown CM, et al. Use of a reduced (4-dose) vaccine schedule for postexposure prophylaxis to prevent human rabies: recommendations of the advisory committee on immunization practices. *MMWR Recomm Rep*. 2010;59(RR-2):1-9.

Appendix B

Infection Control and Isolation Recommendations

Caline Mattar and Stephen Y. Liang

- **Standard Precautions** should be practiced on all patients at all times to minimize the risk of healthcare-associated infection.
  - **Perform hand hygiene** with an alcohol-based hand sanitizer before patient contact, before clean or aseptic procedures, after body fluid exposure, after touching a patient (including after gloves are removed), and after touching patient surroundings. (Figure B-1, Table B-1) Soap and water should be used to clean visibly contaminated hands and after contact with patients with confirmed or suspected *Clostridium difficile* infection if the alcohol-based preparation used is not active against *C. difficile* spores.
  - **Wear gloves** when direct contact with body secretions or blood is anticipated.
  - **Wear a gown** when clothing may be in contact with body fluids.
  - **Wear a surgical mask** when prolonged procedures, including puncture of the spinal canal, are performed (e.g., myelography, epidural anesthesia, intrathecal chemotherapy).
  - **Wear a surgical mask and protective eyewear** when splashes of body fluid are possible.
  - **Use proper respiratory hygiene and cough etiquette** (applies to health-care workers as well as all patients and visiting family or friends). Mouth and nose must be covered when coughing, and tissues must be disposed of properly. Hand hygiene must be performed after contact with respiratory secretions.
  - **Safely dispose** of sharp instruments, needles, wound dressings, and disposable gowns.
- **Transmission-Based Precautions** supplement Standard Precautions for patients with documented or suspected infection or colonization depending on the major mode of microorganism transmission in health-care settings.
  - **Contact Precautions** are used when micro-organisms can be transmitted via direct contact between patients and health-care workers or by contact between patients and contaminated objects and/or environments. In addition to Standard Precautions, the following must be done:
    - Assign the patient to a **private room** if possible. Cohorting is allowed if necessary.
    - **Wear gown and gloves** to enter the room; remove them before leaving the room.
    - Use a **dedicated stethoscope and thermometer.**
    - Minimize environmental contamination during patient transport (e.g., patient can be placed in a gown).
  - **Droplet Precautions** are used when micro-organisms can be transmitted by respiratory droplets (>5 μm). Droplets remain suspended in the air for limited periods, and exposure of ≤3 feet (1 m) is usually required for human-to-human transmission. In addition to Standard Precautions, the following must be done:
    - Assign the patient to a **private room**. The door must be kept closed as much as possible. Rooms with special air handling systems are **not** required.
    - Wear a **surgical mask** within 6 feet of patients.
    - Limit patient transport and activity outside their room. If transporting the patient outside the room is necessary, the patient must wear a surgical mask.
  - **Airborne precautions** must be used when microorganisms can be transmitted by respiratory droplet nuclei (<5 μm). These droplet nuclei remain suspended in the air for extended periods. In addition to Standard Precautions, the following must be done:
    - Assign the patient to a **negative-pressure airborne infection isolation room**. Doors must remain closed.

Your 5 moments for HAND HYGIENE

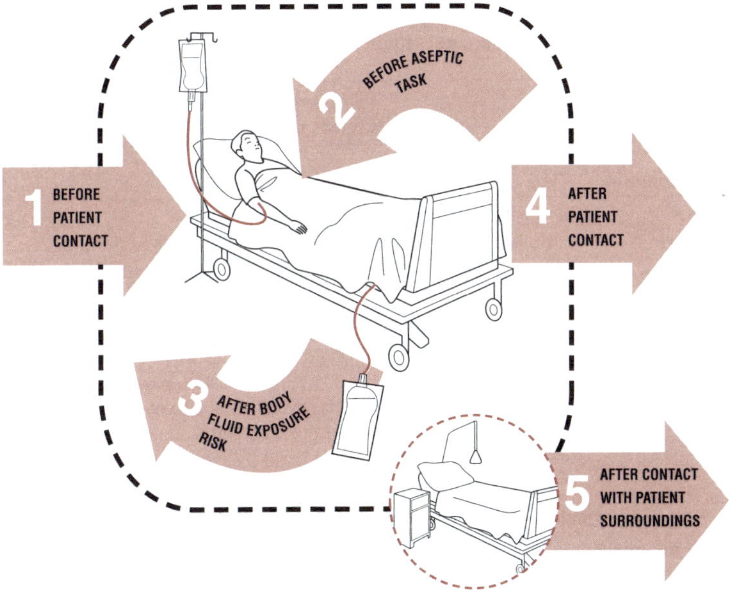

1 BEFORE PATIENT CONTACT	WHEN?	Clean your hands before touching a patient when approaching him or her
	WHY?	To protect the patient against harmful germs carried on your hands
2 BEFORE AN ASEPTIC TASK	WHEN?	Clean your hands immediately before any aseptic task
	WHY?	To protect the patient against harmful germs, including the patient's own germs, entering his or her body
3 AFTER BODY FLUID EXPOSURE RISK	WHEN?	Clean your hands immediately after an exposure risk to body fluids (and after glove removal)
	WHY?	To protect yourself and the healthcare environment from harmful patient germs
4 AFTER PATIENT CONTACT	WHEN?	Clean your hands after touching a patient and his or her immediate surroundings when leaving
	WHY?	To protect yourself and the healthcare environment from harmful patient germs
5 AFTER CONTACT WITH PATIENT SURROUNDINGS	WHEN?	Clean your hands after touching any object or furniture in the patient's immediate surroundings, when leaving–even without touching the patient
	WHY?	To protect yourself and the healthcare environment from harmful patient germs

World Health Organization

Figure B-1. World Health Organization's My Five Moments for Hand Hygiene. From World Health Organization's 5 Moments for Hand Hygiene in acute care settings. Reproduced, with permission of the publisher, from "*Five Moments for Hand Hygiene,*" World Health Organization; 2009. https://www.who.int/gpsc/tools/5momentsHandHygiene_A3.pdf?ua=1. Accessed January 2019.

- Wear a **tightly fitting respirator** that covers the nose and mouth with a filtering capacity of 95% (e.g., N95 mask) to enter the room. Susceptible individuals should not enter the room of patients with confirmed or suspected measles or chicken pox.
- Limit patient transport and activity outside their room. If transporting the patient outside the room is necessary, the patient must wear a surgical mask. Higher level respirator masks (e.g., N95) are **not** required for the patient.

TABLE B-1 Health-Care Isolation Recommendations for Specific Infections

Infection/Condition	Type	Duration, Comments
Adenovirus, pneumonia	Droplet, Contact	Duration of illness In immunocompromised hosts, extend duration of precautions owing to prolonged viral shedding.
Anthrax	Standard	Duration of illness Contact precautions indicated if wound with uncontained copious drainage. Alcohol hand rubs ineffective against spores; use soap and water or 2% chlorhexidine gluconate solution for hand hygiene. If aerosolizable spore-containing substance (e.g., powder) is present, wear respirator, protective clothing until decontamination is complete.
Botulism	Standard	Duration of illness
Burkholderia cepacia, pneumonia or colonization	Contact	Unknown Recommendations will vary by institution. Avoid exposure to persons with cystic fibrosis. Private room preferred.
Clostridium difficile	Contact	Duration of hospitalization and future hospitalizations Recommendations for initiation and discontinuation of precautions will vary by institution.
Conjunctivitis, acute viral	Contact	Duration of illness
Diphtheria		
Cutaneous	Contact	Until off antimicrobial treatment and two cultures taken 24 h apart are negative
Pharyngeal	Droplet	Same as for cutaneous diphtheria
Hepatitis, viral	Standard	Duration of illness For hepatitis A and E, contact precautions are indicated for diapered or incontinent individuals.
Herpes simplex virus		
Encephalitis	Standard	Duration of illness
Mucocutaneous, recurrent (skin, oral, genital)	Standard	Duration of illness

(Continued)

TABLE B-1 Health-Care Isolation Recommendations for Specific Infections (Continued)

Infection/Condition	Type	Duration, Comments
Mucocutaneous, severe (disseminated or primary)	Contact	Until lesions dry and crusted
Herpes zoster		See Varicella
Human metapneumovirus	Contact	Duration of illness
Influenza	Droplet	Immunocompetent: 7 d after illness onset or until 24 h after resolution of symptoms, whichever is longer Immunocompromised: Duration of illness Respiratory protection equivalent to an N95 respirator is recommended during aerosol-generating procedures.
Lice		
Head (pediculosis)	Contact	Until 24 h after start of therapy
Body	Standard	Duration of illness Can be transmitted via infested clothing. Wear gown and gloves when handling clothing.
Pubic	Standard	Duration of illness
Measles (rubeola)	Airborne	Immunocompetent: 4 d after onset of rash Immunocompromised: Duration of illness[a]
Meningitis, *Haemophilus influenzae* type B or *Neisseria meningitidis*	Droplet	Until 24 h after start of therapy For other etiologies of meningitis, standard precautions can be used.
Meningococcal disease (*N. meningitidis*)	Droplet	Until 24 h after start of therapy If colonization without active disease, standard precautions can be used.
Middle eastern respiratory syndrome coronavirus (MERS-CoV)	Airborne, Contact	Determine on a case-by-case basis in consultation with local, state, and federal public health authorities
Monkeypox	Airborne, Contact	Airborne: Until monkeypox confirmed and smallpox excluded Contact: Until lesions crusted
Multidrug-resistant organisms, infection or colonization (e.g., MRSA, VRE, ESBL)	Contact	Duration of hospitalization and future hospitalizations Recommendations for initiation and discontinuation of precautions will vary by institution and organism.

(Continued)

TABLE B-1 Health-Care Isolation Recommendations for Specific Infections (Continued)

Infection/Condition	Type	Duration, Comments
Mumps (infectious parotitis)	Droplet	Until 5 d after onset of symptoms[a]
Mycoplasma, pneumonia	Droplet	Duration of illness
Parvovirus B19 (erythema infectiosum)	Droplet	Immunocompromised patient: Duration of hospitalization Transient aplastic crisis or red cell crisis: 7 d
Pertussis (*Bordetella pertussis*, whooping cough)	Droplet	Until 5 d after start of therapy
Plague (*Yersinia pestis*)		
Bubonic	Standard	Duration of illness
Pneumonic	Droplet	Until 48 h after start of therapy
Poliomyelitis	Contact	Duration of illness
Respiratory syncytial virus	Contact	Duration of illness In immunocompromised hosts, extend duration of precautions due to prolonged viral shedding.
Rhinovirus	Droplet	Duration of illness Add contact precautions if copious moist secretions.
Rubella (German measles)	Droplet	Until 7 d after onset of rash[a] Pregnant women who are not immune should not care for these patients.
Scabies	Contact	Until 24 h after start of therapy For Norwegian scabies: 8 d or 24 h after the second treatment with scabicide
Severe acute respiratory syndrome coronavirus (SARS)	Airborne, Droplet, Contact	Duration of illness plus 10 d after resolution of fever if respiratory symptoms are absent or improving Eye protection (goggles, face shield) also recommended.
Smallpox (variola)	Airborne, Contact	Duration of illness; until all scabs have crusted and separated (3–4 wk)[a] For vaccine complications, see Vaccinia.
Streptococcus group A	Droplet	Until 24 h after start of therapy For endometritis or limited skin, wound, or burn infection, standard precautions can be used.

(Continued)

TABLE B-1 Health-Care Isolation Recommendations for Specific Infections (Continued)

Infection/Condition	Type	Duration, Comments
Tuberculosis (*Mycobacterium tuberculosis*)	Recommendations regarding initiation and discontinuation of precautions will vary by institution.	
Extrapulmonary, draining lesion	Airborne, Contact	Until patient is improving clinically and drainage has ceased or there are three consecutive negative cultures of drainage. Rule out active pulmonary disease.
Extrapulmonary, without draining lesion	Standard	Duration of illness Rule out active pulmonary disease.
Pulmonary or laryngeal disease, confirmed	Airborne	Until patient is on effective therapy, is improving clinically, and has three consecutive sputum smears negative for acid-fast bacilli collected on separate days
Pulmonary or laryngeal disease, suspected	Airborne	Until likelihood of infectious tuberculosis is deemed negligible and either there is another diagnosis that explains the clinical syndrome or the results of three sputum smears for AFB are negative Each of the sputum specimens should be collected 8–24 h apart, and at least one should be an early-morning specimen
Tularemia	Standard	Duration of illness
Vaccinia	Standard	Duration of illness[a] Contact precautions recommended for eczema vaccinatum, fetal vaccinia, generalized vaccinia, progressive vaccinia, and blepharitis or conjunctivitis with significant drainage. If unvaccinated, only health care workers without contraindications to vaccine should provide care.
Varicella		
Varicella disease (chickenpox)	Airborne, Contact	Until lesions dry and crusted[a] In immunocompromised host, prolong duration of precautions for duration of illness.
Herpes zoster, localized (shingles)	Standard	Duration of illness[a] In immunocompromised host, use airborne and contact precautions until disseminated disease ruled out.
Herpes zoster, disseminated	Airborne, Contact	Duration of illness[a]

(Continued)

TABLE B-1 Health-Care Isolation Recommendations for Specific Infections (Continued)

Infection/Condition	Type	Duration, Comments
Viral hemorrhagic fevers		
Ebola virus disease	Droplet, Contact	Discontinue only in consultation with local, state, and federal public health officials In addition to droplet and contact precautions, a powered air-purifying respirator (PAPR) or N95 respirator, examination gloves with extended cuffs, and fluid-resistant or impermeable gowns, aprons, and boot covers are recommended. Detailed information and updated recommendations can be found at http://www.cdc.gov/vhf/ebola/healthcare-us/hospitals/infection-control.html
Lassa, Marburg, and Crimean–Congo fever viruses	Droplet, Contact	Duration of illness Single-patient room preferred. Emphasize use of sharps safety devices and safe work practices, hand hygiene, barrier protection against blood and body fluids, including goggles or face shields and appropriate waste handling. Use N95 or higher respirators when performing aerosol-generating procedures.

Adapted from Siegel JD, Rhinehart E, Jackson M, et al. 2007 Guideline for isolation precautions: Preventing transmission of infectious agents in healthcare settings. *Am J Infect Control*. 2007;35:S65–S164. (https://www.cdc.gov/infectioncontrol/guidelines/isolation/index.html)

[a]Susceptible healthcare workers should not enter room if immune caregivers are available.

AFB, acid-fast bacilli; ESBL, extended-spectrum β-lactamase; MRSA, methicillin-resistant *Staphylococcus aureus*; VRE, vancomycin-resistant enterococcus.

Appendix C

Advanced Cardiac Life Support Algorithms

Zachary Crees

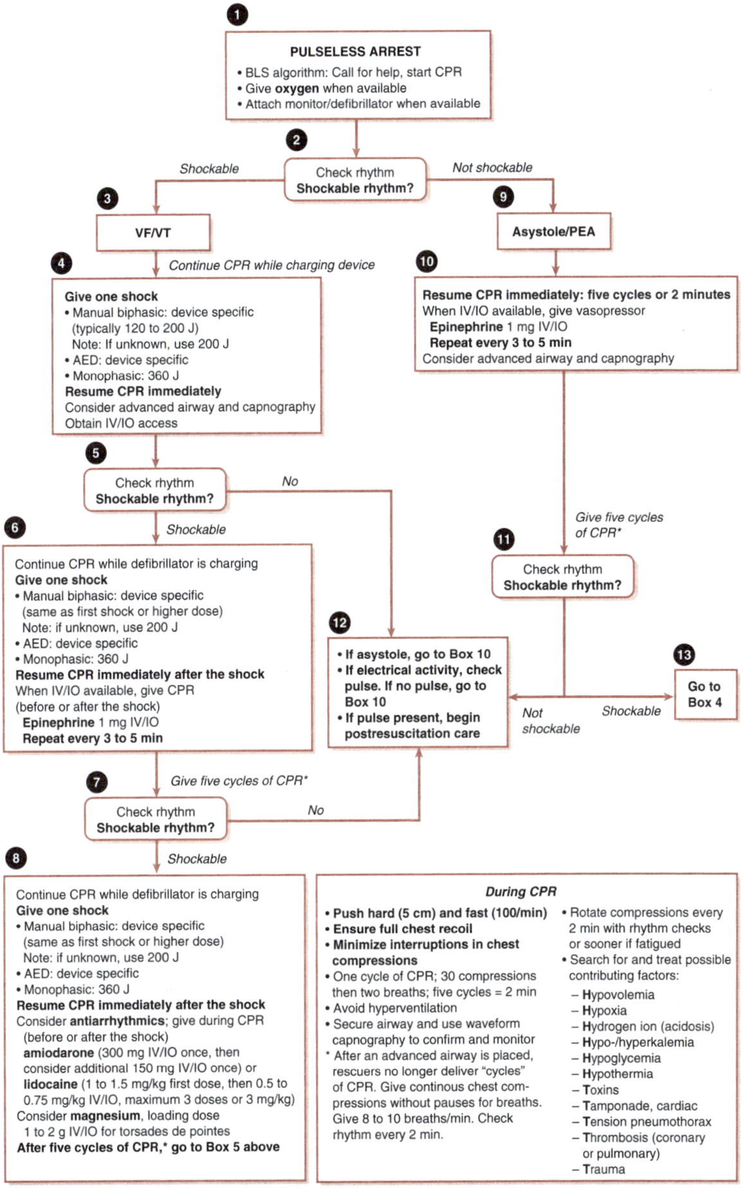

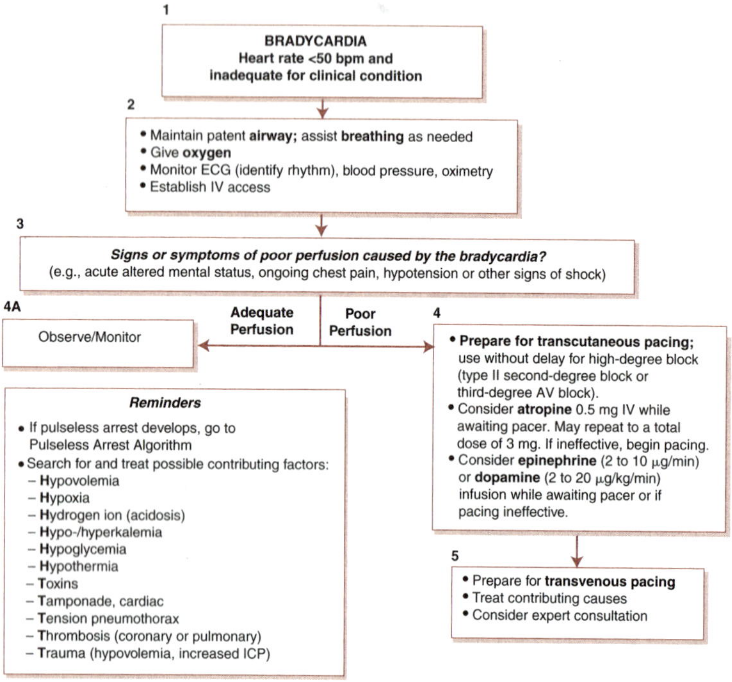

Figure C-2. Bradycardia algorithm. AV, atrioventricular; bpm, beats per minute; ICP, intracranial pressure. From American Heart Association in Collaboration with the International Liaison Committee on Resuscitation. Guidelines 2010 for cardiopulmonary resuscitation and emergency cardiovascular care. *Circulation*. 2010;122:S729–S767 and 2015 American Heart Association guidelines update for cardiopulmonary resuscitation and emergency cardiovascular care. *Circulation*. 2015;132:S315–S518.

Figure C-1. Advanced cardiac life support pulseless arrest algorithm. AED, automated external defibrillator; BLS, basic life support; CPR, cardiopulmonary resuscitation; IO, intraosseous; PEA, pulseless electrical activity; U, unit; VF, ventricular fibrillation; VT, ventricular tachycardia. From American Heart Association in Collaboration with the International Liaison Committee on Resuscitation. Guidelines 2010 for cardiopulmonary resuscitation and emergency cardiovascular care. *Circulation*. 2010;122:S729–S767 and 2015 American Heart Association guidelines update for cardiopulmonary resuscitation and emergency cardiovascular care. *Circulation*. 2015;132:S315–S518.

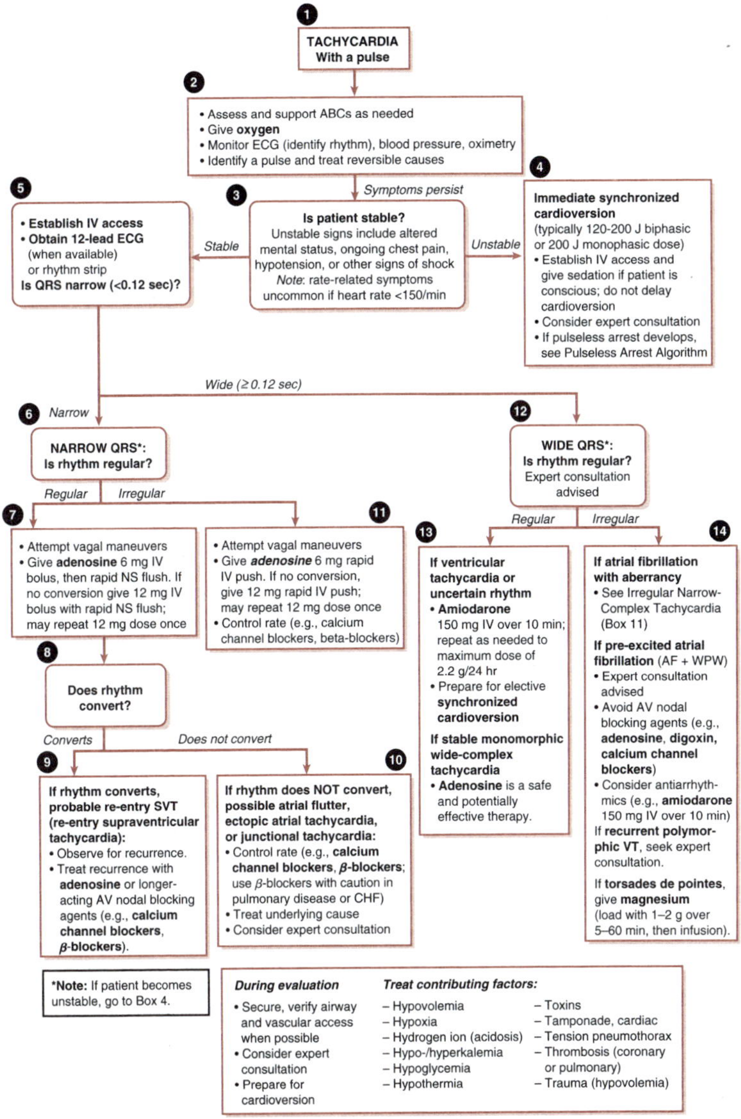

Figure C-3. Advanced cardiac life support tachycardia algorithm. AF, atrial fibrillation; AV, atrioventricular; CHF, congestive heart failure; NS, normal saline; SVT, supraventricular tachycardia; VT, ventricular tachycardia; WPW, Wolff–Parkinson–White syndrome. From American Heart Association in Collaboration with the International Liaison Committee on Resuscitation. Guidelines 2010 for cardiopulmonary resuscitation and emergency cardiovascular care. *Circulation*. 2010;122:S729–S767 and 2015 American Heart Association guidelines update for cardiopulmonary resuscitation and emergency cardiovascular care. *Circulation*. 2015;132:S315–S518.

Index

Note: Page numbers followed by *t* and *f* indicate table and figure respectively.

B

D

F

H

M

N

O

P

W